Osteonecrosis

Kyung-Hoi Koo • Michael A. Mont • Lynne C. Jones
Editors

Osteonecrosis

Springer

Editors
Kyung-Hoi Koo, MD, PhD
Department of Orthopaedic Surgery
Seoul National University College of Medicine
Seoul National University Bundang Hospital
Seongnam, Kyonggi-do
Republic of Korea (South Korea)

Michael A. Mont, MD
Rubin Institute for Advanced Orthopedics
Center for Joint Preservation and Replacement
Sinai Hospital of Baltimore
Baltimore, MD
USA

Lynne C. Jones, PhD, MS
Department of Orthopaedic Surgery
Center for Osteonecrosis Research and Education
Center for Metabolism and Obesity Research
Johns Hopkins University School of Medicine
Baltimore, MD
USA

Johns Hopkins Orthopaedics
Baltimore, MD
USA

ISBN 978-3-662-51154-1 ISBN 978-3-642-35767-1 (eBook)
DOI 10.1007/978-3-642-35767-1
Springer Heidelberg New York Dordrecht London

Printed on acid-free paper

Springer is part of Springer Science+Business Media (www.springer.com)

Preface

Osteonecrosis usually affects adults younger than 50 years and frequently leads to collapse and subsequent osteoarthritis. It is becoming more prevalent because of increasing use of steroids in the management of organ transplantation and adjuvant therapy for leukemia and other myelogenous diseases. In the United States, 10,000–20,000 people are affected with osteonecrosis of the femoral head annually, which accounts for up to 10 % of total hip arthroplasties performed each year. In nationwide surveys from Japan and Korea, the annual prevalence was more than 10,000. In Taiwan, about half of the total hip arthroplasties were done due to femoral head osteonecrosis. Thus, osteonecrosis leads to increasing socioeconomic burden worldwide.

However, the pathogeneses by the various etiologic factors are still unclear and the recommendations for treatment remain controversial.

Since the first meeting in 1973, Association Research Circulation Osseous (ARCO) has been the only international society to continuously bring together basic scientists and clinicians to discuss bone circulation and osteonecrosis. The ARCO histological criteria for diagnosis and staging system of osteonecrosis are used worldwide. In 1998, a textbook *Osteonecrosis: Etiology, Diagnosis and Treatment* was published, which was virtually the first textbook on this subject.

During the last 15 years, there has been enormous amount of investigations on osteonecrosis. We update new knowledge on the basic science, epidemiology, etiology, pathophysiology, diagnosis, imaging, and treatment.

We hope the information in this book will help scientists and physicians in their research on osteonecrosis and in their clinical practice.

We thank ARCO members and other internationally acknowledged authorities who participated in the creation of this book. We also thank Mrs. Ute Heilmann and Mrs. Lauren Kim for their excellent support in publishing this book.

Seongnam, South Korea — Kyung-Hoi Koo, MD, PhD
Baltimore, MD — Michael A. Mont, MD
Baltimore, MD — Lynne C. Jones, PhD, MS

Contents

Part I History

1 **Osteonecrosis: Historical Perspective** 3
Marvin E. Steinberg and David R. Steinberg

Part II Anatomy and Blood Flow

2 **Vascular Anatomy and Blood Supply to the Femoral Head** 19
Marcin Zlotorowicz and Jaroslaw Czubak

3 **Ischemia and Reperfusion Injury in Bone** 27
Howard Winet

Part III Epidemiology

4 **The Prevalence of Osteonecrosis in Different Parts of the World** 35
A.C. Gosling-Gardeniers, W.H.C. Rijnen, and J.W.M. Gardeniers

5 **Epidemiology of Osteonecrosis in the USA** 39
Sameer M. Naranje and Edward Y. Cheng

6 **The Epidemiology of Osteonecrosis in Japan** 47
Takuaki Yamamoto, Ryosuke Yamaguchi, and Yukihide Iwamoto

7 **Epidemiology of Osteonecrosis of the Femoral Head in South Korea** 51
Joon Soon Kang and Kee Hyung Rhyu

8 **Current Trends of Osteonecrosis of the Femoral Head in Taiwan and China** 55
Fang-Tsai Lee, Tso-Chiang Ma, and Mel S. Lee

Part IV Etiology

9 **Genetic Studies in Osteonecrosis of the Femoral Head** 61
Shin-Yoon Kim and Tae-Ho Kim

10 **Osteonecrosis and Intravascular Coagulation Revisited** 71
Lynne C. Jones and Deborah McK. Ciombor

11 **Glucocorticoids (as an Etiologic Factor)** 81
Eun Young Lee and Yun Jong Lee

12 **Corticosteroid Usage and Osteonecrosis of the Hip** 91
Jeffrey J. Cherian, Bhaveen H. Kapadia, Samik Banerjee, Julio J. Jauregui, and Michael A. Mont

13 **Alcohol** 95
Wakaba Fukushima and Yoshio Hirota

14 **Traumatic Avascular Necrosis of the Femoral Head** 101
Simon Damian Steppacher, Pascal Cyrill Haefeli, Helen Anwander, Klaus Arno Siebenrock, and Moritz Tannast

15 **Posttraumatic Osteonecrosis of the Femoral Head** 113
Taek Rim Yoon and Ha Sung Kim

16 **Osteonecrosis in Sickle-Cell Disease** 125
Philippe Hernigou and Gildasio Daltro

17 **Autoimmune Disease (SLE, Antiphospholipid Syndrome), Posttransplantation (Kidney, Liver, Heart, Bone Marrow), and Other Risk Factors (Chemotherapy, Caisson Disease, Radiation, Pancreatitis, Gaucher's Disease)** 133
Jeong Joon Yoo

Part V Pathology

18 **Pathophysiology of Ischemic Diseases of the Hip: Osteonecrosis, Borderline Necrosis, and Bone Marrow Edema Syndrome** 143
Kyung-Hoi Koo, Young-Kyun Lee, and Yun Jong Lee

19 **The Pathology of Osteonecrosis of the Femoral Head** 151
Takuaki Yamamoto

Part VI Clinical Manifestation

20 **Natural History of Osteonecrosis** 161
Samik Banerjee, Bhaveen H. Kapadia, Julio J. Jauregui, Jeffrey J. Cherian, and Michael A. Mont

21 **Causes of Pain in Early and Advanced Stage Osteonecrosis** 165
Vivek S. Jagadale and Edward Y. Cheng

22 **Accumulation of Necrotic Fatty Marrow in Osteonecrotic Hips Mimicking Septic Arthritis** 173
Tae-Young Kim, Kyung-Hoi Koo, and Javad Parvizi

Part VII Imaging Diagnosis

23 **Radiography, MRI, CT, Bone Scan, and PET-CT** 179
Kyung Nam Ryu, Wook Jin, and Ji Seon Park

Part VIII Staging and Classification

24 **Ficat Staging System** 199
Kyung-Hoi Koo

25 **The University of Pennsylvania Classification of Osteonecrosis** 201
David R. Steinberg and Marvin E. Steinberg

26 **Natural Course and the JIC Classification of Osteonecrosis of the Femoral Head** 207
Nobuhiko Sugano and Kenji Ohzono

27 **Modified Kerboul Classification System of Necrotic Extent Using MRI** 211
Yong-Chan Ha, Young-Kyun Lee, and Kyung-Hoi Koo

28 **The ARCO Staging System: Generation and Evolution Since 1991** 215
J.W.M. Gardeniers, A.C. Gosling-Gardeniers, and W.H.C. Rijnen

Part IX Differential Diagnosis

29 **Subchondral Stress Fracture of the Femoral Head** 221
Hee Joong Kim, Jeong Joon Yoo, and Pil Whan Yoon

30 **Bone Marrow Edema Syndrome of the Hip** 231
Young-Kyun Lee and Kyung-Hoi Koo

31 **Distinguishing Bone Marrow Edema Syndrome from Osteonecrosis** 235
Marc W. Hungerford and Kyung-Hoi Koo

Part X Non-surgical Treatments

32 **Treatment of Osteonecrosis of the Hip and Knee with Enoxaparin** 241
Charles J. Glueck, Richard A. Freiberg, and Ping Wang

33 **The Role of Coagulopathy in the Pathogenesis and Prevention of Corticosteroid-Induced Osteonecrosis** 249
Takuaki Yamamoto, Goro Motomura, Ryosuke Yamaguchi, and Yukihide Iwamoto

34 **Lipid-Lowering Agents and Their Effects on Osteonecrosis: Pros and Cons** 255
Abdurrahman Kandil and Quanjun Cui

35 **Is There a Role for BMPs in the Treatment of Osteonecrosis?** 261
Philipp Leucht and Stuart B. Goodman

36 **Alendronate in the Prevention of Collapse of the Femoral Head in Nontraumatic Osteonecrosis** 265
Chung-Hwan Chen and Gwo-Jaw Wang

37 **New Therapies of Bone Necrosis** 273
Wolf Drescher, Matthias Knobe, Wolfgang Wagner, and Thomas Pufe

Part XI Surgical Treatments

38 **Principles of Core Decompression for Osteonecrosis of the Hip** 279
Bhaveen H. Kapadia, Samik Banerjee, Jeffrey J. Cherian, Julio J. Jauregui and Michael A. Mont

39 **Stem Cells in Osteonecrosis: Cons** 285
Anjan P. Kaushik, Anusuya Das, and Quanjun Cui

40 Cement Techniques in Hip Osteonecrosis with Collapse: From Traditional Methyl Methacrylate to Bone Substitutes and Stem Cells 291
Philippe Hernigou and Gildasio Daltro

41 Impaction Bone Grafting 297
Seung-Hoon Baek and Shin-Yoon Kim

42 Principles of Bone Grafting for Osteonecrosis of the Hip 307
Julio J. Jauregui, Samik Banerjee, Bhaveen H. Kapadia, Jeffrey J. Cherian, Kimona Issa, and Michael A. Mont

43 Vascularized Pedicle Iliac Bone Grafting for Osteonecrosis of the Femoral Head 315
Mel S. Lee

44 The Vascularized Fibular Graft in the Treatment of Osteonecrosis: Data, Dogma, and Controversies 321
Will Eward

45 Transtrochanteric Rotational Osteotomy for Femoral Head Osteonecrosis 325
Yong-Chan Ha, Jae-Hwi Nho, and Kyung-Hoi Koo

46 Posterior Rotational Osteotomy for Severe Femoral Head Osteonecrosis 331
Takashi Atsumi

47 Transtrochanteric Curved Varus Osteotomy for the Treatment of Osteonecrosis of the Femoral Head 339
Takuaki Yamamoto, Satoshi Ikemura, and Yukihide Iwamoto

48 Total Hip Arthroplasty Using Ceramic-on-Ceramic Articulation 345
Young-Kyun Lee, Ki-Choul Kim, Bun Jung Kang, and Kyung-Hoi Koo

49 Highly Crosslinked Polyethylene Liners in Patients with Osteonecrosis of the Femoral Head in the United States and Europe 349
Patrick O'Toole and Javad Parvizi

50 Alumina Ceramic-on-Highly Cross-Linked Polyethylene Bearing in Cementless Total Hip Arthroplasty in Young Patients with Osteonecrosis of Femoral Head 355
Young-Hoo Kim

51 Hip Arthroplasty for Osteonecrosis of the Femoral Head 363
Harlan C. Amstutz, Michel J. Le Duff, and Mariam Al-Hamad

52 Resurfacing Arthroplasty for Osteonecrosis of the Femoral Head 375
Bernard N. Stulberg and Jayson D. Zadzilka

Part XII Osteonecrosis in Bones Other than the Hip

53 Multifocal Osteonecrosis 383
Samik Banerjee, Bhaveen H. Kapadia, Jeffrey J. Cherian, Julio J. Jauregui, and Michael A. Mont

54 Osteonecrosis of the Humeral Head 389
Nobuhiko Sugano

55 Knee Osteonecrosis 395
Karthik E. Ponnusamy, Savyasachi Thakkar, and Harpal S. Khanuja

56 Osteonecrosis of the Talus 403
Kyoung Min Lee, Sung Hun Won, and Moon Seok Park

57 Kienböck's Disease of the Lunate 411
Dawn M. LaPorte and Thomas J. Kim

Part XIII Legg-Calvé-Perthes Disease

58 The Epidemiology and Etiology of Perthes' Disease 419
Daniel C. Perry

59 Legg-Calvé-Perthes Disease: Pathology, Pathophysiology, and Pathogenesis of Deformity 427
Harry K.W. Kim

60 Legg-Calvé-Perthes Disease: Diagnosis, Imaging, and Classifications 437
Benjamin Shore and Harry K.W. Kim

61 Legg-Calvé-Perthes Disease: Treatments 451
Benjamin D. Martin and Harry K.W. Kim

62 Developing Medical Therapy for Legg-Calvé-Perthes' Disease 469
Harry K.W. Kim and David G. Little

63 Corticosteroid-Associated Osteonecrosis in Children 479
Scott Rosenfeld and Harry K.W. Kim

Part XIV Animal Models

64 Animal Models of Corticosteroid-Associated Bone Diseases 493
Lynne C. Jones, Michelle A. Tucci, Azeb Haile, and Dongqing Wang

65 Animal Models of Bone Necrosis: An Overview 507
Wagner Drescher, Matthias Knobe, Wolfgang Wagner, and Thomas Pufe

Index 511

Contributors

Mariam Al-Hamad, BS Joint Replacement Institute at St Vincent Medical Center, Los Angeles, CA, USA

Harlan C. Amstutz, MD Joint Replacement Institute at St Vincent Medical Center, Los Angeles, CA, USA

Helen Anwander, MD Department of Orthopaedic Surgery, Inselspital, University of Bern, Bern, Switzerland

Takashi Atsumi, MD, PhD Department of Orthopaedic Surgery, Showa University Fujigaoka Hospital, Showa University School of Medicine, Yokohama, Japan

Seung-Hoon Baek, MD Department of Orthopedic Surgery, School of Medicine Kyungpook National University, Daegu, South Korea

Samik Banerjee, MS (Orth), MRCS (Glasg) Department of Orthopaedic Surgery, Rubin Institute for Advanced Orthopedics, Center for Joint Preservation and Replacement, Sinai Hospital of Baltimore, Baltimore, MD, USA

Chung-Hwan Chen Departments of Orthopedics and Orthopedic Research Center, College of Medicine, Kaohsiung Medical University, Kaohsiung, Taiwan

Departments of Orthopedics, Kaohsiung Medical University Hospital, Kaohsiung Medical University, Kaohsiung, Taiwan

Medical Device Innovation Center, National Cheng-Kung University, Tainan, Taiwan

Skeleton-Joint Research Center, National Cheng-Kung University, Tainan, Taiwan

Edward Y. Cheng, MD Department of Orthopaedic Surgery, University of Minnesota Medical School, Minneapolis, MN, USA

Jeffrey J. Cherian, DO Department of Orthopaedic Surgery, Rubin Institute for Advanced Orthopedics, Center for Joint Preservation and Replacement, Sinai Hospital of Baltimore, Baltimore, MD, USA

Ki-Choul Kim Department of Orthopaedic Surgery, Dankook University College of Medicine, Cheonan, South Korea

Deborah McK. Ciombor, PhD Department of Orthopaedics, Duffy Cell Biology Laboratory, Brown University, Providence, RI, USA

Quanjun Cui, MD Department of Orthopaedic Surgery, University of Virginia School of Medicine, Charlottesville, VA, USA

Jaroslaw Czubak, MD, PhD Department of Orthopaedic, Pediatric Orthopaedic and Traumatology, The Medical Centre of Postgraduate Education in Warsaw, Gruca Teaching Hospital, Otwock, Poland

Gildasio Daltro Department of Orthopaedic Surgery, Hospital Edgar Santos, University Federal of Bahia, Salvador, Brazil

Anusuya Das, PhD Department of Orthopaedic Surgery, University of Virginia School of Medicine, Charlottesville, VA, USA

Wolf Drescher, MD, PhD Department of Orthopaedic Surgery, RWTH University Hospital Aachen, Aachen, Germany

Department of Orthopaedic and Spine Surgery, Agaplesion Ev. Bathildis-Hospital, Bad Pyrmont, Germany

Wagner Drescher Department of Orthopaedic Surgery, RWTH University Hospital Aachen, Aachen, Germany

Department of Orthopaedic and Spine Surgery, Agaplesion Ev. Bathildis-Hospital, Bad Pyrmont, Germany

Michel J. Le Duff, MA Joint Replacement Institute at St Vincent Medical Center, Los Angeles, CA, USA

Will Eward, DVM, MD Department of Orthopaedic Surgery, Duke University Medical Center, Durham, NC, USA

Richard A. Freiberg, MD Orthopedic Surgery Service VA Hospital, Cincinnati, OH, USA

Wakaba Fukushima Department of Public Health, Osaka City University Faculty of Medicine, Osaka, Japan

J.W.M. Gardeniers, MD, PhD Department of Orthopaedics, Radboud University Medical Centre, Nijmegen, The Netherlands

Charles J Glueck, MD The Cholesterol Center, Jewish Hospital of Cincinnati, Cincinnati, OH, USA

Stuart B Goodman, MD, PhD Department of Orthopaedic Surgery and Bioengineering, Stanford University Medical Center Outpatient Center, Redwood City, CA, USA

A.C. Gosling-Gardeniers, MSc Department of Orthopaedics, Radboud University Medical Centre, Nijmegen, The Netherlands

Yong-Chan Ha, MD, PhD Department of Orthopaedic Surgery, Chung-Ang University College of Medicine, Seoul, South Korea

Pascal Cyrill Haefeli, MD Department of Orthopaedic Surgery, Inselspital, University of Bern, Bern, Switzerland

Azeb Haile, MS Department of Orthopaedic Surgery, Center for Metabolism and Obesity Research, Johns Hopkins University School of Medicine, Baltimore, MD, USA

Philippe Hernigou Department of Orthopaedic Surgery, University Paris East, Créteil, France

Yoshio Hirota Department of Public Health, Osaka City University Faculty of Medicine, Osaka, Japan

Marc W. Hungerford, MD Orthopedics and Joint Replacement, Mercy Medical Center, Baltimore, MD, USA

Satoshi Ikemura, MD, PhD Department of Orthopaedic Surgery, Kyushu University, Fukuoka, Japan

Kimona Issa, MD Rubin Institute for Advanced Orthopedics, Center for Joint Preservation and Replacement, Sinai Hospital of Baltimore, Baltimore, MD, USA

Yukihide Iwamoto, MD, PhD Department of Orthopaedic Surgery, Kyushu University, Fukuoka, Japan

Vivek S. Jagadale, MBBS Department of Orthopaedic Surgery, University of Minnesota Medical School, Minneapolis, MN, USA

Julio J. Jauregui, MD Department of Orthopaedic Surgery, Rubin Institute for Advanced Orthopedics, Center for Joint Preservation and Replacement, Sinai Hospital of Baltimore, Baltimore, MD, USA

Wook Jin, MD, PhD Department of Radiology, Kyung Hee University Hospital at Kandong, Seoul, South Korea

Lynne C. Jones, PhD, MS Department of Orthopaedic Surgery, Center for Osteonecrosis Research and Education, Center for Metabolism and Obesity Research, Johns Hopkins University School of Medicine, Baltimore, MD, USA

Johns Hopkins Orthopaedics, Baltimore, MD, USA

Abdurrahman Kandil, MD Department of Orthopaedic Surgery, University of Virginia, Charlottesville, VA, USA

Joon Soon Kang, MD, PhD Department of Orthopaedic Surgery, Inha University Hospital, Incheon, South Korea

Bun Jung Kang Department of Orthopaedic Surgery, Gyeongsang National University School of Medicine, Jinju, South Korea

Bhaveen H. Kapadia, MD Department of Orthopaedic Surgery, Rubin Institute for Advanced Orthopedics, Center for Joint Preservation and Replacement, Sinai Hospital of Baltimore, Baltimore, MD, USA

Anjan P. Kaushik, MD Department of Orthopaedic Surgery, University of Virginia School of Medicine, Charlottesville, VA, USA

Harpal S. Khanuja, MD Department of Orthopaedic Surgery, Johns Hopkins Bayview Medical Center, Johns Hopkins University, Baltimore, MD, USA

Ha Sung Kim Orthopedic Department of Center for Joint Disease, Chonnam National University Hwasun Hospital, Hwasun, South Korea

Hee Joong Kim, MD Department of Orthopedic Surgery, Seoul National University College of Medicine, Seoul, Korea

Young-Hoo Kim The Joint Replacement Center, Ewha Womans University School of Medicine, Seoul, Republic of Korea

The Joint Replacement Center, Ewha Womans University MokDong Hospital, Seoul, South Korea

Shin-Yoon Kim, MD, PhD Department of Orthopedic Surgery, Musculoskeletal Genome Research Center, School of Medicine, Kyungpook National University, Daegu, South Korea

Department of Orthopedic Surgery, Musculoskeletal Genome Research Center, Kyungpook National University, Daegu, South Korea

Tae-Ho Kim, PhD Skeletal Diseases Genome Research Center, Kyungpook National University Hospital, Daegu, South Korea

Tae-Young Kim, MD Department of Orthopaedic Surgery, Hallym University Sacred Heart Hospital, Anyang, South Korea

Thomas J. Kim, MD Resident Department of Orthopaedic Surgery, Johns Hopkins University School of Medicine, Baltimore, MD, USA

Harry K.W. Kim, MD, MS Center for Excellence in Hip Disorders, Texas Scottish Rite Hospital for Children, Dallas, TX, USA

Department of Orthopaedic Surgery, UT Southwestern Medical Center, Dallas, TX, USA

Matthias Knobe, MD Department of Traumatology, RWTH University Hospital, Aachen, Germany

Kyung-Hoi Koo, MD, PhD Department of Orthopaedic Surgery, Seoul National University College of Medicine, Seoul National University Bundang Hospital, Seongnam, Kyonggi-do, Republic of Korea (South Korea)

Dawn M. LaPorte, MD Department of Orthopaedic Surgery, Johns Hopkins University School of Medicine, Baltimore, MD, USA

Eun Young Lee, MD Department of Internal Medicine, Seoul National University College of Medicine, Seoul, South Korea

Department of Internal Medicine, Seoul National University Hospital, Seoul, South Korea

Fang-Tsai Lee, MD, MHA Department of Orthopedics and Administration Center, Kuang-Tien General Hospital and Hung Kuang University, Taichung, Taiwan

Kyoung Min Lee, MD Department of Orthopaedic Surgery, Seoul National University Bundang Hospital, Seongnam, South Korea

Mel S. Lee, MD, PhD Department of Orthopaedic Surgery, Chia-Yi Chang Gung Memorial Hospital, College of Medicine, Chang Gung University, Taoyuan, Taiwan

Young-Kyun Lee, MD, PhD Department of Orthopaedic Surgery, Seoul National University Bundang Hospital, Seongnam, South Korea

Yun Jong Lee, MD Department of Internal Medicine, Seoul National University College of Medicine, Seoul, South Korea

Department of Internal Medicine, Seoul National University Bundang Hospital, Seongnam, South Korea

Philipp Leucht, MD Department of Orthopaedic Surgery, Stanford University Medical Center Outpatient Center, Stanford, CA, USA

David G. Little, MBBS, FRACS (Orth), PhD Department of Orthopaedic Research and Biotechnology, The Children's Hospital at Westmead, University of Sydney, Westmead, NSW, Australia

Tso-Chiang Ma, PhD Department of Health Services Administration, China Medical University, Taichung, Taiwan

Benjamin D. Martin, MD Division of Orthopaedic Surgery and Sports Medicine, Children's National Medical Center, Washington, DC, USA

Michael A. Mont, MD Department of Orthopaedic Surgery, Rubin Institute for Advanced Orthopedics, Center for Joint Preservation and Replacement, Sinai Hospital of Baltimore, Baltimore, MD, USA

Goro Motomura, MD, PhD Department of Orthopaedic Surgery, Kyushu University, Fukuoka, Japan

Sameer M. Naranje, MBBS, MRCS (Glasgow) Department of Orthopaedic Surgery, University of Minnesota, Minneapolis, MN, USA

Jae-Hwi Nho Department of Orthopaedic Surgery, Soonchunhyang University Hospital Cheonan, Cheonan, South Korea

Patrick O'Toole, MD, FRCS (Tr & Orth) The Rothman Institute, Thomas Jefferson University, Philadelphia, PA, USA

Kenji Ohzono, MD, PhD Department of Orthopaedic Surgery, Kansai Rousai Hospital, Amagasaki, Japan

Moon Seok Park, MD Department of Orthopaedic Surgery, Seoul National University Bundang Hospital, Seongnam, Korea

Ji Seon Park, MD, PhD Department of Radiology, Kyung Hee University Hospital, Seoul, South Korea

Javad Parvizi, MD Rothman Institute of Orthopaedics, Thomas Jefferson University Hospital, Philadelphia, PA, USA

Daniel C. Perry, MB ChB (Hons), FRCS (Tr& Orth), PhD Warwick Orthopaedics, Warwick Medical School, Coventry, UK

Karthik E. Ponnusamy, MD Department of Orthopaedic Surgery, Johns Hopkins University, Baltimore, MD, USA

Thomas Pufe, PhD Institute of Anatomy and Cell Biology, RWTH University, Aachen, Germany

Kee Hyung Rhyu, MD, PhD Department of Orthopaedic Surgery, Kyung Hee University Hospital at Gangdong, Seoul, South Korea

W.H.C. Rijnen, MD, PhD Department of Orthopaedics, Radboud University Medical Centre, Nijmegen, The Netherlands

Scott Rosenfeld, MD Pediatric Orthopaedic Surgery, Baylor College of Medicine, Texas Children's Hospital, Houston, TX, USA

Kyung Nam Ryu, MD, PhD Department of Radiology, Kyung Hee University Hospital, Seoul, South Korea

Benjamin Shore, MD, MPH, FRCSC Department of Orthopaedic Surgery, Boston Children's Hospital, Harvard Medical School, Boston, MA, USA

Klaus Arno Siebenrock, MD Department of Orthopaedic Surgery, Inselspital, University of Bern, Bern, Switzerland

David R. Steinberg, MD Department of Orthopaedic Surgery, Perelman School of Medicine, University of Pennsylvania, Philadelphia, PA, USA

Department of Orthopaedic Surgery, Penn Presbyterian Medical Center, Philadelphia, PA, USA

Marvin E. Steinberg, MD Department of Orthopaedic Surgery, Perelman School of Medicine, University of Pennsylvania, Philadelphia, PA, USA

Department of Orthopaedic Surgery, Hospital of the University of Pennsylvania, Philadelphia, PA, USA

Simon Damian Steppacher, MD Department of Orthopaedic Surgery, Inselspital, University of Bern, Bern, Switzerland

Bernard N. Stulberg, MD Orthopaedic and Rheumatologic Institute, Cleveland Clinic, Cleveland, OH, USA

Nobuhiko Sugano, MD, PhD Department of Orthopaedic Medical Engineering, Osaka University Graduate School of Medicine, Suita, Japan

Moritz Tannast, MD Department of Orthopaedic Surgery, Inselspital, University of Bern, Bern, Switzerland

Savyasachi Thakkar, MD Department of Orthopaedic Surgery, Johns Hopkins University, Baltimore, MD, USA

Michelle A. Tucci, PhD Department of Orthopedic Surgery and Rehabilitation, University of Mississippi Medical Center, Jackson, MS, USA

Wolfgang Wagner, MD, PhD Division for Stem Cell Biology and Cellular Engineering, Helmholtz Institute for Biomedical Engineering, RWTH University Hospital, Aachen, Germany

Gwo-Jaw Wang Departments of Orthopedics and Orthopedic Research Center, College of Medicine, Kaohsiung Medical University, Kaohsiung, Taiwan

Department of Orthopedic Surgery, National Cheng-Kung University and Hospital, Tainan, Taiwan

Medical Device Innovation Center, National Cheng-Kung University, Tainan, Taiwan

Skeleton-Joint Research Center, National Cheng-Kung University, Tainan, Taiwan

Department of Orthopedic Surgery, University of Virginia, Charlottesville, VA, USA

Ping Wang, PhD The Cholesterol Center, Jewish Hospital of Cincinnati, Cincinnati, USA

Dongqing Wang, MD, PhD Department of Orthopaedic Surgery, Center for Metabolism and Obesity Research, Johns Hopkins University School of Medicine, Baltimore, MD, USA

Howard Winet Departments of Orthopaedic Surgery and Bioengineering, University of California, Los Angeles, CA, USA

Sung Hun Won, MD Department of Orthopaedic Surgery, Seoul National University Bundang Hospital, Seongnam, Korea

Ryosuke Yamaguchi, MD, PhD Department of Orthopaedic Surgery, Kyushu University, Fukuoka, Japan

Takuaki Yamamoto, MD, PhD Department of Orthopaedic Surgery, Kyushu University, Fukuoka, Japan

Jeong Joon Yoo, MD, PhD Department of Orthopedic Surgery, Seoul National University College of Medicine, Seoul, Korea

Taek Rim Yoon Orthopedic Department of Center for Joint Disease, Chonnam National University Hwasun Hospital, Hwasun, Korea

Pil Whan Yoon, MD, PhD Department of Orthopedic Surgery, Seoul National University Boramae Hospital, Seoul, Korea

Jayson D. Zadzilka, MS Orthopaedic and Rheumatologic Institute, Cleveland Clinic, Cleveland, OH, USA

Marcin Zlotorowicz, MD, PhD Department of Orthopaedic, Pediatric Orthopaedic and Traumatology, The Medical Centre of Postgraduate Education in Warsaw, Gruca Teaching Hospital, Otwock, Poland

Part I

History

1 Osteonecrosis: Historical Perspective

Marvin E. Steinberg and David R. Steinberg

1.1 Introduction

Osteonecrosis, also known as avascular necrosis, ischemic necrosis, and aseptic necrosis, is not a specific disease entity. It is rather a condition in which a circumscribed area of bone becomes necrotic as a result of the loss of its blood supply. The most common cause is trauma, a displaced fracture or dislocation which results in a mechanical injury to the local vessels. However, many etiologic factors unrelated to trauma have also been identified. The femoral head is the region most often affected, but the proximal humerus, femoral condyles, and small bones of the hands and feet may also be involved. Despite considerable progress in the study of this condition, there is still much to be learned about its etiology, pathogenesis, and treatment.

This chapter will attempt to provide an historical perspective on osteonecrosis, starting with the earliest case reports and extending to the present. It will focus on specific developments in regard to etiology and pathogenesis, diagnosis, classification, and management. It will end with some suggested goals for the future. Discussion will essentially be limited to nontraumatic osteonecrosis in the adult and will emphasize the hip, since this joint is the region most frequently affected and the one which has been studied most extensively. The material contained herein was derived from many sources but much additional information exists which was not available for review. We thereby apologize for any significant oversights or omissions.

1.1.1 Early Case Reports

Osteonecrosis was first described in 1738 by Alexander Munro [1]. In 1794, James Russell, Professor of Clinical Surgery in Edinburgh, published his classic essay on necrosis of bone, which was one of the first detailed pathologic descriptions of this condition. A clear distinction between septic and aseptic necrosis was not made at this time and the majority of his cases may have been septic [2]. Between 1829 and 1842, Jean Cruveilhier, the noted French anatomist, described gross deformity of the femoral head as a late complication of trauma, presumably due to vascular injury [3, 4]. Kraglund in 1886 and Konig in 1888 described the condition in more depth [5]. However, Freund in 1936 provided the first detailed description of bilateral aseptic necrosis of the femoral heads [6]. Between 1934 and 1949, Phemister and his associates wrote a series of classical articles on the etiology and pathogenesis of aseptic necrosis [7–9]. Chandler identified the vascular etiology of osteonecrosis in his 1948 article entitled "Coronary Disease of the Hip" [10]. In 1951, deMarneffe published results of his detailed studies on the circulation in long bones [11], and in 1953, Trueta and Harrison described the vascular anatomy of the adult hip which furthered our understanding of the pathogenesis of ON [12].

1.1.2 Increasing Prevalence

In 1962, Mankin and Brower reported five new cases of bilateral idiopathic avascular necrosis of the hip and stated that only 22 additional cases could be found in the English

M.E. Steinberg (✉)
Department of Orthopaedic Surgery,
Perelman School of Medicine,
University of Pennsylvania, Philadelphia, PA, USA

Department of Orthopaedic Surgery,
Hospital of the University of Pennsylvania,
Silverstein 2, 3400 Spruce Street, Philadelphia, PA 19104, USA
e-mail: marvin.steinberg@uphs.upenn.edu

D.R. Steinberg
Department of Orthopaedic Surgery,
Perelman School of Medicine,
University of Pennsylvania, Philadelphia, PA, USA

Department of Orthopaedic Surgery,
Penn Presbyterian Medical Center, 3900 Market Street,
One Cupp Pavilion, Philadelphia, PA 19104, USA
e-mail: david.steinberg@uphs.upenn.edu

K.-H. Koo et al. (eds.), *Osteonecrosis*,
DOI 10.1007/978-3-642-35767-1_1, © Springer-Verlag Berlin Heidelberg 2014

literature [13]. However, over the next several years an increasing number of cases were reported, probably related both to an increased awareness and diagnosis of this condition and to an actual increase in the incidence of ON due in large part to increased use of corticosteroids [1, 3, 14–18]. Although we do not have accurate data on the current incidence of osteonecrosis, it has been estimated that over 20,000 new cases are diagnosed annually and that approximately 10 % of all primary total hip replacements are performed for ON in the United States alone. The incidence is considerably higher in other parts of the world. In Korea and Taiwan, for example, approximately one half of all primary total hip replacements are done for osteonecrosis. The reason for this is not entirely clear, but it may be related to a number of genetic factors which have recently been identified [19–22].

1.1.3 Conferences, Symposia, and Publications

The importance of osteonecrosis and the many unanswered questions surrounding this condition have led to several conferences and symposia on this topic during the past 50 years. In 1964, a conference on aseptic necrosis of the femoral head was held in St. Louis, Missouri, under the auspices of the Surgery Study Sections, National Institutes of Health, United States Public Health Service [23]. A number of distinguished scientists and clinicians participated in a comprehensive 2-day symposium which focused on the etiology and pathogenesis of avascular necrosis. Several diverse topics were covered including the anatomy of the hip, circulation, pathophysiology, and biochemistry. Experimental techniques were described including the use of various isotopes to study blood flow and bone viability. As a result of this conference, the American Orthopaedic Association organized a committee on aseptic necrosis of the femoral head to promote further study of this condition, with the goal of finding means of prevention and cure.

The first international symposium on bone circulation was organized by Professors Paul Ficat and Jacques Arlet and was held in Toulouse, France, in 1973. A number of surgeons and researchers involved in the study of bone circulation took part. The symposium was quite successful and was followed by a second symposium in 1977, a third in 1982, and a fourth in 1987.

1.1.4 Formation of ARCO

A small group of those who had participated in the Toulouse symposia met in London in December of 1989 to found the Association Internationale de Recherche sur la Circulation Osseous (ARCO). Thereafter, international symposia on bone circulation, organized by members of ARCO, were held on a regular basis in various locations in Europe, Asia, Australia, and the United States. The most recent symposium at the time of this publication was held in March of 2013 in Chicago, USA. Papers presented at certain ARCO symposia were compiled and published in 1982 [24], 1987 [25], 1992 [26], 1994, and 2005 [27]. The headquarters of ARCO remained in Toulouse, France, from which its activities were guided by Professors Arlet, Ficat, and Mazieres, who served as Secretary General and Treasurer. In 2000, ARCO moved its headquarters to Baltimore, Maryland. Drs. Hungerford, Mont, and Jones assumed responsibility for the administration and scientific activities and served in various capacities including President, Program Chairman, Executive Director, and Secretary-Treasurer.

1.1.5 National Organizations

In 1996, the American Orthopaedic Association sponsored an international symposium entitled "Osteonecrosis: Etiology, Diagnosis and Management," held at Duke University, Durham, North Carolina, under the direction of James R. Urbaniak. The proceedings were published in 1997 [28].

In addition to ARCO, national organizations concerned with osteonecrosis were also formed. In Japan, under the auspices of the Ministry of Health and Welfare, the Japanese Investigation Committee for Intractable Disease established a section on avascular necrosis of the femoral head [29]. In the United States, the National Osteonecrosis Foundation was founded in Baltimore by David S. Hungerford in 1996. It included patients, physicians, and others interested in finding a cure for osteonecrosis. Its primary mission was to provide support for research and education. Dr. Hungerford served as its first President and Dr. Lynne Jones as Secretary-Treasurer.

1.2 Etiology and Pathogenesis

By the 1960s, several specific etiologic factors were recognized and others were being added steadily. In some cases, the mechanisms by which they led to ON were not entirely clear and they were often referred to as factors "associated with" ON rather than as causes of ON. The role of trauma as the first to be identified was mentioned earlier [30–37].

As early as 1911 [38] and 1913 [39], osteonecrotic lesions were found in divers and tunnel works. This entity became known as "Caisson disease" and later as dysbaric osteonecrosis. Axhausen, in 1928, first suggested thromboembolism as a possible cause of osteonecrosis [40]. Bone changes in patients with sickle cell disease and related hemoglobinopathies were well recognized by the 1930s [41]. The first case of ON reported in association with prolonged corticosteroid administration was published in 1957 by Pietrogrande and Mastromarino [42]. By 1962, it was clear that there was an increased incidence of ON in patients who consumed excessive amount of alcohol, and it soon became apparent that the majority of cases of nontraumatic osteonecrosis were related to either steroid administration or alcohol consumption [4, 17, 43–45].

By 1965, Jones had noted the relationship between fat embolism and osteonecrosis. He concluded that intravascular coagulation could be initiated by a variety of factors, including fat embolism, and suggested that this was perhaps the most frequent pathway leading to osteonecrosis. He and others published several studies in this area [4, 46–48].

In the 1990s, Glueck and his colleagues published a series of papers establishing a relationship between certain coagulation abnormalities, specifically thrombophilia and hypofibrinolysis, and osteonecrosis. In many instances, a familial incidence could be identified. These were later found to be due to specific gene mutations. They concluded that subtle coagulopathies could be found in up to 70 % of patients with ON if the appropriate tests were performed [49, 50].

A number of clinical conditions have been identified in association with osteonecrosis. The pathologic mechanisms involved have not been clear. In many instances, prolonged treatment with corticosteroid was involved, and this may play a greater role in the development of ON than the underlying condition for which it was prescribed. Examples are ON following organ transplantation, lupus erythematosus and other collagen-vascular disorders, severe acute respiratory syndrome (SARS), various allergic states, and HIV infection [4, 51]. Increased intraosseous pressure is often present in the femoral head and neck of hips with ON. It was initially felt that this was an etiologic factor causing vascular compromise [43]; however, it is also present in hips with other disorders, such as osteoarthritis. It is now felt by some to be the result of the osteonecrosis rather than the cause, although it may contribute to the pathogenesis. It is probable that multiple factors often act in concert in causing ON, leading to the concept that this is a multifactorial condition [52, 53].

During the past several years, there has been a significant increase in the number of studies on etiologic factors related to osteonecrosis. With improvements in technology and developments in molecular biology, biochemistry, and genetics, investigations have begun to shift away from the classical studies of anatomy and histology. It has been recognized that the prevalence of osteonecrosis in populations in China, Korea, and Taiwan has been considerably higher than in other areas of the world. The explanation was not initially apparent. However, recent studies have identified a number of genetic abnormalities in patients with ON which might in large part account for this [19–22]. Some of these directly affect coagulation mechanisms and result in a tendency towards hypercoagulation, particularly in the presence of other initiating factors, such as corticosteroids, alcohol, and increased circulating lipids. Vascular endothelial growth factor polymorphism has also been identified in patients with steroid induced osteonecrosis. The resulting decrease in VEGF activity increases the risk for osteonecrosis [20]. Another genetic abnormality associated with osteonecrosis involves endothelial nitric oxide synthase (eNOS). Decreased production of nitric oxide could affect angiogenesis, thrombus formation, and bone turnover [19]. Other etiologic factors identified recently include cryofibrinogen, P-glycoprotein [22], and certain metabolic effects of adipocytes, osteoblasts, and osteoclasts.

1.3 Diagnosis

Although we do not yet have an entirely satisfactory treatment for osteonecrosis of the femoral head, the best results are obtained when the condition is treated early, ideally before collapse of the femoral head has occurred. Early treatment requires early diagnosis. During the 1960s, there was a growing awareness of the condition, and there was a steady increase in the number of cases reported. The diagnosis depended initially on the history since it was recognized that predisposing factors and conditions could be identified in a majority of cases. A number of cases were considered to be "idiopathic"; however as we learned more about the etiologic factors involved, the numbers assigned to this category diminished steadily. Excessive alcohol consumption and prolonged steroid administration continue to be the most frequently identified predisposing factors and are present in approximately 80 % of cases. The numbers of cases associated with steroid has continued to increase as the administration of steroids for a variety of conditions, such as organ transplantation, increases. The association with sickle cell disorders and dysbarism was also identified early, whereas the role of hyperlipidemias and various coagulation abnormalities was determined somewhat later.

1.3.1 Functional Investigation of Bone

Plain radiographs initially were and continue to be the mainstay in the diagnosis of this condition. Changes are often pathognomonic. However, it was recognized in the 1960s that plain films may initially appear normal. As early as 1964, Arlet and Ficat studied the early stages of ON by means of "functional investigation of bone." This involved a surgical procedure performed either under general or spinal anesthesia. The hemodynamics of bone were investigated by taking pressure measurements and performing intraosseous venography. A core biopsy of bone, and occasionally articular cartilage, was removed and examined histologically. This enabled the authors to diagnose the presence of osteonecrosis prior to its appearance on radiographs. Although this procedure was initially used for the study and diagnosis of osteonecrosis, they found that patients were often relieved of pain and felt that the clinical course in many cases was improved. It was presumed that this was in large part due to a release of the increased intraosseous pressure which was usually present. Thereafter, this procedure was frequently employed in the treatment of osteonecrosis and became known as "core decompression."

The functional evaluation also included the use of various radio isotopes. These were employed to study both the bone circulation and the metabolic status of the necrotic region. These bone-seeking isotopes often identified bone lesions of vascular origin. Initially, 45 and 47 calcium and 42 phosphorus were used. Later, 18 fluoride and 85 and 87 strontium were employed, and more recently 99M technetium diphosphonate. Although these agents often did identify areas of necrosis not seen on plain films, they were neither sensitive nor specific. Theoretically, the necrotic region of bone would not take up the isotope and would therefore appear "cold" on the scan. However, the viable areas of bone surrounding the region of necrosis were engaged in attempts at repair and often showed increased uptake, frequently masking the lack of uptake in the center of the lesion. However, prior to the introduction of MRI, "bone scans" or scintigraphy was an important technique for the early diagnosis of ON, before radiographic changes appeared. These studies were employed by Ficat and Arlet in developing their radiologic classification of ischemic necrosis [15, 54, 55].

Arteriography was used to a limited extent, basically as an investigational tool, and not for clinical diagnosis.

1.3.2 Magnetic Resonance Imaging (MRI)

During the very late 1970s and early 1980s, a new imaging technique was developed using magnetic signals rather than X-rays. This was initially referred to as nuclear magnetic resonance or NMR. Largely because of the concern created by the use of the term "nuclear," it was shortly thereafter referred to as "magnetic resonance imaging" or MRI. It was soon found to be extremely useful in the diagnosis of a variety of pathologic conditions and particularly in the early diagnosis of osteonecrosis. A number of studies confirmed that it was perhaps the most valuable technique for the early diagnosis of osteonecrosis, being both sensitive and specific [56–58]. It can usually detect the presence of necrosis within a few weeks after the insult, well before any changes appear on either X-ray or computerized tomography. Over the years, a number of improvements have been made in the technology, use, and interpretation of MRI. Fortunately, no deleterious effects of MRI have been identified. Its use is now widespread and allows early diagnosis of the condition, thus improving the efficacy of treatment.

Since the development of MRI, CT has played a limited role and scintigraphy is seldom used except perhaps as a tool for whole-body screening. The role of other imaging techniques for the diagnosis of osteonecrosis has not been established. These include positron emission tomography (PET), single-photon emission computerized tomography (SPECT), gadolinium-enhanced MRI, and perfusion MRI. Almost certainly with the passage of time newer and improved techniques will be developed which will allow earlier diagnosis and better evaluation of patients with osteonecrosis.

1.3.3 Differential Diagnosis

As with any new technique, it took a while for the value of MRI in the early diagnosis of osteonecrosis to be recognized. Initially it was used infrequently. However, within a short time its value became widely recognized and it was then used perhaps too frequently. In addition, many other conditions affecting the hip also show MRI abnormalities. Unfortunately, these were often confused with osteonecrosis and misdiagnosed. These include transient osteoporosis of the hip (TOH) or bone marrow edema syndrome (BMES), femoral head cysts, subchondral insufficiency fracture, and rapidly progressive osteoarthritis. Other conditions to be differentiated from osteonecrosis include spontaneous osteonecrosis of the knee, which is most likely an insufficiency fracture, and osteonecrosis of the jaw, which may actually be osteomyelitis.

1.4 Classification Systems

For quite some time, the importance of an effective and uniformly used classification system has been recognized. This would help establish a prognosis, follow improvement or progression of the condition, compare the effectiveness of different methods of treatment, and determine the best method of management for patients with different stages of osteonecrosis. This system should also help to eliminate much of the current confusion about both the natural history and the treatment of ON.

1.4.1 Ficat and Arlet

The first system for classification of osteonecrosis was described in the early 1960s by Arlet and Ficat [59] and included three specific stages. In the 1970s, a fourth stage was added, and this is the version most widely used today, although later Stage 0 and a transitional stage were added [14, 15]. Symptoms and physical findings were in part correlated with radiographic changes and functional evaluation of bone was used to diagnose the early stages. These included bone scans or scintigraphy, but MRI was not included. The Ficat and Arlet classification continues to be popular; however, it has been modified by some to include MRI, and bone biopsies and functional evaluation are no longer used. A major disadvantage of this system is that it does not indicate the size of the necrotic lesion and the extent of joint involvement. Thus, it cannot differentiate between small and large lesions, nor can it indicate with any degree of accuracy whether progression has taken place.

1.4.2 Marcus, Enneking, and Massam

In 1973, Marcus, Enneking, and Massam [60] described six radiographic stages of osteonecrosis. These were correlated with both the gross and histologic findings as well as the patient's symptoms and physical examination. No preradiographic stages were included and MRI was not available at this time. This classification did not attempt to quantitate the extent of involvement. However, it was subsequently modified by Urbaniak et al. and Enneking to include MRI and later to include quantitative measurements [60–63].

1.4.3 Sugioka

In 1976, Sugioka [64] outlined a simple radiographic rating for hips with osteonecrosis that placed hips into four separate categories. Although this classification did not indicate lesion size, he did describe a method for measuring the extent of the lesion as seen on lateral radiographs, as this measurement was an important predictor of outcome in hips being considered for his rotational osteotomy [65]. The location of the lesion was used to determine whether an anterior or a posterior rotational osteotomy should be performed, depending on which would better shift an intact articular surface into the region of major weight bearing.

1.4.4 The University of Pennsylvania

The University of Pennsylvania classification was developed in the early 1980s and identified seven clearly defined radiographic stages. Initially, it incorporated technetium bone scans, but these were supplemented and replaced soon thereafter by magnetic resonance imaging. An indication of the size of the necrotic lesion and the extent of joint involvement were integral parts of this classification and subdivided each of the stages into a mild, moderate, and severe category. The patient's symptoms and physical findings were not included as part of the classification, but they were considered important in determining management. The two most important features of this classification are that it was the first to include measurement of lesion size and joint involvement as an integral part of the system and the first to employ MRI as a specific modality for determining stage [66, 67].

1.4.5 The Japanese Investigation Committee for Avascular Necrosis

In 1987, the Japanese Investigation Committee for Avascular Necrosis described a new classification [68, 69]. Hips were initially evaluated using the four-part Ficat and Arlet classification. Hips in Stages II and III were further divided by the type, location, and extent of the lesion. It did not specifically evaluate Stages I or IV nor the amount of femoral head collapse or joint involvement. It has been used primarily in Japan.

1.4.6 The Association Research Circulation Osseous (ARCO)

The Committee on Nomenclature and Staging of the Association Research Circulation Osseous (ARCO) met in 1991 to establish uniform terminology, a set of diagnostic criteria, and a classification of osteonecrosis. The Committee endorsed the University of Pennsylvania Staging System [70]. In 1992, the location of the lesion, as described by the Japanese Investigating Committee, was added [71, 72]. However, this addition was found to have made the system too complex, and in 1993, Stages III and IV and Stages V and VI were combined to provide five rather than seven stages [73]. Subsequently, there was concern that the system no longer provided a separate category for the hip with a crescent sign without femoral head flattening and that it remained unnecessarily complicated by adding a separate category for localization in addition to lesion size.

1.4.7 Other Methods of Evaluation

In addition to the classification systems described, a number of investigators have used specific methods of indicating lesion size which are not part of a classification system. In 1974, Kerboul et al. [74] noted that the outcome of proximal femoral osteotomies for osteonecrosis was related to location and extent of necrosis. This was determined by measuring the arc of the articular surface overlying the lesion on both AP and lateral radiographs, referred to as the "combined necrotic angle" [75]. The authors found a rough correlation between the size and location and the results following a flexion-adduction osteotomy. Wagner and Zeiler [76] reported similar observations. In 1995, Koo and Kim [77] also used angular measurements made on MRIs rather than radiographs to predict outcome. This measurement was referred to as the "index of necrotic extent" or "index of necrosis." It was correlated with the percentage of the articular surface involved. These measurements were used to classify hips as having small, medium, or large lesions. In 2003, Cherian et al. modified this technique slightly by using MRI images which showed the maximum lesion size rather than using midsagittal images. They referred to this as the "modified index of necrotic extent" [78]. In 2006, Ha et al. reported on the use of a modified Kerboul method of measurements using MRI images rather than radiographs. The sums of the arcs measured on midcoronal and midsagittal sections were added together and placed the hip into four separate grades [79].

These and other methods of using angular measurements as a rough approximation of lesion size were relatively simple to use and demonstrated at least some degree of correlation with prognosis and outcome in hips treated either nonoperatively or by core decompression [80].

1.4.8 Ongoing Evaluation

In March of 2013 in conjunction with its international symposium on osteonecrosis, ARCO held a workshop on classification. It was agreed that much could be gained in the evaluation and treatment of patients with osteonecrosis if there were uniform use by the international community of an effective system of classification. It suggested that further study and development were required, and a number of individuals expressed interest in resolving this problem.

A recent review of articles on the treatment of osteonecrosis, published during the past 25 years, showed that although nonquantitative classifications are still frequently used and the four-part classification of Ficat and Arlet is the most often cited, there has been a steady trend towards the use of more comprehensive, quantitative systems of staging including the classifications of ARCO and the University of Pennsylvania [81, 82].

1.5 Management

Although small areas of necrosis may remain asymptomatic and resolve spontaneously, up to 80 % of clinically diagnosed cases involving the hip progress without treatment to collapse and eventual arthroplasty. Our goal therefore is to prevent femoral head collapse and to preserve rather than to replace the joint.

1.5.1 Prevention

A number of risk factors have been identified, and these should be eliminated or minimized to the extent possible. This applies to steroid administration, alcohol ingestion, smoking, and exposure to hyperbaric conditions. The protocol for treating organ transplant patients has changed considerably over the years, and accordingly, the incidence of osteonecrosis in these patients has diminished dramatically. Guidelines for divers and others working under hyperbaric conditions have been established, and when followed, they diminish the incidence of osteonecrosis in this population. The recognition of a variety of genetic factors in the past several years has identified a group of patients at risk for developing osteonecrosis. In this particular population, efforts should be redoubled to minimize factors which could lead to this clinical syndrome. This includes patients with underlying coagulation abnormalities and those with a tendency towards hyperlipidemia.

1.5.2 Nonoperative Management

Initially, many patients with osteonecrosis were treated with non-weight bearing or limited weight bearing in the hope that spontaneous healing would take place. Unfortunately, the results with this approach were usually poor, and there was no conclusive evidence that progression could be retarded by eliminating weight bearing. However, as mentioned, small necrotic lesions, especially those located in areas of minimal weight bearing, have a good prognosis and can be treated with close observation alone. Limited weight bearing can be employed for the symptomatic management of patients who are waiting for prophylactic surgery, those not yet ready for arthroplasty, and as part of the postoperative management following procedures designed to preserve the femoral head.

Various physical modalities of treatment have been employed for the treatment of ON, including different types of electrical stimulation and ultrasound. These have been used either alone or as adjuncts to operative procedures, such as core decompression. Although the initial results were promising, at the present time these modalities are used only infrequently and further evaluation and development may be indicated [83, 84]. Since hyperbaric oxygen therapy has been found useful in the treatment of certain conditions, such as infection and poorly healing skin grafts, there was some early enthusiasm about its role in the treatment of osteonecrosis [85]. Unfortunately, there is little definitive evidence that it is effective and it is rarely used at the present time.

Medical management has included the use of anticoagulants in patients with known coagulopathy and lipid-lowering agents in patients with hyperlipidemia. Although the use of anticoagulants has been recommended in patients with hypercoagulable states [50], it should be noted that this is not a benign form of treatment and should not be employed until there is further evidence of their effectiveness. Bisphosphonates have been administered to slow the process of bone resorption which is felt to be a deleterious component in the pathogenesis of this disorder. A limited number of studies showed promising early results. It is uncertain whether these can be maintained over a longer period of time [86]. Other agents have been considered in the treatment of osteonecrosis, such as vasodilators and fullerol, but their clinical effectiveness has yet to be established.

1.5.3 Preservation of the Femoral Head

If the condition is diagnosed early, before there is any evidence of femoral head collapse, a number of operative procedures have been advocated in an attempt to retard or halt progression and encourage healing.

1.5.3.1 Core Decompression

During the early 1960s, Arlet and Ficat used core decompression as a method to study the earliest changes in osteonecrosis and to diagnose the condition prior to its appearance on X-rays [14, 15, 59]. Following this procedure, patients reported a marked decrease in hip pain which was felt to be due to a decrease in the abnormally elevated intraosseous marrow pressure. Subsequently, this technique was used quite widely as a method of treating early cases of osteonecrosis. Classically, the channel created is left open to allow adequate decompression. However, the procedure has been modified by the insertion of loosely fitted cancellous bone grafts and the introduction of various agents to stimulate healing, such as bone morphogenetic protein (BMP) and demineralized bone matrix (DBM). It has also been supplemented by the addition of various forms of electrical stimulation [84, 87]. Another modification is to use a series of small holes drilled into the necrotic lesion rather than a single large channel. Although core decompression remains one of the most popular procedures for the treatment of early osteonecrosis, there have been some differences of opinion as to its safety and effectiveness. Most studies report a very low incidence of complications if the procedure is performed correctly and results significantly better than with symptomatic management [88–91]. Although theoretically one would think that the addition of various growth stimulating factors to the classical core decompression would improve the results, to date this has not been demonstrated with most techniques. An exception to this is the introduction of mesenchymal stem cells into the core tract. This technique will be discussed later.

1.5.3.2 Osteotomies

Various types of osteotomies have been described for the treatment of osteonecrosis of the femoral head during the past 40 years. The rationale for their efficacy is the biomechanical effect of moving the necrotic segment from a region of major weight bearing to an area that bears less weight and replacing it with a relatively normal segment of the femoral head. These involve varus/valgus, flexion/extension, and rotation. Varying degrees of success have been reported after short- and intermediate-term follow-up for varus or valgus osteotomies, occasionally combined with extension and supplemented with curettage and bone grafting [92, 93]. In 1974, Kerboul et al. reported the relationship between outcome and the location and size of the lesion which they referred to as "the combined necrotic angle" [74]. The effectiveness of varus or valgus osteotomies is necessarily limited by the amount that one can alter the normal neck-shaft angle.

To overcome this limitation transtrochanteric anterior rotational osteotomies were devised by Sugioka [64]. These were later modified by Atsumi to include posterior rotation, which allows a greater degree of rotation and is therefore able to be used for especially large necrotic lesions [94, 95]. These procedures are technically demanding and careful attention must be paid to the indications for surgery, preoperative planning, and postoperative care. Good results have been reported by surgeons experienced in performing these procedures, and they have enjoyed a reasonable degree of popularity in Asia, though less in other regions.

1.5.3.3 Bone Grafting

Various techniques have been described for the use of cortical and cancellous bone grafts. Grafts can be inserted into a channel extending from the lateral femoral cortex to the necrotic region of the femoral head, through a window in the anterior aspect of the femoral neck, or directly through a trap door made in the articular cartilage of the femoral head. Cancellous bone can be combined with cortical grafts which may be harvested along with a muscle pedicle to provide some degree of vascularity. Osteochondral grafts have also been used to replace both necrotic bone as well as a depressed portion of the femoral head overlying the lesion. Long-term success with these techniques has generally not been observed and they are less often used today [96–100].

As early as 1934, Phemister described a procedure in which a channel was created extending from the lateral femoral cortex into the region of necrosis. Dead bone was removed and a cortical graft was inserted [7, 9]. This technique was later modified by Bonfiglio and associates [100, 101] and served as a precursor to free vascularized fibular grafting, which was introduced later [61, 102–105].

1.5.3.4 Free Vascularized Fibular Grafting (FVFG)

With advances in surgical technique, it became possible to harvest a fibular graft together with its vascular supply and to introduce this directly into the necrotic lesion of the femoral head via a channel through the lateral femoral cortex. A microvascular anastomosis is then performed to local vessels. The goals of this procedure are to decompress the femoral head, to remove a significant portion of necrotic bone, to fill this defect with osteo-inductive cancellous bone, to support the subchondral bone with a cortical strut, and to enhance the revascularization process by means of the vascular anastomoses. This procedure was introduced simultaneously in the United States and in Italy by Brunelli and Brunelli and by Urbaniak in 1979, and by Gilbert et al. in France. Although experience with this technique is somewhat limited, those centers with sufficient experience with its use have reported encouraging results. In a symposium on osteonecrosis which was sponsored by the American Academy of Orthopaedic Surgeons and the American Orthopaedic Association and held at Duke University in 1997, a large portion of the proceedings was devoted to FVFG. Eight authors presented their experience with this technique [105]. However, FVFG is a technically difficult procedure which requires a well-trained staff who are experienced in microvascular surgery. In general, two teams operate simultaneously and there is a steep learning curve. The complication rate is not insignificant, and later conversion to total hip replacement may be more difficult. Rigid indications are to be followed. Because of these factors, there is less enthusiasm for performing this procedure today than there was perhaps 10–15 years ago. Some feel that the theoretical advantages of FVFG may not be warranted by the disadvantages [61, 102–105].

1.5.3.5 Mesenchymal Stem Cell Introduction

The treatment of osteonecrosis with autologous bone marrow grafting was developed by Hernigou et al. at the Henri Mondur Hospital (Creteil, France) in 1990 [106]. Since then a limited number of publications regarding the various facets of this technique and the results have appeared. This method of treatment was also the topic of a number of presentations at the international symposia on bone circulation held by ARCO in 2012 and 2013. Promising results with this technique have been reported by Hernigou, Gangji, and others [107, 108]. Various techniques for obtaining, processing, and inserting the marrow into the femoral head were described. Experience with this technique now exceeds 20 years and several hundred patients have been treated to date. This is perhaps the most promising of the newer techniques designed for the early treatment of osteonecrosis, and we will look forward to continued research and development and to additional experience with the use of stem cells in the treatment of ON.

1.5.3.6 Miscellaneous Procedures

Other approaches to the early treatment of osteonecrosis have been reported. Hernigou et al. described the use of acrylic cement injection directly into the femoral head to retard collapse in patients with ON secondary to sickle cell disease [109]. This can be done either with or without curettage of the necrotic segment and elevating a minimally collapsed joint surface. In some reports the early results were promising, but intermediate results appeared to diminish with the passage of time. The use of this technique to date is limited, and further studies will be required to determine whether it can play a role in the treatment of ON.

Another procedure designed to retard or prevent femoral head collapse is the insertion of a porous tantalum rod. Early results were promising, but recent reports have indicated that less than 50 % of patients obtained acceptable results. It is therefore not considered a viable option at this time [110].

1.5.4 Arthroplasty

Prior to the development of total hip replacement, there were a limited number of options for the treatment of patients with advanced stages of avascular necrosis of the femoral head. During the 1950s and 1960s, a number of these patients underwent cup arthroplasty. This often provided a reasonable degree of pain relief and improved function but the results as compared to modern techniques were inconsistent and mediocre at best [111]. With the development of femoral endoprostheses, these devices began to replace cup arthroplasty. Results were variable. In some cases satisfactory outcomes were obtained and survivorship of these devices could exceed 15 or more years. However, in many cases, the results were poor and were accompanied by degenerative changes on the acetabular side and protrusio acetabuli, as well as loosening of the femoral component. Results with bipolar femoral endoprostheses were only slightly better than with the original unipolar devices.

Other choices included hip fusion or resection arthroplasty. Fusion was of particular concern and limited use both because of the incidence of bilateral disease and the high failure rate of the procedure. Resection arthroplasty could produce pain relief but resulted in shortening, instability, and poor function.

1.5.4.1 Total Hip Replacement

In the later 1960s in Europe and in the early 1970s in the United States total hip replacement became available. There was considerable reluctance to use these devices in patients with osteonecrosis, particularly because of their young age. In five reports published between 1981 and 1984 on total hip arthroplasty in younger patients, good to excellent results were obtained in approximately 81 % of patients with 5-year follow-up and the mean incidence of revision was 13 %. Salvati and Cornell [112] reported an overall failure rate of 37 % at a mean follow-up of 8 years (range 5–10 years). Since that time considerable advancements in surgical technique, materials, and design, and manufacture of total hip replacements have taken place. These have led to considerable improvements in function and survivorship and to a significant decrease in complications. Initially it was felt that the results in ON would be considerably inferior to those in patients with DJD, both because of the age differential and other factors. However, recent studies have found that the results in patients with ON are approaching those in patients with other conditions. Improvements in design have resulted in firm and durable component fixation with both cementless and cemented components. The use of ceramic bearing surfaces and highly cross-linked polyethylene has led to a marked decrease in wear and in wear particles, thus in turn markedly diminishing osteolysis and prosthesis loosening. Improved surgical techniques have decreased infection and dislocation. It is therefore not unreasonable to anticipate 25 or more years of survivorship even for young patients with osteonecrosis who undergo modern total hip replacement. However, it is important that we continue to follow these patients to be sure that these results will be as durable as anticipated [113, 114].

1.5.4.2 Surface Replacement Arthroplasty (SRA)

In the 1970s the reluctance to performed standard total hip replacement on patients with osteonecrosis was in part responsible for the development of surface replacement arthroplasty. Initially it was felt that this was a much more conservative procedure, especially in the younger patient. However, within a relatively short period of time the failure rate with these early designs was excessive, and by 1982 it was recognized that their use should be severely limited. At that time a high percentage of failures were related to the necessity of using a very thin polyethylene acetabular component anchored to bone by an equally thin layer of cement. Thus, the acetabular side was most often the reason for failure. However, failure was not limited here and continued necrosis of the femoral head under the metal cap as well as femoral neck fracture also occurred [115]. Research and development on surface replacement continued, and metal acetabular components were designed to replace the earlier polyethylene components. Initially these metal-on-metal surface replacements gave excellent results, and their popularity increased, not only in patients with osteonecrosis but also in patients with other conditions [116]. Where the pathology was limited to the femoral head, the use of hemi-surface replacement arthroplasty was introduced. Here the femoral head was resurfaced with a metal component which was then allowed to articulate with the native acetabulum. Unfortunately the survivorship of these devices was limited as degeneration of acetabular cartilage often followed within a few years. This was not entirely surprising as studies showed that in virtually all hips with symptoms severe enough to require replacement, there was already damage to the acetabular cartilage at the time of arthroplasty, despite normal appearing X-rays [117]. In addition, one would not expect even normal acetabular cartilage to withstand for long articulating with a metal prosthesis. Thus, hemiarthroplasty was considered to be only a temporizing procedure and its use diminished considerably [118]. However, the use of metal-on-metal surface replacements continued.

1.5.4.3 Bearing Surfaces

By 2008 reports of problems began to appear concerning both standard and surface replacement arthroplasties with metal-on-metal bearing surfaces. Pseudotumors and various soft tissue reactions around some of these prostheses developed, resulting in pain, loosening, and the necessity for revision [119, 120]. This was particularly true in younger females and in small males. There was also increasing concern regarding the long term effects of metal ions. At one point nearly one third of all total hip replacements performed on younger patients in the United States employed metal-on-metal bearing surfaces, but within a short period of time this diminished to 10 % or less. It is uncertain how this will be resolved. At the present time, results with ceramic on ceramic and with metal or ceramic on highly cross-linked polyethylene have shown acetabular and femoral components to be well fixed by bone ingrowth with little evidence of either osteolysis or component loosening at a follow-up of more than 11 years. Much longer follow-ups are required to determine the ultimate survivorship of these components, but there is currently considerable optimism about the future role of modern total hip replacement for patients with osteonecrosis [121].

1.6 Future Goals

A number of future goals can be identified. We should continue to search for an appropriate experimental model of osteonecrosis which will facilitate the study of this disorder. We will increase our understanding of the etiology and pathogenesis of osteonecrosis and, in particular, will learn more about the genetic factors that are involved. With increased awareness of the existence of ON and with the development of improved imaging techniques, osteonecrosis is being diagnosed earlier than it had been and this trend will continue. This is important since earlier diagnosis leads to earlier treatment and improved results. Nearly 30 years ago, we saw the introduction of more effective methods of evaluation and classification of osteonecrosis. These classification systems are being used with increasing frequency by the orthopedic community, and this trend should continue. In addition, we are currently reaching out to our colleagues in musculoskeletal radiology to encourage them to follow a similar path. We must reevaluate the current classification systems and strive for further improvements to increase their effectiveness and ease of use. We must also continue to examine and compare the various operative procedures currently being employed to preserve the femoral head so as to determine more accurately the results of and the indications for each of these. Newer and more effective methods of management must be developed. One of the promising new developments in this area is treatment with mesenchymal stem cells. We anticipate that with further research and development and more experience with this technique, it will prove its effectiveness and will enjoy wider use in the future. In addition, the role of growth factors, including bone morphogenetic protein (BMP), transforming growth factor-beta (TGF-beta), and vascular endothelial growth factor (VegF), will be evaluated. It is particularly important for us to strive for the prevention of osteonecrosis whenever possible, rather than waiting for it to develop and then require treatment. The role of anticoagulants and other agents is still being evaluated. As we learn more about the genetic predispositions in certain groups, it is quite possible that in the future gene therapy for those at high risk may become a reality.

And finally, for those patients in whom severe joint damage cannot be prevented, developments in total joint replacement are extremely promising. Many of the initial problems which led to early component failure in the young, active patient with osteonecrosis seem to have been at least partially resolved. With continued improvement in technology, materials, and component design and manufacture, this trend will undoubtedly continue. When we achieve a mean survivorship of 25 or more years for joint replacement in patients with osteonecrosis, we will have reached a very gratifying solution to a most difficult and challenging problem.

References

1. Luck JV. Bone and joint diseases. Springfield: Charles C Thomas; 1950.
2. Russell J. An essay on necrosis. Section I. General remarks and description of appearances. Clin Orthop. 1978;130:5.
3. Dubois EL, Cozen L. Avascular (aseptic) bone necrosis associated with systemic lupus erythematosus. JAMA. 1960;174:108.
4. Jones Jr JP, Engleman EP. Osseous avascular necrosis associated with systemic abnormalities. Arthritis Rheum. 1966;9:728.
5. Konig F. Ueber freie korper in der gezenken z. Beitrage Zoe Aetiologic Der Cordora Mobilia. Entstehung Derselben Durch Osteochondritis Dissecans. Dtsch Z Chir. 1988;27:99.
6. Freund E. Bilateral aseptic necrosis of the femoral head. Ann Surg. 1936;104:100.
7. Phemister DB. Fractures of neck of femur, dislocations of hip, and obscure vascular disturbances producing aseptic necrosis of head of femur. Surg Gynecol Obstet. 1934;59:415.
8. Phemister DB. Changes in bones and joints resulting from interruption of circulation. I. General consideration and changes resulting from injury. Arch Surg. 1940;41:436.
9. Phemister DB. Treatment of the necrotic head of the femur in adults. J Bone Joint Surg Am. 1949;31:55.
10. Chandler FA. Coronary disease of the hip. J Int Coll Surg. 1948;11:34.
11. deMarneffe R. The circulation in long bones. In: Schoutens A, Arlet J, Gardeniers JWM, Hughes SPF, editors. Bone circulation and vascularization in normal and pathological conditions. New York/London: Plenum Press; 1993. p. 7–18.
12. Trueta J, Harrison MHM. The normal vascular anatomy of the femoral head in adult man. J Bone Joint Surg Br. 1953;39:442.
13. Mankin HJ, Brower TD. Bilateral idiopathic aseptic necrosis of the femur in adults: "Chandler's disease". Bull Hosp Joint Dis. 1962;23:42.
14. Ficat RP. Idiopathic bone necrosis of the femoral head: early diagnosis and treatment. J Bone Joint Surg Br. 1985;67:3–9.
15. Ficat RP, Arlet J. Necrosis of the femoral head. In: Hungerford DS, editor. Ischemia and necrosis of bone. Baltimore: Williams & Wilkins; 1980. p. 53–74.
16. Ficat P, et al. Resultats thérapeutiques du forage biopsie dans les ostéonécroses femoro capitals primitives (idocas). Rev Rheum Mal Osteoartic. 1971;38:269.
17. Heimann WG, Frieberger RH. Avascular necrosis of the femoral and humeral heads after high-dosage corticosteroid therapy. N Engl J Med. 1960;263:672.
18. Merle d'Aubigne R, Postel M, Mazabraud A, et al. Idiopathic necrosis of the femoral head in adults. J Bone Joint Surg Br. 1965;47:612.
19. Koo K-H, Lee J-A, Lee Y-S, et al. Endothelial nitric oxide synthase gene polymorphisms in patients with non-traumatic femoral head osteonecrosis. J Orthop Res. 2006;24(8):1722–8.
20. Kim T-H, Hong J-M, Lee J-Y, et al. Promoter polymorphisms of the vascular endothelial growth factor gene is associated with osteonecrosis of the femoral head in the Korean population. Osteoarthritis Cartilage. 2008;16(3):287–91.
21. Chang JD, Hur M, Lee SS, et al. Genetic background of nontraumatic osteonecrosis of the femoral head in the Korean population. Clin Orthop Relat Res. 2008;466(5):1041–6.
22. He W, Li K. Incidence of genetic polymorphisms involved in lipid metabolism among Chinese patients with osteonecrosis of the femoral head. Acta Orthop. 2009;80(3):325–9.
23. Aaron RK, Ciombor DM. Electrical stimulation, demineralized bone matrix and bone morphogenic protein. Semin Arthroplasty. 1998;9:221.
24. Arlet J, Ficat RP, Hungerford DS, editors. Bone circulation. Baltimore/London: Williams & Wilkins; 1982. (Papers presented at the Third International Symposium on Circulation in Bone. Toulouse: University of Paul Sabatier; 1982).
25. Arlet J, Mazieres B, editors. Bone circulation and bone necrosis. Proceedings of the IVth International Symposium on Bone Circulation, Toulouse; 1987 Sept 17–19. Berlin: Springer; 1990.
26. Schoutens A, Arlet J, Gardeniers JWM, Hughes SPF, editors. Bone circulation and vascularization in normal and pathological conditions. New York/London: Plenum Press; 1993. (Proceedings of a NATO Advanced Research Workshop on Bone and Bone Marrow Circulation in Normal and Pathological Conditions; 1992 Sept 25–26, Brussels).

27. J Bone Joint Surg. 2006;88-A Suppl 3. Selected papers from the ARCO 13th International Symposium on Bone Circulation. 15–17 Sep 2007. London: Imperial College. p. 1–179
28. Urbaniak JR, Jones JP, editors. Osteonecrosis: etiology, diagnosis and treatment. American Academy of Orthopaedic Surgeons, Developed by the American Orthopaedic Association; Rosemont, IL, USA; 1997.
29. Sugano N, Takoka K, Chzono K, et al. Prognostication of non-traumatic avascular necrosis of the femoral head. Clin Orthop Relat Res. 1994;303:155–64.
30. Bauer TW, Plenk Jr H. The pathology of early osteonecrosis of the femoral head. Semin Arthroplasty. 1998;9(3):192–202.
31. Glimcher MJ, Kenzora JE. The biology of osteonecrosis of the human femoral head and its clinical implications. I. Tissue biology. Clin Orthop. 1979;138:284–309.
32. Glincher MJ, Kenzora JE. The biology of osteonecrosis of the human femoral head and its clinical implications. II. The pathological changes in the femoral head as an organ and in the hip joint. Clin Orthop. 1979;139:283–312.
33. Catto M. A histological study of avascular necrosis of the femoral head after transcervical fracture. J Bone Joint Surg Br. 1965; 47:749.
34. Catto M. The histological appearances of late segmental collapse of the femoral head after transcervical fracture. J Bone Joint Surg Br. 1965;47:777.
35. Arlet J, Durroux R, Fauchier C, Thiẽchart C. Histopathology on the non-traumatic necrosis of the femoral head: topographic and evolutive aspects. In: Arlet J, Ficat P, Hungerford DS, editors. Bone circulation. Baltimore: Williams and Wilkins; 1984. p. 296.
36. Ficat RP, Arlet J. Ischemia and necrosis of bone. Hungerford DS, editor. Baltimore/London: Williams and Wilkins; 1980. p. 85–92.
37. Steinberg ME, Mont MA. Chapter 125 Osteonecrosis. In: Chapman MW, editor. Chapman's orthopaedic surgery. 3rd ed. Philadelphia: Lippincott-Raven Publ.; 2001. p. 3263–308.
38. Bornstein A, Plate E. Uber chronische Gelenkveranderungen, entstanden durch Presslufterkrangkung. Fortschr Geb Roentgenstr. 1911;18:197.
39. Bassoe P. The late manifestations of compressed air disease. Am J Med Sci. 1913;145:526.
40. Axhausen G. Uber Anamische Inkarkte am Knochensystem und ihre Bedeutung fur dies Lehre von den primaren Epiphyseonekrosen. Arch Klin Chir. 1928;151:71.
41. Chung SMK, Ralston EL. Necrosis of the femoral head associated with sickle-cell anemia and its genetic variants. J Bone Joint Surg Am. 1969;51:33.
42. Pietrogrande V, Mastromarino R. Osteopatia da prolunga trattamento cortisonico. ORTOP Traumatol. 1957;25:791.
43. Hungerford DS, Zizic TM. Alcoholism associated ischemic necrosis of the femoral head. Clin Orthop Relat Res. 1978;130:144–53.
44. Arlet J. Nontraumatic avascular necrosis of the femoral head. Clin Orthop Relat Res. 1992;277:12–21.
45. Zinn WM, editor. Idiopathic ischemia necrosis of the femoral head in adults. Stuttgart: George Thieme Publishers; 1971.
46. Jones Jr JP, Sakovich L. Fat embolism of bone. J Bone Joint Surg Am. 1966;48:149.
47. Jones Jr JP. Alcoholism, hypercortisonism, fat embolism and osseous avascular necrosis of the femoral head. In: Zinn WM, editor. Idiopathic ischemic necrosis of the femoral head in adults. Stuttgart: Georg Thieme; 1971. p. 112.
48. Jones JP. Intravascular coagulation and osteonecrosis. Clin Orthop. 1992;277:41–53.
49. Glueck CJ, Freiberg R, Gruppo R, et al. Chapter 14. Thrombophilia and hypofibrinolysis: reversible pathogenetic etiologies of osteonecrosis. In: Urbaniak JR, Jones JP, editors. Osteonecrosis: etiology, diagnosis, and treatment. Chicago: American Academy of Orthopaedic Surgeons, Developed by the American Orthopaedic Association; 1997. p. 105–10.
50. Glueck CJ, Freiberg RA, Fontaine RC, et al. Hypofibrinolysis, thrombophilia, osteopenia. Clin Orthop Relat Res. 2001;386:19–33.
51. Catto M. Pathology of aseptic bone necrosis. In: Davidson JK, editor. Aseptic necrosis of bone. Amsterdam: Excerpta Medica; 1976.
52. Kenzora JE, Glimcher MJ. Accumulative cell stress: the multifactorial etiology of idiopathic osteonecrosis. Orthop Clin North Am. 1985;16:669.
53. Cheras PA. Chapter 13. Role of hyperlipidemia, hypercoagulability and hypofibrinolysis in osteonecrosis and osteoarthritis. In: Urbaniak JR, Jones JP, editors. Osteonecrosis: etiology, diagnosis and treatment. American Academy of Orthopaedic Surgeons, Developed by the American Orthopaedic Association; Rosemont, IL, USA; 1997. p. 97–104.
54. Alavi A, McCloskey JR, Steinberg ME. Early detection of avascular necrosis of the femoral head by 99m technetium diphosphonate bone scan: a preliminary report. Clin Orthop. 1977;127:137.
55. Schoutens A, Stallenberg B, Hauzeur JP, et al. Scintigraphy in osteonecrosis of the hip. In: Urbaniak JR, Jones JP, editors. Osteonecrosis, Chap 29. American Academy of Orthopaedic Surgeons, Developed by the American Orthopaedic Association; Rosemont, IL, USA; 1997. p. 209–12.
56. Mitchell MD, Kundel HL, Steinberg ME, et al. Avascular necrosis of the hip: comparison of MRI, CT, and scintigraphy. Am J Radiol. 1986;147:67.
57. Mitchell DG, Rao VM, Dalinka MK, et al. Avascular necrosis of the femoral head: MRI appearance correlated with radiographic staging and radionuclide, histologic and clinical findings. Radiology. 1987;162:709–15.
58. Lang P, Genant HK, Jergesen HF, et al. Imaging of the hip joint: computed tomography versus magnetic resonance imaging. Clin Orthop Relat Res. 1992;157:751–6.
59. Arlet J, Ficat RP. Forage-biopsie de la tete femorale dans l'osteonecrose primitive. Observations histopathologiques portant sur huit foranes. Rev Rheum. 1964;31:257–64.
60. Marcus ND, Enneking WF, Massam RA. The silent hip in idiopathic aseptic necrosis: treatment by bone grafting. J Bone Joint Surg Am. 1973;55:1351–66
61. Urbaniak JR, Coogan PG, Gunneson EB, Nunley JA. Treatment of osteonecrosis of the femoral head with free vascularized fibular grafting. J Bone Joint Surg Am. 1995;77:681–94.
62. Enneking WF. Classification of nontraumatic osteonecrosis of the femoral head. In: Urbaniak JR, Jones JP, editors. Osteonecrosis: etiology, diagnosis and treatment. Rosemont: American Academy of Orthopaedic Surgeons, Developed by the American Orthopaedic Association; 1997. p. 269–75.
63. Berend KR, Gunneson EE, Urbaniak JR. Free vascularized fibular grafting for the treatment of post collapse osteonecrosis of the femoral head. J Bone Joint Surg Am. 2003;85:987–93.
64. Sugioka Y. Transtrochanteric anterior rotational osteotomy of the femoral head in the treatment of osteonecrosis affecting the hip. Clin Orthop. 1978;130:191–201.
65. Sugioka Y, Katsuki I, Hotokebechi T. Transtrochanteric rotational osteotomy of the femoral head for the treatment of osteonecrosis: follow-up statistics. Clin Orthop. 1982;169:115–26.
66. Steinberg ME, Hayken GD, Steinberg DR. A quantitative system for staging avascular necrosis. J Bone Joint Surg Br. 1995;77:34–41.
67. Steinberg ME, Hayken GD, Steinberg DR. A new method for evaluation and staging of avascular necrosis of the femoral head. In: Arlet J, Ficat RP, Hungerford DS, editors. Bone circulation. Baltimore: Williams & Wilkins; 1984. p. 398–403.
68. Ono K. Diagnostic criteria, staging system and roentgenographic classification of avascular necrosis of the femoral head (steroid induced, alcohol associated or idiopathic nature (in Japanese). In: Ono K, editor. Annual report of Japanese investigation committee for intractable disease, avascular necrosis of the femoral head. Tokyo: Ministry of Health and Welfare; 1987. p. 331–6.

69. Sugano N, Takaoka K, Ohzono K, Matsui M, Masuhara K, Ono K. Prognostication of non-traumatic avascular necrosis of the femoral head: significance of location and size of the necrotic lesion. Clin Orthop. 1994;303:155–64.
70. Gardeniers J. ARCO committee on terminology and staging. A new proposition of terminology and an international classification of osteonecrosis. ARCO Newslett. 1991;3:153–9.
71. Gardeniers JWM. A new international classification of osteonecrosis of the ARCO committee on terminology and classification. ARCO Newslett. 1992;4:41–6.
72. Gardeniers JWM. The ARCO perspective for reaching one uniform staging system of osteonecrosis. In: Schoutens A, Arlet J, Gardiniers JWM, Hughs SPF, editors. Bone circulation and vascularization in normal and pathological conditions. New York: Plenum Press; 1993. p. 375–80.
73. Gardeniers JWM, ARCO Committee on Terminology and Staging. Report on the committee meeting at Santiago de Compostella. ARCO Newslett. 1993;5:79–82.
74. Kerboul M, Thomine J, Postel M, Merle D'Aubigne R. The conservative surgical treatment of idiopathic aseptic necrosis of the femoral head. J Bone Joint Surg Br. 1974;56:291–6.
75. Mont MA, Jones LC, Pacheo I, Hungerford DS. Radiographic predictors of outcome of core decompression for osteonecrosis stage III. Clin Orthop. 1998;354:159–68.
76. Wagner H, Zeiler G. Idiopathic necrosis of the femoral head: results of intertrochanteric osteotomy and joint resurfacing. In: Weill U, editor. Segmental idiopathic necrosis of the femoral head: progress in orthopaedic surgery. Berlin: Springer; 1981. p. 87–116.
77. Koo K-H, Kim R. Quantifying the extent of osteonecrosis of the femoral head: a new method using MRI. J Bone Joint Surg Br. 1995;77:875–80.
78. Cherian SF, Laorr A, Saleh KJ, et al. Quantifying the extent of femoral head involvement in osteonecrosis. J Bone Joint Surg. 2003;85-A:309–15.
79. Ha Y-C, Jung WH, Kim J-R, et al. Prediction of collapse in femoral head osteonecrosis: a modified Kerboul method with use of magnetic resonance images. J Bone Joint Surg. 2006;88-A Suppl 3:35–40.
80. Steinberg DR, Steinberg ME, Garino JP, et al. Determining lesion size in osteonecrosis of the femoral head. J Bone Joint Surg. 2006;88-A Suppl 3:27–34.
81. Lee G-C, Steinberg ME. Are we evaluating osteonecrosis adequately? Int Orthop (SICOT). 2012;36:2433–9.
82. Mont MA, Marulanda GA, Jones LC, et al. Systematic analysis of classification systems for osteonecrosis of the femoral head. J Bone Joint Surg. 2006;88-A Suppl 3:16–26.
83. Massari L, Fini M, Cadossi R, et al. Biophysical stimulation with pulsed electromagnetic fields in osteonecrosis of the femoral head. J Bone Joint Surg. 2006;88-A Suppl 3:56–60.
84. Ciombor DMK, Aaron RK. Electric, electromagnetic and acoustic treatment for avascular necrosis of the femoral head. Tech Orthop. 2008;23(1):11–7.
85. Reis ND, Schwartz O, Militianu D, et al. Hyperbaric oxygen therapy as a treatment for stage-I avascular necrosis of the femoral head. J Bone Joint Surg. 2003;85B:371–5.
86. Nishi T, Sugano N, Mike H, et al. Does alendronate prevent collapse in osteonecrosis of the femoral head? Clin Orthop Relat Res. 2006;443:273–9.
87. Steinberg ME, Brighton CT, Corces A, et al. Osteonecrosis of the femoral head: results of core decompression and grafting with and without electrical stimulation. Clin Orthop. 1989;249:199–208.
88. Hungerford DS, Jones LC. Core decompression. Tech Orthop. 2008;23(1):26–34.
89. Hungerford DS, Mont MA. Chapter 39. The role of core decompression in the treatment of osteonecrosis of the femoral head. In: Urbaniak JR, Jones JP, editors. Osteonecrosis: etiology, diagnosis and treatment. American Academy of Orthopaedic Surgeons, Developed by the American Orthopaedic Association; Rosemont, IL, USA; 1997. p. 287–92.
90. Mont MA, Carbone JJ, Fairbank AC. Core decompression versus nonoperative management for osteonecrosis of the hip. Clin Orthop. 1996;324:169.
91. Fairbank AC, Bhatia D, Jinnah RH, Hungerford DS. Long-term results of core decompression for ischemic necrosis of the femoral head. J Bone Joint Surg Br. 1995;77:42.
92. Maistrelli G, Fusco U, Avai A, Bombelli R. Osteonecrosis of the hip treatment by intertrochanteric osteotomy. A four to fifteen year follow up. J Bone Joint Surg Br. 1988;70:761.
93. Scher MA, Jakim I. Intertrochanteric osteotomy and autogenous bone grafting for avascular necrosis of the femoral head. J Bone Joint Surg Am. 1993;75:1119.
94. Atsumi T, Kajiwara T, Hiranuma Y, et al. Posterior rotation osteotomy for nontraumatic osteonecrosis with extensive collapse in young patients. J Bone Joint Surg. 2006;88-A Suppl 3:42–7.
95. Atsumi T, Hosalkar H. Proximal femoral osteotomies. Tech Orthop. 2008;23(1):54–64.
96. Meyers MH. The treatment of osteonecrosis of the hip with fresh osteochondral allografts and with the muscle pedicle graft technique. Clin Orthop. 1978;130:202.
97. Meyers MH, Convery FR. Grafting procedures in osteonecrosis of the hip. Semin Arthroplasty. 1991;3:189.
98. Mont MA, Einhorn TA, Sponseller PD, Hungerford DS. The trapdoor procedure using autogenous cortical and cancellous bone grafts in the treatment of osteonecrosis of the femoral head. J Bone Joint Surg Br. 1998;80:56.
99. Rosenwasser MP, Garino JP, Kiernan HA, Michelson CB. Long-term followup of thorough debridement and cancellous bone grafting of the femoral head for avascular necrosis. Clin Orthop. 1994;306:17.
100. Boettcher WB, Bonfiglio M, Smith K. Non-traumatic necrosis of the femoral head. Part II. Experiences in treatment. J Bone Joint Surg Am. 1970;52:322.
101. Bonfiglio M, Bardenstein MD. Treatment by bone grafting of aseptic necrosis of the femoral head and non-union of the femoral neck (Phemister Technique). J Bone Joint Surg Am. 1958;40:1329.
102. Gilbert A, Judet H, Judet J, Agatti A. Microvascular transfer of the fibula for necrosis of the femoral head. Orthopedics. 1986;9:885.
103. Aldridge III JM, Urbaniak JR. Free vascularized fibular grafting for the treatment of osteonecrosis of the femoral head. Tech Orthop. 2008;23(1):44–53.
104. Judet H, Gilbert A. Long term results of free vascularized fibular grafting for femoral head necrosis. Clin Orthop Relat Res. 2001;386:114–9.
105. Coogan PG, Urbaniak JR. , Chapter 45. Multicenter experience with free vascularized fibular grafts for osteonecrosis of the femoral head. In: Urbaniak JR, Jones JP, editors. Osteonecrosis: etiology, diagnosis and treatment. American Academy of Orthopaedic Surgeons, Developed by the American Orthopaedic Association; Rosemont, IL, USA; 1997. p. 327–46.
106. Hernigou P, Zilber S, Filippini P, Rouard H, Mathieu G, Poignard A. Bone marrow injection in hip osteonecrosis. Tech Orthop. 2008;23(1):18–25.
107. Hernigou P, Beaujean F. Treatment of osteonecrosis with autologous bone marrow grafting. Clin Orthop. 2002;405:14–23.
108. Gangji V, Hauzeur JP. Treatment of osteonecrosis of the femoral head with implantation of autologous bone-marrow cells. J Bone Joint Surg. 2005;87(A):106–12.
109. Hernigou P, Bachir D, Galacteros F. Avascular necrosis of the femoral head in sickle-cell disease: treatment of collapse by the injection of acrylic cement. J Bone Joint Surg Br. 1993;75(B):875–80.

110. Veillette CJ, Mehdian H, Schemitsch EH, et al. Survivorship analysis and radiographic outcome following tantalum rod insertion for osteonecrosis of the femoral head. J Bone Joint Surg. 2006;88-A Suppl 3:48–55.
111. Sedel L, Travers V, Witvoet J. Spherocylindric (Luck) cup arthroplasty for osteonecrosis of the hip. Clin Orthop. 1987;219:127.
112. Salvati EA, Cornell CN. Long-term follow-up of total hip replacements in patients with avascular necrosis. Instr Course Lect. 1988;37:67. American Academy of Orthopaedic Surgeons.
113. Mont MA, Seyler TM, Plate JF. Uncemented total hip arthroplasty in young adults with osteonecrosis of the femoral head: a comparative study. J Bone Joint Surg. 2006;88-A Suppl 3:104–9.
114. Seyler TM, Bonutti PM, Shen J, et al. Use of alumina-on-alumina bearing system in total hip arthroplasty for osteonecrosis of the hip. J Bone Joint Surg. 2006;88A Suppl 3:116–25.
115. Steinberg ME. Summary and conclusions. The Orthopaedic Clinics of North America. Surf Replacement Arthroplasty Hip. 1982;13(4):895–902.
116. Revell MP, McBryde CW, Bhatnagar S, et al. Metal-on-metal resurfacing in osteonecrosis of the femoral head. J Bone Joint Surg. 2006;88-A Suppl 3:98–103.
117. Steinberg ME, Corces A, Fallon M. Acetabular involvement in osteonecrosis of the femoral head. J Bone Joint Surg. 1999;81-A: 60–5.
118. Mont MA, Delanois RE, Quesada MJ, Childress L. Femoral and acetabular surface replacement and hemi-surface replacement for osteonecrosis of the hip. Tech Orthop. 2008;23(1):65–73.
119. Huo MH, Stockton KO, Mont MA, Bucholz RW. What's new in total hip arthroplasty. J Bone Joint Surg. 2012;94A: 1721–7.
120. Glyn-Jones S, Roques A, Taylor A, et al. The in vivo linear and volumetric wear of hip resurfacing implants revised for pseudotumor. J Bone Joint Surg. 2011;93-A:2180–8.
121. Hannouche D, Zaoui A, Sedel L, Nizard R. Thirty years experience with alumina-on-alumina bearings in total arthroplasty. Int Orthop. 2011;35(2):207–13.

Part II

Anatomy and Blood Flow

Vascular Anatomy and Blood Supply to the Femoral Head

2

Marcin Zlotorowicz and Jaroslaw Czubak

2.1 Introduction

The vascular anatomy of the femoral head has been already described in many textbooks and studies.

First descriptions of vascular anatomy came from the seventeenth century, when Hunter described *circulus articuli vasculosus*—the vascular ring at the base of the femoral neck [1]. Many other studies from the twentieth century have assessed the vascular anatomy of the femoral head in classical anatomical studies [2–5] and in angiographic studies [6–8].

Several studies during the last 15 years have demonstrated new concepts in the vascularization of the femoral head. Recent studies have used different methods of visualization of the arteries: classical anatomical dissections preserved in formaldehyde [9], classical anatomical dissections of fresh cadavers after intra-arterial injections of colored silicone [10–12], and visualization using contrast-enhanced magnetic resonance imaging [13] or contrast-enhanced computed tomography (CT) [14].

2.2 Nomenclature

While all authors use the same nomenclature to describe the medial femoral circumflex artery (MFCA), lateral femoral circumflex artery (LFCA), and superficial femoral and deep femoral arteries, the nomenclature of nutrient arteries is controversial. Some authors name the vessels retinacular arteries because of the neighboring retinacular fibers [6, 10–12, 15]. Other authors name the vessels according to the growth period, when the epiphysis and metaphysis are supported by different arteries and the epiphyseal plate constitutes a barrier to the circulation within the epiphysis and metaphysis [8]. Crock and Chung described the arteries of the proximal end of the femur as an extracapsular and intracapsular arterial ring of the femoral neck with ascending cervical branches (anterior, posterior, lateral, and medial) and arteries of the round ligament [3, 4]. Howe described the terminal branches as the posterior superior and posterior inferior capital arteries arising from the MFCA and the foveal artery [2]. Judet named these vessels as superior and inferior groups of arteries supplying the femoral head [5].

The anastomosis of the MFCA with the inferior gluteal artery (IGA) was described in the early edition of Gray's Anatomy [16] as the anastomotic and articular branches, Jedral described it as a terminal branch of the IGA [17], while Gautier and Grose characterized it as the piriformis branch of the IGA [10, 18].

In our opinion, the most descriptive nomenclature names the vessels as nutrient arteries of the femoral head, which are delineated as posterior superior, posterior inferior, anterior, and the artery of ligamentum teres [9, 14]. For the anastomosis with the IGA we used the nomenclature by Gautier and Grose—the piriformis branch of the IGA [10, 18].

2.3 Blood Supply to the Femoral Head During Growth Phase

The vascular anatomy of the femoral head is very specific because the vascular patterns established during the growth phases do not change at maturity and persist throughout life [3, 4, 8]. The epiphysis and metaphysis have their own blood supply, and the arteries supporting them during the growth phase are called the epiphyseal arteries and metaphyseal arteries, respectively. Based on their sites of entry into the bone, the epiphyseal arteries are referred to as lateral and medial, and the metaphyseal arteries are indicated as superior and inferior. Lateral epiphyseal and superior metaphyseal arteries enter the bone at the superior and posterior-superior aspect of the femoral neck, near the

M. Zlotorowicz (✉) • J. Czubak
Department of Orthopaedic, Pediatric Orthopaedic and Traumatology, The Medical Centre of Postgraduate Education in Warsaw, Gruca Teaching Hospital, Konarskiego 13, Otwock 05-400, Poland
e-mail: m.zlotorowicz@wp.pl; jarek@czubak.neostrada.pl

K.-H. Koo et al. (eds.), *Osteonecrosis*,
DOI 10.1007/978-3-642-35767-1_2, © Springer-Verlag Berlin Heidelberg 2014

margin of the articular cartilage. The inferior metaphyseal arteries enter the bone close to the inferior margin of the articular cartilage. The lateral epiphyseal and both groups of the metaphyseal arteries arise from the MFCA. The medial epiphyseal artery is a continuation of the artery within the ligamentum teres, arising from the acetabular branch of the obturator artery. Injections to the femoral head proved that the lateral epiphyseal arteries predominate in the epiphysis and the inferior metaphyseal arteries in the metaphysis, and any contribution to vascularization by the artery of the ligamentum teres may be negligible or absent in some cases [8].

2.4 Blood Supply to the Femoral Head

The femoral head is supplied by vessels arising mainly from the MFCA and IGA. Other vessels with lesser contribution arise from the LFCA, obturator artery, superior gluteal artery, and the first perforating branch of the deep femoral artery.

Most authors agree that there are three main groups of arteries supplying the femoral head: the group of posterior superior nutrient arteries of the femoral head arising from the deep branch of the MFCA, a posterior inferior nutrient artery also arising from the main trunk of the MFCA, and the piriformis branch of the IGA [2–6, 9, 10, 14].

2.4.1 MFCA with Terminal Branches

The MFCA arises either from the deep femoral artery (65–81 %) (Fig. 2.1) or, less commonly, from the femoral artery (6,4–34 %) [12, 19–22]. It can also arise as two branches, as noted in a single case example in one study [20], or there may be no main trunk of the MFCA present, as noted in a single case example in another study [14]. From this point, the MFCA travels through the space between the pectineus and iliopsoas muscles, changing course in direction to the lesser trochanter. During its course, it branches off superficially and these branches anastomose with the obturator artery in the space between the adductor longus and adductor brevis muscles [2, 9, 10]. A superficial branch, usually single, is observed in 98 % of cases and its diameter is 1.4 mm (0.7–3.5 mm) [19]. When the main trunk of the MFCA is kinked or otherwise occluded, the superficial branch may play a crucial role in supplying blood to the deep branch of the MFCA [19]. Anterior to the lesser trochanter and distal to the distal margin of the obturator externus muscle, the main trunk of the MFCA gives rise to the posterior inferior nutrient artery of the femoral head (Fig. 2.2). At approximately 53 mm (31–87 mm) from the origin of its course, the main trunk of the MFCA bifurcates into a deep branch and a descending branch. This typical bifurcation of the main trunk of the MFCA is characteristic of 96 % of the cases [9, 14, 19] (Figs. 2.3, 2.4, and 2.5).

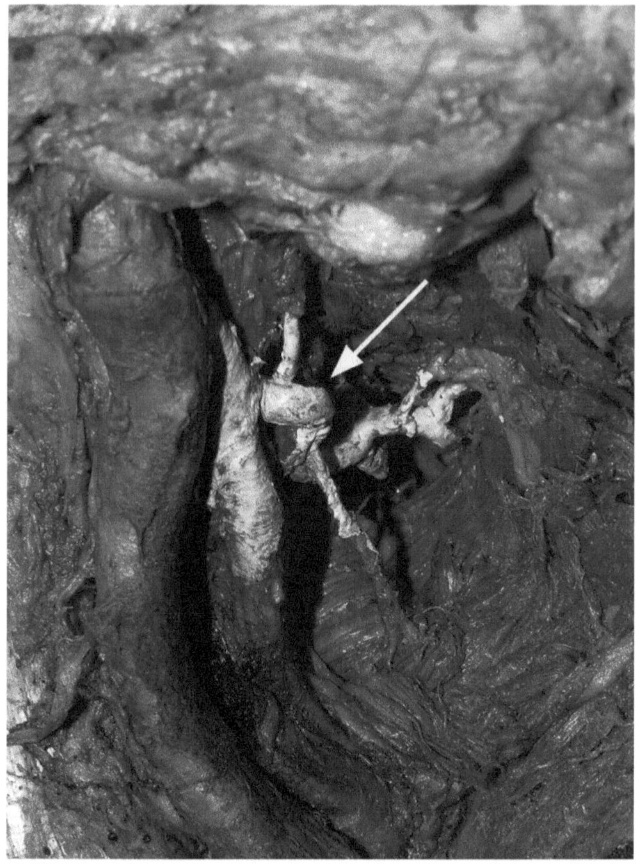

Fig. 2.1 Photograph during cadaver dissection showing the anterior view of the right inguinal region, with the main trunk of the medial femoral circumflex artery (*arrow*) originating from the deep femoral artery. (Reproduced with permission and copyright © of the *British Editorial Society of Bone and Joint Surgery* [9])

The main trunk bifurcates into the descending branch, usually single with a diameter of 1.7 mm (0.8–3.6 mm) that divided into two branches, which supply the muscles of the posterior compartment of the thigh. The deep branch, with a diameter of 1.6 mm (1.1–2.7 mm), follows a course directed to the femoral head [7, 9, 14, 19] (Figs. 2.3, 2.4, and 2.5).

2.4.1.1 Posterior Inferior Nutrient Artery

The posterior inferior nutrient artery of the femoral head is not present in all cases. Incidence of appearance depends on the method of visualization used by different authors; it is observed in 11 % of cases by angiographic CT examination [14] compared to 100 % of cases in a classical anatomical study with colored silicone injection [6, 11–13, 15]. Its diameter has been estimated in a microangiographic study to be approximately 0.4 mm (0.1–0.6 mm) [6]. In its intra-articular

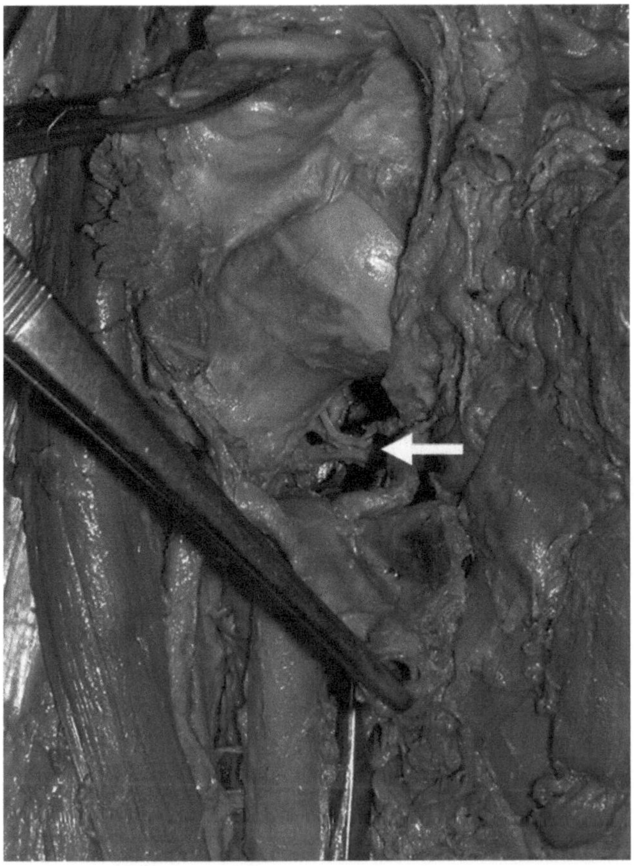

Fig. 2.2 Photograph during cadaver dissection of the anterior view with the right femoral head partly exposed and the femoral neck showing the posterior inferior femoral head nutrient artery (*white arrow*) (Reproduced with permission and copyright © of the *British Editorial Society of Bone and Joint Surgery* [9])

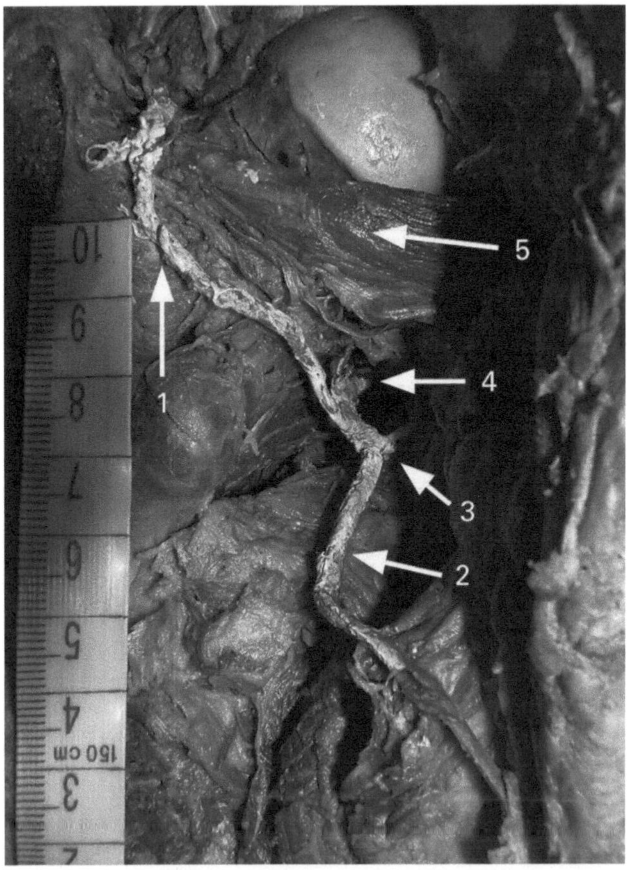

Fig. 2.3 Photograph during cadaver dissection of the posterior view of the left hip joint with the femoral head partly exposed, showing the main branches of the medial femoral circumflex artery (MFCA): *1* deep branch, *2* descending branch, *3* bifurcation of the MFCA, *4* posterior inferior femoral head nutrient artery, and *5* obturator externus muscle (Reproduced with permission and copyright © of the *British Editorial Society of Bone and Joint Surgery* [9])

course, it runs proximally on the medial aspect of the neck toward the femoral head on top of the mobile fold of tissue commonly referred to as the Weitbrecht ligament [12] (Figs. 2.2, 2.3, and 2.5). During the growth phase, the posterior inferior nutrient artery—under the name "inferior metaphyseal artery"—was found to supply approximately two-thirds of the metaphyseal tissue of the femoral head [8]. Almost 18 % of the vascular foramina around the head are located in the posterior inferior aspect of the femoral head in comparison to approximately 80 % located in the posterior superior and anterior superior quadrants of the femoral head [23].

2.4.1.2 The Deep Branch with Posterior Superior Nutrient Arteries

After bifurcation, the deep branch arises proximally, posterior to the obturator externus muscle and anterior to the quadratus femoris muscle. It is easily identifiable in the adipose tissue between these two muscles and is usually closely associated with two veins [9]. In this area, the deep branch of the MFCA can rupture during traumatic hip dislocation when the obturator externus tendon ruptures. The obturator externus muscle and its tendon protects the vessel [10, 24] (Fig. 2.6). In that area, the deep branch is also at risk of iatrogenic damage during posterior exposure of the hip. During the Kocher-Langenbeck approach, division of the tendon of the obturator externus should be avoided. It is also unsafe to divide the distal part of the conjoined tendon comprised of the gemellus inferior and fibers of the obturator internus muscle [10]. After bypassing the obturator externus, the deep branch goes into the trochanteric fossa where it gives off trochanteric branches toward the greater trochanter [2, 10]. In this region, the deep branch of the MFCA anastomoses with the piriformis branch of the IGA. Moving in a cranial direction toward the femoral head, it lies anterior to the conjoined tendon of gemelli and obturator internus and enters the hip joint

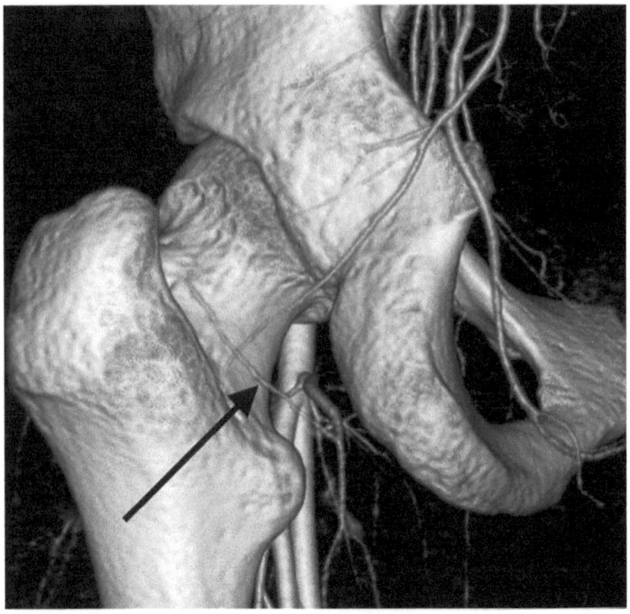

Fig. 2.4 Volume rendering image of the angio-CT scans showing the deep branch of the medial femoral circumflex artery (*arrow*) from its bifurcation to its division into the posterior superior nutrient arteries (Reproduced with permission and copyright © of the *British Editorial Society of Bone and Joint Surgery* [14])

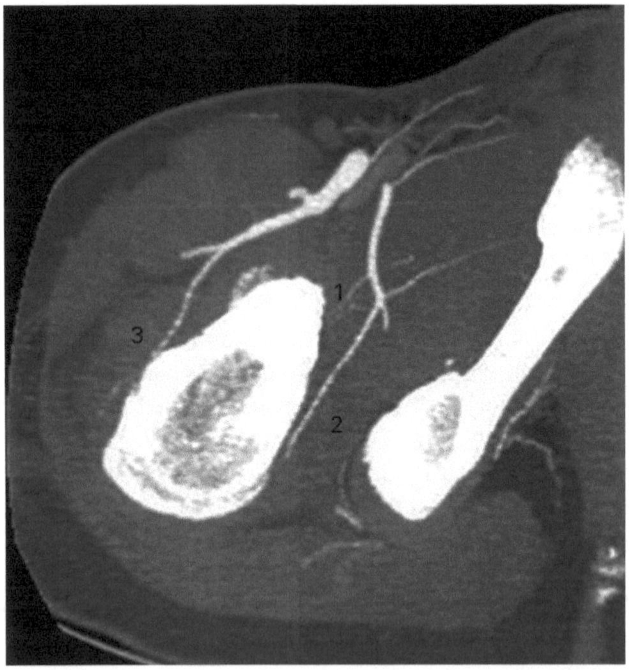

Fig. 2.5 Maximum intensity projection image of the angio-CT scans showing the posterior inferior nutrient artery (*1*), the deep branch of the medial femoral circumflex artery (*2*), and the anterior nutrient artery of the femoral neck (*3*) (Reproduced with permission and copyright © of the *British Editorial Society of Bone and Joint Surgery* [14])

through a femoral attachment of the posterior capsule, superior to the insertion of gemellus superior and distal to the insertion of the piriformis [2, 9–11, 23]. On this course,

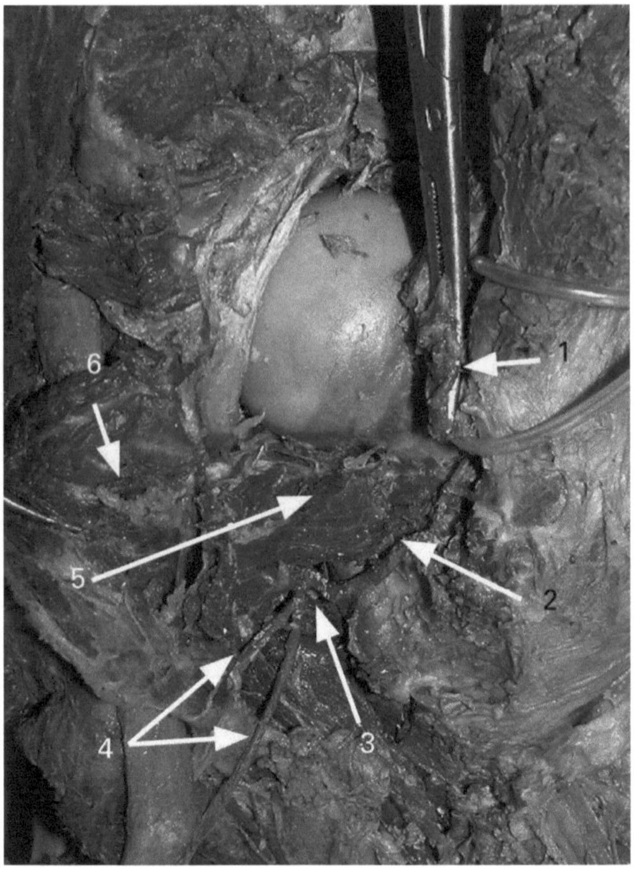

Fig. 2.6 Photograph during cadaver dissection of the posterior view of the right hip joint, showing the topography of the deep branch of the medial femoral circumflex artery (MFCA): *1* conjoined tendon of the gemellus superior, gemellus inferior, and obturator internus muscles (after tenotomy near its femoral attachment), *2* deep branch of the MFCA, *3* bifurcation of the MFCA, *4* descending branches of the MFCA, *5* obturator externus muscle, and *6* quadratus femoris muscle (turned medially) (Reproduced with permission and copyright © of the *British Editorial Society of Bone and Joint Surgery* [9])

it becomes intracapsular, obliquely through the capsule. To protect the deep branch of the vessel, approximately 1.5 cm of the conjoined tendon and capsule should be left undivided from the trochanteric crest during posterior exposure of the hip [10]. During its intracapsular and intra-articular courses, the deep branch is at risk of stretching and increased vessel resistance because of intra-articular pressure [25].

Intra-articularly, it travels subsynovially along the femoral neck within the retinacular fibers.

In its intra-articular course, it divides into 1–5 posterior superior nutrient arteries of the femoral head, continuing within the retinaculum toward the femoral head [9, 10, 12] (Fig. 2.7a, b). Many authors agree that the deep branch divides into the terminal nutrient arteries in all cases [2–15]. Posterior superior nutrient arteries are the most important source of blood supply; they can completely perfuse the femoral head without any other vascular input [15]. The

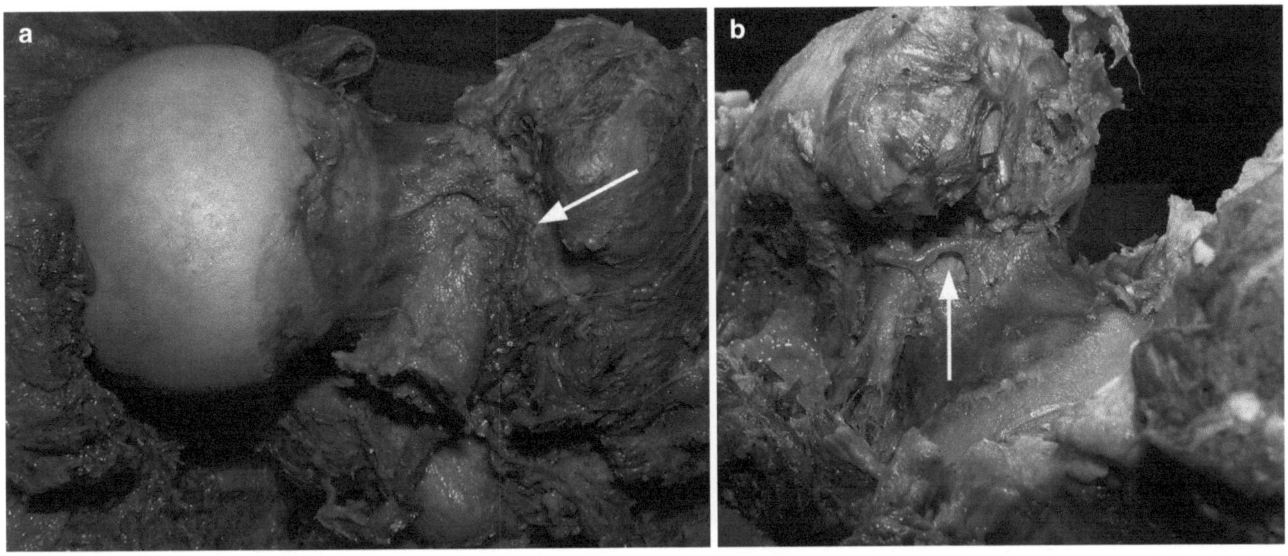

Fig. 2.7 Photographs during cadaver dissection of (**a**) a posterior view of the right hip joint with the femoral head exposed, showing the terminal branch of the medial femoral circumflex artery (*arrow*), which we consider to be the posterior superior femoral head nutrient artery, and (**b**) a posterior view of the left hip joint showing the terminal branches of the medial femoral circumflex artery (*arrow*), which we consider to be the three posterior superior femoral head nutrient arteries (Reproduced with permission and copyright © of the *British Editorial Society of Bone and Joint Surgery* [9])

estimated size, via microangiographic studies, of a nutrient artery from the group of posterior superior nutrient arteries of the femoral head in adults is 0.8 mm (0.3–1.6 mm) [6]. Zlotorowicz found that the deep branch was absent in 1/55 cases—the femoral head then being supplied by a well-defined piriformis branch of the IGA—using angiographic CT [14].

Based on the examination of 150 dried cadaveric specimens, Lavigne stated that 80 % of the vascular foramina on the bone were located in the posterior superior and anterior superior quadrants of the femoral head, where the posterior superior nutrient arteries enter the femoral head [23].

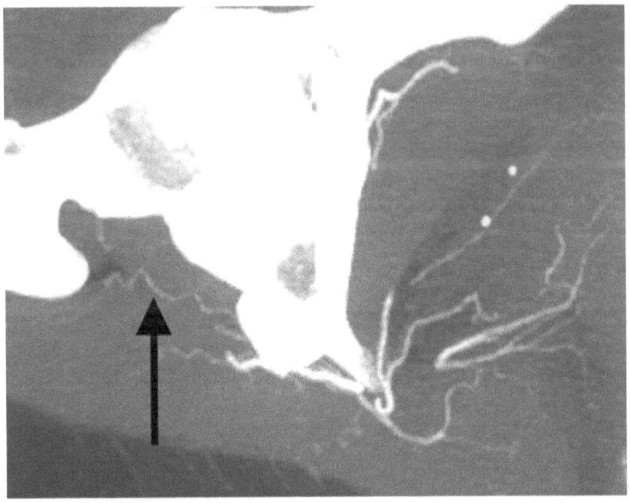

Fig. 2.8 Maximum intensity projection image of the angio-CT scans showing the piriformis branch (*arrow*) of the inferior gluteal artery (Reproduced with permission and copyright © of the *British Editorial Society of Bone and Joint Surgery* [14])

2.4.2 Inferior Gluteal Artery

The IGA also plays a crucial role in blood supply to the femoral head. Although all agree that the deep branch of the MFCA is a dominant vessel supplying the femoral head, the IGA was found to be a dominant vessel supplying the femoral head in >50 % of human fetuses aged 16–29 weeks of intrauterine life [17]. Kalhor found the piriformis branch of the IGA to be the main vessel supplying the femoral head in 6/35 specimens [12]. In another study, the piriformis branch of the IGA was also found to be the main vessel supplying the femoral head in the absence of the deep branch of the MFCA [14]. The most precise description of the anastomosis is given by Grose. In 7/8 specimens examined, constant anastomosis between the deep branch of the MFCA and the terminal branches of the IGA, called the piriformis branch, was observed. In this study, in all seven specimens observed, it was possible to inject the posterior superior nutrient arteries and posterior inferior nutrient artery via the IGA [18]. The piriformis branch of the IGA travels posteriorly across the piriformis and conjoined tendons, meeting the MFCA in the interval space between the inferior gemellus and the tendon of obturator externus (Figs. 2.8 and 2.9). The incidence of the piriformis branch varies depending on which method was used to visualize the vessel. Incidence varies from 49 % in

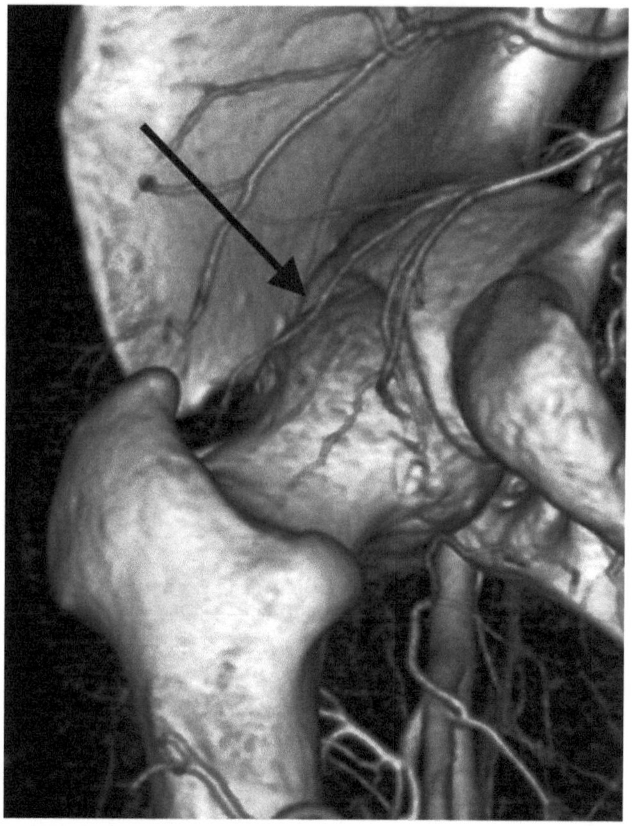

Fig. 2.9 Volume rendering image of the angio-CT scans showing the piriformis branch (*arrow*) of the inferior gluteal artery with the terminal nutrient arteries supplying the femoral head in the absence of the deep branch of the medial femoral circumflex artery. The main trunk takes the direction of the descending branch (Reproduced with permission and copyright © of the *British Editorial Society of Bone and Joint Surgery* [14])

CT angiography, with the size 1.0 mm (0.5–1.8 mm), to 100 % in an anatomical study involving injection of the arteries with colored silicone [14, 18].

2.4.3 Lateral Femoral Circumflex Artery

The LFCA arises from the deep femoral artery or, less commonly, from the femoral artery. It contributes to the femoral head and neck blood supply by a single artery with mean diameter 0.25–1.1 mm [6, 19]. This artery was found in 25–88 % of specimens [4, 6, 11, 12].

The anterior nutrient artery of the femoral neck is the vessel supplying the femoral neck rather than the femoral head. The vessel enters the bone at the anterior aspect of the femoral neck and is located at many different levels. In 39 % of specimens, it enters the bone immediately after piercing the capsule, in the middle of the neck in another 42 %, and near the articular rim in only 18 % [2]. In another study, the anterior nutrient artery enters the bone at a 22 mm distal to a 24 mm proximal point from the top of the lesser trochanter (mean distance, 4.5 mm proximal) (Fig. 2.5) [19].

The extracapsular and intracapsular arterial ring described by Chung, which is formed by the LFCA and MFCA, was not found by other authors [4, 7, 8, 10–12, 14].

Microangiographic studies showed that the anterior nutrient artery of the femoral neck does not supply the cancellous portion of the bone, but ends into the cortex forming a thicker peripheral meshwork [5, 15]. Some authors, in assessing the blood supply to the femoral head, do not describe the anterior nutrient artery as the vessel supplying the femoral head [2, 8].

2.4.4 Obturator Artery with Terminal Artery of the Ligamentum Teres

The artery of the ligamentum teres arises either from the obturator or MFCA, or from both [6]. Although it functions during the growth phase as a medial epiphyseal artery, most authors agree that its contribution to the femoral head blood supply is minimal [2, 8, 10–12, 15]. On the other hand, studies show that the artery of the ligamentum teres anastomoses with the intraosseous arteries of the femoral head. The size of the anastomosis is estimated to be 0.33 mm (0.07–0.62 mm) and the incidence is approximately 70 % [6].

The passage of one or, less frequently, two small arteries through the ligamentum teres toward the femoral head is usually too small in diameter to permit demonstration of their passage to the femoral head in anatomical studies [2]. Experimental divisions of the ligamentum teres showed that cutting this ligament has no effect on the capital arterial pattern including the subfoveal part of the head.

When the artery of the ligamentum teres was considered the only vessel supplying the femoral head, contrast medium was not taken up by the capital vessels in 35 % of specimens; another 35 % showed uptake in a small subfoveal area, and 29 % in other capital arteries (one or two arteries from the posterior superior nutrient arteries). In one preparation, only 6 % of normal area of the head was observed [15].

Experimental studies, therefore, showed that the ligamentum teres artery is unimportant as a supply vessel in most femoral heads, but can occasionally provide supporting blood supply to the femoral head in some individuals.

2.4.5 Superior Gluteal Artery

A branch of the superior gluteal artery descending toward the top of the greater trochanter, alongside the gluteus medius and minimus muscles, could potentially be a vessel anastomosing with the deep branch of the MFCA or with the piriformis branch of IGA. In 16 % of injected specimens, contrast penetrated to the top of the greater trochanter; however, the anastomosis was not visualized [11, 14]. Most authors do not consider the superior gluteal artery a main source of blood supply.

2.4.6 Transcervical Arteries from the First Perforator Artery

Most authors agree that vessels inside the marrow cavity of the femoral shaft and more proximally in the femoral neck are of no importance in blood supply to the femoral head [2, 8, 15]. On the other hand, it was possible for some authors to inject the nutrient arteries of the femoral head via the nutrient artery of the femoral shaft and vice versa [6, 26]. It is estimated that the anastomosis between a nutrient artery of the femoral shaft and nutrient arteries of the femoral head is 0.1–0.25 mm in diameter [6]. It is not possible to quantify the frequency at which the anastomosis occurs because of the presence of red marrow and a dense cloud of capillaries, making visibility poor in some specimens [6].

2.5 Summary

The femoral head receives blood supply mostly from the MFCA, with the deep branch of this artery being the most important. The deep branch of the MFCA terminates in the group of posterior superior nutrient arteries of the femoral head. The posterior superior nutrient arteries enter the femoral head via the vascular foramina in the posterior superior and anterior superior quadrants of the femoral head and neck. In these quadrants, 80 % of all femoral head vascular foramina are localized. The deep branch of the MFCA along with the terminal posterior superior nutrient arteries of the femoral head can support all, or nearly all, of the blood supply to the femoral head. Another source of blood supply, also originating from the MFCA, is the posterior inferior nutrient artery. From the anastomoses that contribute to the blood supply of the femoral head, the most important is the anastomosis with the IGA via the piriformis branch, which can also be a dominant vessel supplying the femoral head. The anterior nutrient artery of the femoral neck—originating from the lateral circumflex artery—and the obturator artery, via the artery of the ligamentum teres, constitute a minor component of the blood supply to the femoral head.

References

1. Hunter W. Of the structure and diseases of articulating cartilages. Philos Trans R Soc. 1743;43:514–21.
2. Howe W, Lacey T, Schwartz R. A study of the gross anatomy of the arteries supplying the proximal portion of the femur and the acetabulum. J Bone Joint Surg Am. 1950;32-A:856–66.
3. Crock H. A revision of the anatomy of the arteries supplying the upper end of the human femur. J Anat. 1965;99:77–88.
4. Chung S. The arterial supply of the developing proximal end of the human femur. J Bone Joint Surg Am. 1976;58-A:961–70.
5. Judet J, Judet R, Lagrange J, Dunoyer J. A study of the arterial vascularization of the femoral neck in adult. J Bone Joint Surg Am. 1955;37-A:663–80.
6. Tucker F. Arterial supply of the femoral head and its clinical importance. J Bone Joint Surg Br. 1949;31-B:82–93.
7. Müssbichler H. Arteriographic investigations of the normal hip in adults. Evaluation of methods and vascular finding. Acta Radiol. 1971;11:195–215.
8. Trueta J. The normal vascular anatomy of the femoral head in adult man. 1953. Clin Othop Relat Res. 1997;334:6–14.
9. Zlotorowicz M, Szczodry M, Czubak J, Ciszek B. Anatomy of the medial femoral circumflex artery with respect to the vascularity of the femoral head. J Bone Joint Surg Br. 2011;93-B:1471–4.
10. Gautier E, Ganz K, Krugel N, Gill TJ, Ganz R. Anatomy of the medial femoral circumflex artery and surgical implications. J Bone Joint Surg Br. 2000;82-B:679–83.
11. Kalhor M, Beck M, Huff T, Ganz R. Capsular and pericapsular contributions to acetabular and femoral head perfusion. J Bone Joint Surg Am. 2009;91-A:409–18.
12. Kalhor M, Horowitz K, Gharehdaghi J, Beck M, Ganz R. Anatomic variations in femoral head circulation. Hip Int. 2012;22(3):307–12.
13. Boraiah S, Dyke J, Hertrich C, Parker R, Miller A, Helfet D, Lorich D. Assessment of vascularity of the femoral head using gadolinium (Gd-DTPA) – enhanced magnetic resonance imaging. A cadaver study. J Bone Joint Surg Br. 2009;91-B:131–7.
14. Zlotorowicz M, Czubak J, Kozinski P, Boguslawska-Walecka R. Imaging the vascularisation of the femoral head by CT angiography. J Bone Joint Surg Br. 2012;94-B:1176–9.
15. Sewitt S, Thompson RG. The distribution and anastomoses of arteries supplying the head and neck of the femur. J Bone Joint Surg Br. 1965;47-B:560–73.
16. Gray H. Anatomy of the human body. 20th ed. Philadelphia: Lea and Febiger; 1918.
17. Jedral T, Anyzewski P, Ciszek B, Benke G. Vascularization of the hip joint in the human fetuses. Folia Morphol (Warsz). 1996;4: 293–4.
18. Grose A, Gardner M, Sussmann P, Helfet D, Lorich D. The surgical anatomy of the blood supply to the femoral head. Description of the anastomosis between the medial femoral circumflex artery and inferior gluteal arteries at the hip. J Bone Joint Surg Br. 2008;90-B:1298–303.
19. Zlotorowicz M, Czubak J. The anatomy of the medial femoral circumflex artery – chances for microsurgical reconstruction. Thesis. Medical Centre of Postgraduate Education, Warsaw, 2010.
20. Tanieli E, Üzel M, Yildirim M, Çelik H. An anatomical study of the origins of the medial circumflex femoral artery in the Turkish population. Folia Morphol. 2006;65:209–12.
21. Siddharth P, Smith NL, Mason RA, Giron F. Variational anatomy of the deep femoral artery. Anat Rec. 1985;212:206–9.
22. Massoud T, Fletcher E. Anatomical variants of the profunda femoris artery: an angiographic study. Surg Radiol Anat. 1997;19:99–103.
23. Lavigne M, Kalhor M, Beck M, Ganz R, Leunig M. Distribution of vascular foramina around the femoral head and neck junction: relevance for conservative intracapsular procedures of the hip. Orthop Clin North Am. 2005;36:171–6.
24. Zlotorowicz M, Czubak J, Caban A, Kozinski P, Boguslawska-Walecka R. The blood supply to the femoral head after posterior fracture/dislocation of the hip, assessed by CT angiography. Bone Joint J. 2013;95-B:1453–7.
25. Beck M, Siebenrock K, Affolter B, Nötzli H, Parvizi J, Ganz R. Increased intracapsular pressure reduces blood flow to the femoral head. Clin Orthop Relat Res. 2004;424:149–52.
26. Wolcott WE. The evolution of the circulation in the developing femoral head and neck. An anatomic study. Surg Gynecol Obstet. 1943;77:61–8.

3 Ischemia and Reperfusion Injury in Bone

Howard Winet

3.1 Introduction

Bone cells may be killed in a variety of ways, from radiation to poison. But the clinical phenomenon that has become most identified with the term "osteonecrosis" is associated with ischemia. Ischemic osteonecrosis (ION) is the preferred term, although clinicians traditionally use AVN (avascular necrosis) in spite of the fact that the absence of vessels has never been histologically confirmed (ischemic vessels are still vessels just as a dead body is still a body). It is generally agreed that ION results from two main causes of ischemia: (1) hypercoagulation that is associated with a wide range of diseases, leading to the name of this category as "idiopathic" ION, and (2) physical damage to bone blood vessels resulting from impact—high energy or compression—known as "traumatic" ION. This review is divided into three sections: (a) idiopathic ION, (b) traumatic ION and reperfusion, and (c) intravital microscopic investigation of both.

3.2 Idiopathic ION

Since the early 1990s a consensus has been building that the ischemia associated with idiopathic ION is caused by hypercoagulation [1–3]. Unfortunately, the number of pathophysiological roads to hypercoagulation is so great that one can find published data correlating a large fraction of them with clinical presentations [4].

Since ION of the femoral head is by far the highest in incidence [5, 6], it is logical to ask if there is a circulatory basis for such a bias. Why does ION not occur as frequently in other joints? For that matter, why does it not frequently occur elsewhere in the femur? Of course it occurs in any bone if the conditions stated in the first paragraph are met. But ION does not progress to bone collapse in other bones as often as it does in the hip.

Since pathology is a deviation from normal physiology, one cannot expect to understand circulatory pathophysiology without understanding normal circulatory physiology of the femur. The human femur is normally fed by two nutrient arteries from the femoral profunda that enter the upper diaphyseal cortex through foramina. They then branch just central to the endosteum into ascending and descending tributaries. These in turn send centrifugal branches into adjacent cortical bone and centripetal branches toward sinusoids in the medullary canal as the tributaries continue toward the metaphysis. There is a net centrifugal pressure drop across the diaphyseal cortex and a net movement of its interstitial fluid (bone fluid flow) toward the periosteum [7]. However, pressure changes in the medullary canal are not well translated into pressure changes within the cortex, suggesting that septi—anatomical or functional—exist interrupting any continuous medullary canal-to-periosteum fluid flow [7].

In most limbs the ascending nutrient artery branch eventually reaches metaphyseal cancellous bone where it appears to form anastomoses with metaphyseal arteries. Metaphyseal arteries often anastomose with epiphyseal arteries. Epiphyseal and metaphyseal bones typically have a more direct supply. Separate perforating arteries enter the subcondylar region at two or more foramina and after branching may anastomose.

Metaphyseal-epiphyseal blood supply to the proximal femur is different. Vessels enter at the femoral neck, superior to the greater trochanter and inferior to the capsule of the hip joint. There are two tributaries from the femoral profunda that circle the bone, the medial (MFCA) and lateral circumflex arteries. The lateral circumflex supplies the inferior bone at the level of the trochanter and the MFCA supplies the superior femoral head. There is variation between individuals. In some cases the inferior gluteal artery contribution dominates the MFCA [8, 9]. There is also evidence for anastomoses between the MFCA and inferior gluteal artery [10]. After penetrating the joint

H. Winet
Departments of Orthopaedic Surgery and Bioengineering,
University of California, Los Angeles, CA, USA
e-mail: hwinet@ucla.edu

K.-H. Koo et al. (eds.), *Osteonecrosis*,
DOI 10.1007/978-3-642-35767-1_3, © Springer-Verlag Berlin Heidelberg 2014

capsule, the MFCA runs along the posterosuperior aspect of the femoral neck sending subsynovial retinacular branches caudad [10]. One of the most interesting findings of Crock is the presence of sinusoids at the tips of these retinacular branches [11]. Other investigators do not seem to have been able to get their injected media to penetrate to vessels small enough to confirm or disprove this observation, although Figs 7 and 8 of Sevitt and Thompson's report suggest a similar result [12].

In adults some of the femoral head blood supply may come from the ligamentum teres artery [12, 13]. It enters the femoral head apex and its distal branches anastomose with the retinacular arteries [14].

The diaphyseal periosteum of the femur is fed by periosteal arteries that branch from arteries in tendons connected to the cortex by Sharpey's fibers. These vessels supply not only the periosteum but up to 1/3 of the outer cortical bone under normal conditions [15]. When medullary nutrient artery tributaries are damaged as occurs when the canal is reamed, periosteal circulation increases its supply to the cortex [16]. There do not appear to be any studies of contributions of femoral neck periosteal blood supply to the neck cortex, although this bone is well vascularized [17]. This circulation may be a factor in healing of the osteonecrotic head.

When blood reaches the end of its retinacular artery, it flows into increasingly smaller-diameter branches regressing from terminal branches (down to 60 μm) to arterioles (down to 20 μm) to capillaries (down to 8 μm). All of these vessels are lined with endothelial cells (ECs). Precapillary vessels are surrounded with smooth muscle. As arterioles become capillaries, they are increasingly surrounded with pericytes that are not muscles but can change the vessel diameter by coiling actin of their intracellular matrix. Capillaries are one EC thick and surrounded with a laminin-plus-collagen IV basement membrane and an occasional pericyte. There are three general types of capillaries:

1. Continuous: with continuous basement membranes and ECs overlapping at junctions
2. Fenestrated: with continuous basement membranes and ECs with pores up to 1,000 Å wide at junctions
3. Discontinuous: with holes in basement membranes and clear fissures in EC junctions, sinusoids

In some tissues there are shunts called metarterioles from precapillary vessels to pre-venular capillaries. Should smaller capillaries become plugged, blood would divert across these shunts.

Systemic pathologies like disseminated intravascular coagulation (DIC) cannot by themselves explain a tendency for ischemia to occur in a femoral head [18]. Accordingly, one must determine if there is some basis for hypothesizing that head vasculature has an inherent tendency to be thrombogenic. Blood vessel function is essentially EC function, and if the microcirculation is to experience the hypercoagulation required for ION [3], ECs must be, logically, integral components of the thrombogenic process.

Table 3.1 Regulators of thrombosis and hemostasis in endothelium

EC Features	Antithrombotic	Prothrombotic
Coagulation protein binding sites	Glycosaminoglycans/ATIII	Binding sites for fibrin, FIX, IXa, X, Xa, FXII, kallikrein
	TFPI	Tissue factor
	Thrombomodulin	Thrombin receptor
		Receptor for protein C/APC
Products produced and/or stored by platelets	PGI_2	vWF
	NO	PAF
	ADPase	Fibrinogen
		FV
		FXI
Fibrinolytic factors	t-PA production	PAI-1, PAI-2
	u-PA expression	PAI-3 (protein C Inhibitor)
	u-PAR	TAFI activation
	Plasminogen binding sites	
	Annexin II	
Vasomotor factors	NO	TxA_2
	PGI_2	Endothelin-1

From Cines et al. [42]

EC agents, binding sites, receptors, and actions that control coagulation in blood vessels

Abbreviations: *ATIII* antithrombin III, *PGI_2* prostacyclin, *TFPI* tissue factor pathway inhibitor, *APC* activated protein C, *PAF* platelet activating factor, *t-PA* tissue plasminogen activator, *u-PA* urokinase plasminogen activator, *u-PAR* urokinase plasminogen activator receptor, *PAI* plasminogen activator inhibitor, *TAFI* thrombin-activatable fibrinolysis inhibitor, *TxA_2* thromboxane A_2

ECs are not the same in all tissues. Those lining capillaries of different organs are arranged differently [19]. Consider those in brain with its blood–brain barrier vs. those in marrow sinusoids. The size of the vessel makes a difference (Kumar [20]). Endothelial cells from microcirculatory vessels express more MHC I and II as well as adhesion molecules than do those from larger vessels [21, 22]. In fact the surface proteins vary sufficiently to allow immunological differentiation of ECs by organ [22]. Pathologies that reflect this organ-to-organ variation are classified as regional endothelial dysfunctions or RED [18]. Such heterogeneity is not unique to humans. It is at least chordate phylum wide [23].

Is the heterogeneity that leads to RED reflected in thrombogenicity? Table 3.1 summarizes various EC components that influence the clotting process. Each component can induce or inhibit thrombosis by secreting or activating various agents that control clotting. Tissue factor, PAI-1, vWF, and protease-activated receptors vary in circulatory

Table 3.2 Extracellular signals that regulate procoagulant or anticoagulant mRNA expression in endothelial cells

Source of signal	Effect
TNFα	Decreases expression of thrombomodulin
	Increases expression of plasminogen-activator inhibitor type 1 and tissue factor
IL-1	Decreases expression of thrombomodulin
TGF-β	Decreases expression of thrombomodulin
	Increases expression of plasminogen-activator inhibitor type 1
VEGF	Increases expression of thrombomodulin, plasminogen-activator inhibitor type 1, and tissue-type plasminogen activator
PDGF	Increases expression of von Willebrand factor
Shear stress	Increases expression of thrombomodulin, tissue-type plasminogen activator, tissue factor, and nitric oxide synthase
Hypoxia	Increases expression of plasminogen-activator inhibitor type 1
	Decreases expression of tissue-type plasminogen activator

From Rosenberg et al. [24]

beds from organ to organ [24, 25]. Tissue factor expression is heterogeneous over the body [26]. Thrombomodulin and endothelial protein C receptors are expressed heterogeneously in different vascular beds [27]. There is circulatory heterogeneity as well. Venular valves are more frequent in bone than in skeletal muscle vessels [28]. It has been postulated that individuals with poor circulation to femoral head retinaculars are at high risk for thrombi and EC apoptosis resulting from reduced fluid shear in their microvasculature [1]. Signals that affect thrombogenesis are summarized in Table 3.2.

Does the heterogeneity in EC MHCII antigens contribute directly to RED and thrombogenicity? ECs present MHCII antigens to CD4⁺ T cells—more in micro- than macrovasculature [21, 22]—and some express CD40 (in dendritic cells this marker interacts with T cells), CD80, and CD86 (both T cell costimulatory) suggesting presentation to CD8⁺ T cells as well [28]. There are conflicting data on the extent to which these interactions anergize the T cells [29, 30]. But there is support for the conclusion that CD8⁺ T cells can activate and induce proinflammatory changes in ECs [31, 32].

Dendritic cells (DCs) may have a role in multifoci ION. Their role in DIC begins with systemic challenge to the innate immune system. In experiments with lipopolysaccharide (LPS), the challenge begins with detection of the immunogen by DC TLR4. In the lymph nodes LPS activates DC TLR4 that in turn upregulates its protease-activated receptor 1 (PAR1). Through an internal cascade, PAR1 activates sphingosine-phosphate 3 receptor (S1P3R) that initiates secretion of TF and IL-1β. In lymph circulation this TF has little effect. But the continuous LPS signal eventually stimulates migration of DCs from the lymph nodes to lymph vessels that carry them to ducts that drain into the blood circulation. As the DCs circulate they secrete TF stimulating receptive ECs to secrete thrombin and form local thrombi. Thrombin directly stimulates DC PAR1 to complete the autocrine cycle, further amplifying DIC [33].

Local thrombosis may be stimulated by LPS in vessels like the retinacular microcirculation as well. Endothelial cells have TLR4s [34], S1P3R [35], Waeber [36] and PAR1 [37]. This effect has apparently been demonstrated by Okazaki et al. [38] who challenged mice with LPS and were able to produce femoral ION and cytokines associated with TLR4 stimulation.

3.3 Traumatic ION

Thrombogenesis is not necessary for ION if vessels are simply destroyed as is the case for traumatic ION. But bone not directly made ischemic via traumatic destruction of feeder vessels may become ischemic as the result of reperfusion injury. Compartment syndrome would likely produce the necessary ischemia, as would a crush injury of limited force.

Endothelial cells normally control both upstream and downstream vessel diameters by converting L-arginine to NO that is delivered countercurrently or downstream to sphincters. They also normally oxidize their purines using xanthine oxidase to produce superoxide anions, which at physiologic pH dismutates (via superoxide dismutases) to H_2O_2 and in the presence of ferrous ions and peroxidases to H_2O and ferric ions.

During ischemia blood flow in microvasculature stops and neutrophils that have become trapped are no longer stimulated by blood flow shear to remain in the vessel lumen. They upregulate their L-selectin and seek to extravasate through the nearest endothelium. Meanwhile, ECs, in the absence of flow and O_2, are increasingly exposed to an anaerobic and decreasing pH environment. As a result NO production and peroxidase activity stops, allowing accumulation of superoxide anion. Accumulation of these free radicals damages ECs, primarily by lipid peroxidation [39].

As tissue adjacent to that made necrotic directly by the trauma proceeds through a wound healing inflammatory phase, constricted vessels upstream begin to relax and blood is shunted to the patent ischemic vasculature. When the highly oxygenated reperfusing blood meets a lumen with neutrophils lining the walls and free radicals and inflammatory cytokines (some from adjacent mast cells) in high concentration, incoming platelets are activated and, in the absence of NO, thrombosis and vessel constriction condemn the flow to stasis.

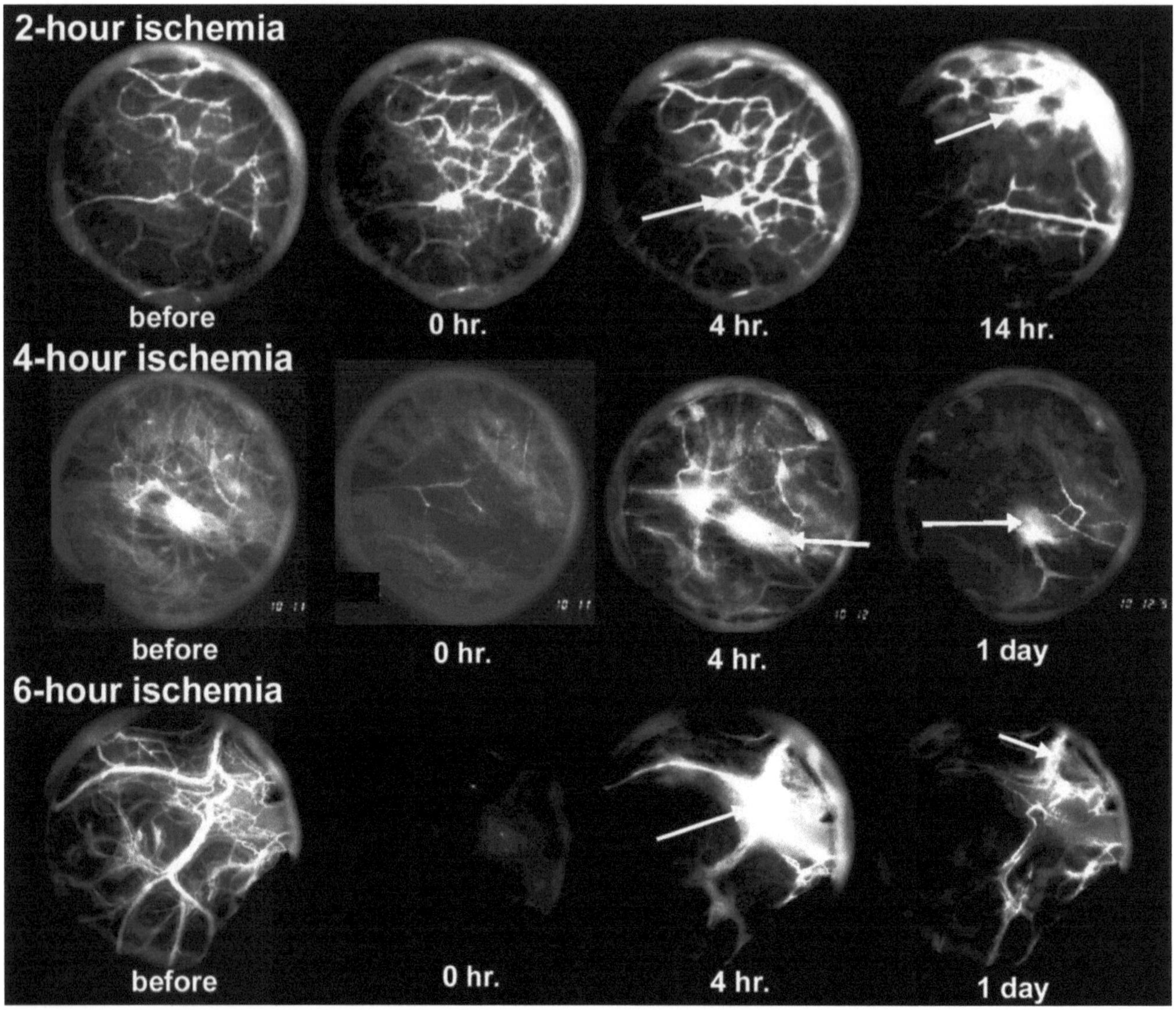

Fig. 3.1 Examples of reperfusion phase vascularity for three ischemia durations. Each circle has a diameter of about 2 mm (disregarding the outer ring of reflected light). Visible vessels show circulating FITC-D70 which normally leaks only through so-called large pores (according to the two-pore permeability model; few in number in tissue at equilibrium). Baseline vascularity is shown at far left. Reperfusion at zero hours (0 H) is photographed 10 min after cuff deflation and shows a pattern suggesting an inverse relationship between duration and initial reperfusion. At 4 h vessels exhibit abnormal leakage which appears to increase with ischemia duration. At 14 per day, reperfusion has decreased from its 4-h value for all three treatments. Also, leakage at this time is less for the higher durations, probably because so little plasma is circulating (From Hsieh et al. [40] with permission)

Selection of vessels that undergo reperfusion injury first is probably not as important for the progress of ION as is the ischemia length of time. We have found significant effects at 2 h [40] as can be seen in Fig. 3.1. These events probably occur at different points and times in the femoral head, depending on local conditions. Diffusion through the extracellular matrix of cytokines and other agents—from mast cells in particular—will spread signals to adjoining tissue. Of particular interest is the source of macrophages, ECs, and fibroblasts that will form the repair tissue of early healing. Unlike idiopathic ION wherein the pathological agent often persists, the trauma source is usually gone when repair begins.

3.4 Intravital Microscopy for Assessing Bone Microcirculatory Pathology

If one wishes to directly view microcirculatory events in vivo and in situ in an intact animal, it is usually necessary to expose the organ and place it in a special microscope. The observing instrument is called an intravital microscope (IVM). P.I. Brånemark developed it for use in bone by adding a window implant in 1964 [41]. In order to give direct visual access to bone cortex, medullary canal, and their vasculature, Albrektsson modified the window into a surgically implanted optical bone chamber. The images in Fig. 3.1 were obtained with a horizontal modification of the original vertical IVM. The horizontal IVM allows the animal being observed to be upright and free of clamping pressure on the bone being observed.

The bone chamber used for intravital microscopy is usually implanted in the tibial medial cortex immediately distal of the medial collateral ligament insertion. It is permanently exposed and is managed for infection prevention by daily peroxide lavage. It has been designed to perforate both cortices so that transmitted light may pass into the lateral end and illuminate bone that is growing and has grown into a 100 μm deep × 2 mm wide discoid chamber. Vessels are illuminated by fluorescence. Fluorescent objects may range from molecules small enough to trace nutrient exchange through capillary walls to microspheres large enough to observe as discrete points, but small enough to not significantly alter vessel fluid mechanics.

If transmitted light is not required, the chamber may be redesigned to extend no further than the nearest medullary canal. Such a short chamber may be implanted nearer the joint and possibly serve in a model for ION of the knee. Unless an endoscopic form of the chamber were developed, its implantation near the femoral head would be problematic because of musculature surrounding the femur. The chamber is designed for chronic studies (18 months has been achieved). Thus, it would be suitable for experiments testing hypotheses about the effects of long-term exposure to an agent on microcirculation. Fluorescent dyes for bone could be added to evaluate its growth and viability.

The reader is encouraged to "google" "intravital microscopy" to gain an appreciation of the current use of this technique in microcirculation research, particularly in the area of cancer.

References

1. Kerachian MA, Harvey EJ, Cournoyer D, Chow TYK, Séguin C. Avascular necrosis of the femoral head: vascular hypothesis. Endothelium. 2006;13:237–44.
2. Glueck CJ, Freiberg RA, Boppana S, Wang P. Thrombophilia, hypofibrinolysis, the eNOS T-786C polymorphism, and multifocal osteonecrosis. J Bone Joint Surg. 2008;90:2220–9.
3. Lykissas MG, Gelalis ID, Kostas-Agnatis IP, Vozonelos G, Korompilas AV. The role of hypercoagulability in the development of osteonecrosis of the femoral head. Orthop Rev. 2012;4:73–7.
4. Jones JP. Concepts of etiology and early pathogenesis of osteonecrosis. In: Schafer M, editor. Instructional course lectures. Chicago: American Academy of Orthopaedic Surgeons; 1994. p. 499–512.
5. Bose VC, Baruah BD. Resurfacing arthroplasty of the hip for avascular necrosis of the femoral head: a minimum follow-up of four years. J Bone Joint Surg. 2010;92B:922–8.
6. Steffen RT, Athanasou NA, Gil HS, Murray DW. Avascular necrosis associated with fracture of the femoral neck after hip resurfacing: histological assessment of femoral bone from retrieval specimens. J Bone Joint Surg. 2010;92B:787–93.
7. Winet H. Blood flow in bone. In: Cowin S, editor. Bone mechanics handbook. Boca Raton: CRC Press; 2001. p. 21.21–7.
8. Kalhor M, Horowitz K, Gharehdaghi J, Beck M, Ganz R. Anatomic variations in femoral head circulation. Hip Int. 2012;22:307–12.
9. Grose AW, Gardner MJ, Sussman PS, Helfet DL, Lorich DG. The surgical anatomy of the blood supply to the femoral head: description of the anastomosis between the median femoral circumflex and inferior gluteal arteries at the hip. J Bone Joint Surg. 2008;90B: 1298–303.
10. Gautier E, Ganz K, Krügel N, Gill T, Gaz R. Anatomy of the medial femoral circumflex artery and its surgical implications. J Bone Joint Surg. 2000;82B:679–83.
11. Crock HV. A revision of the anatomy of the arteries supplying the upper end of the human femur. J Anat. 1965;99:77–88.
12. Sevitt S, Thompson RG. The distribution and anastomoses of arteries supplying the head and neck of the femur. J Bone Joint Surg. 1965;47B:560–73.
13. Trueta J. The normal vascular anatomy of the human femoral head during growth. J Bone Joint Surg. 1957;39B:358–94.
14. Wertheimer LG, Lopes SL. Arterial supply of the femoral head. J Bone Joint Surg. 1971;53A:545–56.
15. Rhinelander FW. The normal microcirculation of diaphyseal cortex and its response to fracture. J Bone Joint Surg. 1968;50A: 784–800.
16. Grundnes O, Gjerdet NR, Utvåg SE, Reikerås O. Vascular and structural changes in rat femora following nailing and intramedullary occlusion. J Orthop Res. 1998;16:293–9.
17. Shea JE, Hallows RK, Ricks S, Bloebaum RD. Microvascularization of the hypermineralized calcified fibrocartilage and cortical bone in the sheep proximal femur. Anat Rec. 2002;268:365–70.
18. Séguin C, Kassis J, Busque L, Bestawros A, Theodoropoulos J, Alonso M-L, Harvey EJ. Non-traumatic necrosis of bone (osteonecrosis) is associated with endothelial cell activation but not thrombophilia. Rheumatology. 2008;47:1151–5.
19. Craig LE, Spelman JP, Strandberg JD, Zink MC. Endothelial cells from diverse tissues exhibit differences in growth and morphology. Microvasc Res. 1998;55:65–76.
20. Kumar S, West DC, Ager A. Heterogeneity in endothelial cells from large vessels and microvessels. Different. 1987;36:57–70
21. Beilke MA. Vascular endothelium in immunology and infectious disease. Rev Infect Dis. 1989;11:273–83.
22. Page C, Rose M, Yacoub M, Pigott R. Antigenic heterogeneity of vascular endothelium. Am J Pathol. 1992;141:673–83.
23. Yano K, Gale D, Massberg S, Cheruvu PK, Monohan-Early P, Morgan ES, Haig D, von Andrian H, Dvorak AM, Aird WC. Phenotypic heterogeneity is an evolutionary conserved feature of the endothelium. Blood. 2007;109:613–5.
24. Rosenberg RD, Aird WC. Vascular bed-specific hemostasis and hypercoagulable states. N Engl J Med. 1999;340:1555–64.
25. Aird WC. Phenotypic heterogeneity of the endothelium I. Structure, function and mechanisms. Circ Res. 2007;100:158–73.
26. Edelberg JM, Christie PD, Rosenberg RD. Regulation of vascular bed-specific prothrombic potential. Circ Res. 2001;89:117–24.
27. Franscini N, Bachli EB, Blau N, Leikauf M-S, Schaffner A, Schoedon G. Gene expression profiling of inflamed human endothelial cells and influence of activated protein C. Circulation. 2004; 110:2903–9.
28. Aird WC. Phenotypic heterogeneity of the endothelium II. Representative vascular beds. Circ Res. 2007;100:174–90.
29. Firner S, Onder L, Nindl V, Ludewig B. Tight control – decision-making during T cell-vascular endothelial cell interaction. Front Immunol. 2012;3:1–6.
30. Rothermel AL, Wang Y, Schechner J, Mook-Kanamori B, Aird WC, Pober JS, Tellidides G, Johnson DR. Endothelial cells present antigens *in vivo*. BMC Immunol. 2004;5:1–15.
31. Celik S, Shankar V, Rchter A, Hippe H-J, Akhavanpoor M, Bea F, Erbel C, Urban S, Blank N, Wambsgans N, et al. Proinflammatory and prothrombotic effects in human vascular endothelial cells of immune cell-derived LIGHT. Eur J Med Res. 2009;14:147–56.

32. Kish DD, Volokh N, Baldwin WMI, Fairchhild RL. Hapten application to the skin induces an inflammatory program directing hapten-primed effector CD8 T cell interaction with hapten-presenting endothelial cells. J Immunol. 2011;186:2117–26.
33. Niessen F, Schaffler F, Furlan-Freguia C, Pawlinski R, Bhattacharjee G, Chun J, Derian CK, Andrade-Gordon P, Rosen H, Ruf W. Dendritic cell PAR1-S1P3 signalling couples coagulation and inflammation. Nature. 2008;452:654–8.
34. Dauphinee SM, Karsan A. Lipopolysaccharide signaling in endothelial cells. Lab Invest. 2006;86:9–22.
35. Swan DJ, Kirby JA, Ali S. Vascular biology: the role of sphingosine 1-phosphate in both the resting state and inflammation. J Cell Mol Med. 2001;14:2211–22.
36. Waeber C, Blondeau N, Salamone S. Vascular sphingosine-1-phosphate $S1P_1$ and $S1P_3$ receptors. Drug News Persp. 2004;17: 365–82.
37. Feistritzer C, Riewald M. Endothelial barrier protection by activated protein C through PAR1-dependent sphingosine 1-phosphate receptor-1 crossactivation. Blood. 2005;105:3178–84.
38. Okazaki S, Nishitani Y, Nagoya S, Kaya M, Yamashita T, Matsumoto H. Femoral head osteonecrosis can be caused by disruption of the systemic immune response via toll-like receptor 4 signalling pathway. Rheumatology. 2009;48:227–32.
39. Hunt BJ, Jurd K. Endothelial function in inflammation, sepsis, reperfusion and vasculitides. In: Halliday A, Hund BJ, Poston L, Schachter M, editors. An introduction to vascular biology. Cambridge: Cambridge University Press; 1998. p. 225–47.
40. Hsieh AS, Winet H, Bao JY, Glas H, Plenk H. Evidence for reperfusion injury in cortical bone as a function of crush injury ischemia duration: a rabbit bone chamber study. Bone. 2001;28: 94–103.
41. Winet H. A horizontal intravital microscope bone chamber system for observing microcirculation. Microvasc Res. 1989;37:105–14.
42. Cines DB, Pollak ES, Buck CA, Loscalzo J, Zimmerman GA, McEver RP, Pober JS, Wick TM, Konkle BA, Schwartz BS, et al. Endothelial cells in physiology and in the pathophysiology of vascular disorders. Blood. 1998;91:3527–61.

Part III

Epidemiology

4 The Prevalence of Osteonecrosis in Different Parts of the World

A.C. Gosling-Gardeniers, W.H.C. Rijnen, and J.W.M. Gardeniers

4.1 Introduction

Osteonecrosis is a major increasing health problem all over the world. Osteonecrosis is the final stage of a number of conditions leading to bone death [1]. It has undergone several name changes. Several used synonyms are avascular necrosis, idiopathic avascular necrosis, aseptic necrosis, and ischemic necrosis of bone. Aseptic necrosis was initially used to differentiate the condition of osteonecrosis from bone infections. Avascular or ischemic necrosis presumed a homogeneous etiology and pathogenesis. The term osteonecrosis describes the main common aspect of bone death and is more neutral in its assumption of causation [2].

Many studies have consistently observed that more patients with osteonecrosis are younger and have a longer life expectancy [3]. This is mainly due to the fact that osteonecrosis is associated with alcoholism, hyperlipemia, an increasing number of transplant recipients, corticosteroid usage, and long-term survival with a better quality of life of patients with chronic diseases [2–4]. These different conditions are presumed causes of osteonecrosis, and it is difficult to assess the frequency and causative impact of each different cause. Demographic data are reported differently in many health centers worldwide. The Osaka University of Japan reported that 23 % of the osteonecrosis of the femoral head cases has been associated with alcohol and 37 % with corticosteroids [2, 5]. The Johns Hopkins University in the United States reported approximately 10,000–20,000 new cases of osteonecrosis of the femoral head each year [5–7].

Most of the studies reported rough estimates of the frequency of osteonecrosis over the world. However, specific information concerning the frequency of osteonecrosis is indeed a very important subject. In some small countries with a centralized health service, such as the Netherlands, it might in fact be possible that the diagnosis of osteonecrosis is listed among the demographic records. This study is performed to examine the magnitude of the problem of osteonecrosis in different parts of the world. What is the frequency of osteonecrosis in Europe, the United States, and Japan? Is there anything known about the increasing morbidity connected to this disorder for both men and women?

4.2 Methods

First, more precise demographic data of osteonecrosis are obtained by a detailed literature search and a summary. Different terms and authors were used in PubMed database to find scientific articles about the magnitude of the problem of osteonecrosis worldwide. In particular, the chapter on osteonecrosis in the US book, The Adult Hip (new version for 2006), is used to discuss difficulties establishing prevalence numbers of ON worldwide.

Second, a research on the Internet is done to find health organizations and to try to obtain the prevalence numbers of osteonecrosis in the Netherlands. Contacts were made by phone and/or email with different health organizations, CBS (Central Office for Statistics), WHO (World Health Organization), VWS (Ministry of Public health and Sports), RIVM (Institute for Health and Environment), and NVZ (Association for Hospitals), finally leading to Prismant (Dutch Research Databank).

Finally, a research on the Internet is done to find health organizations worldwide and to try to obtain more specific demographic information of osteonecrosis over the world. Contact by email with the WHO Europe/United States/Southeast Asia has been made. Important orthopedic surgeons and researchers from different universities in the United States, Japan, Korea, and Europe were contacted by email to obtain answers to our questions.

A.C. Gosling-Gardeniers • W.H.C. Rijnen • J.W.M. Gardeniers (✉)
Department of Orthopaedics,
Radboud University Medical Centre, Geert Grooteplein zuid 10, 9101, Nijmegen 6500 HB, The Netherlands
e-mail: wim.rijnen@radboudumc.nl; jeanwmgardeniers@me.com

K.-H. Koo et al. (eds.), *Osteonecrosis*,
DOI 10.1007/978-3-642-35767-1_4, © Springer-Verlag Berlin Heidelberg 2014

Table 4.1 Demographic data of osteonecrosis in the Netherlands in 2003

	Gender		Type of age (years)			Total
	Men	Women	0–16	17–35	>35	
Aseptic bone necrosis	14	11	4	12	12	25
Chronic osteomyelitis	25	23	15	15	18	48
Total osteonecrosis	39	34	19	27	30	**73**

Table 4.2 Demographic data of osteonecrosis in the Netherlands in 2004

	Gender		Type of age (years)			Total
	Men	Women	0–16	17–35	>35	
Aseptic bone necrosis	14	14	3	10	12	28
Chronic osteomyelitis	28	20	14	14	20	48
Total osteonecrosis	42	34	17	24	32	**76**

4.3 Results

4.3.1 The Netherlands

The Dutch population living in the Netherlands counts about 15 million people. Prevalence numbers of osteonecrosis in the Netherlands have been reported by Prismant, a Dutch Research Databank. Demographic data of osteonecrosis in the Netherlands from the years 2003 and 2004 are given to Radboud Academic Hospital, Department of Orthopaedics, and used subsequently in this report. Two differentiations are made for registrations of the different stages of osteonecrosis, aseptic bone necrosis and chronic osteomyelitis (septic necrosis), both for men and women. Type of age was categorized into 0–16, 17–35, and >35 years old.

Table 4.1 shows the demographic data of osteonecrosis in the Netherlands in 2003. In this sample, osteonecrosis was more often reported in men (53.4 %). Osteonecrosis was also more frequently found in adults aged above 35 years. The total number of 73 patients with osteonecrosis was reported in 2003. Patients with chronic osteomyelitis, septic necrosis, were more often found (65.8 %) than patients with aseptic bone necrosis (34.2 %).

Table 4.2 shows the demographic data of osteonecrosis in the Netherlands in 2004. In this sample, 55.3 % of the diagnosis osteonecrosis was found in men. Again, osteonecrosis was more frequently reported in adults aged above 35 years. The total number of osteonecrosis in the year 2004 was 76 patients. Chronic osteomyelitis, septic necrosis, was more often found (63.2 %) than aseptic bone necrosis (36.8 %). The number of patients with osteonecrosis has increased in 2004 compared with 2003. The number of men with osteonecrosis has increased, while the number of women with osteonecrosis remains the same. In addition there has been a small increase in the number of patients in each age category in 2004 compared with 2003. The same data of osteonecrosis for 2005 will be available next year, probably in May 2006.

4.3.2 Europe

There are about 370 million people living in Europe. Information on demographic data of osteonecrosis is unknown for the rest of Europe. There is no centralized health service in Europe to collect and report these data on osteonecrosis. Some countries in Europe have more precise data but only data on their own country.

4.3.3 The United States

There are approximately 295 million people living in the United States. Demographics of osteonecrosis in the United States are not collected with very much precision and not kept up to date. There is published information that would indicate that there is an estimate of approximately 20,000 new cases of osteonecrosis of the hip in the United States every year [6]. The accumulated numbers of ON is between 0.3 million and 0.6 million people. However, that information is based upon several large series of total hip replacements in which 10 % of the patients had a total hip replacement because of osteonecrosis. Not taken into account are all the new cases of osteonecrosis which do not have a hip replacement. This could probably add another 5 or 10 % to the mix. The estimate is calculated at approximately 22,000 new cases of osteonecrosis of the hip in the United States every year [6]. These numbers are indeed very "soft" numbers.

In the United States the diagnosis of osteonecrosis is not listed among general demographic records and a research has to deal with rough estimates only. As mentioned before, it might only be possible in a small country with a centralized health service, such as the Netherlands and maybe Hong Kong and Japan, to get more precise demographic data.

4.3.4 Asia

Several reports state that the numbers of osteonecrosis are increasing and the disorder becomes more and more serious in Asia and other continents. The total population living in China is approximately 1.3 billion people. About 127 million people live in Japan and about 70 million people in Korea. In 1994, Japan had an appearance of 4,000 new cases of ON every year (Wang, G.). Recently, reports show a frequency of 1/10,000 patients as a low number. Recently, this estimate certainly has been doubled to 2/10,000 (Prof. Atsumi, T. and Dr. Yamano, K.). This gives a low estimate of 12,000 and a high estimate of 24,000 patients per year. Based on the report of Hong Kong, the prevalence of osteonecrosis is much higher in Asia [5]. Chang J. et al. reported several years ago that osteonecrosis was the reason for total hip replacement in 50 % of the cases (Chang, J.).

In Hong Kong and China there is a high estimated prevalence and asymptomatic presentation of osteonecrosis in adults. In China, the number of new appearance is about 75,000–150,000 per year. The accumulated numbers of ON is between 1.5 and 3 million people (Wang, G.). No data on its prevalence are known in children [8].

4.4 Discussion

This study tried to examine the magnitude of the problem of osteonecrosis in different parts of the world. The complexity of this disorder is enormous. The different stages of osteonecrosis and the different root causes make it really difficult to give a good overall estimate rate of osteonecrosis. Early stages of osteonecrosis with still intact femoral heads and functionary hip joints are not reported at all. Many doctors do not recognize the disease, and if they do, they "wait and see" till the disease progresses into the final stages. These late stages get secondary osteoarthritis and need a total hip replacement. However, the early stage can be treated successfully and the femoral heads can be preserved for at least 10 years [3, 9, 10]. In the Netherlands with a centralized health service, demographic reported data are differentiated into only two stages of osteonecrosis, chronic osteomyelitis and aseptic bone necrosis. This shows the great complexity of collecting and reporting overall data of osteonecrosis even for small countries.

No centralized health services exist to report reliable data for the different continents, Europe, the United States, Asia, and in more detail the large Asian countries, such as Japan and China. Only rough estimates on the rate of osteonecrosis are reported. Therefore no hard information on the magnitude of the problem all over the world can be obtained. Most information collected and reported worldwide is not scientific provided evidence. No scientific articles are published with exact numbers of osteonecrosis in each country or continent. Rough estimates are made through detailed literature research and by contacts with orthopedic surgeons in this specific field all over the world.

However, what is clear and hard evidence is the fact that osteonecrosis becomes more prevalent in a younger age group and it has more impact in the patient's quality of daily life. More specific information about the frequency of osteonecrosis is needed to identify the real magnitude of this disorder worldwide. It is important for patients, especially these younger patients with a longer life expectancy, that more precise data becomes available and the magnificence of the problem gets more attention to implement new treatment techniques to preserve the hip joint and to improve the quality of life [3, 10, 11].

In conclusion, this study shows a considerable lack of hard evidence and detailed knowledge of the prevalence of osteonecrosis worldwide. All continents need centralized health services to report several disorders, such as osteonecrosis. Osteonecrosis becomes more and more important in daily life every year and in younger patients. We should look for long-term prevalence rates of osteonecrosis in each continent and report it to pinpoint the magnitude of the problem of osteonecrosis worldwide.

References

1. Pavelka K. Osteonecrosis. Baillieres Best Pract Res Clin Rheumatol. 2000;14(2):399–414.
2. Aaron RK, Gray RRL. The adult hip. 2nd ed. Philadelphia: Lippincott Williams & Wilkins; 2005.
3. Gardeniers JWM. Treatment of osteonecrosis by joint replacement. Hip Int. 1998;8(3):159–66.
4. Assouline-Dayan Y, Chang C, Greenspan A, Shoenfeld Y, Gershwin ME. Pathogenesis and natural history of osteonecrosis. Semin Arthritis Rheum. 2002;32(2):94–124.
5. Ono K, Sugioka Y. Epidemiology and risk factors in avascular necrosis of femoral head. In: Schoutens A et al., editors. Bone circulation and vascularization in normal and pathologic conditions. New York: Plenum Press; 1993. p. 301–12.
6. Hungerford DS. Osteonecrosis: avoiding total hip arthroplasty. J Arthroplasty. 2002;17(4):121–4.
7. Hungerford DS, Jones LC. Asymptomatic osteonecrosis: should it be treated? Clin Orthop Relat Res. 2004;429:124–30.
8. Chan CW, Chiu WK, Chan CC, Chow EY, Cheung HM, Ip PL. Osteonecrosis in children with severe acute respiratory syndrome. Pediatr Infect Dis J. 2004;23(9):888–90.
9. Wang Y, Zhao D, Wang J, Lu S, Zhu S. Memorial metal ball for the treatment of avascular necrosis of femoral head. Zhonghua Wai Ke Za Zhi. 1998;36(10):579–81, 117.
10. Rijnen WH, Gardeniers JW, Buma P, Yamano K, Slooff TJ, Schreurs BW. Treatment of femoral head osteonecrosis using bone impaction grafting. Clin Orthop Relat Res. 2003;417:74–83.
11. Rijnen WH, Gardeniers JW, Westrek BL, Buma P, Schreurs BW. Sugioka's osteotomy for femoral-head necrosis in young Caucasians. Int Orthop. 2005;29(3):140–4.

Epidemiology of Osteonecrosis in the USA

5

Sameer M. Naranje and Edward Y. Cheng

5.1 Introduction

Osteonecrosis (ON) is an uncommon disease. It is therefore important to know the populations at high risk for ON and the anatomic sites most frequently involved in order to improve diagnostic acumen. Knowledge of the risk factors and etiology of ON lends insight into management and potentially prevention. Furthermore, the differences in the distribution of ON internationally may help highlight important topics for research and identify key areas of intervention to prevent the occurrence of disease.

5.2 Types of Osteonecrosis

5.2.1 Traumatic Osteonecrosis

The fractures most commonly associated with the subsequent development of ON are fractures of the femoral neck, scaphoid, and talus. The blood supply to these bones is unique in that one end portion of the bone is highly dependent upon vascular flow through a single, more central portion of the bone, and a fracture may disrupt this flow.

A major complication of femoral neck fractures is development of ON. This leads to revision surgery or hip arthroplasty. The major determinants of whether or not ON occurs are fracture displacement and, to a lesser degree, age, excessive valgus reduction, and timing of reduction of dislocation. The incidence of ON has been reported to be 50 % higher for displaced versus undisplaced fractures [1, 2]. In a series of 73 femoral neck fractures in patients between the ages of 15 and 50 years treated at a single institution, Haidukewych et al. found an overall frequency of osteonecrosis of 23 % [3] over a mean follow-up period of 6.6 years. Osteonecrosis developed in 27 % of displaced fractures and 14 % of nondisplaced fractures. Initial fracture displacement and the quality of reduction were found to affect results. In younger patients (ages 15–50 years) with femoral neck fractures, the overall incidence of osteonecrosis is reported to be 20–36 % over a mean follow-up period of 3–7 years [4, 5]. In older patients (65 years or older) with displaced femoral neck fractures, osteonecrosis is reported to be 15–33 % [6]. When evaluating healed fractures only, the reported incidence of ON is 12 % in displaced fractures versus 7 % in undisplaced fractures over a mean follow-up of greater than 2 years [1, 7]. Excessive valgus reduction has been associated with ON [8]. Bunata [9] found that excessive valgus reduction was associated with four times increased incidence of ON (42 %) as compared to those without excessive valgus.

The incidence of necrosis with nonunions has been reported to be four times greater than for united femoral neck fractures [10], while the incidence of ON was found to be about doubled for delayed unions [8]. Incidence of ON with nonunions is reported to be 60 % [11].

The incidence of anterior dislocation is far below that of the posterior variety, and there is a similar contrast in the incidence of associated necrosis. The reported incidence of osteonecrosis with anterior dislocations has been 3–9 %, whereas that for posterior dislocation has been 13–26 % over a mean follow-up period of 5 years [12]. Certain fracture-dislocation patterns increase the likelihood of osteonecrosis. Epstein [12] reported 11 % necrosis with type 1 dislocations (with, or without, minor fracture) as opposed to 42 % with type 4 injuries (with acetabular rim or floor fractures).

The relationship between the timing of reduction and the incidence of osteonecrosis has been very well documented [13, 14]. Stewart et al. [14] found ON in 14 (15.5 %) out of the 90 patients treated by closed reduction and in 11 (40 %)

S.M. Naranje
Department of Orthopaedic surgery,
University of Minnesota, 2512 South 7th Street R200,
Minneapolis, MN 55454, USA
e-mail: sameernaranje@gmail.com

E.Y. Cheng (✉)
Department of Orthopaedic surgery,
University of Minnesota Medical School, 2512 South 7th Street R200,
Minneapolis, MN 55454, USA
e-mail: cheng002@umn.edu

K.-H. Koo et al. (eds.), *Osteonecrosis*,
DOI 10.1007/978-3-642-35767-1_5, © Springer-Verlag Berlin Heidelberg 2014

out of 28 patients in those treated surgically. The interval between the time of injury and close reduction averaged to 3 days, whereas that between injury and surgery averaged to 21 days. In a prospective study by McKee et al. [13] on 25 patients with irreducible dislocations of hip, ON was found to be associated with delay in reduction. Brav [15] reported 18 % ON for hips reduced within 12 h when compared to 57 % for hips subjected to greater delay.

The scaphoid is second only bone to the femoral head in its overall incidence of posttraumatic osteonecrosis [16–18]. Osteonecrosis is thought to occur in 13–40 % of all scaphoid fractures. The reported incidence varies according to the fracture location and amount of displacement. Fractures of the proximal third have the highest incidence of ON (14–100 % in different series) than the fractures of the middle third (30–50 % cases). Osteonecrosis develops in nearly all fractures of the proximal pole that involve the proximal one-fifth of the bone. Fracture displacement more than 1 mm has been associated with ON which occur in up to 50 % of such cases [16–18].

Osteonecrosis of the talus is a complication of talar neck fractures [19]. Nondisplaced talar neck fractures have an approximately 10 % chance of developing osteonecrosis, whereas displaced fractures have an associated disruption of the subtalar articulation, carrying an approximate 40 % risk of osteonecrosis. Displaced fractures with incongruity of both the ankle and subtalar joints have an approximate 90 % incidence of osteonecrosis [20]. Canale and Kelly [21] further reported that extrusion of the talar body and subluxation of the talonavicular joint virtually guarantees osteonecrosis.

5.2.2 Nontraumatic Osteonecrosis

The epidemiology of nontraumatic ON is completely different than traumatic ON. As the etiology is unrelated to a precipitating traumatic fracture, the affected populations, risk factors, and demographic distribution are all different.

5.3 Epidemiology of Nontraumatic Osteonecrosis in the USA

The risk factors associated with ON are slightly different comparing Asian to North American and Western European populations. In several studies, the proportion of patients with ethanol-related disease is higher in Asian populations [22, 23].

5.3.1 Incidence

The epidemiology of nontraumatic ON is variable according to the risk factors of the disease. It is difficult to describe the exact incidence of nontraumatic osteonecrosis in the USA because many early asymptomatic cases are not diagnosed or reported. However, there have been few studies that have attempted to study the occurrence of ON. Various described risk factors for osteonecrosis include corticosteroids, alcohol intake, systemic lupus erythematosus (SLE), organ transplantation, chemotherapy and/or radiation, human immunodeficiency virus (HIV) infection, hemoglobinopathies, pancreatitis, hyperuricemia or gout, and childhood history of slipped capital femoral epiphysis (SCFE). Other miscellaneous causes include decompression sickness, autoimmune diseases causing vasculitis, coagulopathy such as thrombophilia or disseminated intravascular coagulation, Gaucher's disease, hyperlipidemia, fat embolus syndrome, treatment of developmental hip dysplasia, and chronic liver disease. In one-fourth of the cases, no associated conditions or diseases can be found [24, 25].

5.3.2 Steroids and Osteonecrosis

Steroids have been known to be a risk factor for ON since 1957 [26]. The incidence of ON is thought to vary with the dose of steroids given; therefore, the prevalence varies from 10 to 60 % of patients in multiple large demographic studies [24, 27]. This variance is likely due to the different populations of patients commonly receiving large doses of steroids either sporadically or on a long-term basis [28, 29].

5.3.2.1 Steroid Immunosuppression for Solid Organ Transplantation

The reported incidence of ON after renal transplantation is 4–37 % [30–34]. The highest reported incidence was 37 % reported by Cruess et al. [30] who have since found a drastic reduction by changing from divided to single dose steroids. In a study carried by Martson et al. [35] on fifty-two patients (103 hips) who had undergone a solid organ transplant, survivorship analysis revealed that, at 1 year after the transplant, 89 % ± 7 % of the hips and 80 % ± 13 % of the patients were free of osteonecrosis of the femoral head. The prevalence of osteonecrosis 1 year after transplantation was 11 % or 20 %, respectively. Using an abbreviated screening MRI, Mulliken et al. [36] found a prevalence of ON of the femoral head of 7.6 %. This prevalence of 7.6 % agrees closely with that reported recently by Tervonen et al. [37], who discovered 6.0 % of asymptomatic renal transplants had ON using a similar abbreviated MRI. Both of these figures are lower than previous reports, possibly due to decreased steroid dosing or other factors. Kopecky et al. [38] studied MR findings in 104 patients up to 24 months after transplantation and found that MR lesions in seven hips (in five asymptomatic patients) regressed in size; in six hips, the MR images returned to normal. They suggested that some patients with MR evidence of ON of the hip have spontaneous improvement.

5.3.2.2 Steroid Treatment for Acute Lymphoblastic Leukemia

The incidence of ON related to allogeneic bone marrow transplant or acute lymphoblastic leukemia (ALL) varies from about 1–72 % [39–41] based on study design, primary diagnosis, symptomatic versus asymptomatic cases, and osteonecrosis definition used. Reports based on symptomatic cases [39–41] and those using radiographic evaluation typically report a lower incidence of osteonecrosis than those prospectively monitoring its development with contemporary MR techniques [40]. In the Childhood Cancer Survivor Study consisting of 9,261 patients and a random sample of 2,872 siblings, 52 (0.56 %) survivors of childhood cancer self-reported osteonecrosis developing in 78 joints; 60 % reported multiple joint involvement [39]. The reported incidence of symptomatic ON in ALL in a study by Mattano et al. [41] ranged from 1.8 % 5-year cumulative incidence to a 3-year life-table incidence of 9.3 %. Kawedia et al. [40] reported a cumulative incidence of osteonecrosis involvement in hips or knees in 72 % of prospectively monitored patients with ALL while on therapy, irrespective of symptoms. ON appears to involve the periarticular knee sites more commonly than the femoral head.

5.3.2.3 Steroid Immunosuppression After Bone Marrow Transplantation

Osteonecrosis is a potentially persistent and debilitating complication after allogeneic bone marrow transplantation (alloBMT) [42, 43]. The reported incidence of ON in alloBMT of any joint ranges from 3.9 to 44.2 % [44–46]. Recently, nearly 22 % of prospectively monitored pediatric patients, irrespective of clinical symptoms, were found to have MR-documented osteonecrosis of the hips or knees. Nearly 50 % of those with osteonecrosis had at least one third of the epiphysis involved [46]. The probable risk factors, such as acute or chronic graft versus host disease (GvHD) requiring steroids, increasing age, and a primary diagnosis of aplastic anemia or acute leukemia, have been documented in post-BMT settings in mixed populations [42].

5.3.2.4 Steroids in Other Medical Conditions

There is no definitive evidence to suggest that steroid inhalers used for chronic obstructive pulmonary disease, occasional Medrol Dosepak for rash or other inflammatory conditions, and locally administered steroids (e.g., steroid injections) cause osteonecrosis. However, oral intake of steroids above certain dose and duration is a risk factor for ON. Straightforward dose dependent association with steroid intake and ON has been demonstrated. Cumulative intravenous methylprednisolone, at doses of >2 g for >3 months, significantly increased the risk for ON [47]. More recently, a statistically significant association was described between ON incidence and the total dose of steroids during the first 2 months after renal transplantation [48].

5.3.3 Alcohol and Osteonecrosis

Ethanol abuse was described as a risk factor in osteonecrosis of the femoral head in 1922. In one study of 57 patients, the incidences of alcohol-associated osteonecrosis of the femoral head and of idiopathic osteonecrosis were 29 and 12 %, respectively [49]. Orlic et al. [50] studied risk factors in a total of 172 patients for the development and progression of osteonecrosis after alcohol use and idiopathic osteonecrosis. They found that patients with alcohol-induced osteonecrosis were significantly older than patients with idiopathic osteonecrosis (average age, 49 years versus 40 years), were men (97 %), and presented with collapsed femoral heads (90 %). In another study group, 164 patients with alcohol-induced osteonecrosis were analyzed for different factors [51]. The average duration of alcohol abuse was 9.5 years, 28 % of patients were younger than 40 years of age, and 76 % were younger than 50 years. Bilateral necrosis of femoral heads was present in 45 % of patients, and within 3 years of the diagnosis, multifocal osteonecrosis became evident in 23 cases at distant sites (shoulders and knees). Elevated cholesterol and triglyceride levels were found in 38 % of cases. Serum amylase was elevated in 33 (20 %) patients, liver dysfunction was present in 50 (30 %), hepatomegaly was found in 32 (20 %), and biopsy-confirmed cirrhosis was present in 22 (13 %) cases.

5.3.4 Systemic Lupus Erythematosus and Osteonecrosis

The incidence of ON in systemic lupus erythematosus (SLE) has been reported to occur in 40 % of patients if silent cases are included. Approximately 15 % of patients develop symptomatic osteonecrosis [4, 52]. Weiner and Abeles [53] reported on 28 of 172 patients (16 %) with SLE who developed ON. Cozen and Wallace [54] reported on their experience over 47 years. ON was found in 26 of 488 (5 %) patients with SLE. In a review of the Hopkins Lupus Cohort, Petri [55] noted a prevalence of ON of 14.5 %. One possible explanation for the differences in these percentages may be the variability of severity of SLE, ranging from mild cases in a private practice setting to severe cases in tertiary referral centers. Glucocorticoid use is considered a risk factor for the occurrence of osteonecrosis in general, but particularly in patients with SLE [56]. Other factors may also be implicated in its development, as osteonecrosis has been described in SLE patients who have not received glucocorticoids [57]. Additional risk factors have been variably identified by different investigators [54, 56, 58]; these include a Cushingoid body habitus, smoking, thrombophlebitis, vasculitis, Raynaud's phenomenon, arthritis, presence of certain autoantibodies (antiphospholipid, anti-Ro plus anti-RNP, or anti-topoisomerase I), or disease-related fibrinolytic abnormalities.

5.3.5 Human Immunodeficiency Virus Infection and Osteonecrosis

Recent retrospective case studies of human immunodeficiency virus (HIV)-infected patients have reported incidences ranging from 0.03 to 0.37 cases per 100 person-years [59, 60]. The true incidence of symptomatic osteonecrosis, however, has not been well defined. Morse et al. [61] found an incidence of ON in HIV to be 0.65 cases per 100 patient-years for asymptomatic patients and 0.26 cases per 100 patient-years for symptomatic patients. This is 100-fold higher than the estimated incidence in the general population [62, 63]. They also found a rapid progression of disease in symptomatic patients (59 %) needing THR [61]. In a study by Assouline-Dayan et al. [57], the prevalence of osteonecrosis in the initial cohort of 339 asymptomatic patients who were evaluated by MRI was found to be extraordinarily high at 5.6 %. In another study by Wallis et al. [64], osteonecrosis was identified by MRI in 2 (18 %) of 11 asymptomatic patients, highlighting the potential risks in this population and further emphasizing how corticosteroids must be used cautiously in HIV-infected patients.

5.3.6 Hematologic Conditions and Osteonecrosis

Osteonecrosis has been associated with several hemoglobinopathies (hemoglobin SS, hemoglobin SC, and sickle thalassemia) and coagulation disorders (thrombophilia and hypofibrinolysis). The reported prevalence of osteonecrosis in these populations has been 4–20 % [24, 65, 66]. At least one coagulation factor abnormality was found in 82 % of patients with osteonecrosis of the femoral head compared with 30 % of controls ($p<.0001$). Two or more abnormalities were identified in 21 patients (47 %) compared with 2.5 % of controls ($p<.0001$) [65]. Glueck et al. [66] found a high prevalence of plasminogen activator inhibitor-1 coagulation abnormalities in patients with osteonecrosis. In a study [67] on multifocal ON, rate of coagulation disorders was found to be similar to rates reported in the literature. Eighty percent to 90 % of patients tested with osteonecrosis had hypofibrinolysis and thrombophilia or both. Patients with single joint involvement are just as likely to have a coagulation disorder as are patients with more joint involvement [67].

5.3.7 Rare Disorders and Osteonecrosis

Additional rare disorders may be associated with ON. As these diseases occur infrequently, the exact incidence of ON among these populations is difficult to discern. Report indicates that ON may be seen with hyperlipidemia (9 %), liver disease (4 %), Gaucher's disease (2 %), and dysbarism (2 %) of all the ON cases [24].

5.4 Age Distribution

The age range of patients is reported from 15 to 83 years, with the vast majority under 50 years for overall nontraumatic osteonecrosis. For alcohol-associated ON, age at the time of diagnosis is reported from 19 to 67 years with 72 % less than 50 years of age [24, 49, 50]. For steroid-related ON, age at diagnosis of ON is reported from 15 to 63 years with 60 % below 50 years of age [24, 63, 68]. The mean age of patients with SLE first diagnosed with ON generally ranges from 25 to 35 years [56, 69]. In a study [24] on US population, pancreatitis-associated ON was found in age group 36–61 years with 82 % less than 50 years of age. For hyperuricemia-associated ON, age at the time of diagnosis of ON ranged from 19 to 81 years with 57 % less than 50 years of age. All patients with sickle cell ON were reported to be less than 50 years at the time of diagnosis [24]. Ages ranged from 31 to 62 years in ON associated with liver disease with the majority less than 50 years old. For hyperlipidemia, ages at the time of diagnosis of ON ranged from 32 to 67 years and 52 % were less than 50 years old. Sixty-seven percent of patients were under 50 years of age when ON was apparent for Gaucher's disease. For multifocal osteonecrosis, a mean age at presentation of 36 years (range, 15–75 years) has been reported [24, 67].

5.5 Gender Distribution

There has been male dominance with ratio of around 4:1 as compared to females for overall osteonecrosis [24, 57, 70]. In a study of 75 patients with steroid-associated ON, 31 % were found to be females [24]. In other series of 72 steroid-treated patients, Fisher and Bickel [68] observed a higher incidence of female involvement (44 %).

SLE-associated ON shows a female preponderance when compared with other risk factors [4, 58, 69, 71]. In the multicenter study on multifocal ON, there was a trend toward a greater proportion of women versus men in the systemic lupus erythematosus group (32 women, 6 men) as compared with the remaining study group (43 women, 20 men) ($p=0.076$) [67]. This is similar to numbers of women in other studies, which are weighted toward patients with systemic lupus erythematosus and other inflammatory disorder [58], but dissimilar to incidences reported in studies [51] where there is a preponderance of patients who use alcohol, in which more men are seen. Complete (100 %) male dominance was reported for pancreatitis- and sickle cell-associated ON [24]. For hyperuricemia, hyperlipidemia, and Gaucher's disease, 83 % male dominance has been reported [24]. In case of liver disease-associated ON, 60 % patients were found to be males [24].

5.6 Race Distribution

Overall, a white versus black predominance exceeding 3:1 has been reported [24, 70, 72]. The reported distribution among patients with steroid-associated ON was 84 % whites in contrast to 64 % blacks for pancreatitis-associated ON. Race distribution also showed 77, 60, 87, and 100 % white dominance for hyperuricemia, liver disease, hyperlipidemia, and Gaucher's disease, respectively [24].

5.7 Anatomical Location

5.7.1 Bilateral Osteonecrosis

Symptomatic osteonecrosis is often unilateral although when asymptomatic disease is considered, bilateral disease is common. The likelihood of bilateral disease, regardless of the presence of symptoms, has been studied in specific patient populations and in the femoral head, ranges from 34 to 80 % [24, 68, 72–74]. In an abbreviated MRI screening study of renal transplant patients' hips, lesions were bilateral 50 % of the time [36]. In other disease cohorts, symmetrical bilateral disease developed in 90 % (SLE), 36 % (pancreatitis and hyperuricemia), 13 % (sickle cell disease), 30 % (liver disease), 17 % (hyperlipidemia), and 17 % (Gaucher's disease) [24].

5.7.2 Multifocal Osteonecrosis

In contrast to bilateral involvement of a single joint, when a patient has diffuse, multifocal ON (i.e., three or more disease sites), the presence of bilateral disease is markedly increased. A multicenter study of multifocal ON revealed bilateral involvement in 98 % (femoral heads), 87 % (knees, distal femur, or proximal tibia), 83 % (proximal humerii), 61 % (distal tibia or talus), and 42 % (peri-elbow) [67]. The overall distribution of disease sites found in this multicenter study is shown in Table 5.1. Common risk factors for the presence of multifocal disease are a history of SLE (20 %) [58], ALL (74 %) [41], or bone marrow transplantation (44 %) [45]. When ON affects knee, shoulder, and ankle joints, multifocal disease should be suspected [75].

Table 5.1 Distribution of multifocal osteonecrotic lesions [67]

Anatomical location	Frequency (%)
Hip	200 (99)
Knee	179 (87)
Shoulder	146 (72)
Ankle	71 (35)
Elbow	17 (8)
Wrist	8 (4)
Calcaneus	6 (3)
Tarsal navicular	2 (1)
Cuneiform	1 (0.5)
Cuboid	1 (0.5)
Metacarpal head	1 (0.1)

5.8 Stage Distribution at Time of Presentation

In a study on multifocal osteonecrosis [67], plain radiography or MRI revealed that most (69 %) joints presented in a precollapse stage. Eighty-five of 200 (43 %) hips had collapse (59 hips) or osteoarthritis (26 hips). Only 17 % of 179 knees, 38 % of 146 shoulders, and 24 % of 71 ankles had collapse or arthritis. Approximately 30 % of the lesions were diagnosed solely by MRI. There was a higher incidence of these asymptomatic lesions in the knee (38 %), shoulder (30 %), and ankle (44 %) than in the hip (18 %). The incidence of negative radiographic findings but positive MRI scans was highest in the ankle (44 %) and knee (38 %) and lower in the shoulder (30 %) and hip (18 %).

5.9 Summary

In summarizing the epidemiology of osteonecrosis in the USA, it is evident that the prevalence and incidence vary according to the risk factor of disease and the population being studied. Traumatic osteonecrosis is associated with specific fractures, and the incidence depends upon many factors such as age, displacement, type of fracture, and method of treatment. Nontraumatic ONFH can be idiopathic but is usually associated with corticosteroid usage, ethanol abuse, systemic lupus erythematosus, barotrauma, or marrow packing disorders such as sickle cell disease and Gaucher's disease. The proportion of patients with steroid-related ONFH is increasing as solid organ and bone marrow transplantation are becoming more commonplace.

References

1. Cleveland M, Fielding JW. A continuing end-result study of intracapsular fracture of the neck of the femur. J Bone Joint Surg Am. 1954;36-A:1020–30.
2. Massie WK. Treatment of femoral neck fractures emphasizing long term follow-up observations on aseptic necrosis. Clin Orthop Relat Res. 1973;92:16–62.
3. Haidukewych GJ, Rothwell WS, Jacofsky DJ, Torchia ME, Berry DJ. Operative treatment of femoral neck fractures in patients between the ages of fifteen and fifty years. J Bone Joint Surg Am. 2004;86-A:1711–6.
4. Dubois EL, Cozen L. Avascular (aseptic) bone necrosis associated with systemic lupus erythematosus. JAMA. 1960;174:966–71.
5. Swiontkowski MF, Winquist RA, Hansen Jr ST. Fractures of the femoral neck in patients between the ages of twelve and forty-nine years. J Bone Joint Surg Am. 1984;66:837–46.
6. American Academy of Orthopaedic Surgeons. Orthopaedic Knowledge Update 7. Rosemont IL. AAOS 2002. p. 410–2.
7. Crawford HB. Conservative treatment of impacted fractures of the femoral neck. A report of fifty cases. J Bone Joint Surg Am. 1960; 42-A:471–9.
8. Arnold WD, Lyden JP, Minkoff J. Treatment of intracapsular fractures of the femoral neck. With special reference to percutaneous Knowles pinning. J Bone Joint Surg Am. 1974;56:254–62.
9. Bunata RE, Fahey JJ, Drennan DB. Factors influencing stability and necrosis of impacted femoral neck fractures. JAMA. 1973;223:41–4.
10. Phemister DB. Treatment of the necrotic head of the femur in adults. J Bone Joint Surg Am. 1949;31A:55–66.
11. Chapman MW, Stehr JH, Eberle CF, Bloom MH, Bovill Jr EG. Treatment of intracapsular hip fractures by the Deyerle method. A comparative review of one hundred and nineteen cases. J Bone Joint Surg Am. 1975;57:735–44.
12. Epstein HC. Traumatic dislocations of the hip. Clin Orthop Relat Res. 1973;92:116–42.
13. McKee MD, Garay ME, Schemitsch EH, Kreder HJ, Stephen DJ. Irreducible fracture-dislocation of the hip: a severe injury with a poor prognosis. J Orthop Trauma. 1998;12:223–9.
14. Stewart MJ, Milford LW. Fracture-dislocation of the hip; an end-result study. J Bone Joint Surg Am. 1954;36:315–42.
15. Brav EA. Traumatic dislocation of the hip. J Bone Joint Surg. 1962;44A:1115.
16. Cooney III WP, Dobyns JH, Linscheid RL. Nonunion of the scaphoid: analysis of the results from bone grafting. J Hand Surg Am. 1980;5:343–54.
17. Green DP. The effect of avascular necrosis on Russe bone grafting for scaphoid nonunion. J Hand Surg Am. 1985;10:597–605.
18. Mack GR, Bosse MJ, Gelberman RH, Yu E. The natural history of scaphoid non-union. J Bone Joint Surg Am. 1984;66:504–9.
19. Haliburton RA, Sullivan CR, Kelly PJ, Peterson LF. The extra-osseous and intra-osseous blood supply of the talus. J Bone Joint Surg Am. 1958;40-A:1115–20.
20. Hawkins LG. Fractures of the neck of the talus. J Bone Joint Surg Am. 1970;52:991–1002.
21. Canale ST, Kelly Jr FB. Fractures of the neck of the talus. Long-term evaluation of seventy-one cases. J Bone Joint Surg Am. 1978;60:143–56.
22. Fukushima W, Fujioka M, Kubo T, Tamakoshi A, Nagai M, Hirota Y. Nationwide epidemiologic survey of idiopathic osteonecrosis of the femoral head. Clin Orthop Relat Res. 2010;468:2715–24.
23. Kang JS, Moon KH, Kwon DG, Shin BK, Woo MS. The natural history of asymptomatic osteonecrosis of the femoral head. Int Orthop. 2013;37:379–84.
24. Jacobs B. Epidemiology of traumatic and nontraumatic osteonecrosis. Clin Orthop Relat Res. 1978;130:51–67.
25. Lopez-Ben R, Mikuls TR, Moore DS, Julian BA, Bernreuter WK, Elkins M, Saag KG. Incidence of hip osteonecrosis among renal transplantation recipients: a prospective study. Clin Radiol. 2004;59:431–8.
26. Singh JM, Palda VA, Stanbrook MB, Chapman KR. Corticosteroid therapy for patients with acute exacerbations of chronic obstructive pulmonary disease: a systematic review. Arch Intern Med. 2002;162:2527–36.
27. Aaron RK, Lennox D, Bunce GE, Ebert T. The conservative treatment of osteonecrosis of the femoral head. A comparison of core decompression and pulsing electromagnetic fields. Clin Orthop Relat Res. 1989;249:209–18.
28. Meyers MH. Osteonecrosis of the femoral head treated with the muscle pedicle graft. Orthop Clin North Am. 1985;16:741–5.
29. Powell C, Chang C, Naguwa SM, Cheema G, Gershwin ME. Steroid induced osteonecrosis: an analysis of steroid dosing risk. Autoimmun Rev. 2010;9:721–43.
30. Cruess RL, Blennerhassett J, MacDonald FR, MacLean LD, Dossetor J. Aseptic necrosis following renal transplantation. J Bone Joint Surg Am. 1968;50:1577–90.
31. Griffiths HJ, Ennis JT, Bailey G. Skeletal changes following renal transplantation. Radiology. 1974;113:621–6.
32. Harrington KD, Murray WR, Kountz SL, Belzer FO. Avascular necrosis of bone after renal transplantation. J Bone Joint Surg Am. 1971;53:203–15.
33. Ibels LS, Alfrey AC, Huffer WE, Weil III R. Aseptic necrosis of bone following renal transplantation: experience in 194 transplant recipients and review of the literature. Medicine (Baltimore). 1978;57:25–45.
34. Nelson CL, Evarts CM, Popowniak K. Musculoskeletal complications of renal transplantation. Surg Clin North Am. 1971;51: 1205–9.
35. Marston SB, Gillingham K, Bailey RF, Cheng EY. Osteonecrosis of the femoral head after solid organ transplantation: a prospective study. J Bone Joint Surg Am. 2002;84-A:2145–51.
36. Mulliken BD, Renfrew DL, Brand RA, Whitten CG. The prevalence and natural history of early osteonecrosis (ON) of the femoral head. Iowa Orthop J. 1994;14:115–9.
37. Tervonen O, Mueller DM, Matteson EL, Velosa JA, Ginsburg WW, Ehman RL. Clinically occult avascular necrosis of the hip: prevalence in an asymptomatic population at risk. Radiology. 1992;182: 845–7.
38. Kopecky KK, Braunstein EM, Brandt KD, Filo RS, Leapman SB, Capello WN, Klatte EC. Apparent avascular necrosis of the hip: appearance and spontaneous resolution of MR findings in renal allograft recipients. Radiology. 1991;179:523–7.
39. Kadan-Lottick NS, Dinu I, Wasilewski-Masker K, Kaste S, Meacham LR, Mahajan A, Stovall M, Yasui Y, Robison LL, Sklar CA. Osteonecrosis in adult survivors of childhood cancer: a report from the childhood cancer survivor study. J Clin Oncol. 2008;26: 3038–45.
40. Kawedia JD, Kaste SC, Pei D, Panetta JC, Cai X, Cheng C, Neale G, Howard SC, Evans WE, Pui CH, Relling MV. Pharmacokinetic, pharmacodynamic, and pharmacogenetic determinants of osteonecrosis in children with acute lymphoblastic leukemia. Blood. 2011;117:2340–7.
41. Mattano Jr LA, Sather HN, Trigg ME, Nachman JB. Osteonecrosis as a complication of treating acute lymphoblastic leukemia in children: a report from the Children's Cancer Group. J Clin Oncol. 2000;18:3262–72.
42. Enright H, Haake R, Weisdorf D. Avascular necrosis of bone: a common serious complication of allogeneic bone marrow transplantation. Am J Med. 1990;89:733–8.
43. Mattano L. The skeletal remains: porosis and necrosis of bone in the marrow transplantation setting. Pediatr Transplant. 2003;7(3): 71–5.

44. Balduzzi A, Gooley T, Anasetti C, Sanders JE, Martin PJ, Petersdorf EW, Appelbaum FR, Buckner CD, Matthews D, Storb R, Sullivan KM, Hansen JA. Unrelated donor marrow transplantation in children. Blood. 1995;86:3247–56.
45. Kaste SC, Shidler TJ, Tong X, Srivastava DK, Rochester R, Hudson MM, Shearer PD, Hale GA. Bone mineral density and osteonecrosis in survivors of childhood allogeneic bone marrow transplantation. Bone Marrow Transplant. 2004;33:435–41.
46. Sharma S, Yang S, Rochester R, Britton L, Leung WH, Yang J, Neel MD, Ness KK, Kaste SC. Prevalence of osteonecrosis and associated risk factors in children before allogeneic BMT. Bone Marrow Transplant. 2011;46:813–9.
47. Saisu T, Sakamoto K, Yamada K, Kashiwabara H, Yokoyama T, Iida S, Harada Y, Ikenoue S, Sakamoto M, Moriya H. High incidence of osteonecrosis of femoral head in patients receiving more than 2 g of intravenous methylprednisolone after renal transplantation. Transplant Proc. 1996;28:1559–60.
48. Shibatani M, Fujioka M, Arai Y, Takahashi K, Ueshima K, Okamoto M, Yoshimura N, Hirota Y, Fukushima W, Kubo T. Degree of corticosteroid treatment within the first 2 months of renal transplantation has a strong influence on the incidence of osteonecrosis of the femoral head. Acta Orthop. 2008;79:631–6.
49. Rico H, Gomez-Castresana F, Cabranes JA, Almoguera I, Lopez DL, Matute JA. Increased blood cortisol in alcoholic patients with aseptic necrosis of the femoral head. Calcif Tissue Int. 1985;37:585–7.
50. Orlic D, Jovanovic S, Anticevic D, Zecevic J. Frequency of idiopathic aseptic necrosis in medically treated alcoholics. Int Orthop. 1990;14:383–6.
51. Jacobs B. Alcoholism-induced bone necrosis. N Y State J Med. 1992;92:334–8.
52. Zizic TM, Hungerford DS, Stevens MB. Ischemic bone necrosis in systemic lupus erythematosus. II. The early diagnosis of ischemic necrosis of bone. Medicine (Baltimore). 1980;59:134–42.
53. Weiner ES, Abeles M. Aseptic necrosis and glucocorticosteroids in systemic lupus erythematosus: a reevaluation. J Rheumatol. 1989; 16:604–8.
54. Cozen L, Wallace DJ. Avascular necrosis in systemic lupus erythematosus: clinical associations and a 47-year perspective. Am J Orthop (Belle Mead NJ). 1998;27:352–4.
55. Petri M. Musculoskeletal complications of systemic lupus erythematosus in the Hopkins Lupus Cohort: an update. Arthritis Care Res. 1995;8:137–45.
56. Mont MA, Glueck CJ, Pacheco IH, Wang P, Hungerford DS, Petri M. Risk factors for osteonecrosis in systemic lupus erythematosus. J Rheumatol. 1997;24:654–62.
57. Assouline-Dayan Y, Chang C, Greenspan A, Shoenfeld Y, Gershwin ME. Pathogenesis and natural history of osteonecrosis. Semin Arthritis Rheum. 2002;32:94–124.
58. Zizic TM, Marcoux C, Hungerford DS, Dansereau JV, Stevens MB. Corticosteroid therapy associated with ischemic necrosis of bone in systemic lupus erythematosus. Am J Med. 1985;79:596–604.
59. Scribner AN, Troia-Cancio PV, Cox BA, Marcantonio D, Hamid F, Keiser P, Levi M, Allen B, Murphy K, Jones RE, Skiest DJ. Osteonecrosis in HIV: a case-control study. J Acquir Immune Defic Syndr. 2000;25:19–25.
60. Brown P, Crane L. Avascular necrosis of bone in patients with human immunodeficiency virus infection: report of 6 cases and review of the literature. Clin Infect Dis. 2001;32:1221–6.
61. Morse CG, Mican JM, Jones EC, Joe GO, Rick ME, Formentini E, Kovacs JA. The incidence and natural history of osteonecrosis in HIV-infected adults. Clin Infect Dis. 2007;44:739–48.
62. Mont MA, Hungerford DS. Non-traumatic avascular necrosis of the femoral head. J Bone Joint Surg Am. 1995;77:459–74.
63. Bauer M, Thabault P, Estok D, Christiansen C, Platt R. Low-dose corticosteroids and avascular necrosis of the hip and knee. Pharmacoepidemiol Drug Saf. 2000;9:187–91.
64. Wallis RS, Kalayjian R, Jacobson JM, Fox L, Purdue L, Shikuma CM, Arakaki R, Snyder S, Coombs RW, Bosch RJ, Spritzler J, Chernoff M, Aga E, Myers L, Schock B, Lederman MM. A study of the immunology, virology, and safety of prednisone in HIV-1-infected subjects with CD4 cell counts of 200 to 700 mm(-3). J Acquir Immune Defic Syndr. 2003;32:281–6.
65. Jones LC, Hungerford DS. Osteonecrosis: etiology, diagnosis, and treatment. Curr Opin Rheumatol. 2004;16:443–9.
66. Glueck CJ, Fontaine RN, Gruppo R, Stroop D, Sieve-Smith L, Tracy T, Wang P. The plasminogen activator inhibitor-1 gene, hypofibrinolysis, and osteonecrosis. Clin Orthop Relat Res. 1999; 366:133–46.
67. Symptomatic multifocal osteonecrosis. A multicenter study. Collaborative Osteonecrosis Group. Clin Orthop Relat Res. 1999; 312–326.
68. Fisher DE, Bickel WH. Corticosteroid-induced avascular necrosis. A clinical study of seventy-seven patients. J Bone Joint Surg Am. 1971;53:859–73.
69. Cozen L, Wallace DJ. Risk factors for avascular necrosis in systemic lupus erythematosus. J Rheumatol. 1998;25:188.
70. Patterson RJ, Bickel WH, Dahlin DC. Idiopathic avascular necrosis of the head of the femur. A study of fifty-two cases. J Bone Joint Surg Am. 1964;46:267–82.
71. Calvo-Alen J, McGwin G, Toloza S, Fernandez M, Roseman JM, Bastian HM, Cepeda EJ, Gonzalez EB, Baethge BA, Fessler BJ, Vila LM, Reveille JD, Alarcon GS. Systemic lupus erythematosus in a multiethnic US cohort (LUMINA): XXIV. Cytotoxic treatment is an additional risk factor for the development of symptomatic osteonecrosis in lupus patients: results of a nested matched case-control study. Ann Rheum Dis. 2006;65:785–90.
72. McCollum DE, Mathews RS, O'Neil MT. Aseptic necrosis of the femoral head: associated diseases and evaluation of treatment. South Med J. 1970;63:241–53.
73. Coventry MB, Beckenbaugh RD, Nolan DR, Ilstrup DM. 2,012 total hip arthroplasties. A study of postoperative course and early complications. J Bone Joint Surg Am. 1974;56:273–84.
74. Boettcher WG, Bonfiglio M, Hamilton HH, Sheets RF, Smith K. Non-traumatic necrosis of the femoral head. I. Relation of altered hemostasis to etiology. J Bone Joint Surg Am. 1970;52:312–21.
75. Mont MA, Hungerford DS. Osteonecrosis of the shoulder, knee, and ankle. In: Urbaniak J, Jones JP, editors. Osteonecrosis. Rosemont: American Academy of Orthopaedic Surgeons; 1997. p. 429–36. 2013.

The Epidemiology of Osteonecrosis in Japan

6

Takuaki Yamamoto, Ryosuke Yamaguchi, and Yukihide Iwamoto

6.1 Introduction (Background of the Epidemiology of Osteonecrosis)

The incidence of a disease is an important parameter for epidemiological research. For example, the incidence of rheumatoid arthritis is estimated to be 23.7 cases per 100,000 person-years [1], while that of osteoarthritis in the hip joint to be 47.3–88 cases per 100,000 person-years in the United States [2, 3]. These data have been adopted to elucidate the burden, risks, and trends of the disease in a general population [1, 4].

Nontraumatic osteonecrosis (ON) of the femoral head is a pathologic process that often progresses to a subchondral collapse, following femoral head deformity and eventually resulting in hip joint destruction. Many studies have been performed to elucidate its etiology, such as the association with corticosteroid usage or alcohol abuse [5, 6]. However, regarding the incidence of nontraumatic ON in any general population, only a few detailed data are available.

6.2 Incidence of Osteonecrosis in Japan [7]

In Japan, nontraumatic ON is designated as an intractable disease by the Specified Disease Treatment Research Program, which is a subsidy program under the Japanese Ministry of Health, Labour and Welfare (secondary ON associated with femoral neck fracture, capital femoral epiphysis, irradiation, dysbarism, or Perthes' disease is not included in this subsidy program). Based on the registration data of this program, the incidence of nontraumatic ON in Japan was calculated.

Nontraumatic ON patients who were newly identified under the Specified Disease Treatment Research Program in Fukuoka Prefecture between 1999 and 2008 were investigated. Fukuoka Prefecture continuously had populations of almost five million (5,004,276–5,050,216) in this 10-year period. The crude incidence rates were calculated as the number of nontraumatic ON patients divided by the total population of Fukuoka Prefecture.

A total of 1,244 nontraumatic ON patients were newly registered in Fukuoka Prefecture, during this 10-year period, including 758 men (61 %) and 486 women (39 %). The gender ratio (men/women) was 1.6. The mean age was 48 (17–85) years for men, and the peak age ranged in the 40s and 50s. On the other hand, the mean age for women was 56 (13–92) years, and a bimodal peak distribution was seen in their 50s and 70s. The crude incidence rate during the 10-year period was 2.58 cases per 100,000 person-years, with a range of 1.54–3.66 (Table 6.1). The age-adjusted incidence rates were 1.56–3.71 cases per 100,000 person-years, and the average of age-adjusted incidence rates was 2.51 cases. Based on the data from Fukuoka Prefecture, the number of newly registered patients with nontraumatic ON of the femoral head in Japan (population, ~120 million) was estimated to be 3,200 cases per year [7].

6.3 Other Data on the Incidence of Osteonecrosis

The Research Committee on Idiopathic Avascular Necrosis of the Femoral Head was established in 1975. The committee has reported five nationwide surveys on the prevalence

T. Yamamoto (✉) • R. Yamaguchi • Y. Iwamoto
Department of Orthopaedic Surgery,
Kyushu University, 3-1-1 Maidashi, Higashi-ku,
Fukuoka 812-8582, Japan
e-mail: yamataku@ortho.med.kyushu-u.ac.jp;
yamaryo@ortho.med.kyushu-u.ac.jp;
yiwamoto@ortho.med.kyushu-u.ac.jp

K.-H. Koo et al. (eds.), *Osteonecrosis*,
DOI 10.1007/978-3-642-35767-1_6, © Springer-Verlag Berlin Heidelberg 2014

Table 6.1 Incidence of nontraumatic ON of the femoral head per 100,000 person-years in Fukuoka Prefecture

	Year										
	1999	2000	2001	2002	2003	2004	2005	2006	2007	2008	
Age at identified	Incidence rate/100,000 person-years										All years
–20	0.18	0.18	0.00	0.19	0.49	0.20	0.20	0.00	0.11	0.32	0.19
20–29	1.43	0.78	1.08	1.22	2.48	1.12	1.82	1.36	1.23	1.41	1.39
30–39	1.97	2.62	2.37	1.85	3.45	3.96	4.10	3.54	3.25	2.41	2.95
40–49	2.42	2.98	4.44	3.62	6.76	2.94	4.24	4.86	4.83	3.31	4.04
50–59	2.25	2.96	2.15	2.94	6.20	4.23	4.90	5.04	4.55	4.17	3.94
60–69	2.52	2.34	2.59	2.56	4.92	3.51	4.34	4.25	3.44	3.43	3.39
70–79	1.04	1.30	2.18	1.63	4.55	3.34	4.89	4.91	3.98	2.50	3.03
80–	0.54	2.15	1.45	0.00	0.44	1.65	2.89	2.58	2.80	2.67	1.72
Crude rate	1.54	1.91	2.03	1.75	3.66	2.62	3.42	3.32	3.02	2.53	2.58
Age-adjusted rate	1.56	1.80	1.92	1.81	3.71	2.57	3.26	3.18	2.89	2.43	**2.51**

Reproduced from Ref. [7]

Table 6.2 Reported incidence of nontraumatic ON of the femoral head

Population	Reference	Year of publishing	Diagnostic method	No. of people	Incidence (per 100 person-years)
SLE (high dose)	Nakamura et al. [12]	2010	MRI	169	34.6
	Nagasawa et al. [10]	2005	MRI	45	31.1
	Oinuma et al. [13]	2001	MRI	72	44.4
(Low dose)	Aranow et al. [14]	1997	MRI	66	12.1
Renal transplantation	Shibatani et al. [15]	2008	MRI	150	24.7
	Lopez-Ben et al. [16]	2004	MRI	49	8.2
	Kubo et al. [11]	1997	MRI	51	25.5
	Metselaar et al. [17]	1985	X-ray	248	13
Bone marrow transplantation	Torii et al. [18]	2001	MRI	100	19
Liver transplantation	Lieberman et al. [19]	2000	MRI	203	0.48
Cardiac transplantation	Bradbury et al. [20]	1994	MRI	168	5.38
Child ALL	Patel et al. [21]	2008	X-ray or MRI	1,088	2.9
	Arico et al. [22]	2003	N/A	1,421	1.6
Sickle cell disease	Milner et al. [23]	1993	X-ray	2,524	2.92
	Milner et al. [24]	1991	X-ray	2,590	2.88
HIV	Morse et al. [25]	2007	MRI	239	0.65
	Ho et al. [26]	2007	N/A	967	0.34
Neurosurgical patients	Wong et al. [27]	2005	MRI	1,352	0.1
General	Yamaguchi et al. [7]		X-ray and MRI	Five million	0.00258

Reproduced from Ref. [7]

of ON in Japan, which showed an annual increase. The prevalence was 6,700–8,200 (95 % confidence interval) in 1994 [8] and 10,100–12,800 (95 % confidence interval) in 2004 [9].

Previously, the incidence of nontraumatic or steroid-associated ON has been reported in disease-limited populations, such as systemic lupus erythematosus (SLE), organ transplantation, and sickle cell disease. Those reported data are summarized in Table 6.2. For example, in SLE patients, an MRI study showed the incidence of ONFH to be 31.1 % (14 of 45 patients) in 1 year [10], while in renal allograft recipients, osteonecrotic changes on MRI have been detected in 25.5 % of the patients (13 of 51 patients) [11].

References

1. Jacobson DL, Gange SJ, Rose NR, Graham NMH. Epidemiology and estimated population burden of selected autoimmune diseases in the United States. Clin Immunol Immunopathol. 1997;84(3):223–43.
2. Oliveria SA, Felson DT, Reed JI, Cirillo PA, Walker AM. Incidence of symptomatic hand, hip, and knee osteoarthritis among patients in a health maintenance organization. Arthritis Rheum. 1995;38(8):1134–41.
3. Arden N, Nevitt MC. Osteoarthritis: epidemiology. Best Pract Res Clin Rheumatol. 2006;20(1):3–25.
4. Marrack P, Kappler J, Kotzin BL. Autoimmune disease: why and where it occurs. Nat Med. 2001;7(8):899–905.
5. Mankin HJ. Nontraumatic necrosis of bone (osteonecrosis). N Engl J Med. 1992;326(22):1473–9.

6. Mont MA, Hungerford DS. Nontraumatic avascular necrosis of the femoral-head. J Bone Joint Surg Am. 1995;77A(3):459–74.
7. Yamaguchi R, Yamamoto T, Motomura G, Ikemura S, Iwamoto Y. Incidence of nontraumatic osteonecrosis of the femoral head in the Japanese population. Arthritis Rheum. 2011;63:3169–73.
8. Hirota Y, Hotokebuchi T, Sugioka Y. Idiopathic osteonecrosis of the femoral head; nationwide epidemiologic studies in Japan. In: Urbaniak JR, Jones Jr JP, editors. Osteonecrosis-etiology, diagnosis and treatment. Rosemont: American Academy of Orthopaedic Surgeons; 1997. p. 51–8.
9. Fukushima W, Fujioka M, Kubo T, Tamakoshi A, Nagai M, Hirota Y. Nationwide epidemiologic survey of idiopathic osteonecrosis of the femoral head. Clin Orthop Relat Res. 2010;468(10):2715–24.
10. Nagasawa K, Tada Y, Koarada S, Horiuchi T, Tsukamoto H, Murai K, et al. Very early development of steroid-associated osteonecrosis of femoral head in systemic lupus erythematosus: prospective study by MRI. Lupus. 2005;14(5):385–90.
11. Kubo T, Yamazoe S, Sugano N, Fujioka M, Naruse S, Yoshimura N, et al. Initial MRI findings of non-traumatic osteonecrosis of the femoral head in renal allograft recipients. Magn Reson Imaging. 1997;15(9):1017–23.
12. Nakamura J, Saisu T, Yamashita K, Suzuki C, Kamegaya M, Takahashi K. Age at time of corticosteroid administration is a risk factor for osteonecrosis in pediatric patients with systemic lupus erythematosus: a prospective magnetic resonance imaging study. Arthritis Rheum. 2010;62(2):609–15.
13. Oinuma K, Harada Y, Nawata Y, Takabayashi K, Abe I, Kamikawa K, et al. Osteonecrosis in patients with systemic lupus erythematosus develops very early after starting high dose corticosteroid treatment. Ann Rheum Dis. 2001;60(12):1145–8.
14. Aranow C, Zelicof S, Leslie D, Solomon S, Barland P, Norman A, et al. Clinically occult avascular necrosis of the hip in systemic lupus erythematosus. J Rheumatol. 1997;24(12):2318–22.
15. Shibatani M, Fujioka M, Arai Y, Takahashi K, Ueshima K, Okamoto M, et al. Degree of corticosteroid treatment within the first 2 months of renal transplantation has a strong influence on the incidence of osteonecrosis of the femoral head. Acta Orthop. 2008;79(5):631–6.
16. Lopez-Ben R, Mikuls TR, Moore DS, Julian BA, Bernreuter WK, Elkins M, et al. Incidence of hip osteonecrosis among renal transplantation recipients: a prospective study. Clin Radiol. 2004;59(5):431–8.
17. Metselaar HJ, Van Steenberge EJP, Bijnen AB. Incidence of osteonecrosis after renal transplantation. Acta Orthop Scand. 1985;56(5):413–5.
18. Torii Y, Hasegawa Y, Kubo T, Kodera Y, Minami S, Morishita Y, et al. Osteonecrosis of the femoral head after allogeneic bone marrow transplantation. Clin Orthop Relat Res. 2001;382:124–32.
19. Lieberman JR, Scaduto AA, Wellmeyer E. Symptomatic osteonecrosis of the hip after orthotopic liver transplantation. J Arthroplasty. 2000;15(6):767–71.
20. Bradbury G, Benjamin J, Thompson J, Klees E, Copeland J. Avascular necrosis of bone after cardiac transplantation. Prevalence and relationship to administration and dosage of steroids. J Bone Joint Surg Am. 1994;76(9):1385–8.
21. Patel B, Richards SM, Rowe JM, Goldstone AH, Fielding AK. High incidence of avascular necrosis in adolescents with acute lymphoblastic leukaemia: a UKALL XII analysis. Leukemia. 2008;22(2):308–12.
22. Arico M, Boccalatte MFP, Silvestri D, Barisone E, Messina C, Chiesa R, et al. Osteonecrosis: an emerging complication of intensive chemotherapy for childhood acute lymphoblastic leukemia. Haematologica. 2003;88(7):747–53.
23. Milner PF, Kraus AP, Sebes JI, Sleeper LA, Dukes KA, Embury SH, et al. Osteonecrosis of the humeral head in sickle cell disease. Clin Orthop Relat Res. 1993;289:136–43.
24. Milner PF, Kraus AP, Sebes JI, Sleeper LA, Dukes KA, Embury SH, et al. Sickle cell disease as a cause of osteonecrosis of the femoral head. N Engl J Med. 1991;325(21):1476–81.
25. Morse CG, Mican JM, Jones EC, Joe GO, Rick ME, Formentini E, et al. The incidence and natural history of osteonecrosis in HIV-infected adults. Clin Infect Dis. 2007;44(5):739–48.
26. Ho Y, Shih TTF, Lin Y, Hsiao C, Chen M, Hsieh S, et al. Osteonecrosis in patients with human immunodeficiency virus type 1 infection in Taiwan. Jpn J Infect Dis. 2007;60(6):382–6.
27. Wong GK, Poon WS, Chiu KH. Steroid-induced avascular necrosis of the hip in neurosurgical patients: epidemiological study. ANZ J Surg. 2005;75(6):409–10.

Epidemiology of Osteonecrosis of the Femoral Head in South Korea

7

Joon Soon Kang and Kee Hyung Rhyu

7.1 Introduction

Osteonecrosis of the femoral head (ONFH) is known to be related to decreased blood supply to the femoral head [1–3]. This may be primary, or idiopathic, in which no clear etiological factor can be established or secondary to several known causative factors [4, 5]. Underlying causes of ONFH can include alcohol abuse, systemic steroid use, Caisson disease, Gaucher's disease, and sickle cell anemia [4, 5]. Regardless of etiology, the histological picture includes death of osteocytes and structural changes in the femoral head, leading to osteoarthritis of the hip [6]. However, apart from these few facts, we still do not understand the exact epidemiology, patho-mechanism, or natural history of the disease.

According to the various literature reports, ONFH accounts for up to 10 % of total hip arthroplasties (THAs) performed in the United States [7–9]. Although the exact number may differ, this pattern is similar in Japan [10, 11]. However, according to most reports from heavy burden hospitals, it is estimated that ONFH is involved in 50–70 % of THAs performed in Korea [12, 13]. Other than this estimate, there are hardly any truly national epidemiological data in the English language literature.

To our knowledge, only two countries have reported nationwide surveys: Japan and Korea [14, 15]. In Japan, the Research Committee on Idiopathic Avascular Necrosis of the Femoral Head was established in 1975. Since then, they have made five surveys. Because directly surveying all medical providers was not possible, they chose stratified random sampling as a sampling method. In their fourth survey, in 1994, they estimated the annual prevalence as 6,700–8,200 (95 % confidence intervals, CI) [14]. In the final survey in 2004, estimated cases increased to 10,100–12,800 (95 % CI) [16]. The Korean Hip Society constituted a research committee to investigate the national epidemiology of ONFH in Korea in 2006. The committee included six orthopedic surgeons, one senior researcher from the National Health Insurance Corporation, one medical statistician, and several researchers in public health matters. The main purposes of this committee were to (1) investigate the annual prevalence of ONFH, (2) examine the influence of causative factors, and (3) provide baseline data for the further establishment of a national registry.

J.S. Kang (✉)
Department of Orthopaedic Surgery, Inha University Hospital, Incheon, Korea
e-mail: kangjoon@inha.ac.kr

K.H. Rhyu
Department of Orthopaedic Surgery, Kyung Hee University Hospital at Gangdong, Seoul, Korea
e-mail: khrhyu@empas.com

7.2 Study of Annual Prevalence in Korea

The Korean government has been operating a public health insurance system since 1989. The National Health Insurance (for people who have regular income) and the National Medical Aid System (for those who need financial support) cover every medical issue for all people registered in Korea [17]. Reimbursement data from the National Health Insurance Corporation is kept and checked for its adequacy by the Health Insurance Review and Assessment Service. Because of these systems, we can obtain all legitimate diagnostic data for the entire country. The only possible problem involves the accuracy of the initial diagnosis. A false diagnosis can occur for various reasons other than a lack of medical or scientific knowledge on the part of the physicians. One known cause is the system for registering a diagnosis. Reimbursement under the Korean National Health Insurance scheme is based on the initial diagnosis. That is, once the initial diagnosis is ONFH, the diagnosis for reimbursement of all medical claims during a given period is ONFH unless the surgeon changes the diagnosis. Suppose the surgeon tentatively enters the diagnosis as ONFH because it *is* the most common hip disease in Korea. If they later realize that the diagnosis was not correct after subsequent examinations, most of them would prefer to add a new diagnosis, or to do

K.-H. Koo et al. (eds.), *Osteonecrosis*,
DOI 10.1007/978-3-642-35767-1_7, © Springer-Verlag Berlin Heidelberg 2014

nothing, rather than delete or correct the initial (incorrect) diagnosis. Because we were aware of this problem, we aimed to perform a direct investigation of medical records and radiographs to clarify diagnostic accuracy. Detailed methods for the entire survey were described in our previous report [15].

7.2.1 Gathering of Diagnostic Data

As a first step, we reviewed medical claims and population data from the Health Insurance Review and Assessment Service from 2002 to 2006. We identified cases that contained ONFH for any reason as a principal diagnosis (M8705, M8715, M8725, M8735, M8785, M8795, M9035, M9045, and M9055 in the ICD-10 list).

The term "a medical claim" was defined as an individual (not a reimbursement issue) who was examined or treated under the diagnosis of ONFH in a given year. Thus, bilateral disease or more than one issue per each individual in a given year was counted as one medical claim. An individual who received services under the same diagnosis during different years was counted as a claim for each year.

Because we expected that there might be some inaccurate diagnoses, we established validation data by randomly sampling the cases. For these samples, actual medical records were reviewed and a true diagnosis of ONFH was confirmed. We used a simple random sampling scheme, instead of the stratified or cluster sampling used in the Japanese survey. The sample was selected from all study years. Data included age, gender, region, type of institute, and number of requests. As a result, 382 patients were randomly selected from 25 different cities or districts in Korea. The sample size was designed to estimate a population proportion with a 5 % margin of error at 95 % confidence level under the most conservative assumption for a true population proportion of $p=0.50$ [18].

7.2.2 Investigating Diagnostic Accuracy

For the direct investigation, we divided Korea into five areas by geography. At least one hip specialist on the committee took responsibility for reviewing the records and images issued in each area. They visited the corresponding hospitals and conducted direct reviews. A structured sheet with three major categories (in addition to the basic demographic data) of information was used for the review. In each category of the questionnaire, a multiple-choice form with check boxes was provided for recording each patient's entire history. The first part consisted of the diagnostic criteria or the definition of a true diagnosis (Table 7.1). At least one (except scintigraphy alone) of the given criteria was required to confirm the diagnosis. If none of the criteria were satisfied, the dataset was classified as incomplete and the diagnosis was considered to be false. The next category contained the past history of the patient. This included any history of exposure to known predisposing factors. The last one focused on the history of treatment. We tried to include every possible treatment method in the time period. We categorized the modalities, including nonoperative treatments, decompression procedures, bone graft procedures, osteotomy, hemiarthroplasty, THA, resurfacing arthroplasty, and cell therapy.

Table 7.1 The criteria to confirm the diagnosis of ONFH in this study

Tools	Findings
Plain radiograph	(a) Ill-defined mottling/mixed sclerosis of the trabeculae
	(b) Geographic and/or band-like sclerosis with or without (c, d, e)
	(c) Crescent sign with (a) or (b)
	(d) Microfracture with (a) or (b)
	(e) Femoral head collapse with or without arthritis
MRI	(a) Geographic region of decreased marrow signal within normal fatty marrow
	(b) Surrounding dense low-intensity line in all views
	(c) White inner line (or double-line sign) in T2-weighted images
Scintigraphy[a]	Abnormal (cold spots and adjacent hot areas) uptake of the radioisotope
Pathology	Microscopically confirmed pathology

[a]Any one of these findings is required to diagnose as ONFH, except for the single (+) findings in scintigraphy, which is considered as additive sign

The confirmed status of diagnosis was used as a binary variable, and a multiple logistic regression was used to calculate the probability of the diagnostic accuracy. Factors considered to affect the accuracy were gender, age, type of medical service (clinic, hospital, general hospital, university hospital), region (Seoul, metropolitan, others), and hospitalization. After correcting the diagnostic accuracy, the estimated nationwide prevalence of ONFH is presented as total counts and per 100,000 persons for each year from 2002 to 2006. The total number of beneficiaries of the National Medical Aid and National Health Insurance programs in Korea was used as the annual population.

7.2.3 Descriptive Epidemiology

The numbers of medical claims of ONFH from 2002 to 2006 were 15,683, 20,746, 22,304, 27,204, and 31,432, respectively. Among the 382 validation samples, 273 (71.5 %) were men and 109 (28.5 %) were women. In total, 209 (54.7 %) patients were hospitalized, while 173 (45.3 %) were treated as outpatients. The number of correct diagnoses among the medical claims was 274 (71.7 %). Significantly lower diagnostic accuracies were found for female patients and nonhospitalized patients (Table 7.2). Overall, 60.3 % of the total claims during 5 years were predicted to be true after regression analysis. The estimated prevalences of true ONFH from 2002 to 2006 constantly increased as 9,870, 12,394, 13,329, 16,230, and 18,691, respectively (Table 7.3). The prevalence per 100,000 population increased during this time period, from 20.53 to 37.96. The average annual prevalence was estimated at 14,103, corresponding to 28.91 per 100,000 population (Table 7.3). The ratio differed from that reported in other studies [19–21]. A male predominance, with a ratio of 3.9:1, was found. Bilateral involvement was found to be relatively low (37.1 %) versus the generally accepted view (50–60 %).

7.2.4 Analysis of Risk factors and Treatment

The exact amount of alcohol or steroids needed to cause the disease has not been established. In our study, we defined "alcohol abuse" as the intake of more than 400 mL of pure alcohol per week for more than 10 years. "Steroid user" was defined as a daily dose of >30 mg/kg or a cumulative dose of >2,000 mg. These definitions were the same as those used in the Japanese survey [14].

Because a detailed history is usually taken after hospitalization for treatment, the analysis was made only for confirmed and hospitalized patients in the validation sample set. Among the 185 samples who meet the criteria, the most frequent risk factors were a history of alcohol abuse (32.4 %), a history of steroid use (14.6 %), and a history of hip fracture (1.6 %). Because we set the criteria conservatively, most of the prevalence of each causative factor was relatively low. However, the proportions themselves were comparable to those reported previously for Korea [22, 23]. Like the proportion of the diagnosis of this disease leading to THA, the prevalence of causative factors was quite different from those reported in other countries [21, 24, 25]. In the Japanese data, the most common risk factor was steroid use (51 % of all cases) [16]. In France, steroid use is also the leading cause and accounts for 30 % of all ONFH cases [25].

In terms of treatment methods, various modalities have been tried. Primary treatments for the 274 confirmed patients were THA (63.9 %), decompression (11.3 %), nonsurgical treatment (10.2 %), bone-grafting procedures (6.6 %), hemiarthroplasty (3.3 %), osteotomy (2.6 %), and other procedures (2.1 %). Other than THA, decompression was the most frequently chosen method in this population group. One interesting point is that nonsurgical treatment (just a regular follow-up) represented more than 10 % of cases. Another noticeable pattern was that of emerging new treatment modalities such as stem cell therapy and resurfacing arthroplasty.

Table 7.2 Factors affecting the diagnostic accuracy of ONFH

Variables		Odds ratio[a] (95 % confidence interval)
Gender	Male	1.00
	Female	0.40[a] (0.23–0.68)
Age (years)	<39	1.00
	40–59	1.36 (0.63–2.94)
	60+	0.83 (0.40–1.75)
Type of medical service	Clinic	1.00
	Hospital	1.04 (0.37–2.89)
	General hospital	0.88 (0.38–2.04)
	University hospital	0.77 (0.36–1.64)
Region	Seoul	1.00
	Metropolitan	1.84 (0.91–3.71)
	Others	0.78 (0.37–1.65)
Hospitalized	Outpatient	1.00
	Inpatient	7.06[a] (3.99–12.52)

[a]Statistically significant in 95 % confidence interval

7.3 Summary

The average estimated prevalence was 14,103 cases in a year, corresponding to 28.91 per 100,000 population. The ratio of male predominance was 3.9:1.

The prevalence increased annually. However, great care should be taken in assessing this result. Because the numbers of medical institutions and medical claims for MRI have also been increasing, we cannot tell from this result alone that the prevalence is truly increasing. An absolute male dominance

Table 7.3 Estimated nationwide prevalence of ONFH in Korea

	Men		Women		Total	
Year	Number	Per 100,000 men	Number	Per 100,000 women	Number	Per 100,000 population
2002	8.28 (8.11–8.46)	34.35 (33.61–35.10)	1.59 (1.51–1.67)	6.62 (6.30–6.95)	9.87 (9.68–10.07)	20.53 (20.13–20.94)
2003	9.88 (9.69–10.08)	40.49 (39.70–41.30)	2.52 (2.42–2.62)	10.41 (10.01–10.83)	12.39 (12.18–12.61)	25.52 (25.07–25.97)
2004	10.61 (10.41–10.82)	43.16 (42.34–43.99)	2.72 (2.62–2.82)	11.17 (10.75–11.60)	13.33 (13.10–13.56)	27.26 (26.80–27.73)
2005	12.83 (12.61–13.05)	51.92 (51.03–52.83)	3.40 (3.29–3.52)	13.91 (13.45–14.39)	16.23 (15.98–16.48)	33.02 (32.51–33.53)
2006	14.65 (14.41–14.89)	59.23 (58.27–60.20)	4.04 (3.92–4.17)	16.49 (15.99–17.01)	18.69 (18.43–18.96)	37.96 (37.42–38.51)

( ): Limits in 95 % confidence interval

was observed. In contrast to reports from other countries, alcohol abuse was the leading cause in Korea.

This study was initially planned to investigate the prevalence and demographics of ONFH in Korea. During its setup, we added analysis of causative factors and choices of primary treatment. Because we have entire "raw" data from the National Health Insurance Company, descriptive epidemiology can be conducted reliably and readily with a sufficient number of validated samples.

References

1. Jones Jr JP. Fat embolism, intravascular coagulation, and osteonecrosis. Clin Orthop Relat Res. 1993;292:294–308.
2. Matsuo K, Hirohata T, Sugioka Y, Ikeda M, Fukuda A. Influence of alcohol intake, cigarette smoking, and occupational status on idiopathic osteonecrosis of the femoral head. Clin Orthop Relat Res. 1988;234:115–23.
3. Matsui M, Saito S, Ohzono K, Sugano N, Saito M, Takaoka K, et al. Experimental steroid-induced osteonecrosis in adult rabbits with hypersensitivity vasculitis. Clin Orthop Relat Res. 1992;277:61–72.
4. Assouline-Dayan Y, Chang C, Greenspan A, Shoenfeld Y, Gershwin ME. Pathogenesis and natural history of osteonecrosis. Semin Arthritis Rheum. 2002;32(2):94–124.
5. Jones LC, Hungerford DS. The pathogenesis of osteonecrosis. Instr Course Lect. 2007;56:179–96.
6. Bullough PG. The morbid anatomy of subchondral osteonecrosis. In: Urbaniak JR, Jones JP, editors. Osteonecrosis – etiology, diagnosis, and treatment. Rosemont: American Academy of Orthopaedic Surgeons; 1997.
7. Coventry MB, Beckenbaugh RD, Nolan DR, Ilstrup DM. 2,012 total hip arthroplasties. A study of postoperative course and early complications. J Bone Joint Surg Am. 1974;56(2):273–84.
8. Mankin HJ. Nontraumatic necrosis of bone (osteonecrosis). N Engl J Med. 1992;326(22):1473–9.
9. Mont MA, Hungerford DS. Non-traumatic avascular necrosis of the femoral head. J Bone Joint Surg Am. 1995;77(3):459–74.
10. Akiyama H, Hoshino A, Iida H, Shindo H, Takakura Y, Miura H, et al. A pilot project for the Japan arthroplasty register. J Orthop Sci. 2012;17(4):358–69.
11. Fujita H, Katayama N, Iwase T, Otsuka H. Multi-center study of use of the Exeter stem in Japan: evaluation of 1000 primary THA. J Orthop Sci. 2012;17(4):370–6.
12. Yoo MC, Cho YJ, Ghanem E, Ramteke A, Kim KI. Deep vein thrombosis after total hip arthroplasty in Korean patients and D-dimer as a screening tool. Arch Orthop Trauma Surg. 2009;129(7):887–94.
13. Kang BJ, Lee YK, Kim HJ, Ha YC, Koo KH. Deep venous thrombosis and pulmonary embolism are uncommon in East Asian patients after total hip arthroplasty. Clin Orthop Relat Res. 2011;469(12):3423–8.
14. Hirota Y, Hotokebuchi T, Sugioka Y. Idiopathic osteonecrosis of the femoral head; nationwide epidemiologic studies in Japan. In: Urbaniak JR, Jones Jr JP, editors. Osteonecrosis-etiology, diagnosis and treatment. Rosemont: American Academy of Orthopaedic Surgeons; 1997. p. 51–8.
15. Kang JS, Park S, Song JH, Jung YY, Cho MR, Rhyu KH. Prevalence of osteonecrosis of the femoral head: a nationwide epidemiologic analysis in Korea. J Arthroplasty. 2009;24(8):1178–83.
16. Fukushima W, Fujioka M, Kubo T, Tamakoshi A, Nagai M, Hirota Y. Nationwide epidemiologic survey of idiopathic osteonecrosis of the femoral head. Clin Orthop Relat Res. 2010;468(10):2715–24.
17. Lee JY, Kim CY. 2006 National Health Insurance statistical yearbook. Beneficiaries of health insurance. Seoul: National Health Insurance Corporation, Health Insurance Review and Assessment Service; 2007. p. 5–35.
18. Cochran WG. Sampling techniques. 2nd ed. New York: Wiley; 1963.
19. Jacobs B. Epidemiology of traumatic and nontraumatic osteonecrosis. Clin Orthop Relat Res. 1978;130:51–67. Epub 1978/01/01.
20. Patterson RJ, Bickel WH, Dahlin DC. Idiopathic avascular necrosis of the head of the femur. A study of fifty-two cases. J Bone Joint Surg Am. 1964;46:267–82.
21. Boettcher WG, Bonfiglio M, Hamilton HH, Sheets RF, Smith K. Non-traumatic necrosis of the femoral head. I. Relation of altered hemostasis to etiology. J Bone Joint Surg Am. 1970;52(2):312–21.
22. Yoo MC, Kim BK, Kim KT, Kin KH. An epidemiologic study of osteonecrosis in femoral head. J Korean Orthop Assoc. 1986;21(5):781–90.
23. Chang JD, Lee SH, Oh SY, Wi YH, Lee JS. The risk factors associated with alcohol-induced osteonecrosis of the femoral head. J Korean Orthop Assoc. 2004;39(6):692–9.
24. Hirota Y, Hirohata T, Fukuda K, Mori M, Yanagawa H, Ohno Y, et al. Association of alcohol intake, cigarette smoking, and occupational status with the risk of idiopathic osteonecrosis of the femoral head. Am J Epidemiol. 1993;137(5):530–8.
25. Merle D'Aubigne R, Postel M, Mazabraud A, Massias P, Gueguen J, France P. Idiopathic necrosis of the femoral head in adults. J Bone Joint Surg Br. 1965;47(4):612–33.

Current Trends of Osteonecrosis of the Femoral Head in Taiwan and China

8

Fang-Tsai Lee, Tso-Chiang Ma, and Mel S. Lee

8.1 Background

Osteonecrosis of the femoral head (ONFH) is a disabling condition characterized by disruption of intravascular blood flow, direct cellular toxicity, and impaired mesenchymal cellular differentiation with subsequent bone death [1–3]. Collapse of the normal spherical head contour with progression to secondary arthritis occurs along a continuum of disease progression. There are an estimated 20,000–30,000 new cases of ONFH diagnosed annually in the USA, with the preponderance among young, active men between the ages of 20 and 50 years [4]. It is evident that ethnic differences in the index diagnosis for hip arthroplasty do exist. In a comparative study by Hoaglund, the incidence of ONFH as indication for THR in Japanese patients, an Asian population, was four times that of American Caucasian patients [5]. Therefore, because the population size of China, for example, is four and one-half times that of the USA, it is reasonable to conclude that there may be 360,000–540,000 new cases diagnosed in China annually. Osteoarthritis is the main indication for THRs performed in Caucasian populations [6], but ONFH is the main indication for hip arthroplasty in Asian populations. For instance, in Hong Kong, 45.6 % of THRs were performed under the diagnosis of ONFH [7], while only 3 % of THRs in the UK [8] and 10 % of THRs in the USA [9] are performed for ONFH. In addition, patients with ONFH are usually young men of working age; therefore, the socioeconomic impact of ONFH is great in Asian countries.

8.2 Risk Factors and Associated Conditions

Though there are many etiologies of ONFH, the major pathogenic parameters can be classified into two categories: arterial compromise and high intraosseous pressure. Arterial supply may be compromised by femoral neck fracture (FNF) or arterial thrombosis/embolism (e.g., HIV, lupus erythematosus, and hemoglobinopathies such as sickle cell disease) [10]. High intraosseous pressure resulting from steroid and ethanol abuse also obstructs blood flow when pressure in the femoral head exceeds the capillary pressure subsequent to increased marrow fat cellularity [11, 12]. Additional genetic and ethnic predispositions have also been observed [13, 14], although trauma and steroid/ethanol abuse account for more than 90 % of ONFH cases [15].

Lee et al. studied the natural history of ONFH in Taiwan by following precollapse lesions in the contralateral hip of 100 patients in whom total hip arthroplasties were performed for the advanced collapse side. Follow-up ranged from 6 to 202 months (mean, 31 months) [16]. The most common etiology was alcohol-induced (58 %) followed by idiopathic (27 %), steroid-induced (13 %), and radiation osteonecrosis (1 %). Overall, 78 % of the hips collapsed within 2 years, i.e., 83 % alcohol related, 78.6 % steroid induced, 100 % radiation, and 68.8 % idiopathic. Genetic studies of ONFH are less reported in the Chinese population. Liu et al. reported higher association of vascular endothelial growth factor −634G/C polymorphism in a cohort of 220 patients in China [17]. Chen and associates reported type II collagen (COL2A1) mutation in two Taiwanese pedigrees as the candidate gene for the development of ONFH [18]. However, controversies on the results of COL2A1 polymorphisms were reported. COL2A1 mutation can be found in familial

F.-T. Lee
Department of Orthopedics and Administration Center, Kuang-Tien General Hospital and Hung Kuang University, Taichung, Taiwan

T.-C. Ma
Department of Health Services Administration, China Medical University, Taichung, Taiwan

M.S. Lee (✉)
Department of Orthopaedic Surgery, Chia-Yi Chang Gung Memorial Hospital, College of Medicine, Chang Gung University, No. 5, Fu-Hsin Street, Kweishan, Taoyuan 333, Taiwan
e-mail: bone@doctor.com

K.-H. Koo et al. (eds.), *Osteonecrosis*,
DOI 10.1007/978-3-642-35767-1_8, © Springer-Verlag Berlin Heidelberg 2014

cases in Japan and Canada [19, 20] but cannot be found in a larger cohort with definite diagnosis in other countries [21].

In Taiwan and China, steroid may account for more than 10 % of the causes in ONFH. Around 58–80 % of the patients will develop ONFH after 3 years of steroid initiation [22, 23]. It was observed in SARS patients that the dosage summation of corticosteroids and the length of therapy were closely related to the ONFH development [23, 24]. Other conditions such as sickle cell disease, coagulation abnormalities, storage disorders, and marrow infiltrating diseases were less reported from Taiwan or China. However, liver cirrhotic patients in Taiwan had been reported to have higher risk for occurrence of ONFH than non-cirrhotic patients [25].

8.3 Current Practice

Several nonoperative treatment modalities were reported from Taiwan and China. Oral alendronate 70 mg per week for 24 weeks had been reported to successfully prevent femoral head collapse in 27 of the 29 hips with a minimal follow-up of 2 years in a randomized clinical trial [26]. Although the short-term results are promising, its use in the treatment of ONFH is not approved and covered by the health insurance policy. The use of alendronate in ONFH remains anecdote in clinical practice. Extracorporeal shock wave therapy was compared with alendronate or in combination with hyperbaric oxygen as a cocktail modality [27–29]. The authors found shock wave alone produced comparable results as compared with its combination of alendronate or hyperbaric oxygen in early ONFH. However, neither shock wave nor hyperbaric oxygen is approved or covered by insurance for ONFH.

Surgical treatments include femoral head-sparing or arthroplasty procedures. From the NHI databank at the Taiwan National Health Research Institutes between January 1997 and December 2004, a total of 25,337 cases of ONFH were identified. Among them, 8,424 (33.25 %) cases were treated by hemiarthroplasty (HA), 14,393 (56.81 %) cases were treated by THR, 1,420 (5.6 %) cases were treated by core decompression (CD), and 1,100 (4.34 %) were treated by other head-preservation surgeries. Those patients who received THR, HA, or CD (n=24,327) were further analyzed. The majority of ONFH patients were male (n=19,596, 80.85 %); accordingly, the gender ratio for this disease is about 4 to 1. More than half of the cases were between the fourth and fifth decades of life (n=12,760, 52.50 %), with the peak incidence in the fifth decade (41–50 years of age, 29.15 %). Among the surgeries, 42.64 % were performed in medical centers, 30.38 % in district hospitals, and 26.69 % in regional hospitals. ONFH accounts for 55 % of nontraumatic hip arthroplasty in Taiwan, and 90 % of ONFH cases were treated by hip arthroplasty. The median survival rates at 8 years were 98.14 % (95 % confidence interval (CI), 99.87, 94.71) and 97.95 % (95 % CI, 99.88, 94.94) for THR and HA, respectively (Table 8.1). The median survival rate at 8 years for the CD procedure was 70.77 % (95 % CI: 99.60, 52.52). The practice pattern with large number of HA performed for ONFH in Taiwan is very unique and different from the general consensus that HA is not recommended for ONFH. However, before 2004, THA was not allowed for early-collapse ONFH in the national health insurance reimbursement plan. Only HA could be performed in those early-collapse cases. The unique situation provides a chance to access the feasibility of using HA in early-collapse ONFH. Based on the NHI database and other reports, HA had non-inferior survival rate as compared with that of THA in a 3–9 years follow-up [30, 31]. A longer term of follow-up should be needed to determine the usefulness of HA in early-collapse ONFH.

Table 8.1 Kaplan-Meier survivorship and log-rank test for THR and/or HA in ONFH with failure defined by NHI registry parameters

Parameter	Available N	Median survival rate (%; range: 1–8 years)	P value
THR by gender			
Male	9,814	96.80 (99.03–93.80)	0.2050
Female	2,641	97.36 (98.65–94.43)	
THR by age			
<30	519	95.18 (98.84–92.68)	0.2841
30–50	6,422	95.97 (98.99–94.18)	
>50	5,525	96.05 (98.64–94.79)	
HA by gender			
Male	6,165	97.96 (99.69–94.29)	0.57
Female	1,266	97.64 (99.92–94.02)	
HA by age			
<30	474	96.20 (99.58–95.36)	0.1855
30–50	4,448	96.08 (98.83–94.72)	
>50	2,495	95.43 (98.60–94.11)	
THR vs. HA, n=19,873			
THR	12,466	98.14 (99.87–94.71)	0.071
HA	7,407	97.95 (99.88–94.94)	

Vascularized iliac grafting or vascularized fibular grafting was less performed as compared with the CD. Vascularized iliac grafting was reported to have 80 % successful clinical results and 70 % successful radiologic results in precollapse cases [32]. It was decreased to 24 % in segmental collapse cases [33]. Alternatively, other salvage procedures such as osteotomy, multiple drilling, or implantation of wire coils were reported in some small case series from Taiwan or China [34–38].

8.4 Summary

The true incidence of ONFH in Taiwan or China has not been reported in the literature. In Canada, ONFH has been reported to account for 11 % of the THR surgeries performed [39]. Other authors have estimated that 10,000–20,000 cases of ONHF are diagnosed in the USA each year and that this diagnosis accounts for between 5 and 18 % of the annual THR procedures [40]. In a smaller comparative study, the incidence of ONFH as the index diagnosis of THR in Japanese population was 4 times higher than that of Caucasian population [5]. Although there are no data on the actual incidence of hip disease in Han Chinese, one study in Hong Kong involving 647 cases of THR revealed that ONFH constituted 45.6 % of all cases of hip replacement procedures [7]. By using the NHI database in Taiwan, ONFH accounted for 55 % of nontraumatic hip arthroplasty procedures in Taiwan, which is close to that of Hong Kong. Genetic and ethnic predisposition to the development of ONFH may explain the disparity between Asian and Caucasian populations. Demographically, men account for 80 % of ONFH cases, and the peak age incidence falls in the fifth decade of life (41–50 years of age). With these demographic features, ONFH may cause great socioeconomic impact.

Based on the NHI database, the most commonly performed procedures were THR, HA, and CD, with the proportions 56.81, 33.25, and 5.6 %, respectively. Joint replacement other than femoral head salvage procedures was performed in more than 90 % of the cases. Some of the disparity may be the delay in diagnosis of early-stage ONFH or the overzealous use of HA in Taiwan. HA carries the risk of periprosthetic osteolysis by polyethylene wear and high incidence of groin pain [41]. HA is not recommended for ONFH as a general consensus in most countries. However, the NHI database and some reports from Taiwan suggested HA had an 8-year survivorships of 94.94 % that was not inferior to 94.71 % for THR [30, 31].

In conclusion, ONFH accounts for the majority of joint replacement cases in Taiwan and China. Although steroid and alcohol are commonly reported as the risk factors, genetic predilections might play an important role in the pathogenesis of ONFH. The awareness of ONFH and to encourage early diagnosis and treatment should be a task of the orthopedic surgeons and their affiliated medical professionals.

Acknowledgments We thank to the research staffs at the Center for Health Policy Research and Development, National Health Research Institutes, for their support in retrieving and cleaning data from the NHI database and to the staff at the Department of Health Services Administration, China Medical University, for data management.

References

1. Jones LC, Hungerford DS. Osteonecrosis: etiology, diagnosis, and treatment. Curr Opin Rheumatol. 2004;16:443–9.
2. Lieberman JR, Berry DJ, Mont MA, et al. Osteonecrosis of the hip: management in the 21st century. Instr Course Lect. 2003;52: 337–55.
3. Lavernia CJ, Sierra RJ, Grieco FR. Osteonecrosis of the femoral head. J Am Acad Orthop Surg. 1999;7:250–61.
4. Hungerford DS, Jones LC. Asymptomatic osteonecrosis: should it be treated? Clin Orthop Relat Res. 2004;429:124–30.
5. Hoaglund FT, Shiba R, Newberg AH, et al. Disease of the hip: a comparative study of Japanese Orientals and American white patients. J Bone Joint Surg. 1985;67-A(9):1376–83.
6. Merx H, Dreinhöfer K, Schräder P, et al. International variation in hip replacement rates. Ann Rheum Dis. 2003;62:222–6.
7. Chiu KY, Ng TP, Poon KC, et al. Primary total hip replacement in Hong Kong Chinese – A review of 647 hips. Hong Kong J Ortho Surg. 1998;1:114–9.
8. National joint registry for England and Wales, 4th annual report. 2006. www.njrcentre.org.uk. Accessed 26 Oct 2008.
9. Hungerford DS. Perspectives on osteonecrosis. Presented at Biennial Meeting of Johns Hopkins Medical/Surgical Association, Baltimore, 2 May 2003.
10. Mankin HJ. Nontraumatic necrosis of bone (osteonecrosis). N Engl J Med. 1992;326:1473–9.
11. Drescher W, Bunger MH, Weigert K, et al. Methylprednisolone enhances contraction of porcine femoral head epiphyseal arteries. Clin Orthop Relat Res. 2004;423:112–7.
12. Drescher W, Li H, Lundgaard A, et al. Endothelin-1-induced femoral head epiphyseal artery constriction is enhanced by long-term corticosteroid treatment. J Bone Joint Surg Am. 2006;88 Suppl 3:173–9.
13. Koo KH, Lee JS, Lee YJ, et al. Endothelial nitric oxide synthase gene polymorphisms in patients with nontraumatic femoral head osteonecrosis. J Orthop Res. 2006;24:1722–8.
14. Baldwin C, Nolan VG, Wyszynski DF, et al. Association of klotho, bone morphogenic protein 6, and annexin A2 polymorphisms with sickle cell osteonecrosis. Blood. 2005;106:372–5.
15. Schroer WC. Current concepts on the pathogenesis of osteonecrosis of the femoral head. Orthop Rev. 1994;23:487–97.
16. Lee MS, Chang YH, Chao EK, Shih CH. Conditions before collapse of the contralateral hip in osteonecrosis of the femoral head. Chang Gung Med J. 2002;25:228–37.
17. Liu B, Cao Y, Wang D, Yao G, Bi Z. Vascular endothelial growth factor -634G/C polymorphism associated with osteonecrosis of the femoral head in a Chinese population. Genet Test Mol Biomarkers. 2012;16(7):739–43.
18. Chen WM, Liu YF, Lin MW, Chen IC, Lin PY, Lin GL, Jou YS, Lin YT, Fann CSJ, Wu JY, Hsiao KJ, Tsai SF. Autosomal dominant avascular necrosis of femoral head in two Taiwanese pedigrees and linkage to chromosome 12q13. Am J Genet. 2004;75:310–7.
19. Miyamoto Y, Matsuda T, Kitoh H, Haga N, Ohashi H, Nishimura G, Ikegawa S. A recurrent mutation in type II collagen gene causes Legg-Calvé-Perthes disease in a Japanese family. Hum Genet. 2007;121:625–9.
20. Kannu P, Irving M, Aftimos S, Savarirayan R. Two Novel COL2A1 mutations associated with a Legg-Calvé-Perthes disease-like presentation. Clin Orthop. 2011;469:1785–90.
21. Kenet G, Ezra E, Wientroub S, Steinberg DM, Rosenberg N, Waldman D, Hayek S. Perthes' disease and search for genetic associations. Collagen mutations, Gaucher's disease, and thrombophilia. J Bone Joint Surg. 2008;90B:1507–11.
22. Zhao FC, Li ZR, Guo KJ. Clinical analysis of osteonecrosis of the femoral head induced by steroids. Orthop Surg. 2012;4(1): 28–34.
23. Lv H, de Vlas SJ, Liu W, Wang TB, Cao ZY, Li CP, Cao WC, Richardus JH. Avascular osteonecrosis after treatment of SARS: a 3-year longitudinal study. Trop Med Int Health. 2009;14 Suppl 1:79–84.
24. Li YM, Wang SX, Gao HS, Wang JG, Wei CS, Chen LM, Hui WL, Yuan SL, Jiao ZS, Yang Z, Su B. Factors of avascular necrosis of femoral head and osteoporosis in SARS patients' convalescence. Zhonghua Yi Xue Za Zhi. 2004;84(16):1348–53.

25. Hung TH, Hsieh YH, Tsai CC, Tseng CW, Tseng KC, Tsai CC. Is liver cirrhosis a risk factor for osteonecrosis of the femoral head in adults? A population-based 3-year follow-up study. Intern Med. 2011;50(21):2563–8.
26. Lai KA, Shen WJ, Yang CY, Shao CJ, Hsu JT, Lin RM. The use of alendronate to prevent early collapse of the femoral head in patients with nontraumatic osteonecrosis. A randomized clinical study. J Bone Joint Surg. 2005;87A(1):2155–9.
27. Wang CJ, Wang FS, Yang KD, Huang CC, Lee MS, Chan YS, Wang JW, Ko JY. Treatment of osteonecrosis of the hip: comparison of extracorporeal shockwave with shockwave and alendronate. Arch Orthop Trauma Surg. 2008;128:901–8.
28. Wang CJ, Ko JY, Chan YS, Lee MS, Chen JM, Wang FS, Yang KD, Huang CC. Extracorporeal shockwave for hip necrosis in systemic lupus erythematosus. Lupus. 2009;18:1082–6.
29. Hsu SL, Wang CJ, Lee MS, Chan YS, Huang CC, Yang KD. Cocktail therapy for femoral head necrosis of the hip. Arch Orthop Trauma Surg. 2010;130:23–9.
30. Chan YS, Shih CH. Bipolar versus total hip arthroplasty for hip osteonecrosis in the same patient. Clin Orthop. 2000;379:169.
31. Lee MS, Chen AC, Kuo CH, Senan V, Shih HN, Tai CL, Shih CH. The position of the bipolar cup reflects the direction of the hip contact force pivoting on it. J Arthroplasty. 2007;22(2):189–94.
32. Yen CY, Tu YK, Ma CH, Yu SW, Kao FC, Lee MS. Osteonecrosis of the femoral head: comparison of clinical results for vascularized iliac and fibular bone grafting. J Reconstr Microsurg. 2006;22:21–4.
33. Chen CC, Lin CL, Chen WC, Shih HN, Ueng SWN, Lee MS. Vascularized iliac bone-grafting for osteonecrosis with segmental collapse of the femoral head. J Bone Joint Surg Am. 2009;91:2390–4.
34. Lee MS, Hsieh PH, Chang YH, Chan YS, Agrawal S, Ueng SWN. Elevated intraosseous pressure in the intertrochanteric region is associated with poorer results in osteonecrosis of the femoral head treated by multiple drilling. J Bone Joint Surg Br. 2008;90: 852–7.
35. Chen WP, Tai CL, Shih CH, Leou MC, Lee MS. Selection of fixation devices in proximal femur rotational osteotomy: clinical complications and finite element analysis. Clin Biomech. 2004;19: 255–62.
36. Lee MS, Tai CL, Senan V, Shih CH, Lo SW, Chen WP. The effect of necrotic lesion size and rotational degree on the stress reduction in transtrochanteric rotational osteotomy for femoral head osteonecrosis – a three-dimensional finite-element simulation. Clin Biomech. 2006;21:969–76.
37. Wang Y, Chai W, Wang ZG, Zhou YG, Zhang GQ, Chen JY. Superelastic cage implantation. A new technique for treating osteonecrosis of the femoral head with mid-term follow ups. J Arthoplast. 2009;24:1006–14.
38. Chang YH, Hu CC, Chen DW, Ueng SW, Shih CH, Lee MS. Local cancellous bone grafting for osteonecrosis of the femoral head. Surg Innov. 2009;16(1):63–7.
39. Canadian Institute for Health Information (CIHI). Canadian Joint Replacement Registry (CJRR) Bulletin: surgical and orthopaedic implant information for total hip and total knee replacement procedures performed in Canada. Bulletin, May 2001–2002. Toronto: CIHI; 2002.
40. Vail TP, Covington DB. The incidence of osteonecrosis. In: Urbaniak JR, Jones JP, editors. Osteonecrosis: aetiology, diagnosis, treatment. Rosemont: American Academy of Orthopaedic Surgeons; 1997. p. 43–9.
41. Schmalzried TP, Jasty M, Harris WH. Periprosthetic bone loss in THA: polyethylene wear debris and the concept of the effective joint space. J Bone Joint Surg. 1992;74-A:849–63.

Part IV

Etiology

9 Genetic Studies in Osteonecrosis of the Femoral Head

Shin-Yoon Kim and Tae-Ho Kim

9.1 Introduction

Osteonecrosis of the femoral head (ONFH) is a complex, polygenic, or multifactorial disease which is caused by a number of genetic factors of relatively smaller effects and environmental factors. Diverse conditions have been implicated in the development of ONFH. There are several well-accepted common associations: corticosteroids use [1], alcohol abuse [2], systemic lupus erythematosus [3], Legg-Calvé-Perthes disease [4], sickle cell disease [5], radiation [6], cytotoxic agents [7], Gaucher disease [8], dysbarism [9], HIV [10], hyperlipidemia [11], pancreatitis [12], and gout [13]. Idiopathic ONFH defines only when there are no identifiable factors identified.

The etiology of ONFH involves (1) vascular insult by trauma such as femoral neck fracture or hip dislocation, (2) intravascular coagulation, and (3) fat emboli by alcohol or corticosteroids. The pathogenesis involves vascular interruption by trauma, thrombotic occlusion by intravascular coagulation, and extravascular compression by fat emboli. Steroids enhance adipogenesis and hinder osteogenesis as well as angiogenesis by marrow stem cells [14]. Alcohol stimulates adipogenesis and inhibits osteogenesis by marrow stromal cells [15]. The pathophysiology involves decreased blood flow and ischemia by the above pathogenesis. Ischemia leading to death of osteocytes followed by repairing process, subsequent structural changes, and progressive collapse of the femoral head followed by degenerative arthritis of the hip joint (Fig. 9.1). In this chapter, we are going to review the genetic studies performed by a few technology in literatures and introduce future genetic studies by recent developed techniques to identify more gene variants associated with ONFH. These findings will help the early diagnosis and appropriate therapeutics of ONFH also.

S.-Y. Kim (✉)
Department of Orthopedic Surgery, Musculoskeletal Genome Research Center, School of Medicine, Kyungpook National University, 130 Dongdeok-ro, Jung-gu, Daegu 700-721, South Korea
e-mail: syukim@knu.ac.kr

T.-H. Kim
Skeletal diseases Genome Research Center, Kyungpook National University Hospital, 130 Dongdeok-ro, Jung-gu, Daegu 700-721, South Korea
e-mail: kim.taeho@me.com

9.2 Methods of Genetic Study

Various genetic studies had been developed and changed rapidly to identify disease-associated loci or to identify causal variation for specific disease. Single nucleotide polymorphisms (SNPs) are the most common form of DNA sequence variations. They can be very useful markers to map genes that modify the susceptibility of specific disease or those related drug responsiveness or side effect. Discovery of large numbers of SNPs is necessary to narrow down the genetic loci of specific disease susceptibility to small region of one gene by linkage disequilibrium mapping. Over the last few decades, genetic studies performing linkage analysis by positional cloning have identified about 3,000 genes as being inherited causing diseases. Linkage analysis which requires family pedigree is good for initial detection and, especially, is powerful for rare variants. To the contrary, candidate gene approach for association analysis was done to identify less than 1,000 SNPs using genotyping technology between a few hundred disease cases and controls under the concept of common variants implicated as common diseases. It is good for fine mapping, but poor for initial detection, and powerful for common variants.

Human genome project (HGP) identified 3,000,000,000 base pair DNA sequence. The reference sequence of genome constructed by the HGP is very informative about the vast majority of bases that are invariant across individuals.

K.-H. Koo et al. (eds.), *Osteonecrosis*,
DOI 10.1007/978-3-642-35767-1_9, © Springer-Verlag Berlin Heidelberg 2014

Fig. 9.1 Common pathway of developing osteonecrosis of the femoral head

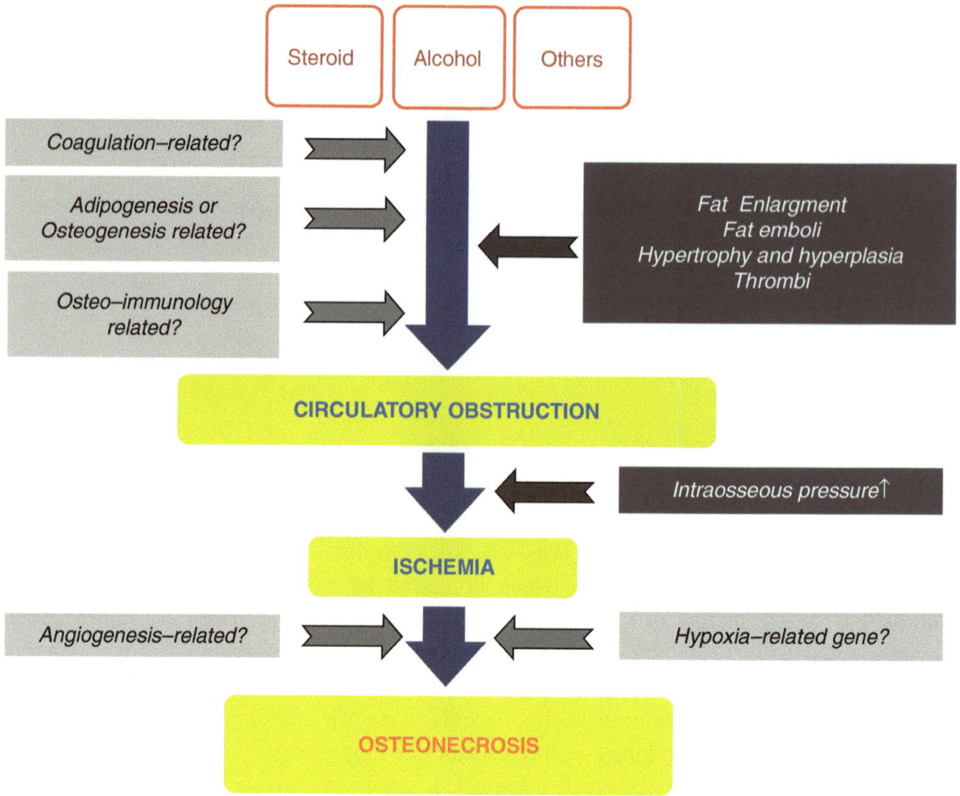

Subsequently, HapMap focusing on DNA sequence differences among individuals could inform substantial correlations of SNPs with many of their neighbors by recombination of linkage disequilibrium and low haplotype diversity. After international HapMap projects (Phase 1), genome-wide association study (GWAS) was used extensively through the world. GWAS enabled high-throughput genotyping more than 500,000 SNPs to identify disease-associated loci and rarely to identify causal variation of disease. It consisted of phenotyping (recruitment of thousands of cases and controls), genotyping of SNPs of individuals, and mapping to determine linkage disequilibrium block by statistical analysis. GWAS mapped a huge number of susceptibility genes for common diseases. However, because the proportion of heritability explained by GWAS was relatively low for common diseases, it had many false positives, and genetic markers applied in GWAS are common variants with minor allele frequency (MAF) greater than 5 % and odds ratio of phenotype less than 1.5. Genome-wide association meta-analysis (GWA MA) imputed 1.5–3 million genotyped SNPs. Next-generation sequencing (NGS) such as targeted resequencing for disease loci, whole-exome sequencing (WES) selective capturing and sequencing of all annotated protein-coding genes of whole exons, and whole-genome sequencing are expected to find to identify low-frequency (0.5 % < MAF <5 %) or rare (MAF <0.5 %) variants and high odds ratio for phenotype of disease in the near future(Table 9.1).

Table 9.1 Development of method in genomic research

Year	Method	Technology	Main purpose
–	Linkage analysis	Positional cloning	Identification of rare variation for disease
2005	Candidate gene approach for association analysis	Genotyping (1–1,000 SNPs)	Identification of disease-associated loci Identification of causal variation for disease
2007	GWAS[a]	High-throughput genotyping (>500 K SNPs)	Identification of disease-associated loci
2011	GWA MA[b]	Imputation/ meta-analysis (>1.5–3 M imputed/ genotyped SNPs)	Identification of causal variation for disease(rarely)
2011	Targeted resequencing for disease loci	NGS[d]	Identification of causal variation for disease
2012	Exome sequencing		
Future	WGS[c]		

[a]*GWAS* genome-wide association study
[b]*GWA MA* genome-wide association meta-analysis
[c]*WGS* whole-genome sequencing
[d]*NGS* next-generation sequencing

9.3 Genetic Studies in Osteonecrosis of the Femoral Head

The cause of ONFH is multifactorial. Both genetic predisposition and exposure to certain environmental factors are associated. The incidence or prevalence of idiopathic ONFH reflects ethnic differences [16]. Some patients who have taken high dose of corticosteroids or excessive alcohol intake for long period develop ONFH, but rare cases of ONFH occur after short corticosteroid treatment indicating the presence of differences in susceptibility to risk factors as well as genetic predisposition to ONFH between individuals [17, 18]. Particularly, idiopathic ONFH in identical twins or a clustering of cases in families implicates involvement of genetic factors [19, 20].

9.3.1 Hypercoagulopathy and Genetic Alteration

Increased intravascular coagulation, hypercoagulability, seems to be associated with the development of ON [11]. The role of sickle cell disease and other hemoglobinopathies in the development of ONFH had been documented as undergoing the pathway of intravascular coagulation.

There were two studies using pedigrees linkage analysis followed by positional cloning on familial autosomal-dominant ONFH in Taiwanese. Chen et al. mapped the presence of mutations in the protein C, protein S, and PAI-1 protein to the 2q14-q14, 3q11.1-q11.2, and 7q21.3-q22 chromosomal segments, respectively. Liu et al. showed that the mutation in COL2A2 (mapped on chromosome 12q13) is associated with the genetic cause of ONFH. COL2A2 mutation, a major structural protein in the extracellular matrix of cartilage, was identified in three families with idiopathic ONFH showing autosomal-dominant inheritance [21].

Thrombophilia due to protein C and protein S deficiency was reported to have an association with ONFH. Pierre-Jacques et al. reported a familial heterozygous protein S deficiency in a patient with multifocal ON [22].

Factor V Leiden (G1691A, Arg506Gln) through generation of coagulation factor V results in a hypercogulable state. Homozygosity in the mutation is associated with much higher increase in the lifetime risk of venous thrombosis than heterozygosity in the mutation(100-fold versus 7-8 fold) [23].

Mutations in the factor V Leiden (FVL; G1691A) were significantly more common in patients with idiopathic ON than in a healthy population. Glueck et al. compared the prevalence of heterozygote for the FVL mutation between 244 ON patients (161 idiopathic and 83 secondary ON) and 104 controls [24]. Twenty-three of 244 patients with ON (9.4 %) had heterozygote for FVL, whereas 2 of 104 (1.9 %) controls had heterozygote for it. Fifteen of 161 patients with idiopathic ON (9.3 %) and 8 of 83 (9.6 %) patients with secondary ON had heterozygote for FVL. In contrast with this study, our study comparing the incidence of heterozygote in Korean population (423 patients with ON versus 348 controls), however, could not find significant difference (unpublished data). Therefore, the prevalence of the FVL mutation seems to be different in ethnic groups.

The substitution of G for A at nucleotide position 20210 in prothrombin gene (PTG) which results in increased plasma prothrombin levels has been reported to be associated with increased risk of thrombosis [25]. Almost all of studies reported negative association between G20210A and primary ON [26–30], only one reported the presence of G20210A associated with ON of knee with an OR of 3.6 compared with control subjects [31].

Plasminogen-activating inhibitor-1 (PAI-1) is a critical factor that regulates coagulation and fibrinolytic systems. Homozygosity or heterozygosity for 4G allele (4G/4G) has been reported to increase the levels of PAI-I levels, and this leads to reduced plasma fibrinolytic activity [29, 32]. PAI-1 gene is reported to be polymorphic, especially in rs1799889 (−675 4G/5G SNP) of the promoter region. Homozygosity for the 4G allele (4G/4G) has been reported to significantly increase the plasma PAI-1. Recently, Kim et al. reported prevalence of rs1799889 (−675; 4G/5G) and rs2227631 (−844G/A) in the promoter, and +107009 C/T in the 3′UTR (rs11178) SNP of PAI-1was significantly high in 206 patients with ONFH than that of 251 controls [33]. PAI-1 4G/5G polymorphism, particularly 4G allele, may be a risk factor for ON [29, 30, 33].

The 5,10-methylenetetrahydrofolate reductase (MTHFR) is the metabolic enzyme involved in the conversion of homocysteine to methionine via the remethylation pathway. Reduced levels of MTHFR activity lead to elevated plasma concentrations of homocysteine, a condition referred to as hyperhomocysteinemia. Hyperhomocysteinemia has also been identified as an independent risk factor for thrombotic events and ON [30]. Several case-control studies have examined the association between the C677T polymorphism in MTHFR and ONFH. However, reports concerning the role of this polymorphism in the pathogenesis ONFH have been inconsistent [29, 34, 35]. The association between the MTHFR C677T gene polymorphism and the development of ON was reported in a small number of Caucasian people [29, 34, 35]; we could not find any association between the MTHFR C677T gene polymorphism and the development of ON in 443 Korean patients with ONFH and 273 controls [35]. Recent meta-analysis with eight study samples reported that there was an association between MTHFR C677T polymorphism and ONFH in non-Asian population, but not for Asian population, although study samples were not considered etiology [36].

Tissue factor pathway inhibitor (TFPI) is an important regulator of blood coagulation pathway, and mutations of TFPI genes can increase the risk of thrombin generation and venous thrombosis. The haplotypes of AAAT and GAAT of TFPI were associated with the risk of ONFH in 474 Korean population with ONFH compared with 349 normal controls [37].

9.3.2 Genetic Risk Factors for Glucocorticoid-Induced Osteonecrosis

The high-dose corticosteroid use (~2 g of prednisone within 2–3 months) is the most common risk factor accounting for almost 10–30 % of ON cases [1, 38, 39]. However, only 8–10 % of patients exposed to corticosteroid therapy may develop ON [1]. Since not all patients who are treated with steroids develop ONFH, the presence of additional risk factors or individual variation of sensitivity for glucocorticoids has been suggested. However, no definite risk factor has been confirmed to date [40]. Genetic studies in subgroups of patients with steroid-induced ON first focused on coagulation, fibrinolytic factors, and homocysteine metabolism. Some authors reported a positive association of PAI and MTHFR [30] or factor V Leiden [31] polymorphisms with steroid-induced ON, but these studies included a relatively small number of patients. Moreover, results in these studies were not replicated in other studies [27, 34].

The 3435TT genotype and homozygosity in the mutant 2677T/A variants in the multidrug resistance gene 1(ABCB1; MDR1) had a protective effect against the development of ONFH after renal transplantation. These two polymorphisms were found to be in linkage dis-equilibrium [41]. The ABCB1 polymorphism was associated with ONFH in patients with SLE in Chinese people [42]. The 3435TT genotype individuals had increased pump activity of P-gp which might prevent the accumulation of steroids in bone cells. These results suggested genes related to steroid metabolism might influence sensitivity for steroid in patients with ONFH. However, polymorphisms in the CYP3A4, CYP2D6, and CYP2C19 isoforms and the CYP3A4 promoter region of cytochrome P450, participating in the drug metabolism of steroid, had not been associated with the increased risk of ON [43].

The development of ONFH increases in renal transplanted patients treated with glucocorticoids [43, 44]. Ferrari et al. reported a positive association of PAI 4G/4G genotype with ON [32]. However, other studies have not replicated this result [44, 45].

Recent meta-analysis showed there was no evidence for significant association between MTFHR C677T and ABCB1 G2677/A polymorphisms and risk of steroid-induced ON. However, the PAI-1 4G/5G and ABCB1 C3435T may be risk factors for steroid-induced ON.

9.3.3 Genetic Risk Factors for Alcohol-Induced Osteonecrosis

Liver alcohol dehydrogenase (ADH) and aldehyde dehydrogenase (ALDH) converts ethanol to acetic acid. Acetaldehyde quickly forms free radicals which are highly toxic to the kidney and liver. The liver ADH, ALDH, and cytochrome P4502E1 are polymorphic at the ADH2, ADH3, ALDH2 loci, and the 5′-flank region of the P4502E1. Individuals with ADH2 2/2 genotypes were reported to have faster rates of alcohol metabolism. The ADH2*1 allele was lower in the ONFH patients than in the cirrhosis subgroup [46].

9.3.4 Other Genetic Abnormalities

In recent years, we have focused on new candidate genes participating in hypoxia, angiogenesis, adipogenesis, and osteogenesis for genetic association with ONFH.

A vascular hypothesis is considered to be the most persuasive in explaining pathogenesis of ONFH. It assumes that if thrombosis occurs, it is followed by a sequential process of blood flow obstruction, increased venous pressure, impaired arterial flow, osseous hypoxia, and bone death [27, 31], which appear to be important in ONFH development; hypoxia-inducible factor 1 (HIF1) [47], vascular endothelial growth factor (VEGF) [40, 48], annexin 6 [49], and catalase (CAT) [50] showed significant and meaningful association with risk of ONFH.

Hypoxia can induce both apoptosis as well as necrosis of cells and is associated with vascular disease. HIF1 is a master transcription regulator induced by hypoxia and critically acts in a wide range of cellular regulation processes including glycolysis, apoptosis, erythropoiesis, and angiogenesis [51]. We firstly examined association between polymorphisms of HIF1-α and ONFH using 384 ONFH patients and 237 normal controls. Our study suggested that genetic variations in HIF1 alpha (−89A/T, −20T > C, +3033C/T, +14539A > T, +22348C > T, +244413T > C) were associated with the risk of ONFH in 443 Korean population with ONFH compared with 273 normal controls [47].

Oxidative stress is one of the factors inducing vascular injury and apoptosis. Alcohol promotes the generation of ROS resulting in oxidative stress. Steroid-induced ON in the rabbit demonstrated that administration of steroids promotes to the development of oxidative stress and oxidative injury in bone tissue soon thereafter [52]. A number of polymorphisms in the CAT have been described as being associated with several diseases, such as osteoporosis, hypertension, diabetes mellitus, Alzheimer's disease, and vitiligo. Six polymorphisms (−89A/T, −20T > C, +3033C/T, +14539A > T, +22348C > T) of CAT gene were associated with the risk of ONFH in 443 Korean population with ONFH compared with 273 normal controls [50]. These results suggest that oxidative stress may play an important role in the pathogenesis of ONFH.

Nitric oxide synthesized by eNOS has vasodilatory effects on vascular tone, inhibits platelet aggregation, and modulates smooth muscle proliferation [53]. Many studies have been carried out to determine the associations between genetic polymorphisms in the eNOS gene and vascular diseases, including coronary artery disease or myocardial infarction, hypertension, stroke, and renal diseases. A few studies have showed an association between eNOS polymorphisms and ONFH. Allele 4a of a VNTR polymorphism in intron 4 and T-786C polymorphism in the eNOS gene were associated with idiopathic ONFH [54, 55]. Furthermore, we also found that Asp258Asp (rs1549758) and Glu298Asp (rs1799983) polymorphisms of eNOS gene were significantly associated with the risk of ONFH in Korean SLE patients [56].

VEGF, a major inducer of angiogenesis, is important for bone formation processes, such as normal growth plate morphogenesis, including blood vessel invasion and cartilage remodeling [57], and it has also been implicated in bone repair [58]. During hypoxia, HIF binds to the hypoxia-responsive elements and the expression of *VEGF* can be induced. This leads to the stimulation of angiogenesis [59]. The *VEGF* gene was reported to be polymorphic, especially in the promoter region (−2578, −1154, etc.), the 5′-UTR (−634, −7), and the 3′-UTR (+936). Several studies have shown that polymorphisms within the 5′-UTR have led to differences in *VEGF* expression and that they could influence the etiology of a variety of pathological conditions such as diabetic retinopathy, prostate cancer, and breast cancer. Our study showed that the −634G > C polymorphism in the *VEGF* promoter was significantly associated with an increased susceptibility of ONFH in 317 Korean patients with ONFH compared with 497 normal controls. Lee et al. also found that −1154A/G in promoter was associated with 74 steroid-induced ONFH compared with 160 age- and gender-matched normal controls [40]. Additionally, Liu et al. reported the VEGF −634G/C polymorphism was associated with ONFH in 220 Chinese patients with ONFH compared with 220 normal controls [60]. Also, rs1485766 and rs3775203 SNPs of VEGF-C gene were associated with the risk of ONFH in 460 Korean patients with ONFH compared with 300 normal controls, especially in idiopathic and steroid-induced ON [61].

Annexins have been implicated in inhibition of coagulation and have been reported as major components of matrix vesicles. SNPs and haplotypes of annexin A2 were associated with sickle cell necrosis [5]. rs9324679, rs9324677, rs10037814, and rs11960458 SNPs of annexin A6 gene were associated with the risk of ONFH in 443 Korean population with ONFH compared with 273 normal controls [48].

Recently, Hirata et al. examined the differences of gene polymorphism frequencies of apolipoprotein B (ApoB) and apolipoprotein A1 (ApoA1), which are important proteins for lipid transport, as well as of lipid parameters, between ONFH cases and referent patients among those who were subjected to renal transplantation [62]. The results showed that a higher frequency of 7623TT or CT of the ApoB gene was observed in ONFH cases than in referent patients. Regarding lipid parameters, a higher value of ApoB/ApoA1 ratio was observed in cases. Miyanishi et al. also reported the relationship between ONFH and serum ApoB/ApoA1 ratio in a study of Japanese subjects [63].

Peroxisome proliferator-activated receptor-gamma (PPAR-γ) is predominantly expressed in adipose tissue. It regulates the lipid homeostasis and angiogenesis. −769 > G, +34C > G, and +82466c > T SNPs of PPAR-γ gene were associated with the risk of ONFH in 448 Korean population with ONFH compared with 336 normal controls [64].

SREBP-2 plays central role in the maintenance of lipid homeostasis through stimulating expression of genes associated with cholesterol biosynthetic pathway. rs2267439, rs2269567, rs1052717, and rs2267443 SNPs of SREBP-2 were significantly associated with the risk of ONFH in 443 Korean population with ONFH compared with 273 normal controls [65].

SREBP-1, sterol regulatory element-binding protein, activates genes regulating lipid biosynthesis. IVS7 + 117A > G SNPs of SREBP-1 genes were significantly associated with the risk of ONFH in 423 Korean population with ONFH compared with 348 normal controls, especially in male [15].

We investigate SNPs of other genes relating angiogenesis and hypoxia. rs1880669, rs2692695, and rs2718806 SNPs of transferring (TF) gene were significantly associated with the risk of ONFH in 460 Korean population with ONFH compared with 300 normal controls, especially in idiopathic ON. rs4309, rs4344, and rs4461142 SNPs of angiotensin-1-converting enzyme gene were associated with the risk of ONFH in 460 Korean population with ONFH compared with 300 normal controls, especially in steroid-induced ON. The most significant association with risk of ONFH was an SNP (rs2453839) of the insulin-like growth factor binding protein-3, especially in idiopathic and alcohol-induced ON. Two SNPs (rs6837735 and rs1870377) of kinase insert domain receptor and three SNPs (rs12573218, rs12358370, rs2269091) of neutrophilin 1 were associated with the reduction of ONFH risk [61].

Immunologic factors involving interleukins and cytokines might influence the development of ONFH [66]. Also autoimmune disorders including SLE, polymyalgia rheumatica, rheumatoid arthritis, and ulcerative colitis are related to the development of osteonecrosis. Kim et al. reported that three SNPs (rs4655686, rs1569922, and rs7539625) of IL-23

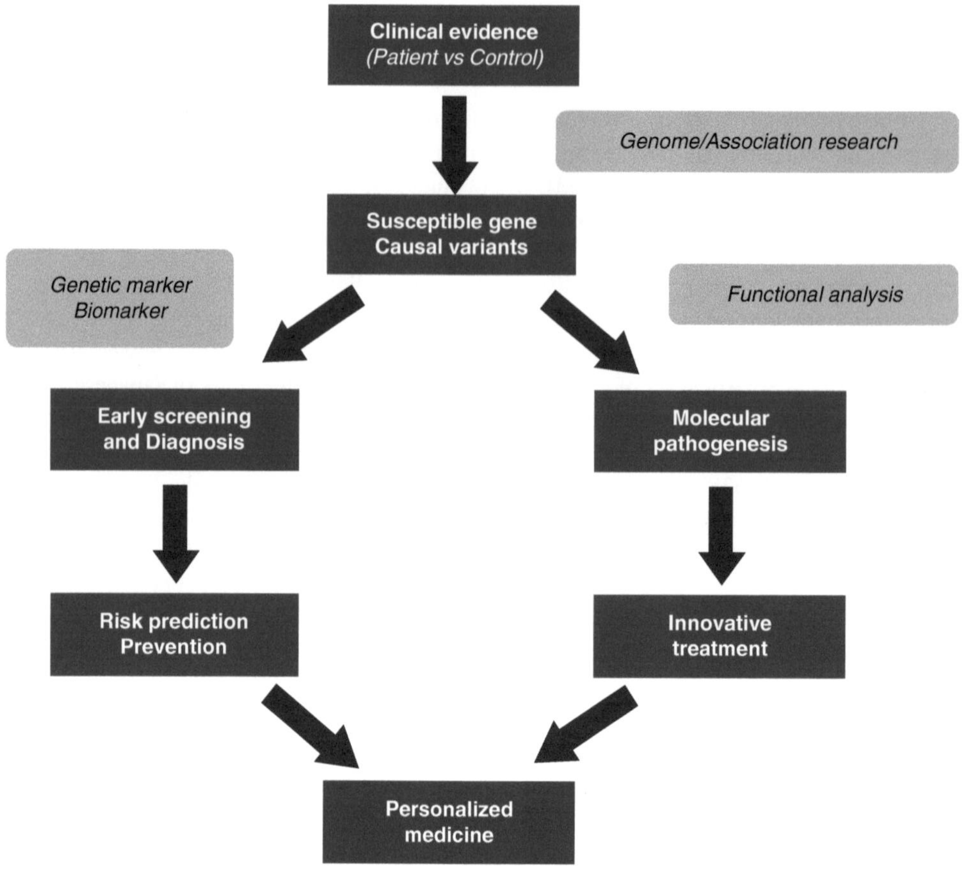

Fig. 9.2 Present and future application of genetic research for personalized medicine

receptor gene were significantly associated with the risk of ONFH in 443 Korean population with ONFH compared with 273 normal controls, especially idiopathic ON [67].

Samara et al. reported the CT and GA genotypes of the IL-1A (−889) and TNF-a genes were higher and the G to C polymorphism in the homozygous state in TGF-b codon 25 and GC genotype of IL-10 (−1082) gene were lower in 112 ON patients than 438 healthy donors [68].

In addition to mentioned above, many genetic association studies have been reported about ON in sickle cell disease patients, Legg-Calvé-Perthes disease, and malignancy such as acute leukemia or acute lymphoblastic lymphoma [69].

9.4 Future Genetic Study of ONFH

We are living in era of genome, and the recent advent of next-generation sequencing technologies has dramatically changed the nature of biomedical research. ONFH is believed to be a multifactorial disease associated in some cases with both genetic predilection and exposure to certain risk factors (environmental factors). The genetic studies about ONFH had been performed using linkage analysis on familial ONFH and candidate genes approach identifying the difference of SNPs between patients with ONFH and controls in limited numbers. The genetic susceptibility to ONFH probably involves many genes, most of which have very small effects. This fact represents the importance of the identification of large numbers of SNPs throughout the genome. Traditionally, the use of linkage analysis of families with extreme disease phenotypes has been successful in gene mutation discovery in ONFH. GWAS provides an important method for undertaking an evaluation of the association between common genetic variants and risk of disease. However, GWAS explained only a small fraction of the disease risk and showed problems of false-positive or false-negative [70]. As a result, a greater attention has been drawn to profiling rare variants. Advent of next-generation sequencing (NGS) such as targeted resequencing for disease loci, whole-exome sequencing (WES) selective capturing and sequencing of all annotated protein-coding genes of whole exons, and whole-genome sequencing are expected to find to identify low-frequency (0.5 % < MAF < 5 %) or rare (MAF < 0.5 %) variants and high odds ratio for phenotype of disease in the near future (Table 9.1). This approach would not be limited by the choice of candidate genes and cover the complete spectrum of coding and noncoding variants. Unlike GWASs, it would be able to test both rare and common variants for roles in ONFH.

Next, to study the genetic basis of disease, it is essential to determine the appropriate sample size and sampling design for well-designed study. Genetic associations can be real but nonetheless not reproducible if the underlying genetic effect is weak. As summarized in reported genetic associations with ONFH have become numerous but are mostly of small sample sizes. Even some association studies about same gene showed conflicting results. Increasing the size of the patient cohort will strengthen the power to discover variants. The lack of consistency across these studies may be the result of the geographic and ethnic variability of populations or the probability of a type II error resulting from small sample sizes.

Lastly, population stratification, which occurs when the cases and controls are unintentionally drawn from two or more ethnic groups or subgroups, also linked to false appearance of association [71]. Possible approach is to reevaluate the clinical diagnosis in the cohort by correlating subtle differences of clinical measurements and genetic variants in order to focus the analysis on a more clinically homogeneous set of patients as a separate cohort.

Furthermore, replication of findings in independent data sets is now widely regarded as a prerequisite for convincing evidence of association. Systematic reviews and meta-analyses have become a common approach to summarize gene-disease associations [72].

Therefore, genetic studies in the future should be performed in a cohort with more clinically homogeneous set of patients and normal controls and should be well designed. Global collaboration is essential to replicate the results across the ethnics. Next generation sequencing will provide tremendous genetic information about ONFH which can be applied to early diagnosis, prediction of the disease, reinvention of treatment practice, and the development of personalized medicine (Fig. 9.2).

References

1. Koo KH, Kim R, Kim YS, Ahn IO, Cho SH, Song HR, Park YS, Kim H, Wang GJ. Risk period for developing osteonecrosis of the femoral head in patients on steroid treatment. Clin Rheumatol. 2002;21(4):299–303.
2. Jones Jr JP. Alcoholism, hypercortisonism, fat embolism and osseous avascular necrosis. 1971. Clin Orthop Relat Res. 2001;393:4–12.
3. Mont MA, Glueck CJ, Pacheco IH, Wang P, Hungerford DS, Petri M. Risk factors for osteonecrosis in systemic lupus erythematosus. J Rheumatol. 1997;24(4):654–62.
4. Koo KH, Song HR, Ha YC, Kim JR, Kim SJ, Kim KI, Chang KC, Ahn IO, Cho SH. Role of thrombotic and fibrinolytic disorders in the etiology of Perthes' disease. Clin Orthop Relat Res. 2002;399:162–7.
5. Baldwin C, Nolan VG, Wyszynski DF, Ma QL, Sebastiani P, Embury SH, Bisbee A, Farrell J, Farrer L, Steinberg MH. Association of klotho, bone morphogenic protein 6, and annexin A2 polymorphisms with sickle cell osteonecrosis. Blood. 2005;106(1):372–5.
6. Morrish Jr RB, Chan E, Silverman Jr S, Meyer J, Fu KK, Greenspan D. Osteonecrosis in patients irradiated for head and neck carcinoma. Cancer. 1981;47(8):1980–3.
7. Hancock BW, Huck P, Ross B. Avascular necrosis of the femoral head in patients receiving intermittent cytotoxic and corticosteroid therapy for Hodgkin's disease. Postgraduate medical journal. 1978;54(634):545–6.
8. Amstutz HC. The hip in Gaucher's disease. Clin Orthop Relat Res. 1973;90:83–9.
9. Slichter SJ, Stegall P, Smith K, Huang TW, Harker LA. Dysbaric osteonecrosis: a consequence of intravascular bubble formation, endothelial damage, and platelet thrombosis. J Lab Clin Med. 1981;98(4):568–90.
10. Glesby MJ, Hoover DR, Vaamonde CM. Osteonecrosis in patients infected with human immunodeficiency virus: a case-control study. J Infect Dis. 2001;184(4):519–23.
11. Jones Jr JP. Fat embolism and osteonecrosis. Orthop Clin North Am. 1985;16(4):595–633.
12. Koseki H, Tsurumoto T, Osaki M, Shindo H. Multifocal osteonecrosis caused by traumatic pancreatitis in a child. A case report. J Bone Joint Surg Am. 2009;91(9):2229–31.
13. Hungerford DS, Lennox DW. The importance of increased intraosseous pressure in the development of osteonecrosis of the femoral head: implications for treatment. Orthop Clin North Am. 1985;16(4):635–54.
14. Kawai K, Tamaki A, Hirohata K. Steroid-induced accumulation of lipid in the osteocytes of the rabbit femoral head. A histochemical and electron microscopic study. J Bone Joint Surg Am. 1985;67(5):755–63.
15. Lee HJ, Choi SJ, Hong JM, Lee WK, Baek JI, Kim SY, Park EK, Kim SY, Kim TH, Kim UK. Association of a polymorphism in the intron 7 of the SREBF1 gene with osteonecrosis of the femoral head in Koreans. Ann Hum Genet. 2009;73(1):34–41.
16. Kim S-Y, Rubash HE. Avascular necrosis of the femoral head: the Korean experience. In: The adult hip. 2nd ed. Philadelphia: Lippincott Williams & Wilkins; 2006. p. 1078–86.
17. Orlic D, Jovanovic S, Anticevic D, Zecevic J. Frequency of idiopathic aseptic necrosis in medically treated alcoholics. Int Orthop. 1990;14(4):383–6.
18. Jones LC, Hungerford DS. The pathogenesis of osteonecrosis. Instr Course Lect. 2007;56:179–96.
19. Glueck CJ, Glueck HI, Welch M, Freiberg R, Tracy T, Hamer T, Stroop D. Familial idiopathic osteonecrosis mediated by familial hypofibrinolysis with high levels of plasminogen activator inhibitor. Thromb Haemost. 1994;71(2):195–8.
20. Nobillot R, Le Parc JM, Benoit J, Paolaggi JB. Idiopathic osteonecrosis of the hip in twins. Ann Rheum Dis. 1994;53(10):702.
21. Liu YF, Chen WM, Lin YF, Yang RC, Lin MW, Li LH, Chang YH, Jou YS, Lin PY, Su JS, Huang SF, Hsiao KJ, Fann CS, Hwang HW, Chen YT, Tsai SF. Type II collagen gene variants and inherited osteonecrosis of the femoral head. N Engl J Med. 2005;352(22):2294–301.
22. Pierre-Jacques H, Glueck CJ, Mont MA, Hungerford DS. Familial heterozygous protein-S deficiency in a patient who had multifocal osteonecrosis. A case report. J Bone Joint Surg Am. 1997;79(7):1079–84.
23. Koster T, Rosendaal FR, de Ronde H, Briet E, Vandenbroucke JP, Bertina RM. Venous thrombosis due to poor anticoagulant response to activated protein C: Leiden Thrombophilia Study. Lancet. 1993;342(8886–8887):1503–6.
24. Glueck CJ, Freiberg RA, Boriel G, Khan Z, Brar A, Padda J, Wang P. The role of the factor V Leiden mutation in osteonecrosis of the hip. Clin Appl Thromb Hemost. 2013;19(5):499–503.
25. Poort SR, Rosendaal FR, Reitsma PH, Bertina RM. A common genetic variation in the 3′-untranslated region of the prothrombin

gene is associated with elevated plasma prothrombin levels and an increase in venous thrombosis. Blood. 1996;88(10):3698–703.

26. Bjorkman A, Burtscher IM, Svensson PJ, Hillarp A, Besjakov J, Benoni G. Factor V Leiden and the prothrombin 20210A gene mutation and osteonecrosis of the knee. Arch Orthop Trauma Surg. 2005;125(1):51–5.
27. Bjorkman A, Svensson PJ, Hillarp A, Burtscher IM, Runow A, Benoni G. Factor V leiden and prothrombin gene mutation: risk factors for osteonecrosis of the femoral head in adults. Clin Orthop Relat Res. 2004;425:168–72.
28. Chang JD, Hur M, Lee SS, Yoo JH, Lee KM. Genetic background of nontraumatic osteonecrosis of the femoral head in the Korean population. Clin Orthop Relat Res. 2008;466(5):1041–6.
29. Glueck CJ, Fontaine RN, Gruppo R, Stroop D, Sieve-Smith L, Tracy T, Wang P. The plasminogen activator inhibitor-1 gene, hypofibrinolysis, and osteonecrosis. Clin Orthop Relat Res. 1999;366:133–46.
30. Glueck CJ, Freiberg RA, Fontaine RN, Tracy T, Wang P. Hypofibrinolysis, thrombophilia, osteonecrosis. Clin Orthop Relat Res. 2001;386:19–33.
31. Zalavras CG, Vartholomatos G, Dokou E, Malizos KN. Genetic background of osteonecrosis: associated with thrombophilic mutations? Clin Orthop Relat Res. 2004;422:251–5.
32. Ferrari P, Schroeder V, Anderson S, Kocovic L, Vogt B, Schiesser D, Marti HP, Ganz R, Frey FJ, Kohler HP. Association of plasminogen activator inhibitor-1 genotype with avascular osteonecrosis in steroid-treated renal allograft recipients. Transplantation. 2002;74(8): 1147–52.
33. Kim H, Cho C, Cho Y, Cho S, Yoon K, Kim K. Significant associations of PAI-1 genetic polymorphisms with osteonecrosis of the femoral head. BMC Musculoskelet Disord. 2011;12:160.
34. Zalavras CG, Malizos KN, Dokou E, Vartholomatos G. The 677C->T mutation of the methylene-tetrahydrofolate reductase gene in the pathogenesis of osteonecrosis of the femoral head. Haematologica. 2002;87(1):111–2.
35. Kim TH, Hong JM, Kim HJ, Park EK, Kim SY. Lack of association of MTHFR gene polymorphisms with the risk of osteonecrosis of the femoral head in a Korean population. Molecules and cells. 2010;29(4):343–8.
36. Shang X-f, Su H, Chang W-w, Wang C-c, Han Q, Xu Z-w. Association between MTHFR C677T polymorphism and osteonecrosis of the femoral head: a meta-analysis. Mol Biol Rep. 2012;39(6):7089–94.
37. Dai XL, Hong JM, Oh B, Cho YS, Lee JY, Park EK, Kim CY, Kim SY, Kim TH. Association analysis of tissue factor pathway inhibitor polymorphisms and haplotypes with osteonecrosis of the femoral head in the Korean population. Mol Cells. 2008;26(5):490–5.
38. Griffith JF, Antonio GE, Kumta SM, Hui DS, Wong JK, Joynt GM, Wu AK, Cheung AY, Chiu KH, Chan KM, Leung PC, Ahuja AT. Osteonecrosis of hip and knee in patients with severe acute respiratory syndrome treated with steroids. Radiology. 2005;235(1): 168–75.
39. Wang GJ, Cui Q, Balian G. The Nicolas Andry award. The pathogenesis and prevention of steroid-induced osteonecrosis. Clin Orthop Relat Res. 2000;370:295–310.
40. Lee YJ, Lee JS, Kang EH, Lee YK, Kim SY, Song YW, Koo KH. Vascular endothelial growth factor polymorphisms in patients with steroid-induced femoral head osteonecrosis. J Orthop Res. 2012;30(1):21–7.
41. Asano T, Takahashi KA, Fujioka M, Inoue S, Okamoto M, Sugioka N, Nishino H, Tanaka T, Hirota Y, Kubo T. ABCB1 C3435T and G2677T/A polymorphism decreased the risk for steroid-induced osteonecrosis of the femoral head after kidney transplantation. Pharmacogenetics. 2003;13(11):675–82.
42. Yang XY, Xu DH. MDR1(ABCB1) gene polymorphisms associated with steroid-induced osteonecrosis of femoral head in systemic lupus erythematosus. Pharmazie. 2007;62(12):930–2.
43. Asano T, Takahashi KA, Fujioka M, Inoue S, Satomi Y, Nishino H, Tanaka T, Hirota Y, Takaoka K, Nakajima S, Kubo T. Genetic analysis of steroid-induced osteonecrosis of the femoral head. J Orthop Sci. 2003;8(3):329–33.
44. Celik A, Tekis D, Saglam F, Tunali S, Kabakci N, Ozaksoy D, Manisali M, Ozcan MA, Meral M, Gulay H, Camsari T. Association of corticosteroids and factor V, prothrombin, and MTHFR gene mutations with avascular osteonecrosis in renal allograft recipients. Transplant Proc. 2006;38(2):512–6.
45. Asano T, Takahashi KA, Fujioka M, Inoue S, Ueshima K, Hirata T, Okamoto M, Satomi Y, Nishino H, Tanaka T, Hirota Y, Kubo T. Relationship between postrenal transplant osteonecrosis of the femoral head and gene polymorphisms related to the coagulation and fibrinolytic systems in Japanese subjects. Transplantation. 2004;77(2):220–5.
46. Chao YC, Wang SJ, Chu HC, Chang WK, Hsieh TY. Investigation of alcohol metabolizing enzyme genes in Chinese alcoholics with avascular necrosis of hip joint, pancreatitis and cirrhosis of the liver. Alcohol Alcohol. 2003;38(5):431–6.
47. Hong JM, Kim TH, Chae SC, Koo KH, Lee YJ, Park EK, Choi JY, Ryoo HM, Kim SY. Association study of hypoxia inducible factor 1alpha (HIF1alpha) with osteonecrosis of femoral head in a Korean population. Osteoarthritis Cartilage. 2007;15(6): 688–94.
48. Kim TH, Hong JM, Lee JY, Oh B, Park EK, Lee CK, Bae SC, Kim SY. Promoter polymorphisms of the vascular endothelial growth factor gene is associated with an osteonecrosis of the femoral head in the Korean population. Osteoarthritis Cartilage. 2008;16(3):287–91.
49. Kim TH, Hong JM, Shin ES, Kim HJ, Cho YS, Lee JY, Lee SH, Park EK, Kim SY. Polymorphisms in the Annexin gene family and the risk of osteonecrosis of the femoral head in the Korean population. Bone. 2009;45(1):125–31.
50. Kim TH, Hong JM, Oh B, Cho YS, Lee JY, Kim HL, Shin ES, Lee JE, Park EK, Kim SY. Genetic association study of polymorphisms in the catalase gene with the risk of osteonecrosis of the femoral head in the Korean population. Osteoarthritis Cartilage. 2008;16(9):1060–6.
51. Semenza GL. HIF-1 and human disease: one highly involved factor. Genes Dev. 2000;14(16):1983–91.
52. Ichiseki T, Kaneuji A, Katsuda S, Ueda Y, Sugimori T, Matsumoto T. DNA oxidation injury in bone early after steroid administration is involved in the pathogenesis of steroid-induced osteonecrosis. Rheumatology (Oxford). 2005;44(4):456–60.
53. Cooke JP, Dzau VJ. Nitric oxide synthase: role in the genesis of vascular disease. Annu Rev Med. 1997;48:489–509.
54. Koo KH, Lee JS, Lee YJ, Kim KJ, Yoo JJ, Kim HJ. Endothelial nitric oxide synthase gene polymorphisms in patients with nontraumatic femoral head osteonecrosis. J Orthop Res. 2006;24(8):1722–8.
55. Glueck CJ, Freiberg RA, Oghene J, Fontaine RN, Wang P. Association between the T-786C eNOS polymorphism and idiopathic osteonecrosis of the head of the femur. J Bone Joint Surg Am. 2007;89(11):2460–8.
56. Kim HS, Bae SC, Kim TH, Kim SY. Endothelial nitric oxide synthase gene polymorphisms and the risk of osteonecrosis of the femoral head in systemic lupus erthematosus. Int Orthop. 2013;37(11):2289–96.
57. Schipani E, Ryan HE, Didrickson S, Kobayashi T, Knight M, Johnson RS. Hypoxia in cartilage: HIF-1alpha is essential for chondrocyte growth arrest and survival. Genes Dev. 2001;15(21): 2865–76.
58. Komatsu DE, Hadjiargyrou M. Activation of the transcription factor HIF-1 and its target genes, VEGF, HO-1, iNOS, during fracture repair. Bone. 2004;34(4):680–8.
59. Treins C, Giorgetti-Peraldi S, Murdaca J, Van Obberghen E. Regulation of vascular endothelial growth factor expression by

advanced glycation end products. J Biol Chem. 2001;276(47):43836–41.
60. Liu B, Cao Y, Wang D, Yao G, Bi Z. Vascular endothelial growth factor -634G/C polymorphism associated with osteonecrosis of the femoral head in a Chinese population. Genet Test Mol Biomarkers. 2012;16(7):739–43.
61. Hong JM, Kim TH, Kim HJ, Park EK, Yang EK, Kim SY. Genetic association of angiogenesis- and hypoxia-related gene polymorphisms with osteonecrosis of the femoral head. Exp Mol Med. 2010;42(5):376–85.
62. Hirata T, Fujioka M, Takahashi KA, Arai Y, Asano T, Ishida M, Kuribayashi M, Akioka K, Okamoto M, Yoshimura N, Satomi Y, Nishino H, Fukushima W, Hirota Y, Nakajima S, Kato S, Kubo T. ApoB C7623T polymorphism predicts risk for steroid-induced osteonecrosis of the femoral head after renal transplantation. J Orthop Sci. 2007;12(3):199–206.
63. Miyanishi K, Yamamoto T, Irisa T, Noguchi Y, Sugioka Y, Iwamoto Y. Increased level of apolipoprotein B/apolipoprotein A1 ratio as a potential risk for osteonecrosis. Ann Rheum Dis. 1999;58(8):514–6.
64. Kim TH, Hong JM, Park EK, Kim SY. Peroxisome proliferator-activated receptor-gamma gene polymorphisms are not associated with osteonecrosis of the femoral head in the Korean population. Mol Cells. 2007;24(3):388–93.
65. Kim TH, Baek JI, Hong JM, Choi SJ, Lee HJ, Cho HJ, Park EK, Kim UK, Kim SY. Significant association of SREBP-2 genetic polymorphisms with avascular necrosis in the Korean population. BMC Med Genet. 2008;9:94.
66. Boss JH. Experimental models of osteonecrosis of the femoral head. J Orthop Sci. 2004;9(5):533–4.
67. Kim TH, Hong JM, Oh B, Cho YS, Lee JY, Kim HL, Lee JE, Ha MH, Park EK, Kim SY. Association of polymorphisms in the Interleukin 23 receptor gene with osteonecrosis of femoral head in Korean population. Exp Mol Med. 2008;40(4):418–26.
68. Samara S, Kollia P, Dailiana Z, Chassanidis C, Papatheodorou L, Koromila T, Malizos KN. Predictive role of cytokine gene polymorphisms for the development of femoral head osteonecrosis. Dis Markers. 2012;33(4):215–21.
69. Hadjigeorgiou G, Dardiotis E, Dardioti M, Karantanas A, Dimitroulias A, Malizos K. Genetic association studies in osteonecrosis of the femoral head: mini review of the literature. Skeletal Radiol. 2008;37(1):1–7.
70. Gibson G. Rare and common variants: twenty arguments. Nat Rev Genet. 2011;13(2):135–45.
71. Hirschhorn JN, Lohmueller K, Byrne E, Hirschhorn K. A comprehensive review of genetic association studies. Genet Med. 2002;4(2):45–61.
72. Ioannidis JP, Gwinn M, Little J, Higgins JP, Bernstein JL, Boffetta P, Bondy M, Bray MS, Brenchley PE, Buffler PA, Casas JP, Chokkalingam A, Danesh J, Smith GD, Dolan S, Duncan R, Gruis NA, Hartge P, Hashibe M, Hunter DJ, Jarvelin MR, Malmer B, Maraganore DM, Newton-Bishop JA, O'Brien TR, Petersen G, Riboli E, Salanti G, Seminara D, Smeeth L, Taioli E, Timpson N, Uitterlinden AG, Vineis P, Wareham N, Winn DM, Zimmern R, Khoury MJ. A road map for efficient and reliable human genome epidemiology. Nat Genet. 2006;38(1):3–5.

Osteonecrosis and Intravascular Coagulation Revisited

10

Lynne C. Jones and Deborah McK. Ciombor

10.1 Introduction

The primary pathophysiologic feature of advanced osteonecrosis is a zone of necrotic bone containing trabeculae with dead osteocytes associated with marrow necrosis and fibrosis [1]. This pathognomonic feature led to the use of the expression "avascular necrosis," although the international society for the study of the circulation to bone and its disorders, ARCO International (Association Internationale pour la Recherche sur la Circulation Osseuse), recommends using the term "osteonecrosis." There are several theories regarding the pathogenesis of osteonecrosis [ON], as discussed in several outstanding review articles [2–6]. These can be categorized as (1) extraosseous, (2) intraosseous, or (3) direct cellular. There are many other theories as well, such as intravascular or extravascular pathologies. John Paul Jones, Jr., suggested that multiple etiologies may lead to a final common pathway of intravascular coagulation. He hypothesized that intravascular coagulation is an "intermediary mechanism" in the development of ON [7]. The evidence that intravascular coagulation plays an integral role in the pathogenesis of ON is both direct and indirect and will be the focus of this chapter.

L.C. Jones (✉)
Department of Orthopaedic Surgery,
Center for Osteonecrosis Research and Education,
Center for Metabolism and Obesity Research,
Johns Hopkins University School of Medicine,
Baltimore, MD, USA

Johns Hopkins Orthopaedics,
601 N. Caroline St., JHOC 5255, Baltimore, MD 21287, USA
e-mail: ljones3@jhmi.edu

D.M. Ciombor
Department of Plastic Surgery, Lifespan Academic Medical Center,
The Warren Alpert Medical School of Brown,
239 Multiphasic Building, 593 Eddy St.,
Providence, RI 02903, USA

10.2 Clinical Laboratory Assessments

In 1970, Boettcher et al. reported the results of clinical and laboratory testing of 50 patients with nontraumatic osteonecrosis [8]. The patients underwent a battery of hematological and coagulation tests including ESR (erythrocyte sedimentation rate), platelet number, thrombin time, and prothrombin utilization. Direct evidence of a clotting abnormality was detected in 26 patients and indirect evidence in 48 patients. However, no specific test was "consistently abnormal." For example, for platelet counts, 16 patients were normal, 15 patients had low counts (thrombocytopenic), and 6 patients had elevated counts (thrombocythemia). The authors propose that any of the vascular abnormalities could "cause circulatory disturbance and infarction when anastomoses are insufficient to maintain viability of the head" [8]. Using the clot lysis test, Pósán et al. observed a significantly lower "speed of the lysis" for patients with either primary or secondary ON [9]. Using an assay for beta-thromboglobulin, they also noted significantly higher platelet activation in the ON patients compared to controls.

Thrombophilia (increased clots in blood vessels) and hypofibrinolysis (decreased ability to break down clots) have both been implicated as "causative factors" for osteonecrosis [5]. Several investigators have identified thrombi within the arterial and venous circulation of diseased femoral heads (Table 10.1). In their evaluation of human biopsy samples, Ficat and Arlet frequently observed sinusoidal distension, thickening of the arteriolar walls, and arteriolar thrombosis [1]. In three cases of osteonecrosis, Jones observed fibrin thrombi in the subchondral Haversian capillaries, arterioles, and marrow sinusoids [14]. He also noted microfocal marrow hemorrhages with extravasated erythrocytes. Jones suggested that the intravascular thrombosis of the intraosseous arterioles was initiated by lipid embolism and endothelial damage [7, 22]. Saito et al. also observed thrombosed intraosseous arterioles associated with damage to the

K.-H. Koo et al. (eds.), *Osteonecrosis*,
DOI 10.1007/978-3-642-35767-1_10, © Springer-Verlag Berlin Heidelberg 2014

Table 10.1 Evidence of clotting and thrombi in patients with osteonecrosis

Citation	Observation	Types of patients
Bonfiglio [10]	Thrombosed arteries	Dysbaric osteonecrosis
Ficat and Arlet [1]	Arteriolar thromboses	Etiology not noted
Spencer and Brookes [11]	Thrombus observed in multiple intraosseous vessels of *one* patient; associated with degenerative changes of the blood vessels within the femoral head	5 corticosteroid-treated (for 3 months to 4 years after transplant) transplant recipients
Saito et al. [12]	One figure of a Haversian vessel (arrow), showing damaged vascular wall and thrombosis in the lumen; fibrosis in the Haversian canal	Osteonecrosis (1° and 2°)
Asherson et al. [13]	Vasculitis and arterial thrombosis	Lupus patients
Jones [14]	Focal anemic infarctions associated with subchondral necrosis and adjacent extravasation of blood into fatty marrow	1. Kissing bug 2. Trauma 3. Alcohol-associated ON
Cheras et al. [15]	"Established" intraosseous thrombosis of the femoral head	Various etiologies
Egan and Munn [16]	Widespread infarction of the marrow elements and bony trabeculae; multiple thrombin thrombi in nasal septum	Antiphospholipid antibody syndrome (case report)
Starklint et al. [17]	(a) Vessels packed with erythrocytes and fibrin thrombi	(c) Osteonecrosis (1°and 2°); 14 femoral heads from 12 patients
Laroche et al. [18]	(b) Vascular thrombosis in femoral heads of 4 of 20 patients	(d) Osteonecrosis (1° and 2°)
Saito et al. [19, 20]	Thrombosed arterioles but fewer than in their animal models. Based on their observations, they have concluded that arteriopathy is "essential"	2° Osteonecrosis
Aaron [21]	Microcirculatory thrombus in the subchondral cancellous bone	2° ON

vascular wall [12]. Starklint and colleagues observed dilated veins and venules within the transitional zone between the necrotic lesion and the "normal" bone [17]. Using the Martius Scarlet Blue stain, tightly packed erythrocytes and fibrin thrombi were detected within these blood vessels, suggesting that the dilated vessels are a consequence of thrombi in other areas. There is, however, considerable debate as to the role of thrombi in the pathogenesis of ON and whether, if it exists at all, it is a primary or secondary event [23]. The lack of thrombi in some histological sections has been explained away by some as a result of the delay in the timing of histological sampling from the onset of disease and that thrombolysis had removed the implicating stimulus [14].

Many of the comorbidities associated with osteonecrosis are also associated with vascular pathologies (Table 10.2). For example, systemic lupus erythematosus (SLE) is associated with vasculitis, premature atherosclerosis, and hypercoagulability. The incidence of thrombosis in patients with SLE is 2 per 100 person-years of follow-up [39]. There are also several reports of intraosseous thrombi in ON cases associated with dysbarism [40], antiphospholipid antibody syndrome [41, 42], and Crohn's disease [43, 44]. It should be noted here that many of these conditions result in corticosteroid therapy. The association of corticosteroids to ON will be discussed thoroughly later in the chapter.

10.3 Coagulation Cascade and Regulation

Every basic physiology and hematology textbook describes the physiologic mechanisms involved in the formation and the resolution of blood clots [45, 46]. While it is not the intention of this chapter to provide a detailed description of the pathways involved (e.g., extrinsic vs. intrinsic pathways), it is important to understand the complexity of the coagulation factors involved in both coagulation and fibrinolysis.

Blood clots form via one of the two pathways based upon whether the inciting event is tissue factor (TF) pathway (extrinsic) or amplification by the formation of a primary complex of factors in contact with collagen in the endothelium of damaged vessel walls (intrinsic) [45]. While some of the factors involved in the cascades are the same (e.g., factor X), others are different [factor VII (extrinsic) vs. factor XII (intrinsic)] (Fig. 10.1). In both pathways, the final step is the conversion of prothrombin to thrombin by prothrombin activator in the presence of calcium ions. Thrombin converts fibrinogen to fibrin monomers, which, in turn, polymerize into long fibrin threads. The clot acts to entrap platelets, blood cells, and plasma [48]. A thrombus is established when a blood clot attaches and remains stationary along the wall of a blood vessel, impairing blood flow and, in some cases, totally obscuring lumen [48]. The downregulation of coagulation is effected by proteolytic inactivation of specific coagulation factors [49]. These factors include antithrombin III, protein C, protein S, and others.

As with the coagulation cascades, the fibrinolytic system is built upon a system of activators and inhibitors [50]. The induction of fibrinolysis is dependent on the formation of the active enzyme, proplasmin, a serine protease that degrades fibrin clots. Plasminogen is released as a zymogen and converted to plasmin by one of two activators: tissue plasminogen activator (tPA) and urokinase plasminogen activator (u-PA) – based upon whether fibrin is in the circulation or cell bound, respectively. Inhibitors of the fibrinolytic system

Table 10.2 Abnormal factor levels (serology)

	Patients	s-tPA-Fx	PAI-Fx	Lp(a)	RAPC	aCL	Protein C	Protein S	HCY	aPL	Factor VIII	Factor V Leiden	vWF	Apo B	Homocysteine	AT III (Ag and fct)	Beta-globulin	plasminogen	Anti-p53	crosslaps
Asherson et al. [13]	37 ON									X										
Björkman et al. [24, 25]	38 knee; 63 hip											x								
Cenni et al. [26]	36 ON		X (smokers + I ON)				x											X		
Chotanaphuti et al. [20]	55 ONFH						x	x			x									
Glueck et al. [27]	30 ON;18 2° ON; 12 I ON	x	x	x [27, 28]										X (I ON)						
Glueck et al. [28]	31 ON; 13 2° ON; 18 I ON	x		x	x		x													
Glueck et al. [29]	50 ONFH	x	x [29–31]	x																
Glueck et al. [31]	36 ONFH		x	x				x							x					
Glueck et al. [32]	133 ON; 62 2° ON; 71 I ON			X (I ON)	X (2° ON)						X	X (2° ON)								
Gruppo [33]	55 ON of the jaw	X	X	X	X	X														
Jones et al. [34]	45 ONFH	x	x			x														
Korompilias et al. [35]	40 ONFH					X														
Korompilias et al. [36]	216 ONFH			x	x	x														
Pósán et al. [9]	49 adults			x													X			
Tan et al. [37]	12 ONFH	X	X																X	X
Zalavras et al. [38]	68 ON; 17 I ON; 51 2° ON			X			X	X (2° ON)					X	X (I ON)			X (also α1 & α2)			

I idiopathic, 2° *ON* secondary osteonecrosis, *ONFH* osteonecrosis of the femoral head, *TO* transient osteoporosis
[a]Results from a selected group of the patient cohort that received a full coagulation profile

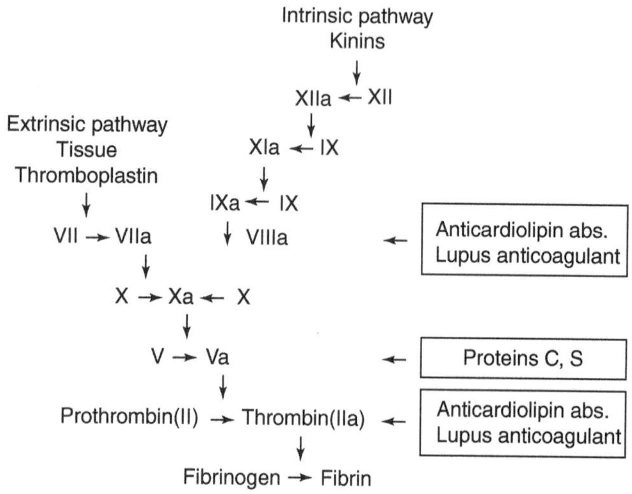

Fig. 10.1 The intrinsic and extrinsic coagulation pathways (Published with permission Aaron and Ciombor [47])

include α2-macroglobluin (A2M) and α1 antitrypsin as well as the plasminogen activator inhibitors (PAI-1 and PAI-2) [51].

10.4 Osteonecrosis and Coagulation Factors

The literature is replete with reports of an association between osteonecrosis and abnormalities of the factors participating in both the coagulation and fibrinolytic pathways. Many studies have focused on the circulating levels of these factors, while others have evaluated whether there is an association with inherited thrombophilia or hypofibrinolysis. While a genetic abnormality may lead to unusually high or low circulating levels of a specific coagulation factor, this may not always be the case. It is, therefore, important to conduct both genetic and serologic studies to explore this association. Several external factors such as corticosteroid therapy and alcoholism have also been associated with abnormal circulating levels of these factors and increased risk of thromboembolism [52–54]. Unfortunately, many of these associations have been based on case reports or small series [14, 55–67]. The following discussion will address the results of the larger studies.

10.4.1 Thrombophilia

Thrombophilia is the increased tendency towards intravascular thrombosis [28]. Elevations in anticardiolipin antibodies, anti-β-GPI antibodies, homocysteine and activated protein C resistance have been observed with thrombophilia [34, 46, 68]. Inherited thrombophilia is associated with mutations in the genes for factor V (factor V Leiden, a mutation in the F5 gene at position 1691), prothrombin (prothrombin G20210A, at position 20210 in the 3′ untranslated region of the gene), factor XIII, methylenetetrahydrofolate reductase (MTHFR), and abnormal fibrinogen [46, 68]. When factor V is mutated, it is unable to bind to protein C so that factor V is more resistant to inactivation by protein C [28, 47]. Deficiencies in antithrombin III, protein C, or protein S are also associated with thrombophilia [28, 46]. As proteins C and S are involved in the activation of factor V, decreased levels of these proteins result in an increased tendency to form thrombi [47]. As shown in Tables 10.2 and 10.3, numerous reports have indicated an association between osteonecrosis and abnormal levels of specific factors or gene mutations involved with thrombophilia.

- Glueck and colleagues have studied the association between osteonecrosis and coagulopathies for over 20 years. They have reported higher resistance to activated protein C [28], low protein C [28], low protein S [30, 31], high anticardiolipin antibodies [34], high homocysteine levels [30, 31, 34], and high factor VIII [30]. Korompilias et al. have also reported increased resistance to activated protein C, high levels of anticardiolipin antibody, and low levels of protein S in some osteonecrosis patients [35, 36]. Deficiencies in antithrombin III, protein C, and protein S are associated with deep venous thrombosis of the extremities [73].

Heritable thrombophilia has also been investigated, especially in regard to mutations in genes for MTHFR, V Leiden, and prothrombin. The mutant form of MTHFR, the C677T polymorphisms, decreases the activity of the enzyme and interferes with the intracellular metabolism of homocysteine, resulting in an elevated plasma homocysteine level [74, 75]. Elevated levels of homocysteine are associated with thrombophilia [76]. As shown by Glueck et al. [31], osteonecrosis patients were more likely to have the heterozygous for the MTHFR mutation (64 %) than were controls (38 %) ($p=0.014$). This was associated with elevated homocysteine levels in this patient cohort ($p=0.05$). Resistance to activated protein C (RAPC) is associated with the Arg506Gln mutation in factor V (factor V Leiden) [24]. In a study of 68 patients with osteonecrosis, Björkman and colleagues reported 13.2 % of the patients with the factor V Leiden mutation, while the idiopathic group exhibited a 22.9 % rate [24]. In a study of 244 ON patients, Glueck et al. found that 9.4 % of the patients were heterozygous for factor V Leiden; the rates were similar for both idiopathic (9.3 %) and secondary (9.6 %) osteonecroses [71].

Thrombin plays a critical role in the conversion of fibrinogen to fibrin in the coagulation pathway (Fig. 10.1). Prothrombin is enzymatically cleaved by activated factor X to form thrombin, and this action is further enhanced in the presence of factor V. The mutation in prothrombin

Table 10.3 Genes associated with hypofibrinolysis and thrombophilia

Protein encoded	Gene(s)	Coagulopathy	References
Plasminogen activator inhibitor-1	4G/4G; 4G/5G alleles in the promoter region	Hypofibrinolysis	Glueck et al. [29] Glueck et al. [31] Ferrari et al. [69]
Plasminogen activator inhibitor-1	SNP rs1799889 (promoter region; −675, 4G/5G), rs2227631, (promoter region; −844 G/A), and rs11178 (3′ UTR region, +10700C/T)	Hypofibrinolysis	Kim et al. [70]
Methylenetetrahydrofolate reductase	C677T polymorphism	Thrombophilia	Glueck et al. [31]
Factor V Leiden	Mutation of F5	Thrombophilia	Glueck et al. [71]
Factor V Leiden	Arg506Gln mutation	Thrombophilia	Gillespie et al. [72]
Prothrombin	20210A gene mutation	Thrombophilia	Bjorkman et al. [24]

Table 10.4 Risk factors for osteonecrosis associated with thrombophilic and hypofibrinolytic abnormalities

Lupus	Adams et al. [77], Palatinus and Adams [78]
Sickle cell	Nsiri et al. [79]
Caisson disease	Candito et al. [80]
Alcoholism with liver disease	Tran-Thang et al. [81]
Inflammatory bowel disease	Koutroubakis et al. [82]
End-stage renal disease/renal transplant	Klai et al. [83]
Antiphospholipid antibody syndrome	Reshetniak et al. [84]
Pregnancy	Factor V Leiden, prothrombin 20210G --> A, methylenetetrahydrofolate reductase 677C --> T and plasminogen activator inhibitor 4G/5G polymorphism in women with pregnancy-related venous thromboembolism (Glueck et al. [85]).

(20210A) causes increased circulating levels and therefore predisposes to thrombotic events [24, 75]. While Glueck et al. found no difference in the presence of prothrombin gene heterozygosity between osteonecrosis cases (3.4 %) and controls (2.9 %) [71], Björkman et al. reported a 5.9 % incidence of heterozygosity for the prothrombin 20210A mutation [24].

10.4.2 Hypofibrinolysis

Markers of hypofibrinolysis have also been identified in some patients with osteonecrosis (Tables 10.3 and 10.4). Plasminogen activator inhibitor-1 (PAI-1) acts to inhibit tissue plasminogen activator (tPA) which is an activator of plasminogen (Fig. 10.2). When plasminogen becomes activated, it is converted to plasmin which then acts to dissolve the fibrinogen fibers within a blood clot (fibrinolysis). An increase in PAI-1 activity suppresses the generation of plasmin resulting in hypofibrinolysis [47]. Several studies have documented elevated levels of plasminogen activator

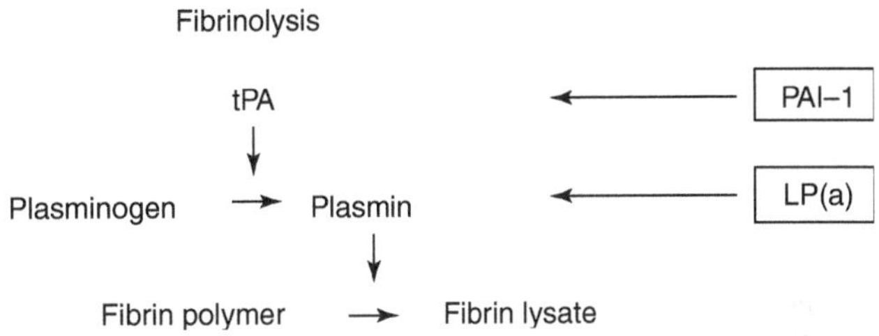

Fig. 10.2 The fibrinolytic pathway (Aaron and Ciombor [47])

inhibitor 1 (PAI-1) and/or low levels of tissue plasminogen activator [27–29, 31, 33, 34, 86].

Glueck et al. found differences in the basal and stimulated levels of tPA-Fx, tPA-Ag, PAI-Fx, and PAI-Ag between patients with idiopathic ON and secondary ON [27]. (These abbreviations need to be defined and explained here.) Three secondary ON patients had basal tPA-Fx outside of the normal range (elevated), while only one idiopathic patient was outside of the range (low). Most of the 2° ON patients had stimulated levels within the normal range (only 4 patients elevated), while 9/12 idiopathic patients had levels below the range of normal. Furthermore, the majority of the 2° ON patients had basal and stimulated PAI-Fx and PAI-Ag within normal range, while two thirds of the idiopathic patients had elevated PAI-Fx and PAI-Ag levels as compared to the normal controls. They also noted that patients with 2° ON had markedly lower basal and stimulated PAI-Fx and PAI-Ag than patients with idiopathic osteonecrosis.

Lipoprotein(a) Lp(a) has also been associated with hypofibrinolysis and hypercoagulability [75, 76]. One of the subunits of Lp(a), apolipoprotein(a), contains domains with extensive homology to plasminogen [36]. Apo(a) inhibits the conjunction of plasminogen and tPA at the surface of fibrin, thereby interrupting fibrinolysis [76]. Elevated levels of Lp(a) have been observed in osteonecrosis patients in numerous studies [9, 27, 28, 30, 31, 33, 36, 38, 87]. Glueck et al. [27] observed that the mean Lp(a) level was within the normal range for the idiopathic patients, while it was elevated for the secondary osteonecrosis patients. While they did not note any elevated levels of Apo A1 for either group as compared to controls, a significant elevation Apo B for the idiopathic group was observed. Apo B is a major component in the formation of low density lipoprotein (LDL) and is responsible for carrying into the tissues. Hirata et al. [88] found that there was a strong association between the low molecular weight phenotype of apolipoprotein (a) and ON in renal transplant patients (adjusted odds ratio 5.75). Furthermore, Korompilias et al. reported an association between anticardiolipin antibody and Lp(a) [36].

Heritable hypofibrinolysis has also been studied extensively. The mutated 4G/4G genotype for PAI-1 was more prevalent in patients with AVN (61.5 %) than in control patients without ON (clinical, 20.7 %; radiological, 17.3 %) [69]. In another study, Kim et al. reported that three single nucleotide polymorphisms (SNP) [rs1799889 (4G allele), rs2227631 (A allele), and rs11178 (C allele)] were associated with increased risk of ON [70]. Asano et al. reported that plasma PAI-1 levels were the highest in ON patients with the 4G/4G genotype [89]. However, univariate analysis demonstrated no significant difference in the incidence of ON between patients with different genotypes of PAI-1. Whether their results reflect the etiology (renal transplant) or ethnicity (Japanese) of the patient population requires further evaluation.

10.4.3 No Association

A number of studies have reported no association between thrombophilic and fibrinolytic factors and osteonecrosis. However, it is important to appreciate that this conclusion is based on a selective analysis of factors known to be thrombophilic and hypofibrinolytic. Furthermore, as stated previously, lack of evidence for gene mutations associated with heritable hypofibrinolysis or thrombophilia does not necessarily mean that there are no abnormalities in the local and systemic levels of the gene products, i.e., the proteins and enzymes involved in the coagulation and fibrinolytic cascades.

In a prospective case-controlled study, Mehsen et al. reported no significant difference in the frequency of thrombosis risk factors between aseptic osteonecrosis patients (56.4 %) and their matched controls (48.7 %) [90]. Assessment of thrombosis was based on circulating levels of protein S, homocysteine level, anticardiolipin Ab, β2 glycoprotein I Ab, and antiprothrombin. Seventy-one percent of the patients presented with at least one risk factor vs. 38 % of the controls. However, no significant difference was shown between the ON patients and the matched controls. They did find a significant association between smoking and risk for developing ON. Séguin et al. [91] also found no association between osteonecrosis of the femoral head and any specific marker for thrombophilia (antithrombin III, protein C, protein S, anticardiolipin Ab). Although deficiencies were observed in a few patients, their frequency was within the expected range published for healthy controls. Furthermore, there is no allelic or genotypic association or trend found for each PAI-1 genotype analyzed. Studies have also reported no association between osteonecrosis and antiphospholipid antibodies [92, 93].

In genetic studies, Celik et al. [94] reported no significant difference in the presence of factor V Leiden, prothrombin G20210A, and MTHFR C677T mutations between osteonecrosis (renal transplant patients) and volunteer controls. One limitation of this study was the relatively small numbers of patients ($n=11$, ON; $n=39$ controls). In a study of 31 Japanese osteonecrosis patients (renal transplant patients), Asano et al. did not find a correlation between osteonecrosis and the distribution of different genotypes for PAI-1 (4G/5G) or MTHFR C677T [89]. Kim et al. [95] evaluated 443 Korean patients with osteonecrosis and compared their results to that obtained for 273 controls. Genotyping using 15 single nucleotide polymorphisms (SNPs) for MTHFR, they found no significant difference in frequencies of the MTHFR polymorphisms and haplotypes. Cenni et al. detected homozygosity or heterozygosity for factor V Leiden in two corticosteroid-associated patients and no idiopathic ON patients [26]. While they state that the frequency of thrombophilia was not different than controls, more steroid-associated ON patients had 4G/5G (50 %) and fewer had 4G/4G (22 %) as compared to the idiopathic (39 %/33 %) or control (36 %/43 %) groups. In a study of post-severe acute respiratory distress syndrome patients with osteonecrosis, Sun et al. did not detect any mutations of factor V Leiden or prothrombin G20210A [96]. With respect for the gene for PAI-1, Asano et al. suggest that the differences between published results may reflect differences in the genetic backgrounds and frequency of thrombotic diseases in different ethnic groups [89].

10.4.4 Intravascular Coagulation and Pathogenesis

In order to understand the potential role that thrombophilia and hypofibrinolysis may play in the pathogenesis of osteonecrosis, one should appreciate the concept of intravascular coagulation as proposed by John Paul Jones, Jr. In 1974, he hypothesized that intravascular osteonecrosis is the final common pathway in the early pathogenesis of osteonecrosis [97]. He expanded on this to emphasize that he did not believe that intravascular coagulation was the cause of osteonecrosis but that it was an intermediary event initiated by an underlying etiologic factor, i.e., a factor associated with an underlying disease [7, 14, 98, 99]. The list of comorbidities that could potentially activate intravascular coagulation is extensive and includes both genetic (e.g., familial thrombophilia, Gaucher's disease, hemoglobinopathies) and nongenetic (hyperlipemia, fat emboli, hypercortisonism, alcoholism, dysbaric phenomenon, hypersensitivity reactions, allograft organ rejection, endotoxic (Shwartzman) reactions, proteolytic enzyme). Other prothrombotic and hypofibrinolytic conditions, tissue factors such as TNF, antiphospholipid Ab, pancreatitis, malignancies, collagen vascular diseases, pregnancy, and immune complex disorders must also be considered [4, 98]. Intraosseous fat embolism as an initiator of intravascular coagulation was proposed by Jones [7, 14] and supported by others [47, 100]. Once triggered, intravascular coagulation may then result in irreversible cell injury with ATP depletion and cell membrane damage, leading to ischemic osteocytic and adipocytic necrosis [6]. Jones also suggests that many of the factors associated with the underlying disease or disorder lead to intravascular coagulation as well as "rapid endothelial sloughing, exposure of subendothelial collagen, and release of tissue thromboplastin" [14]. Endothelial damage has been suggested by others as an underlying mechanism in the pathogenesis of osteonecrosis [73, 101–103]. Corticosteroids have also been shown to directly injure endothelial cells [104]. Jones proposed, "There is upregulation of procoagulant activity, because the perturbed endothelial cell surface represents a binding site for Factor VIIa mediating the activation of the extrinsic pathway of coagulation. There is downregulation of anticoagulant activity, because the perturbed endothelial cell loses its thrombomodulin membrane receptor and the protein C pathway is not activated." This would create a vicious cycle where the prothrombotic response becomes amplified.

Jones proposed the concept of an "ischemic threshold" [7]. In relation to the theory of fat emboli, Jones proposed that an ischemic threshold could develop when the intravascular fat load exceeds or overwhelms the anti-lipemic and anticoagulant clearance mechanisms. Below the threshold level, there is fatty degeneration of subchondral and subperiosteal osteocytes and osteoblasts; above the threshold, there is free fatty acid production, no clearance of procoagulant factors, leading to bony ischemia. Increased circulating free fatty acids were observed by Kabata et al. in an animal model of corticosteroid-induced osteonecrosis [100].

10.5 Corticosteroid Therapy

One of the major risk factors for osteonecrosis is high-dose corticosteroid therapy. There are several mechanisms by which corticosteroid therapy may have an impact on the incidence of hypercoagulability in patients with ON. Corticosteroids may directly injure endothelial cells and thereby initiate the coagulation cascade [73, 101, 105, 106]. Corticosteroids may act to increase PAI-1 activity [5, 69] as well as decrease tPA activity [5, 106]. Of particular note, in a systemic review of the literature, Van Zaane et al. reported there was an increase in the activity of factors VII, VIII, and XI following corticosteroid treatment; this was found to be exacerbated during active inflammation [107].

Although one study reported no significant difference in the frequency of genetic mutations for factor V, prothrombin, or MTHFR [94], this does not preclude the possibility that the corticosteroid treatment had an effect on the circulating levels of the gene products for these are other procoagulants.

Conclusions

Hypercoagulability and hypofibrinolysis have both been implicated in the pathogenesis of osteonecrosis. Both may be inherited or acquired. Acquired coagulation abnormalities are related to external factors such as corticosteroid therapy, smoking, or excessive alcohol consumption. In contradistinction, genetic studies have identified inherited abnormalities in the genes coding for a number of different coagulation factors in both the coagulation and fibrinolytic pathways. Understanding the clinical ramifications of these findings is complicated. *There is no one abnormality which is common to all patients with osteonecrosis.* In fact, some of the most frequent abnormalities have included abnormal RAPC levels (50 %) [28, 32, 33, 36], elevated PAI-1 [26, 27, 33, 34, 86], and Lp (a) [9, 33, 36, 38] of ON patients. A major confounding factor is that many of the studies proposing a link between osteonecrosis and specific coagulation factors have either limited numbers of ON patients or have not included adequate controls. Individual orthopedic surgeons often do not see sufficient numbers of osteonecrosis patients to be able to conduct a statistically robust study. Furthermore, a complete battery of serologic and genetic markers is expensive, and external funding is frequently lacking. While some investigators have made an effort to age and sex/gender match their controls, more appropriate disease-matched controls would provide additional information. A study evaluating lupus patients with and without steroid therapy and with or without osteonecrosis is a perfect example but extremely difficult to undertake and complete with adequate follow-up. A third major factor adding to the complexity of risk assessment in ON is that the abnormal coagulation factors may be associated with diverse etiologic factors already identified for osteonecrosis – this may be particularly true for those diseases associated with autoimmune disorders such as lupus erythematosus (Table 10.4). It is these associations between coagulation abnormalities and the comorbidities that may help to define which patients are more truly at risk to develop osteonecrosis. Finally, as we continue to increase our knowledge of the regulation and interrelationships between different modulators of the coagulation and fibrinolytic cascades, new associations will emerge. There may be factors upstream or downstream of those already identified that play a critical role and may eventually unify the pathogenetic mechanisms involved.

A number of studies have shown a high percentage of patients with at least one coagulation factor abnormality [20, 28, 34, 36, 38]. Several of these studies show similar rates between patients with idiopathic and secondary ON [34, 38]. In a previous study, our group has shown that while 82.2 % of the patients with ON had at least one coagulopathy, 46.7 % had two or more abnormal tests (as compared to 2.5 % of controls) [34]. This could have implications regarding specific patients.

Previous investigators have suggested the multihit theory of osteonecrosis [4, 47, 106, 108]. There may be a genetic predisposition for osteonecrosis that may or may not be related to a hypercoagulable state. The individual may then experience external factors (such as alcoholism, corticosteroids therapy, hyperbaric exposure, or smoking) or develop a comorbidity (such as hemoglobinopathies, Gaucher's disease, autoimmune diseases, and pregnancy) that act to "push them over" the threshold of disease [36]. Cosgriff [109] and Jones [7] have also suggested that steroid treatment may place some patients in a "prothrombotic state." Without question, further study is needed to resolve these issues.

References

1. Ficat RP, Arlet J. Ischemia and Necroses of Bone. In: Hungerford DS, editor. Baltimore: Williams & Wilkins; 1980. p. 196.
2. Schroer WC. Current concepts on the pathogenesis of osteonecrosis of the femoral head. Orthop Rev. 1994;23(6):487–97.
3. Jones LC, Hungerford DS. The pathogenesis of osteonecrosis. Instr Course Lect. 2007;56:179–96.
4. Assouline-Dayan Y, et al. Pathogenesis and natural history of osteonecrosis. Semin Arthritis Rheum. 2002;32(2):94–124.
5. Powell C, Chang C, Gershwin ME. Current concepts on the pathogenesis and natural history of steroid-induced osteonecrosis. Clin Rev Allergy Immunol. 2011;41(1):102–13.
6. Jones JJP. Etiology and pathogenesis of osteonecrosis. Semin Arthroplasty. 1991;2(3):160–8.
7. Jones Jr JP. Intravascular coagulation and osteonecrosis. Clin Orthop Relat Res. 1992;277:41–53.
8. Boettcher WG, et al. Non-traumatic necrosis of the femoral head. I. Relation of altered hemostasis to etiology. J Bone Joint Surg Am. 1970;52(2):312–21.
9. Posan E, et al. Thrombotic and fibrinolytic alterations in the aseptic necrosis of femoral head. Blood Coagul Fibrinolysis. 2003;14(3): 243–8.
10. Bonfiglio M. Development of bone necrosis lesions. In: Lambertsen C, editor. 5th symposium underwater physiology. Bethesda: Fed Am Soc Exp Biol; 1976. p. 117–32.
11. Spencer JD, Brookes M. Avascular necrosis and the blood supply of the femoral head. Clin Orthop Relat Res. 1988;235:127–40.
12. Saito S, et al. Long-term results of total hip arthroplasty for osteonecrosis of the femoral head. A comparison with osteoarthritis. Clin Orthop Relat Res. 1989;244:198–207.
13. Asherson RA, et al. Avascular necrosis of bone and antiphospholipid antibodies in systemic lupus erythematosus. J Rheumatol. 1993;20(2):284–8.
14. Jones Jr JP. Fat embolism, intravascular coagulation, and osteonecrosis. Clin Orthop Relat Res. 1993;292:294–308.
15. Cheras PA, Freemont AJ, Sikorski JM. Intraosseous thrombosis in ischemic necrosis of bone and osteoarthritis. Osteoarthritis Cartilage. 1993;1(4):219–32.
16. Egan RM, Munn RK. Catastrophic antiphospholipid antibody syndrome presenting with multiple thromboses and sites of avascular necrosis. J Rheumatol. 1994;21(12):2376–9.
17. Starklint H, Lausten GS, Arnoldi CC. Microvascular obstruction in avascular necrosis. Immunohistochemistry of 14 femoral heads. Acta Orthop Scand. 1995;66(1):9–12.
18. Laroche M, et al. Histological appearance of the intra-osseous vessels of the femoral head in aseptic osteonecrosis of the hip, with or without antiphospholipid antibodies. Clin Rheumatol. 1997;16(4):367–71.
19. Saito S, Ohzono K, Matsui M. Early arteriopathy and hemorrhage in osteonecrosis of the femoral head. In: Urbaniak JR, Jones JPJ, editors. Osteonecrosis: etiology, diagnosis, and treatment. Rosemont: AAOS; 1997. p. 81–5.
20. Chotanaphuti T, et al. The prevalence of thrombophilia in idiopathic osteonecrosis of the hip. J Med Assoc Thai. 2009;92 Suppl 6:S141–6.
21. Aaron R. Osteonecrosis: etiology, pathophysiology, and diagnosis. In: Callaghan T, editor. The adult hip. Philadelphia: Lippincott Raven; 1998. p. 451–66.
22. Jones Jr JP. Fat embolism and osteonecrosis. Orthop Clin N Am. 1985;16(4):595–633.
23. Atsumi T, Kuroki Y, Yamano K. A microangiographic study of idiopathic osteonecrosis of the femoral head. Clin Orthop Relat Res. 1989;246:186–94.
24. Bjorkman A, et al. Factor V leiden and prothrombin gene mutation: risk factors for osteonecrosis of the femoral head in adults. Clin Orthop Relat Res. 2004;425:168–72.
25. Bjorkman A, et al. Factor V Leiden and the prothrombin 20210A gene mutation and osteonecrosis of the knee. Arch Orthop Trauma Surg. 2005;125(1):51–5.
26. Cenni E, et al. Idiopathic and secondary osteonecrosis of the femoral head show different thrombophilic changes and normal or higher levels of platelet growth factors. Acta Orthop. 2011;82(1):42–9.
27. Glueck CJ, et al. Hypofibrinolysis: a common, major cause of osteonecrosis. Am J Hematol. 1994;45(2):156–66.
28. Glueck CJ, et al. Thrombophilia and hypofibrinolysis: pathophysiologies of osteonecrosis. Clin Orthop Relat Res. 1997;334:43–56.
29. Glueck CJ, et al. The plasminogen activator inhibitor-1 gene, hypofibrinolysis, and osteonecrosis. Clin Orthop Relat Res. 1999;366:133–46.
30. Glueck CJ, et al. Thrombophilia, hypofibrinolysis, the eNOS T-786C polymorphism, and multifocal osteonecrosis. J Bone Joint Surg Am. 2008;90A(10):2220–9.
31. Glueck CJ, et al. Hypofibrinolysis, thrombophilia, osteonecrosis. Clin Orthop Relat Res. 2001;386:19–33.
32. Glueck CJ, Freiberg RA, Wang P. Heritable thrombophilia-hypofibrinolysis and osteonecrosis of the femoral head. Clin Orthop Relat Res. 2008;466(5):1034–40.
33. Gruppo R, et al. The pathophysiology of alveolar osteonecrosis of the jaw: anticardiolipin antibodies, thrombophilia, and hypofibrinolysis. J Lab Clin Med. 1996;127(5):481–8.

34. Jones LC, et al. Procoagulants and osteonecrosis. J Rheumatol. 2003;30(4):783–91.
35. Korompilias AV, et al. Anticardiolipin antibodies and osteonecrosis of the femoral head. Clin Orthop Relat Res. 1997;345:174–80.
36. Korompilias AV, Ortel TL, Urbaniak JR. Coagulation abnormalities in patients with hip osteonecrosis. Orthop Clin N Am. 2004;35(3): 265–71, vii.
37. Tan X, et al. Comparative analysis of serum proteomes: discovery of proteins associated with osteonecrosis of the femoral head. Trans Res. 2006;148(3):114–9.
38. Zalavras C, et al. Potential aetiological factors concerning the development of osteonecrosis of the femoral head. Eur J Clin Invest. 2000;30(3):215–21.
39. Petri M. Thrombosis and systemic lupus erythematosus: the Hopkins Lupus Cohort perspective. Scand J Rheumatol. 1996;25(4): 191–3.
40. Gertler SL, et al. Mesenteric venous thrombosis as sole complication of decompression sickness. Digest Dis Sci. 1984;29(1):91–5.
41. Yang P, Kruh JN, Foster CS. Antiphospholipid antibody syndrome. Curr Opin Ophthalmol. 2012;23(6):528–32.
42. Taraborelli M, Andreoli L, Tincani A. Much more than thrombosis and pregnancy loss: the antiphospholipid syndrome as a 'systemic disease'. Best Pract Res Clin Rheumatol. 2012;26(1):79–90.
43. Lund KS, et al. Increased risk of venous thromboembolism and arterial cardiovascular events in patients with inflammatory bowel disease. Ugeskr Laeger. 2012;174:3003–6.
44. Papa A, et al. Vascular involvement in inflammatory bowel disease: pathogenesis and clinical aspects. Digest Dis. 2008;26(2):149–55.
45. Hall JE, Guyton AC. Guyton and Hall textbook of medical physiology. 12th ed. Philadelphia: Saunders/Elsevier; 2011. xix, 1091 p.
46. Hoffbrand AV, Moss PAH, Pettit JE. Essential haematology. 6th ed. Malden: Wiley-Blackwell; 2011. xi, 454 p.
47. Aaron RK, Ciombor DM. Coagulapathies and osteonecrosis. Curr Opin Orthop. 2001;12:378–83.
48. Hoffbrand AV, Moss PAH, Pettit JE. Essential haematology. 5th ed. Malden/Oxford: Blackwell; 2006. ix, 380 p.
49. Castoldi E, Rosing J. APC resistance: biological basis and acquired influences. J Thromb Haemostasis JTH. 2010;8(3):445–53.
50. Lijnen HR. Role of fibrinolysis in obesity and thrombosis. Thromb Res. 2009;123 Suppl 4:S46–9.
51. Lijnen HR. Elements of the fibrinolytic system. Ann N Y Acad Sci. 2001;936:226–36.
52. Tran-Thang C, et al. Plasminogen activators and plasminogen activator inhibitors in liver deficiencies caused by chronic alcoholism or infectious hepatitis. Thromb Haemostasis. 1989;62(2): 651–3.
53. Johannesdottir SA, et al. Use of glucocorticoids and risk of venous thromboembolism: a nationwide population-based case–control study. JAMA Int Med. 2013;173(9):743–52.
54. van Zaane B, et al. Systematic review on the effect of glucocorticoid use on procoagulant, anti-coagulant and fibrinolytic factors. J Thromb Haemostasis JTH. 2010;8(11):2483–93.
55. Elishkewich K, et al. Idiopathic osteonecrosis in an adult with familial protein S deficiency and hyperhomocysteinemia. Blood Coagul Fibrinolysis. 2001;12(7):547–50.
56. Glueck CJ, et al. Idiopathic osteonecrosis, hypofibrinolysis, high plasminogen activator inhibitor, high lipoprotein(a), and therapy with Stanozolol. Am J Hematol. 1995;48(4):213–20.
57. Glueck CJ, et al. Estrogen replacement in a protein S deficient patient leads to diarrhea, hyperglucagonemia, and osteonecrosis. JOP J Pancreas. 2001;2(5):323–9.
58. Glueck CJ, et al. Thrombophilia, hypofibrinolysis, the eNOS T-786C polymorphism, and multifocal osteonecrosis. J Bone Joint Surg Am. 2008;90(10):2220–9.
59. Kubo T, et al. Antithrombin III deficiency in a patient with multifocal osteonecrosis. Clin Orthop Relat Res. 2000;378:306–11.
60. Moore J, et al. Bilateral knee osteonecrosis in a patient with thrombotic thrombocytopenic purpura. Aust N Z J Med. 1999;29(1): 88–9.
61. Pierre-Jacques H, et al. Familial heterozygous protein-S deficiency in a patient who had multifocal osteonecrosis. A case report. J Bone Joint Surg Am. 1997;79(7):1079–84.
62. Shahin AA. Arthritis and osteonecrosis in a patient with thrombophilia. Rheumatol Int. 2001;20(6):243–5.
63. Ureten K, et al. Atraumatic osteonecrosis after estrogen replacement therapy associated with low protein S level in a patient with Turner syndrome. Clin Appl Thromb/Hemostasis. 2010;16(5):599–601.
64. Vairaktaris E, et al. Bisphosphonate-induced avascular osteonecrosis of the mandible associated with a common thrombophilic mutation in the prothrombin gene. J Oral Max Surg. 2009;67(9):2009–12.
65. Wermes C, et al. Severe protein C deficiency and aseptic osteonecrosis of the hip joint: a case report. Eur J Pediatr. 1999;158 Suppl 3:S159–61.
66. Zhang H, et al. Proteomic analysis of bone tissues of patients with osteonecrosis of the femoral head. Omics J Integr Biol. 2009;13(6): 453–66.
67. Benbih M, et al. Multiple osteonecroses and venous thrombosis: one case of patient with a novel mutation of protein C (N102S) and heterozygous for FV Leiden. Ann De Biol Clin. 2008;66(4):437–40.
68. Varga EA, et al. Cardiology patient pages. Homocysteine and MTHFR mutations: relation to thrombosis and coronary artery disease. Circulation. 2005;111(19):e289–93.
69. Ferrari P, et al. Association of plasminogen activator inhibitor-1 genotype with avascular osteonecrosis in steroid-treated renal allograft recipients. Transplantation. 2002;74(8):1147–52.
70. Kim H, et al. Significant associations of PAI-1 genetic polymorphisms with osteonecrosis of the femoral head. BMC Musculoskelet Disord. 2011;12:160.
71. Glueck CJ, et al. The role of the factor V Leiden mutation in osteonecrosis of the hip. Clin Appl Thromb Hemost. 2012;19(5): 499–503.
72. Gillespie DL, et al. Resistance to activated protein C: a common inherited cause of venous thrombosis. Ann Vasc Surg. 1996;10(2): 174–7.
73. Kerachian MA, et al. Avascular necrosis of the femoral head: vascular hypotheses. Endothelium. 2006;13(4):237–44.
74. Shang XF, et al. Association between MTHFR C677T polymorphism and osteonecrosis of the femoral head: a meta-analysis. Mol Biol Rep. 2012;39(6):7089–94.
75. Orth P, Anagnostakos K. Coagulation abnormalities in osteonecrosis and bone marrow edema syndrome. Orthopedics. 2013;36(4): 290–300.
76. Lykissas MG, et al. The role of hypercoagulability in the development of osteonecrosis of the femoral head. Orthop Rev (Pavia). 2012;4(2):e17.
77. Adams MJ, Palatinus AA, Harvey AM, Khalafallah AA. Impaired control of the tissue factor pathway of blood coagulation in systemic lupus erythematosus. Lupus. 2011;20(14):1474–83.
78. Palatinus A, Adams M. Thrombosis in systemic lupus erythematosus. Semin Thromb Hemost. 2009;35(7):621–9.
79. Nsiri B, et al. Abnormalities of coagulation and fibrinolysis in homozygous sickle cell disease. Hematol Cell Ther. 1996;38(3): 279–84.
80. Candito M, et al. Homocysteinemia and thrombophilic factors in unexplained decompression sickness. Rev Neurol (Paris). 2006;162(8-9):840–4.
81. Tran-Thang C, et al. Plasminogen activators and plasminogen activator inhibitors in liver deficiencies caused by chronic alcoholism or infectious hepatitis. Thromb Haemost. 1989;62(2):651–3.
82. Koutroubakis IE, Tsiolakidou G, Kouroumalis EA. Inherited thrombophilia and thrombosis in inflammatory bowel disease. Am J Gastroenterol. 2006;101(2):403; author reply 403–4.

83. Klai S, et al. Thrombophilic disorders: a real threat to patients with end-stage renal disease on hemodialysis and at the time of renal transplantation. Blood Coagul Fibrinolysis. 2012;23(5):406–10.
84. Reshetniak TM, Seredavkina NV, Nasonov EL. Cardiovascular aspects of antiphospholipid syndrome. Klin Med (Mosk). 2008;86(9):4–12.
85. Glueck CJ, et al. The 4G/4G polymorphism of the hypofibrinolytic plasminogen activator inhibitor type 1 gene: an independent risk factor for serious pregnancy complications. Metabolism. 2000;49(7):845–52.
86. Tan X, et al. Comparative analysis of serum proteomes: discovery of proteins associated with osteonecrosis of the femoral head. Transl Res. 2006;148(3):114–9.
87. Glueck CJ, et al. Plasminogen activator inhibitor activity: an independent risk factor for the high miscarriage rate during pregnancy in women with polycystic ovary syndrome. Metabolism. 1999;48(12):1589–95.
88. Hirata T, et al. Low molecular weight phenotype of Apo(a) is a risk factor of corticosteroid-induced osteonecrosis of the femoral head after renal transplant. J Rheumatol. 2007;34(3):516–22.
89. Asano T, et al. Relationship between postrenal transplant osteonecrosis of the femoral head and gene polymorphisms related to the coagulation and fibrinolytic systems in Japanese subjects. Transplantation. 2004;77(2):220–5.
90. Mehsen N, et al. Coagulopathies frequency in aseptic osteonecrosis patients. Joint Bone Spine. 2009;76(2):166–9.
91. Seguin C, et al. Non-traumatic necrosis of bone (osteonecrosis) is associated with endothelial cell activation but not thrombophilia. Rheumatology. 2008;47(8):1151–5.
92. Dromer C, et al. No link between avascular necrosis of the femoral head and antiphospholipid antibodies. Rev Rhum Engl Ed. 1997;64(6):382–5.
93. Alarcon-Segovia D, et al. Antiphospholipid antibodies and the antiphospholipid syndrome in systemic lupus erythematosus. A prospective analysis of 500 consecutive patients. Medicine (Baltimore). 1989;68(6):353–65.
94. Celik A, et al. Association of corticosteroids and factor V, prothrombin, and MTHFR gene mutations with avascular osteonecrosis in renal allograft recipients. Transplant Proc. 2006;38(2): 512–6.
95. Kim TH, et al. Lack of association of MTHFR gene polymorphisms with the risk of osteonecrosis of the femoral head in a Korean population. Mol Cells. 2010;29(4):343–8.
96. Sun W, et al. Hematological changes and related gene mutation of post-severe acute respiratory syndrome patients with osteonecrosis. Zhonghua Yi Xue Za Zhi. 2006;86(7):442–5.
97. Jones JPJ, Sakovich L, Andersen CE. Dysbarism-related osteonecrosis. Washington, DC: E. Department of Health, and Welfare, Editor; 1974. p. 117–32.
98. Jones Jr JP. Risk factors potentially activating intravascular coagulation and causing nontraumatic osteonecrosis. In: Urbaniak JR, Jones Jr JP, editors. Osteonecrosis: etiology, diagnosis, and treatment. Rosemont: AAOS; 1997. p. 89–96.
99. Jones Jr JP. Coagulopathies and osteonecrosis. Acta Orthop Belg. 1999;65 Suppl 1:5–8.
100. Kabata T, et al. Onset of steroid-induced osteonecrosis in rabbits and its relationship to hyperlipaemia and increased free fatty acids. Rheumatology (Oxford). 2005;44(10):1233–7.
101. Jacobs B. Epidemiology of traumatic and nontraumatic osteonecrosis. Clin Orthop Relat Res. 1978;130:51–67.
102. Slichter SJ, et al. Dysbaric osteonecrosis: a consequence of intravascular bubble formation, endothelial damage, and platelet thrombosis. J Lab Clin Med. 1981;98(4):568–90.
103. Li Y, et al. The experimental study on treatment of glucocorticoid-induced ischemic necrosis of femoral head by gu fu sheng capsule. J Tradit Chin Med. 2004;24(4):303–7.
104. Nishimura T, et al. Histopathologic study of veins in steroid treated rabbits. Clin Orthop Relat Res. 1997;334:37–42.
105. Boss JH, Misselevich I. Osteonecrosis of the femoral head of laboratory animals: the lessons learned from a comparative study of osteonecrosis in man and experimental animals. Vet Pathol. 2003;40(4):345–54.
106. Kerachian MA, Seguin C, Harvey EJ. Glucocorticoids in osteonecrosis of the femoral head: a new understanding of the mechanisms of action. J Steroid Biochem Mol Biol. 2009;114(3–5): 121–8.
107. van Zaane B, et al. Systematic review on the effect of glucocorticoid use on procoagulant, anti-coagulant and fibrinolytic factors. J Thromb Haemost. 2010;8(11):2483–93.
108. Kenzora JE, Glimcher MJ. Accumulative cell stress: the multifactorial etiology of idiopathic osteonecrosis. Orthop Clin North Am. 1985;16(4):669–79.
109. Cosgriff SW. Thromboembolic complications associated with ACTH and cortisone therapy. J Am Med Assoc. 1951;147(10): 924–6.

11 Glucocorticoids (as an Etiologic Factor)

Eun Young Lee and Yun Jong Lee

11.1 Introduction

Adrenocortical hormones were first prepared from the adrenal gland as a new compound by Kendall in 1935 [1]. Thirteen years later, Hench et al. [2] observed a miraculous effect of cortisone in a patient with severe rheumatoid arthritis, which opened new doors to innovative treatments for a variety of inflammatory diseases. Against this background, Kendall, Hench, and Reichstein were awarded the 1950 Nobel Prize for Physiology or Medicine. Since then, glucocorticoids have been used as a first-line therapy for immune-mediated conditions or as an adjunctive therapy in many inflammatory, infectious, or malignant diseases.

However, the Janus-faced effects of glucocorticoids became apparent a few years after their introduction into clinical practice. Today, it is well known that glucocorticoids can have harmful effects on many tissues and can produce numerous adverse effects throughout the body, mainly depending on the dose, the administration route, and the duration of treatment (Table 11.1). Since 1957 when the first case of glucocorticoid-induced femoral head osteonecrosis (GI-FHON) was reported [3], many human and animal studies have reported an association between glucocorticoids and FHON. To date, glucocorticoids have been considered the most common cause of nontraumatic FHON [4]. Nevertheless, pathophysiological mechanisms and effective preventive or therapeutic strategies against GI-FHON have not yet been completely established.

E.Y. Lee
Department of Internal Medicine, Seoul National University College of Medicine, Seoul, South Korea

Department of Internal Medicine, Seoul National University Hospital, 101 Daehak-ro, Jongno-gu, Seoul 110-744, South Korea
e-mail: elee@snu.ac.kr

Y.J. Lee (✉)
Department of Internal Medicine, Seoul National University College of Medicine, Seoul, South Korea

Department of Internal Medicine, Seoul National University Bundang Hospital, 166 Gumi-ro, Seongnam 463-707, South Korea
e-mail: yn35@snu.ac.kr

11.2 Prevalence

GI-FHON may develop in patients receiving glucocorticoids in short-term high doses or in long-term doses and even after intra-articular injection or application of topical preparations. Since glucocorticoids have been widely used as therapeutic drugs to treat numerous diseases in various regimens, the reported prevalences of GI-FHON differ among investigators. Most reports have documented the prevalences in patients with systemic lupus erythematosus (SLE), renal transplantation, or leukemia. In prospective studies where 50 or more patients were included and an MRI was used for diagnosis [5–23], 14.5–34.6 % of SLE patients were diagnosed as having GI-FHON (Table 11.2). Of patients

Table 11.1 Adverse effects of systemic glucocorticoids

System	Adverse effects
Metabolic/ endocrine	Weight gain/obesity, fluid retention/edema, hypokalemia, diabetes mellitus/insulin resistance, adrenal insufficiency, amenorrhea
Dermatologic	Skin thinning, purpura, Cushingoid appearance, acne, hirsutism
Ophthalmologic	Posterior subcapsular cataract, glaucoma, central serous chorioretinopathy
Cardiovascular	Arrhythmia, hypertension, dyslipidemia, premature atherosclerotic disease
Gastrointestinal	Peptic ulcer disease (especially, concurrent user of NSAIDs), acute pancreatitis, steatohepatitis, visceral perforation
Musculoskeletal	Osteoporosis, osteonecrosis, myopathy, growth retardation
Neuropsychiatric	Mood disorder: depression, mania, anxiety, and emotional irritability; psychosis; insomnia
Immune	Increased risk of infections: bacterial, fungal, parasitic, and viral; reactivation of latent viruses

NSAID nonsteroidal anti-inflammatory drug

K.-H. Koo et al. (eds.), *Osteonecrosis*,
DOI 10.1007/978-3-642-35767-1_11, © Springer-Verlag Berlin Heidelberg 2014

Table 11.2 Prevalence of glucocorticoid-induced femoral head osteonecrosis reported in prospective studies

Authors	Publication year	Underlying disease	Patients	Age	Follow-up period	Prevalence FHON	Total ON	Reference
Zizic et al.	1985	SLE	54	18–67			51.9 %	[5]
Ono et al.	1992	SLE	62	Mean 30.7	≤5 years	14.5 %		[6]
Sugano et al.	1994	SLE	60	14–57	3–7 years	15.0 %		[7]
Oinuma et al.	2001	SLE	72	13–66	≤12 months	31.9 %	44.4 %	[8]
Nakamura et al.	2010	SLE	169			34.6 %	38.5 %	[9]
Shigemura et al.	2011	SLE	173		1 year		37.1 %	[10]
Kopecky et al.	1991	Kidney TPL	97	14–59	24 months	10.3 %		[11]
Tervonen et al.	1992	Kidney TPL	100	24–75	0.5–25.5 years	6.0 %		[12]
Marston et al.	2003	Solid organ TPL	52	24–65	0.3–4.3 years	13.5 %		[13]
Shibatani et al.	2008	Kidney TPL	150	16–36	≤12 months	24.7 %		[14]
Guichelaar et al.	2007	Liver TPL	360		≤8 years	6.1 %	7.5 %	[15]
Ribeiro et al.	2001	ALL, NHL	116			7.8 %	14.7 %	[16]
Tauchmanovà et al.	2003	Stem cell TPL	207	18–59		5.8 %		[17]
Talamo et al.	2005	MM	553	25–77	5–114 months	8.9 %		[18]
Schulte et al.	2005	Stem cell TPL	255	15–59	>5 years	4.3 %		[19]
Niinimäki et al.	2007	ALL	97	1.2–15.3		11.3 %	23.7 %	[20]
te Winkel et al.	2011	ALL	574	Mean 6.4	2.5–3.3 months	4.4 %	6.6 %	[21]
Kawedia et al.	2011	ALL	194				45.9 %	[22]
Wing et al.	1998	Spinal cord injury	59	15–64	6–46 months	0.0 %	0.0 %	[23]
Shigemura et al.	2011	Inflammatory diseases	129		1 year		20.9 %	[10]

SLE systemic lupus erythematosus, *TPL* transplantation, *ALL* acute lymphoblastic leukemia, *NHL* non-Hodgkin's lymphoma, *MM* multiple myeloma, *FHON* femoral head osteonecrosis, *ON* osteonecrosis

undergoing kidney transplantation, 6.0–24.7 % were reported to suffer from GI-FHON. On the other hand, GI-FHON occurred in 4.3–11.3 % of patients with hematologic diseases, including acute lymphoblastic leukemia.

11.3 Risk Factors

Because GI-FHON develops in patients with different underlying conditions, risk factors are not homogeneous in all disease states.

11.3.1 Risk Factors for GI-FHON in Animal Models

The dose of the glucocorticoids has been the primary focus of research on risk factors for GI-FHON. Many human studies have described associations between glucocorticoid doses and the prevalences of GI-FHON, while others have not. For example, a study analyzing 24 cohorts receiving glucocorticoids reported a 4.6 % increase in GI-FHON development as the doses of oral prednisone increase by 10 mg/day [24]. Animal models have shown that higher doses are more likely to develop GI-FHON [25]. It has been reported that rabbits are more susceptible to the development of GI-FHON when treated with methylprednisolone than to prednisolone or triamcinolone in [26], although there is no similar evidence in humans. Among rabbits receiving methylprednisolone, those with increased low-density lipoprotein (LDL) cholesterol to high-density lipoprotein (HDL) cholesterol, increased free fatty acids, or decreased hepatic cytochrome P4503A activity are at high risk of developing GI-FHON [27, 28].

11.3.2 Risk Factors in SLE Patients

In SLE patients, a daily prednisone dose of >30–40 mg has been reported to be associated with GI-FHON [6, 29]. However, cumulative or the highest dose has been heterogeneously reported as a risk factor by different investigators. Additionally, methylprednisolone pulse therapy and cytotoxic agents have also been found to be related to GI-FHON [29–32]. Generally, SLE patients with more active diseases are more likely to receive glucocorticoids in higher doses of methylprednisolone pulse therapy or cytotoxic agents. However, there are discrepancies regarding results on SLE disease activity between patients with and without the development of GI-FHON [33, 34]. The majority of GI-FHON cases develop within 3–12 months of initiation of glucocorticoid treatment [8, 31]. Increases in glucocorticoid doses secondary to a relapse of SLE may be associated with GI-FHON [34].

In addition to the use of glucocorticoids, several features of SLE have been identified as risk factors: thrombophlebitis, vasculitis, Raynaud's phenomenon, renal dysfunction, arthritis, smoking, preeclampsia, and so on [6, 30]. In contrast, nested case-control studies have revealed that the use of glucocorticoids is the only risk factor for GI-FHON [32, 33]. Studies on the association between antiphospholipid antibodies and GI-FHON have reported different results [35–37]. Therefore, a specific manifestation may not be a risk factor for GI-FHON in SLE patients.

Because not all SLE patients do develop GI-FHON when receiving high-dose glucocorticoids, the presence of additional regional risk factors or individual variations of glucocorticoid sensitivity can be involved in the occurrence of GI-FHON. For example, age at the time of initial glucocorticoid administration can affect the development of GI-FHON. A prospective study has revealed that GI-FHON did not develop in SLE patients at the age of <14 years, suggesting that children may tolerate ischemia due to their abundant vascularity with growth plates and red marrow [9]. In addition, posttreatment presentation of Cushingoid body phenotype, which is a characteristic feature of glucocorticoid excess and does not develop in patients with glucocorticoid resistance, is reported to be a risk factor [29, 30, 35].

11.3.3 Risk Factors in Kidney Transplant Patients

Kidney transplantation is the treatment of choice for patients with end-stage renal diseases. Just after transplantation, immunosuppressive therapy, including glucocorticoids, is needed to prevent and treat acute graft rejection and to avoid chronic graft damage. It has been shown that the risk of GI-FHON is associated with glucocorticoid doses [14, 38, 39]. In particular, the total dose of glucocorticoids during the first 7 months can have a significant risk [14, 38]. Introduction of immunosuppressants, such as cyclosporine or tacrolimus, can decrease the incidence of GI-FHON in kidney transplant patients [38] because these immunosuppressants reduce glucocorticoids doses. An association of the incidence of GI-FHON with a history of acute rejection is not consistently reported [14, 39].

Several pretransplantation conditions can impact on the development of GI-FHON: iron overload, hypophosphatemia secondary to hyperparathyroidism, or poor renal function [39–41]. Additionally, apoprotein(a) molecular weight phenotype was reported to be an independent risk factor [42].

11.3.4 Risk Factors in Patients with Hematologic Malignancies

Glucocorticoids successfully treat acute lymphoblastic leukemia (ALL), lymphoma (NHL), and multiple myeloma (MM) because they can kill hematologic malignant cells. Thus, many treatment regimens include glucocorticoids, such as dexamethasone. Since the prevalence of ALL is higher in children than in adults, most GI-FHON studies in ALL patients have been conducted on pediatric patients. ALL patients at the age of >10 years increase the risk of GI-FHON [16, 20–22, 43, 44], and old age is also an independent risk factor in adult patients with MM [18]. Additionally, female patients have a higher risk of GI-FHON than males [20, 21, 43, 44]. Intensive therapy with dexamethasone confers a high incidence of GI-FHON [20, 22], and alternate-week scheduling of dexamethasone can reduce the development of GI-FHON [43, 44]. In some studies, patients receiving dexamethasone more frequently developed FHON than those receiving prednisone [43]. An association between FHON and poor dexamethasone clearance has been reported [22]. In patients undergoing stem cell transplantation, both an episode of graft-versus-host disease (GVHD) and the use of glucocorticoid are risk factors [17]. The incidence of GI-FHON has been reported to be higher in patients receiving unrelated donor transplants than in those receiving allogenic matched related donor or autologous transplants [17, 45].

11.4 Pathogenic Mechanisms

The pathophysiology of GI-FHON is multifactorial, complex, and poorly understood. Although host factors and underlying diseases have been shown to play a significant role in the development of GI-FHON, investigators have failed to explain why only a fraction of patients are at greater risk than others. Additionally, the multisystemic effects of glucocorticoids and their interactions make the pathological mechanisms more complicated. In this context, the multi-hit theory proposed by several investigators is a plausible explanation for the development of GI-FHON [46, 56]. In susceptible patients who have a genetic predisposition or an underlying disease that threatens bone and vascular tissues, the accumulative glucocorticoid effects may result in the occurrence of GI-FHON (Fig. 11.1). Genetic factors will be discussed in another chapter.

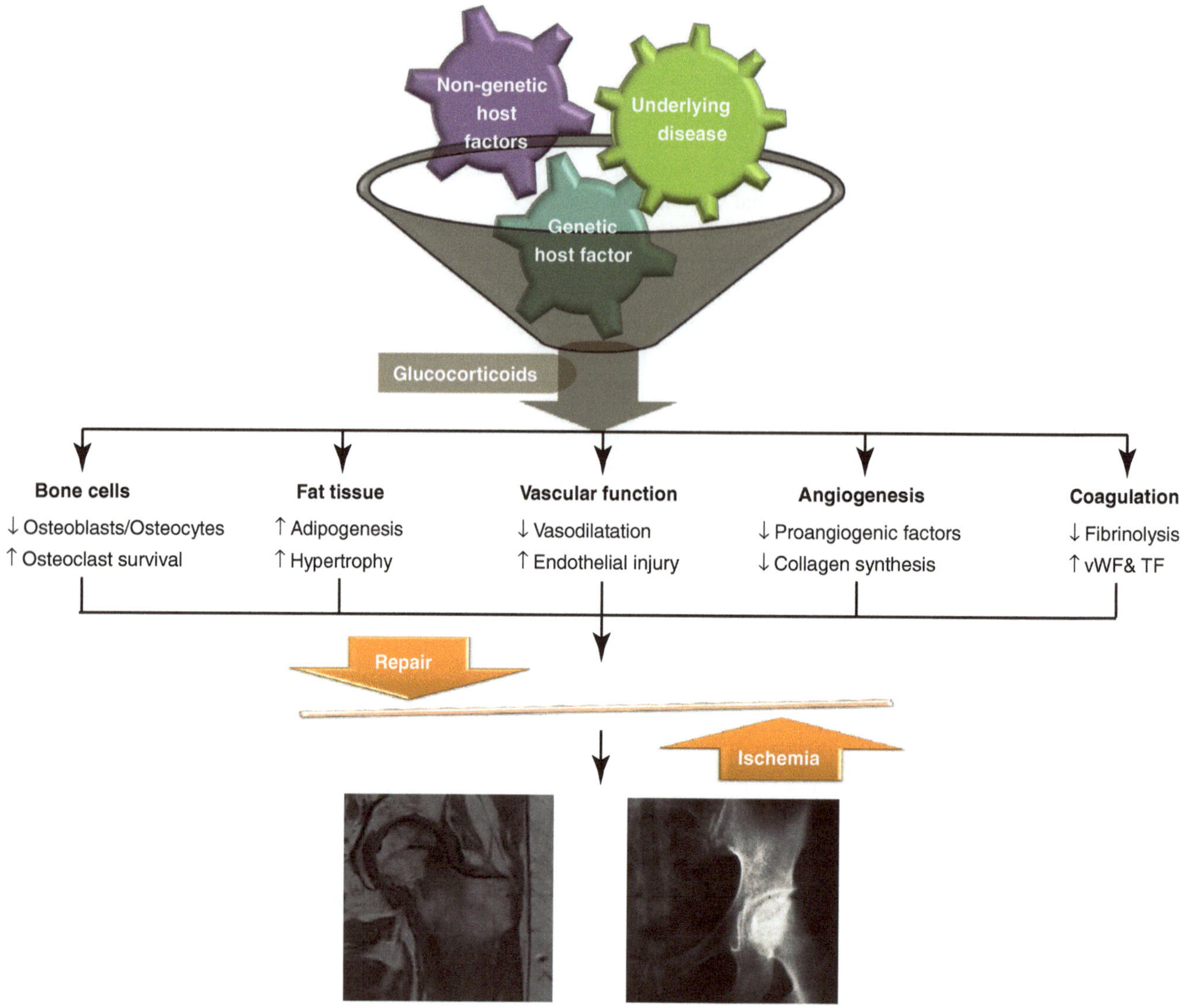

Fig. 11.1 Schematic presentation of the multifactorial pathogenesis of glucocorticoid-induced femur neck osteoporosis. *vWF* von Willebrand factor, *TF* tissue factor

11.4.1 Effects of Glucocorticoids on Bone Cells

Animal and human studies have shown that glucocorticoids can induce apoptosis of osteoblasts and suppress the production of osteoblasts in the bone marrow [47]. Osteoblast-/osteocyte-specific 11β-hydroxysteroid dehydrogenase type 2 (HSD2, the enzyme metabolizes glucocorticoids into inactive metabolites) transgenic mice protect from prednisolone-induced decrease in osteoblast survival, osteoblast number, and bone formation [48]. On the other hand, the survival of osteoclasts can be prolonged by glucocorticoids [49]. The interaction of receptor activator of NF-κB ligand (RANKL) and osteoprotegerin (OPG) is a major determinant of osteoclastogenesis. RANKL and macrophage colony-stimulating factor (M-CSF) are essential for osteoclastogenesis, while OPG prevents RANKL from binding to RANK, resulting in inhibition of osteoclastogenesis. Glucocorticoids increase RANKL and M-CSF expression and decrease OPG expression by human osteoblastic and stromal cells in culture [50, 51]. From the results of studies using mice with conditional osteoclast-specific deletion of glucocorticoid receptors [52], glucocorticoids inhibit proliferation of osteoclast precursors and mature osteoclast-mediated bone resorption. Such glucocorticoid-induced suppression of osteoclasts induces blunting of osteoblast function in the context of osteoclast-osteoblast interactions throughout bone remodeling [53]. Also, glucocorticoids suppress the secretion of sex hormones and the expression of bone morphogenetic protein-2, insulin growth factor 1, and osteocalcin [54, 55]. Furthermore, calcium absorption from the kidney and intestine is disturbed by glucocorticoids [54].

Osteocytes are the most abundant cells (>95 %) in the bone and embedded in mineralized bone matrices. They are thought to play a pivotal role as mechanosensors and initiators of the bone remodeling process [56]. Living osteocytes directly stimulate osteoblastogenesis and inhibit osteoclastic resorption through OPG expression. The femurs from patients with GI-FHON show many apoptotic osteocytes, anatomically juxtaposed to the osteonecrotic fractures [57]. Glucocorticoid-induced osteocyte apoptosis results in the mechanosensory dysfunction of the osteocyte network and consequently leads to impairment of bone repair processes. Additionally, hypoxia-inducible factor (HIF)-1α, a critical regulator of cellular response in hypoxic condition, can alter the mechanosensitivity of osteocytes and suppress load-induced bone formation [58].

11.4.2 Effects of Glucocorticoids on Fat Tissue

Glucocorticoids promote differentiation of preadipocytes to mature adipocytes via upregulation of the peroxisome proliferator-activated receptor (PPAR)-γ and downregulation of runt-related transcription factor 2 (Runx2). In addition, glucocorticoids can cause adipocyte hypertrophy through increased synthesis and storage of lipids [59]. It has been shown that the number and area of fat cells increase in the bone marrow after exposure to glucocorticoids [60, 61]. These changes can generate compression of venous sinusoids and congestion in the bone marrow. As a result, adequate arterial blood flow may not be achieved due to increases in intraosseous pressures, eventually leading to osteonecrosis [62].

11.4.3 Effects of Glucocorticoids on Vascular Functions

Patients with Cushing syndrome have been reported to have increased cardiovascular morbidity and mortality. Chronic administration of glucocorticoids inhibits the synthesis of vasorelaxants, such as prostaglandin E1, prostacyclin, and endothelial nitric oxide (NO), via a suppression phospholipase A2 and endothelial nitric oxide synthase (eNOS) [63]. In addition, glucocorticoids indirectly increase vascular tone through the upregulation of angiotensin II type I receptor and α-1 adrenergic receptors in vascular smooth muscle cells [64]. Furthermore, glucocorticoids can stimulate the synthesis of vasoconstrictor endothelin-1 and potentiate its vasoconstricting effect in vascular smooth muscle cells [65]. There is some evidence that glucocorticoids increase reactive oxidative stress species (ROS) which decrease NO availability [66]. Thus, glucocorticoids can cause dysregulation of endothelium-dependent and endothelium-independent vasodilatation. Furthermore, higher doses of dexamethasone were reported to result in microvascular endothelial cell apoptosis and could lead to capillary rarefaction in a glucocorticoid-induced hypertension model [67]. This may be involved in glucocorticoid-induced hypertension and hypercoagulability. The effect of glucocorticoids on the coagulation system is discussed below.

11.4.4 Effects of Glucocorticoids on Angiogenesis

New blood vessel formation is essential for the repair of ischemia-damaged tissues when FHON develops. However, glucocorticoids have been shown to inhibit angiogenesis. In a dexamethasone-induced FHON rabbit model, vascular endothelial growth factor (VEGF) gene therapy improved the repair process of osteonecrosis [68]. Glucocorticoids suppress expression of VEGF and increase expression of antiangiogenic thrombospondin-1 [69, 70]. Glucocorticoid-induced suppression of matrix metalloproteinases and plasminogen activators may affect the proangiogenic process through impairment of basement membrane turnover [71]. It has also been shown that GCs can inhibit capillary growth by reducing collagen synthesis by myofibroblasts [72]. Because cartilage components released from subchondral fracture sites have been considered antiangiogenic, the negative effects of glucocorticoids on angiogenesis may be potentiated in the subchondral bone tissue in FHON cases [73].

11.4.5 Effects of Glucocorticoids on the Coagulation System

Fibrinolytic activity is balanced by tissue plasminogen activator (t-PA) and plasma plasminogen activator inhibitor-1 (PAI-1). The accumulated evidence of in vitro studies as well as studies of patients with Cushing syndrome suggests that glucocorticoids increase the PAI-1 activity, resulting in a relatively hypercoagulable state [74]. The plasma level of the von Willebrand factor (vWF) is a marker of endothelial cell damage because the vWF is synthesized and stored in the endothelial cells. Plasma vWF levels are reported to increase in subjects with exogenous or endogenous excess glucocorticoids, and dexamethasone induces the expression of vWF, cell adhesion molecules, and tissue factor in vascular endothelial cells [75]. Since vWF is involved in platelet aggregation and adhesion, glucocorticoid-induced endothelial damage may contribute to thrombi formation.

11.5 Clinical Manifestations

The clinical features of GI-FHON are not different from those in other FHON. Patients with GI-FHON usually experience pain primarily in the groin but occasionally the buttocks. The pain onset often can be described as acute. The pain is usually deep and throbbing and becomes worse with ambulation. Patients frequently complain of a catching or popping sensation with motion. In patients with a history of glucocorticoid treatment, especially in higher doses, persistent hip pain with joint movement, tenderness, or reduced range of motions indicates the need for a prompt workup for GI-FHON. On physical examination, limitation of internal rotation in both flexion and extension is observed, with passive internal rotation in extension being particularly painful. A Trendelenburg gait is often present. Additionally, some characteristic features of chronic glucocorticoid users can be seen: moon face, central obesity, and buffalo hump.

Anteroposterior radiographs and frog lateral radiographs of both hips are the primary diagnostic modalities, while plain radiographic findings are frequently normal. Magnetic resonance imaging (MRI) is ideal if x-ray findings are normal and clinical suspicion is high [9, 37]. The sensitivity and specificity of MRI are both greater than 98 % for the diagnosis of osteonecrosis, which is higher than those of other diagnostic modalities. Therefore, MRI should be performed in all patients with osteonecrosis to assess the extent of the disease. Three-dimensional MRI with image registration can be used to assess changes in lesion size [76, 88]. Bone scan may be helpful when x-ray findings are normal and when MRI cannot be performed. It may be low-cost alternative when the suspicion index is low [77, 89].

11.6 Natural Course

Most studies on the natural history of FHON have been conducted on patients with heterogeneous subtypes of nontraumatic FHON. However, the natural history of nontraumatic FHON cannot represent that of GI-FHON because subtypes of nontraumatic FHON may have different pathogenic mechanisms and underlying conditions necessitating glucocorticoids can affect the course of FHON. The results of studies using MRI to diagnose asymptomatic GI-FHON are summarized in Table 11.3 [7, 11, 78–83]. About one-third of patients with asymptomatic early GI-FHON have symptomatic or radiological progression over a period of several years. Thus, clinical progression or subchondral collapse rate seems to be lower than the other subtypes of nontraumatic FHON, especially FHON associated with sickle cell anemia. Sometimes small lesions of GI-FHON are reported to be spontaneously resolved [81–83]. However, as with other subtypes, femoral head collapse develops most often in GI-FHON patients with larger osteonecrosis areas (>15–30 %), lesions occupying the weight-bearing surface, higher radiographic stages, or hip pain [84]. There is no established risk stratification system to exactly estimate outcomes in GI-FHON patients. Because proper therapeutic decisions depend on the natural course of FHON, more extended studies are needed to develop an improved risk classification system.

11.7 Prevention and Treatments

11.7.1 General Guideline

Until now, no specific prevention strategy has been developed. Because the risk of GI-FHON is usually associated with the dose and duration of glucocorticoid treatment, the effort to use the minimal effective dose and to appropriately taper glucocorticoid doses is needed. Because introduction of immunosuppressants may decrease the incidence of GI-FHON in renal transplant patients [38],

Table 11.3 Progression of asymptomatic GI-FHON

Authors	Publication year	Underlying disease	Hip no.	Initial status	Follow-up period		Progression		Reference
					Mean	Range	Symptom	Collapse	
Kopecky et al.	1991	Kidney TPL	25		17 months	9–26	28 %	24 %	[11]
Sugano et al.	1994	SLE	16	Type A/B/C = 6/2/8	60 months	36–84	38 %	38 %	[7]
Kubo et al.	1997	Kidney TPL	23	Type A/B/C = 6/1/16	52 months	30–78	30 %	30 %	[78]
Sakamoto et al.	1997	10 SLE 4 DM/PM 1 MCTD 1 pemphigus 1 lymphoma	31	Grade A/B/C/D = 4/5/11/11	31 months	24–69	13 %	10 %	[79]
Yoshida et al.	2002	SLE	24	Type A/B/C = 8/4/12	51 months	12–95	29 %	4 %	[80]
Cheng et al.	2004	Solid organ TPL	30				37 %	–	[81]
Nakamura et al.	2010	SLE	251	Type A/B/C1/C2 = 6/7/42/42	163 months	120–240	–	35 %	[82]
Zhao et al.	2012	SARS	190	ARCO stage I/II = 168/22	>84 months		35 %	26 %	[83]

SARS severe acute respiratory syndrome, *SLE* systemic lupus erythematosus, *TPL* transplantation, *DM/PM* dermatomyositis/polymyositis, *MCTD* mixed connective tissue disease, *ARCO* Association Research Circulation Osseous, type C2 or grade D lesions extend beyond the acetabular edge early introduction of effective corticosteroid-sparing agents should be considered in such patients.

Once FHON develops, an assessment of FHON staging (refer to Chap. 28) should be made since the choice of treatment depends on the staging. To reduce weight bearing using canes, crutches, or a walker for about 6 weeks is the first acceptable treatment. Simple analgesics or nonsteroidal anti-inflammatory drugs can be prescribed for symptomatic treatments. However, no conservative or medical therapy has been proven to benefit patients with GI-FHON, and surgical treatment is inevitable in most symptomatic cases [84].

11.7.2 Medical Treatment

Based on hypothetical mechanisms, various therapeutic agents have been attempted in GI-FHON animal models. Among them, the preventive effect of statin and warfarin was evaluated in patients receiving glucocorticoids; the results concerning statin effects were controversial [85, 86], and warfarin treatment only tended to decrease symptomatic GI-FHON cases in SLE patients [87]. Additionally, enoxaparin, a low molecular weight heparin, is not helpful in GI-FHON patients [88]. A single-arm study reported that intravenous infusion of prostaglandin I_2 for 5 days decreased pain and radiographic outcomes in patients with bone marrow edema or early nontraumatic FHON [89]. However, some evidence suggests that alendronate is a candidate drug for the treatment of early GI-FHON. Although 7 (18 %) of the 40 study subjects had GI-FHON, a randomized controlled study demonstrated that alendronate (70 mg/week for 25 weeks) could significantly prevent the collapse of the femoral head in FHON patients with Steinberg stage IIC or IIIC [90]. A prospective open-label study, where 28 (47 %) of the 60 patients had GI-FHON, showed symptomatic improvement and minimal or no radiographic progression after 1 year of follow-up [91]. In another prospective study that included 26 (79 %) of the 33 patients with GI-FHON, alendronate (5 mg/day for 1 year) decreased the frequency of the femoral head collapse [92]. When the add-on effect of alendronate was studied for 4 years, combination therapy of multiple drilling and alendronate showed a significant benefit in GI-FHON patients with Ficat stages II and III [93]. However, a 2-year randomized double-blind study where 12 (23 %) of the 52 patients developed GI-FHON reported no significant effects in the 52 patients at stage IIC or IIIC [94]. Thus, further studies are warranted to confirm that alendronate is a potential option to postpone the need for hip surgery in patients with GI-FHON.

Recently, stem cell-based therapy has attracted attention. Because GI-FHON is believed to have limited reparative capacity partially secondary to decreased proliferation of mesenchymal stem cells, the approach could be acceptable [95]. In rabbit GI-FHON models, cell-based therapies using autologous bone marrow or mesenchymal stem cells, peripheral blood-derived mononuclear cells, or endogenital progenitor cells showed beneficial effects on progression prevention, vascularization, and bone regeneration of the femoral head [96–99]. A pilot controlled study was performed using autologous bone marrow mononuclear cells in 18 patients with early stage (I and II) FHON. Direct implantation of bone marrow-derived mononuclear cells into the femoral head resulted in a significant decrease in symptoms and collapse rate at 2 years [100]. In an observational study of SLE patients with GI-FHON, concentrated autologous bone marrow aspirate transplantation improved joint pain and resulted in a 40 % radiographic progression rate over a period of 41 months in patients with type C2 lesions [101]. Although several preclinical results showed promising benefits, cell-based therapies have not been widely used to treat GI-FHON, and there are no long-term and large-scale studies. Further clinical studies are needed to evaluate the availability and safety of the stem cell-based therapies in human patients.

11.7.3 Surgical Treatment

Various joint-preserving treatments have been proposed because of the failure of nonoperative treatments and the limited durability of prosthetics. Core decompression, vascularized fibular grafts, bone grafting, bone marrow grafting, and osteotomy have been applied to delay total hip replacement with variable outcomes (for detailed information, refer to Chap. 28). In advanced or symptomatic GI-FHON, total hip replacement is the treatment of choice.

11.8 Summary

Glucocorticoids are considered the most common cause of nontraumatic FHON and GI-FHON, which can develop in less than 30 % of patients receiving higher doses of glucocorticoids. Although the pathophysiological mechanisms have not yet been fully deduced, accumulation of glucocorticoid effects can lead to the development of GI-FHON in subjects with a genetic predisposition or an underlying disease that threatens bone and vascular tissue. The clinical features of GI-FHON are not different from those of other FHON. Clinical progression or subchondral collapse rates may be similar to or lower in asymptomatic GI-FHON than in other subtypes of nontraumatic FHON. Total hip replacement is eventually needed in many symptomatic cases. Efforts to use the minimal effective dose and to appropriately taper doses of glucocorticoids are essential to preventing GI-FHON. More studies are necessary to establish the effects of pharmacologic and non-pharmacologic joint-preserving therapies in patients with early stage GI-FHON.

References

1. Mason HL, Myers CS, Kendall EC. The chemistry of crystalline substances isolated from the suprarenal gland. J Biol Chem. 1936;114(3):613–31.
2. Hench PS, Kendall EC, Slocumb CH, Polley HF. The effect of a hormone of the adrenal cortex (17-hydroxy-11-dehydrocorticosterone: Compound E) and of pituitary adrenocorticotropic hormone on rheumatoid arthritis. Proc Staff Meet Mayo Clin. 1949;24:181–97.
3. Pietrogrande V, Mastromarino R. Osteopatia da prolongato trattamento cortisono. Orthop e Traumatol dell' Apparto Motore. 1957;25:791–810.
4. Arlet J. Nontraumatic avascular necrosis of the femoral head. Past, present, and future. Clin Orthop Relat Res. 1992;277:12–21.
5. Zizic TM, Marcoux C, Hungerford DS, Dansereau JV, Stevens MB. Corticosteroid therapy associated with ischemic necrosis of bone in systemic lupus erythematosus. Am J Med. 1985;79(5):596–604.
6. Ono K, Tohjima T, Komazawa T. Risk factors of avascular necrosis of the femoral head in patients with systemic lupus erythematosus under high-dose corticosteroid therapy. Clin Orthop Relat Res. 1992;277:89–97.
7. Sugano N, Ohzono K, Masuhara K, Takaoka K, Ono K. Prognostication of osteonecrosis of the femoral head in patients with systemic lupus erythematosus by magnetic resonance imaging. Clin Orthop Relat Res. 1994;305:190–9.
8. Oinuma K, Harada Y, Nawata Y, Takabayashi K, Abe I, Kamikawa K, Moriya H. Osteonecrosis in patients with systemic lupus erythematosus develops very early after starting high dose corticosteroid treatment. Ann Rheum Dis. 2001;60(12):1145–8.
9. Nakamura J, Saisu T, Yamashita K, Suzuki C, Kamegaya M, Takahashi K. Age at time of corticosteroid administration is a risk factor for osteonecrosis in pediatric patients with systemic lupus erythematosus: a prospective magnetic resonance imaging study. Arthritis Rheum. 2010;62(2):609–15.
10. Shigemura T, Nakamura J, Kishida S, Harada Y, Ohtori S, Kamikawa K, Ochiai N, Takahashi K. Incidence of osteonecrosis associated with corticosteroid therapy among different underlying diseases: prospective MRI study. Rheumatology (Oxford). 2011;50(11):2023–8.
11. Kopecky KK, Braunstein EM, Brandt KD, Filo RS, Leapman SB, Capello WN, Klatte EC. Apparent avascular necrosis of the hip: appearance and spontaneous resolution of MR findings in renal allograft recipients. Radiology. 1991;179(2):523–7.
12. Tervonen O, Mueller DM, Matteson EL, Velosa JA, Ginsburg WW, Ehman RL. Clinically occult avascular necrosis of the hip: prevalence in an asymptomatic population at risk. Radiology. 1992; 182(3):845–7.
13. Marston SB, Gillingham K, Bailey RF, Cheng EY. Osteonecrosis of the femoral head after solid organ transplantation: a prospective study. J Bone Joint Surg Am. 2002;84(12):2145–51.
14. Shibatani M, Fujioka M, Arai Y, Takahashi K, Ueshima K, Okamoto M, Yoshimura N, Hirota Y, Fukushima W, Kubo T. Degree of corticosteroid treatment within the first 2 months of renal transplantation has a strong influence on the incidence of osteonecrosis of the femoral head. Acta Orthop. 2008;79(5):631–6.
15. Guichelaar MM, Schmoll J, Malinchoc M, Hay JE. Fractures and avascular necrosis before and after orthotopic liver transplantation: long-term follow-up and predictive factors. Hepatology. 2007;46(4):1198–207.
16. Ribeiro RC, Fletcher BD, Kennedy W, Harrison PL, Neel MD, Kaste SC, Sandlund JT, Rubnitz JE, Razzouk BI, Relling MV, Pui CH. Magnetic resonance imaging detection of avascular necrosis of the bone in children receiving intensive prednisone therapy for acute lymphoblastic leukemia or non-Hodgkin lymphoma. Leukemia. 2001;15(6):891–7.
17. Tauchmanovà L, De Rosa G, Serio B, Fazioli F, Mainolfi C, Lombardi G, Colao A, Salvatore M, Rotoli B, Selleri C. Avascular necrosis in long-term survivors after allogeneic or autologous stem cell transplantation: a single center experience and a review. Cancer. 2003;97(10):2453–61.
18. Talamo G, Angtuaco E, Walker RC, Dong L, Miceli MH, Zangari M, Tricot G, Barlogie B, Anaissie E. Avascular necrosis of femoral and/or humeral heads in multiple myeloma: results of a prospective study of patients treated with dexamethasone-based regimens and high-dose chemotherapy. J Clin Oncol. 2005;23(22):5217–23.
19. Schulte CM, Beelen DW. Low pretransplant bone-mineral density and rapid bone loss do not increase risk for avascular osteonecrosis after allogeneic hematopoietic stem cell transplantation. Transplantation. 2005;79(12):1748–55.
20. Niinimäki RA, Harila-Saari AH, Jartti AE, Seuri RM, Riikonen PV, Pääkkö EL, Möttönen MI, Lanning M. High body mass index increases the risk for osteonecrosis in children with acute lymphoblastic leukemia. J Clin Oncol. 2007;25(12):1498–504.
21. te Winkel ML, Pieters R, Hop WC, de Groot-Kruseman HA, Lequin MH, van der Sluis IM, Bökkerink JP, Leeuw JA, Bruin MC, Egeler RM, Veerman AJ, van den Heuvel-Eibrink MM. Prospective study on incidence, risk factors, and long-term outcome of osteonecrosis in pediatric acute lymphoblastic leukemia. J Clin Oncol. 2011;29(31):4143–50.
22. Kawedia JD, Kaste SC, Pei D, Panetta JC, Cai X, Cheng C, Neale G, Howard SC, Evans WE, Pui CH, Relling MV. Pharmacokinetic, pharmacodynamic, and pharmacogenetic determinants of osteonecrosis in children with acute lymphoblastic leukemia. Blood. 2011;117(8):2340–7.
23. Wing PC, Nance P, Connell DG, Gagnon F. Risk of avascular necrosis following short term megadose methylprednisolone treatment. Spinal Cord. 1998;36(9):633–6.
24. Felson DT, Anderson JJ. Across-study evaluation of association between steroid dose and bolus steroids and avascular necrosis of bone. Lancet. 1987;1(8538):902–6.
25. Motomura G, Yamamoto T, Irisa T, Miyanishi K, Nishida K, Iwamoto Y. Dose effects of corticosteroids on the development of osteonecrosis in rabbits. J Rheumatol. 2008;35(12):2395–9.
26. Miyanishi K, Yamamoto T, Irisa T, Motomura G, Jingushi S, Sueishi K, Iwamoto Y. Effects of different corticosteroids on the development of osteonecrosis in rabbits. Rheumatology (Oxford). 2005;44(3):332–6.
27. Kabata T, Kubo T, Matsumoto T, Hirata T, Fujioka M, Takahashi KA, Yagishita S, Kobayashi M, Tomita K. Onset of steroid-induced osteonecrosis in rabbits and its relationship to hyperlipaemia and increased free fatty acids. Rheumatology (Oxford). 2005;44(10): 1233–7.
28. Masada T, Iwakiri K, Oda Y, Kaneshiro Y, Iwaki H, Ohashi H, Takaoka K. Increased hepatic cytochrome P4503A activity decreases the risk of developing steroid-induced osteonecrosis in a rabbit model. J Orthop Res. 2008;26(1):91–5.
29. Massardo L, Jacobelli S, Leissner M, González M, Villarroel L, Rivero S. High-dose intravenous methylprednisolone therapy associated with osteonecrosis in patients with systemic lupus erythematosus. Lupus. 1992;1(6):401–5.
30. Gladman DD, Urowitz MB, Chaudhry-Ahluwalia V, Hallet DC, Cook RJ. Predictive factors for symptomatic osteonecrosis in patients with systemic lupus erythematosus. J Rheumatol. 2001; 28(4):761–5.
31. Nagasawa K, Tada Y, Koarada S, Horiuchi T, Tsukamoto H, Murai K, Ueda A, Yoshizawa S, Ohta A. Very early development of steroid-associated osteonecrosis of femoral head in systemic lupus erythematosus: prospective study by MRI. Lupus. 2005;14(5): 385–90.
32. Calvo-Alén J, McGwin G, Toloza S, Fernández M, Roseman JM, Bastian HM, Cepeda EJ, González EB, Baethge BA, Fessler BJ,

Vilá LM, Reveille JD, Alarcón GS. LUMINA Study Group. Systemic lupus erythematosus in a multiethnic US cohort (LUMINA): XXIV. Cytotoxic treatment is an additional risk factor for the development of symptomatic osteonecrosis in lupus patients: results of a nested matched case-control study. Ann Rheum Dis. 2006;65(6):785–90.
33. Prasad R, Ibanez D, Gladman D, Urowitz M. The role of non-corticosteroid related factors in osteonecrosis (ON) in systemic lupus erythematosus: a nested case-control study of inception patients. Lupus. 2007;16(3):157–62.
34. Sekiya F, Yamaji K, Yang K, Tsuda H, Takasaki Y. Investigation of occurrence of osteonecrosis of the femoral head after increasing corticosteroids in patients with recurring systemic lupus erythematosus. Rheumatol Int. 2010;30(12):1587–93.
35. Mont MA, Glueck CJ, Pacheco IH, Wang P, Hungerford DS, Petri M. Risk factors for osteonecrosis in systemic lupus erythematosus. J Rheumatol. 1997;24(4):654–62.
36. Sheikh JS, Retzinger GS, Hess EV. Association of osteonecrosis in systemic lupus erythematosus with abnormalities of fibrinolysis. Lupus. 1998;7(1):42–8.
37. Houssiau FA, N'Zeusseu Toukap A, Depresseux G, Maldague BE, Malghem J, Devogelaer JP, Vande Berg BC. Magnetic resonance imaging-detected avascular osteonecrosis in systemic lupus erythematosus: lack of correlation with antiphospholipid antibodies. Br J Rheumatol. 1998;37(4):448–53.
38. Hedri H, Cherif M, Zouaghi K, Abderrahim E, Goucha R, Ben Hamida F, Ben Abdallah T, Elyounsi F, Ben Moussa F, Ben Maiz H, Kheder A. Avascular osteonecrosis after renal transplantation. Transplant Proc. 2007;39(4):1036–8.
39. Patton PR, Pfaff WW. Aseptic bone necrosis after renal transplantation. Surgery. 1988;103(1):63–8.
40. Fink JC, Leisenring WM, Sullivan KM, Sherrard DJ, Weiss NS. Avascular necrosis following bone marrow transplantation: a case-control study. Bone. 1998;22(1):67–71.
41. Inoue S, Horii M, Asano T, Fujioka M, Ogura T, Shibatani M, Kim WC, Nakagawa M, Tanaka T, Hirota Y, Kubo T. Risk factors for nontraumatic osteonecrosis of the femoral head after renal transplantation. J Orthop Sci. 2003;8(6):751–6.
42. Hirata T, Fujioka M, Takahashi KA, Asano T, Ishida M, Akioka K, Okamoto M, Yoshimura N, Satomi Y, Nishino H, Hirota Y, Nakajima S, Kato S, Kubo T. Low molecular weight phenotype of Apo(a) is a risk factor of corticosteroid-induced osteonecrosis of the femoral head after renal transplant. J Rheumatol. 2007;34(3):516–22.
43. Vora A. Management of osteonecrosis in children and young adults with acute lymphoblastic leukaemia. Br J Haematol. 2011;155(5):549–60.
44. Mattano Jr LA, Devidas M, Nachman JB, Sather HN, Hunger SP, Steinherz PG, Gaynon PS, Seibel NL. Children's Oncology Group. Effect of alternate-week versus continuous dexamethasone scheduling on the risk of osteonecrosis in paediatric patients with acute lymphoblastic leukaemia: results from the CCG-1961 randomised cohort trial. Lancet Oncol. 2012;13(9):906–15.
45. Campbell S, Sun CL, Kurian S, Francisco L, Carter A, Kulkarni S, Parker P, Karanes C, Forman SJ, Bhatia S. Predictors of avascular necrosis of bone in long-term survivors of hematopoietic cell transplantation. Cancer. 2009;115(18):4127–35.
46. Kenzora JE, Glimcher MJ. Accumulative cell stress: the multifactorial etiology of idiopathic osteonecrosis. Orthop Clin North Am. 1985;16(4):669–79.
47. Weinstein RS. Glucocorticoid-induced osteoporosis and osteonecrosis. Endocrinol Metab Clin North Am. 2012;41(3):595–611.
48. O'Brien CA, Jia D, Plotkin LI, Bellido T, Powers CC, Stewart SA, Manolagas SC, Weinstein RS. Glucocorticoids act directly on osteoblasts and osteocytes to induce their apoptosis and reduce bone formation and strength. Endocrinology. 2004;145(4):1835–41.
49. Jia D, O'Brien CA, Stewart SA, Manolagas SC, Weinstein RS. Glucocorticoids act directly on osteoclasts to increase their life span and reduce bone density. Endocrinology. 2006;147(12):5592–9.
50. Hofbauer LC, Gori F, Riggs BL, Lacey DL, Dunstan CR, Spelsberg TC, Khosla S. Stimulation of osteoprotegerin ligand and inhibition of osteoprotegerin production by glucocorticoids in human osteoblastic lineage cells: potential paracrine mechanisms of glucocorticoid-induced osteoporosis. Endocrinology. 1999;140(10):4382–9.
51. Rubin J, Biskobing DM, Jadhav L, Fan D, Nanes MS, Perkins S, Fan X. Dexamethasone promotes expression of membrane-bound macrophage colony-stimulating factor in murine osteoblast-like cells. Endocrinology. 1998;139(3):1006–12.
52. Kim HJ, Zhao H, Kitaura H, Bhattacharyya S, Brewer JA, Muglia LJ, Ross FP, Teitelbaum SL. Glucocorticoids suppress bone formation via the osteoclast. J Clin Invest. 2006;116(8):2152–60.
53. Kim HJ. New understanding of glucocorticoid action in bone cells. BMB Rep. 2010;43(8):524–9.
54. Canalis E, Delany AM. Mechanisms of glucocorticoid action in bone. Ann N Y Acad Sci. 2002;966:73–81.
55. Subramaniam M, Colvard D, Keeting PE, Rasmussen K, Riggs BL, Spelsberg TC. Glucocorticoid regulation of alkaline phosphatase, osteocalcin, and proto-oncogenes in normal human osteoblast-like cells. J Cell Biochem. 1992;50(4):411–24.
56. Rochefort GY, Pallu S, Benhamou CL. Osteocyte: the unrecognized side of bone tissue. Osteoporos Int. 2010;21(9):1457–69.
57. Weinstein RS, Nicholas RW, Manolagas SC. Apoptosis of osteocytes in glucocorticoid-induced osteonecrosis of the hip. J Clin Endocrinol Metab. 2000;85(8):2907–12.
58. Riddle RC, Leslie JM, Gross TS, Clemens TL. Hypoxia-inducible factor-1α protein negatively regulates load-induced bone formation. J Biol Chem. 2011;286(52):44449–56.
59. Peckett AJ, Wright DC, Riddell MC. The effects of glucocorticoids on adipose tissue lipid metabolism. Metabolism. 2011;60(11):1500–10.
60. Motomura G, Yamamoto T, Miyanishi K, Yamashita A, Sueishi K, Iwamoto Y. Bone marrow fat-cell enlargement in early steroid-induced osteonecrosis – a histomorphometric study of autopsy cases. Pathol Res Pract. 2005;200(11–12):807–11.
61. Kitajima M, Shigematsu M, Ogawa K, Sugihara H, Hotokebuchi T. Effects of glucocorticoid on adipocyte size in human bone marrow. Med Mol Morphol. 2007;40(3):150–6.
62. Miyanishi K, Yamamoto T, Irisa T, Yamashita A, Jingushi S, Noguchi Y, Iwamoto Y. Bone marrow fat cell enlargement and a rise in intraosseous pressure in steroid-treated rabbits with osteonecrosis. Bone. 2002;30(1):185–90.
63. Girod JP, Brotman DJ. Does altered glucocorticoid homeostasis increase cardiovascular risk? Cardiovasc Res. 2004;64(2):217–26.
64. Ullian ME. The role of corticosteroids in the regulation of vascular tone. Cardiovasc Res. 1999;41(1):55–64.
65. Kanse SM, Takahashi K, Warren JB, Ghatei M, Bloom SR. Glucocorticoids induce endothelin release from vascular smooth muscle cells but not endothelial cells. Eur J Pharmacol. 1991;199(1):99–101.
66. Iuchi T, Akaike M, Mitsui T, Ohshima Y, Shintani Y, Azuma H, Matsumoto T. Glucocorticoid excess induces superoxide production in vascular endothelial cells and elicits vascular endothelial dysfunction. Circ Res. 2003;92(1):81–7.
67. Vogt CJ, Schmid-Schönbein GW. Microvascular endothelial cell death and rarefaction in the glucocorticoid-induced hypertensive rat. Microcirculation. 2001;8(2):129–39.
68. Yang C, Yang S, Du J, Li J, Xu W, Xiong Y. Vascular endothelial growth factor gene transfection to enhance the repair of avascular necrosis of the femoral head of rabbit. Chin Med J (Engl). 2003;116(10):1544–8.
69. Weinstein RS, Wan C, Liu Q, Wang Y, Almeida M, O'Brien CA, Thostenson J, Roberson PK, Boskey AL, Clemens TL,

Manolagas SC. Endogenous glucocorticoids decrease skeletal angiogenesis, vascularity, hydration, and strength in aged mice. Aging Cell. 2010;9(2):147–61.

70. Logie JJ, Ali S, Marshall KM, Heck MM, Walker BR, Hadoke PW. Glucocorticoid-mediated inhibition of angiogenic changes in human endothelial cells is not caused by reductions in cell proliferation or migration. PLoS One. 2010;5(12):e14476.
71. Shikatani EA, Trifonova A, Mandel ER, Liu ST, Roudier E, Krylova A, Szigiato A, Beaudry J, Riddell MC, Haas TL. Inhibition of proliferation, migration and proteolysis contribute to corticosterone-mediated inhibition of angiogenesis. PLoS One. 2012;7(10): e46625.
72. Harada I. The effects of glucocorticoids on angiogenesis in vitro. Nihon Seikeigeka Gakkai Zasshi. 1992;66(7):763–70.
73. Kerachian MA, Séguin C, Harvey EJ. Glucocorticoids in osteonecrosis of the femoral head: a new understanding of the mechanisms of action. J Steroid Biochem Mol Biol. 2009;114(3–5):121–8.
74. van Zaane B, Nur E, Squizzato A, Gerdes VE, Büller HR, Dekkers OM, Brandjes DP. Systematic review on the effect of glucocorticoid use on procoagulant, anti-coagulant and fibrinolytic factors. J Thromb Haemost. 2010;8(11):2483–93.
75. Kerachian MA, Cournoyer D, Harvey EJ, Chow TY, Neagoe PE, Sirois MG, Séguin C. Effect of high-dose dexamethasone on endothelial haemostatic gene expression and neutrophil adhesion. J Steroid Biochem Mol Biol. 2009;116(3–5):127–33.
76. Takao M, Sugano N, Nishii T, Miki H, Sato Y, Tamura S, Yoshikawa H. Longitudinal quantitative evaluation of lesion size change in femoral head osteonecrosis using three-dimensional magnetic resonance imaging and image registration. J Orthop Res. 2006;24(6):1231–9.
77. Mont MA, Ulrich SD, Seyler TM, Smith JM, Marker DR, McGrath MS, Hungerford DS, Jones LC. Bone scanning of limited value for diagnosis of symptomatic oligofocal and multifocal osteonecrosis. J Rheumatol. 2008;35(8):1629–34.
78. Kubo T, Yamazoe S, Sugano N, Fujioka M, Naruse S, Yoshimura N, Oka T, Hirasawa Y. Initial MRI findings of non-traumatic osteonecrosis of the femoral head in renal allograft recipients. Magn Reson Imaging. 1997;15(9):1017–23.
79. Sakamoto M, Shimizu K, Iida S, Akita T, Moriya H, Nawata Y. Osteonecrosis of the femoral head: a prospective study with MRI. J Bone Joint Surg Br. 1997;79(2):213–9.
80. Yoshida T, Kanayama Y, Okamura M, Negoro N, Inoue T, Yoshikawa J. Long-term observation of avascular necrosis of the femoral head in systemic lupus erythematosus: an MRI study. Clin Exp Rheumatol. 2002;20(4):525–30.
81. Cheng EY, Thongtrangan I, Laorr A, Saleh KJ. Spontaneous resolution of osteonecrosis of the femoral head. J Bone Joint Surg Am. 2004;86-A(12):2594–9.
82. Nakamura J, Harada Y, Oinuma K, Iida S, Kishida S, Takahashi K. Spontaneous repair of asymptomatic osteonecrosis associated with corticosteroid therapy in systemic lupus erythematosus: 10-year minimum follow-up with MRI. Lupus. 2010;19(11):1307–14.
83. Zhao FC, Guo KJ, Li ZR. Osteonecrosis of the femoral head in SARS patients: seven years later. Eur J Orthop Surg Traumatol. 2013;23(6):671–7.
84. Mont MA, Zywiel MG, Marker DR, McGrath MS, Delanois RE. The natural history of untreated asymptomatic osteonecrosis of the femoral head: a systematic literature review. J Bone Joint Surg Am. 2010;92(12):2165–70.
85. Ajmal M, Matas AJ, Kuskowski M, Cheng EY. Does statin usage reduce the risk of corticosteroid-related osteonecrosis in renal transplant population? Orthop Clin North Am. 2009;40(2):235–9.
86. Pritchett JW. Statin therapy decreases the risk of osteonecrosis in patients receiving steroids. Clin Orthop Relat Res. 2001;386: 173–8.
87. Nagasawa K, Tada Y, Koarada S, Tsukamoto H, Horiuchi T, Yoshizawa S, Murai K, Ueda A, Haruta Y, Ohta A. Prevention of steroid-induced osteonecrosis of femoral head in systemic lupus erythematosus by anti-coagulant. Lupus. 2006;15(6):354–7.
88. Glueck CJ, Freiberg RA, Sieve L, Wang P. Enoxaparin prevents progression of stages I and II osteonecrosis of the hip. Clin Orthop Relat Res. 2005;435:164–70.
89. Jäger M, Tillmann FP, Thornhill TS, Mahmoudi M, Blondin D, Hetzel GR, Zilkens C, Krauspe R. Rationale for prostaglandin I2 in bone marrow oedema: from theory to application. Arthritis Res Ther. 2008;10(5):R120.
90. Lai KA, Shen WJ, Yang CY, Shao CJ, Hsu JT, Lin RM. The use of alendronate to prevent early collapse of the femoral head in patients with nontraumatic osteonecrosis. A randomized clinical study. J Bone Joint Surg Am. 2005;87(10):2155–9.
91. Agarwala S, Jain D, Joshi VR, Sule A. Efficacy of alendronate, a bisphosphonate, in the treatment of AVN of the hip. A prospective open-label study. Rheumatology (Oxford). 2005;44(3):352–9.
92. Nishii T, Sugano N, Miki H, Hashimoto J, Yoshikawa H. Does alendronate prevent collapse in osteonecrosis of the femoral head? Clin Orthop Relat Res. 2006;443:273–9.
93. Kang P, Pei F, Shen B, Zhou Z, Yang J. Are the results of multiple drilling and alendronate for osteonecrosis of the femoral head better than those of multiple drilling? A pilot study. Joint Bone Spine. 2012;79(1):67–72.
94. Chen CH, Chang JK, Lai KA, Hou SM, Chang CH, Wang GJ. Alendronate in the prevention of collapse of the femoral head in nontraumatic osteonecrosis: a two-year multicenter, prospective, randomized, double-blind, placebo-controlled study. Arthritis Rheum. 2012;64(5):1572–8.
95. Wang BL, Sun W, Shi ZC, Lou JN, Zhang NF, Shi SH, Guo WS, Cheng LM, Ye LY, Zhang WJ, Li ZR. Decreased proliferation of mesenchymal stem cells in corticosteroid-induced osteonecrosis of femoral head. Orthopedics. 2008;31(5):444.
96. Asada T, Kushida T, Umeda M, Oe K, Matsuya H, Wada T, Sasai K, Ikehara S, Iida H. Prevention of corticosteroid-induced osteonecrosis in rabbits by intra-bone marrow injection of autologous bone marrow cells. Rheumatology (Oxford). 2008;47(5):591–6.
97. Matsuya H, Kushida T, Asada T, Umeda M, Wada T, Iida H. Regenerative effects of transplanting autologous mesenchymal stem cells on corticosteroid-induced osteonecrosis in rabbits. Mod Rheumatol. 2008;18(2):132–9.
98. Terayama H, Ishikawa M, Yasunaga Y, Yamasaki T, Hamaki T, Asahara T, Ochi M. Prevention of osteonecrosis by intravenous administration of human peripheral blood-derived CD34-positive cells in a rat osteonecrosis model. J Tissue Eng Regen Med. 2011;5(1):32–40.
99. Sun Y, Feng Y, Zhang C, Cheng X, Chen S, Ai Z, Zeng B. Beneficial effect of autologous transplantation of endothelial progenitor cells on steroid-induced femoral head osteonecrosis in rabbits. Cell Transplant. 2011;20(2):233–43.
100. Gangji V, Hauzeur JP, Matos C, et al. Treatment of osteonecrosis of the femoral head with implantation of autologous bone marrow cells. A pilot study. J Bone Joint Surg Am. 2004;86-A:1153–60.
101. Yoshioka T, Mishima H, Akaogi H, Sakai S, Li M, Ochiai N. Concentrated autologous bone marrow aspirate transplantation treatment for corticosteroid-induced osteonecrosis of the femoral head in systemic lupus erythematosus. Int Orthop. 2011;35(6): 823–9.

Corticosteroid Usage and Osteonecrosis of the Hip

12

Jeffrey J. Cherian, Bhaveen H. Kapadia, Samik Banerjee, Julio J. Jauregui, and Michael A. Mont

12.1 Introduction

The disease process of atraumatic osteonecrosis was first described as ischemic necrosis of the hip [1]. This pathological process can lead to destructive arthritis in multiple joints, most commonly occurring in the hips, knees, shoulders, and ankles [1]. Currently, there is no consensus on the pathophysiological mechanism of osteonecrosis, but it is thought to be multifactorial in nature. However, there are certain direct risk factors implicated in the development of osteonecrosis such as trauma, radiation, Caisson's disease, and sickle cell disease [2]. In addition, various other risk factors have been shown to have a direct correlation with osteonecrosis such as corticosteroids, habitual alcohol intake, hyperlipidemia, chemotherapeutic agents, systemic lupus erythematosus, lipid storage diseases, and inflammatory bowel disease [3, 4].

In 1958, Chandler and Wright described the adverse effects of high-dose intra-articular corticosteroid injection [5]. Later in 1960, Heimann and Freiberger noticed similar results seen with high-dose oral corticosteroids on the femoral and humeral head [6]. Although there are several theories behind corticosteroid-induced osteonecrosis, it is generally thought to be caused by vascular compromise to the femoral head. The most widely accepted mechanism of corticosteroid-induced osteonecrosis results from adipocyte hypertrophy which increases intraosseous pressure causing extramural compression of the vasculature to the femoral head [7]. This leads to a disruption in blood flow, which causes a lack of delivered vital nutrients. In addition, corticosteroids have been found to cause a decrease in osteoclast and osteoblast activity, which subsequently results in decreased bony turnover, trabecular width, density, and formation [8].

Recently, numerous studies have shown there to be a direct correlation between the use of high-dose corticosteroids and the increased risk of osteonecrosis. It is widely accepted that doses greater than 2 g over a 3-month interval impart the greatest risk for the development of corticosteroid-induced osteonecrosis [2]. This chapter therefore aims to evaluate the effects of corticosteroids on the incidence of osteonecrosis of the hip, particularly in relation to dosing, and duration of treatment, and the effects of pulse therapy.

12.2 Treatment Dosing

Current studies demonstrate that there is a direct correlation between the incidence of osteonecrosis and the use of corticosteroids. A recent study by Felson et al. demonstrated that the incidence of corticosteroid-induced osteonecrosis may be increasing due to higher dosing regimens. The authors found there to be a 4.6 % increase in incidence of osteonecrosis with every 10 mg/day increase in corticosteroid use. Additionally, it was seen that the daily dose of corticosteroid may be one of the greatest risk factors for osteonecrosis ($R^2=0.75$) [9]. Similarly, the incidence of osteonecrosis has been reported to be higher with a mean daily dose of >40 mg/day. Shigemura et al. in a prospective randomized study found a fourfold increase in the risk of osteonecrosis with the use >40 mg/day of corticosteroids ($OR=4.2$; $p=0.001$). This study showed that an increase in the mean daily dose may result in an increased incidence of osteonecrosis [10].

In a prospective study of 45 patients diagnosed with systemic lupus erythematosus (SLE), Nagasawa et al. examined the dose–response relationship with development of osteonecrosis over a 5-year period. During this period patients had magnetic resonance imaging (MRI) evaluations every year following initiation of 40 mg/day of corticosteroid therapy. The authors demonstrated that the cohort who developed

J.J. Cherian • B.H. Kapadia • S. Banerjee • J.J. Jauregui
M.A. Mont (✉)
Department of Orthopaedic Surgery, Rubin Institute for Advanced Orthopedics, Center for Joint Preservation and Replacement, Sinai Hospital of Baltimore, 2401 West Belvedere Avenue, Baltimore, MD 21215, USA
e-mail: jjaicherian@gmail.com; bhaveen.k@gmail.com; bashb02@gmail.com; juljau@gmail.com; mmont@lifebridgehealth.org, rhondamont@aol.com

K.-H. Koo et al. (eds.), *Osteonecrosis*,
DOI 10.1007/978-3-642-35767-1_12,

osteonecrosis had a significantly higher proportion of patients who received >1,000 mg/day of corticosteroids than that group of patients who demonstrated no radiographic evidence of the disease (87 % versus 37 %; $p<0.01$) [11].

Studies have also demonstrated that patients receiving a cumulative dose of corticosteroids >2 g are at a higher risk for developing osteonecrosis. A retrospective study by Nakamura et al., who examined 201 SLE patients over a 13-year period, demonstrated that 15 % of patients who received high corticosteroid doses had increased risks of developing osteonecrosis [4].

The cumulative corticosteroid dosage has been shown to have a direct association with the risk of osteonecrosis. In particular, a study by Shjibatani et al. found that patients who have had renal transplantation are at a potentially higher risk of developing osteonecrosis. The authors found that patients who received ≤1,795 mg and >1,795 mg of cumulative steroid dosing over an 8-week period after renal transplantation had higher risks of developing osteonecrosis compared to those who received less than 1,400 mg of corticosteroids (hazards ratio, 2.9 and 3.2, respectively; $p=0.07$ and 0.07, respectively) [12].

Despite the positive correlation seen in the previous studies, a prospective study by Ono et al. showed that there may be no correlation between corticosteroid use and development of osteonecrosis. This study consisted of 62 patients with SLE who were treated with 30 mg/day of corticosteroids for at least 30 days. The authors found no significant correlation between the mean dose, the total cumulative usage, and the duration of high-dose corticosteroids and the subsequent risk of developing osteonecrosis [13]. It is possible that limiting corticosteroid use to the lowest dose possible that is medically effective may minimize the risk of osteonecrosis.

12.3 Treatment Duration

Another independent risk factor associated with an increased risk of osteonecrosis is the duration of corticosteroid treatment. A study by Nakamura et al. observed the risk of osteonecrosis in relation to the dose and duration in 201 SLE (537 joints) patients over a 13-year period [4]. This study demonstrated a direct association between osteonecrosis risk and longer duration of corticosteroid use, as well as with increased doses required for patients who had recurrent episodes. The authors found that 238 out of the 537 joints developed osteonecrosis at an average of 26 years of age. Additionally, a study by Li et al. evaluated the correlation between osteonecrosis and corticosteroid in 539 patients with severe acute respiratory syndrome. In relation to duration of treatment, the authors found that patients who developed osteonecrosis received corticosteroids for a significantly longer duration when compared to patients who did not develop the disease (38 ± 17 versus 27 ± 15 days; $p<0.01$) [14].

However, no studies were found refuting that increased duration of treatment increased the risk of osteonecrosis. It is postulated that this could have been a compounding variable with higher dosages as well. Therefore, it may be important to minimize treatment to the shortest duration feasible.

12.4 Pulsed Therapy

Pulsed therapy refers to the intermittent administration of corticosteroids at suprapharmacologic dosages intravenously [15]. A study by Ce et al. compared 60 patients who had multiple sclerosis and were treated with corticosteroids to a group who had multiple sclerosis but did not receive corticosteroid treatment. The authors found from MRI evaluation that patients had a significantly higher risk for developing osteonecrosis with treatment of >10 g of cumulative pulsed corticosteroid dose, compared to the matched group (15.5 % versus 0 %; $p=0.043$) [16]. However, it is uncertain whether the positive correlation seen in this study is from the treatment with pulsed corticosteroids or the higher cumulative dose. Similarly, a study by Lausten et al. of 374 renal transplant patients found that patients who were treated with pulsed corticosteroid therapy ($n=34$) had a significantly higher rate of osteonecrosis when compared to treatment without pulsed therapy ($n=22$; $p<0.05$) [17].

However, a study by Oinuma et al. of 72 patients with SLE showed that there was no significant difference in the incidence of osteonecrosis with the use of pulsed therapy. The authors found that 45 % (18 of 40) of patients who had osteonecrosis received pulsed corticosteroid therapy when compared to 53 % (17 of 32) of patients without osteonecrosis who received pulsed therapy. However, this study failed to mention the dosage of pulsed corticosteroid therapy [18].

The current use of pulsed therapy has shown to have conflicting results in association with the development of osteonecrosis. Due to a lack of concordance between studies, larger prospective randomized studies are needed to determine a cause-effect relationship between pulsed therapy and osteonecrosis.

Conclusion

Treatment with corticosteroids may have up to a tenfold increase in the risk of developing osteonecrosis. Additionally, patients receiving higher mean doses have been shown to be at an even higher increased risk of osteonecrosis. However, it is uncertain whether corticosteroid duration and cumulative dose have an effect on the incidence of osteonecrosis. It is believed that it may be a compounding factor along with the underlying disease. Furthermore, the reported studies demonstrate the pulsed corticosteroids may also increase the risk of osteonecrosis. Based on the current literature, it is believed that minimizing the dosage and duration of corticosteroid treatment may potentially minimize the risk of developing osteonecrosis. Due to paucity of reports, we believe that larger prospective studies are needed to assess the effects of corticosteroids on the incidence of osteonecrosis. Furthermore, molecular studies may be important in elucidating the pathogenetic mechanism of corticosteroids and osteonecrosis.

References

1. Johnson AJ, Mont MA, Tsao AK, Jones LC. Treatment of femoral head osteonecrosis in the united states: 16-year analysis of the nationwide inpatient sample. Clin Orthop Relat Res. 2013. doi:10.1007/s11999-013-3220-3.
2. Mont MA, Jones LC, Hungerford DS. Nontraumatic osteonecrosis of the femoral head: ten years later. J Bone Joint Surg Am. 2006;88(5):1117–32. doi:10.2106/JBJS.E.01041. 88/5/1117 [pii].
3. Seguin C, Kassis J, Busque L, Bestawros A, Theodoropoulos J, Alonso ML, Harvey EJ. Non-traumatic necrosis of bone (osteonecrosis) is associated with endothelial cell activation but not thrombophilia. Rheumatology (Oxford). 2008;47(8):1151–5. doi:10.1093/rheumatology/ken206.
4. Nakamura J, Harada Y, Oinuma K, Iida S, Kishida S, Takahashi K. Spontaneous repair of asymptomatic osteonecrosis associated with corticosteroid therapy in systemic lupus erythematosus: 10-year minimum follow-up with mri. Lupus. 2010;19(11):1307–14. doi:10.1177/0961203310372951. 0961203310372951 [pii].
5. Chandler GN, Wright V. Deleterious effect of intra-articular hydrocortisone. Lancet. 1958;2(7048):661–3.
6. Heimann WG, Freiberger RH. Avascular necrosis of the femoral and humeral heads after high-dosage corticosteroid therapy. New Engl J Med. 1960;263:672–5. doi:10.1056/NEJM196010062631404.
7. Sheng H, Sheng CJ, Cheng XY, Zhang G, Lee KM, Leung KS, Qu S, Qin L. Pathomorphological changes of bone marrow adipocytes in process of steroid-associated osteonecrosis. Int J Clin Exp Pathol. 2013;6(6):1046–50.
8. Powell C, Chang C, Gershwin ME. Current concepts on the pathogenesis and natural history of steroid-induced osteonecrosis. Clin Rev Allergy Immunol. 2011;41(1):102–13. doi:10.1007/s12016-010-8217-z.
9. Felson DT, Anderson JJ. Across-study evaluation of association between steroid dose and bolus steroids and avascular necrosis of bone. Lancet. 1987;1(8538):902–6.
10. Shigemura T, Nakamura J, Kishida S, Harada Y, Ohtori S, Kamikawa K, Ochiai N, Takahashi K. Incidence of osteonecrosis associated with corticosteroid therapy among different underlying diseases: prospective mri study. Rheumatology (Oxford). 2011;50(11):2023–8. doi:10.1093/rheumatology/ker277.
11. Nagasawa K, Tada Y, Koarada S, Horiuchi T, Tsukamoto H, Murai K, Ueda A, Yoshizawa S, Ohta A. Very early development of steroid-associated osteonecrosis of femoral head in systemic lupus erythematosus: prospective study by MRI. Lupus. 2005;14(5):385–90. doi:10.1191/0961203305lu2103oa.
12. Shibatani M, Fujioka M, Arai Y, Takahashi K, Ueshima K, Okamoto M, Yoshimura N, Hirota Y, Fukushima W, Kubo T. Degree of corticosteroid treatment within the first 2 months of renal transplantation has a strong influence on the incidence of osteonecrosis of the femoral head. Acta Orthop. 2008;79(5):631–6. doi:10.1080/17453670810016641.
13. Ono K, Tohjima T, Komazawa T. Risk factors of avascular necrosis of the femoral head in patients with systemic lupus erythematosus under high-dose corticosteroid therapy. Clin Orthop Relat Res. 1992;277:89–97.
14. Li ZR, Sun W, Qu H, Zhou YX, Dou BX, Shi ZC, Zhang NF, Cheng XG, Wang DL, Guo WS. Clinical research of correlation between osteonecrosis and steroid. Zhonghua wai ke za zhi [Chin J Surg]. 2005;43(16):1048–53.
15. Sinha A, Bagga A. Pulse steroid therapy. Indian J Pediatr. 2008;75(10):1057–66. doi:10.1007/s12098-008-0210-7.
16. Ce P, Gedizlioglu M, Gelal F, Coban P, Ozbek G. Avascular necrosis of the bones: an overlooked complication of pulse steroid treatment of multiple sclerosis. Eur J Neurol. 2006;13(8):857–61. doi:10.1111/j.1468-1331.2006.01375.x.
17. Lausten GS, Jensen JS, Olgaard K. Necrosis of the femoral head after renal transplantation. Acta Orthop Scand. 1988; 59(6):650–4.
18. Oinuma K, Harada Y, Nawata Y, Takabayashi K, Abe I, Kamikawa K, Moriya H. Osteonecrosis in patients with systemic lupus erythematosus develops very early after starting high dose corticosteroid treatment. Ann Rheum Dis. 2001;60(12):1145–8.

13 Alcohol

Wakaba Fukushima and Yoshio Hirota

13.1 Introduction

Osteonecrosis is a condition of bone death leading to joint pain, bone destruction, and loss of function. Nontraumatic osteonecrosis, a disease entity in which the underlying etiology and pathogenesis have not been fully elucidated, commonly involves the femoral heads. Although a wide spectrum of conditions, including systemic steroid administration, that are potentially related to nontraumatic osteonecrosis of the femoral head (ONFH) have been reported so far [1–5], alcohol consumption continues to be important as an environmental factor. In this chapter, we present a summary of the descriptive and analytic epidemiology regarding alcohol-induced ONFH, as well as related issues including potential mechanisms for disease etiology and influences of alcohol-associated factors.

13.2 Descriptive Epidemiology of Alcohol-Induced ONFH

According to published reviews, the association of alcoholism with osteonecrosis was first described in 1922 [1, 4]. Several studies have examined the frequency of ONFH among alcoholics and found that the prevalence was low. A study from the USA assessed 790 patients who were hospitalized for treatment of alcoholism. ONFH was diagnosed in 2 patients, resulting in a prevalence of 0.3 % [6]. In Yugoslavia, among 1,157 patients who had been treated for excessive alcohol consumption, 92 sites in 62 patients (5 %) were diagnosed as nontraumatic osteonecrosis. Of these, 82 sites were found to be ONFH [7].

Some epidemiological studies reported the frequency of alcohol-induced ONFH among all ONFH patients on the basis of country. In Japan, a nationwide survey was conducted by stratified random sampling from all orthopedic departments to estimate the number of patients with ONFH who sought medical care during 2004 and to reveal their basic characteristics [8]. Of 1,502 patients from whom clinical information was obtained, 31 % had a history of habitual alcohol use, 51 % had a history of systemic steroid administration, 3 % had both histories, and 15 % had neither history. After stratification by gender and age group, the proportions of patients with a history of habitual alcohol use were 47 % for males and 6 % for females and 27 % for patients aged <40 years, 36 % for those aged 40–64 years, and 17 % for those aged ≥65 years (Table 13.1). Another nationwide survey in Korea estimated the prevalence of osteonecrosis of the femoral head, including posttraumatic cases, between 2002 and 2006 using medical claims and population data from the National Health Insurance Corporation of Korea [9]. Regarding a subset of the validation data with 185 hospitalized patients for whom a diagnosis was confirmed, 32.4 % had a history of alcohol abuse, 14.6 % had a history of steroid use, and 1.6 % had a history of hip fracture.

Although frequency of alcohol-induced ONFH among all ONFH patients is likely to be described among study participants in clinical studies that evaluated outcomes of operative or therapeutic procedures, this is not always the case. Even when described, the frequency varied across the studies. For example, with respect to several recent reports, the proportion[1] was 27/52 patients (52 %) [10], 6/23 patients (26 %) [11], 5/28 patients (18 %) [12], 18/80 patients (23 %) [13], 1/19 patients (5 %) [14], 37/100 patients (37 %) [15], 26/32 patients (81 %) [16], 16/42 hips (38 %) [17], and 11/71 hips (15 %) [18]. In addition to differences in ethnicity,

[1]Note: If patients with posttraumatic osteonecrosis of the femoral head were included in the study, the authors excluded the subjects and recalculated the proportion of alcohol-induced ONFH patients (hips) among all patients (hips).

W. Fukushima (✉) • Y. Hirota
Department of Public Health,
Osaka City University Faculty of Medicine,
1-4-3, Asahi-machi, Abeno-ku, Osaka 545-8585, Japan
e-mail: wakaba@med.osaka-cu.ac.jp;
hiro8yoshi@med.osaka-cu.ac.jp

K.-H. Koo et al. (eds.), *Osteonecrosis*,
DOI 10.1007/978-3-642-35767-1_13, © Springer-Verlag Berlin Heidelberg 2014

Table 13.1 Distribution of potential causative factors among ONFH patients: a nationwide epidemiological survey in Japan, 2004

	All patients (n = 1,502)	Stratified by gender[a]		Stratified by age (years) at diagnosis[a]		
		Male (n = 885)	Female (n = 612)	<40 (n = 548)	40–64 (n = 706)	≥65 (n = 153)
Variables	n (%)	n (%)	n (%)	n (%)	n (%)	n (%)
Systemic steroid administration	760 (51)	295 (34)	462 (76)	325 (60)	340 (48)	58 (38)
Habitual alcohol use	456 (31)	415 (47)	39 (6)	146 (27)	253 (36)	26 (17)
Both	47 (3)	39 (4)	8 (1)	16 (3)	24 (3)	6 (4)
Neither	225 (15)	127 (15)	98 (16)	59 (11)	85 (12)	62 (41)
Unknown/not filled-in	14	9	5	2	4	1

Reproduced with permission and copyright © of the *Association of Bone and Joint Surgeons* [8; Table 2]
Some totals of "%" do not equal 100 % attributable to rounding
ONFH nontraumatic osteonecrosis of the femoral head
[a]There was no available information regarding gender for five patients and for age at diagnosis for 95 patients

diagnostic criteria, and definitions for eligibility and exclusion in each study, no universal definition regarding alcohol-induced ONFH explains the different frequencies among studies. Some studies defined alcohol-induced ONFH as having a history of greater than 400 mL of pure ethanol consumption per week [16] or equivalent consumption for at least 6 months [10]. However, even less alcohol consumption might increase the risk of ONFH, because a threshold of alcohol consumption for alcohol-induced ONFH is unknown, and the causal mechanisms of alcohol intake have not been fully proven.

13.3 Analytic Epidemiology of Alcohol-Induced ONFH

13.3.1 Alcohol Consumption as a Risk Factor for ONFH

Although cohort, case-control, and cross-sectional studies can all be used to determine the factors associated with ONFH, the case-control approach is particularly suited to evaluate alcohol intake as a risk factor for development of ONFH. Possible reasons for this are that ONFH is an uncommon disease, and it is crucial to obtain a detailed history of alcohol consumption in each subject. Several hospital-based case-control studies have been reported from Japan [19–22]. In all studies, patients with ONFH without a history of systemic steroid treatment and control patients were recruited at departments of orthopedic surgery.

A case-control study by Matsuo et al. recruited 112 cases with ONFH and 168 controls from 4 collaborating hospitals in Western Japan [19]. Later, Hirota et al. reported results from another case-control study in which 118 cases and 236 controls were recruited from 20 collaborating hospitals all over Japan [20]. These two studies are highly comparable with respect to case definition, control selection, matching conditions between cases and controls (gender, age, ethnicity, date of initial examination/diagnosis, and hospital), and statistical analysis. According to the results by Hirota et al.

Table 13.2 Adjusted relative risks of alcohol drinking for ONFH: a case-control study in Japan, 1988–1990

	Cases		Controls			
Characteristics	No.	%	No.	%	Relative odds[a]	95 % CI
Alcohol drinking						
Never	23	19.5	87	36.9	1.0	
Former	4	3.4	10	4.2	1.0	0.2–6.2
Occasional	26	22.0	80	33.9	3.2	1.1–9.2
Regular	65	55.1	59	25.0	13.1	4.1–42.5
					Trend: $p < 0.001$	
Weekly ethanol intake (g/week)						
Nondrinker	27	22.9	97	41.1	1.0	
<320	24	20.3	87	36.9	2.8	1.0–7.8
320–799	49	41.5	45	19.1	9.4	3.0–29.0
≥800	18	15.3	7	3.0	14.8	3.8–57.2
					Trend: $p < 0.001$	
Drink-years						
Never drank	23	19.7	87	37.5	1.0	
<3,200	15	12.8	62	26.7	2.2	0.7–6.9
3,200–7,999	25	21.4	36	15.5	9.7	2.6–36.1
≥8,000	54	46.2	47	20.3	12.9	3.8–43.4
					Trend: $p < 0.001$	

Reproduced with permission and copyright © 1993 by the *Johns Hopkins University School of Hygiene and Public Health* [20;Tables 2 and 3]
ONFH nontraumatic osteonecrosis of the femoral head, *CI* confidence interval
[a]Adjusted for cigarette smoking, occupational energy consumption, body mass index, and liver dysfunction, using conditional logistic regression model

[20], the odds ratios (ORs) of former, occasional, and regular drinkers were 1.0, 3.2, and 13.1, respectively, compared to never drinkers (trend $p < 0.001$). Likewise, elevated ORs with a clear dose–response relationship were observed with respect to weekly ethanol consumption (ORs 2.8, 9.4, and 14.8 for <320, 320–799, and ≥800 g/week, respectively, in comparison to nondrinker; trend $p < 0.001$) and cumulative alcohol consumption (ORs 2.2, 9.7, and 12.9 for <3,200, 3,200–7,999, and ≥8,000 drink-years, respectively, in comparison to never drinker; trend $p < 0.001$) (Table 13.2). Similar findings were also seen in the

Table 13.3 Multiplicative or additive interaction between current drinking status and oral corticosteroid use for ONFH: a case-control study in Japan, 2002–2004

	Never user of oral corticosteroids		User of oral corticosteroids			
Variables	Cases (*n*)/controls (*n*)	Adjusted OR (95 % CI)[a]	Cases (*n*)/controls (*n*)	Adjusted OR (95 % CI)[a]	*p*-value for multiplicative interaction[b]	Synergy index[c] (95 % CI)
Current drinking status						
Nondrinker	4/79	1	22/15	31.5 (9.05–109)		
Drinker	23/122	2.79 (0.89–8.77)	22/11	31.6 (8.67–115)	0.19	0.95 (0.32–2.80)

ONFH nontraumatic osteonecrosis of the femoral head, *OR* odds ratio, *CI* confidence interval
[a]Adjusted for gender, age, smoking, and past history of liver disease, hyperlipidemia, and gout, using logistic regression model
[b]Wald test for each interaction term (DF = 1)
[c]Synergy index >1 indicates additive interaction

earlier study by Matsuo et al. [19]. Later, two case-control studies confirmed the positive association between alcohol intake and ONFH [21, 22].

Because both current consumption and cumulative consumption were positively associated with ONFH, effects of alcohol on ONFH are likely to be immediate, as well as cumulative [20]. However, detailed pathogenesis for alcohol-induced ONFH has not been well established. Some studies observed morphological changes in the bone marrow of the femoral head among alcohol-treated animals: an induced adipogenesis and decreased osteogenesis [23] and an increased fat cell size and higher bone marrow pressure [24]. These studies also reported an elevated serum cholesterol or triglyceride [23, 24]. Likewise, a recent experimental study in rabbits revealed abnormalities in lipid status both in bone marrow and in blood after intragastric administration of different doses of alcohol. In addition, these abnormalities were more pronounced in rabbits with higher doses of alcohol [25]. An increased level of serum cortisol in patients with alcohol-induced ONFH has been reported as another hematological change [26]. With respect to in vitro studies, suggested mechanisms include nitric oxide-mediated apoptosis of osteoblasts and osteocytes [27] and a decreased ability in osteogenic differentiation of mesenchymal stem cells isolated from the bone marrow [28].

13.3.2 Interaction Between Alcohol Consumption and Other Factors

Pathogenesis of ONFH is likely to be multifactorial. However, little is known about the interaction of alcohol consumption with other factors in the development of ONFH.

Recently, we reported results from a hospital-based case-control study that examined the risk of ONFH due to interactions between oral corticosteroid use and alcohol intake [29]. Among 71 cases with ONFH and 227 controls, we evaluated multiplicative interaction and additive interaction, as proposed by Rothman [30], using a two-by-two table of "nondrinker vs. drinker" for alcohol intake and "never user vs. user" for oral corticosteroids. Compared to nondrinkers without steroid use, an elevated but nonsignificant OR was observed for drinkers without steroid use (OR 2.79). In contrast, we found a substantially elevated OR in nondrinkers with steroid use (OR 31.5). However, no further increase in OR was seen for the combined effect of alcohol and steroid use (OR 31.6). As a result, we did not detect any significant multiplicative or additive interaction (Table 13.3). Although pharmacokinetic interaction between steroids and alcohol is possible, the most plausible interpretation may be that the added effect of alcohol intake was too small to make any significant difference in the presence of the overwhelming effect of steroids in the development of ONFH.

Our case-control study also demonstrated the importance of stratification by steroid use [29]. When we evaluated the effects of cumulative alcohol intake on ONFH among all subjects, a positive relationship (OR of the highest category of cumulative consumption: 3.93) was weaker than that in previous reports by Matsuo et al. [19] or Hirota et al. [20]. After we limited the analysis to those subjects who had never used steroids, we obtained a pronounced positive association between cumulative intake and ONFH (OR 11.1), which was comparable to the results from the previous two reports. An association between factors of interest and ONFH may be masked if subjects with a history of steroid administration are included in the study. A similar finding was also observed in a study that evaluated the effect of smoking on the risk of ONFH [31].

13.3.3 Alcohol-Associated Factors and ONFH: Activities of Aldehyde Dehydrogenases and History of Liver Dysfunction

Alcohol consumption can be influenced by the activities of alcohol dehydrogenases and aldehyde dehydrogenases. Aldehyde dehydrogenase 2 (ALDH2), a key enzyme in the elimination of acetaldehyde, has a genetic polymorphism that is prevalent in East Asians, but rare in Caucasians or Africans [32]. The mutant ALDH2*2 allele encodes a catalytically inactive subunit, and the molecules containing 1 or 2 ALDH2*2 allele subunits (i.e., ALDH2*1/*2 or ALDH2*2/*2) are considered to be inactive. Those with inactive ALDH2 are likely to experience facial flushing responses due to acetaldehydemia after drinking alcohol, resulting in reduced alcohol intake with respect to both frequency and amount [33–36]. In a case-control study, Shibata et al. examined whether facial flushing pattern (i.e., flusher or non-flusher), as a proxy measure for sensitivity of alcohol, was independently associated with ONFH among 64 male cases and 128 male controls who were recruited from five collaborating hospitals in Japan [21]. Compared to flushers, the crude OR of non-flushers was significantly elevated (OR 2.08). However, no association was shown after adjustment for several confounders including alcohol consumption (OR 0.73). Sakata et al. directly assayed ALDH2 genotypes among 34 male cases and 68 male controls in a single-center case-control study in Japan [22]. Although the crude OR of ALDH2*1/*1 for ONFH was significantly elevated (OR 3.31) in comparison to ALDH2*1/*2 or ALDH2*2/*2, the authors did not find a significant association in the multivariate analyses (OR 1.51). Because non-flushers or those with active ALDH2 are likely to drink heavily, the findings from these two studies clearly showed that an apparent association in the univariate analysis was confounded by alcohol consumption. Interaction of flushing pattern or ALDH2 polymorphism with alcohol consumption was not evaluated due to the small numbers of subjects.

It has been reported that a history of liver dysfunction was positively associated with ONFH. The OR was increased approximately fivefold after simultaneous adjustment for alcohol consumption, as well as other covariates, in the multivariate analysis [19]. Some studies also found a similar association, although a statistical significance was not achieved [20, 21, 37]. Clinicians may question whether such an association can be substantially attributed to alcohol consumption as a risk factor of ONFH because alcohol consumption per se induces liver dysfunction. However, if a history of liver dysfunction was truly an intermediate step between alcohol consumption and ONFH, the positive association in these studies would disappear in the multivariate analyses due to multicollinearity. Thus, the positive relationship of liver diseases with subsequent ONFH risk is likely to be independent, although the influence of residual confounding cannot be ruled out. It should be noted that, in general, laboratory testing for liver dysfunction as a part of routine medical examinations is rarely performed for control subjects because they have no clinical signs of liver diseases. In some studies, subjects were considered to have a history of liver dysfunction if they had received treatment for three or more months for any diseases of the liver [19, 20, 37]. Self-reported information may be unacceptable as a surrogate for laboratory data in clinical settings. However, this approach would be useful in epidemiological studies in order to retain comparability between cases and controls and thus provide some clues for disease etiology.

13.4 Summary

Alcohol consumption is one of the important underlying factors for the development of ONFH. A history of habitual alcohol use or alcohol abuse was frequently observed among patients with ONFH, although the prevalence of ONFH among alcoholics seemed to be low. Several analytic epidemiological studies have consistently found a strong positive association between alcohol consumption and ONFH. However, compared to steroid-induced ONFH, less is known about the pathogenesis or mechanisms of alcohol-induced ONFH. Exploring possible interactions between alcohol consumption and other potential risk factors also could contribute to a better understanding of the etiology of ONFH. Other issues to be proven include determining a threshold of alcohol consumption, which would lead to the definition of a universal criterion of alcohol-induced ONFH and thus increase comparability across studies.

References

1. Chang CC, Greenspan A, Gershwin ME. Osteonecrosis: current perspectives on pathogenesis and treatment. Semin Arthritis Rheum. 1993;23(1):47–69.
2. Mont MA, Hungerford DS. Non-traumatic avascular necrosis of the femoral head. J Bone Joint Surg Am. 1995;77(3):459–74.
3. Lavernia CJ, Sierra RJ, Grieco FR. Osteonecrosis of the femoral head. J Am Acad Orthop Surg. 1999;7(4):250–61.
4. Assouline-Dayan Y, Chang C, Greenspan A, Shoenfeld Y, Gershwin ME. Pathogenesis and natural history of osteonecrosis. Semin Arthritis Rheum. 2002;32(2):94–124.
5. Mont MA, Jones LC, Hungerford DS. Nontraumatic osteonecrosis of the femoral head: ten years later. J Bone Joint Surg Am. 2006;88(5):1117–32.
6. Gold EW, Cangemi PJ. Incidence and pathogenesis of alcohol-induced osteonecrosis of the femoral head. Clin Orthop Relat Res. 1979;143:222–6.
7. Orlić D, Jovanović S, Anticević D, Zecević J. Frequency of idiopathic aseptic necrosis in medically treated alcoholics. Int Orthop. 1990;14(4):383–6.
8. Fukushima W, Fujioka M, Kubo T, Tamakoshi A, Nagai M, Hirota Y. Nationwide epidemiologic survey of idiopathic osteonecrosis of the femoral head. Clin Orthop Relat Res. 2010;468(10):2715–24.
9. Kang JS, Park S, Song JH, Jung YY, Cho MR, Rhyu KH. Prevalence of osteonecrosis of the femoral head: a nationwide epidemiologic analysis in Korea. J Arthroplasty. 2009;24(8):1178–83.
10. Chen CH, Chang JK, Lai KA, Hou SM, Chang CH, Wang GJ. Alendronate in the prevention of collapse of the femoral head in nontraumatic osteonecrosis: a two-year multicenter, prospective, randomized, double-blind, placebo-controlled study. Arthritis Rheum. 2012;64(5):1572–8.
11. Sen RK, Tripathy SK, Aggarwal S, Marwaha N, Sharma RR, Khandelwal N. Early results of core decompression and autologous

bone marrow mononuclear cells instillation in femoral head osteonecrosis: a randomized control study. J Arthroplasty. 2012; 27(5):679–86.
12. Ito H, Tanino H, Yamanaka Y, Nakamura T, Takahashi D, Minami A, Matsuno T. Long-term results of conventional varus half-wedge proximal femoral osteotomy for the treatment of osteonecrosis of the femoral head. J Bone Joint Surg Br. 2012;94(3):308–14.
13. Zhao D, Cui D, Wang B, Tian F, Guo L, Yang L, Liu B, Yu X. Treatment of early stage osteonecrosis of the femoral head with autologous implantation of bone marrow-derived and cultured mesenchymal stem cells. Bone. 2012;50(1):325–30.
14. Gangji V, De Maertelaer V, Hauzeur JP. Autologous bone marrow cell implantation in the treatment of non-traumatic osteonecrosis of the femoral head: five year follow-up of a prospective controlled study. Bone. 2011;49(5):1005–9.
15. Ha YC, Kim HJ, Kim SY, Kim KC, Lee YK, Koo KH. Effects of age and body mass index on the results of transtrochanteric rotational osteotomy for femoral head osteonecrosis. J Bone Joint Surg Am. 2010;92(2):314–21.
16. Chen CC, Lin CL, Chen WC, Shih HN, Ueng SW, Lee MS. Vascularized iliac bone-grafting for osteonecrosis with segmental collapse of the femoral head. J Bone Joint Surg Am. 2009;91(10): 2390–4.
17. Zhao G, Yamamoto T, Ikemura S, Motomura G, Iwasaki K, Yamaguchi R, Nakashima Y, Mawatari T, Iwamoto Y. Clinico-radiological factors affecting the joint space narrowing after transtrochanteric anterior rotational osteotomy for osteonecrosis of the femoral head. J Orthop Sci. 2012;17(4):390–6.
18. Zhao G, Yamamoto T, Ikemura S, Motomura G, Mawatari T, Nakashima Y, Iwamoto Y. Radiological outcome analysis of transtrochanteric curved varus osteotomy for osteonecrosis of the femoral head at a mean follow-up of 12.4 years. J Bone Joint Surg Br. 2010;92(6):781–6.
19. Matsuo K, Hirohata T, Sugioka Y, Ikeda M, Fukuda A. Influence of alcohol intake, cigarette smoking, and occupational status on idiopathic osteonecrosis of the femoral head. Clin Orthop Relat Res. 1988;234:115–23.
20. Hirota Y, Hirohata T, Fukuda K, Mori M, Yanagawa H, Ohno Y, Sugioka Y. Association of alcohol intake, cigarette smoking, and occupational status with the risk of idiopathic osteonecrosis of the femoral head. Am J Epidemiol. 1993;137(5):530–8.
21. Shibata A, Fukuda K, Inoue A, Higuchi F, Miyake H, Nishi M, Mori M, Ishii S, Nagao M, Yanagawa H. Flushing pattern and idiopathic avascular necrosis of the femoral head. J Epidemiol. 1996;6(1):37–43.
22. Sakata R. A case-control study of association between life-style, alcohol dehydrogenase 2 and aldehyde dehydrogenase 2 genotype and idiopathic osteonecrosis of the femoral head. Kurume Med J. 2003;50(3–4):121–30.
23. Wang Y, Li Y, Mao K, Li J, Cui Q, Wang GJ. Alcohol-induced adipogenesis in bone and marrow: a possible mechanism for osteonecrosis. Clin Orthop Relat Res. 2003;410:213–24.
24. Shih CH, Yang WE, Lee ZL, Kao YL, Hsueh S, Wei JS. Effect of long-term alcohol ingestion on the femoral head of rabbit. J Formos Med Assoc. 1991;90(5):443–7.
25. Ikemura S, Yamamoto T, Motomura G, Iwasaki K, Yamaguchi R, Zhao G, Iwamoto Y. Lipid metabolism abnormalities in alcohol-treated rabbits: a morphometric and haematologic study comparing high and low alcohol doses. Int J Exp Pathol. 2011;92(4):290–5.
26. Rico H, Gomez-Castresana F, Cabranes JA, Almoguera I, Lopez Duran L, Matute JA. Increased blood cortisol in alcoholic patients with aseptic necrosis of the femoral head. Calcif Tissue Int. 1985;37(6):585–7.
27. Calder JD, Buttery L, Revell PA, Pearse M, Polak JM. Apoptosis–a significant cause of bone cell death in osteonecrosis of the femoral head. J Bone Joint Surg Br. 2004;86(8):1209–13.
28. Suh KT, Kim SW, Roh HL, Youn MS, Jung JS. Decreased osteogenic differentiation of mesenchymal stem cells in alcohol-induced osteonecrosis. Clin Orthop Relat Res. 2005;431:220–5.
29. Fukushima W, Yamamoto T, Takahashi S, Sakaguchi M, Kubo T, Iwamoto Y, Hirota Y. The effect of alcohol intake and the use of oral corticosteroids on the risk of idiopathic osteonecrosis of the femoral head: a case-control study in Japan. Bone Joint J. 2013;95-B(3):320–5.
30. Rothman KJ. Epidemiology. An introduction. New York: Oxford University Press; 2002.
31. Takahashi S, Fukushima W, Kubo T, Iwamoto Y, Hirota Y, Nakamura H. Pronounced risk of nontraumatic osteonecrosis of the femoral head among cigarette smokers who have never used oral corticosteroids: a multicenter case-control study in Japan. J Orthop Sci. 2012;17(6):730–6.
32. Goedde HW, Agarwal DP, Fritze G, Meier-Tackmann D, Singh S, Beckmann G, Bhatia K, Chen LZ, Fang B, Lisker R, et al. Distribution of ADH2 and ALDH2 genotypes in different populations. Hum Genet. 1992;88(3):344–6.
33. Harada S, Agarwal DP, Goedde HW. Aldehyde dehydrogenase deficiency as cause of facial flushing reaction to alcohol in Japanese. Lancet. 1981;2(8253):982.
34. Higuchi S, Muramatsu T, Shigemori K, Saito M, Kono H, Dufour MC, Harford TC. The relationship between low Km aldehyde dehydrogenase phenotype and drinking behavior in Japanese. J Stud Alcohol. 1992;53(2):170–5.
35. Tanaka F, Shiratori Y, Yokosuka O, Imazeki F, Tsukada Y, Omata M. Polymorphism of alcohol-metabolizing genes affects drinking behavior and alcoholic liver disease in Japanese men. Alcohol Clin Exp Res. 1997;21(4):596–601.
36. Suzuki K, Matsushita S, Ishii T. Relationship between the flushing response and drinking behavior among Japanese high school students. Alcohol Clin Exp Res. 1997;21(9):1726–9.
37. Sakaguchi M, Tanaka T, Fukushima W, Kubo T, Hirota Y, Idiopathic ONF Multicenter Case-Control Study Group. Impact of oral corticosteroid use for idiopathic osteonecrosis of the femoral head: a nationwide multicenter case-control study in Japan. J Orthop Sci. 2010;15(2):185–91.

Traumatic Avascular Necrosis of the Femoral Head

14

Simon Damian Steppacher, Pascal Cyrill Haefeli, Helen Anwander, Klaus Arno Siebenrock, and Moritz Tannast

14.1 Introduction

Avascular necrosis (AVN) of the femoral head is a rare but devastating complication following fractures of the proximal femur or hip dislocation. Traumatic AVN derives from the interruption of the blood flow to the femoral head, which is mainly supplied by the medial circumflex femoral artery (MCFA) in the adult hip [1, 2]. The incidence of AVN depends on the fracture pattern and the integrity of the deep branch of the MCFA. While fractures with close proximity to the nutrient vessels (femoral head and neck fractures) have a considerable risk for AVN, AVN rarely occurs in fractures which do not interfere with the MCFA (intertrochanteric or femoral shaft fractures). In addition to traumatic interruption of the femoral head blood supply, the MCFA can be injured iatrogenically. Symptoms and radiographic changes in hips with AVN of the femoral head usually occur late and often months after the trauma. There is no curative treatment and therefore prevention is most important.

This article (1) describes the pathophysiology of AVN with a special focus on the vascular anatomy of the femoral head, (2) reports on the different modalities to assess the integrity of the nutrient vessels, (3) compares the different injury patterns and their associated risk of AVN, and (4) provides information to prevent iatrogenic damage to the blood supply of the femoral head.

S.D. Steppacher • P.C. Haefeli • H. Anwander • K.A. Siebenrock
M. Tannast (✉)
Department of Orthopaedic Surgery, Inselspital,
University of Bern, Freiburgstrasse, Bern 3010, Switzerland
e-mail: simon.steppacher@insel.ch; pascal.haefeli@insel.ch; helen.anwander@insel.ch; klaus.siebenrock@insel.ch; moritz.tannast@insel.ch

14.2 Blood Supply to the Femoral Head

14.2.1 Vascular Anatomy of the Femoral Head

Precise knowledge of the vascular anatomy of the femoral head helps to understand the etiology of traumatic AVN. The deep branch of the MCFA provides the main blood supply to the femoral head [1, 2]. Most commonly, it arises from the deep femoral artery or, alternatively, from the common femoral artery (Fig. 14.1). There are five constant branches of the MCFA. Of these, the most relevant for the femoral head perfusion is the deep branch of the MCFA [1, 2]. It runs posteriorly towards the intertrochanteric crest between the pectineus muscle medially and the iliopsoas tendon laterally (Fig. 14.1). The deep branch of the MCFA then runs along the inferior border of the obturator externus muscle, which is the most important structure to protect the course of the MCFA (Fig. 14.1). As long as the obturator externus muscle is in continuity, the deep branch of the MCFA is not under relevant tension even with the femoral head dislocated [1]. After crossing the obturator externus tendon posteriorly, a constant trochanteric branch is given off which runs between the quadratus femoris muscle and the triceps coxae (gemelli and obturator internus muscles; Fig. 14.1). The deep branch of the MCFA continues cranially and ventrally to the triceps coxae muscles and penetrates the joint capsule at the level of the superior border of the gemellus superior muscle (Fig. 14.1). At the posterosuperior aspect of the femoral neck, it splits up into four to five retinacular vessels (Fig. 14.1). The retinacular vessels lie extraosseously but intracapsularly and enter the head 2–4 mm lateral to the bone-cartilage junction.

Multiple anastomoses with the MCFA exist [1]. The most important anastomosis regarding femoral head perfusion is a branch of the inferior gluteal artery, which runs along the

K.-H. Koo et al. (eds.), *Osteonecrosis*,
DOI 10.1007/978-3-642-35767-1_14, © Springer-Verlag Berlin Heidelberg 2014

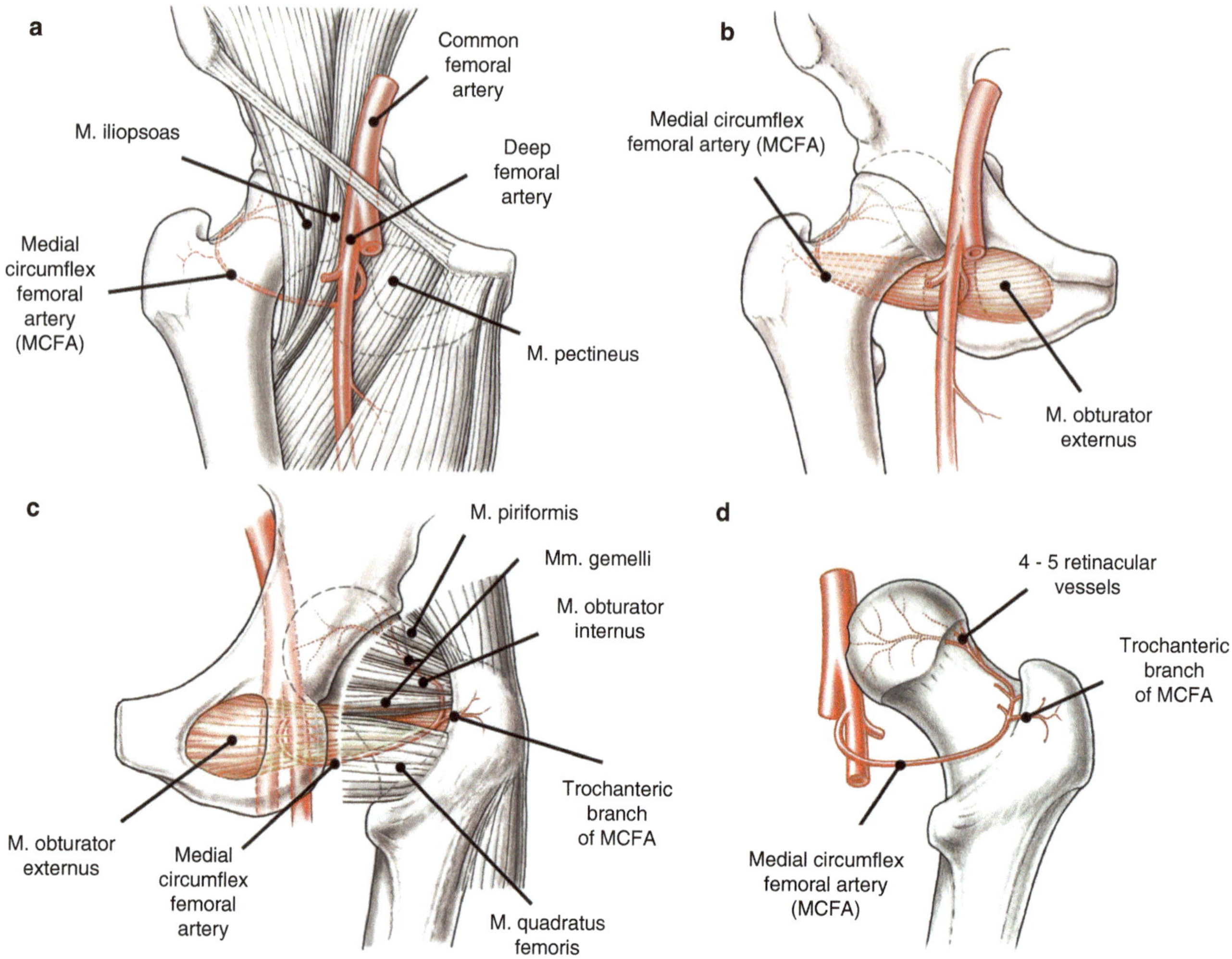

Fig. 14.1 Vascular anatomy of the femoral head. (**a**) The deep branch of the medial circumflex femoral artery (*MCFA*) runs towards the intertrochanteric crest between the pectineus muscle medially and the iliopsoas tendon laterally. (**b**) The MCFA then runs along the inferior border of the obturator externus muscle. (**c**) After crossing the obturator externus tendon posteriorly, a trochanteric branch is given off which runs between the quadratus femoris muscle and the triceps coxae (gemelli and obturator internus muscles). The deep branch of the MCFA continues cranially and ventrally to the triceps coxae muscle and enters the joint capsule at the level of the superior border of the gemellus superior muscle. (**d**) At the posterosuperior aspect of the femoral neck, it splits up into four to five retinacular vessels which enter the head (Reprinted with permission Tannast et al. [3])

piriformis muscle [1, 4]. It could be shown that this vessel has the capacity to compensate for an interruption of the blood supply of the afferent portion of the MCFA [5]. The lateral circumflex femoral artery or the ligamentum teres arteries contribute very little to head perfusion [2]. Usually, the intraosseous blood flow cannot compensate for an intracapsular injury to the deep branch of the MCFA. Therefore, in clinical practice, viability of the femoral head directly depends on the integrity of the MCFA.

14.2.2 Assessment of the Integrity of the Nutrient Vessels of the Femoral Head

Damage to the MCFA can theoretically occur by direct traumatic injury from the accident (i.e., rupture of the vessel), kinking due to fracture and/or joint dislocation, thrombosis, vasospasm, or iatrogenic injury (e.g., forced closed reduction, surgical approach, hardware insertion).

14.2.2.1 Preoperative Modalities for Detection of an Interrupted Blood Supply to the Femoral Head

A reliable, clinically routinely usable, preoperative technique to diagnose an injury of the MCFA with interruption of the blood supply to the femoral head does not exist. Direct visualization of the nutrient vessels to the femoral head is possible by angiography [5, 6]. It can show the interruption of the MCFA but is unable to show the ultimate perfusion of femoral head. Two historic studies [5, 6] tried to correlate the angiographic results in proximal femoral fractures with the occurrence of

AVN at most recent follow-up. In hips with preserved blood supply to the femoral head in the angiography, AVN occurred very rarely. In contrast, if the preoperative blood supply to the femoral head was interrupted in the angiography, this did not necessarily end up in an AVN. In these cases, the blood supply can sometimes even be restored by simple closed internal rotation of the hip in femoral neck fractures or after open reduction and internal fixation [6, 7]. This supports the theory of a transient kinking and/or vasospasm of the nutrient vessels. Despite its utility, angiography has not become part of the routine clinical follow-up. Nowadays, CT angiography may be a promising noninvasive alternative to conventional angiography [8]. The MCFA and its anastomoses can be visualized in detail with this technique [8]. However, similar to classic angiography, the terminal intraosseous blood flow to the femoral head is not visible. The usability of this technique in clinical routine has not yet been proven.

There are two imaging modalities that can show the preoperative femoral head vascularity with proximal femoral fractures. The first modality is the dynamic magnetic resonance imaging (MRI), which monitors quantitatively the flow of an intravenously applied contrast agent in the femoral head [9]. The signal intensity of the fractured side before and after application of gadolinium is then compared to the unaffected side. Similarly, bone scintigraphy (as the second modality) uses an intravenously applied radiographic tracer [10, 11]. Unlike dynamic MRI, this method reveals more qualitative results. Despite relative promising results of these two techniques, neither has found its way into clinical routine use.

14.2.2.2 Intraoperative Assessment

One of the most reliable and technically simple methods to assess femoral head perfusion is intraoperative drilling of the femoral head [7]. After reduction of the fracture, two to four 2.0 mm drill holes are made at the base of the femoral head to assess femoral head bleeding. This requires an open approach to the hip and usually takes up to 2 min until reliable bleeding from the femoral head may be observed. If a closed reduction and percutaneous fixation is attempted, the retrograde blood flow through the cannulated screws can provide a relatively reliable assessment of the femoral head perfusion [12]. More sophisticated methods such as laser Doppler flowmetry [13] and intramedullary oxygen tension measurements [14] have been described but basically offer a lower sensitivity and specificity for prediction of AVN in comparison to direct drilling of the femoral head.

14.3 Injury Patterns of the Proximal Femur

The incidence of traumatic AVN of the femoral head depends on the fracture pattern and its proximity to the deep branch of the MCFA (Table 14.1). While the femoral head and neck fractures have the highest incidence of AVN (up to 40 % [18]), the incidence decreases for intertrochanteric fractures (1–5 % [17, 18, 23]), and AVN rarely occurs in femoral shaft fractures [24] (Table 14.1). Femoral head necrosis has also

Table 14.1 Selected literature reporting on incidence of avascular necrosis of the femoral head following fractures of the proximal femur or traumatic hip dislocation

Study	Fracture pattern	Treatment	Number of hips (patients)	Mean age with range (year)	Incidence of AVN (%)	Results
Giannoudis et al. [15]	Head	23 % nonsurgical 77 % surgical	453 (450)	39 (6–81)	12	Systematic review 3.7 and 2.2 times increased risk for AVN for posterior or trochanteric flip approach compared to anterior approach
Guo et al. [16]	Head	18 % nonsurgical 82 % surgical	176 (176)	n.a.	13	Systematic review Incidence of AVN of 16 % for posterior, 13 % for trochanteric flip, and 8 % for anterior approach
Moon and Mehlmann [17]	Head, neck, intertrochanteric	Surgical and nonsurgical	360 (360)	10 (1–16)	21[a] I: 38 II: 28 III: 18 IV: 5	Systematic review Fracture type[a], displacement, age, and treatment (open vs. closed reduction) are risk factors for AVN
Yeranosian et al. [18]	Head, neck, intertrochanteric	Surgical and nonsurgical	n.a. (935)	n.a. (1–19)	23[a] I: 40 II: 27 III: 20 IV: 5	Systematic review Fracture type[a], treatment (open vs. closed reduction), delay in treatment (>24 h), and use of fixation are risk factors for AVN; no association with decompression

(continued)

Table 14.1 (continued)

Study	Fracture pattern	Treatment	Number of hips (patients)	Mean age with range (year)	Incidence of AVN (%)	Results
Garden [19]	Neck	100 % surgical	406 (n.a.)	n.a.	23	Case series Incidence of AVN depends on quality of reduction; definition of alignment index; no AVN inside normal range of index; 100 % incidence of AVN with varus (<150°) or valgus (>185°) malreduction
Holmberg et al. [20]	Neck	3 % nonsurgical 97 % surgical	2,251 (n.a.)	74 (39–99)	12	Case series Increased incidence of AVN in hips with operative treatment (12 %) compared to nonoperative treatment (2 %)
Johnson and Crothers [21]	Neck	26 % pinning 74 % intramedullary nailing	153	72 (n.a.)	14	Case series Increased incidence of AVN in hips with intramedullary nailing (16 %) compared to pinning (8 %)
Strömqvist et al. [22]	Neck	100 % surgical	n.a. (300)	78 (18–98)	7	Case series Increased incidence of AVN in hips with displaced neck fractures (9 %) compared to non-displaced fractures (3 %)
Aguado-Maestro et al. [23]	Intertrochanteric	100 % PFN	n.a. (200)	n.a.	1	Case series Patient series with intertrochanteric fractures treated with PFN and 1 out of 200 with AVN
Orler et al. [24]	Shaft	100 % intramedullary nailing	17 (17)	13 (8–15)	n.a.	Systematic review of case reports with AVN following intramedullary nailing of femoral shaft fractures
Brav [25]	Dislocation	93 % closed reduction 7 % ORIF	523 (517)	25 (3–75)	26	Case series Incidence of AVN depends on direction of dislocation, associated fractures, delay in treatment (>12 h)
Epstein [26]	Dislocation	Closed reduction and ORIF	242 (242)	n.a.	18	Case series Incidence of AVN depends on associated fractures
Hougaard and Thomsen [27]	Dislocation	Closed reduction and ORIF	100 (98)	39 (16–89)	13	Case series Incidence of AVN depends on delay of treatment (>6 h)

n.a. not available, *AVN* avascular necrosis, *PFN* proximal femoral nailing, *ORIF* open reduction internal fixation
[a]Incidence for the type of Delbet classification [28]: I = head, II = medial neck, III = lateral neck, and IV = intertrochanteric fracture

been reported following traumatic dislocations with an incidence ranging up to 26 % [25–27].

Fractures of the proximal femur are divided into head, neck, intertrochanteric, and femoral shaft fractures. For each fracture pattern, the etiology of AVN, the anatomical relation to the MCFA, and the incidence of AVN reported in literature are summarized.

14.3.1 Femoral Head Fractures

Among the different fracture types of the proximal femur, femoral head fractures have the highest incidence for AVN ranging up to 40 % (Table 14.1) [18]. Femoral head fractures typically are related to direct mechanical damage to the intraosseous blood flow from the retinacular vessels (Fig. 14.2). The vascularity of the femoral head fragment can only be reestablished by diffusion from the viable femoral head portion. Based on two systematic reviews [15, 16], an increased risk for AVN has not been found for a specific subtype of femoral head fracture or concomitant traumatic dislocation. However, in both reviews [15, 16], the risk of AVN was associated with the type of approach used for surgical treatment (Table 14.2). The highest incidence of 16 % was found for the posterior approach, followed by the trochanteric flip approach with 13 % and the anterior approach with 8 % [15, 16]. These results suggest that an iatrogenic lesion to the nutrient vessels of the femoral head may play an important role. The posterior approach to the hip can potentially be dangerous for the blood supply to the femoral head if the topographical course of the MCFA is not fully understood and respected (Fig. 14.1).

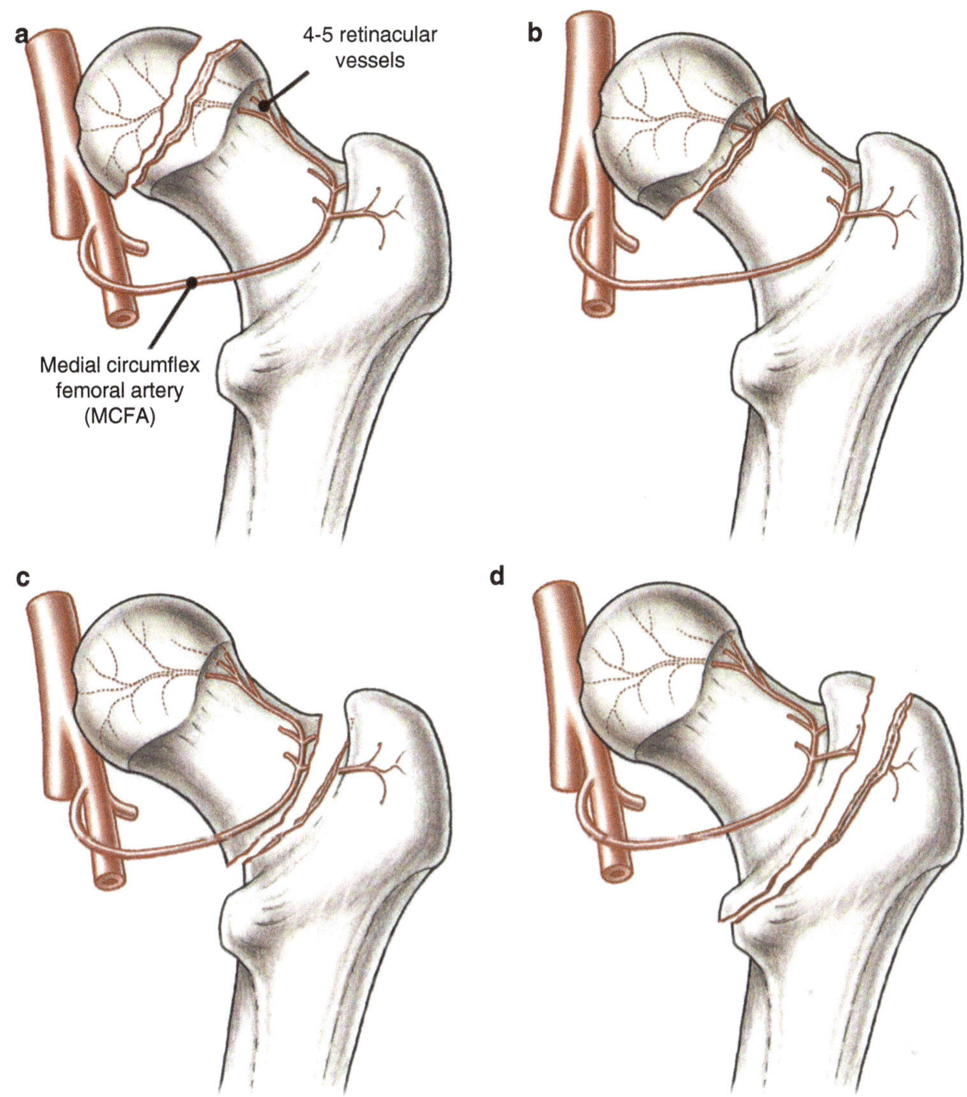

Fig. 14.2 (**a**) Femoral head fractures have the highest incidence of avascular necrosis (AVN) of the femoral head ranging up to 40 % [18] and typically are related to direct mechanical damage to the retinacular vessels. (**b**) In medial neck fractures, direct mechanical trauma to the nutrient vessel results in increased risk for AVN compared to (**c**) lateral neck fractures which less likely interfere with the MCFA. (**d**) AVN rarely occurs in hips with intertrochanteric fractures because these fractures usually do not interfere with the nutrient vessel

If a trochanteric osteotomy is conducted, the osteotomy should exit just anterior to the most posterior insertion of the gluteus medius muscle in order to protect the deep branch of the MCFA [34].

14.3.2 Femoral Neck Fractures

AVN in femoral neck fractures is typically the result of an injured retinaculum (Fig. 14.2). Several risk factors have been reported that can be attributed to the integrity of the retinacular vessels. This includes the location of neck fracture [17, 18], fracture dislocation [13, 17, 22], quality of reduction [19], delay of treatment [18, 29], and type of treatment [17, 18, 20, 21] (Table 14.2).

14.3.2.1 Location of Femoral Neck Fracture

Medial femoral neck fractures have an increased incidence of AVN (28 %) in comparison to lateral neck fractures (18 %, Table 14.1) [17, 18]. The increased incidence for medial neck fractures can be explained by the very close topographical relationship of the retinacular vessels and the fracture (Figs. 14.2 and 14.3). Lateral neck fractures show an increased distance between the fracture and the terminal branches of the MCFA; therefore, the fracture has less potential to damage the vessel (Fig. 14.2).

14.3.2.2 Fracture Dislocation

Fracture dislocations of the femoral neck can be classified as varus/valgus, dorsal/ventral, and rotational (Fig. 14.4).

A varus dislocation without dorsal angulation inevitably causes tension on the retinacular vessels (Fig. 14.4). This can lead to an impairment of the femoral blood supply [6, 13]. Eventually, the vulnerable retinaculum ruptures with large dislocations. A valgus impaction without dorsal angulation theoretically relaxes the retinaculum (Fig. 14.4). Isolated valgus impactions up to 30° do not impair the blood supply to the femoral head [6]. However, large valgus impactions are associated with AVN [19] and attributed to kinking of the retinacular vessels.

Table 14.2 Fracture pattern with corresponding risk factors and incidence of avascular necrosis of the femoral head

Fracture pattern	Risk factor for AVN of femoral head	Description/incidence of AVN
Head	Surgical approach [15, 16]	Posterior approach with incidence of 16 %, trochanteric flip with 13 %, and anterior approach with 8 %
Neck	Location of fracture [17, 18]	Medial neck fractures with incidence of 28 % compared to lateral fractures with 18 %
	Fracture dislocation [13, 17, 22]	Adults: dislocated fractures with incidence of 9 % compared to non-dislocated fractures with 3 %
		Children: dislocated fractures with incidence of 25 % compared to non-dislocated with 9 %
	Quality of reduction [19]	Anatomical reduction with incidence of 7 % compared to severe valgus/varus with 100 %
	Delay of treatment [18, 29]	Adults: increased incidence of 16 vs. 0 % for a delay of >12 h
		Children: four times increased risk for a delay of >24 h
	Type of treatment [17, 18, 20, 21]	Adults: incidence of 12 % for surgical treatment vs. 2 % for nonsurgical treatment, 16 % for open reduction vs. 8 % for closed reduction
		Children: 2.5 times increased risk for surgical vs. nonsurgical treatment, 2.7 times increased risk for open vs. closed reduction
Intertrochanteric	n.a.	
Shaft	Young age [24, 30, 31]	Patients aged between 8 and 15 years; only two case reports with patients older than 20 years
	Antegrade femoral nailing [32]	Nail insertion in the piriformis fossa results in complete disruption of the MCFA in 57 %
		In all case reports nail insertion was performed with reaming of the femoral medullary canal
		Implants designed for adults but used in children
Dislocation	Direction of dislocation [25]	Posterior dislocations with incidence of 29 % compared to 9 % for anterior dislocations
	Concomitant fracture [25, 26]	Dislocation without fracture with incidence of 22 % compared to 60 % for concomitant femoral head or acetabulum fracture
	Delay of reduction [25, 27]	Increased incidence of 59 vs. 5 % for a delay of >6 h or 57 vs. 18 % for a delay of >12 h
	Surgical approach [33]	Three times increased risk for ORIF using posterior vs. anterior approach

AVN avascular necrosis, *MCFA* medial circumflex femoral artery, *ORIF* open reduction internal fixation, *n.a.* not available

A dorsal tilt of the femoral head can lead to a kinking of the posterosuperiorly located retinaculum (Fig. 14.4). A reperfusion of the femoral head can be achieved by simple (closed) internal rotation of the leg [6] or by anatomical open reduction and internal fixation [6, 13]. An additional varus dislocation can aggravate the kinking of the retinacular vessels [6].

Rotational errors at the level of the femoral neck can typically occur when performing closed reduction [35] or by excessive torque from an implant (e.g., a dynamic hip screw [36]). Rotational errors are hard to detect with fluoroscopy or conventional radiographs but can have serious consequences on the retinaculum. A flexion of the head fragment can stretch the retinaculum (Fig. 14.4). However, a large extension of the head fragment may compromise the head vascularity by kinking of the vessel (Fig. 14.4).

14.3.2.3 Quality of Reduction

Quality of reduction was found to be a significant predictor for AVN (Table 14.2) [19]. Severe residual varus and valgus deformities are associated with a higher incidence of AVN [19]. The same principles as mentioned above (see Sect. 14.3.2.2) apply for the integrity of the vascularity.

14.3.2.4 Delay of Treatment and Tamponade Effect

Delay of treatment of more than 12–24 h is associated with a higher risk of AVN (Table 14.2). This could be attributed to a tamponade effect of the retinacular vessels by hemarthrosis. Because the retinacular vessels are extraosseous and intracapsular, they may be compressed by increased hydrostatic pressure resulting from the fracture hematoma. This tamponade effect can occur in both displaced and non-displaced fractures [37–39]. This would explain the presence of AVN in undisplaced fractures [17]. The time limit of 12 h is somewhat arbitrarily chosen but could be reproduced in a canine animal model [40].

14.3.2.5 Type of Treatment

An increased incidence of AVN was found for neck fractures treated surgically compared to hips with nonsurgical treatment (Table 14.2). Additionally, the incidence of AVN was increased in hips with open reduction and internal fixation compared to hips with closed reduction only (Table 14.2). With an open treatment the MCFA can potentially be iatrogenically damaged. However, type of treatment might also be confounding with previously mentioned risk factors such as location of fracture or fracture dislocation.

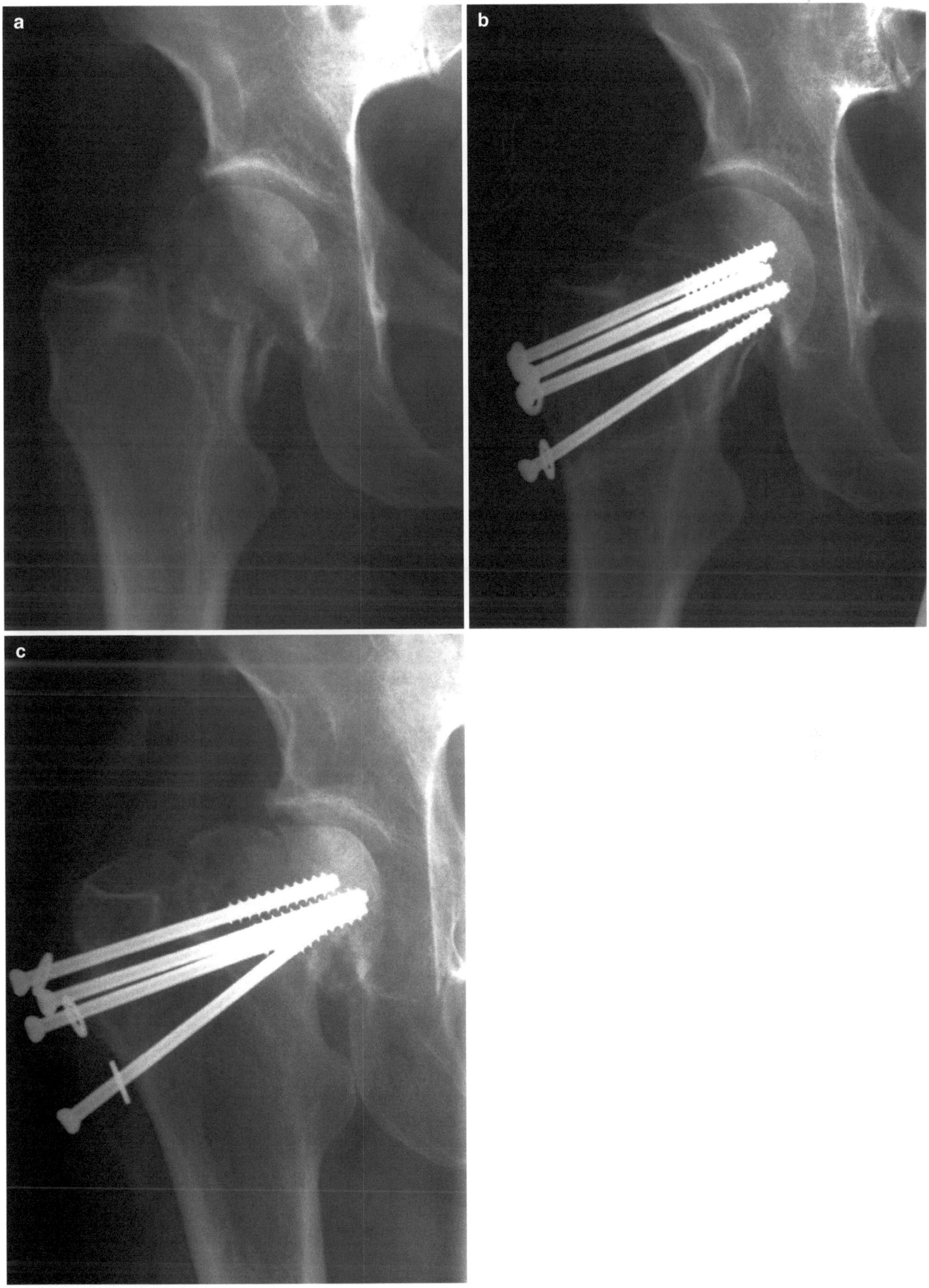

Fig. 14.3 (**a**) A 49-year-old male patient with a medial femoral neck fracture. (**b**) He underwent closed reduction and screw fixation resulting in insufficient reduction and stabilization. (**c**) At a 1.2 year follow-up, avascular necrosis of the femoral head occurred necessitating total hip arthroplasty

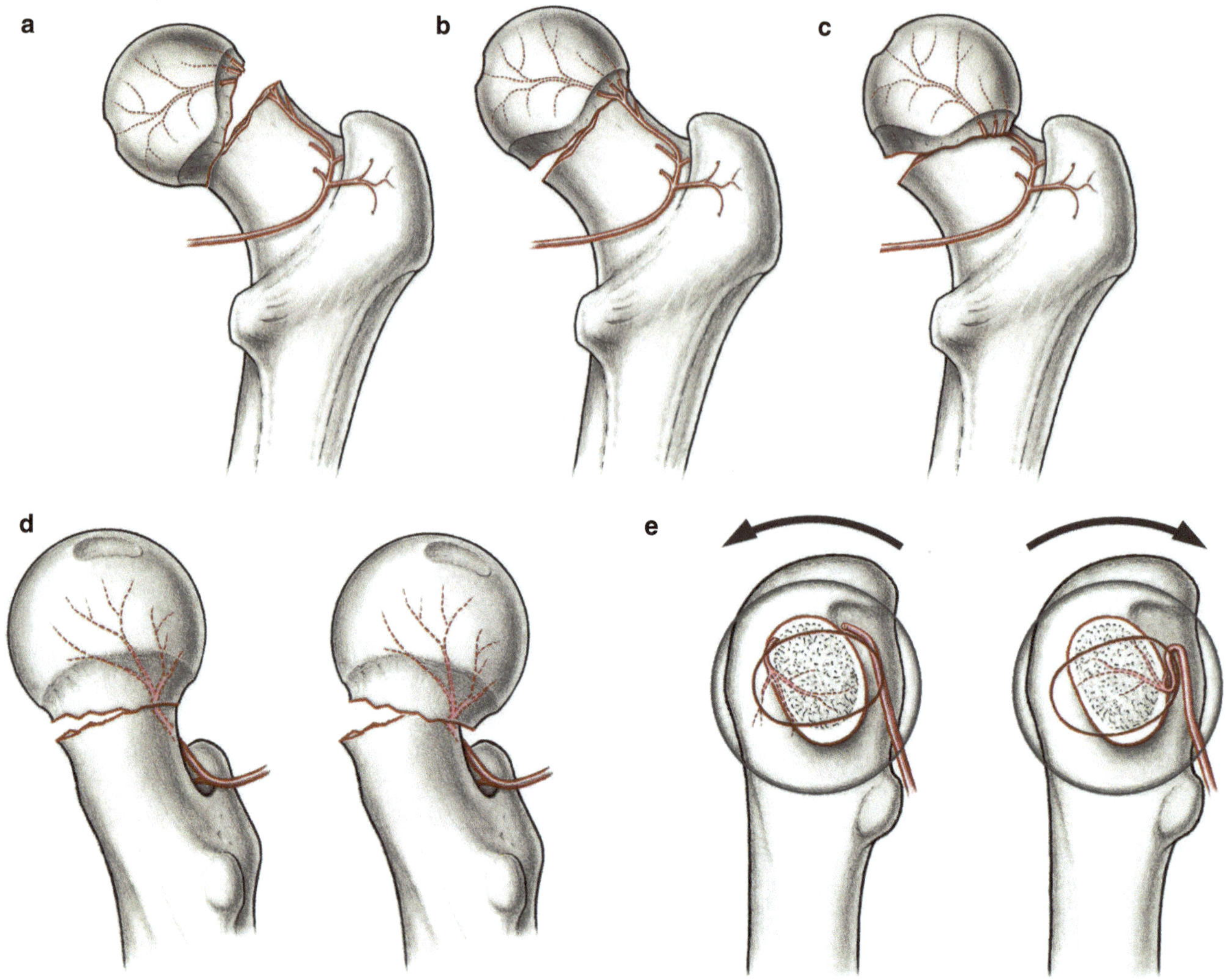

Fig. 14.4 Neck fractures with (**a**) varus dislocation cause tension and possibly rupture of the retinacular vessels. (**b**) A mild valgus dislocation (<30°) relaxes the retinacular vessels and does not impair the blood supply [6]. (**c**) However, a severe valgus dislocation results in kinking of the retinacular vessels and impaired blood supply [19]. (**d**) A mild dorsal tilt usually does not impair perfusion of the femoral head. However, a severe dorsal tilt and, particularly, when in combination with a varus dislocation, leads to impairment of the head perfusion. (**e**) Rotational errors can compromise the head vascularity. Flexion of the head can stretch the retinacular vessels and result in rupture. Extension of the femoral head can result in impaired blood supply by kinking of the vessel

14.3.3 Intertrochanteric and Greater Trochanteric Fractures

Intertrochanteric fractures are rarely associated with AVN, and the incidence ranges from 1 to 5 % (Table 14.1). Generally, these fractures do not interfere directly with the anatomical course of the deep branch of the MCFA in the adult hip (Fig. 14.2). Associated risk factors have therefore not clearly been described based on large patient cohorts. Assumed risk factors that can compromise the vascular supply are high-energy trauma, associated fractures of the base of the femoral neck, and iatrogenic vascular damage [41].

Three case reports exist for isolated fractures of the greater trochanter and femoral head necrosis [42–44]. Two patients were treated conservatively [43, 44], while one patient was treated with open reduction and screw fixation [42]. Interestingly, all cases occurred in children aged between 12 and 13 years. In adults, greater trochanteric fractures typically involve avulsion fractures of the tip. In the pediatric population, the fracture often involves the trochanteric growth plate. This results in a larger fragment of the greater trochanter which extends far medial in the femoral neck [45] and may compromise the blood supply of the MFCA (Fig. 14.5).

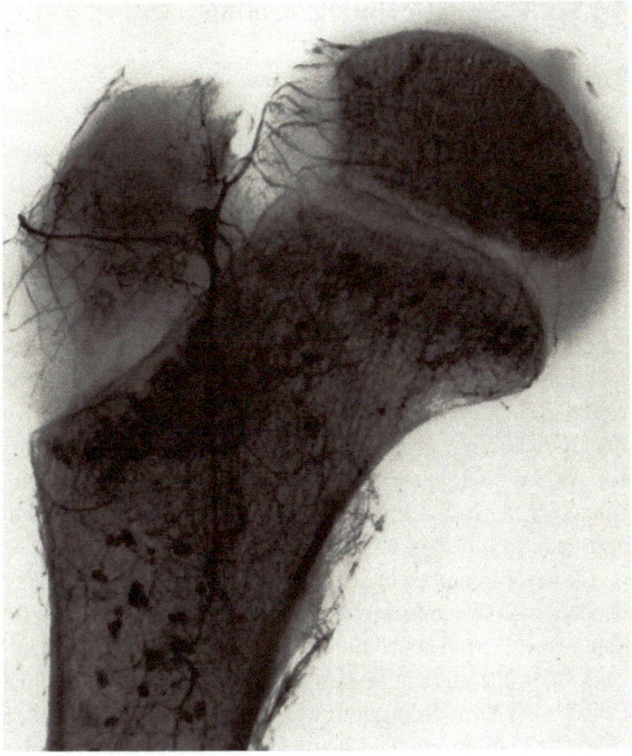

Fig. 14.5 Radiograph of the proximal femur and angiography of the medial circumflex femoral artery (MCFA) of a 6-year-old male. Both the epiphyseal and trochanteric growth plates are clearly visible. All cases of a greater trochanteric fracture resulting in AVN of the femoral head occurred in children. These fractures often involve the trochanteric growth plate. This results in a larger fragment of the greater trochanter which extends far medial in the femoral neck and may compromise the blood supply of the MFCA [45] (Reprinted with permission Trueta [45])

14.3.4 Femoral Shaft Fractures

Although femoral shaft fractures generally do not interfere with the course of the MCFA, a few cases of AVN following antegrade intramedullary nailing of the femur have been reported [24]. In these cases an iatrogenic damage to the MCFA at the location of nail insertion at the proximal femur has been described [32]. For geometrical and biomechanical reasons, the piriformis fossa has been recommended as nail insertion point of straight femoral nails. However, the piriformis fossa has a high risk for iatrogenic damage to the MCFA due to its close proximity (Fig. 14.6). In a cadaver study, nail insertion in the piriformis fossa resulted in damage to the nutrient vessel in all cases with complete disruption of the MCFA in 57 % [32]. In addition, intramedullary femoral reaming may put the vascular supply of the femoral head at risk (Table 14.2). The tip of the greater trochanter was suggested as a more appropriate insertion point with the use of an anatomically shaped femoral nail [32]. The problem

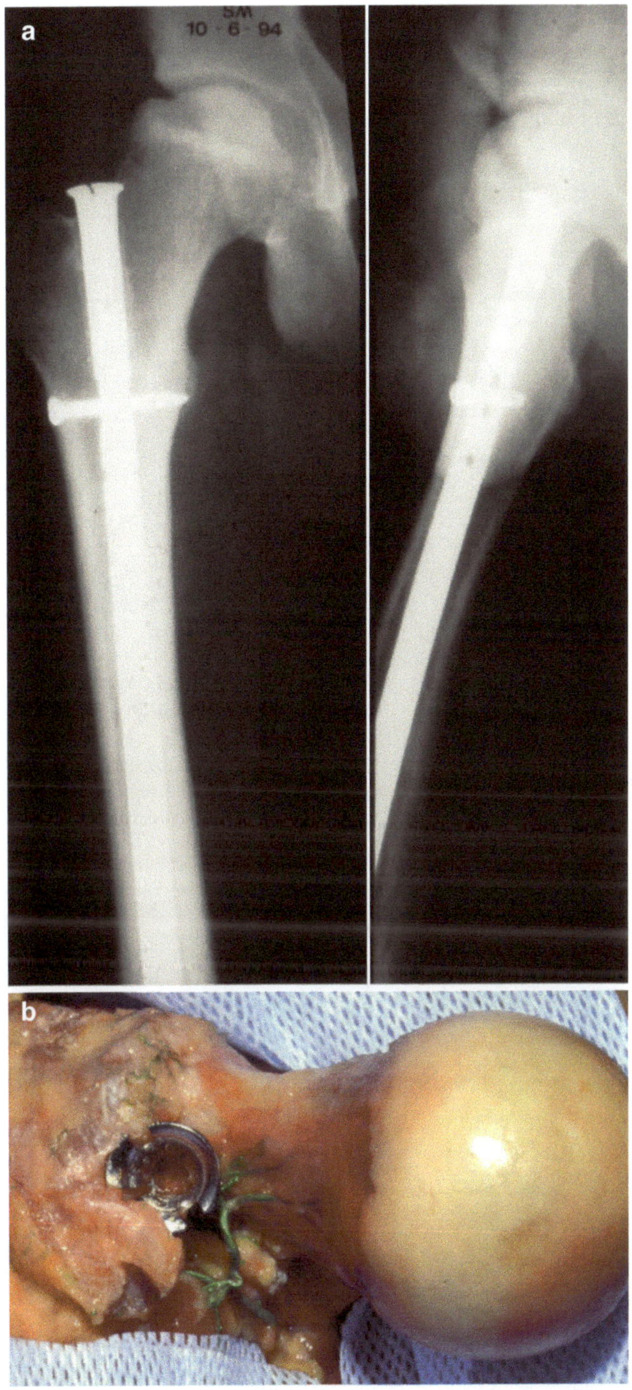

Fig. 14.6 (**a**) Fourteen-year-old male patient who sustained a femoral shaft fracture which was treated with antegrade intramedullary nailing. A very medial nail insertion point was chosen in close proximity to the medial circumflex femoral artery (MCFA). Eight months postoperative, avascular necrosis of the femoral head occurred. (Reprinted with permission Orler et al. [24]) (**b**) The risk of avascular necrosis of the femoral head following antegrade intramedullary nailing of the femur depends on the location of nail insertion [32]. In a cadaver study the use of the piriformis fossa as location of insertion with its close proximity to the MCFA showed damage to the nutrient vessel in all cases with complete disruption of the MCFA in 57% [32] (Reprinted with permission Dora et al. [32])

can be aggravated when oversized implants for adults are used in the pediatric population, which represent the majority of these cases with femoral shaft fractures and AVN of the femoral head [24] (Table 14.2).

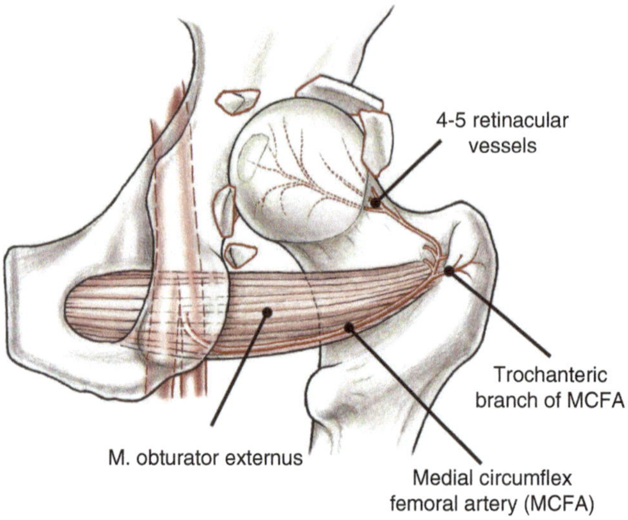

Fig. 14.7 The obturator externus muscle protects the deep branch of the MCFA in hips with traumatic dislocation [1]. Its integrity ascertains blood supply to the femoral head in hips with traumatic dislocation [46]

14.3.5 Traumatic Hip Dislocation

Traumatic hip dislocation is not necessarily associated with AVN. It could be shown that the obturator muscle is the most important structure to protect the MCFA in the dislocated position (Fig. 14.7) [1]. This fact is based on cadaver experiments for surgical hip dislocations [1]. As long as the obturator externus muscle is in continuity, the deep branch of the MCFA is not in danger or under relevant tension even with the femoral head dislocated [34, 47, 48]. Since the obturator externus muscle typically remains intact in traumatic hip dislocations [46], additional factors have to contribute to the reported incidence of AVN up to 26 % (Table 14.1) following traumatic hip dislocations. These additional risk factors for AVN include direction of dislocation [25], concomitant fracture [25, 26], delay of reduction [25, 27], and surgical approach [33] (Table 14.2).

Posterior traumatic hip dislocations have an increased incidence for AVN compared to anterior dislocations (29 vs. 9 %; Table 14.1) [25]. A concomitant femoral fracture may mechanically harm the nutrient vessels to the femoral head. The incidence of AVN for dislocations without fractures is zero to 22 % (Fig. 14.8) [46]. In contrast, the incidence for dislocations with a concomitant femoral head or acetabulum fracture was 66 % [25]. Early reduction may reduce the incidence of AVN [25, 27].

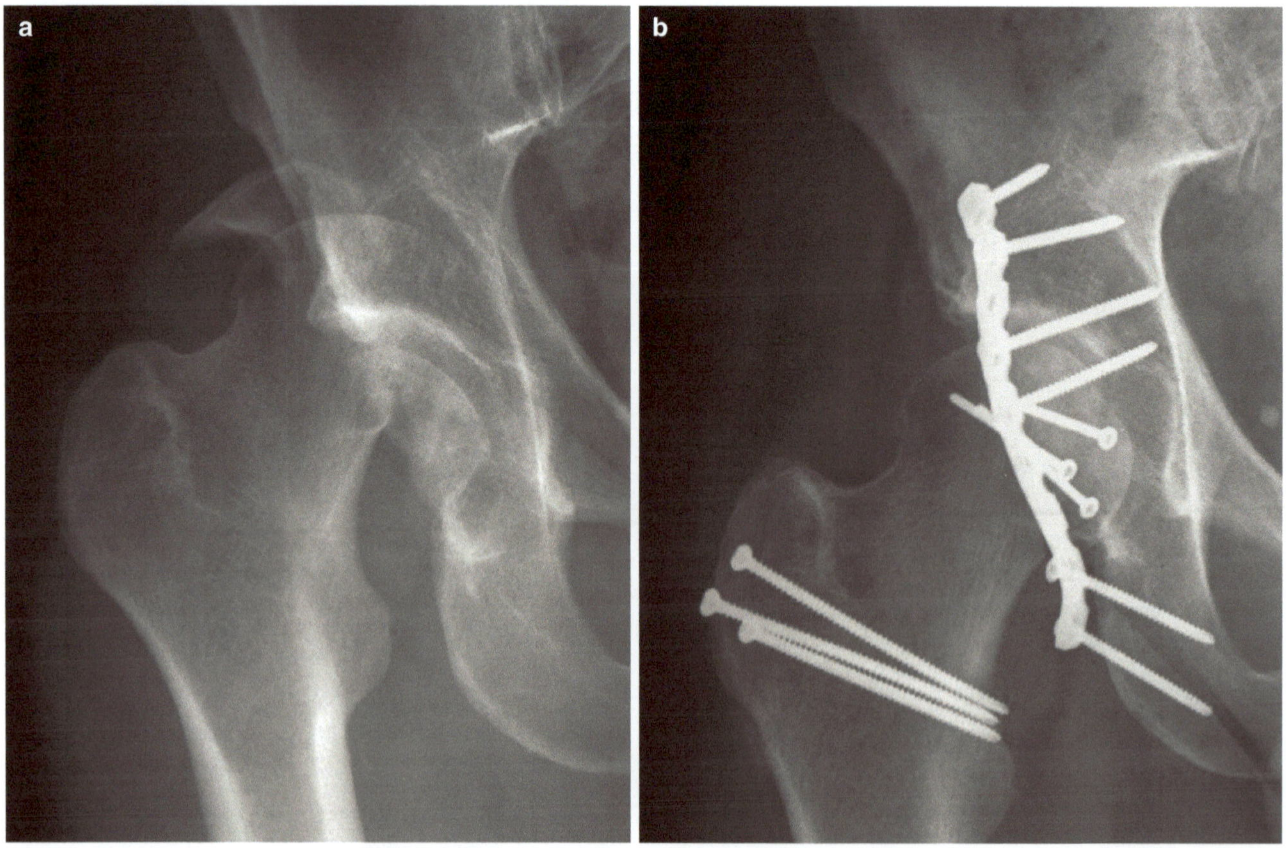

Fig. 14.8 (**a**) A 59-year-old male patient with traumatic posterior hip dislocation with a fracture of the femoral head and posterior acetabular wall. (**b**) Open reduction with internal fixation of the femoral head and posterior wall was performed using a trochanteric flip approach. (**c**) Half a year postoperative, avascular necrosis of the femoral head occurred necessitating total hip arthroplasty

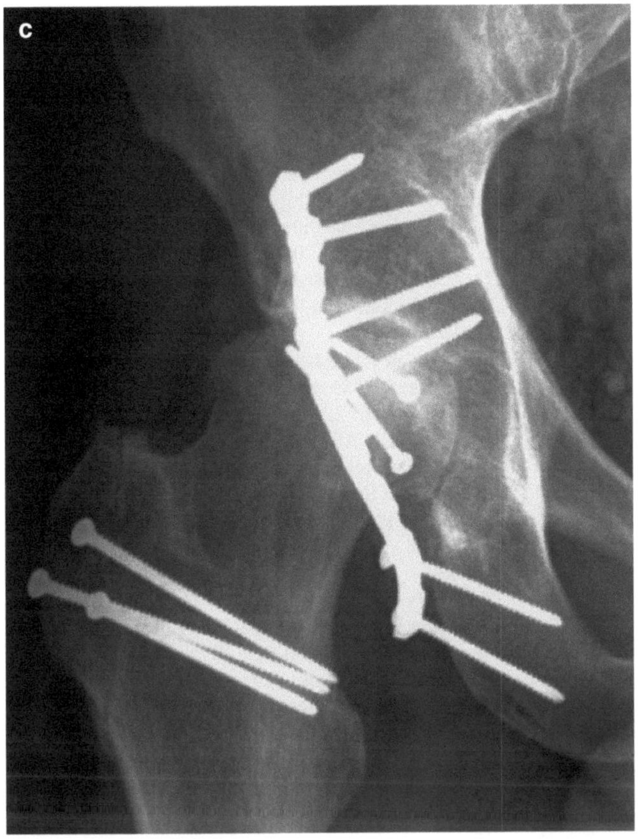

Fig. 14.8 (continued)

Based on laser Doppler studies, the femoral head blood supply can be reduced in the dislocated position, but will normalize after reduction in all hips [47]. With a delay of 6 or 12 h for reduction, the incidence increases from 5 to 59 % [27] or from 18 to 57 % [25], respectively. When performing a standard Kocher-Langenbeck approach (with or without detachment of the short external rotators), the MCFA can potentially be iatrogenically harmed. This could explain the three times higher incidence of AVN in traumatic hip dislocations with a posterior approach for internal fixation in comparison to the anterior approach [33].

14.4 Summary

Traumatic AVN of the femoral head derives from the interruption of the blood supply to the femoral head. The MCFA plays the key role for maintenance of the femoral head viability. The incidence of AVN varies greatly among the different fracture types of the proximal femur. It is directly correlated to the proximity of the fracture site with the topographical course of the MCFA. Preoperative noninvasive assessment of intact vascularity of the femoral head is theoretically possible with various imaging modalities. However, none of these methods has found its way into clinical routine use. The most sensitive and specific method to determine an intact vascularity is bleeding of the femoral head after intraoperative drilling. Lack of bleeding may be due to an interruption of the afferent blood supply to the femoral head, from either a definitive (e.g., rupture) or transient (e.g., vasospasm, kinking) stop of the MCFA.

References

1. Gautier E, Ganz K, Krugel N, Gill T, Ganz R. Anatomy of the medial femoral circumflex artery and its surgical implications. J Bone Joint Surg Br. 2000;82(5):679–83.
2. Sevitt S, Thompson RG. The distribution and anastomoses of arteries supplying the head and neck of the femur. J Bone Joint Surg Br. 1965;47:560–73.
3. Tannast M, Mack PW, Klaeser B, Siebenrock KA. Hip dislocation and femoral neck fracture: decision-making for head preservation. Injury. 2009;40(10):1118–24.
4. Kalhor M, Horowitz K, Gharehdaghi J, Beck M, Ganz R. Anatomic variations in femoral head circulation. Hip Int. 2012;22(3):307–12.
5. Brünner S, Christiansen J, Kristensen JK. Arteriographic prediction of femoral head viability in medial femoral neck fractures. Acta Chir Scand. 1967;133(6):449.
6. Müssbichler H. Arteriographic studies in fractures of the femoral neck and trochanteric region type and incidence of findings in pre- and postoperative examina tions, relation to fracture dislocation and prognostic value. Angiology. 1970;21(6):385–402.
7. Gill TJ, Sledge JB, Ekkernkamp A, Ganz R. Intraoperative assessment of femoral head vascularity after femoral neck fracture. J Orthop Trauma. 1998;12(7):474–8.
8. Zlotorowicz M, Czubak J, Kozinski P, Boguslawska-Walecka R. Imaging the vascularisation of the femoral head by CT angiography. J Bone Joint Surg Br. 2012;94(9):1176–9.
9. Hirata T, Konishiike T, Kawai A, Sato T, Inoue H. Dynamic magnetic resonance imaging of femoral head perfusion in femoral neck fracture. Clin Orthop Relat Res. 2001;393:294–301.
10. Bauer G, Weber DA, Ceder L, Darte L, Egund N, Hansson LI, Strömqvist B. Dynamics of technetium-99m methylenediphosphonate imaging of the femoral head after hip fracture. Clin Orthop Relat Res. 1980;152:85–92.
11. D'Ambrosia RD, Riggins RS, Stadalnik RC, Denardo GL. Vascularity of the femoral head: 99mTc diphosphonate scintigraphy validated with tetracycline labeling. Clin Orthop Relat Res. 1976;121:143–8.
12. Cho M-R, Lee S-W, Shin D-K, Kim S-K, Kim S-Y, Ko S-B, Kwun K-W. A predictive method for subsequent avascular necrosis of the femoral head (AVNFH) by observation of bleeding from the cannulated screw used for fixation of intracapsular femoral neck fractures. J Orthop Trauma. 2007;21(3):158–64.
13. Sugamoto K, Ochi T, Takahashi Y, Tamura T, Matsuoka T. Hemodynamic measurement in the femoral head using laser Doppler. Clin Orthop Relat Res. 1998;353:138–47.
14. Watanabe Y, Terashima Y, Takenaka N, Kobayashi M, Matsushita T. Prediction of avascular necrosis of the femoral head by measuring intramedullary oxygen tension after femoral neck fracture. J Orthop Trauma. 2007;21(7):456–61.
15. Giannoudis PV, Kontakis G, Christoforakis Z, Akula M, Tosounidis T, Koutras C. Management, complications and clinical results of femoral head fractures. Injury. 2009;40(12):1245–51.
16. Guo JJ, Tang N, Yang HL, Qin L, Leung KS. Impact of surgical approach on postoperative heterotopic ossification and avascular

necrosis in femoral head fractures: a systematic review. Int Orthop. 2010;34(3):319–22.
17. Moon ES, Mehlman CT. Risk factors for avascular necrosis after femoral neck fractures in children: 25 Cincinnati cases and meta-analysis of 360 cases. J Orthop Trauma. 2006;20(5):323–9.
18. Yeranosian M, Horneff JG, Baldwin K, Hosalkar HS. Factors affecting the outcome of fractures of the femoral neck in children and adolescents a systematic review. J Bone Joint Surg Am. 2013;95(1):135–42.
19. Garden RS. Malreduction and avascular necrosis in subcapital fractures of the femur. J Bone Joint Surg Br. 1971;53(2):183–97.
20. Holmberg S, Kalén R, Thorngren KG. Treatment and outcome of femoral neck fractures an analysis of 2418 patients admitted from their own homes. Clin Orthop Relat Res. 1987;218:42–52.
21. Johnson JT, Crothers O. Nailing versus prosthesis for femoral-neck fractures. A critical review of long-term results in two hundred and thirty-nine consecutive private patients. J Bone Joint Surg Am. 1975;57(5):686–92.
22. Strömqvist B, Hansson LI, Nilsson LT, Thorngren K-G. Hook-pin fixation in femoral neck fractures a two-year follow-up study of 300 cases. Clin Orthop Relat Res. 1987;218:58–62.
23. Aguado-Maestro I, Escudero-Marcos R, Garcia-Garcia JM, Alonso-Garcia N, Perez-Bermejo DD, Aguado-Hernandez HJ, Nistal-Rodriguez J, Garcia-Alonso M. Results and complications of pertrochanteric hip fractures using an intramedullary nail with a helical blade (proximal femoral nail antirotation) in 200 patients. Rev Esp Cir Ortop Traumatol. 2013;57(3):201–7.
24. Orler R, Hersche O, Helfet DL, Mayo KA, Ward T, Ganz R. Avascular necrosis of the femoral head as a serious complication following femoral nailing in children and adolescents. Unfallchirurg. 1998;101(6):495–9.
25. Brav EA. Traumatic dislocation of the hip: army experience and results over a 12 year period. J Bone Joint Surg Am. 1962;44:1115–34.
26. Epstein HC. Posterior fracture-dislocations of the hip; long-term follow-up. J Bone Joint Surg Am. 1974;56(6):1103–27.
27. Hougaard K, Thomsen PB. Traumatic posterior dislocation of the hip—prognostic factors influencing the incidence of avascular necrosis of the femoral head. Arch Orthop Trauma Surg. 1986; 106(1):32–5.
28. Delbet MP. Fractures du col de femur. Bull Mem Soc Chir. 1907;35:387–9.
29. Jain R, Koo M, Kreder HJ, Schemitsch EH, Davey JR, Mahomed NN. Comparison of early and delayed fixation of subcapital hip fractures in patients sixty years of age or less. J Bone Joint Surg Am. 2002;84(9):1605–12.
30. Pillai A, Little K, Chappell A. Osteonecrosis of the femoral head following medullary nailing of the femur in an adult. Acta orthopaedica belgica. 2007;73(2):258.
31. Wu C-C, Yu C-T, Hsieh C-P, Chen S-J, Chang L. Femoral head avascular necrosis after interlocking nail of a femoral shaft fracture in a male adult: a case report. Arch Orthop Trauma Surg. 2008;128(4):399–402.
32. Dora C, Leunig M, Beck M, Rothenfluh D, Ganz R. Entry point soft tissue damage in antegrade femoral nailing: a cadaver study. J Orthop Trauma. 2001;15(7):488–93.
33. Stannard JP, Harris HW, Volgas DA, Alonso JE. Functional outcome of patients with femoral head fractures associated with hip dislocations. Clin Orthop Relat Res. 2000;377:44–56.
34. Ganz R, Gill TJ, Gautier E, Ganz K, Krugel N, Berlemann U. Surgical dislocation of the adult hip a technique with full access to the femoral head and acetabulum without the risk of avascular necrosis. J Bone Joint Surg Br. 2001;83(8):1119–24.
35. Shan-hong Q. Accuracy of closed reduction for displaced subcapital femoral neck fractures assisted by C-arm X-ray machine. CRTER. 2012;16(9):1643–6.
36. Mohan R, Karthikeyan R, Sonanis SV. Dynamic hip screw: does side make a difference? Effects of clockwise torque on right and left DHS. Injury. 2000;31(9):697–9.
37. Beck M, Siebenrock KA, Affolter B, Nötzli H, Parvizi J, Ganz R. Increased intraarticular pressure reduces blood flow to the femoral head. Clin Orthop Relat Res. 2004;424:149–52.
38. Bonnaire F, Schaefer DJ, Kuner EH. Hemarthrosis and hip joint pressure in femoral neck fractures. Clin Orthop Relat Res. 1998;353:148–55.
39. Crawfurd EJ, Emery RJ, Hansell DM, Phelan M, Andrews BG. Capsular distension and intracapsular pressure in subcapital fractures of the femur. J Bone Joint Surg Br. 1988;70(2):195–8.
40. Woodhouse CF. Dynamic influences of vascular occlusion affecting the development of avascular necrosis of the femoral head. Clin Orthop Relat Res. 1964;32:119–29.
41. Shih L-Y, Chen T-H, Lo W-H. Avascular necrosis of the femoral head-an unusual complication of an intertrochanteric fracture. J Orthop Trauma. 1992;6(3):382–5.
42. Kaweblum M, Lehman WB, Grant AD, Strongwater A. Avascular necrosis of the femoral head as sequela of fracture of the greater trochanter: a case report and review of the literature. Clin Orthop Relat Res. 1993;294:193–5.
43. Linhart W, Stampfel O, Ritter G. Post-traumatic femur head necrosis following trochanter fracture. Z Orthop Ihre Grenzgeb. 1984;122(6):766.
44. Stougard J. Post-traumatic avascular necrosis of the femoral head in children. Report of two cases. J Bone Joint Surg Br. 1969;51(2): 354–5.
45. Trueta J. The normal vascular anatomy of the human femoral head during growth. J Bone Joint Surg Br. 1957;39(2):358–94.
46. Tannast M, Pleus F, Bonel H, Galloway H, Siebenrock KA, Anderson SE. Magnetic resonance imaging in traumatic posterior hip dislocation. J Orthop Trauma. 2010;24(12):723–31.
47. Notzli HP, Siebenrock KA, Hempfing A, Ramseier LE, Ganz R. Perfusion of the femoral head during surgical dislocation of the hip. Monitoring by laser Doppler flowmetry. J Bone Joint Surg Br. 2002;84(2):300–4.
48. Tannast M, Siebenrock KA. Open therapy of femoroacetabular impingement. Oper Orthop Traumatol. 2010;22(1):3–16.

15 Posttraumatic Osteonecrosis of the Femoral Head

Taek Rim Yoon and Ha Sung Kim

15.1 Introduction

The lifetime incidence of hip trauma is about 23.3 % in males and 11.2 % in females [1, 2]. Major complications of hip traumas include nonunion, malunion, and osteonecrosis. Posttraumatic osteonecrosis, which is reported in a range of 4.8–52.9 %, ultimately leads to arthritis unless diagnosed in the initial stage [3, 4]. Patients with hip injuries should be followed closely for the earlier diagnosis of osteonecrosis. Timely treatment can prevent the progression of osteonecrosis and later arthritic changes. After the diagnosis of necrosis, appropriate treatment must be done in early stages if head preservation seems possible.

Treatment in both posttraumatic and nontraumatic osteonecrosis is very similar. The choice of treatment will depend on patient age, gender, extent of necrosis, and location of osteonecrosis.

15.2 Incidence of Posttraumatic Osteonecrosis

Hip trauma is a major risk factor of osteonecrosis together with steroid, alcohol, and connective tissue diseases. The risk increases with the degree of displacement and comminution of fracture and dislocation. The risk of osteonecrosis also increases as the fracture line moves closer to the head, and subcapital fractures have the maximum risk of osteonecrosis [5–10].

The incidence of osteonecrosis after dislocation, which is reported to be in the range of 10–25 %, varies depending on the severity of injury of the associated femoral head or acetabular fractures [11]. Eighty-five to ninety percent of hip dislocations are posterior dislocations with or without other associated femoral head injuries [12]. Hougaahou et al. [4] reported that the incidence of osteonecrosis was 4.8 % when anatomical reduction was performed within 6 h after dislocation, while the percentage rose to 52.9 % when the reduction was performed after 6 h.

The incidence of osteonecrosis after a displaced femoral neck fracture is reported to be 15–20 % [13–16]. The discrepancies in the reported incidence reflect variation with fracture types, accuracy of reduction, and time to reduction.

Osteonecrosis can occur in neck fractures whether the fracture occurs at the intra- and extracapsular level. In general intracapsular fractures are at higher risk compared to extracapsular fractures [17, 18]. The actual incidence may be estimated to be higher considering the possibility of follow-up loss or overlooked reports of osteonecrosis after pertrochanteric fractures in the literature [19].

15.2.1 Factors Related to the Incidence of Osteonecrosis

15.2.1.1 Age

Age is a suspected, but unconfirmed, factor related with the incidence of osteonecrosis [13, 20–23]. Some researchers claimed that the incidence of posttraumatic osteonecrosis is positively correlated with age [20, 21], while another study reported that the incidence decreased after 75 years of age [13]. This may reflect the fact that in younger people these injuries often occur after high-energy trauma, with associated damage to soft tissue and vascularity similar to nontraumatic osteonecrosis, in contrast to more elderly individuals in which injuries typically occur after low-energy trauma. These research findings suggest that the estimated incidence of osteonecrosis is high after intracapsular fractures that occur among adults under 50 years of age. It is very important to determine the best treatment, especially in young patients who have a long life expectancy and high activity level.

T.R. Yoon (✉) • H.S. Kim
Orthopedic Department of Center for Joint Disease, Chonnam National University Hwasun Hospital, 160 Ilsimri, Hwasuneup, Hwasun 519-809, Korea
e-mail: tryoon@jnu.ac.kr; hasskim@naver.com

K.-H. Koo et al. (eds.), *Osteonecrosis*,
DOI 10.1007/978-3-642-35767-1_15, © Springer-Verlag Berlin Heidelberg 2014

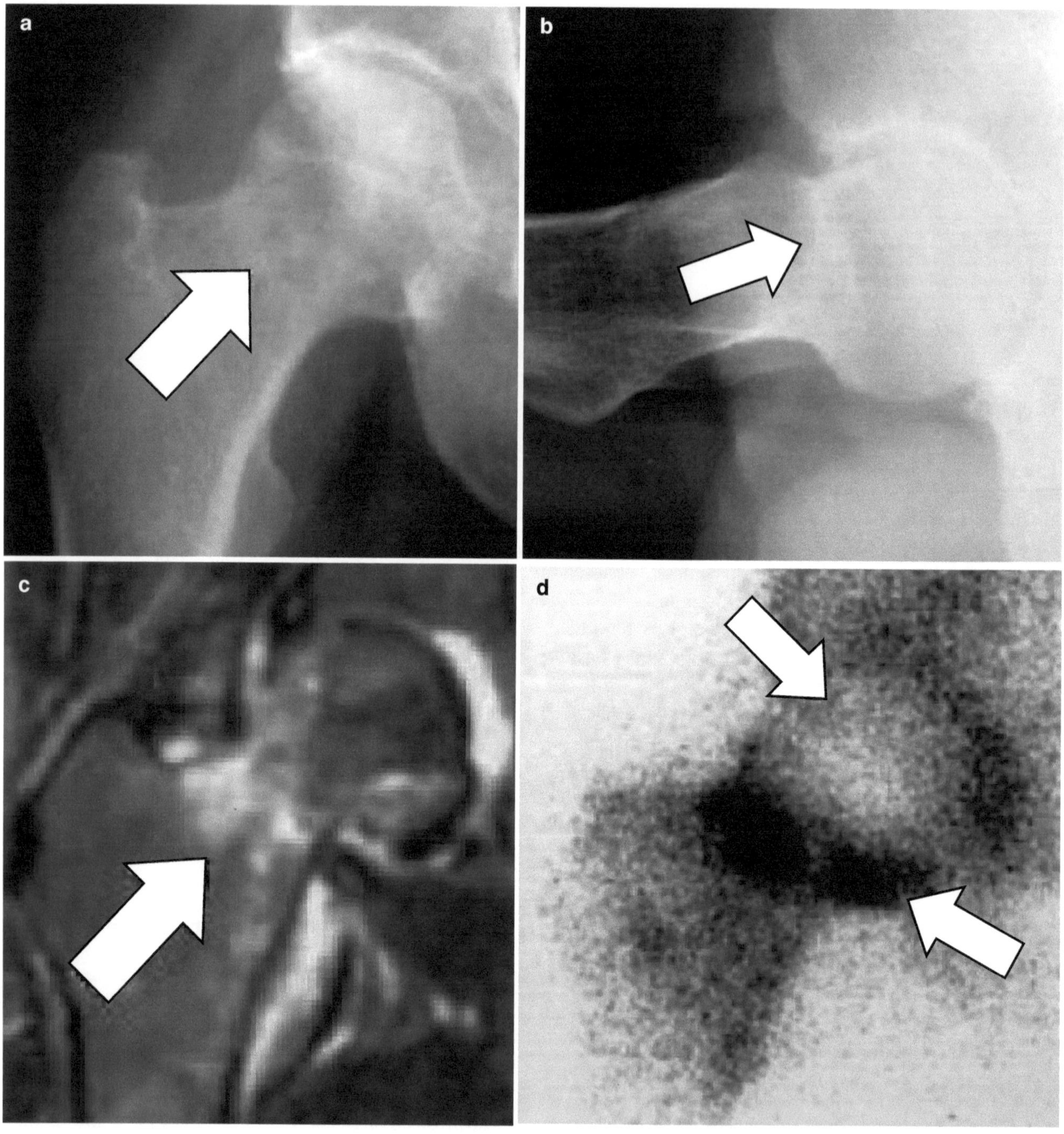

Fig. 15.1 Plain radiographs of a 45-year-old man with right femoral osteonecrosis show linear sclerosis (*arrow*) in the right femoral neck (**a**, **b**). These look like a femoral neck fracture pattern (High signal intensity bandlike lesion, indicated by *arrow*) on MRI image (**c**), but bone scan images show the characteristics of avascular necrosis with photon defect and increased uptake of subcapital area (**d**)

15.2.1.2 Degree of Displacement and Reduction

The degree of displacement in the intracapsular fracture is closely related with the development of osteonecrosis. In Garden's classification, without displacement is classified as Type 1 and 2 and with displacement is classified as Type 3 and 4. This classification helps to predict development of osteonecrosis [14]. Researchers have reported a strong correlation between the development of avascular necrosis and fragment displacement [24]. This suggests that damage in reticular arteries caused by displacement of bone fragments or posterior dislocation plays an important role in the development of posttraumatic osteonecrosis.

The degree of reduction in femur neck fracture is determined based on the Garden's alignment index, which refers to

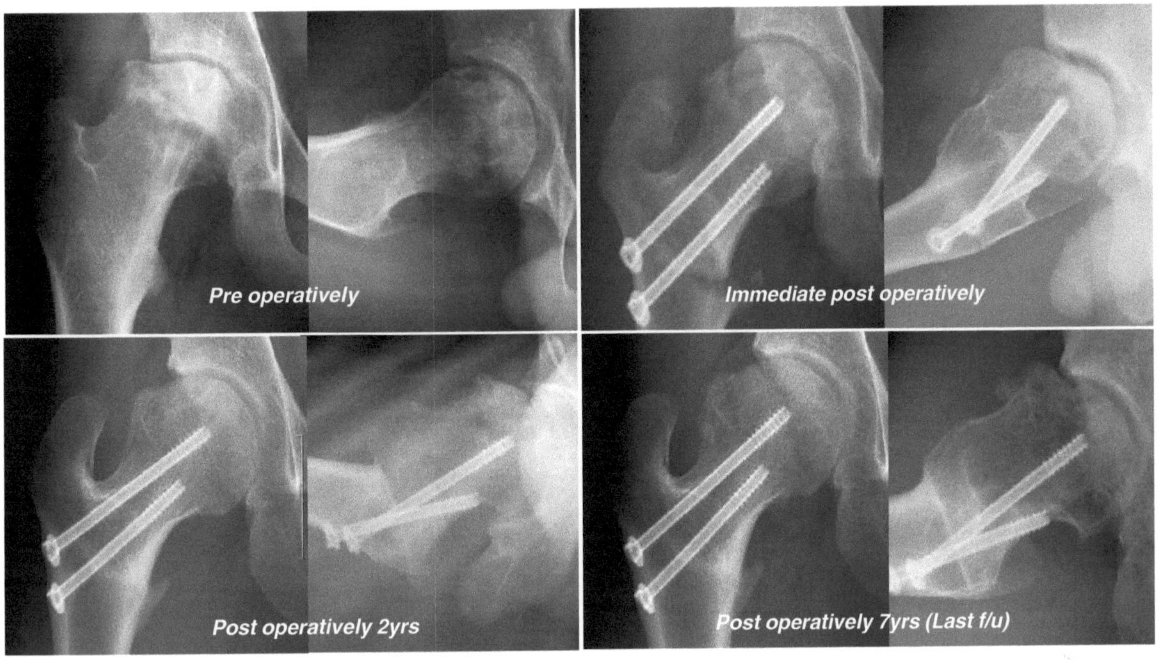

Fig. 15.2 Serial radiographs of anterior rotational trochanteric osteotomy from a 16-year-old man with posttraumatic osteonecrosis of the femoral head are shown

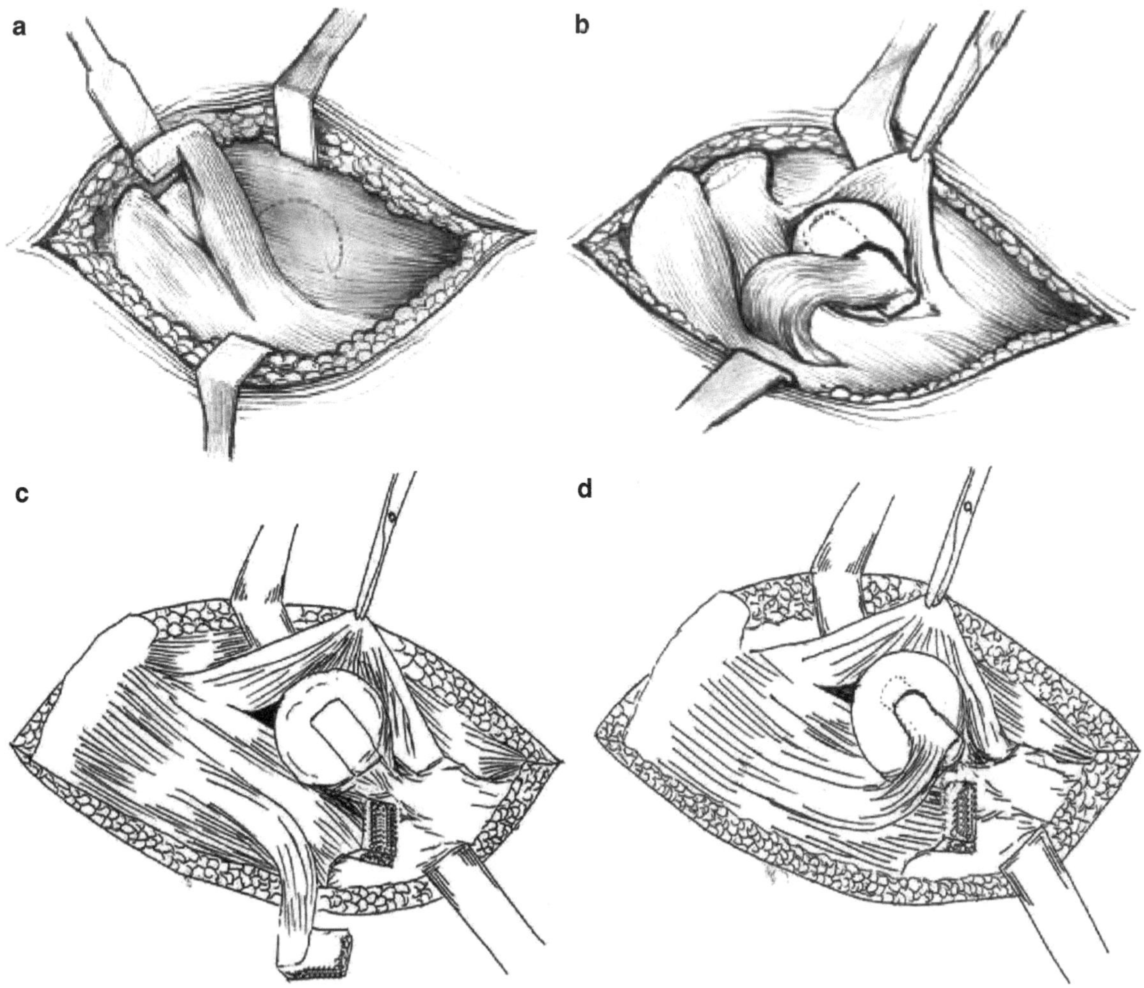

Fig. 15.3 Gluteus medius muscle pedicl bone graft from iliac crest (**a**, **b**) and from greater trochanter (**c**, **d**)

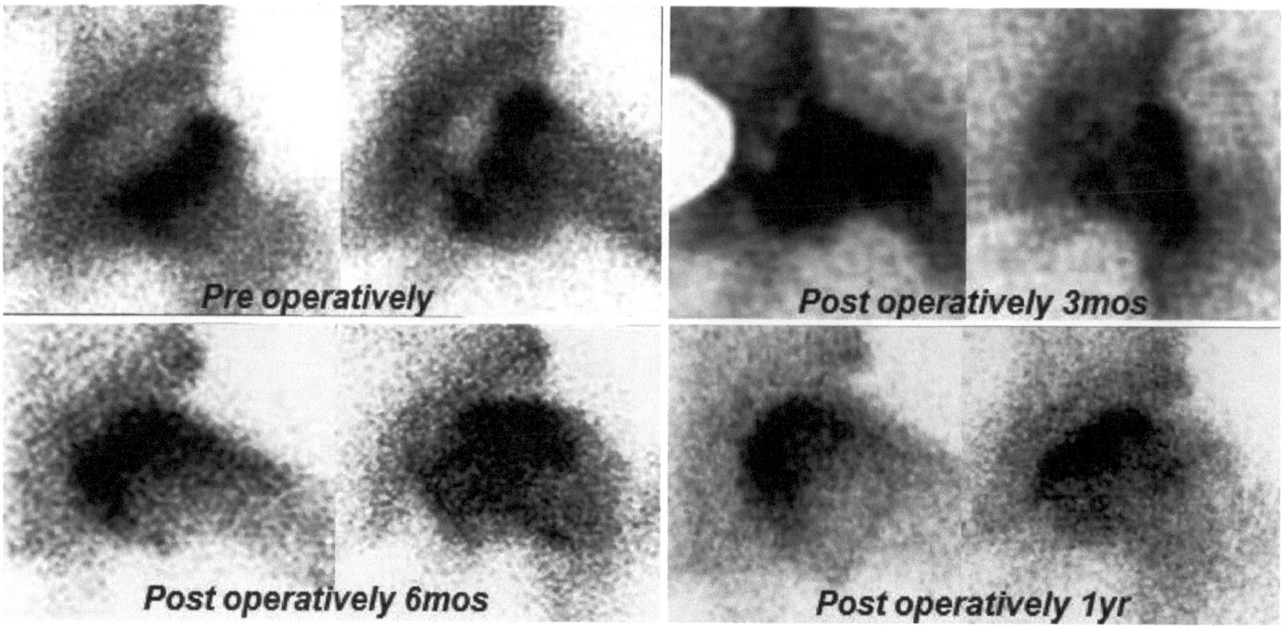

Fig. 15.4 Serial pinhole bone scintigraphy after vessel-pedicle bone graft for osteonecrosis of the femoral head shows gradually increasing uptake in the femoral head

the angles of the medial cortex line and proximal trabeculae bundle axis on a radiograph of the anterior and posterior segments of hip joints. An acceptable range of 150–185° insures maximum chances of union and minimum chances of osteonecrosis [8, 25, 26]. However, severe comminuted fracture of the femoral neck or malrotation and/or unstable fixation may negatively affect revascularization of the head and may lead to osteonecrosis [14]. Sustained traction or excessive internal/external rotation of the hip, especially if maintained for a long time before surgery, may damage the lateral femoral circumflex artery causing osteonecrosis [27–30].

To decrease risk of damage of the major vessels, it is preferable to avoid excessive extension or internal rotation of the hip joint [28–32]. Several reports recommended that the removal of intracapsular hematoma improves blood flow of the femoral head and decreases the development of osteonecrosis [33–35].

Every reduction after traumatic hip dislocation is also important to prevent osteonecrosis. Sanders et al. [9] found that the incidence of osteonecrosis was 4.8 % when reduced within 6 h and 52.9 % when reduced after 6 h. Similarly, Yeranosian et al. [36] also reported that when the reduction was achieved within 24 h, osteonecrosis progression was four times less as compared to patients in whom reduction was achieved after more than 24 h. These findings emphasize the significance of early reduction in hip joint dislocations.

15.2.1.3 Timing of Surgical Intervention

It is still controversial whether delay of surgery increases the incidence of osteonecrosis when treating neck fractures [37, 38]. There is a close correlation between delayed treatment and onset of traumatic osteonecrosis of the hip [39, 40]. It was recommended that traction for the neck fracture should be kept in flexion position to decrease intracapsular pressure before surgery [30]. In contrast, another report claimed that early preoperative reduction of the fracture using splinting or traction of a limb did not affect outcome and no correlation was found between the development of osteonecrosis and the time to surgical intervention after trauma. The authors recommended a good preoperative plan and achievement of a stable and anatomical reduction during operation because these aspects are more important than early surgery [38]. More evidence needs to be collected more a definitive conclusion is reached.

15.2.1.4 Type of Surgery

The type of surgery also affects the development of osteonecrosis. The incidence of posttraumatic osteonecrosis reportedly decreased significantly when less invasive procedure and the accurate reduction was achieved [29]. Garden et al. reported that the results of follow-up of 500 cases of subcapital femoral neck fracture showed a decrease in the incidence of osteonecrosis depending on the skills and experience of the surgeons [14]. The fixation methods affected the incidence of osteonecrosis based on a study of 219 patients with femoral neck fracture in which four different fixation methods were used [37].

The majority of displaced neck fractures require open reduction and internal fixation. However, during the intraoperative femoral head screw fixation, the remaining retinacular vessel can be damaged if the head rotation is not precise. The lateral circumflex artery can be damaged dur-

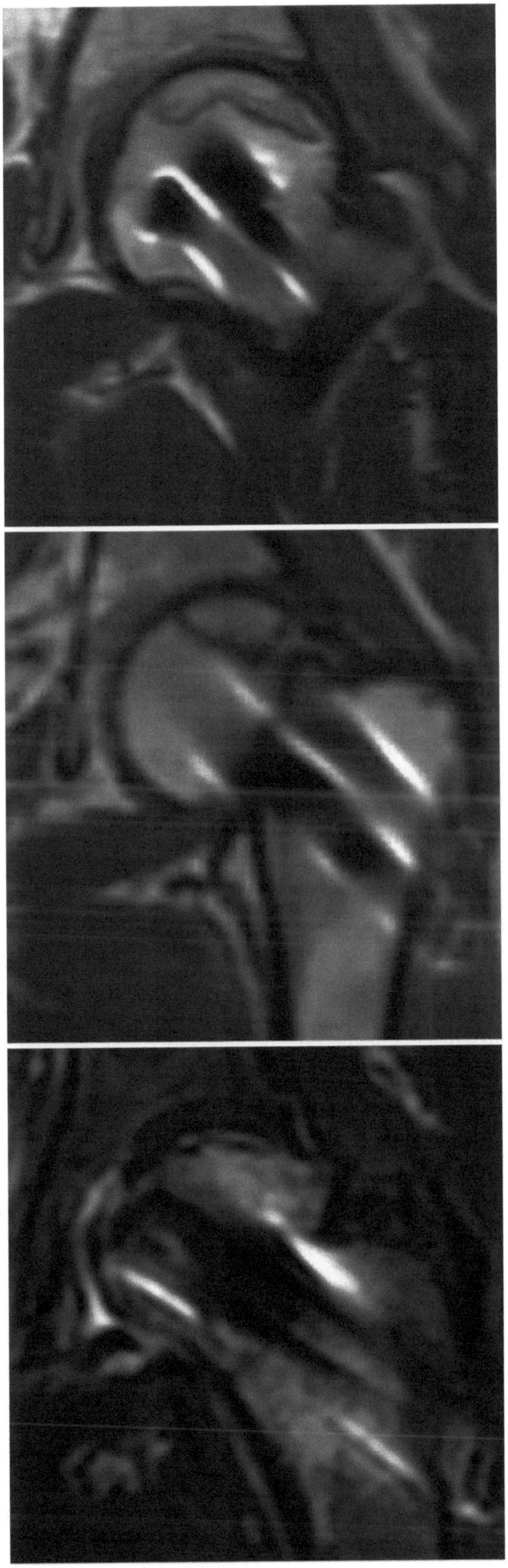

Fig. 15.5 Three cases of posttraumatic osteonecrosis development are shown

ing intramedullary nail insertion in pertrochanteric or subtrochanteric fracture [41]. Thus, at the time of a internal fixation, the surgeon should be careful about malrotation of the femoral head. Attention should be paid to avoid retinacular artery damage when intramedullary nailing is performed.

In older patients with a femoral neck fracture, arthroplasty as a primary treatment has been performed to avoid secondary surgery because of later osteonecrosis or nonunion. Patient's age is one of the crucial factors for the choice of treatment in femoral neck fracture. Primary arthroplasty rather than internal fixation is preferred in older patients with femoral neck fracture [42]. Bipolar hemiarthroplasty has advantages of shorter surgery time and lesser bleeding compared with total hip arthroplasty. However, since some patients complain of groin pain after bipolar hemiarthroplasty, total hip arthroplasty is increasing [43].

15.3 Diagnosis of Posttraumatic Osteonecrosis

15.3.1 Signs and Symptoms

Most patients with osteonecrosis may not present clinically until later stages. Some patients may remain asymptomatic even in the stage of segmental collapse. The pain in osteonecrosis is usually located in the inguinal/gluteal/proximal femoral region. However, it is commonly neglected by patients and wrongly attributed to previous trauma. Therefore it is important that clinician differentiate these symptoms very carefully. Long-term follow-up of these patients is important as segmental collapse can occur as late as 2 years after injury [8, 13]. It is impossible to detect early osteonecrosis in patients with nontraumatic osteonecrosis, while early diagnosis is possible by interval checkup in patients with posttraumatic osteonecrosis. Therefore, compared with patients with nontraumatic osteonecrosis, proper treatment can be provided to patients with posttraumatic osteonecrosis.

15.3.2 Imaging

15.3.2.1 X-ray

X-ray diagnosis of posttraumatic osteonecrosis is very similar to nontraumatic osteonecrosis. When a diagnosis of early stage of osteonecrosis is considered using X-ray, the reported sensitivity of radiologic diagnosis in the early stage is around 41 % [44]. It takes 1–5 years for the pathology of osteonecrosis to progress and produce abnormalities that are apparent on X-ray, and posttraumatic osteonecrosis usually does not appear until 1–2 years after injury. Some reports suggested that most patients show radiologic changes of osteonecrosis within 2–3 years after trauma, while others reported the osteonecrosis was detected at 11–24 months after the internal fixation on plain radiography [7, 13, 14, 16, 45]. Considering these dichotomous reports, osteonecrosis should not be ruled out after a simple check of X-ray with normal appearance, and all patients should be followed up for a protracted time.

If osteoclastic resorption overlaps with new bone formation on the revascularized area, it is evident as mottled density on the X-ray. If the femoral head is collapsed, increased density is evident in the compacted area. Subchondral sclerosis or lucency also suggests osteonecrosis. This may be caused by increased density or osteoporosis in bone tissue where blood is not supplied. In cases of associated nonunion, radiologic changes and late femoral head collapse may be further delayed due to the absence of the revascularization process.

The best view for the femoral neck can be obtained by anteroposterior radiographic view with 15° internal rotation of the hip joint in the supine position. For a clearer view of the femoral head, it is necessary to check the femoral head lateral view, because femoral head collapse and crescent sign (subchondral facture sign) in early stages are mainly detected in the anterosuperior segment of the femoral head. The patient is laid in the supine position with the hip in 90° flexion and 45° abduction. The X-ray beam is directed from anterior to posterior. If the metallic implant blocks the necrotic lesion of interest on the X-ray, the patient's position may be changed to obtain a better view. The radiographic images are only a basic standard for examination. Magnetic resonance imaging (MRI) and bone scan should be added for precise and definite diagnosis.

15.3.2.2 MRI

MRI is considered to be the most effective diagnostic tool for the diagnosis of nontraumatic osteonecrosis and traumatic osteonecrosis because of its specificity and sensitivity [46, 47]. MRI can detect bone marrow change very early and can predict its progression. MRI has a higher sensitivity than computed tomography (CT) or radionuclide bone scintigraphy [48, 49]. Glickstein et al. [46] reported MRI specificity and sensitivity of 98 and 97 %, respectively. Diagnoses can be made on the T1-weighted axial localizer and T1-weighted or T2-weighted spin-echo coronal images. The necrotic margin is evident as a single line on T1-weighted images and a double line on T2-weighted images. The double-line sign is a specific and pathognomonic sign also in nontraumatic osteonecrosis, and it is seen in concentric low- and high-signal-intensity bands on the T2-weighted image [50].

MRI has a 96.7 % accuracy compared with the pathologic diagnosis of core biopsy [47]. Even though MRI patterns do not exactly match radiographic stages, MRI can provide all the information necessary for diagnosis and clinical staging, while the bone scan offers limited information [51, 52].

Contrary to general beliefs, internal metallic fixation does not cause any problems in MRI imaging because most metallic implants do not have a ferromagnetic property. However, metallic implants have different susceptibility between metallic implants and surrounding tissues which could cause a geometric distortion known as the susceptibility artifact. If an internal metallic fixation is in place after the injury, it leads to image distortion making diagnosis difficult [48, 53]. The cause of the problem is the nonlinearity that characterizes metal elements. Nonlinearity resulting from pixel shift and intensity variation can lead to serious distortions in images [46, 49, 51, 52, 54–57].

This susceptibility artifact is determined by the composition of metallic devices and the different MRI parameters such as the orientation of devices in relation to direction of the main magnetic field, type of pulse sequence, voxel size as determined by the field of view, image matrix, section thickness, and echo train length [47, 50, 57–60]. Titanium implants create fewer artifacts than stainless steel implants [47]. Bagheri et al. [61] reported fewer artifacts with increasing duration after surgery with metallic implants. Artifacts remain a significant problem in MRI. Some artifacts remain, even when the implants are removed [62].

There are few reports about the MRI findings in posttraumatic osteonecrosis. Speer et al. [63] reported that a two-dimensional Fourier transform spin-echo technique detected no changes in the first 48 h after intracapsular neck fracture. Along the same line, another study reported that no significant changes or histological necrosis were detected even after the first 65 days. Kamano et al. [64] reported on the three patterns on the T1 and T2 fat saturation images taken 24.5 h after femur transcervical neck fractures. Type I, which revealed non-enhancement, was related to necrosis in all cases, while type III showing a total enhancement was linked to femoral head viability in all patients. Type II which reveals partial enhancement was related with osteonecrosis in five of 12 cases. In the report of Sugano et al., MRI was done 1, 6, and 12 months after internal fixation in 17 cases of femur neck transcervical fracture [65]. At 1 month after the surgery, a low signal was detected in T1 and high signal in T2 in eight cases. The authors identified three different types of images: small upper lateral infarction was classified as type 1, narrow upper lateral lesion extending to the fovea as type 2, and wide lesion taking up most of femoral head as type 3. All 17 cases were observed to have abnormalities on MRI. None of the cases in type 1, 75 % cases in type 2, and all the cases in type 3 progressed to necrosis. In the report of Kawasaki et al. on femur neck transcervical fracture, T1-weighted MRI and plain radiographic images were taken at 1, 2, 6, and 12 months after internal fixation [45]. On the images taken 2 months after the procedure, eight of

31 cases showed band-like images; on the images taken in 6 months, 12 cases showed band-like images. Among the band-like images classified as B1 (lateral), B2 (superficial), B3 (intermediate), and B4 (extensive), necrosis was related to the B2, B3, and B4 bands. It was also related to Garden types 3 and 4. Specificity and diagnosis accuracy was 100 and 87 %, respectively.

15.3.2.3 Bone Scan

Planar scintigraphic imaging has a sensitivity ranging from 47.8 to 78.3 %. Despite the fact that sensitivity is low at stages I and II, planar scintigraphic imaging has several strengths. It has no false-positive imaging and is useful in patients with cardiac pacemakers or intracranial clips or who suffer from claustrophobia, for whom MRI is not indicated [66]. Bone scintigraphy can detect early osteonecrosis even when MRI does not detect the necrotic changes [67, 68]. Maillefert et al. [66] reported that bone scintigraphy with a pinhole collimator has a better sensitivity in diagnosing osteonecrosis compared with bone scintigraphy. Turner et al. [69] reported that technetium-99m antimony colloid as a radionuclide does not stop additional osteogenesis by binding with subendothelial dendritic macrophages. According to the authors, uptake of technetium 99 m antimony colloid decreases after bone fracture and devascularization. The uptake increases as the necrosis progresses, and vascularity and bone activity increases. According to Dong et al. [70], nuclide uptake increases 3–4 months after surgery and peaks 6–12 months after surgery.

A pinhole collimator is a type of a conical collimator having a small circular aperture (3–5 mm). A pinhole collimator produces an inverted image as a photographic camera does. This image can be enlarged so that even a small structure can be detected, contributing to diagnosis of scintigraphic abnormality. A pinhole collimator increases the resolution of circumscribed areas, and its acquisition time is just 15 min, while SPECT scanning takes 45 min. Planar scintigraphic imaging using quantitative bone scanning offers physiologic data not possible in MRI and also makes uptake quantification available at perfusion and static phase. Therefore, when the patients with head-preserving surgery were followed for revascularization, planar scintigraphic imaging is most useful than any other diagnostic tools [66].

15.4 Treatment

15.4.1 General Considerations for Choosing Treatment

As in the treatment of nontraumatic osteonecrosis, the ultimate goal of treatment for posttraumatic osteonecrosis is to preserve the femoral head, especially in young patients. However, arthroplasty has been widely used with great development of surgical procedures, implants and their materials, high survival rates and patient satisfaction. Clear differentiation of indications between arthroplasty and head salvage procedure is still controversial, and a grey zone still persists. Even though arthroplasty shows good prognosis in most cases, there are some related complications that include joint infection, osteolysis, and aseptic loosening. These compromise the longevity of total hip arthroplasty.

Femoral head-preserving surgery should be considered for young patients, especially adolescent patients, when a surgeon decides on treatment of posttraumatic osteonecrosis considering the remaining life expectancy and high activity of patients.

Osteotomy has been one of the methods preserving the femoral head in osteonecrosis. If the necrotic lesion is anteriorly or posteriorly shifted, rotational trochanteric osteotomy may be one choice. If the lesion is medially or laterally shifted, varus osteotomy or valgus osteotomy can be performed.

After the head-preserving surgery, the healing period until ambulation is around 3 months. On the other hand, total hip arthroplasty is usually shorter in the healing period than that of head-preserving surgery. For this reason, there are some patients who prefer total hip arthroplasty because the patients have to return to work soon. If a patient who has suffered osteonecrosis desires an early return to daily life, even if head-preserving surgery is more appropriate for the patient, total hip arthroplasty may be indicated.

Total hip arthroplasty may be considered inevitable in cases with large necrosis or serious collapse. Regarding the bearing surface for total hip arthroplasty, ceramic-on-ceramic surface is recommended to reduce complications such as aseptic loosening or osteolysis, especially in young patients [71].

In determining the surgery for the osteonecrosis, the age of the patient; severity, extent, and location of necrosis; and socioeconomic needs of the patient should be considered carefully. Surgeon's ability to perform head-preserving surgery seems one of the factors to be considered in the decision process.

15.4.2 Head-Preserving Procedures

Electric shock wave shows some effects on the treatment of osteonecrosis but no established conclusion is possible yet. Wang et al. showed that in patients with the ARCO I, II, and III osteonecrosis, treatment with extracorporeal shock wave had better results than treatment with core decompression and nonvascularized fibular grafting. They postulated that shock wave induces hyperstimulation analgesia by increasing threshold of pain and promotes bone healing as a result of microfracture [72]. Further prospective studies with reliable clinical data are required for wide clinical application.

15.4.2.1 Bisphosphonate

Bisphosphonate can be effective for patients with posttraumatic osteonecrosis if it is used together with other means of treatment [72–76].

The use of bisphosphonate for nontraumatic osteonecrosis both enhances the apoptosis of osteoclasts and reduces the apoptosis of osteoblasts, thus blocking the progression of bone resorption and collapse. Similar effects have been observed among posttraumatic osteonecrosis patients. Agarwala et al. [73] reported that the use of bisphosphonate brought about functional improvement and helped prevent osteonecrosis progression in their study based on 69 cases of hip osteonecrosis including five cases of posttraumatic osteonecrosis. However, the study reported that the result was unsatisfactory for the osteonecrosis where collapse was already in progress. Ramachandran et al. [74] also found in their clinical study of 28 posttraumatic hip cases that bisphosphonate led to a delay in osteonecrosis progression.

In recent years, cocktail therapies that use bisphosphonate together with extracorporeal shock wave therapy, electrical shock wave therapy, hyperoxygen therapy, and nonsteroidal anti-inflammatory drug have been suggested for femoral head necrosis of the hip [72, 75]. Bisphosphonate has been avidly investigated. In treatment of osteonecrosis of the hip, comparison of extracorporeal shock wave with shock wave and alendronate and the proper volume of bisphosphonate and period for using are not established yet [76]. But, research on bisphosphonate suggests that its use for the treatment of patients in a relatively early stage of posttraumatic osteonecrosis could be justified.

15.4.2.2 Viable Bone Grafting

Viable bone grafting that has been used for nontraumatic osteonecrosis can also be a good method treating traumatic osteonecrosis. Many reports introduced several bone graft methods including autograft or central decompression combined with allogeneic transplantation. Free vascularized fibular grafting for the treatment of osteonecrosis of the femoral head was first described in the 1970s [77]. Later Phemister [78] reported success rate of 70 % using vascularized fibular graft; Zhang et al. [79] reported that free vascularized fibular grafting was worthwhile for teenagers with posttraumatic osteonecrosis, even though collapse of the femoral head had reported that through this method, pain relief and restoration of the sphericity of the femoral head could be expected. Even though the vascularized fibular grafting had good results in atraumatic osteonecrosis in early stages, recently these methods are not used widely due to the unpredictable results and complicated surgical technique.

Since the early 1980s, vessel-pedicle iliac bone has been used for treatment for avascular necrosis. Patients with up to 2 mm collapse of the femoral head can be considered for surgery. Zhang et al. [79] reported a 72 % success rate of free vascularized fibular grafting in teenaged patients. They suggested that free vascularized fibular grafting is a viable procedure in teenagers with posttraumatic osteonecrosis even when the head has already collapsed. Noguchi et al. [80] suggested that success with this method requires surgeons to pay attention to the size of the bone graft, adequate position of insertion, good circulation to the bone graft, and sufficient varus fixation when there is additional transtrochanteric rotational osteotomy of the femoral head. Once the procedure is successful through a microsurgical technique, quicker and definitive healing can be expected. However, some limitations are long operation time and presence of poor lateral femoral circumflex artery in some patients.

Muscle-pedicle iliac bone graft is a method that can be used for patients with the same indications as vessel-pedicle iliac bone graft. Pallazzi et al. [81] first performed tensor fascia lata muscle-pedicle iliac graft in 1973; Baksi reported sartorius muscle-pedicle iliac graft in 1983 and tensor fascia lata muscle-pedicle iliac graft in 1991. All these muscle-pedicle bone grafts have the merit of not requiring microsurgical skill, faster bony union with more cancellous portion, shorter surgical time, and ease of the technique. However, this therapy is limited in preventing head collapse, and some patients may have poor muscle vascularity or weakness of transferred muscle [82, 83]. In our institution, we use the greater trochanter graft instead of iliac graft attached with gluteus medius muscle. This technique is less invasive, with only a small incision, and preserves the strength of the gluteus medius muscle. Furthermore, it shows good results in patients who have undergone muscle-pedicle bone graft with greater trochanter, similar to the results in those who underwent muscle-pedicle bone graft with ilium [84].

15.4.2.3 Osteotomy

Osteotomy can be used for both nontraumatic or posttraumatic osteonecrosis. The different type are intertrochanteric osteotomy and transtrochanteric rotational osteotomy developed by Sugioka and varus/valgus osteotomy. Intertrochanteric osteotomy rotates the femoral head anteriorly or posteriorly, substituting weight-bearing portion from necrotic lesion to healthy bone and cartilage. This method was first proposed by Wagner and Zeiler in the 1960s [81, 85]. Later, Sugioka et al. [86] tried a new method of transtrochanteric osteotomy; many surgeons subsequently adopted this method. The purpose of the Sugioka transtrochanteric osteotomy is to rotate necrotic lesion of the femoral head from anterosuperior to inferior area, thus removing shearing force transmitted to necrotic lesion, thereby preventing progressive collapse of articular surface in younger patients. This osteotomy is used in lesions that do not proceed to the end stage and which are limited to anterior or posterior of bone head [81]. In their 11-year follow-up, Sugioka et al. reported a success rate of 88 %. Even in stages III and IV where the necrotic area had progressed so as to cause degenerative arthritis, the reported success rates were 73 and 68 %, respectively [86].

The Sugioka osteotomy is done with the patient in the lateral position. An anterolateral approach and capsule incision is used to expose the femoral neck. Two pins are inserted in the basicervical area. Greater trochanteric osteotomy is done perpendicular to the femoral neck long axis, followed by secondary perpendicular osteotomy above the lesser trochanter. By using pin of proximal bone fragment, the femoral head is anteriorly rotated along with necrotic lesion between 70° and 90°, substituting the weight-bearing surface to the non-necrotic portion. Yoon et al. modified the original technique. The quadratus femoris muscle was left attached and the branch of medial circumflex just above the lesser trochanter was identified by Doppler ultrasonography and preserved. After joint capsule incision, osteotomy was then done in the basicervical area perpendicular to the long axis of the neck of femur, without greater trochanteric osteotomy. The femoral neck and head were then rotated using Steinmann pin and fixation accomplished by two or three cannulated cancellous screws. Since Yoon's modified transtrochanteric rotational osteotomy does not involve greater trochanter osteotomy, fixing the greater trochanter is not needed. The advantage of this osteotomy comparing to Sugioka's osteotomy is shorter surgery time, less distortion of the proximal femur, and early rehabilitation. Preservation of the greater trochanter makes total hip arthroplasty easier if required later. However, this method is technically demanding, and therefore good results are possible only in the hands of an experienced surgeon [81].

15.4.3 Hip Joint Arthroplasty

Recently, hip arthroplasty has become the most effective method to treat end-stage osteonecrosis, despite unresolved problems of infection, dislocation, implant failure, osteolysis, and aseptic loosening. Results of total hip arthroplasty for osteonecrosis have varied widely. Ortiguera et al. [87] reported that in the 18-year follow-up of 188 people under the age of 50 who underwent total hip arthroplasty, 79 % of the patients needed revision surgery after primary total hip arthroplasty on osteonecrosis. On the other hand, Kim et al. recently reported no complications, except for one, in a study of 127 cases. They suggested that the cementless metaphyseal-fitting anatomical total hip prosthesis provides outstanding midterm fixation and the alumina-on-alumina ceramic bearing provides a high rate of survivorship without osteolysis. Yoon et al. [88] reported that in a minimum 6-year follow-up of 41 people under the age of 50 who underwent total hip arthroplasty, there were no complications such as osteolysis, femoral stem subsidence, or liner wear at the final follow-up.

When total hip arthroplasty is needed in young patients inevitably, using uncemented stem makes later revision simple [8, 89]. In the past, young and active patients were not recommended for arthroplasty using ceramic-on-ceramic surface because of the problems such as ceramic liner fracture [90]. However, recent development of delta ceramic has provided better longevity by reduced aseptic loosening and osteolysis. Therefore, to reduce incidence of loosening related to osteolysis, the use of ceramic-on-ceramic surface is recommended as the bearing surface choice [91].

15.5 Summary

Posttraumatic osteonecrosis is one of the most unfortunate complications in patients with hip trauma. The most important thing is early detection and getting the best prevention and treatment. At the postoperative follow-up, accurate and fast diagnosis should be performed. Proper decision should be provided with consideration of age, location of necrotic lesion, extent of necrosis, and socioeconomic demand of the patients. Especially in young patients, total hip arthroplasty should be considered as not the best choice of the treatment but as the last choice of the treatment.

References

1. Prasad Antapur NM, Gandhi R. Fractures in the elderly: when is hip replacement a necessity? Clin Interv Aging. 2010;6:1–7.
2. Kanis JA, Johnell O, Oden A, Sembo I, Redlund-Johnell I, Dawson A, De Laet C, Jonsson B. Long-term risk of osteoporotic fracture in Malmo. Osteoporos Int. 2000;11:669–74.
3. Sen RK, Tripathy SK, Gill SS, Verma N, Singh P, Radotra BD. Prediction of posttraumatic femoral head osteonecrosis by quantitative intraosseous aspirate and core biopsy analysis: a prospective study. Acta Orthop Belg. 2010;76:486–92.
4. Hougaard K, Thomsen PB. Traumatic posterior dislocation of the hip–prognostic factors influencing the incidence of avascular necrosis of the femoral head. Arch Orthop Trauma Surg. 1986;106:32–5.
5. McCutchen JW, Carnesale PG. Comparison of fixation in the treatment of femoral neck fractures. Clin Orthop Relat Res. 1982;171: 44–50.
6. Hungerford DS. Early diagnosis of ischemic necrosis of the femoral head. Johns Hopkins Med J. 1975;137(6):270–5.
7. Jacobs B. Epidemiology of traumatic and nontraumatic osteonecrosis. Clin Orthop Relat Res. 1978;130:51–67.
8. Bachiller FG, Caballer AP, Portal LF. Avascular necrosis of the femoral head after femoral neck fracture. Clin Orthop Relat Res. 2002;399:87–109.
9. Sanders S, Tejwani N, Egol KA. Traumatic hip dislocation–a review. Bull NYU Hosp Jt Dis. 2010;68:91–6.
10. Aaron RK, Stulberg BN, Lennox DW. Clinical and radiographic outcomes in untreated symptomatic osteonocrosis of the femoral head. Tech Orthop. 2001;16:1–5.
11. Callaghan JJ, Aaron G, Rubash HE. The adult hip. 2nd ed. Philadelphia, PA: Lippincott Williams & Wilkins; 2007.
12. Kain MS, Tornetta IIIP. Hip dislocations and fractures of the femoral head. Bucholz RW, Heckman JD, Court-Brown CM, Tornetta P,

editors. Rockwood and Green's Fractures in Adults, 7th ed. Philadelphia, PA: Lippincott Williams & Wilkins; 2010.
13. Barnes R, Brown JT, Garden RS, Nicoll EA. Subcapital fractures of the femur. A prospective review. J Bone Joint Surg Br. 1976;58:2–24.
14. Garden RS. Malreduction and avascular necrosis in subcapital fractures of the femur. J Bone Joint Surg Br. 1971;53:183–97.
15. James J, Steijn-Myagkaya GL. Death of osteocytes. Electron microscopy after in vitro ischaemia. J Bone Joint Surg Br. 1986;68:620–4.
16. Sevitt S. Avascular necrosis and revascularisation of the femoral head after intracapsular fractures: a combined arteriographic and histological necropsy study. J Bone Joint Surg Br. 1964;46:270–96.
17. Shin AY, Morin WD, Gorman JD, Jones SB, Lapinsky AS. The superiority of magnetic resonance imaging in differentiating the cause of hip pain in endurance athletes. Am J Sports Med. 1996; 24:168–76.
18. Chen CM, Chiu FY, Lo WH. Avascular necrosis of femoral head after gamma-nailing for unstable intertrochanteric fractures. Arch Orthop Trauma Surg. 2001;121:505–7.
19. Bartonicek J, Fric V, Skala-Rosenbaum J, Dousa P. Avascular necrosis of the femoral head in pertrochanteric fractures: a report of 8 cases and a review of the literature. J Orthop Trauma. 2007;21:229–36.
20. Brown JT, Abrami G. Transcervical femoral fracture. A review of 195 patients treated by sliding nail-plate fixation. J Bone Joint Surg Br. 1964;46:648–63.
21. Graham J. Early or delayed weight-bearing after internal fixation of transcervical fracture of the femur. A clinical trial. J Bone Joint Surg Br. 1968;50:562–9.
22. Protzman RR, Burkhalter WE. Femoral-neck fractures in young adults. J Bone Joint Surg Am. 1976;58:689–95.
23. Stromqvist B, Hansson LI, Nilsson LT, Thorngren KG. Hook-pin fixation in femoral neck fractures. A two-year follow-up study of 300 cases. Clin Orthop Relat Res. 1987;218:58–62.
24. Lu-Yao GL, Keller RB, Littenberg B, Wennberg JE. Outcomes after displaced fractures of the femoral neck. A meta-analysis of one hundred and six published reports. J Bone Joint Surg Am. 1994;76:15–25.
25. Kofoed H. Femoral neck fractures in young adults. Injury. 1982;14:146–50.
26. Lindequist S, Tornkvist H. Quality of reduction and cortical screw support in femoral neck fractures. An analysis of 72 fractures with a new computerized measuring method. J Orthop Trauma. 1995;9:215–21.
27. Arnoldi CC, Lemperg RK. Fracture of the femoral neck. II. Relative importance of primary vascular damage and surgical procedure for the development of necrosis of the femoral head. Clin Orthop Relat Res. 1977;129:217–22.
28. Crawfurd EJ, Emery RJ, Hansell DM, Phelan M, Andrews BG. Capsular distension and intracapsular pressure in subcapital fractures of the femur. J Bone Joint Surg Br. 1988;70:195–8.
29. Gómez-Castresana FB. Fracturas de la extremidad superior del fémur: Estudio de la presión intramedular de la cabeza del fémur y análisis estadístico y valor diagnóstuco de la necrosis avascular. Estudio comparativo con la venografía intraósea [dissertation]. Madrid: Editorial de la Universidad Complutense; 1981.
30. Maruenda JI, Barrios C, Gomar-Sancho F. Intracapsular hip pressure after femoral neck fracture. Clin Orthop Relat Res. 1997;340:172–80.
31. Soto-Hall R, Johnson LH, Johnson RA. Variations in the intra-articular pressure of the hip joint in injury and disease. A probable factor in avascular necrosis. J Bone Joint Surg Am. 1964;46:509–16.
32. Woodhouse CF. Dynamic influences of vascular occlusion affecting the development of avascular necrosis of the femoral head. Clin Orthop Relat Res. 1964;32:119–29.
33. Bonnaire F, Schaefer DJ, Kuner EH. Hemarthrosis and hip joint pressure in femoral neck fractures. Clin Orthop Relat Res. 1998;353:148–55.
34. Harper WM, Barnes MR, Gregg PJ. Femoral head blood flow in femoral neck fractures. An analysis using intra-osseous pressure measurement. J Bone Joint Surg Br. 1991;73:73–5.
35. Laing PG, Ferguson Jr AB. Radiosodium clearance rates as indicators of femoral-head vascularity. J Bone Joint Surg Am. 1959; 41-A:1409–22.
36. Yeranosian M, Horneff JG, Baldwin K, Hosalkar HS. Factors affecting the outcome of fractures of the femoral neck in children and adolescents: a systematic review. Bone Joint J. 2013;95-B:135–42.
37. Holmberg S, Kalen R, Thorngren KG. Treatment and outcome of femoral neck fractures. An analysis of 2418 patients admitted from their own homes. Clin Orthop Relat Res. 1987;218:42–52.
38. Gao YS, Ai ZS, Zhu ZH, Yu XW, Zhang CQ. Injury-to-surgery interval does not affect postfracture osteonecrosis of the femoral head in young adults: a systematic review. Eur J Orthop Surg Traumatol. 2013;23:203–9.
39. Parker MJ, Pryor GA, Myles JW. The value of a special surgical team in preventing complications in the treatment of hip fractures. Int Orthop. 1994;18:184–8.
40. Zuckerman JD, Skovron ML, Koval KJ, Aharonoff G, Frankel VH. Postoperative complications and mortality associated with operative delay in older patients who have a fracture of the hip. J Bone Joint Surg Am. 1995;77:1551–6.
41. Orler R, Hersche O, Helfet DL, Mayo KA, Ward T, Ganz R. Avascular femur head necrosis as severe complication after femoral intramedullary nailing in children and adolescents. Unfallchirurg. 1998;101:495–9.
42. Bhandari M, Devereaux PJ, Tornetta 3rd P, Swiontkowski MF, Berry DJ, Haidukewych G, Schemitsch EH, Hanson BP, Koval K, Dirschl D, Leece P, Keel M, Petrisor B, Heetveld M, Guyatt GH. Operative management of displaced femoral neck fractures in elderly patients. An international survey. J Bone Joint Surg Am. 2005;87:2122–30.
43. Diwanji SR, Kim SK, Seon JK, Park SJ, Yoon TR. Clinical results of conversion total hip arthroplasty after failed bipolar hemiarthroplasty. J Arthroplasty. 2008;23:1009–15.
44. Resnick D, Niwayama G. Osteonecrosis: diagnostic techniques, special situations and complications. Philadelphia: WB Saunders; 1995.
45. Kawasaki M, Hasegawa Y, Sakano S, Sugiyama H, Tajima T, Iwasada S, Iwata H. Prediction of osteonecrosis by magnetic resonance imaging after femoral neck fractures. Clin Orthop Relat Res. 2001;385:157–64.
46. Glickstein MF, Lawrence BD, Scheibler ML, et al. Avascular necrosis versus other diseases of the hip. Radiology. 1988;169: 213–215.
47. Sofka CM. Optimizing techniques for musculoskeletal imaging of the postoperative patient. Radiol Clin North Am. 2006;44:323–9.
48. Hendrick RE. The AAPM/RSNA physics tutorial for residents. Basic physics of MR imaging: an introduction. Radiographics. 1994;14:829–46; Quiz 47–8.
49. Bui FM, Li J, Bott K, Mintchev MP. Volterra series modelling and compensation of non-linear distortions caused by susceptibility difference artefacts related to the presence of ferromagnetic implants in magnetic resonance imaging. Med Eng Phys. 2001;23: 207–15.
50. Laakman RW, Kaufman B, Han JS, Nelson AD, Clampitt M, O'Block AM, Haaga JR, Alfidi RJ. MR imaging in patients with metallic implants. Radiology. 1985;157:711–4.
51. Baldwin LN, Wachowicz K, Thomas SD, Rivest R, Fallone BG. Characterization, prediction, and correction of geometric distortion in 3 T MR images. Med Phys. 2007;34:388–99.
52. Schenck JF. The role of magnetic susceptibility in magnetic resonance imaging: MRI magnetic compatibility of the first and second kinds. Med Phys. 1996;23:815–50.
53. Taber KH, Herrick RC, Weathers SW, Kumar AJ, Schomer DF, Hayman LA. Pitfalls and artifacts encountered in clinical MR imaging of the spine. Radiographics. 1998;18:1499–521.
54. Pauchard Y, Smith M, Mintchev M. Modeling susceptibility difference artifacts produced by metallic implants in magnetic resonance

imaging with point-based thin-plate spline image registration. Conf Proc IEEE Eng Med Biol Soc. 2004;3:1766–9.
55. Beuf O, Briguet A, Lissac M, Davis R. Magnetic resonance imaging for the determination of magnetic susceptibility of materials. J Magn Reson B. 1996;112:111–8.
56. Posse S. Direct imaging of magnetic field gradients by group spin-echo selection. Magn Reson Med. 1992;25:12–29.
57. Lee MJ, Kim S, Lee SA, Song HT, Huh YM, Kim DH, Han SH, Suh JS. Overcoming artifacts from metallic orthopedic implants at high-field-strength MR imaging and multi-detector CT. Radiographics. 2007;27:791–803.
58. Harris CA, White LM. Metal artifact reduction in musculoskeletal magnetic resonance imaging. Orthop Clin North Am. 2006;37:349–59, vi.
59. Suh JS, Jeong EK, Shin KH, Cho JH, Na JB, Kim DH, Han CD. Minimizing artifacts caused by metallic implants at MR imaging: experimental and clinical studies. AJR Am J Roentgenol. 1998;171: 1207–13.
60. Port JD, Pomper MG. Quantification and minimization of magnetic susceptibility artifacts on GRE images. J Comput Assist Tomogr. 2000;24:958–64.
61. Bagheri MH, Hosseini MM, Emami MJ, Foroughi AA. Metallic artifact in MRI after removal of orthopedic implants. Eur J Radiol. 2012;81:584–90.
62. Buckwalter KA. Optimizing imaging techniques in the postoperative patient. Semin Musculoskelet Radiol. 2007;11:261–72.
63. Speer KP, Spritzer CE, Harrelson JM, Nunley JA. Magnetic resonance imaging of the femoral head after acute intracapsular fracture of the femoral neck. J Bone Joint Surg Am. 1990;72:98–103.
64. Kamano M, Narita S, Honda Y, Fukushima K, Yamano Y. Contrast enhanced magnetic resonance imaging for femoral neck fracture. Clin Orthop Relat Res. 1998;350:179–86.
65. Sugano N, Masuhara K, Nakamura N, Ochi T, Hirooka A, Hayami Y. MRI of early osteonecrosis of the femoral head after transcervical fracture. J Bone Joint Surg Br. 1996;78:253–7.
66. Mailletert JF, Toubeau M, Piroth C, Piroth L, Brunotte F, Tavernier C. Bone scintigraphy equipped with a pinhole collimator for diagnosis of avascular necrosis of the femoral head. Clin Rheumatol. 1997;16:372–7.
67. Yoon TR, Rowe SM, Song EK, Mulyadi D. Unusual osteonecrosis of the femoral head misdiagnosed as a stress fracture. J Orthop Trauma. 2004;18:43–7.
68. Yamagata M, Chao EY, Ilstrup DM, Melton 3rd LJ, Coventry MB, Stauffer RN. Fixed-head and bipolar hip endoprostheses. A retrospective clinical and roentgenographic study. J Arthroplasty. 1987;2:327–41.
69. Turner JH. Post-traumatic avascular necrosis of the femoral head predicted by preoperative technetium-99 m antimony-colloid scan. An experimental and clinical study. J Bone Joint Surg Am. 1983;65:786–96.
70. Dong QR, Wang JX, Dong TH. Early diagnosis by scintigraphy of segmental collapse of the femur head following femur neck fracture. J Radiol. 1994;75:423–5.
71. Hungerford DS. Treatment of osteonecrosis of the femoral head: everything's new. J Arthroplasty. 2007;22:91–4.
72. Wang CJ, Wang FS, Huang CC, Yang KD, Weng LH, Huang HY. Treatment for osteonecrosis of the femoral head: comparison of extracorporeal shock waves with core decompression and bone-grafting. J Bone Joint Surg Am. 2005;87:2380–7.
73. Agarwala S, Jain D, Joshi VR, Sule A. Efficacy of alendronate, a bisphosphonate, in the treatment of AVN of the hip. A prospective open-label study. Rheumatology (Oxford). 2005;44:352–9.
74. Ramachandran M, Ward K, Brown RR, Munns CF, Cowell CT, Little DG. Intravenous bisphosphonate therapy for traumatic osteonecrosis of the femoral head in adolescents. J Bone Joint Surg Am. 2007;89:1727–34.
75. Hsu SL, Wang CJ, Lee MS, Chan YS, Huang CC, Yang KD. Cocktail therapy for femoral head necrosis of the hip. Arch Orthop Trauma Surg. 2010;130:23–9.
76. Lai KA, Shen WJ, Yang CY, Shao CJ, Hsu JT, Lin RM. The use of alendronate to prevent early collapse of the femoral head in patients with nontraumatic osteonecrosis. A randomized clinical study. J Bone Joint Surg Am. 2005;87:2155–9.
77. Aldridge 3rd JM, Urbaniak JR. Vascularized fibular grafting for osteonecrosis of the femoral head with unusual indications. Clin Orthop Relat Res. 2008;466:1117–24.
78. Phemister DB. Treatment of the necrotic head of the femur in adults. J Bone Joint Surg Am. 1949;31A:55–66.
79. Zhang CQ, Sun Y, Chen SB, Jin DX, Sheng JG, Cheng XG, Xu J, Zeng BF. Free vascularised fibular graft for post-traumatic osteonecrosis of the femoral head in teenage patients. J Bone Joint Surg Br. 2011;93:1314–9.
80. Noguchi M, Kawakami T, Yamamoto H. Use of vascularized pedicle iliac bone graft in the treatment of avascular necrosis of the femoral head. Arch Orthop Trauma Surg. 2001;121: 437–42.
81. Yoon TR. How do I treat ONFH with medium and large lesion in young patients. In: The 57th Spring Congress of the Korean Orthopaedic Association. Hotel inter-burgo DAEGU. 2013.
82. Baksi DP, Pal AK, Baksi DD. Long-term results of decompression and muscle-pedicle bone grafting for osteonecrosis of the femoral head. Int Orthop. 2009;33:41–7.
83. Baksi DP. Treatment of osteonecrosis of the femoral head by drilling and muscle-pedicle bone grafting. J Bone Joint Surg Br. 1991;73:241–5.
84. Baksi DP. Treatment of post-traumatic avascular necrosis of the femoral head by multiple drilling and muscle-pedicle bone grafting. Preliminary report. J Bone Joint Surg Br. 1983;65:268–73.
85. Wagner H, Zeiler G. Idiopathic avascular necrosis of the femoral head. Results of intertrochanteric osteotomy and resurfacing (author's translation). Orthopade. 1980;9:290–310.
86. Sugioka Y. Transtrochanteric anterior rotational osteotomy of the femoral head in the treatment of osteonecrosis affecting the hip: a new osteotomy operation. Clin Orthop Relat Res. 1978;130:191–201.
87. Ortiguera CJ, Pulliam IT, Cabanela ME. Total hip arthroplasty for osteonecrosis: matched-pair analysis of 188 hips with long-term follow-up. J Arthroplasty. 1999;14:21–8.
88. Byun JW, Yoon TR, Park KS, Seon JK. Third-generation ceramic-on-ceramic total hip arthroplasty in patients younger than 30 years with osteonecrosis of femoral head. J Arthroplasty. 2012;27: 1337–43.
89. Phillips FM, Pottenger LA, Finn HA, Vandermolen J. Cementless total hip arthroplasty in patients with steroid-induced avascular necrosis of the hip. A 62-month follow-up study. Clin Orthop Relat Res. 1994;303:147–54.
90. Hannouche D, Nich C, Bizot P, Meunier A, Nizard R, Sedel L. Fractures of ceramic bearings: history and present status. Clin Orthop Relat Res. 2003;417:19–26.
91. Hamilton WG, McAuley JP, Dennis DA, Murphy JA, Blumenfeld TJ, Politi J. THA with Delta ceramic on ceramic: results of a multicenter investigational device exemption trial. Clin Orthop Relat Res. 2010;468:358–66.

16 Osteonecrosis in Sickle-Cell Disease

Philippe Hernigou and Gildasio Daltro

16.1 Introduction

Sickle-cell disease (SCD), an autosomal recessive disorder, is also called sickle-cell anemia (SCA) due to the hemolytic anemia characterized by abnormally shaped (sickled) red blood cells (RBCs), which are removed from the circulation and destroyed at increased rates, leading to anemia. Of greater clinical importance, the sickled RBCs cause vascular occlusion, which leads to tissue ischemia and infarction. The patients who are homozygous for the sickle-cell gene (hemoglobin SS) have a high risk of bone osteonecrosis [1–3] due to microvascular occlusion in relation to the disturbance in the erythrocyte architecture and the polymerization of hemoglobin S (in a deoxygenated state) producing cells that are crescent- or sickle-shaped with decreased deformability; the decreased deformability results in greater risk for clotting in small vessels. The incidence of osteonecrosis is also high in patients with hemoglobin SC (compound heterozygotes for Hb S- and Hb C-producing alleles: SC) and in the various types of sickle-beta-thalassemia (SThal) population. So, patients with sickle-cell disease often present with orthopedic disease manifestations requiring surgical intervention, with the most common indications being osteonecrosis and osteomyelitis. This article based on the experience of the authors treating more than 2,000 patients with SCD reviews the incidence of multifocal osteonecrosis in this disease, the distribution of the joints concerned by multifocal osteonecrosis, and the clinical consequences in the long term (average 15 years of follow-up) of multifocal osteonecrosis in these patients with sickle-cell disease and includes an approach to the medical and surgical management of patients with orthopedic complications related to sickle-cell disease.

P. Hernigou (✉)
Department of Orthopaedic Surgery,
University Paris East, 51 avenue du Maréchal de Lattre de Tassigny, Créteil 94010 cedex, France
e-mail: philippe.hernigou@wanadoo.fr

G. Daltro
Department of Orthopaedic Surgery, Hospital Edgar Santos,
University Federal of Bahia, Salvador, Brazil
e-mail: gildasio.daltro@yahoo.com.br

16.2 History

This disease was unknown until the explanation of the sickle cells in 1904 by the Chicago cardiologist and professor of medicine James B. Herrick (1861–1954), whose intern Ernest Edward Irons (1877–1959) found "peculiar elongated and sickle-shaped" cells in the blood of Walter Clement Noel, a 20-year-old first-year dental student from Grenada; Noel was admitted to the Chicago Presbyterian Hospital in December 1904 suffering from anemia. Noel was readmitted several times over the next 3 years for "muscular rheumatism" and "bilious attacks." The first published paper of SCD [4] was therefore done by Herrick in 1910, who described the clinical and hematologic manifestations of the disease. Noel completed his studies and returned to the capital of Grenada (St. George's) to practice dentistry. He died of pneumonia in 1916 and was buried in the Catholic cemetery at Sauteurs in the north of Grenada. The disease was named "sickle-cell anemia" by Vernon Mason in 1922 [5]. As more cases began to surface, the mystery of just what this disease was only deepened. It was clear that for whatever reason, it occurred only or primarily in persons of African origin. In 1927, Hahn and Gillespie discovered that red blood cells from persons with the disease could be made to sickle by removing oxygen. Linus Pauling and colleagues were the first, in 1949, to demonstrate that sickle-cell disease occurs as a result of an abnormality in the hemoglobin molecule. This was the first time a genetic disease was linked to a mutation of a specific protein, a milestone in the history of molecular biology, and it was published in their paper "Sickle Cell Anemia." Two years later, in 1951, the famous Nobel Prize-winning chemist Dr. Linus Pauling and his colleague Dr. Harvey Itano discovered that the red, oxygen-carrying protein called "hemoglobin" had a different chemical structure in persons with SCD.

K.-H. Koo et al. (eds.), *Osteonecrosis*,
DOI 10.1007/978-3-642-35767-1_16, © Springer-Verlag Berlin Heidelberg 2014

This led Dr. Pauling [6] to coin the term "molecular disease" for disorders that resulted from proteins with abnormal chemical structures. Today, thousands of such diseases are known, but in 1951, SCD was the first. The details of the abnormality were worked out by Dr. Vernon Ingram [7] in 1956. In the 1970s, more details of how this abnormal structure affects the red blood cells were revealed, and better tests for the detection of the disease were developed.

16.3 Geography and Epidemiology

The origin of the mutation that led to the sickle-cell gene was initially thought to be in the Arabian Peninsula, spreading to Asia and Africa. It is now known, from evaluation of chromosome structures [8], that there have been at least four independent mutational events, three in Africa and a fourth in either Saudi Arabia or central India. These independent events occurred between 3,000 and 6,000 generations ago, approximately 70,000–150,000 years. The global distribution of Hb S is indicative of two factors: selection for carriers through their survival advantage in malaria-endemic regions and subsequent migration. Four region-specific African haplotypes (the Senegal, Benin, Bantu, and Cameroon haplotypes) and one Asian haplotype (the Arab-India haplotype) have been defined, providing support for the hypothesis that the mutation-causing Hb S has occurred, and been locally amplified, on at least two, and possibly several, separate occasions. In addition to the close geographic correlation between the frequency of the Hb S gene in populations and the historic incidence of malaria, evidence for the partial resistance of carriers to all forms of *Plasmodium falciparum* malaria [9] has been reported in many populations. The prevalence of sickle-cell disease is highest in sub-Saharan Africa. Although the scarcity of diagnostic facilities means that precise data are not available, a recent estimate suggests that it concerns 0.74 % of the births in sub-Saharan Africa. By comparison, approximately 0.15 % of the black population in the United States and Europe is afflicted with SCD. Sickle-cell disease is also an important cause of osteonecrosis affecting persons in the Indian subcontinent, in the Persian Gulf, in South America, in the Mediterranean countries and those from the Caribbean, and Central America. SCD is prevalent in other ethnic groups as well, including those from Mediterranean area countries as North Africa, Turkey, Spain, and Italy.

16.4 Basic Science of Sickle-Cell Disease

16.4.1 Molecular Genetics

The normal human hemoglobin molecule consists of four globin chains: two α chains and two ß chains. When α and ß chains are normal, this is abbreviated Hb A. The genetic basis of sickle-cell disease is a mutation on chromosome 11 that results in an amino acid substitution of valine for glutamic acid at the sixth position of the beta-globin subunit of hemoglobin. This results in hemoglobin S (Hb S). Diagnosis of the disease is confirmed by hemoglobin electrophoresis. Abnormal hemoglobin is designated by the type of abnormality in the globin chain. For example, the presence of one sickle-cell (S) ß chain and one C ß chain is abbreviated Hb SC. Homozygous sickle-cell disease is designated Hb SS. Abnormal hemoglobin, such as Hb SS, is usually the result of an abnormality in the ß (not α) chains. The term *sickle-cell disease* applies to all patients with at least a single Hb S chain and one other abnormal ß globin chain, which may be another sickle-cell ß chain (in which case the patient is homozygous Hb SS and by definition has sickle-cell anemia), Hb SC, or one of the thalassemias (Hb S-thal). Overall, Hb SS accounts for 60–70 % of the cases of sickle-cell disease in the United States and has the severest clinical manifestations of any of the sickle-cell disease variants. Sickle-cell trait (the heterozygous Hb SA, with one abnormal sickle gene designated S and one normal hemoglobin gene designated A) is a benign condition from an orthopedic point of view, with no propensity for vaso-occlusive complications, no osteomyelitis, and no osteonecrosis. Sickle-cell trait is however associated with an increased risk of a rare renal tumor, medullary carcinoma [10]. The importance of sickle-cell trait lies also with its implications for genetic counseling [8].

16.4.2 Anemia

The term sickle-cell disease is used to refer to all the different genotypes that cause the characteristic clinical syndrome, whereas sickle-cell anemia, the most common form of sickle-cell disease, refers specifically to homozygosity for the βS allele. In populations of African ethnic origin, sickle-cell anemia typically accounts for 70 % of cases of sickle-cell disease, with most of the remainder having hemoglobin SC disease (Hb SC disease) owing to the coinheritance of the βS and βC alleles. The third major type of sickle-cell disease occurs when βS is inherited with a β-thalassemia allele, causing Hb S/β-thalassemia. Sickle-cell anemia (SCA) is the most important syndrome of sickle-cell disease [11, 12]. This hemolytic anemia is characterized by abnormally shaped (sickled) red blood cells (RBCs), which are destroyed and removed from the circulation, leading to anemia.

16.4.3 Cellular Abnormalities in Sickle-Cell Disease

Hemoglobin S has a tendency to polymerize with relative ease in a deoxygenated state. This leads to a disturbance in erythrocyte architecture, producing cells that are crescent or sickle-shaped in appearance and have decreased deformability. Factors that increase the rate of polymerization include high Hb S concentration, deoxygenation, lower pH, and a decrease in fetal hemoglobin (HbF). RBCs in SCA also appear to have an increased binding affinity for vascular endothelium [13, 14]. The degree of affinity correlates strongly with the severity of clinical disease. Several molecular interactions are likely to contribute to this endothelial affinity [15, 16]. One is a surface complex on reticulocytes that binds to endothelium. Another mechanism is a complex present on both reticulocytes and endothelium that binds thrombospondin (secreted by activated platelets).

16.4.4 Physiopathology of Osteonecrosis

Hb S is caused by a mutation in the β-globin gene. This mutation produces a hydrophobic motif in the deoxygenated Hb S tetramer that results in binding between β1 and β2 chains of two hemoglobin molecules [17]. This crystallization produces a polymer nucleus, which grows and fills the erythrocyte, disrupting its architecture and flexibility and promoting cellular dehydration, with physical and oxidative cellular stress.

16.4.5 Diagnosis and Screening

Diagnosis of sickle-cell disease is based on analysis of hemoglobin [18]. Typically, this analysis involves protein electrophoresis or chromatography, which are cheap techniques and widely available worldwide, although hemoglobin mass spectrometry and DNA analysis are being increasingly used because these techniques enable high-throughput testing. Antenatal screening is available to women in some countries to help to identify couples who are at risk of having a baby with sickle-cell disease and to offer prenatal diagnosis. Universal neonatal screening programs are established in the United States and England, with other programs being developed in Europe and Africa. Some of the improvement in survival in sickle-cell disease over the past few decades has been attributed to neonatal screening, facilitating early access to prophylaxis with penicillin, comprehensive care, and parental education on the early detection of complications such as acute splenic sequestration.

16.5 Frequency of Osteonecrosis

Multifocal osteonecrosis [19, 20] is the most common situation in SCD. It is defined as a disease of three or more anatomic sites. For example, a patient with osteonecrosis of one hip, one knee, and one shoulder would meet the criteria; a patient with three osteonecroses but not three separate sites involved would not be considered as multifocal osteonecrosis (e.g., two hips and one knee). Multifocal osteonecrosis is very frequent in SCD. For example, in a series of 200 patients with sickle-cell disease with a follow-up of 15 years [21], the occurrence of osteonecrosis was 158 lesions of the proximal femur associated with 151 proximal humerus osteonecroses, 33 lateral femoral condyle osteonecroses, 28 distal femoral metaphysic osteonecroses, 27 medial femoral condyle osteonecroses, 23 tibial plateau osteonecroses, 21 upper tibial metaphysic osteonecroses, and 14 ankle osteonecroses. The total number of osteonecrosis was 455 in these 87 patients. The epiphyseal lesions were more frequent than the metadiaphyseal lesions excepted in the proximal tibia. This means that in patients with hip osteonecrosis, the other joints [22] should be evaluated with radiograph and MRI if the joint is symptomatic. In reverse for patients with osteonecrosis of the knee, shoulder or ankle, the patients' hip should be evaluated by radiographs or MRI, regardless of whether the hip is symptomatic.

16.6 Natural Evolution and Consequence of Hip Osteonecrosis in Children

The contribution of synovial fluid to epiphyseal nutrition may offer some protection against infarction in children, among whom there is a lower prevalence of that complication (27 %) than in adults [23, 24].

16.6.1 Epiphyseal Infarction

Frequently, initial radiographs appear normal, and the earliest signs of avascular necrosis are seen on MR images (in particular, T2-weighted inversion recovery images), which show regions of high signal intensity indicative of bone marrow edema. Often, a serpiginous double line that consists of a hyperintense inner border and hypointense periphery can be seen at T2-weighted imaging. The "double line" sign results from the high-signal-intensity inflammatory response of bone with granulation tissue, inside the low-signal-intensity reactive bone interface. As osteonecrosis progresses, changes become evident at radiography. Early radiographic signs include lucency and sclerosis within the epiphysis; subsequently, crescent-shaped subchondral lucencies develop; and eventually, depression of the articular surface, collapse, and fragmentation occur.

16.6.2 Growth Plate

The effects of sickle-cell anemia on growth are thought to result from bone infarction. Epiphyseal shortening arises from vascular compromise, which causes damage to the growth plate, slowing or halting cartilage growth and leading to shortened bone. Premature fusion of growth plates often occurs centrally because of the ingrowth of metaphyseal vessels. Epiphyseal deformities [23] with cupping of adjacent metaphyses have been described in sickle-cell anemia but also may occur in other childhood disorders, such as infection [24].

16.7 Natural Evolution and Consequence of Hip Osteonecrosis in Adults

The description of hip osteonecrosis was reported in the 1960s [25]. The prevalence of osteonecrosis in patients with sickle-cell disease is as high as 37–50 %. Osteonecrosis most commonly occurs in the humeral and femoral heads, due to their limited arterial network, which can easily succumb to occlusion by sickled cells. In both the hip and shoulder joints, the disease is bilateral in approximately 30 % of patients.

16.7.1 Symptomatic Hip Osteonecrosis

Extensive reports [26, 27] on the natural history of the symptomatic hip with osteonecrosis of the femoral head in adults with sickle-cell disease have been reported. Collapse of the femoral head [28] tends to occur early and at a high rate within 5 years after the diagnosis. No significant risk factors that could cause collapse, such as stage or size, were identified possibly because the rate of collapse was so high. This finding suggests that conservative operative procedures should be instituted early to try to prevent a poor outcome in hips with stage II disease.

16.7.2 Asymptomatic Hip Osteonecrosis

The same authors reported their evaluation of asymptomatic hip osteonecrosis [28]. The unfavorable outcome for most patients with an asymptomatic hip and osteonecrosis of the femoral head in the contralateral hip related to sickle-cell disease suggests that careful screening of the asymptomatic hip should be performed on a regular basis. They recommend that the asymptomatic hip be screened at 6-month intervals after presentation of the symptomatic hip, particularly when the volume of the osteonecrosis is large and when there has been collapse of the contralateral hip, because these two factors have been found to be associated with the rate of clinical and radiographic progression in the asymptomatic hip in patients with osteonecrosis of the femoral head associated with corticosteroid use or alcohol abuse. They also recommend evaluating the patient as soon as possible after the onset of pain because symptoms always preceded collapse. The intervals between the onset of pain and collapse may be as short as 3 months, and in the present study, the mean time between pain and collapse was only 35 months.

16.8 Preoperative Evaluation and Management

The complication rate for patients with sickle-cell disease undergoing orthopedic procedures is significantly higher [29, 30] than that for patients without sickle disease undergoing similar procedures, and these patients are more likely to have an extended inpatient hospital stay. Optimal perioperative management with a multidisciplinary approach should decrease the overall morbidity of these patients.

16.8.1 Preoperative Transfusion

The medical status [31] and attempts to prevent medical complications should be monitored by a specific medical team who has experience in preoperative management of patients with SCD undergoing orthopedic procedures [29]. We have experience of management of surgical procedure and medical complications of 2,300 patients with SCD. Part of the routine evaluation of patients with sickle-cell disease should include laboratory tests consisting of serial hemoglobin, Hb S%, renal function, liver function, and oxygen saturation. Based on these laboratory tests, the need for preoperative transfusion can be determined. All patients had a preoperative evaluation including hematologic consultation. Given the frequency of antigen mismatch between mostly Caucasian donors and African-origin recipients and in an attempt to prevent alloimmunization, we used, since 20 years, blood products which are phenotypically typed for ABO, Rhesus (Cc, D, Ee), and Kell. All the patients have antibody screening before surgery. The donor registry for the entire country is used as a resource when necessary. Red blood cell exchange to decrease the hemoglobin S level to less than 30 % was not performed before surgery except for 25 patients with a history of severe acute chest syndrome or a previous cerebrovascular episode or a severe anemia with hemoglobin less than 5 g/dL. For the other patients, acute simple transfusions were performed during and after surgery to maintain a level of hemoglobin between 8 and 10 g/dL. There is a general trend toward a conservative rather than aggressive transfusion regimen [32]. By adopting a simple transfusion therapy, transfusion-related complications in patients are decreased. All the patients had oxygen saturation during 3 days and were managed with anticoagulants postoperatively for 1 month when THA and only 1 week when core decompression.

16.8.2 Prevention of Infection

We prevent infection before, during, and after surgery. All patients with gallbladder stones had their gallbladder removed before hip surgery because gallbladder infection is a major source of secondary bone infection. Antibiotics (first- and second-generation cephalosporins; 2.5 g per day) were administrated during and after surgery (3 days). Furthermore, all the patients had their implants fixed with cement containing antibiotics (Palacos Genta). Patients had surgery only when white blood cell count, erythrocyte sedimentation rate, and C-reactive protein values were within normal limits (according to the disease). According to the frequency of osteomyelitis in SCD, intraoperatively aspirates, smears, and excised specimens were collected before antibiotic administration and cultured for growth of aerobic and anaerobic bacilli. Histologic sections were examined for evidence of bacterial infection. After the operation, the antibiotics were continued for 3 days if intraoperative cultures were negative and for 1 month if the cultures or histologic examination were positive.

16.9 Intraoperative Management

Since there is a constant need for meticulous control of oxygenation and fluid hydration, general anesthesia [33] often is administered for these patients during orthopedic procedures. The most common intraoperative complications are excessive blood loss (53 %), followed by hypothermia (11 %). Therefore, patients require extensive monitoring of cardiac rhythm, blood pressure, temperature, and oxygen saturation. They also need active intraoperative warming, which usually consists of a combination of a warming blanket, humidifier, and blood/fluid warmer.

Patients with sickle-cell disease tend to contain latent Staphylococcus and Salmonella organisms in the infarcted bone due to the frequency of osteomyelitis in childhood. To identify latent infection and determine appropriate antibiotic therapy, culture of the femoral head bone chips and histology of all surgical specimens should be obtained during THA.

16.10 Postoperative Management

Postoperative management consists of intravenous hydration, supplemental oxygen, intravenous antibiotics, chest physiotherapy, and incentive spirometry. Common complications encountered in the early postoperative period include acute chest syndrome, vaso-occlusive crisis, and, less commonly, neurological and renal events.

16.10.1 Acute Chest Syndrome

Acute chest syndrome [34, 35] is characterized by some combination of respiratory symptoms, pain in the thorax or abdomen, fever, an abnormal chest exam, and eventual development of an infiltrate on chest radiograph. Although there is great variability in outcome, acute mortality is a risk. Furthermore, acute chest syndrome is a major risk factor for chronic lung disease. The etiology of this syndrome is a complex interplay of cruoric and/or fat embolism, infection, and in situ microvascular plugging by sickled red cells. Acute chest syndrome has a multifactorial etiology that includes rib infarction [36], infection, pulmonary infarction, and fat embolism. The pathophysiology of acute chest syndrome in sickle-cell disease is due to regional hypoxia leading to vasoconstriction. This results in increased polymerization of Hb S that leads to greater sickling and endothelial activation, with subsequent occlusion of the pulmonary vasculature. This triggers intrapulmonary shunting, which worsens the desaturation. Risks are increased in certain orthopedic procedures, particularly those that involve intramedullary canal reaming of long bones, by increasing the risk of fat embolism. Treatment of acute chest syndrome consists of hemoglobin levels, blood cultures, arterial blood gases, chest radiograph, spiral computed tomography scan of thorax, and exams to rule out pulmonary embolism and deep vein thrombosis. Treatment consists of blood transfusions, supplemental oxygen, adequate pain management, and empirical antibiotics (cephalosporin and macrolide).

16.10.2 Vaso-occlusive Crisis

Vaso-occlusive crisis, experienced by approximately 9 % of patients with sickle-cell disease, is defined as nonsurgical pain lasting >24 h and requiring opioid analgesia. Standard treatment consists of administering continuous IV opioid drug, typically morphine.

16.10.3 Transfusion-Related Complications

Due to large transfusions, patients may develop complications such as new alloantibody formation and immediate or delayed hemolytic reaction. As previously discussed, these complications are more often seen in patients who receive aggressive transfusion regimens.

16.10.4 Thromboembolic Prophylaxis in Sickle-Cell Disease

Little data exist about the risk of thromboembolic events in patients with SCD after THA and the best prophylaxis. Risk factors associated with venous occlusion include activation of the clotting cascade that can facilitate thrombus formation and hyperviscosity as a complication of transfusion [37]. Thrombin induces endothelial retraction resulting in the exposure of proadhesive extracellular components. It also upregulates endothelial expression of P-selectin, which increases binding among platelets and endothelial cells. Our experience with more than 600 patients with THA or revision of THA in SCD has only four documented deep vein thrombosis and/or one documented nonfatal pulmonary embolism. All the patients had a prophylactic anticoagulant for 1 month postoperatively without any routine screening procedure (such as Doppler). Thromboembolism did not appear as a clinical problem in this population of patients. With warfarin, the frequency of hematoma was higher than with low-molecular-weight heparin (HPBM). The problem with HPBM is the risk of thrombocytopenia. In sickle-cell disease, platelets do not contribute to the pathophysiology of microvascular arterial occlusion. However, due to splenic sequestration, patients with sickle-cell disease often have thrombocytopenia. Although it occurs very rarely in adulthood, splenomegaly may be present and induce thrombopenic hypersplenism. After surgery, the high hematopoietic activity and the inflammatory response may induce noticeable thrombocytosis. We did not observe complications related to HPBM such as thrombopenia.

References

1. Miller ST, Sleeper LA, Pegelow CH, et al. Prediction of adverse outcomes in children with sickle cell disease. N Engl J Med. 2000;342:83–9.
2. Mont MA, Hungerford DS. Non-traumatic avascular necrosis of the femoral head. J Bone Joint Surg Am. 1995;77:459–74.
3. Mukisi-Mukaza M, Elbaz A, Samuel Leborgne Y, et al. Prevalence, clinical features, and risk factors of osteonecrosis of the femoral head among adults with sickle cell disease. Orthopedics. 2000;23:357–63.
4. Herrick JB. Peculiar elongated and sickle-shaped red blood corpuscles in a case of severe anemia. Arch Intern Med. 1910;6:517–21.
5. Steinberg B. Sickle cell anemia. Arch Pathol. 1930;9:876–97.
6. Pauling L, Itano HA, Singer SJ, Wells IC. Sickle-cell anemia: a molecular disease. Science. 1949;110:543–9.
7. Ingram VM. Gene mutations in human haemoglobin: the chemical difference between normal and sickle cell haemoglobin. Nature. 1957;180:326–8.
8. Bowman JE, Murray RFJ. Genetic variation in peoples of African origin. Baltimore: Johns Hopkins University Press; 1990. p. 196–201.
9. Aluoch JR. Higher resistance to *Plasmodium falciparum* infection in patients with homozygous sickle cell disease in western Kenya. N Engl J Med. 1997;317:781–7.
10. Davis CJ, Mostofi FK, Sesterhenn IA. Renal medullary carcinoma: the seventh sickle cell nephropathy. Am J Surg Pathol. 1995;19:1–11.
11. Steinberg MH. Modulation of fetal hemoglobin in sickle cell anemia. Hemoglobin. 2001;25:195–211.
12. Steinberg MH, Nagel RL, Higgs D, editors. Disorders of hemoglobin: genetics, pathophysiology, and clinical management. New York: Cambridge University Press; 2001.
13. Hebbel RP, Boogaerts MA, Eaton JW, Steinberg MH. Erythrocyte adherence to endothelium in sickle-cell anemia. A possible determinant of disease severity. N Engl J Med. 1980;302:992–5.
14. Hebbel RP, Vercelotti GM. The endothelial biology of sickle cell disease. J Lab Clin Med. 1997;129:288–93.
15. Manodori AB, Matsui NM, Chen JY, Embury SH. Enhanced adherence of sickle erythrocytes to thrombin-treated endothelial cells involves interendothelial cell gap formation. Blood. 1998;92:3445–54.
16. Michaels LA, Ohene-Frempong K, Zhao H, Douglas SD. Serum levels of substance P are elevated in patients with sickle cell disease and increase further during vaso-occlusive crisis. Blood. 1998;92:3148–51.
17. Hawker H, Neilson H, Hayes RJ, Sergeant GR. Haematological factors associated with avascular necrosis of the femoral head in homozygous sickle cell disease. Br J Haematol. 1982;50:29–34.
18. Wethers DL. Sickle cell disease in childhood. I. Laboratory diagnosis, pathophysiology, and health maintenance. Am Fam Phys. 2000;62:1013–20.
19. Hernigou P, Daltro G, Sobrinho UB, Sberge F. Manifestações osteoarticulares na anemia falciforme. Gaz Méd Bahia. 2010;80(3):74–9.
20. Mukisi Mukaza M, Manicom O, Fillipini P, Hernigou P. Elbow osteonecrosis in sickle cells anemia: a study of six cases. Orthop Traumatol Surg Res. 2009;95(1):82–4.
21. Flouzat-Lachaniete CH, Roussignol X, Poignard A, Mukasa MM, Manicom O, Hernigou P. Multifocal joint osteonecrosis in sickle cell disease. Op Orthop J. 2009;3:32–5.
22. Poignard A, Flouzat-Lachaniette CH, Amzallag J, Galacteros F, Hernigou P. The natural progression of symptomatic humeral head osteonecrosis in adults with sickle cell disease. J Bone Joint Surg Am. 2012;94(2):156–62.
23. Hernigou P, Galacteros F, Bachir D, Goutallier D. Deformities of the hip in adults who have sickle-cell disease and had avascular necrosis in childhood. A natural history of fifty-two patients. J Bone Joint Surg Am. 1991;73:81–92.
24. Hernigou P, Daltro G, Flouzat-Lachaniette CH, Roussignol X, Poignard A. Septic arthritis in adults with sickle cell disease often is associated with osteomyelitis or osteonecrosis. Clin Orthop Relat Res. 2010;468(6):1676–81.
25. Chung SM, Ralston EL. Necrosis of the femoral head associated with sickle-cell anemia and its genetic variants. A review of the literature and study of thirteen cases. J Bone Joint Surg Am. 1969;51:33–58.
26. Daltro G, de Alencar Daniel F, Sobrinho UB, Guedes A, Fortuna VA. Osteonecrose da cabeça femoral na anemia falciforme. Gaz Méd Bahia. 2010;80(3):29–32.
27. Diggs LW. Bone and joint lesions in sickle-cell disease. Clin Orthop Relat Res. 1967;52:119–43.
28. Hernigou P, Bachir D, Galacteros F. Avascular necrosis of the femoral head in sickle-cell disease. Treatment of collapse by the injection of acrylic cement. J Bone Jt Surg Br. 1993;75:875–80.
29. Hernigou P, Zilber S, Filippini P, Mathieu G, Poignard A, Galacteros F. THA in adult osteonecrosis related to sickle cell disease. Clin Orthop Relat Res. 2008;466(2):300–8.
30. Vichinsky EP, Neumayr LD, Haberkem C, et al. The perioperative complication rate of orthopedic surgery in sickle cell disease: report of the National Sickle Cell Surgery Study Group. Am J Hematol. 1999;62:129–38.
31. Serjeant GR. Natural history and determinants of clinical severity of sickle cell disease. Curr Opin Hematol. 1995;2:103–8.
32. Castro O. Management of sickle cell disease: recent advances and controversies. Br J Haematol. 1999;107:2–11.
33. Garden MS, Grant RE, Jebraili S. Perioperative complications in patients with sickle cell disease. An orthopedic perspective. Am J Orthop. 1996;25:353–6.
34. Aldrich TK, Dhuper SK, Patwa NS, et al. Pulmonary entrapment of sickle cells: the role of regional alveolar hypoxia. J Appl Physiol. 1996;80:531–9.
35. Vichinsky EP, Neumayr LD, Earles AN, et al. Causes and outcomes of the acute chest syndrome in sickle cell disease. National Acute

Chest Syndrome Study Group. N Engl J Med. 2000;342: 1855–15865.

36. Gelfand MJ, Daya SA, Rucknagel DL, Kallinyak KA, Paltiel HJ. Simultaneous occurrence of rib infarction and pulmonary infiltrates in sickle cell disease patients with acute chest syndrome. J Nucl Med. 1993;34:614–8.

37. Rodgers GP. Overview of pathophysiology and rationale for treatment of sickle cell anemia. Semin Hematol. 1997;34:2–7.

17 Autoimmune Disease (SLE, Antiphospholipid Syndrome), Posttransplantation (Kidney, Liver, Heart, Bone Marrow), and Other Risk Factors (Chemotherapy, Caisson Disease, Radiation, Pancreatitis, Gaucher's Disease)

Jeong Joon Yoo

17.1 Introduction

The pathogenesis of osteonecrosis (ON) is unclear, although it is known that it results in bone death [1]. ON is associated with a wide spectrum of systemic disorders [1], and corticosteroid use [2], alcohol consumption [3], cigarette smoking [3], intravascular coagulation [4], and trauma [5] are well-known risk factors. In this chapter, we discuss other risk factors of ON, namely, autoimmune disease (systemic lupus erythematosus, antiphospholipid syndrome) [6–9], transplantation (kidney, liver, heart, bone marrow) [10–16], and others (chemotherapy, radiation, caisson disease, pancreatitis, and Gaucher's disease) [1, 17–23].

17.2 Autoimmune Disease

17.2.1 Systemic Lupus Erythematosus (SLE)

Osteonecrosis (ON) is a rather common manifestation of SLE and requires surgical therapy in most cases. The condition was first reported in 1960 by Dubois and Cozen [24]. The reported prevalence of symptomatic ON in patients with SLE ranges from 3 to 30 %, which is higher than the prevalence of general ON [6, 25–28]. In a cohort of 407 patients with SLE, Petri reported a 14.5 % prevalence of ON [25]. Gladman et al. reported that among 744 patients with SLE followed for a mean 8 years, 13 % developed ON [26]. Cozen et al. reported a lower prevalence of 5 % among 488 patients with SLE [27], and similarly, Sayarlioglu et al. reported that among 868 patients with SLE, 6 % developed ON [6]. However, asymptomatic ON was not included in these two studies, and thus, the true prevalence of ON in SLE is much higher. In another study, 12 % of 66 SLE patients were found to have asymptomatic ON of the femoral head by magnetic resonance imaging (MRI) [29].

However, the majority of studies on the subject did not report the annual incidence of ON in SLE. In fact, the risk of ON development varies during the disease course of SLE. Abeles et al. found that the incidence of osteonecrosis increased constantly during the first 5 years from diagnosis [30].

A number of clinical features have been described in association with ON in SLE, and it appears that the etiology of ON in SLE is probably multifactorial. Several clinical risk factors have been proposed, such as the use of corticosteroids [28, 31–34], the presence of Raynaud's phenomenon [35, 36], vasculitis [28, 35], thrombophlebitis, preeclampsia [28], and arthritis [32]. However, the use of corticosteroids remains the only major factor associated with ON in SLE [32], and the roles of other clinical variables remain unclear. These observations were based on small numbers of SLE patients that developed ON, and much of the data reported were derived by univariate analyses. Furthermore, logistic regression models have failed to confirm the link between ON and clinical variables, with the exception of corticosteroids use [32].

ON occurs mainly in SLE patients being treated with corticosteroids and only rarely in SLE patients who had never received corticosteroids [32]. All of the 11 SLE patients reported by Dubois had received adrenal corticosteroids [24]. In another study, the use of corticosteroids was found to be associated with an 18-fold increased risk of ON in SLE patients [32]. Furthermore, several studies have found associations between steroid dosage [28], cumulative dose [30], duration of steroid therapy [32], and mode of therapy [34]

J.J. Yoo
Department of Orthopedic Surgery,
Seoul National University College of Medicine,
101 Daehak-ro, Jongno-gu, Seoul 110-744, Korea
e-mail: jjyos@snu.ac.kr

K.-H. Koo et al. (eds.), *Osteonecrosis*,
DOI 10.1007/978-3-642-35767-1_17,

and the development of ON. Overall, available data suggest that ON tends to develop in SLE patients administered high doses of steroids early during the disease course and particularly in those patients that develop a Cushingoid appearance [28]. It has also been suggested that ON in SLE may be related to the use of pulse therapy [34].

Several pathogenic factors are probably associated with ON in SLE and more than one mechanism may be involved. The strong link between ON and corticosteroid therapy suggests a crucial pathogenic role for steroids. However, even the mechanism by which corticosteroids trigger ON is unclear. Chronic corticosteroid therapy may suppress osteoblastic activity and result in an impaired ability to repair microfractures [37, 38]. Zizac et al. theorized that corticosteroid therapy results in an increase in the size and numbers of intramedullary lipocytes and that this increases bone marrow pressure [35], which in turn causes vascular compression and reduced perfusion to the bone tissue leading to bone ischemia and infarction. Vasculitis and vasospasm of the blood vessels that supply the bone tissues are also factors that probably contribute to the pathogenesis of ON in SLE [28]. Furthermore, hypercoagulopathy can trigger ON in SLE patients in the absence of corticosteroid therapy, and ON can develop as a result of arterial or venous thrombosis of bone blood vessels and subsequent ischemia and infarction in bone tissues [39].

17.2.2 Antiphospholipid Syndrome

Antiphospholipid syndrome (APS) is an autoimmune disease characterized by multiple thrombotic episodes and fetal loses in the presence of anticardiolipin antibodies (aCLs) and/or lupus anticoagulant (LA) [6–9, 40]. APS is classified as "primary" when it occurs in the absence of any other underlying disease [41] and as "secondary" when it is associated with other autoimmune diseases, especially with SLE. The clinical presentation and evolution of APS can vary markedly and range from a mild sporadic event to a recurrent or catastrophic event [9, 42].

aCLs and LA belong to a family of autoantibodies called antiphospholipid antibodies once thought to be directed against negatively charged phospholipids [43]. However, their true antigenic targets were found to be more complex and to include plasma proteins, such as beta2-glycoprotein I and prothrombin [43, 44].

These antibodies are associated with vessel thromboses of all sizes at multiple organ sites [45]. aCL antibodies are associated with thrombosis of a variety of vessels at multiple sites, which probably include bone vasculature [45]. In SLE, the prevalence of previous thrombosis (at any site) was found to be three- to fourfold higher in patients positive for LA and two- to fourfold higher in those positive for aCL [46]. Thus, a thrombotic microvasculopathy at the terminal arteries of the bone supports the role of antiphospholipid antibodies in the pathogenesis of ON.

Antiphospholipid antibodies have recently been associated with ON in SLE. However, this association is controversial as some reports support an association [28, 47, 48], while others do not [49]. A retrospective study by Asherson et al. showed that the prevalence of antiphospholipid antibodies (aCLs or LA) was higher in SLE patients with ON than in those without [47]. Moreover, no significant difference in corticosteroid use was found between patients with or without APS who developed ON. Nagasawa et al. retrospectively investigated 111 SLE patients for ON and found the percentage of patients positive for LA was greater among those with ON ($n=24$) [48].

Tektonidou et al. reported that 20 % of patients (6 of 30) with primary APS had evidence of asymptomatic ON (in the absence of corticosteroid use) by magnetic resonance imaging [50]. The increased incidence of ON among primary APS patients, in the absence of other predisposing factors, suggests that antiphospholipid antibodies play a role in the pathogenesis of ON. In fact, ON might represent an additional clinical feature of APS.

In summary, ON has been observed in patients with antiphospholipid antibodies, with and without a history of corticosteroid treatment. Moreover, thrombosis in APS has been described in the vessels of multiple organs, and thus, the occlusion of bone subchondral arterioles might be expected.

17.3 Posttransplantation

Advances in transplantation technology provided great benefits to patients suffering from organ failure, but the complications induced by steroid used for posttransplant immunosuppression are problematic, and of these side effects, nontraumatic ON constitutes a serious problem.

Organ transplantation requires steroid administration for immune suppression, and there is general agreement that the use of steroids is a risk factor of the development of ON. Traditionally, the incidence of ON of the hip in patients that have undergone renal, liver, or cardiac transplant has been reported to be between 3 and 24 % [1–8, 10–14, 51–62]. In general, patients that undergo renal transplantation are at greater risk of developing ON than patients who undergo cardiac or liver transplantation [12–14, 52, 63, 64]. It has been hypothesized that higher rates of ON after renal transplantation are in some way related to underlying metabolic problems exacerbated by chronic steroid use. Furthermore, new transplant protocols requiring lower steroid use have been associated with lower rates of ON [10, 52, 65].

17.3.1 Renal Transplantation

ON is a major postoperative complication that develops within 12 weeks of renal transplantation [66, 67] with an incidence of 3–40 % [10, 11, 54–58, 68]. There are many potential reasons for this wide range, such as differences in steroid immunosuppressive regimens and in the sensitivities of screening modalities for ON. However, the primary reasons for this wide variation are the retrospective nature of many of these studies and an inability to obtain data on asymptomatic patients [69].

It has been shown that total steroid dosage over 1 year and average daily dose are related to the risk of ON development [54, 55, 70–72]. Recently, Shibatani et al. reported that the risk of developing ON depends on the steroid dose administered at as early as 8 weeks after transplantation, which prompted the suggestion that a reduction in total dose during the first 8 weeks after transplantation could reduce the risk of ON [10]. Duration of dialysis before transplantation [72], number of acute rejection episodes [54], hyperparathyroidism [71], and hypophosphatemia [73] have also been reported to be risk factors of ON after renal transplantation.

Since cyclosporine was introduced as an immunosuppressive agent after renal transplantation, steroid dose, the incidence of acute rejection, and the incidence of ON have reduced [10, 65]. Today, the use of tacrolimus (a potent immune suppressor) has reduced steroid dosages and the incidence of acute rejection further [10]. It has also been reported that tacrolimus may suppress the development of ON [74].

17.3.2 Liver Transplantation

Liver transplantation has become a common procedure for treating patients with severe chronic hepatic disorders, and like allogenic renal transplantation, postoperative immunosuppressive regimens are required for the survival and normal function of transplanted livers. However, increased liver survival rates post transplantation means more patients are at a high risk of developing ON, especially in the femoral head, due to immunosuppressive treatment.

The prevalence of ON after liver transplantation (1.3–9 %) is lower than that after renal transplantation [12, 13, 59, 75, 76]. Papagelopoulos et al. reported that 23 (8.1 %) of 285 liver transplant recipients developed symptomatic ON after surgery, and seven patients required joint arthroplasty [59]. Lieberman et al. reported that 4 (2 %) of 203 liver transplant patients were diagnosed with ON of the hip and commented that due to the rarity of the condition, routine MRI screening is not required [75]. Horiuchi et al. reported despite the use of high-dose corticosteroids for immunosuppression, none of their patients presented with symptomatic ON and that only 1 (2.8 %) of 36 hips in 18 patients developed asymptomatic ON of the hip by MRI screening [13]. Recently, Li et al. reported an incidence of symptomatic ON of the femoral head of 1.3 % among 226 liver transplant recipients under an immunosuppressive protocol consisting mainly of methylprednisolone and calcineurin inhibitors (tacrolimus or cyclosporine A) [12]. They concluded that symptomatic ON does not commonly occur after liver transplantation when current individual immunosuppressive protocols are used. They proposed that the lower prevalence of ON after liver transplant may be explained in part by underlying metabolic bone disease associated with chronic renal failure [12]. Clearly, the organ-specific incidence of ON requires closer examination.

17.3.3 Heart Transplantation

Symptomatic ON does not occur frequently after heart transplantation [14, 60, 62]. Danzig et al. was the first to report ON of the hip in a 28-year-old man after cardiac transplantation, and subsequently, Bradbury et al. retrospectively analyzed the relationship between the development of ON and steroid dosage in 168 patients that had undergone heart transplantation (156 patients) or heart and lung transplantation (12 patients). Five patients (3 %) were diagnosed with symptomatic ON at an average of 5 months after transplantation (range, 2–11 months), and a strong association was noted between the cumulative dose of pulsed intravenous methylprednisolone during the first month post transplantation and the development of ON [60].

Recently, Lieberman et al. retrospectively evaluated 204 patients that underwent cardiac transplantation and noted that only 6 (3 %) developed symptomatic ON of the hip or knee at an average of 38.5 months (range, 21–52 months) after transplantation. However, unlike Bradbury et al., they found no association between steroid dose and the development of symptomatic ON.

17.3.4 Bone Marrow Transplantation

The issue of ON after bone marrow transplantation has attracted little interest until recently because mortality after this procedure is high. However, survival after bone marrow transplantation is increasing rapidly, and it is clear that this complication interferes with return to society, but unfortunately, relatively few reports have been published on the subject [15, 16, 77–79].

Atkinson et al. reported of 50 patients that survived 2 years or more after human leukocyte antigen identical sibling bone marrow transplantation, 5 (10 %) developed ON of the femoral head and that all 5 had graft-versus-host disease

(GVHD). They postulated that the steroid used to treat graft-versus-host disease might have been a causative factor [77]. Other authors have also reported prevalences of 3–10 % among bone marrow transplant patients, particularly in those with steroid-treated GVHD [78, 79].

Tauchmanova et al. reported that symptomatic ON occurred in 12 (5.8 %) of 207 long-term survivors after bone marrow transplantation within 3–114 months (median, 26 months) after grafting and that 10 of the 12 had received allogeneic bone marrow. Furthermore, significant associations were found between the development of ON and the following risk factors: allogeneic transplant, presence and grade of GVHD, and steroid treatment duration and cumulative dose [15].

Allogeneic and autologous-transplanted patients are often pooled in clinical studies on bone complications after bone marrow transplantation. However, Tauchmanova et al. suggested that there could be considerable differences between these two settings, because allografts compromise the host immune system more severely than autografts, due to the intense immunosuppressive effects of the conditioning regimens used to avoid graft rejection and to the prolonged administration of multiple immunosuppressive drugs to prevent GVHD [15].

GVHD is a specific immunologic response whereby mature T lymphocytes from the donor site attack recipient tissues, including the liver, skin, or intestines, and chronic GVHD may be similar to the autoimmune diseases that damage multiple organs. Moreover, in recent pathologic reviews the microangiopathies associated with bone marrow transplantation have been linked with the etiology of ON [16]. In fact, the frequent development of acute or chronic GVHD after allogeneic bone marrow transplantation induces additional alterations in the immune system.

The pathogenesis of ON after bone marrow transplantation is probably multifactorial and the precipitating conditions various. Corticosteroid treatment probably contributes to the development of ON, but strong relationships between ON, allogeneic bone marrow transplantation, and GVHD recurrence suggest that immune-mediated mechanisms also underlie ON development after bone marrow transplantation.

17.4 Other Risk Factors

17.4.1 Chemotherapy

Nontraumatic ON of the bone is a known complication in solid-tumor cancer patients on cytotoxic chemotherapy [17, 80]. Shim et al. summarized recent reports regarding ON associated with chemotherapy in cancer patients. In this study, 54 reported cases of nontraumatic ON in adult patients with solid tumors receiving chemotherapy were identified in the medical literature. ON was observed most commonly in men receiving chemotherapy for testicular cancer but was also observed in patients receiving chemotherapy for breast, ovarian, and small-cell lung cancer and osteosarcoma. Most of the patients affected had received corticosteroids and had delayed onset of ON with femoral head involvement [80].

As the long-term survival of patients with a solid tumor receiving chemotherapy increases, the prevalence of treatment-related ON may also increase. Patients should be informed that ON is a potential complication of cancer treatment [17, 80]; however, the low incidence of ON and the lack of a proven benefit for early intervention weigh against screening for ON in this population. On the other hand, a high index of clinical suspicion in patients at risk supports early intervention.

17.4.2 Radiation

The mechanism of radiation-induced ON has been theoretically attributed to injury of vessel walls or to the application of external pressure to the vessels [81]. Radiologically, ON has only rarely been identified in patients administered megavoltage radiation to a total dose of 45 Gy over 5 weeks [82]. Jenkins et al. identified ON of the hip in 2 of 35 patients undergoing chemoradiation therapy for anal cancer [83] and proposed that sensitization of the microvasculature to radiation by cytotoxic agents explains the apparently high prevalence of symptomatic ON. On the other hand, Dzik-Jurasz et al. found no MRI or clinical evidence of ON in 34 anal cancer patients treated by chemoradiation [18]. Thus, although a relationship between radiotherapy and the occurrence of ON has been proposed by several authors [83–86], more investigation is needed to confirm causality.

17.4.3 Caisson Disease

Dysbaric ON, known as caisson disease, is associated with exposure to large ambient pressure changes. The disease was first reported in tunnel construction worker exposed routinely to compressed air [1, 19]. Furthermore, symptomatic decompression sickness affecting the hip is radiographically consistent with ON [1]; in some communities, such as Turkish sponge divers and Japanese diving fisherman, the prevalence of dysbaric ON reaches 50–85 % [19].

Dysbaric ON may occur months or years after hyperbaric exposure and most commonly affects femoral and humeral heads and femoral and tibial shafts [1]. Its pathogenesis involves the formation of intravascular gas bubbles during decompression that occlude end arterioles. Additional factors include (1) the accumulation of nitrogen gas in the bone marrow; (2) fatty infiltration in bone marrow, leading to microarteriole occlusion [87]; and (3) platelet aggregation and thrombogenesis [88]. However, the critical pressure level required for the development of ON and the optimal decompression conditions required to avoid this serious complication of hyperbaric exposure have not been determined.

17.4.4 Pancreatitis

Proteolytic enzymes generated during pancreatitis may trigger intravascular coagulation and ON [1, 21]. And an association between pancreatic disease and ON has been documented [89]. It is generally believed that fat embolism or fat infiltration in the bone may underlie the pathogenesis of pancreatitis-associated ON. Baron et al. reported a syndrome of ON in association with pancreatitis, subcutaneous fat necrosis, and arthritis [90]. Furthermore, elevated levels of serum pancreatic lipolytic enzymes in pancreatitis increase unbound free fatty acids levels, which could lead to bone necrosis [91].

17.4.5 Gaucher's Disease

Gaucher's disease is an autosomal recessive metabolic disorder characterized by abnormal accumulations of glucocerebroside in macrophages throughout the reticuloendothelial system caused by a deficiency in glucosylceramide ß-glucosidase activity [1, 22, 23].

Infiltration of bone marrow by Gaucher cells has multiple skeletal manifestations, including bone pain and ON, which is one of the most common skeletal manifestations of Gaucher's disease and occurs in up to 60 % of patients [92]. Amstutz and Carey reported that 15 of 20 patients with skeletal manifestations had ON of the femoral head [93]. Gaucher's disease appears to cause ON by causing vascular compromise secondary to mass compression resulting from bone marrow infiltration by lipid-laden Gaucher cells [1, 94]. Enzyme release from damaged macrophages has also been reported to cause bone necrosis [94].

17.5 Summary

Autoimmune diseases, such as systemic lupus erythematosus and antiphospholipid syndrome, and posttransplantation, chemotherapy, radiation, caisson disease, pancreatitis, and Gaucher's disease are potential risk factors of osteonecrosis. A high index of clinical suspicion in patients with these conditions may allow prompt diagnosis, early intervention, and joint preservation.

References

1. Chang CC, Greenspan A, Gershwin ME. Osteonecrosis: current perspectives on pathogenesis and treatment. Semin Arthritis Rheum. 1993;23(1):47–69.
2. Cruess RL. Steroid-induced avascular necrosis of the head of the humerus. Natural history and management. J Bone Joint Surg Br. 1976;58(3):313–7.
3. Matsuo K, Hirohata T, Sugioka Y, Ikeda M, Fukuda A. Influence of alcohol intake, cigarette smoking, and occupational status on idiopathic osteonecrosis of the femoral head. Clin Orthop Relat Res. 1988;234:115–23.
4. Jones Jr JP. Intravascular coagulation and osteonecrosis. Clin Orthop Relat Res. 1992;277:41–53.
5. Swiontkowski MF, Hansen Jr ST. Percutaneous Neufeld pinning for femoral neck fractures. Clin Orthop Relat Res. 1986;206:113–6.
6. Sayarlioglu M, Yuzbasioglu N, Inanc M, Kamali S, Cefle A, Karaman O, et al. Risk factors for avascular bone necrosis in patients with systemic lupus erythematosus. Rheumatol Int. 2012;32(1):177–82. doi:10.1007/s00296-010-1597-9.
7. Abu-Shakra M, Buskila D, Shoenfeld Y. Osteonecrosis in patients with SLE. Clin Rev Allergy Immunol. 2003;25(1):13–24. doi:10.1385/CRIAI:25:1:13. CRIAI:25:1:13 [pii].
8. Rueda JC, Duque MA, Mantilla RD, Iglesias-Gamarra A. Osteonecrosis and antiphospholipid syndrome. J Clin Rheumatol. 2009;15(3):130–2. doi:10.1097/RHU.0b013e31819dbd20.
9. Tektonidou MG, Moutsopoulos HM. Immunologic factors in the pathogenesis of osteonecrosis. Orthop Clin North Am. 2004;35(3): 259–63, vii. 10.1016/j.ocl.2004.02.003. S0030589804000045 [pii].
10. Shibatani M, Fujioka M, Arai Y, Takahashi K, Ueshima K, Okamoto M, et al. Degree of corticosteroid treatment within the first 2 months of renal transplantation has a strong influence on the incidence of osteonecrosis of the femoral head. Acta Orthop. 2008;79(5):631–6. doi:10.1080/17453670810016641. 903404227 [pii].
11. Hedri H, Cherif M, Zouaghi K, Abderrahim E, Goucha R, Ben Hamida F, et al. Avascular osteonecrosis after renal transplantation. Transplant Proc. 2007;39(4):1036–8. doi:10.1016/j.transproceed.2007.02.031. S0041-1345(07)00202-3 [pii].
12. Li H, Zhang J, He JW, Wang K, Wang GS, Jiang N, et al. Symptomatic osteonecrosis of the femoral head after adult orthotopic liver transplantation. Chin Med J (Engl). 2012;125(14):2422–6.
13. Horiuchi H, Hashikura Y, Hisa K, Saito N, Ikegami T, Nakazawa Y, et al. Osteonecrosis of the femoral head in Japanese adults after liver transplantation: a preliminary report. J Orthop Sci. 2004;9(2):119–21. doi:10.1007/s00776-003-0757-0.
14. Lieberman JR, Roth KM, Elsissy P, Dorey FJ, Kobashigawa JA. Symptomatic osteonecrosis of the hip and knee after cardiac transplantation. J Arthroplasty. 2008;23(1):90–6. doi:10.1016/j.arth.2007.01.006. S0883-5403(07)00045-9 [pii].
15. Tauchmanova L, De Rosa G, Serio B, Fazioli F, Mainolfi C, Lombardi G, et al. Avascular necrosis in long-term survivors after allogeneic or autologous stem cell transplantation: a single center experience and a review. Cancer. 2003;97(10):2453–61. doi:10.1002/cncr.11373.
16. Torii Y, Hasegawa Y, Kubo T, Kodera Y, Minami S, Morishita Y, et al. Osteonecrosis of the femoral head after allogeneic bone marrow transplantation. Clin Orthop Relat Res. 2001;382:124–32.
17. Winquist EW, Bauman GS, Balogh J. Nontraumatic osteonecrosis after chemotherapy for testicular cancer: a systematic review. Am J Clin Oncol. 2001;24(6):603–6.
18. Dzik-Jurasz AS, Brooker S, Husband JE, Tait D. What is the prevalence of symptomatic or asymptomatic femoral head osteonecrosis in patients previously treated with chemoradiation? A magnetic resonance study of anal cancer patients. Clin Oncol (R Coll Radiol). 2001;13(2):130–4.

19. Toklu AS, Cimsit M. Dysbaric osteonecrosis in Turkish sponge divers. Undersea Hyperb Med. 2001;28(2):83–8.
20. Hutter CD. Dysbaric osteonecrosis: a reassessment and hypothesis. Med Hypotheses. 2000;54(4):585–90. doi:10.1054/mehy.1999.0901. S0306-9877(99)90901-5 [pii].
21. Jones JP. Epidemiological risk factors for non-traumatic osteonecrosis. Orthopade. 2000;29(5):370–9.
22. Rodrigue SW, Rosenthal DI, Barton NW, Zurakowski D, Mankin HJ. Risk factors for osteonecrosis in patients with type 1 Gaucher's disease. Clin Orthop Relat Res. 1999;362:201–7.
23. Katz K, Horev G, Grunebaum M, Yosipovitch Z. The natural history of osteonecrosis of the femoral head in children and adolescents who have Gaucher disease. J Bone Joint Surg Am. 1996;78(1):14–9.
24. Dubois EL, Cozen L. Avascular (aseptic) bone necrosis associated with systemic lupus erythematosus. JAMA. 1960;174:966–71.
25. Petri M. Musculoskeletal complications of systemic lupus erythematosus in the Hopkins Lupus Cohort: an update. Arthritis Care Res. 1995;8(3):137–45.
26. Gladman DD, Chaudhry-Ahluwalia V, Ibanez D, Bogoch E, Urowitz MB. Outcomes of symptomatic osteonecrosis in 95 patients with systemic lupus erythematosus. J Rheumatol. 2001; 28(10):2226–9.
27. Cozen L, Wallace DJ. Avascular necrosis in systemic lupus erythematosus: clinical associations and a 47-year perspective. Am J Orthop. 1998;27(5):352–4.
28. Mont MA, Glueck CJ, Pacheco IH, Wang P, Hungerford DS, Petri M. Risk factors for osteonecrosis in systemic lupus erythematosus. J Rheumatol. 1997;24(4):654–62.
29. Aranow C, Zelicof S, Leslie D, Solomon S, Barland P, Norman A, et al. Clinically occult avascular necrosis of the hip in systemic lupus erythematosus. J Rheumatol. 1997;24(12):2318–22.
30. Abeles M, Urman JD, Rothfield NF. Aseptic necrosis of bone in systemic lupus erythematosus. Relationship to corticosteroid therapy. Arch Intern Med. 1978;138(5):750–4.
31. Mok CC, Lau CS, Wong RW. Risk factors for avascular bone necrosis in systemic lupus erythematosus. Br J Rheumatol. 1998;37(8): 895–900.
32. Gladman DD, Urowitz MB, Chaudhry-Ahluwalia V, Hallet DC, Cook RJ. Predictive factors for symptomatic osteonecrosis in patients with systemic lupus erythematosus. J Rheumatol. 2001; 28(4):761–5.
33. Zonana-Nacach A, Barr SG, Magder LS, Petri M. Damage in systemic lupus erythematosus and its association with corticosteroids. Arthritis Rheum. 2000;43(8):1801–8. doi:10.1002/1529-0131(200008)43:8<1801::AID-ANR16>3.0.CO;2-O.
34. Massardo L, Jacobelli S, Leissner M, Gonzalez M, Villarroel L, Rivero S. High-dose intravenous methylprednisolone therapy associated with osteonecrosis in patients with systemic lupus erythematosus. Lupus. 1992;1(6):401–5.
35. Zizic TM, Marcoux C, Hungerford DS, Dansereau JV, Stevens MB. Corticosteroid therapy associated with ischemic necrosis of bone in systemic lupus erythematosus. Am J Med. 1985;79(5):596–604. 0002-9343(85)90057-9 [pii].
36. Klipper AR, Stevens MB, Zizic TM, Hungerford DS. Ischemic necrosis of bone in systemic lupus erythematosus. Medicine (Baltimore). 1976;55(3):251–7.
37. Weinstein RS. Glucocorticoid-induced osteonecrosis. Endocrine. 2012;41(2):183–90. doi:10.1007/s12020-011-9580-0.
38. Calder JD, Buttery L, Revell PA, Pearse M, Polak JM. Apoptosis–a significant cause of bone cell death in osteonecrosis of the femoral head. J Bone Joint Surg Br. 2004;86(8):1209–13.
39. Seleznick MJ, Silveira LH, Espinoza LR. Avascular necrosis associated with anticardiolipin antibodies. J Rheumatol. 1991;18(9): 1416–7.
40. Wilson WA, Gharavi AE, Koike T, Lockshin MD, Branch DW, Piette JC, et al. International consensus statement on preliminary classification criteria for definite antiphospholipid syndrome: report of an international workshop. Arthritis Rheum. 1999;42(7):1309–11. doi:10.1002/1529-0131(199907)42:7<1309::AID-ANR1>3.0.CO;2-F.
41. Asherson RA, Khamashta MA, Ordi-Ros J, Derksen RH, Machin SJ, Barquinero J, et al. The "primary" antiphospholipid syndrome: major clinical and serological features. Medicine (Baltimore). 1989;68(6):366–74.
42. Tektonidou MG, Ioannidis JP, Boki KA, Vlachoyiannopoulos PG, Moutsopoulos HM. Prognostic factors and clustering of serious clinical outcomes in antiphospholipid syndrome. QJM. 2000;93(8): 523–30.
43. Roubey RA. Autoantibodies to phospholipid-binding plasma proteins: a new view of lupus anticoagulants and other "antiphospholipid" autoantibodies. Blood. 1994;84(9):2854–67.
44. McNeil HP, Simpson RJ, Chesterman CN, Krilis SA. Antiphospholipid antibodies are directed against a complex antigen that includes a lipid-binding inhibitor of coagulation: beta 2-glycoprotein I (apolipoprotein H). Proc Natl Acad Sci U S A. 1990;87(11): 4120–4.
45. Hughes GR. Thrombosis, abortion, cerebral disease, and the lupus anticoagulant. Br Med J (Clin Res Ed). 1983;287(6399):1088–9.
46. Love PE, Santoro SA. Antiphospholipid antibodies: anticardiolipin and the lupus anticoagulant in systemic lupus erythematosus (SLE) and in non-SLE disorders. Prevalence and clinical significance. Ann Intern Med. 1990;112(9):682–98. S0022214302000896 [pii].
47. Asherson RA, Liote F, Page B, Meyer O, Buchanan N, Khamashta MA, et al. Avascular necrosis of bone and antiphospholipid antibodies in systemic lupus erythematosus. J Rheumatol. 1993;20(2): 284–8.
48. Nagasawa K, Ishii Y, Mayumi T, Tada Y, Ueda A, Yamauchi Y, et al. Avascular necrosis of bone in systemic lupus erythematosus: possible role of haemostatic abnormalities. Ann Rheum Dis. 1989;48(8):672–6.
49. Mok MY, Farewell VT, Isenberg DA. Risk factors for avascular necrosis of bone in patients with systemic lupus erythematosus: is there a role for antiphospholipid antibodies? Ann Rheum Dis. 2000;59(6):462–7.
50. Tektonidou MG, Malagari K, Vlachoyiannopoulos PG, Kelekis DA, Moutsopoulos HM. Asymptomatic avascular necrosis in patients with primary antiphospholipid syndrome in the absence of corticosteroid use: a prospective study by magnetic resonance imaging. Arthritis Rheum. 2003;48(3):732–6. doi:10.1002/art.10835.
51. Felson DT, Anderson JJ. Across-study evaluation of association between steroid dose and bolus steroids and avascular necrosis of bone. Lancet. 1987;1(8538):902–6.
52. Lopez-Ben R, Mikuls TR, Moore DS, Julian BA, Bernreuter WK, Elkins M, et al. Incidence of hip osteonecrosis among renal transplantation recipients: a prospective study. Clin Radiol. 2004;59(5):431–8. doi:10.1016/j.crad.2003.11.001. S0009926003004987 [pii].
53. Abbott KC, Koff J, Bohen EM, Oglesby RJ, Agodoa LY, Lentine KL, et al. Maintenance immunosuppression use and the associated risk of avascular necrosis after kidney transplantation in the United States. Transplantation. 2005;79(3):330–6. 00007890-200502150-00011 [pii].
54. Harrington KD, Murray WR, Kountz SL, Belzer FO. Avascular necrosis of bone after renal transplantation. J Bone Joint Surg Am. 1971;53(2):203–15.
55. Tang S, Chan TM, Lui SL, Li FK, Lo WK, Lai KN. Risk factors for avascular bone necrosis after renal transplantation. Transplant Proc. 2000;32(7):1873–5. S0041-1345(00)01471-8 [pii].
56. Julian BA, Quarles LD, Niemann KM. Musculoskeletal complications after renal transplantation: pathogenesis and treatment. Am J Kidney Dis. 1992;19(2):99–120. S0272638692000246 [pii].
57. Ibels LS, Alfrey AC, Huffer WE, Weil 3rd R. Aseptic necrosis of bone following renal transplantation: experience in 194 transplant

recipients and review of the literature. Medicine (Baltimore). 1978;57(1):25–45.
58. Gustafsson LA, Meyers MH, Berne TV. Total hip replacement in renal transplant recipients with aseptic necrosis of the femoral head. Lancet. 1976;2(7986):606–8.
59. Papagelopoulos PJ, Hay JE, Galanis EC, Morrey BF. Total joint arthroplasty in orthotopic liver transplant recipients. J Arthroplasty. 1996;11(8):889–92.
60. Bradbury G, Benjamin J, Thompson J, Klees E, Copeland J. Avascular necrosis of bone after cardiac transplantation. Prevalence and relationship to administration and dosage of steroids. J Bone Joint Surg Am. 1994;76(9):1385–8.
61. Monegal A, Navasa M, Guanabens N, Peris P, Pons F, Martinez de Osaba MJ, et al. Bone mass and mineral metabolism in liver transplant patients treated with FK506 or cyclosporine A. Calcif Tissue Int. 2001;68(2):83–6.
62. Danzig LA, Coutis RD, Resnick D. Avascular necrosis of the femoral head following cardiac transplantation: report of a case. Clin Orthop Relat Res. 1976;117:217–20.
63. Parfrey PS, Farge D, Parfrey NA, Hanley JA, Guttman RD. The decreased incidence of aseptic necrosis in renal transplant recipients–a case control study. Transplantation. 1986;41(2):182–7.
64. Inoue S, Horii M, Asano T, Fujioka M, Ogura T, Shibatani M, et al. Risk factors for nontraumatic osteonecrosis of the femoral head after renal transplantation. J Orthop Sci. 2003;8(6):751–6. doi:10.1007/s00776-003-0716-9.
65. Landmann J, Renner N, Gachter A, Thiel G, Harder F. Cyclosporin A and osteonecrosis of the femoral head. J Bone Joint Surg Am. 1987;69(8):1226–8.
66. Kubo T, Yamazoe S, Sugano N, Fujioka M, Naruse S, Yoshimura N, et al. Initial MRI findings of non-traumatic osteonecrosis of the femoral head in renal allograft recipients. Magn Reson Imaging. 1997;15(9):1017–23. S0730-725X(97)00159-8 [pii].
67. Fujioka M, Kubo T, Nakamura F, Shibatani M, Ueshima K, Hamaguchi H, et al. Initial changes of non-traumatic osteonecrosis of femoral head in fat suppression images: bone marrow edema was not found before the appearance of band patterns. Magn Reson Imaging. 2001;19(7):985–91. S0730-725X(01)00424-6 [pii].
68. Bradford DS, Janes PC, Simmons RS, Najarian JS. Total hip arthroplasty in renal transplant recipients. Clin Orthop Relat Res. 1983;181:107–14.
69. Marston SB, Gillingham K, Bailey RF, Cheng EY. Osteonecrosis of the femoral head after solid organ transplantation: a prospective study. J Bone Joint Surg Am. 2002;84-A(12):2145–51.
70. Pierides AM, Simpson W, Stainsby D, Alvarez-ude F, Uldall PR. Avascular necrosis of bone following renal transplantation. Q J Med. 1975;44(175):459–80.
71. Chatterjee SN, Massry SG, Friedler RM, Singer FR, Berne TV. The high incidence of persistent secondary hyperparathyroidism after renal homotransplantation. Surg Gynecol Obstet. 1976;143(3): 440–2.
72. Patton PR, Pfaff WW. Aseptic bone necrosis after renal transplantation. Surgery. 1988;103(1):63–8.
73. Briggs WA, Hampers CL, Merrill JP, Hager EB, Wilson RE, Birtch AG, et al. Aseptic necrosis in the femur after renal transplantation. Ann Surg. 1972;175(2):282–9.
74. Sakai T, Sugano N, Kokado Y, Takahara S, Ohzono K, Yoshikawa H. Tacrolimus may be associated with lower osteonecrosis rates after renal transplantation. Clin Orthop Relat Res. 2003;415:163–70. doi:10.1097/01.blo.0000093908.26658.df.
75. Lieberman JR, Scaduto AA, Wellmeyer E. Symptomatic osteonecrosis of the hip after orthotopic liver transplantation. J Arthroplasty. 2000;15(6):767–71. doi:10.1054/arth.2000.6635. S0883-5403(00)32853-4 [pii].
76. Guichelaar MM, Schmoll J, Malinchoc M, Hay JE. Fractures and avascular necrosis before and after orthotopic liver transplantation: long-term follow-up and predictive factors. Hepatology. 2007;46(4):1198–207. doi:10.1002/hep.21805.
77. Atkinson K, Cohen M, Biggs J. Avascular necrosis of the femoral head secondary to corticosteroid therapy for graft-versus-host disease after marrow transplantation: effective therapy with hip arthroplasty. Bone Marrow Transplant. 1987;2(4):421–6.
78. Enright H, Haake R, Weisdorf D. Avascular necrosis of bone: a common serious complication of allogeneic bone marrow transplantation. Am J Med. 1990;89(6):733–8.
79. Socie G, Selimi F, Sedel L, Frija J, Devergie A, Esperou Bourdeau H, et al. Avascular necrosis of bone after allogeneic bone marrow transplantation: clinical findings, incidence and risk factors. Br J Haematol. 1994;86(3):624–8.
80. Shim K, MacKenzie MJ, Winquist E. Chemotherapy-associated osteonecrosis in cancer patients with solid tumours: a systematic review. Drug Saf. 2008;31(5):359–71. 3151 [pii].
81. Mankin HJ. Nontraumatic necrosis of bone (osteonecrosis). N Engl J Med. 1992;326(22):1473–9. doi:10.1056/NEJM199205283262206.
82. Howland WJ, Loeffler RK, Starchman DE, Johnson RG. Postirradiation atrophic changes of bone and related complications. Radiology. 1975;117(3 Pt 1):677–85.
83. Jenkins PJ, Montefiore DJ, Arnott SJ. Hip complications following chemoradiotherapy. Clin Oncol (R Coll Radiol). 1995;7(2):123–6.
84. Csuka M, Brewer BJ, Lynch KL, McCarty DJ. Osteonecrosis, fractures, and protrusio acetabuli secondary to x-irradiation therapy for prostatic carcinoma. J Rheumatol. 1987;14(1):165–70.
85. Sciascia R, Albisinni U, Ammendolia I, Barbieri E, Tondi L. Femoral osteonecrosis in patients treated with radiochemotherapy of Hodgkin's lymphoma. Radiol Med. 1989;77(4):336–41.
86. Delaere O, Orloff S, Autrique JC, Nyssen-Behets C, Dambrain R, Dhem A. Long-term sequelae of pelvis irradiation: histological and microradiographical study of a femoral head. Clin Rheumatol. 1991;10(2):206–10.
87. Rozsahegyi I. Chronic osteoarthropathy of caisson workers. Arch Gewerbepathol Gewerbehyg. 1956;14(5):483–510.
88. Kawashima M, Hayashi K, Torisu T, Kitano M. Histopathology of the early stage of osteonecrosis in divers. Undersea Biomed Res. 1977;4(4):409–17.
89. Immelman EJ, Bank S, Krige H, Marks IN. Roentgenologic and clinical features of intramedullary fat necrosis in bones in acute and chronic pancreatitis. Am J Med. 1964;36:96–105.
90. Baron M, Paltiel H, Lander P. Aseptic necrosis of the talus and calcaneal insufficiency fractures in a patient with pancreatitis, subcutaneous fat necrosis, and arthritis. Arthritis Rheum. 1984;27(11): 1309–13.
91. Wilson HA, Askari AD, Neiderhiser DH, Johnson AM, Andrews BS, Hoskins LC. Pancreatitis with arthropathy and subcutaneous fat necrosis. Evidence for the pathogenicity of lipolytic enzymes. Arthritis Rheum. 1983;26(2):121–6.
92. Goldblatt J, Sacks S, Beighton P. The orthopedic aspects of Gaucher disease. Clin Orthop Relat Res. 1978;137:208–14.
93. Amstutz HC, Carey EJ. Skeletal manifestations and treatment of Gaucher's disease. Review of twenty cases. J Bone Joint Surg Am. 1966;48(4):670–701.
94. Goldblatt J, Sacks S, Dall D, Beighton P. Total hip arthroplasty in Gaucher's disease. Long-term prognosis. Clin Orthop Relat Res. 1988;228:94–8.

Part V

Pathology

18 Pathophysiology of Ischemic Diseases of the Hip: Osteonecrosis, Borderline Necrosis, and Bone Marrow Edema Syndrome

Kyung-Hoi Koo, Young-Kyun Lee, and Yun Jong Lee

18.1 Introduction

Osteonecrosis (ON) of the femoral head is an evolutionary process involving (1) marrow necrosis and osteocytic death, (2) reparative process around the necrotic zone, and (3) collapse of necrotic bone and subsequent degenerative arthritis of the hip [1–3].

Except for radiation necrosis [4] and cytotoxic necrosis [5], which are caused by direct cellular injury, ischemia after a disruption of blood flow seems to be the most probable cause of ON [1–3]. Over the past 50 years, various theories have been developed to explain the pathogenesis of nontraumatic ON. Early hypotheses included intraosseous hypertension of the proximal femur leading to a compartment syndrome [6], intravascular coagulation triggered by fat embolism [7], and hypertrophy of marrow fat cell [8]. However, none of them could explain the pathophysiology independently. They are mutually interactive with each other and seem to play roles together in the development of ON [9–11].

During the past two decades, there has been an enormous progress in our understanding of the puzzling pathomechanism of ON. Currently, three concepts are generally accepted. First, the ischemia occurs through one common pathway, intravascular coagulation [9]. Second, both of marrow mechanisms and intravascular mechanisms are involved in the occurrence of intravascular coagulation [9–12]. Third, ON has a multifactorial etiology. Although certain etiologic factors might be able to cause the disease by virtue of their action alone, underlying genetic predispositions and acquired risk factors have synergistic action in the pathogenesis of most cases [13–20]. This role of genetic predispositions could explain why some chronic users of steroids or alcohol do not acquire the disease. Alcoholics and steroid users with thrombophilia/hypofibrinolysis and/or impaired angiogenesis may have a greater susceptibility for developing ON.

Doctor John Paul Jones Jr. developed a comprehensive concept on the pathomechanism of ON [9–11]. He also suggested that an acute ischemia might lead to various results: nonprogressive marrow necrosis (borderline necrosis), bone marrow edema syndrome, or irreversible ON [10]. The fate of ischemia depends on the restoration of vascular perfusion by fibrinolysis and reparative angiogenesis, which affects the viability of osteocytes [9–11].

In this chapter, the current knowledge on pathomechanism of ON was reviewed and described according to the concept of Doctor Jones.

18.2 Histologic Criteria of ON

The earliest histologic criteria of ON was made by Arlet and Durroux [21]: Type 1, disappearance of hematopoietic marrow; Type 2, necrosis of the fatty marrow; Type 3, complete medullary and trabecular necrosis; and Type 4, complete necrosis with marginal fibrosis and new bone formation. They defined Type 2 lesion as the diagnostic criterion of ON. However, there has been confusion and debate about this criterion because the Type 2 lesion is also observed in BMES [22, 23]. This lesion is also seen in the contralateral femoral heads in patients who have unilateral ON [24] and the femoral heads of patients who are treated with steroid [25, 26]. Moreover, the Type 2 lesion does not progress to Type 4 lesion [10, 27].

To distinguish ON from BMES and to avoid confusion in their respective diagnoses, Type 4 lesion has been suggested for the criterion of ON [10]. Currently, this criterion is the most widely accepted histologic criterion for ON [28].

K.-H. Koo (✉) • Y.-K. Lee
Department of Orthopaedic Surgery,
Seoul National University College of Medicine, Seoul National University Bundang Hospital, 82 Gumi-ro, 173 Beon-gil, Seongnam 463-707, South Korea
e-mail: khkoo@snu.ac.kr

Y.J. Lee
Department of Internal Medicine,
Seoul National University College of Medicine, Seoul, South Korea

Department of Internal Medicine, Seoul National University Bundang Hospital, 166 Gumi-ro, Seongnam 463-707, South Korea
e-mail: yn35@snu.ac.kr

K.-H. Koo et al. (eds.), *Osteonecrosis*,
DOI 10.1007/978-3-642-35767-1_18, © Springer-Verlag Berlin Heidelberg 2014

18.3 Femoral Head Blood Supply: An Ischemia-Vulnerable Vasculature

The blood supply to the femoral head is derived from the lateral epiphyseal artery and the medial epiphyseal artery (a small subsidiary vessel in the ligamentum teres). Actually, the lateral epiphyseal artery is the single main blood supplier to the femoral head in adults. This artery is the intraosseous continuation of the superior retinacular artery, which is derived from the medial femoral circumflex artery [29]. When the lateral epiphyseal artery, the superior retinacular artery, or the medial femoral circumflex artery is disrupted, a precarious state of an ischemia develops in the femoral head. A "watershed cerebral infarct" is an ischemic lesion due to blood flow blockage at the peripheral zones of the territories of cerebral arteries. Thus, this ischemic lesion is frequently located at the cerebral cortex and usually wedge-shaped [30]. Like the watershed cerebral infarct, the ischemia of the femoral head occurs at the peripheral zone of the lateral epiphyseal artery. Thus, femoral head ON is located at the subchondral bone in the anterolateral quadrant of the femoral head and is usually wedge-shaped.

18.4 Pathomechanism

18.4.1 Fat Accumulation and Hematopoietic Cell Depletion in the Marrow and Intraosseous Hypertension

Chandler called the femoral head ON as "the coronary disease of the hip" as he thought the disease simulates the ischemic condition in the heart [31]. However, unlike the coronary artery, the lateral epiphyseal vessels are housed with a closed chamber of the femoral head, which is filled with marrow cells. Steroids and alcohol stimulate the differentiation of bone marrow stem cells into fat cells and induce hypertrophy of fat cell. The diameter of the marrow fat cells increases by more than 10 μm [32]. The marrow space is filled with large round or ovoid fat cells, and hematopoietic cells are depleted (Arlet and Durroux Type 1 lesion) (Fig. 18.1). The proximal femoral metaphysis shows a high signal intensity almost comparable to that of the greater trochanter on T1-weighted MR image, which indicates fatty marrow conversion [33].

This increase in fat cell volume leads to an intraosseous hypertension in the proximal femur [6, 8]. The intraosseous hypertension can cause venous sinusoidal compression, impaired arterial flow, and microvascular coagulation in the proximal femur [6].

A decrease of intramedullary blood flow induces a conversion of hematopoietic marrow to fatty marrow

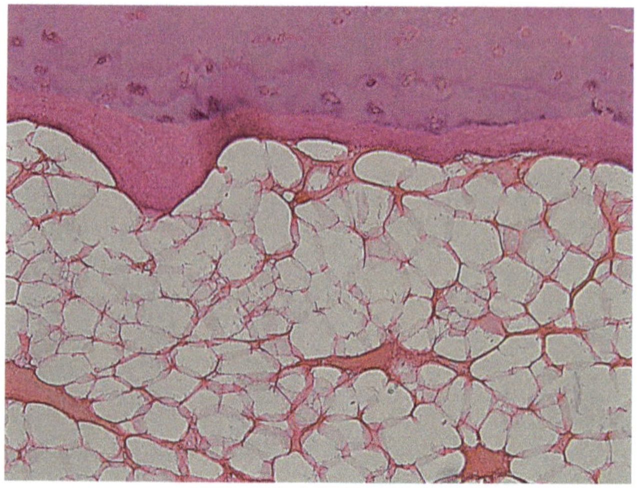

Fig. 18.1 Hematopoietic cells are depleted, and the marrow space is filled with large round or ovoid fat cells. Lacunae are filled with viable osteocytes (Arlet and Durroux Type 1 lesion) (hematoxylin and eosin stain, original magnification ×100)

probably because fatty marrow can survive even with a limited vascular supply relative to hematopoietic marrow [33, 34].

Thus, marrow ischemia and fat marrow conversion mutually interact forming a vicious cycle. Regions composed of fatty marrow have a stronger predilection for ON than do areas of hematopoietic marrow. The femoral head, one of the first places to convert to fatty marrow, is at risk for ON [33, 34].

In Gaucher disease, a fatty substance "glycosphingolipid" is stored in marrow cells, which leads to an intraosseous hypertension [35].

18.4.2 Marrow Necrosis

Intravascular coagulation leads to an acute ischemia in the femoral head.

Individual marrow cells have different sensitivities to ischemia [36–38].

The hematopoietic cells are most sensitive and are the first to die after the ischemia, usually within 12 h [39]. The marrow fat cells die, and their nucleus disappears from the second day of ischemia [40]. Thus, the earliest microscopic signs indicative of bone ischemia are seen in the marrow spaces. The hematopoietic cells disappear, and there is loss of nuclear staining of marrow fat cells. The fatty marrow becomes necrotic (Arlet and Durroux Type 2 lesion) (Fig. 18.2). Necrotic lesions are scattered and patchily distributed in the marrow space. However, most lacunae (more than 50 %) are filled with viable osteocytes. Occasionally, some empty lacunae are seen at this stage probably due to a diminished blood supply, even though technical artifacts

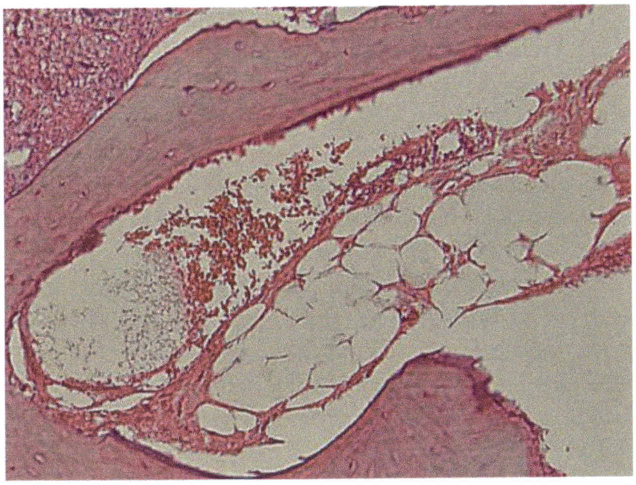

Fig. 18.2 Nuclear staining of marrow fat cells is not seen and the marrow space is necrotic. However, most lacunae (more than 50 %) are filled with viable osteocytes (Arlet and Durroux Type 2 lesion) (hematoxylin and eosin stain, original magnification ×100)

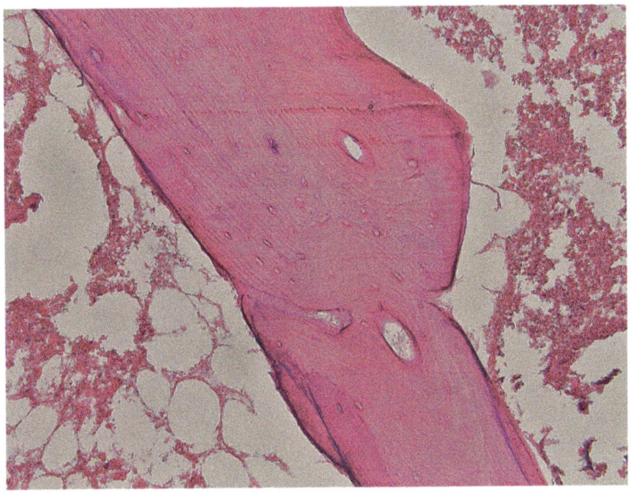

Fig. 18.3 The marrow space is necrotic and most lacunae are empty (Arlet and Durroux Type 3 lesion) (hematoxylin and eosin stain, original magnification ×100)

(suboptimal tissue fixation or decalcification) or aging phenomenon may result in the loss of staining of osteocytic nuclei [40].

In this stage, sequestrum, a focal lesion of completely dead marrow cells and osteocytes, is not formed, and there is no evidence of reparative processes at the periphery of the necrotic zone. Thus, MRI shows no focal lesion in the femoral head. However, angiography shows an arterial interruption, and bone scan shows a cold lesion in the femoral head [26].

When the duration of ischemia is temporary and shorter than the threshold for complete osteocytic death, this lesion is not progressive and remains as so-called borderline necrosis [10].

However, when the ischemia is prolonged with a total lack of perfusion beyond the threshold of osteocytic death, the ischemic lesion progresses to ON.

18.4.3 Thrombophilia and Hypofibrinolysis

Various hereditary and genetic conditions, which cause increased thrombosis and/or impaired fibrinolysis, accentuate and prolong microvascular coagulation.

Protein C has an anticoagulant function by degrading procoagulant factors Va and VIIIa. Protein S serves as cofactor for activated protein C [41]. Protein C and protein S deficiencies [41–43] as well as mutations in the factor V Leiden or the prothrombin 20210A gene [44, 45] increase thrombosis. Polymorphisms of the plasminogen activator inhibitor-1 gene (PAI-1) are associated with hypercoagulable state [41, 46, 47].

Positivity of antiphospholipid antibodies [48, 49], sickle cell disease [50, 51], and inflammatory bowel disease [52, 53] also increases the risk of microvascular thrombi.

18.4.4 Impaired Angiogenesis

The marrow necrosis triggers a reparative process including reactive angiogenesis. An impairment of angiogenesis, as well as thrombophilia/hypofibrinolysis, has been proposed as a mechanism for developing ON. Nitric oxide, which was originally discovered as a vasodilator product of the endothelium, promotes angiogenesis and bone formation. Polymorphism in the nitric oxide synthase gene is associated with idiopathic ON [15, 19]. Vascular endothelial growth factor (VEGF), which is induced by hypoxia, is a strong angiogenic protein and also plays a role in the formation of cartilage and bone. Genetic polymorphisms of VEGF are associated with the development of steroid-induced ON [17, 20]. Steroids also impair angiogenesis by suppressing the production of VEGF [54].

18.4.5 Osteocytic Death and Sequestrum Formation

Thrombophilia/hypofibrinolysis and impaired angiogenesis may lead to a prolonged anoxia and sequestrum formation in the femoral head.

After the onset of ischemia, osteocytes begin to disappear within 2–5 days and completely disappear within 2–4 weeks [39, 40, 55–58].

Once most osteocytes die and a sequestrum is formed, the lesion is irreversible and progresses to definite ON (Arlet and Durroux Type 3 lesion) (Fig. 18.3). However, if the necrotic region is small (<1 cm), it may heal spontaneously.

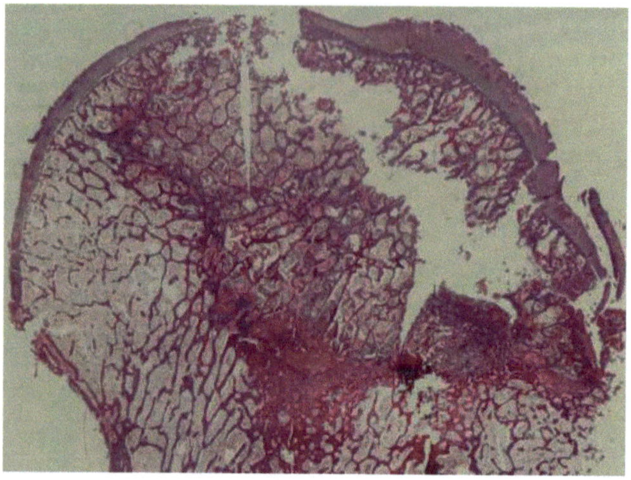

Fig. 18.4 A foreign body reaction is seen at the peripheral portion of the sequestrum. Histiocytes and giant cells aggregate forming a fibrous capsule (Arlet and Durroux Type 4 lesion) (hematoxylin and eosin stain, original magnification ×100)

18.4.6 Reparative Process at the Margin of the Sequestrum

In a usual reparative process such as fracture healing, a fibrous vascular ingrowth occurs in the necrotic region. Vascular canals penetrate the medullary canals of the cancellous bone and the Haversian canals in the overlying cortical bone. Primitive mesenchymal cells infiltrate into the necrotic portion, which differentiate into osteoblasts and osteoclasts. Immature woven bone is deposited on the dead trabecular bone, which is slowly resorbed by the process of so-called creeping substitution [59].

However, creeping substitution does not occur after the formation of sequestrum. Instead, a foreign body reaction occurs at the peripheral portion of the sequestrum. Histiocytes and giant cells aggregate around the sequestrum, forming a fibrous capsule (Arlet and Durroux Type 4 lesion) (Fig. 18.4). This capsule is called a reactive zone, which appears as a band lesion on MRI. A definite diagnosis of ON can be made when there is a focal sequestrum surrounded by a peripheral reactive zone [10]. At this stage, the reactive band appears on MRI.

Around this reactive zone, marrow edema often occurs. During the presence of edema, bone marrow pressure is elevated and patients have hip pain [60].

Although vessels penetrate into the fibrotic capsule, the angiogenesis is blocked at the margin of sequestrum [61], and reparative fibrovascular tissue cannot penetrate into the marrow space of the sequestrum. Thus, no biological repair process occurs in the necrotic portion. The fibrotic capsule is gradually substituted by newly formed bone by osteoblasts and osteocytes, which appears as a sclerotic rim on radiographs.

18.4.7 Saponification and Collapse of Necrotic Bone

Although there is no biological reaction in the necrotic portion, dead marrow undergoes a chemical change. Dead adipocytes release fatty acids, which saponify with extracellular calcium to form insoluble soaps [62–64]. Saponified fats and other necrotic areas eventually calcify, which appear as Mitchell class D lesion (dark signal on T1- and T2-weighted images) on MRI [65]. The dead trabeculae and saponified marrow do not attain the previous mechanical strength and structural integrity. Even with protected weight-bearing load, fatigue fracture occurs at the subchondral portion, which appears as a crescent sign on the radiograph, leading to collapse of the femoral head. Ultimately, this leads to a depression of articular cartilage and degenerative arthritis of the hip.

18.5 Borderline Necrosis

After an intravascular coagulation and marrow necrosis, a complete fibrinolysis and sufficient compensatory angiogenesis may occur within the critical ischemic period. In this situation, most osteocytes (>50 %) remain viable (Arlet and Durroux Type 2 or 3 lesion). The ischemic insult does not form a sequestrum and does not trigger a peripheral reparative process. This lesion is called "borderline necrosis" [10]. Borderline necrosis is seen in the femoral head of patients who have been exposed to risk factors without developing ON and in the contralateral femoral head of patients who have osteonecrosis in one hip.

In borderline necrosis, the reactive band, which is the earliest MR finding for ON, is not seen. The only nonspecific MR finding is an increase of signal intensity of the proximal femoral metaphysis in T1-weighted image, which means a conversion of hematopoietic to fatty marrow and increase of fat content. Angiography shows interruption of superior retinacular artery or medial femoral circumflex artery. Bone marrow pressure is slightly elevated, and bone scan shows decrease of radionuclide uptake. Although some patients have mild hip pain at the initial period of ischemia, most patients are asymptomatic.

The borderline necrosis does not progress to ON (Fig. 18.5).

18.6 Bone Marrow Edema Syndrome

Bone marrow edema syndrome (BMES) is a rare disease of the hip, which regresses spontaneously within several months [23, 66–71].

Although the exact etiology is unknown, ischemia seems to be the most probable cause because histologic findings are similar to those of early-stage ON [23, 67, 68].

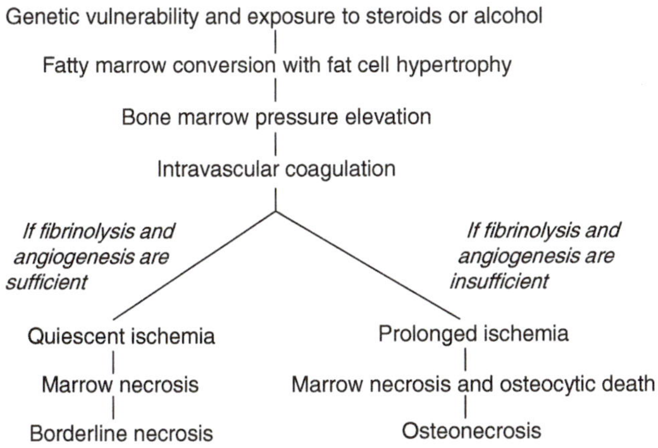

Fig. 18.5 Pathways of borderline necrosis and osteonecrosis

It frequently affects pregnant women in their third trimester [66, 69], and an association with hypofibrinolysis was reported in familial BMES [70, 71]. However, most patients with BMES do not have risk factors for ON [23, 58–68].

Intravascular coagulation and marrow necrosis may occur in the absence or paucity of risk factors. In this situation, the subsequent events after the ischemia are quite different from ON. Complete fibrinolysis and reactive vasodilatation occur [72]. Thus, there is only a brisk period of subthreshold ischemic hypoxia. Reactive hyperemia and increased permeability lead to an interstitial edema in the marrow space.

Although the marrow is necrotic, most osteocytes remain viable, and most lacunae are filled with osteocyte, because the ischemia is not so severe to induce complete bone death. There is no sequestrum formation and no reactive zone around the necrotic portion [23, 68].

A creeping substitution occurs in the regions of marrow necrosis. Fibrovascular tissue and dilated vessels are seen in the medullary cavity. Immature woven bone is deposited on the surface of trabecular bone. The marrow space is filled with fluid. By the Arlet and Durroux classification, these lesions are Type 2 or Type 3 lesions (Fig. 18.6).

During the edema, bone marrow pressure is elevated. Most patients suffer hip pain and are diagnosed at this stage. MRI shows findings of edema in the marrow space. Angiography shows arterial dilatation, and bone scan shows increased uptake in the proximal femur.

The increased perfusion induces transient demineralization of the trabeculae and cortical bone of the proximal femur. When the demineralization is severe, a nonspecific radiolucency of the proximal femur appears on the radiograph. However, the bone trabeculae have normal volume density and no signs of "osteoporosis." Because of this, Wilson et al. proposed to use the term "transient BMES" instead of "transient osteoporosis" [73].

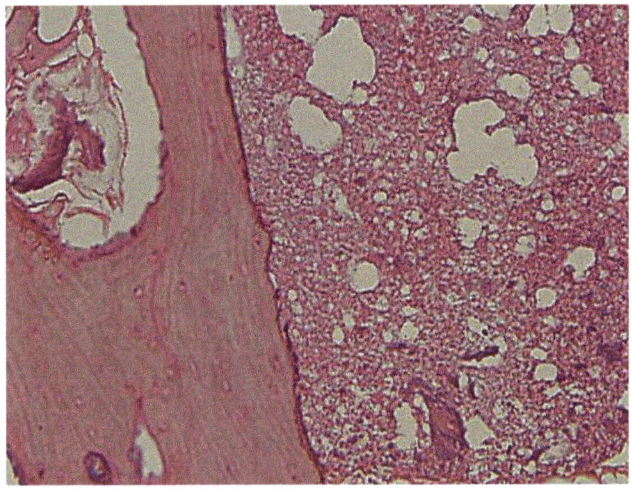

Fig. 18.6 The marrow space is filled with fluid. Fibrovascular tissue and dilated vessels are seen in the marrow space. Immature woven bone is deposited on the surface of trabecular bone. Although the marrow is necrotic, most osteocytes remain viable and most lacunae are filled with osteocytes (hematoxylin and eosin stain, original magnification ×100)

As the intraosseous vascularity and perfusion return to normal, the osteoid mineralizes and the lesion is spontaneously healed.

Bone marrow edema syndrome is a self-limiting disease and does not progress to ON.

References

1. Arlet J. Nontraumatic avascular necrosis of the femoral head. Past, present, and future. Clin Orthop Relat Res. 1992;277:12–21.
2. Mont MA, Hungerford DS. Non-traumatic avascular necrosis of the femoral head. J Bone Joint Surg Am. 1995;77(3):459–74.
3. Jones LC, Hungerford DS. Osteonecrosis: etiology, diagnosis, and treatment. Curr Opin Rheumatol. 2004;16(4):443–9.
4. Prosnitz LR, Lawson JP, Friedlaender GE, Farber LR, Pezzimenti JF. Avascular necrosis of bone in Hodgkin's disease patients treated with combined modality therapy. Cancer. 1981;47(12):2793–7.
5. Shim K, MacKenzie MJ, Winquist E. Chemotherapy-associated osteonecrosis in cancer patients with solid tumours: a systematic review. Drug Saf. 2008;31(5):359–71.
6. Hungerford DS, Lennox DW. The importance of increased intraosseous pressure in the development of osteonecrosis of the femoral head: implications for treatment. Orthop Clin North Am. 1985;16(4): 635–54.
7. Jones Jr JP, Engleman EP, Najarian JS. Systemic fat embolism after renal homotransplantation and treatment with corticosteroids. N Engl J Med. 1965;273(27):1453–8. doi:10.1056/nejm196512302732703.
8. Wang GJ, Sweet DE, Reger SI, Thompson RC. Fat-cell changes as a mechanism of avascular necrosis of the femoral head in cortisone-treated rabbits. J Bone Joint Surg Am. 1977;59(6):729–35.
9. Jones Jr JP. Concepts of etiology and early pathogenesis of osteonecrosis. Instr Course Lect. 1994;43:499–512.
10. Koo KH, Jeong ST, Jones Jr JP. Borderline necrosis of the femoral head. Clin Orthop Relat Res. 1999;358:158–65.
11. Jones Jr JP. Alcoholism, hypercortisonism, fat embolism and osseous avascular necrosis. 1971. Clin Orthop Relat Res. 2001;393:4–12.

12. Seamon J, Keller T, Saleh J, Cui Q. The pathogenesis of nontraumatic osteonecrosis.Arthritis.2012;2012:601763.doi:10.1155/2012/601763.
13. Asano T, Takahashi KA, Fujioka M, Inoue S, Okamoto M, Sugioka N, et al. ABCB1 C3435T and G2677T/A polymorphism decreased the risk for steroid-induced osteonecrosis of the femoral head after kidney transplantation. Pharmacogenetics. 2003; 13(11):675–82. doi:10.1097/01.fpc.0000054135.14659.65.
14. Chao YC, Wang SJ, Chu HC, Chang WK, Hsieh TY. Investigation of alcohol metabolizing enzyme genes in Chinese alcoholics with avascular necrosis of hip joint, pancreatitis and cirrhosis of the liver. Alcohol Alcohol. 2003;38(5):431–6.
15. Koo KH, Lee JS, Lee YJ, Kim KJ, Yoo JJ, Kim HJ. Endothelial nitric oxide synthase gene polymorphisms in patients with nontraumatic femoral head osteonecrosis. J Orthop Res. 2006;24(8):1722–8. doi:10.1002/jor.20164.
16. Chang JD, Hur M, Lee SS, Yoo JH, Lee KM. Genetic background of nontraumatic osteonecrosis of the femoral head in the Korean population. Clin Orthop Relat Res. 2008;466(5):1041–6. doi:10.1007/s11999-008-0147-1.
17. Kim T, Hong JM, Lee J, Oh B, Park EK, Lee C, et al. Promoter polymorphisms of the vascular endothelial growth factor gene is associated with an osteonecrosis of the femoral head in the Korean population. Osteoarthritis Cartilage. 2008;16(3):287–91. doi:10.1016/j.joca.2007.06.017.
18. Kim TH, Hong JM, Oh B, Cho YS, Lee JY, Kim HL, et al. Genetic association study of polymorphisms in the catalase gene with the risk of osteonecrosis of the femoral head in the Korean population. Osteoarthritis Cartilage. 2008;16(9):1060–6. doi:10.1016/j.joca.2008.02.004.
19. Glueck CJ, Freiberg RA, Boppana S, Wang P. Thrombophilia, hypofibrinolysis, the eNOS T-786C polymorphism, and multifocal osteonecrosis. J Bone Joint Surg Am. 2008;90(10):2220–9. doi:10.2106/JBJS.G.00616. 90/10/2220 [pii].
20. Lee YJ, Lee JS, Kang EH, Lee YK, Kim SY, Song YW, et al. Vascular endothelial growth factor polymorphisms in patients with steroid-induced femoral head osteonecrosis. J Orthop Res. 2012;30(1):21–7. doi:10.1002/jor.21492.
21. Arlet J, Durroux R, Fauchier C, Thiechart M. Histopathology of the nontraumatic necrosis of the femoral head: topographic and evaluative aspect. In: Bone circulation. Baltimore: Williams & Wilkins; 1984.
22. Hauzeur JP, Perlmutter N, Appelboom T, Pasteels JL. Medullary impairment at early stage of non-traumatic osteonecrosis of the femoral head. Rheumatol Int. 1991;11(4–5):215–7.
23. Hofmann S, Engel A, Neuhold A, Leder K, Kramer J, Plenk Jr H. Bone-marrow oedema syndrome and transient osteoporosis of the hip. An MRI-controlled study of treatment by core decompression. J Bone Joint Surg Br. 1993;75(2):210–6.
24. Hauzeur JP, Sintzoff Jr S, Appelboom T, De Maertelaer V, Bentin J, Pasteels JL. Relationship between magnetic resonance imaging and histologic findings by bone biopsy in nontraumatic osteonecrosis of the femoral head. J Rheumatol. 1992;19(3):385–92.
25. Hauzeur JP, Pasteels JL, Orloff S. Bilateral non-traumatic aseptic osteonecrosis in the femoral head. An experimental study of incidence. J Bone Joint Surg Am. 1987;69(8):1221–5.
26. Koo KH, Kim R, Cho SH, Song HR, Lee G, Ko GH. Angiography, scintigraphy, intraosseous pressure, and histologic findings in high-risk osteonecrotic femoral heads with negative magnetic resonance images. Clin Orthop Relat Res. 1994;308:127–38.
27. Sugano N, Nishii T, Shibuya T, Nakata K, Masuhara K, Takaoka K. Contralateral hip in patients with unilateral nontraumatic osteonecrosis of the femoral head. Clin Orthop Relat Res. 1997;334:85–90.
28. Goetz JE, Robinson DA, Pedersen DR, Conzemius MG, Brown TD. Cryoinsult parameter effects on the histologically apparent volume of experimentally induced osteonecrotic lesions. J Orthop Res. 2011;29(6):931–7. doi:10.1002/jor.21342.
29. Tucker FR. Arterial supply to the femoral head and its clinical importance. J Bone Joint Surg Br. 1949;31B(1):82–93.
30. Torvik A. The pathogenesis of watershed infarcts in the brain. Stroke. 1984;15(2):221–3.
31. Chandler FA. Coronary disease of the hip. J Int Coll Surg. 1948;11(1):34–6.
32. Miyanishi K, Yamamoto T, Irisa T, Yamashita A, Jingushi S, Noguchi Y, et al. Bone marrow fat cell enlargement and a rise in intraosseous pressure in steroid-treated rabbits with osteonecrosis. Bone. 2003;30(1):185–90. http://dx.doi.org/10.1016/S8756-3282(01)00663-9.
33. Koo KH, Dussault R, Kaplan P, Kim R, Ahn IO, Christopher J, et al. Age-related marrow conversion in the proximal metaphysis of the femur: evaluation with T1-weighted MR imaging. Radiology. 1998;206(3):745–8.
34. Kricun ME. Red-yellow marrow conversion: its effect on the location of some solitary bone lesions. Skeletal Radiol. 1985;14(1): 10–9.
35. Amstutz HC, Carey EJ. Skeletal manifestations and treatment of Gaucher's disease. Review of twenty cases. J Bone Joint Surg Am. 1966;48(4):670–701.
36. Humphreys S, Spencer JD, Tighe JR, Cumming RR. The femoral head in osteonecrosis. A quantitative study of osteocyte population. J Bone Joint Surg Br. 1989;71(2):205–8.
37. James J, Steijn-Myagkaya GL. Death of osteocytes. Electron microscopy after in vitro ischaemia. J Bone Joint Surg Br. 1986; 68(4):620–4.
38. Nadel SN, Debatin JF, Richardson WJ, Hedlund LW, Senft C, Rizk WS, et al. Detection of acute avascular necrosis of the femoral head in dogs: dynamic contrast-enhanced MR imaging vs spin-echo and STIR sequences. AJR Am J Roentgenol. 1992;159(6):1255–61. doi:10.2214/ajr.159.6.1442396.
39. Fondi C, Franchi A. Definition of bone necrosis by the pathologist. Clinical Cases Miner Bone Metab. 2007;4(1):21–6.
40. Catto M. Pathology of aseptic bone necrosis. In: Davidson JK, editor. Aseptic necrosis of bone. Amsterdam: Excepta Medica; 1976. p. 3–100.
41. Glueck CJ, Freiberg R, Tracy T, Stroop D, Wang P. Thrombophilia and hypofibrinolysis: pathophysiologies of osteonecrosis. Clin Orthop Relat Res. 1997;334:43–56.
42. Jones LC, Mont MA, Le TB, Petri M, Hungerford DS, Wang P, et al. Procoagulants and osteonecrosis. J Rheumatol. 2003;30(4):783–91.
43. Pierre-Jacques H, Glueck CJ, Mont MA, Hungerford DS. Familial heterozygous protein-S deficiency in a patient who had multifocal osteonecrosis. A case report. J Bone Joint Surg Am. 1997;79(7):1079–84.
44. Zalavras CG, Vartholomatos G, Dokou E, Malizos KN. Genetic background of osteonecrosis: associated with thrombophilic mutations? Clin Orthop Relat Res. 2004;422:251–5. 00003086-200405000-00040 [pii].
45. Bjorkman A, Svensson PJ, Hillarp A, Burtscher IM, Runow A, Benoni G. Factor V leiden and prothrombin gene mutation: risk factors for osteonecrosis of the femoral head in adults. Clin Orthop Relat Res. 2004;425:168–72. 00003086-200408000-00023 [pii].
46. Glueck CJ, Fontaine RN, Gruppo R, Stroop D, Sieve-Smith L, Tracy T, et al. The plasminogen activator inhibitor-1 gene, hypofibrinolysis, and osteonecrosis. Clin Orthop Relat Res. 1999;366: 133–46.
47. Glueck CJ, Freiberg RA, Fontaine RN, Tracy T, Wang P. Hypofibrinolysis, thrombophilia, osteonecrosis. Clin Orthop Relat Res. 2001;386:19–33.
48. Seleznick MJ, Silveira LH, Espinoza LR. Avascular necrosis associated with anticardiolipin antibodies. J Rheumatol. 1991;18(9): 1416–7.
49. Korompilias AV, Gilkeson GS, Ortel TL, Seaber AV, Urbaniak JR. Anticardiolipin antibodies and osteonecrosis of the femoral head. Clin Orthop Relat Res. 1997;345:174–80.

50. Golding JS. Conditions of the hip associated with hemoglobinopathies. Clin Orthop Relat Res. 1973;90:22–8.
51. Hernigou P, Galacteros F, Bachir D, Goutallier D. Deformities of the hip in adults who have sickle-cell disease and had avascular necrosis in childhood. A natural history of fifty-two patients. J Bone Joint Surg Am. 1991;73(1):81–92.
52. Vakil N, Sparberg M. Steroid-related osteonecrosis in inflammatory bowel disease. Gastroenterology. 1989;96(1):62–7. S0016508589000302 [pii].
53. Hauzeur JP, Malaise M, Gangji V. Osteonecrosis in inflammatory bowel diseases: a review of the literature. Acta Gastroenterol Belg. 2009;72(3):327–34.
54. Kabata T, Matsumoto T, Yagishita S, Wakayama T, Iseki S, Tomita K. Vascular endothelial growth factor in rabbits during development of corticosteroid-induced osteonecrosis: a controlled experiment. J Rheumatol. 2008;35(12):2383–90. doi:10.3899/jrheum.070838.
55. Frost HM. In vivo osteocyte death. J Bone Joint Surg Am. 1960; 42-A:138–43.
56. Catto M. A histological study of avascular necrosis of the femoral head after transcervical fracture. J Bone Joint Surg Br. 1965;47(4): 749–76.
57. Young MH. Epiphysial infarction in a growing long bone. An experimental study in the rabbit. J Bone Joint Surg Br. 1966;48(4): 826–40.
58. McCarthy EF. Aseptic necrosis of bone. An historic perspective. Clin Orthop Relat Res. 1982;168:216–21.
59. Day SM, Ostrum RF, Chao EYS, Rubin CT, Aro HT, Einhorn TA. Bone injury. Regeneration and Repair In: Buckwalter JA, Ein-horn T, Simon S, eds. Orthopaedic Basic Science - The Biology and Biomechanics of the Musculoskeletal System. Rosemont IL: America Academy of Orthopaedic Surgeons. 2000:371–400.
60. Koo KH, Ahn IO, Kim R, Song HR, Jeong ST, Na JB, et al. Bone marrow edema and associated pain in early stage osteonecrosis of the femoral head: prospective study with serial MR images. Radiology. 1999,213(3):715–22.
61. Atsumi T, Kuroki Y, Yamano K. A microangiographic study of idiopathic osteonecrosis of the femoral head. Clin Orthop Relat Res. 1989;246:186–94.
62. Glimcher MJ, Kenzora JE. The biology of osteonecrosis of the human femoral head and its clinical implications: II. The pathological changes in the femoral head as an organ and in the hip joint. Clin Orthop Relat Res. 1979;139:283–312.
63. Glimcher MJ, Kenzora JE. Nicolas Andry award. The biology of osteonecrosis of the human femoral head and its clinical implications: 1. Tissue biology. Clin Orthop Relat Res. 1979;138: 284–309.
64. Glimcher MJ, Kenzora JE. The biology of osteonecrosis of the human femoral head and its clinical implications. III. Discussion of the etiology and genesis of the pathological sequelae; comments on treatment. Clin Orthop Relat Res. 1979;140:273–312.
65. Mitchell DG, Rao VM, Dalinka MK, Spritzer CE, Alavi A, Steinberg ME, et al. Femoral head avascular necrosis: correlation of MR imaging, radiographic staging, radionuclide imaging, and clinical findings. Radiology. 1987;162(3):709–15.
66. Curtiss Jr PH, Kincaid WE. Transitory demineralization of the hip in pregnancy. A report of three cases. J Bone Joint Surg Am. 1959;41-A:1327–33.
67. Hayes CW, Conway WF, Daniel WW. MR imaging of bone marrow edema pattern: transient osteoporosis, transient bone marrow edema syndrome, or osteonecrosis. Radiographics. 1993;13(5): 1001–11; discussion 12.
68. Kim SY, Koo KH, Suh KT, Kim YS, Cho YJ, Min BW, et al. Fatty marrow conversion of the proximal femoral metaphysis in transient bone marrow edema syndrome. Arch Orthop Trauma Surg. 2005;125(6):390–5. doi:10.1007/s00402-005-0824-4.
69. Willis-Owen CA, Daurka JS, Chen A, Lewis A. Bilateral femoral neck fractures due to transient osteoporosis of pregnancy: a case report. Cases J. 2008;1(1):120. doi:10.1186/1757-1626-1-120.
70. Van Veldhuizen PJ, Neff J, Murphey MD, Bodensteiner D, Skikne BS. Decreased fibrinolytic potential in patients with idiopathic avascular necrosis and transient osteoporosis of the hip. Am J Hematol. 1993;44(4):243–8.
71. Berger CE, Kluger R, Urban M, Kowalski J, Haas OA, Engel A. Elevated levels of lipoprotein(a) in familial bone marrow edema syndrome of the hip. Clin Orthop Relat Res. 2000;377:126–31.
72. Koo KH, Ahn IO, Song HR, Kim SY, Jones Jr JP. Increased perfusion of the femoral head in transient bone marrow edema syndrome. Clin Orthop Relat Res. 2002;402:171–5.
73. Wilson AJ, Murphy WA, Hardy DC, Totty WG. Transient osteoporosis: transient bone marrow edema? Radiology. 1988;167(3): 757–60.

19 The Pathology of Osteonecrosis of the Femoral Head

Takuaki Yamamoto

19.1 Introduction

Although the precise etiology of nontraumatic osteonecrosis of the femoral head (ON) is still unclear, this condition has generally been considered to result from an ischemia to the bone and bone marrow tissues. The first pathologic description of the femoral head osteonecrosis was reported in a case of caisson disease in 1888 [1]. In 1915, the microscopic appearances of the necrotic bone caused by a circulatory disturbance (ischemia) were described by Phemister [2], who also described that reparative process was observed around the dead bone (creeping substitution) [3]. Thereafter, both alcohol- and corticosteroid-related osteonecrosis have been reported clinically, and their pathologic appearances have also been described based on the histological examinations [4, 5].

19.2 Pathologic Characteristics of Osteonecrosis

One of the most characteristic pathology in ON is a zone formation, comprising necrotic, reparative, and viable tissue (Fig. 19.1) [6]. A wedge-shaped necrotic area is seen in a subchondral area, which is surrounded by the reparative tissue. This reparative tissue continues to the normal viable bone and bone marrow tissue. This zone formation is quite similar such as seen in myocardial infarction and brain infarction, and thus osteonecrosis is also recognized as bone infarction [4, 5].

In the early phase of ON, the reparative tissue generally consists of infiltration macrophage, granulation tissue, and fibrous tissue (cellular repair tissue), which can only be recognized on MRI. Thereafter, bony repair such as an appositional bone formation or creeping substitution occurs, when radiograph can detect these bony changes as a sclerotic change (Fig. 19.1). MRI is thus useful for the detection of ON in the early phase. In another word, MRI is useful for the detection of early reparative tissue formed around ON [7].

19.3 Pathology of Osteonecrosis

Macroscopically, the articular surface generally undergoes flattening (Fig. 19.2). On the cut section, opaque yellow, wedge-shaped osteonecrosis is observed in a subchondral region, which is bordered by an irregular reparative zone, comprising granulation and fibrous tissue as well as the sclerotic cancellous bone (Fig. 19.3). In general, a fracture (crescent sign) is present at the subchondral region [8].

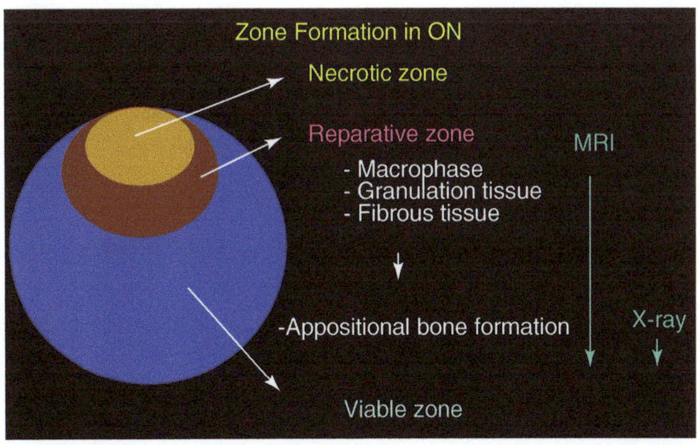

Fig. 19.1 Zone formation in ON. A wedge-shaped necrotic area is seen in a subchondral area, which is surrounded by the reparative tissue. This reparative tissue continues to the normal viable bone and bone marrow tissue. In the early phase of ON, the reparative tissue generally consists of infiltration macrophage, granulation tissue, and fibrous tissue, which can only be recognized on MRI. Thereafter, bony repair such as an appositional bone formation or creeping substitution occurs, when radiograph can detect these bony changes as a sclerotic change

T. Yamamoto
Department of Orthopaedic Surgery,
Kyushu University, 3-1-1 Maidashi, Higashi-ku,
Fukuoka 812-8582, Japan
e-mail: yamataku@ortho.med.kyushu-u.ac.jp

K.-H. Koo et al. (eds.), *Osteonecrosis*,
DOI 10.1007/978-3-642-35767-1_19, © Springer-Verlag Berlin Heidelberg 2014

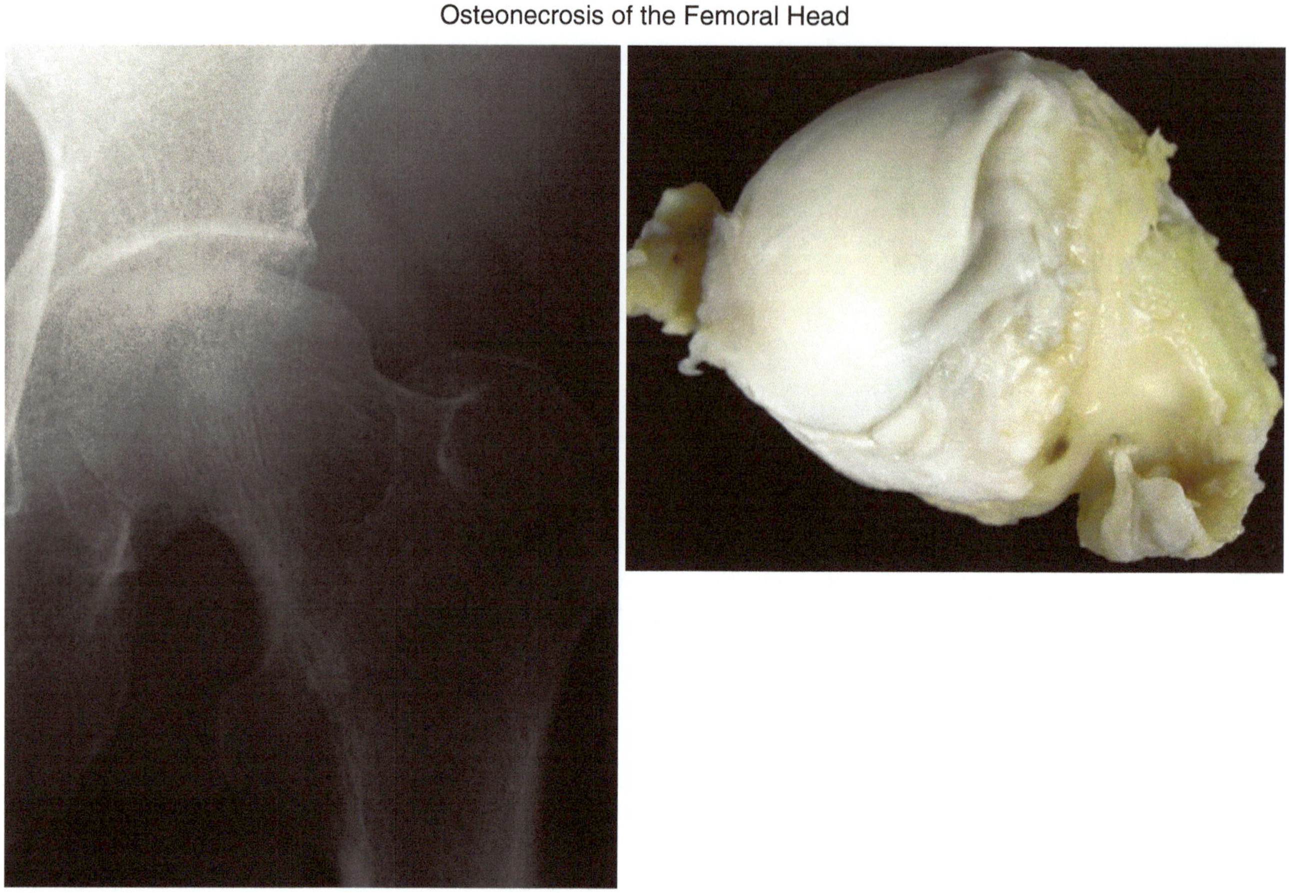

Fig. 19.2 ON often undergoes subchondral collapse, and the resected femoral head also shows the collapsed lesion at the lateral portion of the femoral head

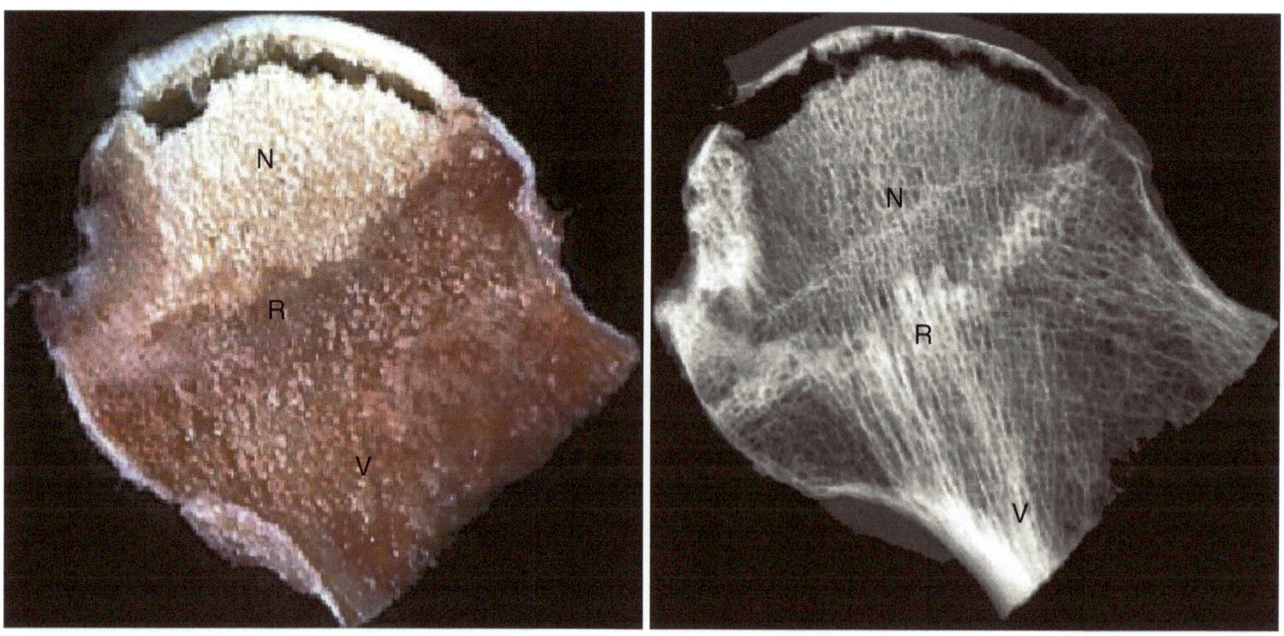

Fig. 19.3 The cut section shows wedge-shaped yellowish necrotic area (N), which is surrounded by the somewhat whitish reparative tissue (R). The reparative tissue continues to the viable normal area (V). The specimen radiograph also demonstrates the zone formation, comprising necrotic (*N*), reparative (*R*), and viable area (*V*)

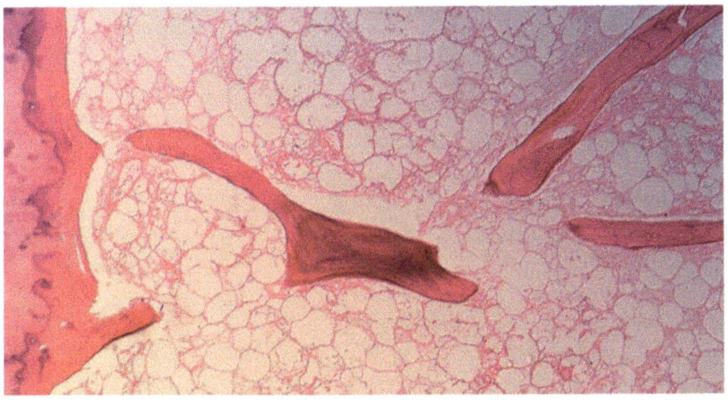

Fig. 19.4 Histology of the necrotic area. Necrotic area shows an accumulation of bone marrow cell debris and bone trabeculae demonstrating empty lacunae occasionally containing some pycnotic nuclei of osteocytes (HE ×100)

Microscopically, typical necrotic area shows an accumulation of bone marrow cell debris and bone trabeculae demonstrating empty lacunae occasionally containing some pycnotic nuclei of osteocytes (Fig. 19.4). At the periphery of this necrotic lesion, repair process such as vascular-rich granulation tissue and appositional bone formation is observed. This appositional bone formation caused the thickening of the bone trabeculae in the reparative area (Fig. 19.5) [5, 6].

19.4 Crescent Sign

In ON, a subchondral fracture is often observed, which is generally called as a "collapse" or "crescent sign" [8]. This sign pathologically corresponds to a space formed between the fractured lesion (Fig. 19.6). Histologically, the fractures generally occur at the junction between the thickened trabecula associated with appositional bone formation and the necrotic bone trabecula [9].

As to the mechanisms of a collapse, the following three causes are proposed: (1) the cumulative effect of microfractures induced by fatigue within the necrotic zone, (2) weakness of trabeculae in the reparative front due to osteoclastic activity, or (3) focal concentration of stress at the junctions between the thickened sclerotic trabecula of the reparative zone and the necrotic trabecula [5].

19.5 Initial Sign of ON

There has been a confusion regarding the initial sign of ON on MRI. Some reports describe that bone marrow edema pattern is the early finding of ON [10, 11]; however, it should be noted that an initial MR finding of ON is a low-intensity band on the T1-weighted images (Fig. 19.7) [7]. In the early phase of ON, the repair tissue formed around the necrotic area consists of accumulation of serofibrinous exudate and cellular-rich granulation tissue, which can be recognized as a band-like lesion surrounding the necrotic area [6, 7].

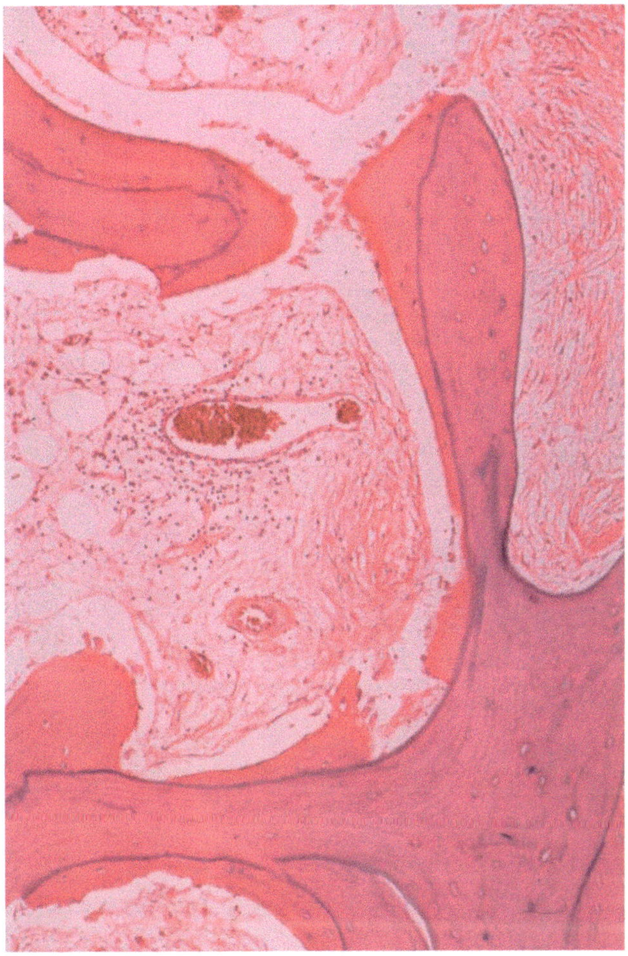

Fig. 19.5 Histology of the reparative zone. In the repair zone, appositional bone formation is seen along the necrotic bone trabeculae, and vascular-rich granulation tissue is seen in the marrow space (HE ×200)

19.6 Bone Marrow Edema in ON

Bone marrow edema is frequently associated around the necrotic zone. This lesion histologically corresponds to fluid collection and hemorrhage in the marrow space [12]. The edema is seen not only in the femoral head but also in the intertrochanteric area. Based on the fine-slice pathologic examination, recurrent ON due to repeated ischemic attack, which results in a voluminous increment of necrotic lesion, is 0.3 % [6]. Therefore, the edematous lesion around the band-like reactive lesion does not progress to necrosis.

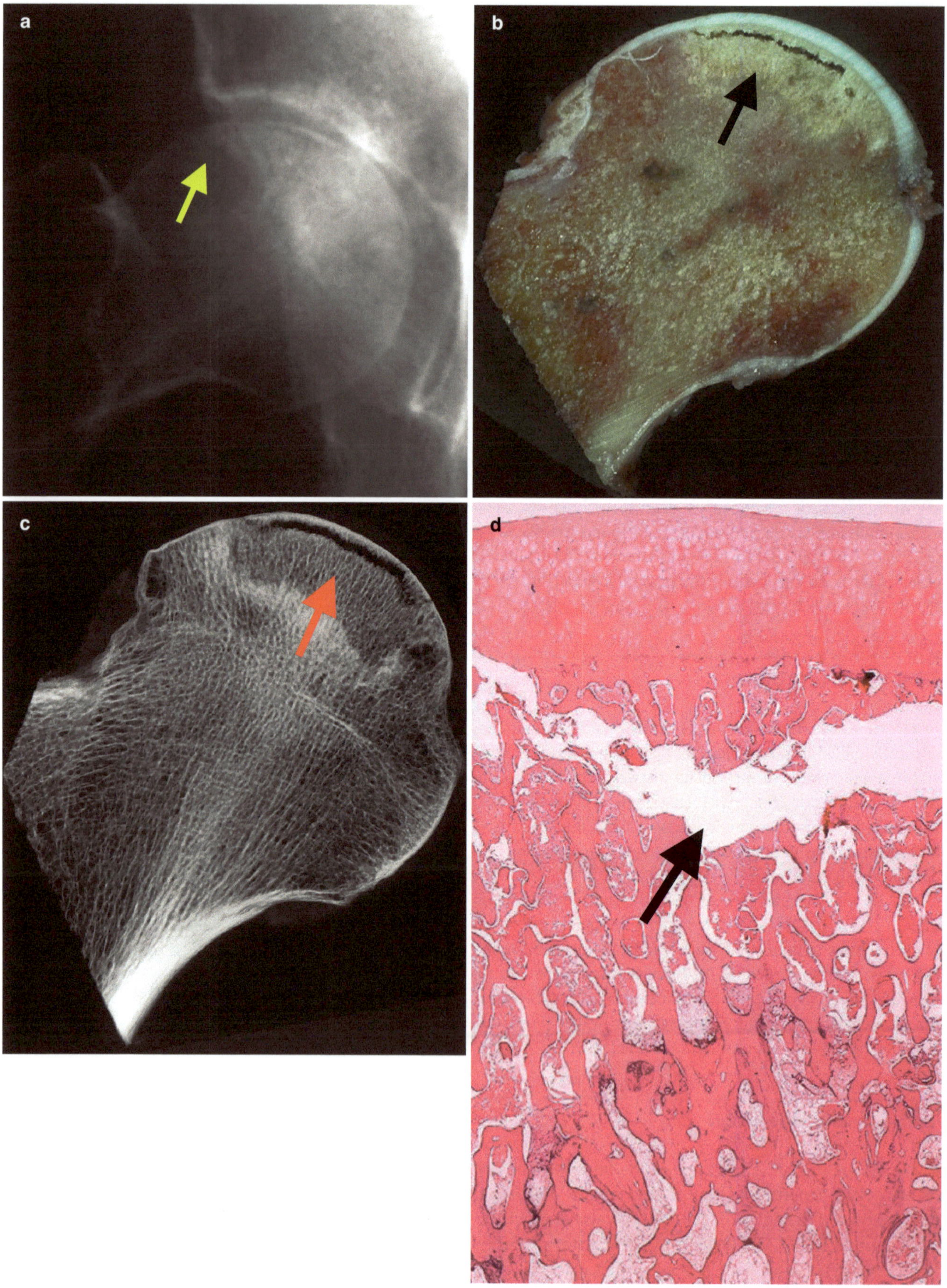

Fig. 19.6 (**a**) Radiographic appearance of subchondral collapse or so-called crescent sign (*arrow*). (**b**, **c**) On the cut section, subchondral collapse is seen just beneath the articular cartilage (*black arrow*), and on the specimen radiograph a subchondral fracture is clearly seen in the corresponding area (*red arrow*). (**d**) This area pathologically corresponds to a space formed between the fractured lesion

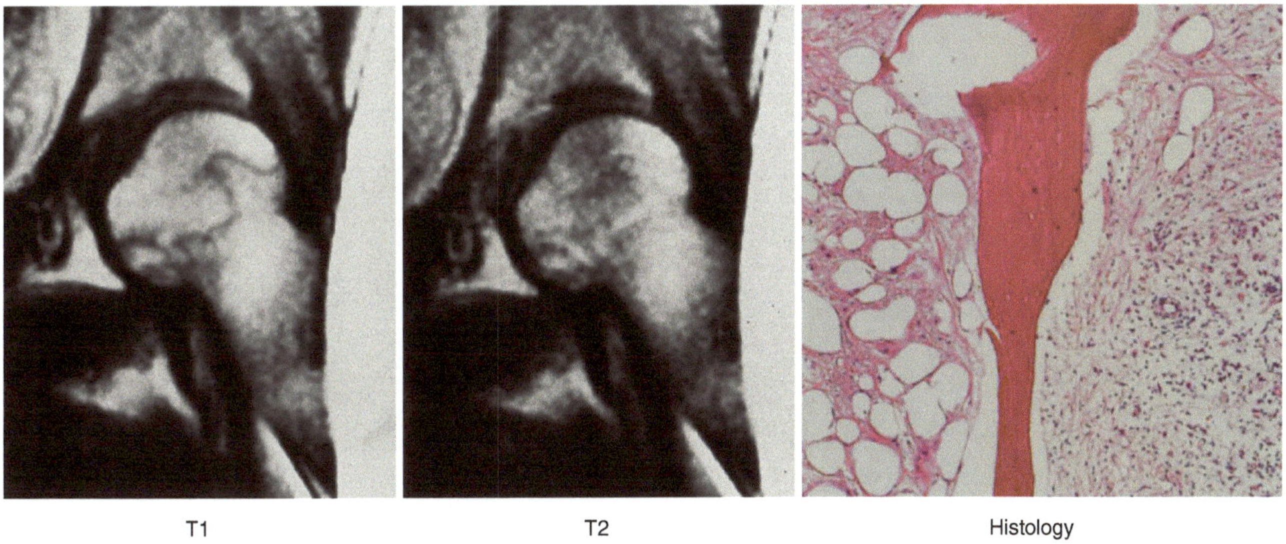

Fig. 19.7 Initial sign of ON. The low-intensity band on T1 is the initial finding. On T2, this band shows high signal intensity, because the repair tissue consists of vascular-rich granulation tissue. Histologically, vascular-rich granulation tissue is seen in the marrow space, where appositional bone formation is not yet observed (HE ×150)

19.7 Differential Diagnosis

19.7.1 Subchondral Insufficiency Fracture

The entity of a primary subchondral insufficiency fracture (SIF) has been described in both the osteoporotic elderly and renal transplant recipients [13, 14].

At the onset of pain, plain radiographs show no obvious findings, but MR imaging reveals a bone marrow edema pattern with an associated irregular serpiginous low signal intensity line on the T1-weighted images. This irregular low-intensity line is one of the characteristic appearances of this condition, which histologically corresponds to a fracture line and an associated repair tissue such as callus and granulation tissue [15]. Before the pathologic concept of SIF was first introduced in 2000 [16], the majority of SIF cases would have been diagnosed histologically as ON, presumably based on small foci of necrosis caused by the fracture. It should be noted that since all fractures lead to some bone and bone marrow necrosis on either side of the fracture line, small segments of necrotic bone trabeculae may be observed. However, such necrotic regions will be observed only around the fracture line and such should not be diagnosed as primary ON [16].

Histopathological criteria for the diagnosis of subchondral fractures have been established [16]. On gross examination, a linear, narrow, irregular whitish-gray zone in the bone marrow space parallel to the subchondral bone end plate is generally seen. Microscopically, this area consists of irregularly arranged fracture callus, reactive cartilage, and granulation tissue (Fig. 19.8).

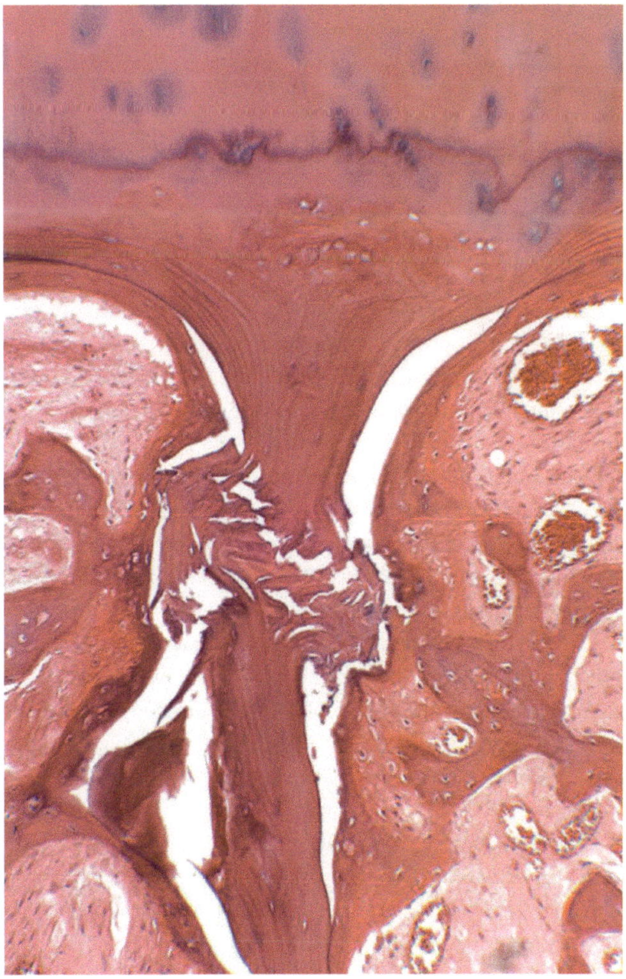

Fig. 19.8 Histology of SIF. The fractured area consists of irregularly arranged fracture callus, reactive cartilage, and granulation tissue (HE ×400)

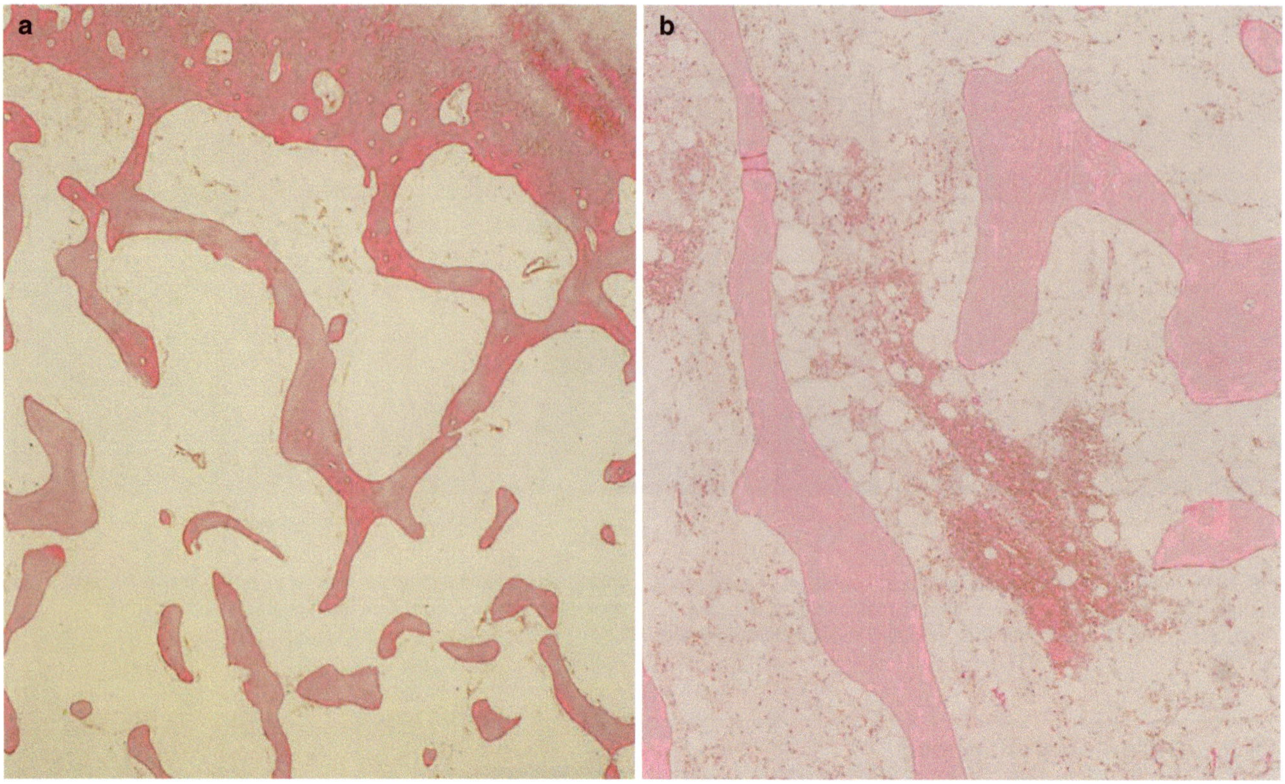

Fig. 19.9 Histology of TOH. (**a**) Bone trabeculae are thin, disconnected, and sparsely arranged. Creeping bone substitution is not recognized (HE ×100). (**b**) In the bone marrow spaces, exudative fluid frequently associated with congestion and interstitial hemorrhage is seen (HE ×200)

19.8 Transient Osteoporosis

Transient osteoporosis of the hip (TOH) is a relatively rare disease seen in pregnant women and middle-aged men. It is characterized clinically by severe pain without an obvious antecedent cause and is considered as a self-limiting disease [17].

The radiological characteristics of the affected femoral head are a focal loss of radiodensity, a diffuse homogeneous uptake on bone scintigram, and a bone marrow edema pattern on MR imaging, often involving the femoral head, neck, and sometimes intertrochanteric region.

The histopathology of the affected area shows nonspecific edematous changes in the marrow space with associated hemorrhage and infiltration of vascular tissue. None of the TOH cases shows an opaque yellow osteonecrotic region or zone formation comprising necrotic, reparative, and viable zone.

Microscopically, bone trabeculae in the affected area are thin, disconnected, and sparsely arranged (osteopenic) (Fig. 19.9). These osteopenic bone trabeculae are variously covered with the osteoid seams and active osteoblasts, but creeping bone substitution is not recognized. In the bone marrow spaces, exudative fluid frequently associated with congestion and interstitial hemorrhage is seen (Fig. 19.9). In TOH cases, a wedge-shaped osteonecrotic region is not observed [18].

References

1. Twynham GE. A case of caisson disease. Br Med J. 1988;1:190–1.
2. Phemister DB. Necrotic bone and subsequent changes which it undergoes. JAMA. 1915;64:211–6.
3. Phemister DB. Repair of bone in the presence of aseptic necrosis resulting from fractures, transplantations, and vascular obstruction. J Bone Joint Surg. 1930;12A:769–87.
4. Mankin HJ. Nontraumatic necrosis of bone. New Engl J Med. 1992;326:1473–9.
5. Bullough PG, DiCarlo EF. Subchondral avascular necrosis: a common cause of arthritis. Ann Rheum Dis. 1990;49:412–20.
6. Yamamoto T, DiCarlo EF, Bullough PG. The prevalence and clinicopathological appearance of extension of osteonecrosis in the femoral head. J Bone Joint Surg. 1999;81B:328–32.

7. Kubo T, Yamazoe S, Sugano N, Fujioka M, Naruse S, Yoshimura N, Oka T, Hirasawa Y. Initial MRI findings of non-traumatic osteonecrosis of the femoral head in a renal allograft recipients. Magn Reson Imaging. 1997;15:1017–23.
8. Norman A, Bullough P. The radiolucent crescent line: an early diagnostic sign of avascular necrosis of the femoral head. Bull Hosp Joint Dis. 1963;24:99–104.
9. Motomura G, Yamamoto T, Yamaguchi R, Ikemura S, Nakashima Y, Mawatari T, Iwamoto Y. Morphological analysis of collapsed regions in osteonecrosis of the femoral head. J Bone Joint Surg. 2011;93B:184–7.
10. Hofmann S, Engel A, Neuhold A, Leder K, Kramer J, Plenk Jr H. Bone-marrow edema syndrome and transient osteoporosis of the hip. J Bone Joint Surg Br. 1993;75B:210–6.
11. Hofmann S, Kramer J, Schneider W, Plenk Jr H. Transient osteoporosis may represent a reversible early form of avascular necrosis of the hip joint. Curr Orthop. 1997;11:164–72.
12. Kubo T, Yamamoto T, Inoue S, Horii M, Ueshima K, Iwamoto Y, Hirasawa Y. Histological findings of bone marrow edema pattern on MRI in osteonecrosis of the femoral head. J Orthop Sci. 2000;5:520–3.
13. Vande Berg B, Malghem J, Goffin EJ, Duprez TP, Maldague BE. Transient epiphyseal lesions in renal transplant recipients: presumed insufficiency stress fractures. Radiology. 1994;191:403–7.
14. Yamamoto T, Bullough PG. Subchondral insufficiency fracture of the femoral head. A differential diagnosis in acute onset of coxarthrosis in the elderly. Arthritis Rheum. 1999;42:2719–23.
15. Yamamoto T, Schneider R, Bullough PG. Subchondral insufficiency fracture of the femoral head. Histopathologic correlation with MRI. Skeletal Radiol. 2001;30:247–54.
16. Yamamoto T, Schneider R, Bullough PG. Insufficiency subchondral fracture of the femoral head. Am J Surg Pathol. 2000;24:464–8.
17. Curtiss Jr PH, Kincaid WE. Transitory demineralization of the hip in pregnancy. J Bone Joint Surg Am. 1959;41A:1327–33.
18. Yamamoto T, Kubo T, Hirasawa Y, Noguchi Y, Iwamoto Y, Sueishi K. A clinicopathologic study of transient osteoporosis of the hip. Skeletal Radiol. 1999;28:621–7.

Part VI

Clinical Manifestation

20 Natural History of Osteonecrosis

Samik Banerjee, Bhaveen H. Kapadia, Julio J. Jauregui, Jeffrey J. Cherian, and Michael A. Mont

20.1 Introduction

Osteonecrosis is an incapacitating disorder of bone circulation that is insidious in onset and affects predominantly the younger population in the second to sixth decade of their lives. In about 75 % of cases, the disease occurs between the third and the sixth decade and is bilateral in about 50 % of the cases. Various terms have been used in literature to describe this condition, such as aseptic necrosis, avascular necrosis, subchondral avascular necrosis, and avascular necrosis. Although both traumatic and nontraumatic disorders have been associated with its development, the final common pathway involves interruption in the vascular supply. This disruption in the blood flow causes bone cell death, leading to collapse of the bony architecture (Table 20.1). Although cell death is a nonspecific marker of major cell stress and is found to occur in a variety of conditions such as fractures, tumors, infections, and osteoarthritis, it is only in osteonecrosis that the predominant abnormality is massive necrosis of the bone and its marrow.

The disruption of the vascular supply in osteonecrosis can result from extra- (e.g., elevated marrow pressure, increased marrow fat) or intraluminal vascular obstruction (e.g., microscopic emboli, sickle cells, nitrogen bubbles) or focal clotting abnormalities (e.g., proteins C and S or antithrombin III deficiency) leading to reduction in the blood flow. Various genetic factors (e.g., polymorphisms of endothelial nitric oxide synthetase) and cytotoxic factors have also been postulated to play a role in its development. When this condition affects the subchondral region, it often leads to subsidence of the overlying articular cartilage causing joint incongruity and subsequent development of end-stage arthritis. Although the vascular disruption is obvious in traumatic cases, the underlying etiopathogenesis in nontraumatic osteonecrosis is often not clear. It is commonly agreed upon that once extensive collapse occurs, total joint arthroplasty remains the only reasonable treatment option. The following sections provide an overview of the natural history of both symptomatic and asymptomatic disease.

S. Banerjee • B.H. Kapadia • J.J. Jauregui • J.J. Cherian
M.A. Mont (✉)
Department of Orthopaedic Surgery, Rubin Institute for Advanced Orthopedics, Center for Joint Preservation and Replacement, Sinai Hospital of Baltimore, 2401 West Belvedere Avenue, Baltimore, MD 21215, USA
e-mail: bashb02@gmail.com; bhaveen.k@gmail.com; juljau@gmail.com; jjaicherian@gmail.com; mmont@lifebridgehealth.org, rhondamont@aol.com

Table 20.1 Risk factors for development of osteonecrosis

Risk factors associated with the development of osteonecrosis
1. Traumatic conditions
2. Nontraumatic conditions
(a) Corticosteroid use (dose >0.5 mg/kg)
(b) Alcohol abuse
(c) HIV
(d) Radiation therapy
(e) Systemic lupus erythematosus
(f) Sickle cell disease (SS or SC or Sβ^+)
(g) Dyslipidemia (hypertriglyceridemia)
(h) Caisson disease
(i) Gaucher's disease
(j) Fat embolism
(k) Organ transplantation (glucocorticoid mediated mostly)
(l) Endogenous hypercorticolism (rare)
(m) Renal failure
(n) Pancreatitis
(o) Cancer chemotherapy
(p) Idiopathic
(q) Hypercoagulable conditions (proteins C and S and antithrombin III deficiency)

K.-H. Koo et al. (eds.), *Osteonecrosis*,
DOI 10.1007/978-3-642-35767-1_20, © Springer-Verlag Berlin Heidelberg 2014

20.2 Natural History of Symptomatic Osteonecrosis

The natural history of symptomatic osteonecrosis and its progression is probably better understood than the multitude of early triggering factors that are responsible for its development. It is often surprising that in some patients osteonecrosis often develops within 1–6 months of exposure to a known risk factor, while in others it never develops despite being exposed to the same risk factor. Analysis of the natural history of symptomatic disease provides a basis for comparison of the efficacy of treatment interventions in nonrandomized studies, allows patients to be informed about prognosis and expected outcomes, and enables assessment of whether nonoperative or surgical treatment will provide better outcomes in a given clinical scenario.

Previous studies have reported that symptomatic osteonecrotic lesions occurring in the weight-bearing regions of the femoral head have a high rate of collapse. Moreover, it was also found that development of subchondral fracture was an early predictor of future collapse (Ficat-Arlet stage III and Steinberg stage IV). Articular surface collapse is considered an irreversible turning point in the natural history of osteonecrosis. This is strongly associated with pain, future development of osteoarthritis, and a poor eventual outcome. It has been found in various studies that once radiographic diagnosis of osteonecrosis is made, collapse usually occurs within 2 years in 32–79 % of patients. Shimuzu et al., in a MRI study, evaluated the risk of progression to collapse for early-stage lesions in 66 hips [1]. At a mean follow-up of 49 months, the authors found that 74 % of the hips that had osteonecrotic involvement of at least 25 % of the head diameter stage I lesions had progressed to stage II disease, while 21 % had progressed beyond stage II. Forty-eight percent of the hips that had stage II disease on presentation had progressed to stage III at final follow-up.

It was initially believed that if no radiographic progression occurs after 3 years from diagnosis, further risk of deterioration is considered to be low. However, Hernigou et al. reported delayed progression of pain and collapse in lesions involving less than 10 % of the femoral head, at an approximate follow-up of 7 years. This suggests that there may be a possibility of inevitable progression of disease once radiographic diagnosis is made. In a separate study Hernigou et al. evaluated the natural history of 92 symptomatic hips in 64 sickle cell patients, at a mean follow-up of 17 years [2]. Of these 92 hips, there were 32 hips in Steinberg stage I, 43 in stage II, 2 in stage III, and 15 in stage IV disease. The authors found that 65 of the 75 hips (87 %) with radiographic evidence of disease on diagnosis sustained collapse within 5 years of diagnosis. The mean time to collapse from diagnosis was 30 months for stage II hips and 42 months for hips in stage I. The authors also found that the size of the lesion had a significant effect on the duration of survival, with mild involvement having a longer survivorship compared to moderate or severe involvement irrespective of the stage of the disease ($p = 0.01$).

Similarly, poor outcomes were reported by Gutierez et al. who in a multicenter study evaluated the natural history of 54 symptomatic osteonecrotic hips secondary to HIV infection. The authors reported that 37 % (20 out of 54 hips) of patients had clinical progression of the disease requiring surgical intervention at a median interval of 12.7 months following diagnosis. The authors also found that male sex ($p = 0.03$) and a relatively high CD4 ($p = 0.03$) were significantly associated with the risks of disease progression requiring surgery.

Improvement of radiographically obvious lesions is exceedingly rare and is currently controversial. Limited studies have evaluated the changes in dimension of osteonecrotic lesions. A few studies have reported that in 23–45 % of cases, a moderate decrease in size of the lesions can occur. Kopecky et al. in a study of 104 renal transplant recipients found MRI changes in 25 hips [3]. During follow-up evaluation these changes were found to reduce in 7 hips and improve in 6 hips. Other authors have reported no progression in the size of the lesions [1, 4]. However, none of the studies were designed to evaluate changes in lesion size over time.

In summary, multiple factors influence the natural history of symptomatic osteonecrosis. A slightly more favorable prognosis occurs in patients who have no radiographic abnormalities at presentation compared to patients who present with radiographic stage II lesions, although the general consensus is that once clinical and radiographic evidence of osteonecrosis occurs, gradual progression to collapse and development of arthritis occurs if no intervention is undertaken. Most authors believe that size has a profound effect on the prognosis of these lesions. Small lesions involving less than 10 % of the head have better outcomes in terms of longer survival and less chance of progression, compared to lesions that involve more than 25 % of the head size. In addition, the proportion of involvement of the weight-bearing area (stage A, <1/3rd; stage B, 1/3rd to 2/3rd; stage C, >2/3rd) of the head affects the rate of progression to collapse. It has been found that the rate of progression to Ficat-Arlet stage III varies from 0 % in stage A and increases to 70 % with stage C disease. Moreover, risk factors such as alcohol abuse, corticosteroid use, presence of radiographic evidence of effusion, and marrow edema underlying the necrotic region have been associated with increased risks of disease progression [5]. Current evidence suggests that size of the lesion usually remains stable over time, although a modest decrease in size can occur. However, complete resolution of osteonecrotic lesions is extremely rare.

Table 20.2 Risk of disease progression of asymptomatic hip involvement in various studies reported in literature

Author/year	Location	Number	Follow-up (in years)	Risk factors	Risk of symptomatic progression (%)	Risk of collapse
Kang et al. (2013) [7]	Hip	68	2.3	Idiopathic, steroid use, alcohol abuse	55.9	NS
Nakamura et al. (2010) [8]	Hip and knee	537	13.6	SLE	14	22
Mont et al. (2010) [6]	Hip	664	3.3	Multiple risk factors	59	49
Min et al. (2008) [9]	Hip	81	8.3	Idiopathic, steroid use, alcohol abuse	38	32
Nam et al. (2008) [10]	Hip	105	8.6	Multiple risk factors	59	59
Morse et al. (2007) [11]	Hip	22	5.7	HIV	9	NS
Hernigou et al. (2006) [12]	Hip	121	14	Sickle cell disease	91	77

20.3 Natural History of Asymptomatic Disease

Many patients are diagnosed when the disease presents itself with gradual onset of pain in the hip, buttock, or groin region which often increases on weight bearing, at least initially, and then progresses to constant rest pain. However, during screening of at-risk populations, often asymptomatic disease is found on the contralateral side. The progression of asymptomatic disease is often uncertain leading to some surgeons recommending a "watchful-waiting" policy for small- or medium-sized lesions, while others believe that many of these asymptomatic patients will ultimately progress and early treatment with joint-preserving procedures may forestall further progression and future need for a total joint arthroplasty. Still others believe that an individualized approach based on various risk factors (e.g., demographic, epidemiological, and radiographic) for disease progression may be needed, rather than a "blanket approach" for treatment of these lesions.

In a systematic review of 16 studies, Mont et al. evaluated the natural history of 664 asymptomatic osteonecrotic hips [6]. The authors found that 394 hips (59 %) had progression to development of symptoms or collapse at a mean follow-up of 39 months (range, 1–134 months) while 49 % of patients had femoral head collapse at a mean follow-up of 49 months (range, 2–143 months). The authors also found that substantial differences were found in the outcomes based on location, size, radiographic stage, and risk factors. The lowest progression (10 %) was found with small medially based lesions and in patients with systemic lupus erythematosus, while disease progression was marked in patients who had sickle cell disease and large- and medium-sized lesions located in the weight-bearing dome of the femoral head. Based on these observations the authors recommended that medium- and large-sized laterally based lesions in asymptomatic patients may benefit from joint preservation procedures.

Similar adverse outcomes of large- and medium-sized lesions and laterally located lesions have been reported by other authors (Table 20.2) [7, 9, 10]. Min et al., in a study of 81 asymptomatic osteonecrotic hips at a mean follow-up of 8.3 years, found that the size of the lesions had a substantial effect on the survival of the hips [9]. The survival rate decreased from 100 % with small lesions to 34 % with medium and 0 % with large-sized lesions. The small and medium lesions had significantly longer duration of survival compared to larger lesions. Similarly, Kang et al., in a study of 68 patients with asymptomatic involvement of the hip, found that approximately 56 % (38 out of 56 hips) of patients had disease progression and developed symptoms at a mean follow-up of 2.3 years after diagnosis [7]. A higher incidence of disease progression was found in patients with alcohol-related disease (64 %), followed by steroid-induced osteonecrosis (57 %) and idiopathic disease (46 %). However, no significant association was found between presence of risk factors such as idiopathic disease, alcohol induced, and steroid-related osteonecrosis, and development of symptoms. Similar to the study by Mont et al., these authors reported that 76 % of patients who had laterally located lesions had progression of disease, compared to 38 % with central lesions and 10 % with medial lesions. It was also reported that 84 % of large-sized lesions had disease progression, compared to 69 % with medium-sized lesions and 10 % with small-sized lesions. Similar to other reports, the authors found that age, gender, body mass index, cholesterol level, and smoking did not correlate with disease progression [9].

Similarly, Hernigou et al. in a study of 121 hips evaluated the natural history of asymptomatic disease in 121 sickle cell patients, who had contralateral symptomatic disease [12]. There were 56 hips in Steinberg stage 0, 42 in stage I, and 23 hips in stage II. At a mean follow-up of 14 years, the authors found 91 % (110 out of 121 hips) developed pain, while 77 % had collapse at final follow-up. In stage 0, 84 % hips developed pain and 61 % had radiographic evidence of collapse, while pain and collapse developed in 95 % and 86 % of the hips in Steinberg stage I.

However, improved outcomes have been reported in renal transplant recipients and HIV-infected patients with early-stage disease. Mulliken et al. studied 11 hips in early-stage osteonecrosis (stage 0) in renal transplant recipients. At a mean follow-up of 22 months, the authors found that only 9 % (1 out of 11 hips) had radiographic progression of the disease beyond stage 0, suggesting against bone-preserving procedures in this group of patients. Similarly Morse et al., in a prospective study, evaluated the natural history of asymptomatic osteonecrotic hips secondary to HIV infection [11]. The authors reported that 64 % (14 out of 22 hips) remained radiographically stable, while 18 % of the hips were found to have radiographic improvement or had resolution of the disease at a mean follow-up of 5.7 years.

20.4 Summary

In summary, current evidence in literature suggests that there is high risk of progression to development of symptoms and femoral head collapse in asymptomatic osteonecrosis of the hip and this varies between 50 and 90 %. The risk of progression in asymptomatic osteonecrotic hips appears to be higher in patients with sickle cell disease compared to patients with lupus-related osteonecrosis, renal transplant recipients, and patients with HIV infection, although there appear to be no considerable differences in the risks of progressions between osteonecroses associated with alcohol abuse, steroid use, and idiopathic disease. Large lesions involving more than 50 % of the head size and laterally located lesions (stage B and stage C hips) have a higher incidence of collapse compared to small (<25 %) and medially located (stage A) lesions. Although the risk of progression appears to be low for stage 0 disease in some reports, it increases substantially from 50 % in stage I to as high as 96 % in stage III osteonecrosis. A low threshold for joint-preserving surgical procedures in these patients may provide substantial benefits in preventing disease progression in contrast to a policy of watchful waiting. However, demographic factors such as age, gender, body mass index, smoking history, and cholesterol levels do not appear to affect the risks of development of symptoms or femoral head collapse.

References

1. Shimizu K, Moriya H, Akita T, Sakamoto M, Suguro T. Prediction of collapse with magnetic resonance imaging of avascular necrosis of the femoral head. J Bone Joint Surg Am. 1994;76:215–23.
2. Gutierrez F, Padilla S, Masia M, et al. Osteonecrosis in patients infected with HIV: clinical epidemiology and natural history in a large case series from Spain. J Acquir Immune Defic Syndr. 2006;42:286–92.
3. Kopecky KK, Braunstein EM, Brandt KD, et al. Apparent avascular necrosis of the hip: appearance and spontaneous resolution of MR findings in renal allograft recipients. Radiology. 1991;179:523–7.
4. Hernigou P, Lambotte JC. Bilateral hip osteonecrosis: influence of hip size on outcome. Ann Rheum Dis. 2000;59:817–21.
5. Iida S, Harada Y, Shimizu K, et al. Correlation between bone marrow edema and collapse of the femoral head in steroid-induced osteonecrosis. AJR Am J Roentgenol. 2000;174:735–43.
6. Mont MA, Zywiel MG, Marker DR, McGrath MS, Delanois RE. The natural history of untreated asymptomatic osteonecrosis of the femoral head: a systematic literature review. J Bone Joint Surg Am. 2010;92:2165–70.
7. Kang JS, Moon KH, Kwon DG, Shin BK, Woo MS. The natural history of asymptomatic osteonecrosis of the femoral head. Int Orthop. 2013;37:379–84.
8. Nakamura J, Harada Y, Oinuma K, Iida S, Kishida S, Takahashi K. Spontaneous repair of asymptomatic osteonecrosis associated with corticosteroid therapy in systemic lupus erythematosus: 10-year minimum follow-up with MRI. Lupus. 2010;19:1307–14.
9. Min BW, Song KS, Cho CH, Lee SM, Lee KJ. Untreated asymptomatic hips in patients with osteonecrosis of the femoral head. Clin Orthop Relat Res. 2008;466:1087–92.
10. Nam KW, Kim YL, Yoo JJ, Koo KH, Yoon KS, Kim HJ. Fate of untreated asymptomatic osteonecrosis of the femoral head. J Bone Joint Surg Am. 2008;90:477–84.
11. Morse CG, Mican JM, Jones EC, et al. The incidence and natural history of osteonecrosis in HIV-infected adults. Clin Infect Dis. 2007;44:739–48.
12. Hernigou P, Habibi A, Bachir D, Galacteros F. The natural history of asymptomatic osteonecrosis of the femoral head in adults with sickle cell disease. J Bone Joint Surg Am. 2006;88:2565–72.

Causes of Pain in Early and Advanced Stage Osteonecrosis

21

Vivek S. Jagadale and Edward Y. Cheng

21.1 Introduction

The natural history, pathophysiology, and etiology of pain in nontraumatic osteonecrosis (ON) are poorly understood. In most clinical scenarios, a patient presents with pain which then leads to imaging examinations that identify the ON. Therefore, it is difficult to determine the frequency of asymptomatic disease. Nonetheless, it is clear that asymptomatic disease occurs as it is often identified incidentally, either in a contralateral site or when imaging is performed for unrelated reasons.

A better understanding of both when symptoms occur and how they are temporally related to the onset of disease is important as pain may be erroneously attributed to ON that is seen on imaging when the true etiology of pain lies elsewhere. In addition, the causes of pain are important to identify in order to provide treatment that effectively resolves the pain. There are numerous potential causes for pain that vary with the stage of ON.

21.2 Natural History

Prospective, longitudinal, observational studies are rare in ON. Nonetheless, several screening studies using magnetic resonance imaging (MRI) have revealed that findings of ON usually precede pain [1–6]. Pain rarely occurs at the time of disease onset. The best predictor of disease progression is the extent of involvement, regardless of how this is quantified. Plain radiographs are not as sensitive as MRI for the detection of ON; therefore, MRI imaging is essential for detecting this disease in an asymptomatic patient. In many scenarios, a patient may not have pain until subchondral collapse occurs. As any intervention attempting to salvage the native femoral head is more successful prior to subchondral collapse, understanding the natural history and relationship between pain and disease onset is crucial.

21.3 Possible Causes of Pain

21.3.1 Increased Marrow Pressure and Edema

There are several aspects of the pathophysiology of ON that may result in increased marrow pressure. These are related to (1) mechanical blockage of the microvasculature as seen in sickle cell disease, Gaucher's disease, hyperlipidemia syndromes, as well as thromboembolic disorders; (2) disruption of the blood supply to the bone marrow due to any of the above diseases; (3) bone marrow infarct and cellular necrosis secondary to the disruption of the blood supply that eventually leads to bone marrow edema and intraosseous compartment syndrome (normal pressure is 20–30 mm of Hg); (4) localized osteopenia and osteoporosis; and (5) direct cellular toxicity possibly secondary to medications or abnormal metabolites [7].

The most striking example of pain from bone marrow edema is the entity bone marrow edema syndrome (BMES) in which patients have marked, severe groin pain demonstrated with increased tracer uptake in the femoral head on Tc-99 bone scan and MRI findings of diffuse, regional marrow edema (Figs. 21.1, 21.2) [2].

In ON, edema at the hyperintense T2 band on the edge of necrosis may also potentially cause pain as opposed to the diffuse, regional marrow edema seen in BMES. However, in ON, this pain may or may not correlate with the stage or extent of anatomic involvement of the bone [1]. Patients with these symptoms typically have diffuse, polyostotic ON involving both subchondral and large metaphyseal infarcts and present with diffuse bone pain, analogous to sickle cell

V.S. Jagadale • E.Y. Cheng (✉)
Department of Orthopaedic Surgery,
University of Minnesota Medical School,
2450 Riverside Ave, R 200, Minneapolis, MN 55454, USA
e-mail: jagadalevs@gmail.com; cheng002@umn.edu

K.-H. Koo et al. (eds.), *Osteonecrosis*,
DOI 10.1007/978-3-642-35767-1_21, © Springer-Verlag Berlin Heidelberg 2014

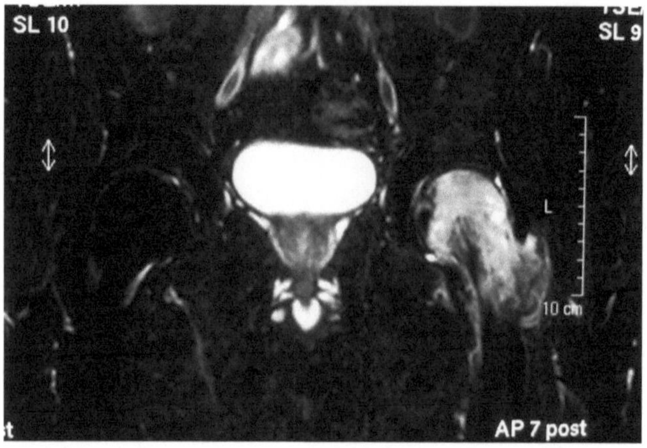

Fig. 21.1 MRI findings (fat suppression, fluid sensitive sequence) of bone marrow edema syndrome showing marked, bright, hyperintense signal in left femoral head and neck

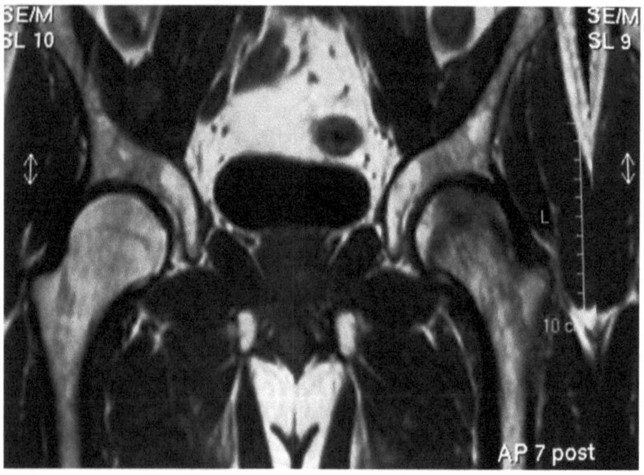

Fig. 21.2 MRI findings (T1 sequence) of bone marrow edema syndrome showing dark, hypointense signal in left femoral head and neck

disease patients. Commonly, this will occur in ON related to steroid usage for either bone marrow transplantation or treatment of acute lymphoblastic leukemia (Fig. 21.3).

21.3.2 Subchondral Fractures

These are the fractures through the necrotic subchondral bone which most often occurs in the superolateral aspect of the femoral head [8]. This classical finding is seen as a "crescent sign" on radiographs in ARCO stage 3 disease and is responsible for increasing pain with activity in stage 3 of the disease process. These fractures may also lead to instability of the overlying articular cartilage with loss of fixation to the subchondral bone occurring (Fig. 21.4a, b). At times a gap may develop between the subchondral bone and overlying cartilage leading to a joint effusion (Fig. 21.5).

21.3.3 Degenerative Joint Disease

The unstable articular cartilage eventually will fracture at the margin of the subchondral bone depression resulting in a loose flap of cartilage. This is associated with flattening of the femoral head and the loss of contour initiates the early degenerative cascade with subsequent advanced degenerative changes responsible for pain either at rest or with minimal activity [2]. The etiology of persistent disabling pain in late stages of ON involves degenerative joint disease that is a combination of joint effusion, synovitis, osteochondral fragments, and a bone-on-bone erosive process that is similar to the end-stage osteoarthritis from any other cause.

21.4 Causes of Pain in Different Stages of Disease

As there are multiple causes for pain in ON, they may vary depending upon the specific stage of disease (ARCO staging Table 21.1) [9].

21.4.1 ARCO Stage 1

By definition, there is no subchondral fracture. Most of the patients are asymptomatic. If a patient has pain, it is likely due to the onset of intraosseous hypertension because of abnormally high content of fluid in the bone marrow secondary to acute bone marrow ischemia. In this stage mild pain can also be perceived as severe by some patients [5].

21.4.2 ARCO Stage 2

Localized osteopenia, marrow necrosis, and bone infarcts are possibly responsible for the dull aching pain in this stage [2]. Patients that have polyostotic disease with large metaphyseal infarcts typically have diffuse poorly localized, vague, non-activity-related pain. This likely is due to elevated intraosseous pressure and/or marrow edema accentuated by the large infarcts. In some patients, a synovial effusion is present despite the absence of a demonstrable subchondral fracture (Fig. 21.3). As is typical for any synovial effusion, the distended joint capsule is symptomatic. Some patients with ARCO stage 2 ONFH may be asymptomatic as well. During this stage, in the absence of a synovial effusion, determining whether or not a patient's pain is due to ON or some other etiology can be challenging (Fig. 21.6a–c).

21.4.3 ARCO Stage 3

Onset of subchondral collapse, flattening of the articular surface, and bone impaction resulting in increased intraosseous pressure are the main causes of pain with activity [2, 10]. In

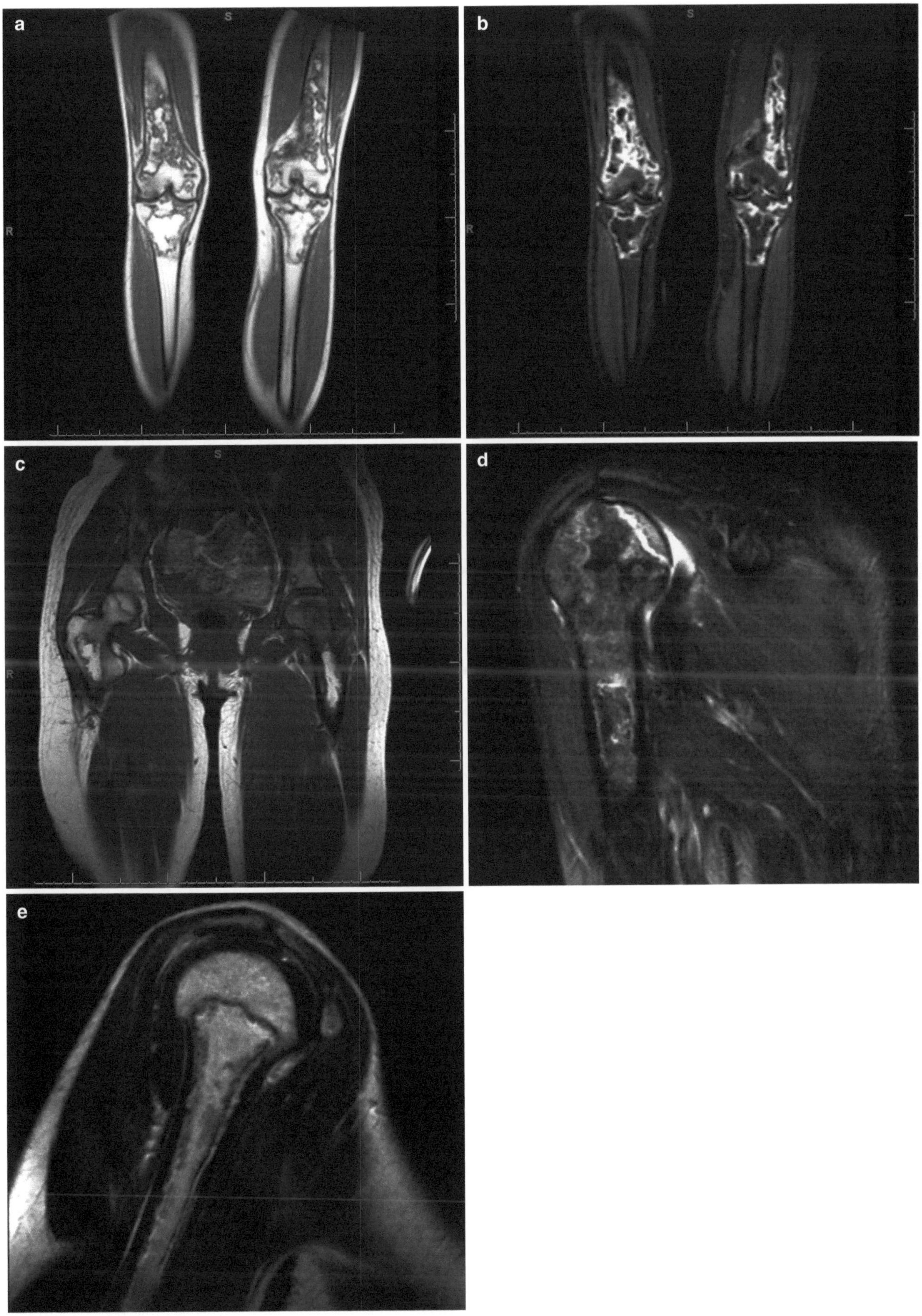

Fig. 21.3 A case example of polyostotic ON involving bilateral distal femur and proximal tibia (**a**, **b**), femoral head and proximal femora (**c**), and proximal humerus (**d**, **e**) as seen on MR

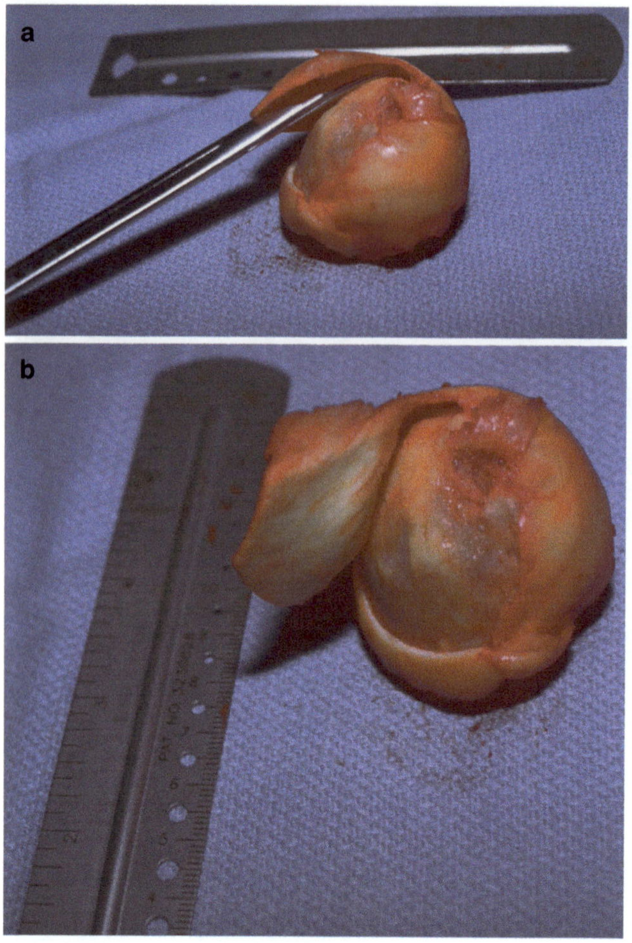

Fig. 21.4 (a, b) A case example of underlying detachment of the cartilage from the bone in the femoral head seen during hip replacement surgery

addition, a synovial effusion is usually present when a joint incongruity is present.

21.4.4 ARCO Stage 4

The irregularity of the articular surface initiates fissures in the cartilage, subsequently followed by onset of advanced degenerative joint disease with corresponding changes on both sides of a joint (e.g., acetabulum) and worsening pain both at rest and with activity [2].

21.5 Clinical Features and Presentation

The most accurate clinic-radiological data comes from prospective screening studies performed in high-risk patient groups [1, 11–14].

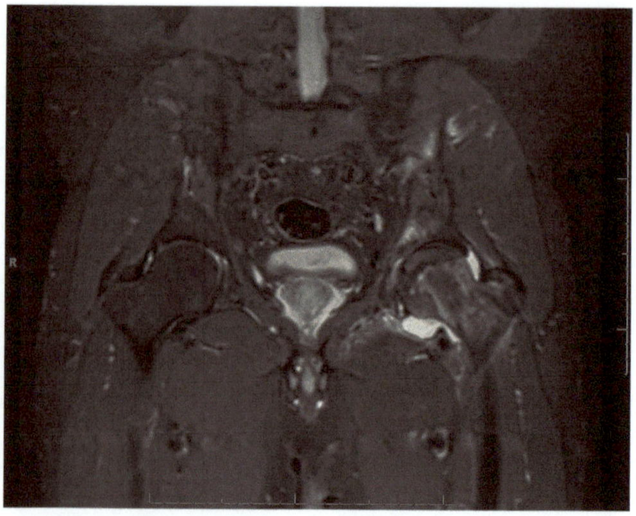

Fig. 21.5 MRI STIR sequence with contrast showing ON with subchondral fracture in the pre-collapse stage. Note the unilateral synovial effusion in the left symptomatic hip and absence of effusion in the right asymptomatic hip

21.5.1 Temporal Relationship Between Diagnosis and Pain

The majority of patients have no pain in the early stages of ON. Marston and Cheng prospectively followed 103 asymptomatic hips in solid organ transplant patients with serial MR imaging, and at 1 year after transplant, life table analysis revealed that 11 % of hips developed ON. Overall, 7 of the 8 hips in patients that developed ON were asymptomatic at the time of diagnosis. Kopecky et al. also prospectively followed 64 renal transplant patients for at least 1 year with serial MR imaging and seven hips had ON that eventually became symptomatic. In each of these hips, the MRI demonstrated ON before the onset of symptoms by a minimum of 3 months (range 3–10). In a mixed population of patients with ethanol- and steroid-related ON, Kang et al. in 2013 found that 38/68 (56 %) hips that were diagnosed initially with asymptomatic disease became painful at a mean of 2.27 years (range 0.5–6.5 years). Therefore, these prospective studies clearly show that ON usually develops in an occult manner and patients are usually asymptomatic at disease onset.

21.5.2 Temporal Relationship Between Pain and Collapse

Several studies have shown that pain precedes collapse. Min et al. in 2008 prospectively followed 81 asymptomatic hips

Table 21.1 Schematic modified outline of the five-stage Association Research Circulation Osseous (ARCO) international classification for osteonecrosis of the femoral head (Reproduced with permissions ARCO [9])

ARCO INTERNATIONAL CLASSIFICATION OF OSTEONECROSIS

STAGE	0	1	2	3	4
FINDINGS	All present techniques normal or non-diagnostic	X-ray and CT are normal at least ONE of the below mentioned is positive	NO CRESCENT SIGN! X-RAY ABNORMAL: sclerosis, osteolysis, focal porosis	CRESCENT SIGN! on the X-ray and/or flattening of articular surface of femoral head	OSTEOARTHRITIS! joint space narrowing, acetabular changes, joint destruction
TECHNIQUES	X-ray, CT Scintigraph MRI	Scintigraph MRI *QUANTITATE on MRI	X-ray, CT Scintigraph MRI *QUANTITATE MRI & X-ray	X-ray, CT ONLY * QUANTITATE on X-ray	X-ray ONLY
SUBCLASSIFICA-TION	NO	LOCATION 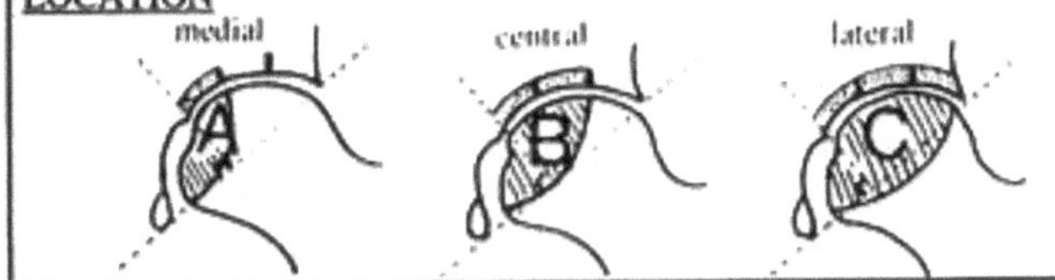			NO
QUANTITATION	NO	QUANTITATION % AREA INVOLVEMENT minimal A < 15% moderate B 15% - 30% extensive C > 30%	LENGTH of CRESCENT A < 15% B 15% - 30% C > 30%	% SURFACE COLLAPSE & DOME DEPRESSION 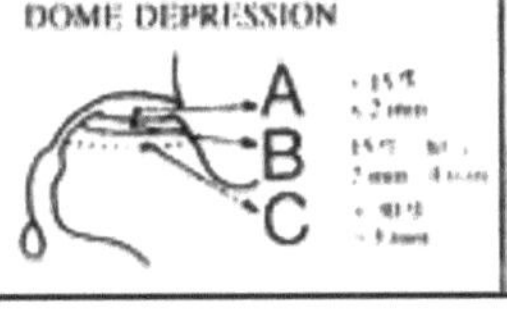	NO

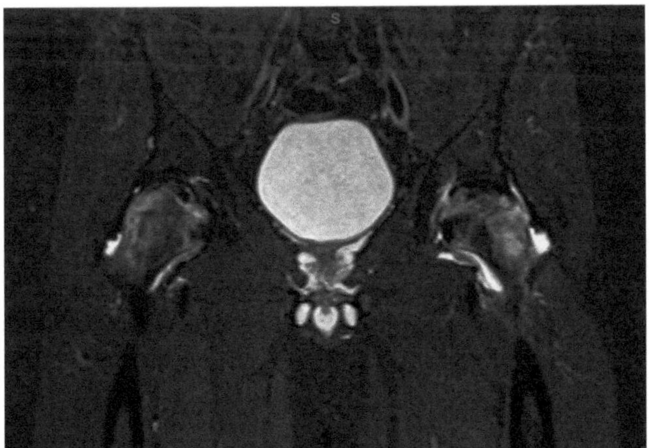

Fig. 21.6 ARCO stage 2 bilateral disease of femoral head that with bilateral small effusions on MR but symptomatic on only one side

for a minimum of 5 years. The mean interval from diagnosis to onset of pain was 3.4 years (range 0.7–8.9) and 31/81 (38 %) of hips became symptomatic. The mean interval from diagnosis to collapse was 4.1 years (range 1.2–11.9) and pain always preceded collapse by a mean of 8 months (range 1–36). Hernigou et al. analyzed 121 asymptomatic hips in patients with sickle cell disease using radiographs. They found that 110 hips (91 %) became painful and collapse occurred in 93 (77 %). In all cases, pain preceded collapse. Although the study populations are different in these two studies, the finding that pain precedes collapse is consistent.

21.5.3 Duration of the Asymptomatic Period

The exact duration of the asymptomatic period in nontraumatic ON is variable. Studies to date have revealed that the time from MR diagnosis to onset of pain varies from 3 months to over 3 years (Table 21.2). This variance is probably due to differences in the cohort population, lesion size, and timing of diagnosis.

21.5.4 Risk Factors for Developing Pain

Pain characteristics are based mainly on the size and location of the lesion with larger size and lateral location being at

Table 21.2 Studies showing the timing of the onset of pain from the initial MRI diagnosis

Study author	Mean time to onset of pain from initial radiological diagnosis (in months)	Maximum range (in months)
Hernigou et al.	64	20–204
Min et al.	40	7–99
Kopecky et al.	3	3–10

greatest risk for becoming symptomatic [13]. Kang et al. studied 68 patients with asymptomatic osteonecrosis of the femoral head and found out that the lesion size and location were significantly associated with symptom development. In their study of 20 hips with small lesions, 10 % became symptomatic; out of 29 hips with medium lesion, 69 % became symptomatic; and out of 19 hips with large lesion, 84.2 % became symptomatic. Also symptoms developed in 76.3 % of their hips with lateral location of the lesion on the femoral head, in 38.1 % of hips with central lesion, and in 10 % of hips with medial lesion.

21.5.5 Time from Risk Factor Insult to MR Diagnosis of Osteonecrosis

The time to development of disease cannot be assessed for risk factors such as sickle cell disease or ethanol usage or coagulopathies. However, the date of administration of steroids related to chemotherapy or immunosuppression can be identified and provide some information about the time to onset of disease. Kubo et al. studied 51 renal allograft recipients and detected abnormal MRI findings in 18 femoral heads of 10 patients at 6–16 weeks (average 10 weeks) from transplantation [15]. Sakaia et al. in their study on rabbit serum sickness model also concluded that ON could be detected very early within 1–12 weeks (average 6 weeks) on conventional MRI [16].

21.5.6 Characteristics of Pain in the Hip in Early, Precollapse Stages of ON (ARCO 1 and 2)

As patients with early precollapse ON may or may not have pain, it is a challenge to know whether or not to attribute pain to the presence of ON on imaging. In the absence of pathology or a pain-generating entity elsewhere, ON demonstrated on imaging is usually identified as the etiology for pain. The onset is usually insidious and sporadic in majority of the patients. The quality of the pain is typically similar to intra-articular pain of the affected joint that might be due to any other cause. If a joint effusion is present with imaging findings of ON, one can be confident that the ON is the cause of the symptoms.

In patients with polyostotic ON involving metaphyseal and subchondral sites, patient may complain of diffuse bone pain in all extremities. The quality of the pain is dull, aching, and mild or at times may seem out of proportion to findings on plain radiographs; however, the MR imaging usually shows bilateral, diffuse skeletal involvement (Fig. 21.4). Management of the pain in these patients is problematic due to the chronicity and severity of the symptoms that usually require narcotic analgesia.

21.5.7 Characteristics of Pain in the Hip in Late, Post-collapse Stages of ON (ARCO 3 and 4)

Pain at this stage is usually typical of degenerative arthritis. It is aggravated by joint motion and activities. In the lower extremity, an abnormal gait is present. Patients have difficulty sleeping and performing daily activities. In patients with bilateral joint involvement, their function may be severely curtailed.

21.6 Summary

Patients diagnosed with nontraumatic ON are usually asymptomatic initially. The duration of asymptomatic disease is variable [1]. In many cases, pain ensues and probably is related to elevation in the intraosseous pressure. The risk factors for developing pain are mainly the extent of disease and, when in the femoral head, the lateral location within the head. Pain usually precedes a subchondral fracture. The most likely pathophysiologies that cause pain are related to increased intraosseous pressure (from marrow edema and/or large infarcts), synovial effusion, or degenerative arthritis after joint incongruity from subchondral collapse. An accurate assessment of the etiology of pain in the setting of osteonecrosis is challenging but essential in order to optimize the successful resolution of pain after any treatment intervention.

References

1. Marston SB, Cheng EY. Osteonecrosis of the femoral head after solid organ transplant-A prospective study. J Bone Joint Surg Am. 2002;84-A(12):2145–51.
2. Mitchell DG, Rao VM, Dalinka MK, Spritzer CE, Alavi A, Steinberg ME, Fallon M, Kressel HY. Femoral head avascular necrosis: correlation of MR imaging, radiographic staging, radionuclide imaging, and clinical findings. Radiology. 1987;162:709–15.

3. Stulberg BN, Levine M, Bauer TW, Belhobek GH, Pflanze W, Feiglin DH, Roth AI. Multimodality approach to osteonecrosis of the femoral head. Clin Orthop. 1989;240:181–93.
4. Mont MA, Hungerford DS. Current concepts review: non-traumatic avascular necrosis of the femoral head. J Bone Joint Surg Am. 1995;77:459.
5. Bassett LW, Gold RH, Reicher M, Bennett LR, Tooke SM. Magnetic resonance imaging in the early diagnosis of ischemic necrosis of the femoral head. Preliminary results. Clin Orthop. 1987;214:237–48.
6. Marcus ND, Enneking WF, Massam RA. The silent hip in idiopathic aseptic necrosis. Treatment by bone-grafting. J Bone Joint Surg Am. 1973;55:1351–66.
7. Jones LC, Hungerford MW, et al. Outcome measures for evaluation of treatments for osteonecrosis. Orthop Clin North Am. 2009;40(2):179–91.
8. Buttaro M, Della Valle AG, Morandi A, Sabas M, Pietrani M, Piccaluga F. Insufficiency subchondral fracture of the femoral head. J Arthroplasty. 2003;18(3):377–82.
9. ARCO (Association Research Circulation Osseous). Committee on terminology and classification. ARCO News. 1992;4:41–6.
10. Soucacos PN, Urbaniak JR. Osteonecrosis of the human skeleton. Orthop Clin North Am. 2004;35(3):xiii–xv.
11. Kopecky KK, Braunstein EM. Apparent avascular necrosis of the hip: appearance and spontaneous resolution of MR findings in renal allograft recipients. Radiology. 1991;179(2):523–27.
12. Min BW, Song KS, Cho CH, Lee SM, Lee KJ. Untreated asymptomatic hips in patients with osteonecrosis of the femoral head. Clin Orthop Relat Res. 2008;466:1087–92.
13. Kang JS, et al. The natural history of asymptomatic osteonecrosis of the femoral head. Int Orthop (SICOT). 2013;37:379–84.
14. Hernigou P, Habibi A, et al. The natural history of asymptomatic osteonecrosis of the femoral head in adults with sickle cell disease. J Bone Joint Surg Am. 2006;88(12):2565–72.
15. Kubo T, Yamazoe S, Sugano N, Fujioka M, Naruse S, Yoshimura N, Oka T, Hirasawa Y. Initial MRI findings of non-traumatic osteonecrosis of the femoral head in renal allograft recipients. Magn Reson Imaging. 1997;15:1017–23.
16. Sakaia T, Sugano N. Serial magnetic resonance imaging in a non-traumatic rabbit osteonecrosis model: an experimental longitudinal study. Magn Reson Imaging. 2000;18(7):897–905.

22 Accumulation of Necrotic Fatty Marrow in Osteonecrotic Hips Mimicking Septic Arthritis

Tae-Young Kim, Kyung-Hoi Koo, and Javad Parvizi

22.1 Introduction

Osteonecrosis (ON) of the femoral head can lead to development of arthritis of the hip necessitating a total hip arthroplasty (THA). The process of degeneration of the femoral head can result in generation of liquefied fat which combined with joint fluid may resemble pus. It is common practice to withhold performing THA in patients with septic arthritis of the joint to avoid periprosthetic joint infection [1–3]. It is thus plausible that the presence of liquefied fat in patients with ON of the femoral head may lead surgeons to erroneously make a diagnosis of septic arthritis and delay THA. This in turn can lead to a socioeconomic burden and increased morbidity for the patient. In this chapter, the relationship between the presence of pseudopus and osteonecrosis of the femoral head is explored [3].

22.2 Osteonecrotic Femoral Head Mimicking Joint Infection

Based on a previous study, the incidence of pseudopus resembling septic arthritis in patients with ON of the femoral head is around is 1.4 % (7/486) [3].

T.-Y. Kim
Department of Orthopaedic Surgery,
Hallym University Sacred Heart Hospital,
896 Pyeongchon-dong, Anyang 431-070, South Korea
e-mail: tykim@hallym.ac.kr

K.-H. Koo (✉)
Department of Orthopaedic Surgery,
Seoul National University College of Medicine, Seoul National University Bundang Hospital, 166 Gumi-ro,
Seongnam 463-707, South Korea
e-mail: khkoo@snu.ac.kr

J. Parvizi
Department of Orthopaedic Surgery,
Rothman Institute at Thomas Jefferson University Hospital,
925 Chestnut Street, Philadelphia, PA 19107, USA
e-mail: parvj@aol.com

22.3 Clinical Presentation and Laboratory Findings

Patients with ON, unlike those with septic arthritis, usually have no systemic symptoms (fever, lassitude, and so on) or local findings (erythema and extreme pain with joint movement) suggestive of infection. The peripheral blood leukocyte counts, C-reactive protein levels, and erythrocyte sedimentation rates are also usually normal in patients with ON of the femoral head and almost always elevated in patients with septic arthritis.

22.4 Operative Findings

The hip joint capsule is ballooned. When hip joint capsule is incised, yellowish turbid fluid gushes out. Joint fluid has an appearance of pus (Fig. 22.1). The femoral head has an osteochondral crack at the surface of the necrotic portion.

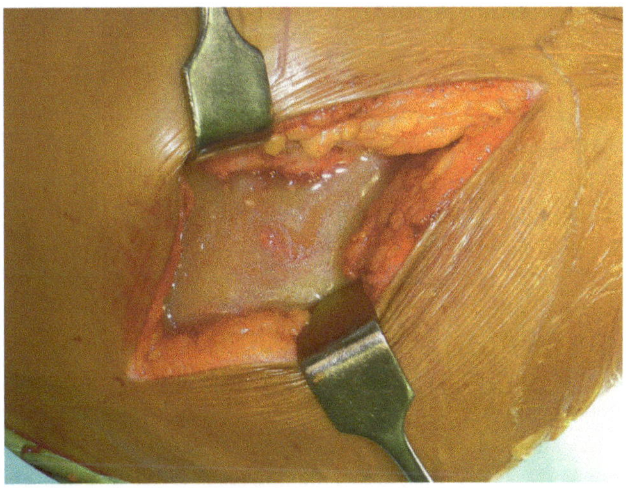

Fig. 22.1 An intraoperative photograph shows the pus-like (yellowish and turbid) joint fluid gushed from the hip joint (Reprint permission for Springer-Verlag)

K.-H. Koo et al. (eds.), *Osteonecrosis*,
DOI 10.1007/978-3-642-35767-1_22, © Springer-Verlag Berlin Heidelberg 2014

Liquefied fat from necrotic marrow leaks into the joint space through this osteochondral crack.

22.5 Erroneous Leukocytosis of Joint Fluid by Automated Cell Counter

When an infection is suspected during operation, the joint aspirate is sent to laboratory for WBC count and neutrophil differential as well as culture. Most of the currently used automated cell counters use electrical impedance or light scattering to obtain a WBC count. The electrical impedance-based technology determines the number and size of cells by detecting and measuring the changes in electrical resistance when a cell in a conductive liquid passes through a small aperture. These cells are analyzed in an electro-optical flow cell. The cell volume is determined by the impedance. The light scattering-based technology determines the cell number and size by detecting the forward angle scatter of a laser-generated monochromatic light [4].

The size of the normal marrow fat cell is approximately 76 μm, which is much larger than that of the leukocytes ranging from 10 to 20 μm [5]. However, the fat cell membrane is ruptured in necrotic marrow and fat globules are released from the fat cells. Some shrunken fat cells and released fat globules are similar in size to leukocytes, which might be counted as leukocytes by automated cell counters [6]. Thus, most of automated cell counters, which are currently in use, may not be able to differentiate necrotic marrow fat from the leukocytes.

22.6 Distinguishing the Accumulation of Necrotic Marrow Fat from a True Septic Arthritis by Microscopic Examination

To avoid a false diagnosis of septic arthritis, microscopic examination of the smear must be performed with a hematoxylin and eosin stain. When only necrotic fat materials are observed and there is no aggregation of neutrophils in the microscopic examination of the smears (Fig. 22.2), THA can be done as scheduled regardless of automated WBC counts.

Concomitant septic arthritis of the hip can occur in patients with ON of the femoral head [7], especially when the patient is immunocompromised or has sickle cell disease [7, 8]. When septic arthritis is confirmed under microscopic identification of an aggregation of neutrophils (Fig. 22.3), THA should be delayed until septic arthritis is treated. It is not known how long THA should be delayed in a patient with prior septic arthritis. The optimal timing of THA in patients with prior septic arthritis is not known. We usually delay the elective arthroplasty in patients with septic arthritis for a period of 1 year.

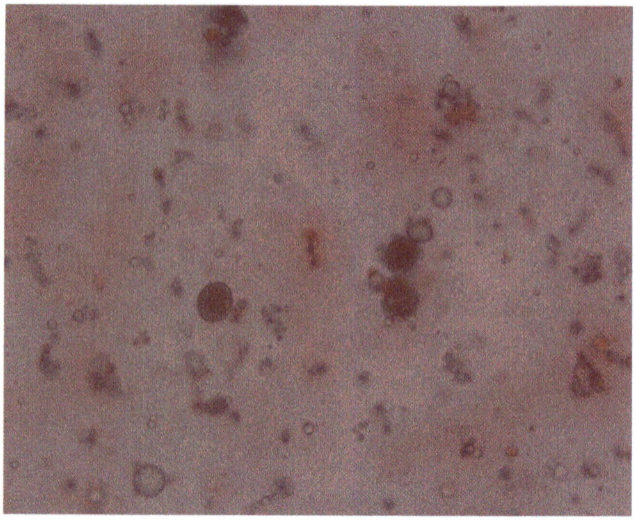

Fig. 22.2 An intraoperative smear of the liquefied fatty marrow from osteonecrotic hip shows fat globules and fat cells. No leukocytes are seen (stain, hematoxylin and eosin, original magnification, 9,400) (Reprint permission for Springer-Verlag)

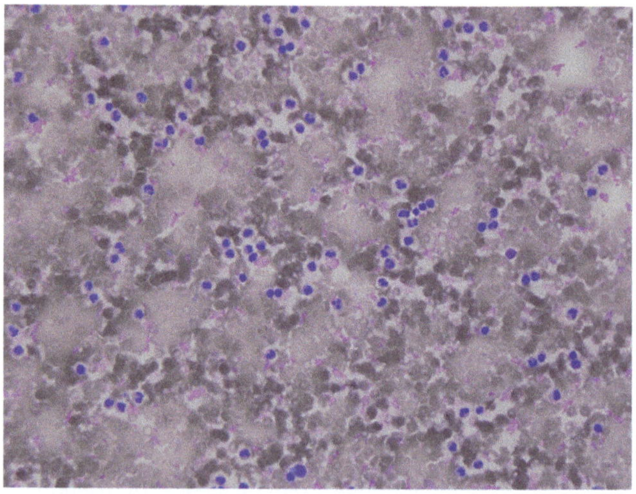

Fig. 22.3 An intraoperative smear of aspirate from septic hip shows numerous neutrophils (stain, Diff-Quik; original magnification, 9,400) (Reprint permission for Springer-Verlag)

22.7 Summary

The presence of liquefied fat combined with joint fluid in patients with osteonecrosis of the femoral head, resembling septic arthritis, can occur in up to 1.4 % of patients undergoing THA. The neutrophil count of the liquid in these patients, when performed using automated systems, may be erroneously high. We recommend that manual cell count of the joint fluid and histological examination of the tissue be performed to avoid unnecessary deferral of THA in these patients. Some patients with ON of the femoral head and concomitant immunocompromising conditions may have coexistent septic arthritis. These patients usually exhibit systemic and local signs of infection and diagnosis of septic arthritis should be suspected in this patient group. In other patients with ON of the femoral head and pseudopus, all efforts should be made to rule out septic arthritis in order not to delay elective THA and cause morbidity to the patient.

References

1. Bittar ES, Petty W. Girdlestone arthroplasty for infected total hip arthroplasty. Clin Orthop Relat Res. 1982;170:83–7.
2. Ghanem E, Restrepo C, Joshi A, Hozack W, Sharkey P, Parvizi J. Periprosthetic infection does not preclude good outcome for revision arthroplasty. Clin Orthop Relat Res. 2007;461:54–9. doi:10.1097/BLO.0b013e318073c246.
3. Sanchez-Sotelo J, Berry DJ, Hanssen AD, Cabanela ME. Midterm to long-term followup of staged reimplantation for infected hip arthroplasty. Clin Orthop Relat Res. 2009;467(1):219–24. doi:10.1007/s11999-008-0480-4.
4. McPherson RA, Pincus MR. Henry's clinical diagnosis and management by laboratory methods, Basic examination of blood and bone marrow. 21st ed. Philadelphia: Saunders; 2007.
5. Motomura G, Yamamoto T, Miyanishi K, Yamashita A, Sueishi K, Iwamoto Y. Bone marrow fat-cell enlargement in early steroid-induced osteonecrosis–a histomorphometric study of autopsy cases. Pathol Res Pract. 2005;200(11–12):807–11. doi:1016/j.prp.2004.10.003. S0344-0338(04)00187-6 [pii].
6. Whiteway AJ, Bain BJ. Artefactual elevation of an automated white cell count following femoral vein puncture. Clin Lab Haematol. 1999;21(1):65–8.
7. Hernigou P, Daltro G, Flouzat-Lachaniette CH, Roussignol X, Poignard A. Septic arthritis in adults with sickle cell disease often is associated with osteomyelitis or osteonecrosis. Clin Orthop Relat Res. 2010;468(6):1676–81. doi:10.1007/s11999-009-1149-3.
8. Phillips FM, Pottenger LA. Acute septic arthritis in chronic osteonecrosis of the hip. J Rheumatol. 1988;15(11):1713–6.

Part VII

Imaging Diagnosis

23 Radiography, MRI, CT, Bone Scan, and PET-CT

Kyung Nam Ryu, Wook Jin, and Ji Seon Park

23.1 Introduction

Imaging diagnosis of osteonecrosis uses various modalities such as plain radiograph, magnetic resonance imaging (MRI), computed tomography (CT), radionuclide examination, and PET-CT [1, 2]. Plain radiograph and MRI are frequently used for diagnostic purposes during the examination. When unilateral osteonecrosis is shown on plain radiograph, radionuclide examination is used to determine whether there is involvement of the contralateral femoral head or not [3–6].

Plain radiograph is generally used as first diagnostic tool for osteonecrosis because of easy availability and low economic costs. It can visualize the characteristic features for osteonecrosis and differentiate the status of disease progression. So, the plain radiograph has been responsible for classifying the stages of osteonecrosis, even though diagnostic limitation for preradiographic stage. MRI is expensive, but has relatively high sensitivity and specificity so that it makes detection on early diagnosis stage possible. CT is more delicate than a plain radiograph, but it has a lower sensitivity than MRI and is not appropriate during the preradiographic stage. Radionuclide examination has a high sensitivity but also a high false-positive rate. Positron emission tomography-computed tomography (PET-CT) is not used to diagnose osteonecrosis, but patients examined by PET-CT for osteonecrosis may show local uptake of FDG. In this case, discrimination between osteonecrosis of the femoral head and metastasis is needed [7, 8].

K.N. Ryu (✉) • J.S. Park
Department of Radiology, Kyung Hee University Hospital, 1, Hoeki-dong, Dongdaemun-gu, Seoul 130-702, South Korea
e-mail: t2star@naver.com; francesca@daum.net

W. Jin
Department of Radiology, Kyung Hee University Hospital at Kandong, 149, Sangil-dong, Gangdong-gu, Seoul 134-727, South Korea
e-mail: jinooki@daum.net

23.2 Imaging

23.2.1 Radiography

In osteonecrosis (ON) of the femoral head shown at preradiographic stage on a plain radiograph, the sensitivity is relatively low that dead bone can be seen as normal with no shaded area. However, plain radiograph may be helpful to grasp the overall structure of the surrounding area and can be used as an imaging examination to monitor progress of the lesion with repeated examinations.

Staging of osteonecrosis of the femoral head is described by plain radiographic findings, MRI, or CT. These are the Arlet-Ficat staging system [9, 10] divided in four stages; the Marcus and Enneking system [11]; and the Steinberg staging system [12], divided in six stages including radiographic findings, clinical signs, and symptoms, which are classified based on plain radiographic findings. Radiographic location with staging system of osteonecrosis is suggested by the Japanese Investigation Committee [13, 14].

Recently, ARCO staging system including plain radiograph, MRI, radionuclide examination, and histological findings is frequently used [15].

The anteroposterior view and the frog leg lateral view are the basic plain radiograph views for diagnosis of osteonecrosis of the femoral head. On anteroposterior view, osteonecrosis of the femoral head usually affects the anterosuperior portion and the lesion is usually overlapped with the acetabulum. However, on frog leg lateral view, the contour of the anterosuperior portion of the femoral head can be seen [15] (Fig. 23.1).

On preradiographic stage of osteonecrosis, plain radiograph can be seen normal (ARCO stage I) even if histopathological osteonecrosis exists. To identify osteonecrosis in this stage, MRI or radionuclide examination might be helpful (Fig. 23.2). After this stage, mottled radiodense and radiolucent areas are noticeable on the subchondral portion of the anterosuperior part of the femoral head (ARCO stage II) (Fig. 23.3). However, the abnormal density of this area must

K.-H. Koo et al. (eds.), *Osteonecrosis*,
DOI 10.1007/978-3-642-35767-1_23, © Springer-Verlag Berlin Heidelberg 2014

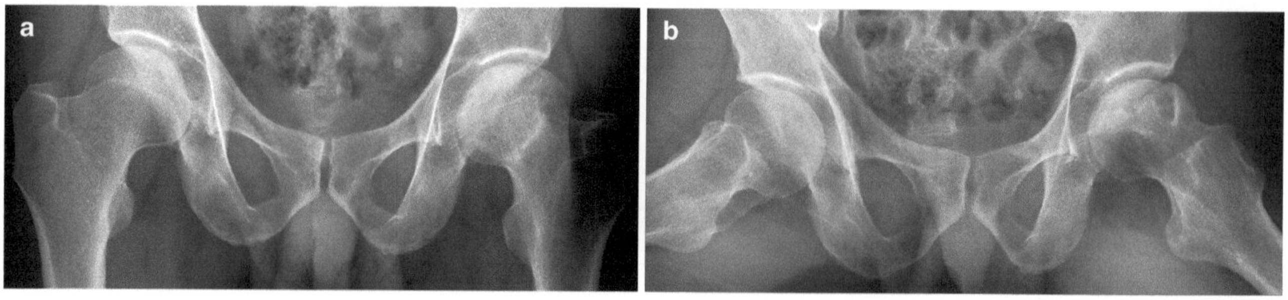

Fig. 23.1 ON in a 44-year-old male patient. (**a**) Anteroposterior view of the hip shows ON of the left femoral head. (**b**) Frog leg lateral view shows clear delineation of ON with subchondral collapse

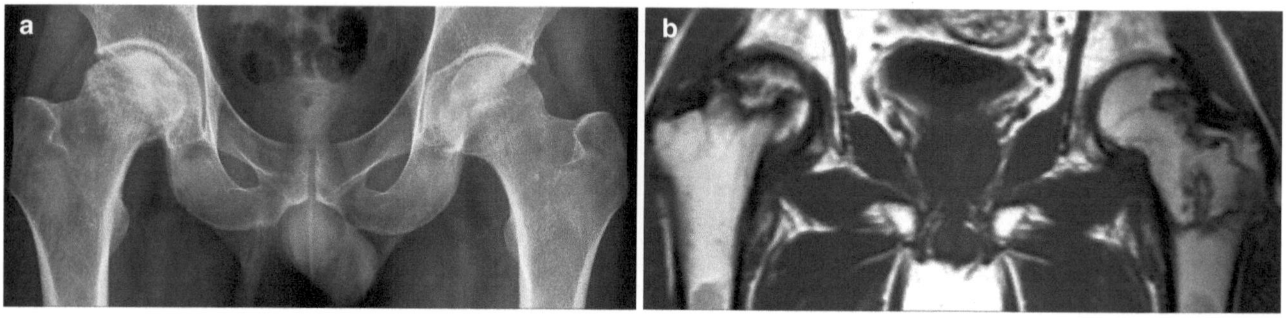

Fig. 23.2 Early stage of ON in a 36-year-old male patient. (**a**) The right femoral head shows ON with subchondral collapse, and marginal sclerosis along the lesion is seen. The left femoral head shows suspicious sclerosis. (**b**) T1-weighted coronal image shows ON of both femoral heads. ON of the left femur shows involvement of the head and intertrochanteric portion

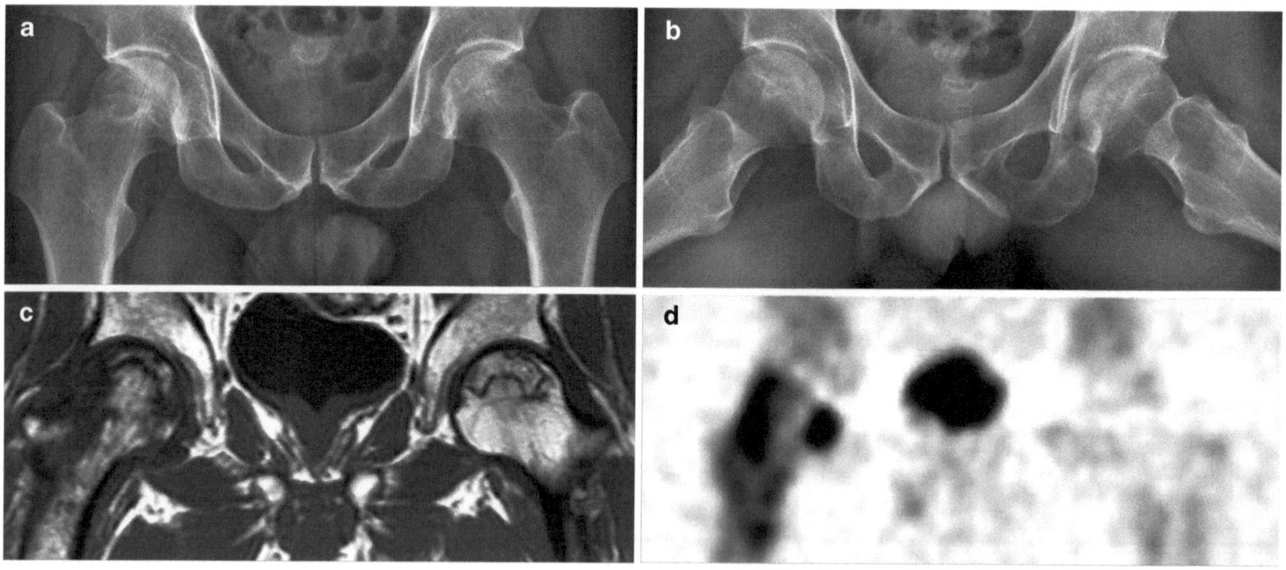

Fig. 23.3 ON (ARCO stage II) of both femoral heads in a 55-year-old male patient. (**a**) Anteroposterior view of hip joints shows radiolucencies of both femoral heads with curvilinear sclerosis. (**b**) Frog leg lateral view shows round contours of both femoral heads. (**c**) T1-weighted coronal image shows ON of both femoral heads. Unlike plain radiographs, diffuse marrow edema at the right femoral head and neck is seen. (**d**) SPECT image shows photon defects at both femoral heads. Hot uptake foci are seen at the right femoral head and neck

be differentiated from the normally heterogeneous density caused by the overlapped shadow of the anterior and posterior columns of the acetabulum. Increased densities on the femoral head show revascularization and osseous repair [10–12].

As osteonecrosis of the femoral head progresses, fibrotic band formed on the border of the dead bone and the live bone cannot be observed on plain radiograph. However, when marginal sclerosis occurs along the band, it can be detected

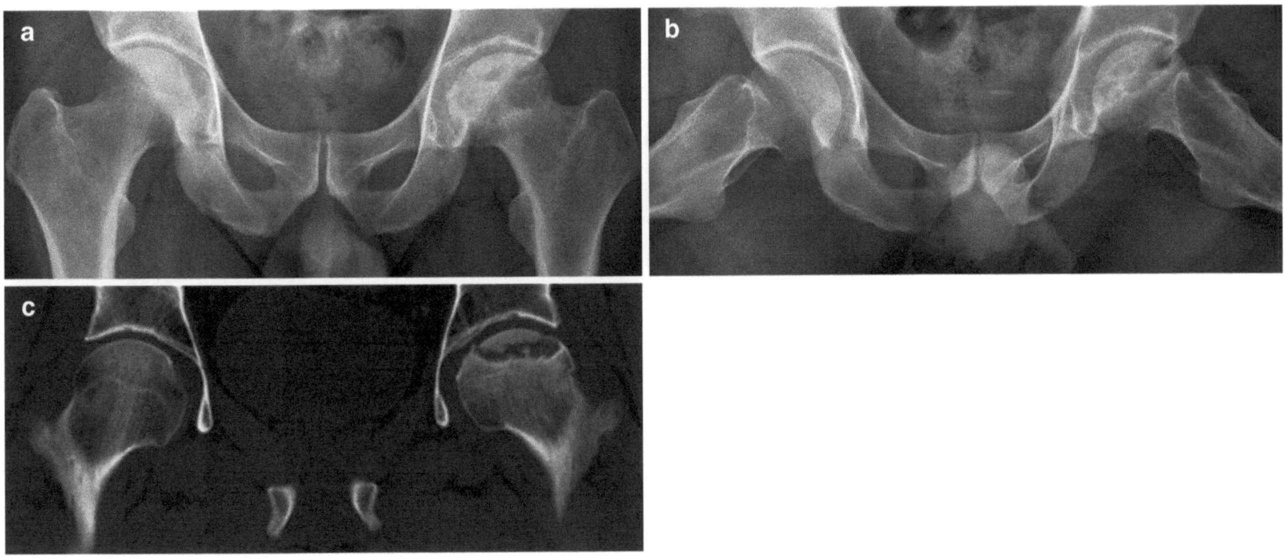

Fig. 23.4 ON (ARCO stage IV) of the left femoral head in a 49-year-old male patient. (**a**) Anteroposterior view of hip joints shows subchondral collapse of the left femoral head with radiolucent and sclerotic lesions. (**b**) Radiolucent lesions are prominent at the superolateral portion of the left femoral head. (**c**) CT coronal image shows subchondral collapse of the left femoral head

on plain radiographs as radiolucent lesion on inner section. Radiolucency is mostly seen on the subchondral portion of the femoral head and in the frog leg lateral view. The radio lucency along the subchondral portion of the femoral head is called the crescent sign (ARCO stage III). The changes affect only the femoral head, and the contour of the femoral head is maintained so that the joint space appears normal and can be distinguished from articular disease. The femoral head starts to collapse and this makes changes to the contour of the femoral head (ARCO stage IV) (Fig. 23.4).

Subchondral fractures are seen as subchondral collapse and sclerosis, mostly on frog leg lateral view. When it starts to collapse, marginal sclerosis along the border of osteonecrosis fades in and reactive sclerosis around the affected area increases. If the lesion progresses continuously, secondary osteoarthritic changes such as joint space narrowing, marginal osteophytes, and subchondral sclerosis on hip joints including defect of articular cartilage appear. The progression of osteonecrosis is mostly influenced by extent, part, and the patient's age [16].

Collapse shows rapid progress as the affected area gets wider. It can be seen as the same condition for several years without collapse if it is not located on the anterosuperior or weight-bearing portion. Osteonecrosis can be limited only to the femoral head, and in this case, no progress would be detected for long periods of time (Fig. 23.5). If osteonecrosis is observed on one femoral head, the contralateral femoral head should also be examined closely.

If the lesion affects not only the anterosuperior portion of femoral head but also the greater part of the femoral head, it shows the form of rapidly destructive hip disease (RDHD) [17]. There has been a reported case of rapid collapse on the femoral head in which the normal contour collapsed only in a few weeks (Fig. 23.6). When collapse proceeds, collapsed bone fragments can be seen on the inner portion of the joint cavity. Bone erosion of the acetabulum is accompanied by an irregular margin of the femoral head. In this case, distinction between RDHDs by other causing factors is necessary and the presence of ON on the contralateral femoral head is a favorable finding to ON-related RDHD.

In patients with large extent of ON, it is possible that pathologic fracture is seen on the border along the lesion instead of collapse of the femoral head (Fig. 23.7). Opposite to RDHD, if the osteonecrosis region is small or if the lesion is located in non-weight-bearing portion, it shows no additional changes for several years.

23.2.2 MRI

MRI is considered as the method of choice for detecting and staging ON due to its multiplanar imaging, excellent soft tissue contrast, and ability to discriminate fat from other tissues in the bony marrow [18]. MRI achieves excellent sensitivity for early ON detection [19, 20] (Fig. 23.8). In one study, MRI achieved a sensitivity of 100 % as opposed to 81 % for scintigraphy [21]. More recent data have shown that MRI may improve staging, investigate radiologically occult collapse, depict other causes of disability and pain, assess prognosis, and evaluate treatment [22]. Also, MRI is effective in assessing joint effusions and bone marrow edema, which has a strong association with hip pain [23, 24]. However,

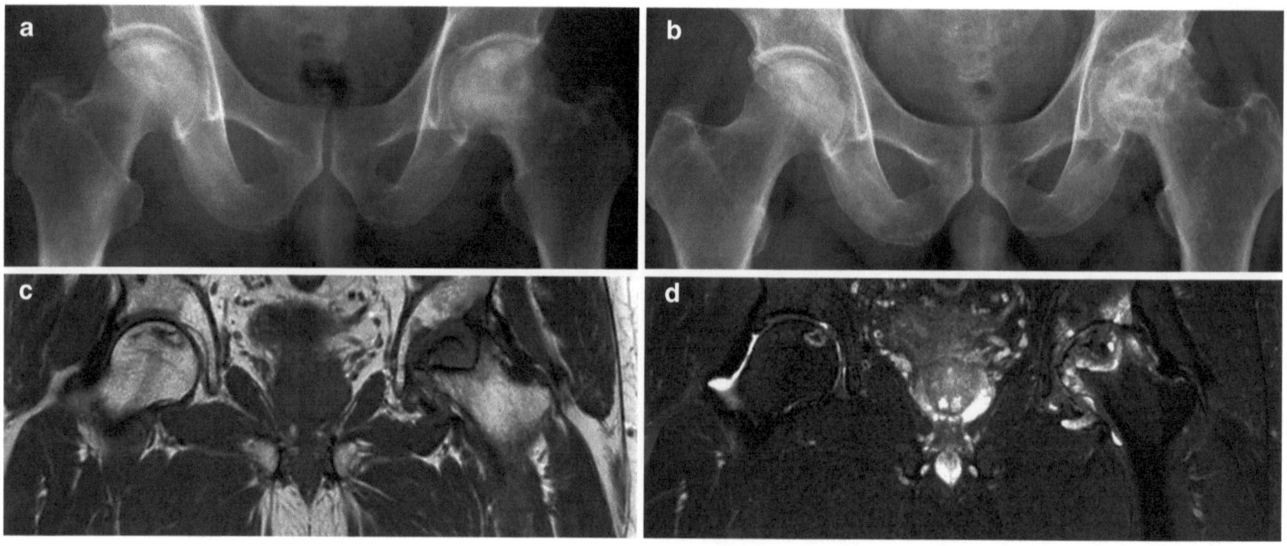

Fig. 23.5 Intraosseous location of ON in a 54-year-old woman. (**a**) Plain radiograph of hip shows ON of both femoral heads. The right femoral head shows normal contour; however, the left femoral head shows subchondral collapse. (**b**) Six months later, the left femoral head shows progression of subchondral collapse. The right femoral head has no change in contour. (**c**) T1-weighted coronal image shows intraosseous location of ON in the right femoral head. The left femoral head shows subchondral collapse with secondary degeneration of the acetabulum. (**d**) T2-weighted fat-saturated coronal image shows typical double-line sign of ON in the right femoral head

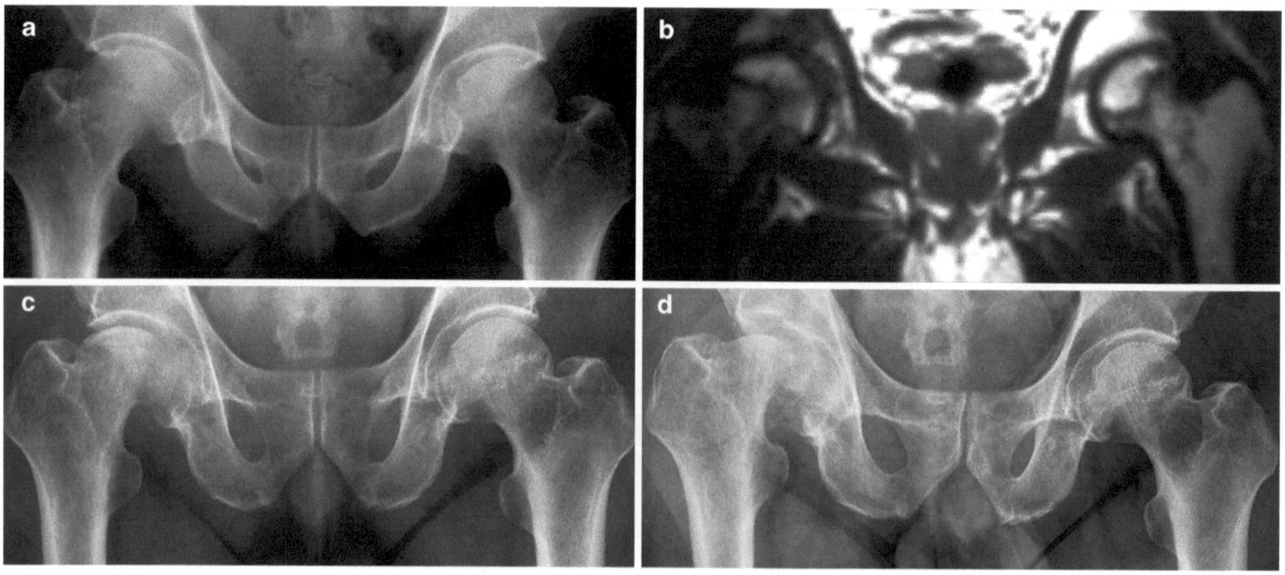

Fig. 23.6 Rapidly destructive hip disease in a 63-year-old male patient. (**a**) Plain radiograph of the hip shows ON of both femoral heads. Contours of femoral heads are relatively preserved. (**b**) T1-weighted coronal image shows ON of both femoral heads. (**c**) Two months later from (a), the right femoral head shows subchondral collapse with contour deformity. The left femoral head is not changed. (**d**) Two weeks later from (c), progression of collapse of the right femoral head is seen with bone fragments. The contour of the right acetabulum is changed with erosion

a negative MRI for ON does not exclude the possibility of ON, especially in patients with corticosteroid treatment such as renal transplant recipients [25].

Imaging protocols for evaluation of patients with ON can include combinations of variable multiplanes and sequences. T1-weighted sagittal imaging may be helpful in defining early changes of cortical flattening associated with subchondral collapse. And T2-weighted fat-saturated imaging or STIR (short tau inversion recovery) imaging can provide excellent contrast for the detection of marrow replacement, fluid, and necrotic tissue [26].

General magnetic resonance (MR) characteristics of ON include the following:

- On T1-weighted MR images, a circumscribed subchondral "band-like" lesion with low signal intensity is pathognomonic [5] (Fig. 23.9a). This lesion outlining a central

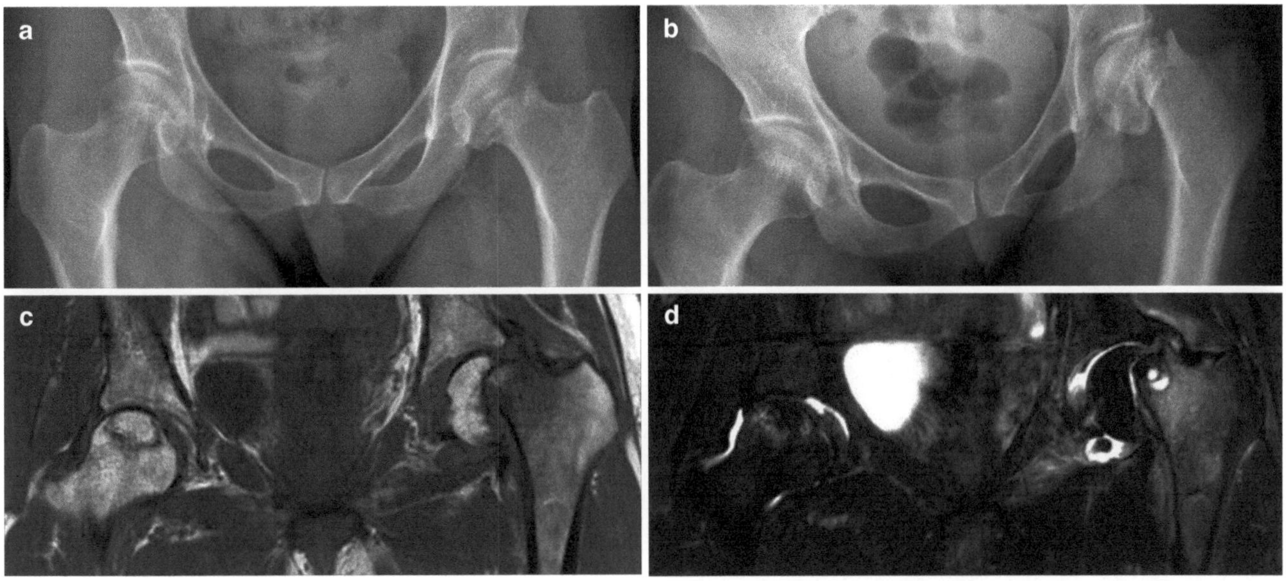

Fig. 23.7 Pathologic fracture of ON in a 45-year-old female patient. (**a**) Both femoral heads show amorphous sclerosis. The junction of the left femoral neck and the head shows acute angulation. (**b**) Two months later, the left femoral head shows pathologic fracture with inferomedial displacement of the femoral head. (**c**) T1-weighted coronal image shows fatty marrow change with diffuse low signal intensity of the femoral head. The right femoral head shows early change of ON. (**d**) T2-weighted fat-saturated image shows diffuse marrow edema of the left femoral neck with cystic changes

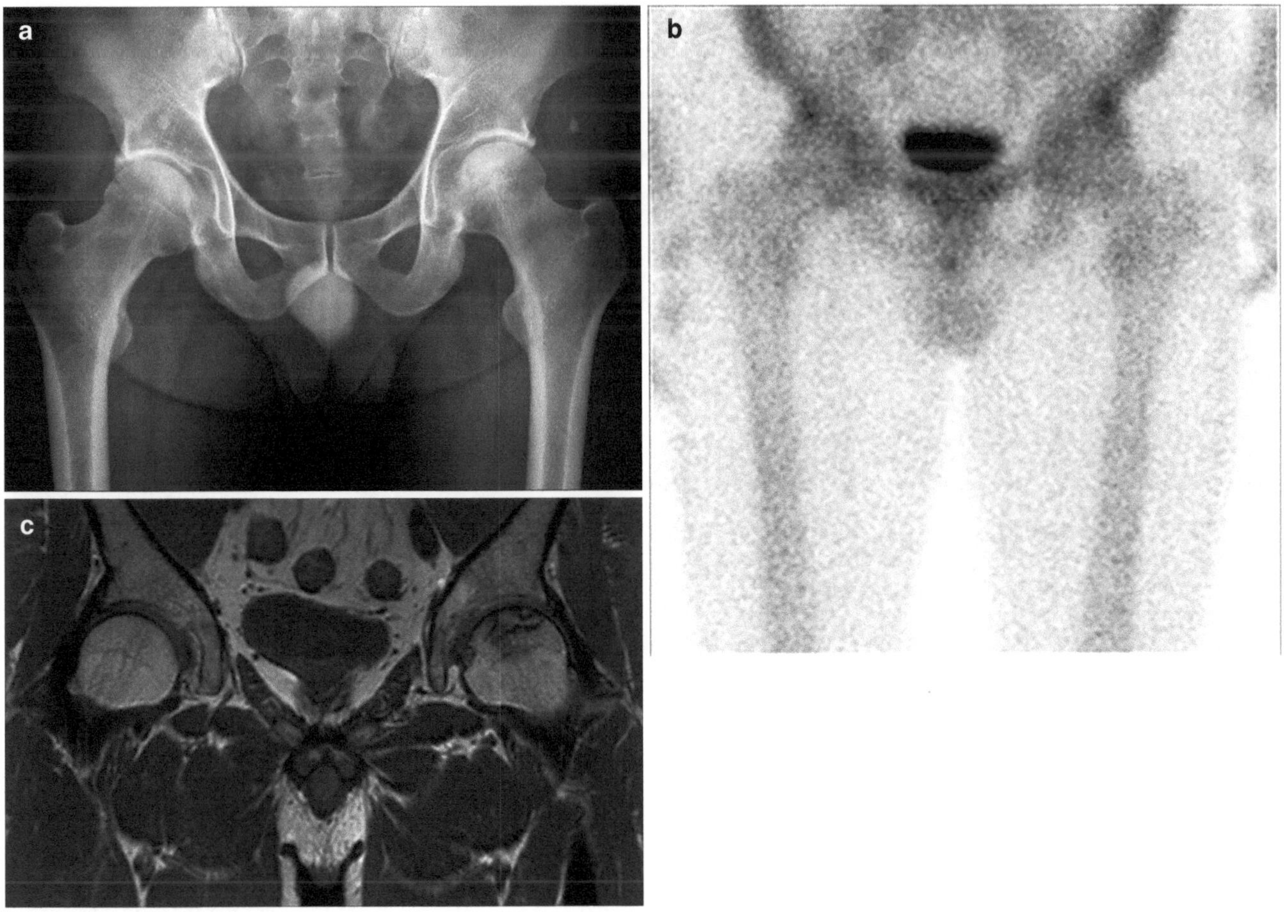

Fig. 23.8 ON of the left femoral head. (**a**) The hip anteroposterior radiograph was interpreted as normal. (**b**) Minimally increased uptakes of the radionuclide are noted at the lateral margins of both acetabula on bone scan (^{99m}Tc-DPD). (**c**) On T1-weighted MR image, low-signal band-like lesion is noted in the left femoral head

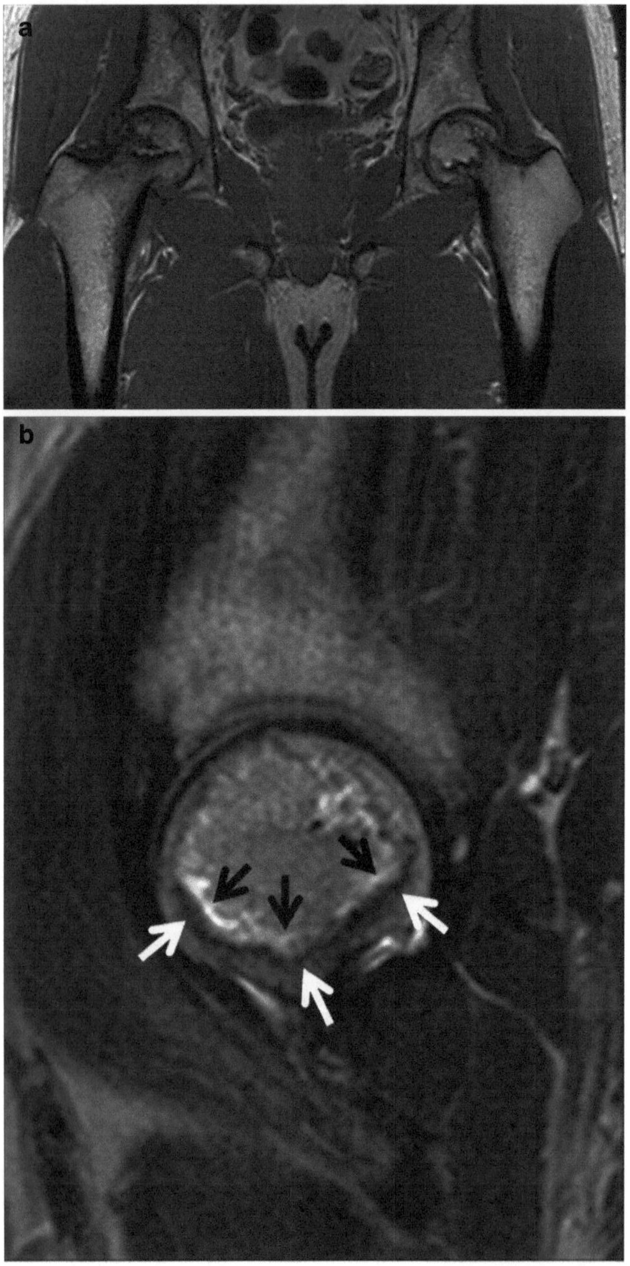

Fig. 23.9 ON of both femoral heads. (**a**) On T1-weighted coronal MR image, circumscribed "band-like" lesions with low signal intensity are noted in both femoral heads. (**b**) On T2-weighted sagittal MR image of the left hip, the "double-line" sign is well noted. This sign consists of a low-signal-intensity outer rim (*white arrows*) and a high-signal-intensity inner rim (*black arrows*)

region of bone marrow represents the reactive interface between necrotic and reparative areas. This finding is not dependent on the plain radiograph being normal or suggesting ON [3].

- On T2-weighted or fluid-sensitive MR images, the "double-line" sign is seen and consists of a low-signal-intensity outer rim and a high-signal-intensity inner rim (Fig. 23.9b). This sign was present in 80 % of the lesions, but in that study, no correlation with the radiographic stage was attempted. This sign was introduced by Mitchell et al. [5] and was considered pathognomonic for ON since the outer rim represents the reactive bone and the inner rim the vascular and repair tissue at the necrotic-viable osseous interface. However, the etiology of the "double line" has been challenged in the literature. It has been reported that a transposition of the frequency and phase-encoding axis results in reversal of the positions of the bright and dark rims, suggesting the presence of a chemical shift misregistration artifact [27–29]. The region within the "double-line" sign may demonstrate hypo-, iso-, and hyperintensity relative to the normal marrow.

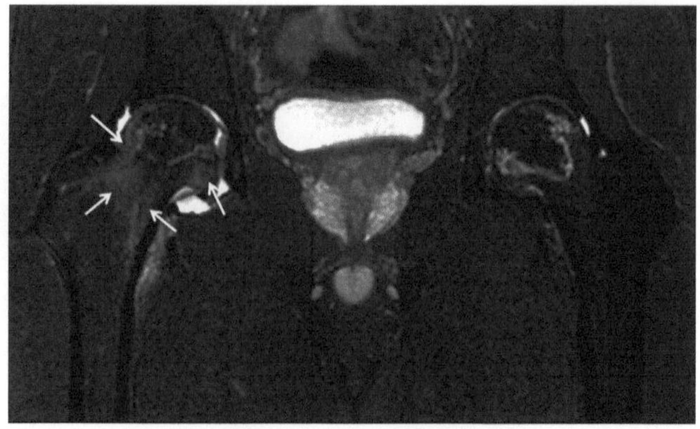

Fig. 23.10 ON of both femoral heads. The patient has ON of both femoral heads. The right hip is painful, but the left hip is asymptomatic. Joint effusion at the right hip joint and diffuse bone marrow edema (*arrows*) of the right femoral head and neck are demonstrated on T2-weighted fat-suppressed coronal MR image

- A joint effusion may be seen and is hypointense on T1-weighted images and hyperintense on fluid-sensitive images. Joint effusions are seen in about half the patients with ON regardless of the presence of articular surface collapse [30]. Although not yet clarified, joint effusion might result from an ON-related synovitis. Joint effusions are correlated with pain and are commonly found together with bone marrow edema [23] (Fig. 23.10).
- Bone marrow edema (BME) in MRI has been a source of controversy in the literature. Distinction between reversible and ON-related BME is of essential importance because ON is a progressive clinical disease requiring a joint-preserving treatment, whereas transient osteoporosis resolves spontaneously without requiring surgical treatment. The presence of BME in ON seems to correlate highly with pain [24] (Fig. 23.10). Further studies showed that BME is a poor prognostic sign since it develops after the onset or worsening of hip pain and correlates with the subsequent collapse of the femoral head suggesting progression to advanced ON [23, 31, 32] (Fig. 23.11).
- Post-contrast enhancement corresponds to a reparative zone, seen as a hypointense band. There may be decreased

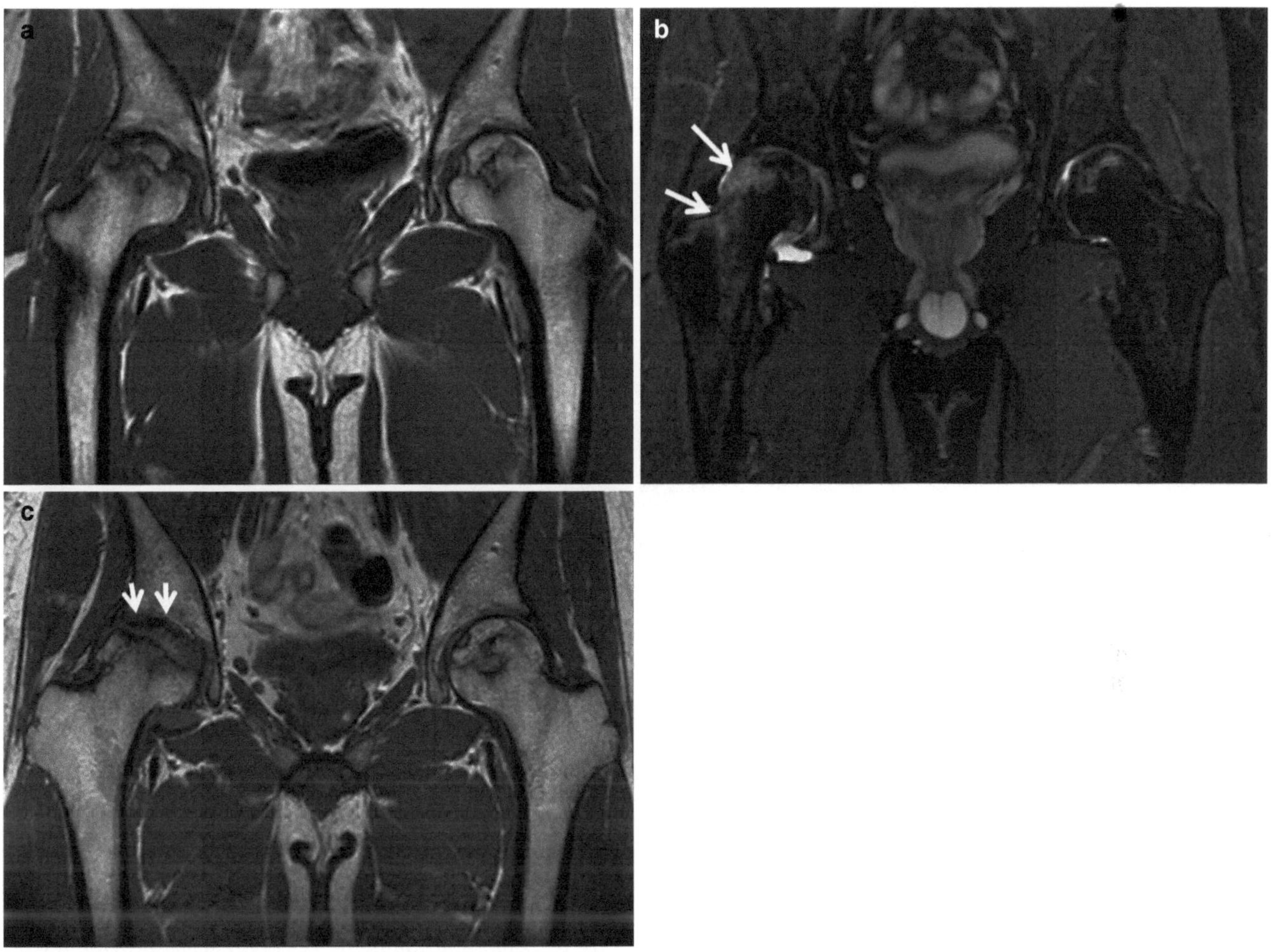

Fig. 23.11 ON of both femoral heads. (**a**) At both femoral heads, ON with band-like low signals is noted with similar involving areas on T1-weighted coronal MR image. (**b**) In the right femoral head and intertrochanteric area, bone marrow edema (*arrows*) is noted on T2-weighted fat-suppressed coronal MR image. In contrast, there is no significant bone marrow edema in the left proximal femur. (**c**) Nine months later, significant collapse (*arrows*) of the superolateral aspect of the right femoral head is identified on T1-weighted coronal MR image. At the left femoral head, there is no significant collapse

enhancement with gadolinium in early ON, and there is no enhancement with nonviable trabeculae and marrow. But, this was not widely accepted as an additional imaging finding of ON at the femoral head [33, 34]. Recent studies with dynamic contrast-enhancing MR (DCE-MR) or perfusion MR have been performed for early evaluation of the blood flow at the femoral head and neck after femoral neck fracture or steroid therapy [35–38]. MRI with these sequences is expected to be a guideline to predict the possibility and prognosis of ON at the femoral head before and after treatment.

23.2.3 CT

On axial images of CT, a star-shaped structure made by radial condensation composed of the primary compressive and primary tensile trabeculae which intersect the central area of femoral head is seen. This figure is called the asterisk sign [39]. In the cases with prominent trabeculae and physeal scar in the femoral head, axial CT image scanned at femoral head level shows that sclerotic raylike branchings from the central dense band representing physeal scar extend to the upper surface of the femoral head. It should not be mistaken for osteonecrosis (Fig. 23.12).

CT shows diagnostic findings on advanced stage but less sensitive to the preradiographic stage. On the early stage of osteonecrosis, bone resorption zones can be detected and no more asterisk sign is seen. Normal forms of bone trabeculae are shown on the upper part and it shows the forms of patch sclerosis and osteoporosis. Axial CT scans show that the lesions appear as round or wedge radiolucency with peripheral sclerotic lines suggesting the border of ON. On the advanced stage, the subchondral fracture or collapse accompanied by extensive sclerosis on the living bone is more clearly visualized

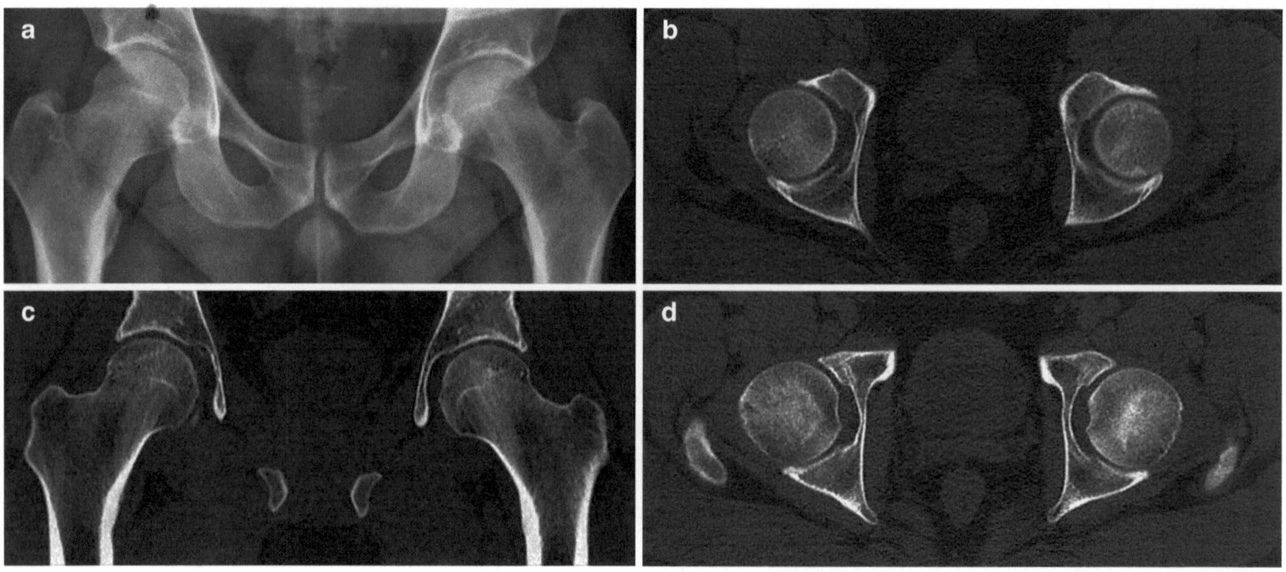

Fig. 23.12 CT findings of ON occurred in a 36-year-old female patient. (**a**) Plain radiograph of the hip shows indistinct sclerosis at the superolateral portions of both femoral heads. (**b**) Axial CT image shows linear sclerosis crossing the central portions of both femoral heads with decreased bone densities. (**c**) Coronal CT image shows curvilinear sclerosis with decreased bone densities at the superolateral portions of both femoral heads. Epiphyseal scars are prominent. (**d**) Axial CT image shows sclerosis caused by epiphyseal scars

than those of radiographs. Following this, secondary osteoarthritic findings of narrowing of the joint space, subchondral sclerosis, and marginal osteophyte from sagittal and coronal images can be identified clearly and easily [40, 41] (Fig. 23.13).

23.2.4 Radionuclide Examinations

23.2.4.1 Bone Scan

Radionuclide bone scintigraphy using technetium-labeled phosphate analogs such as methylene disphosphonate ($^{99mTc\text{-}MDP}$) and dicarboxypropane diphosphonate (^{99m}Tc-DPD) may be used for the early diagnosis of ON of the femoral head [5]. Also, scintigraphy may be useful in evaluating the contralateral asymptomatic hip in patients with apparent unilateral ON of the femoral head. Although bone scans can detect ON earlier than conventional radiography, they are not sensitive as MRI. In acute phase of ON, decreased or absent uptake of bone tracer ("cold" lesion) can be revealed. After weeks or months, increased accumulation of bone tracer occurs ("hot" lesion) with chronic vascular stasis in repair and in revascularization (Fig. 23.14).

23.2.4.2 SPECT

Single-photon emission computed tomography (SPECT) may improve radionuclide sensitivity for the diagnosis of ON [42]. SPECT can contribute to the accurate diagnosis of ON by identifying photopenic defects on serial images that may not be evident on bone scans. On bone scan, increased accumulation of bone tracer from osteoarthritic change in the posterior rim of the acetabulum may in part obscure a photopenic defect from femoral ON [43].

23.2.4.3 PET-CT

Positron emission tomography (PET) scans provide a real-time image of physiology based on the type of radiolabeled marker used. PET imaging has been utilized extensively in orthopedic skeletal disease assessment as well as in cases where interference from implants inhibits the use of other imaging modalities [44, 45]. On PET or PET-CT, ON is seen as a photopenic area.

It may be possible that PET scans detect ON earlier than MRI and SPECT scans and predict the progression as well as outcome of ON [7].

23.3 Postoperative Imaging

Patients who undergone hip surgery for ON present symptomatic hips during follow-up period; postoperative status must be evaluated with imaging studies in addition to physical examination [46, 47]. In contrast to physical examination which is limited to establish the cause of symptomatic hip, the imaging studies including plain radiograph, CT, ultrasound, and MRI are helpful in diagnosing the various postoperative complications and differentiating among them.

Generally, serial plain radiographs are most commonly used for the evaluation of postoperative hip because of the ability of basic overview for hip and pelvic area, low

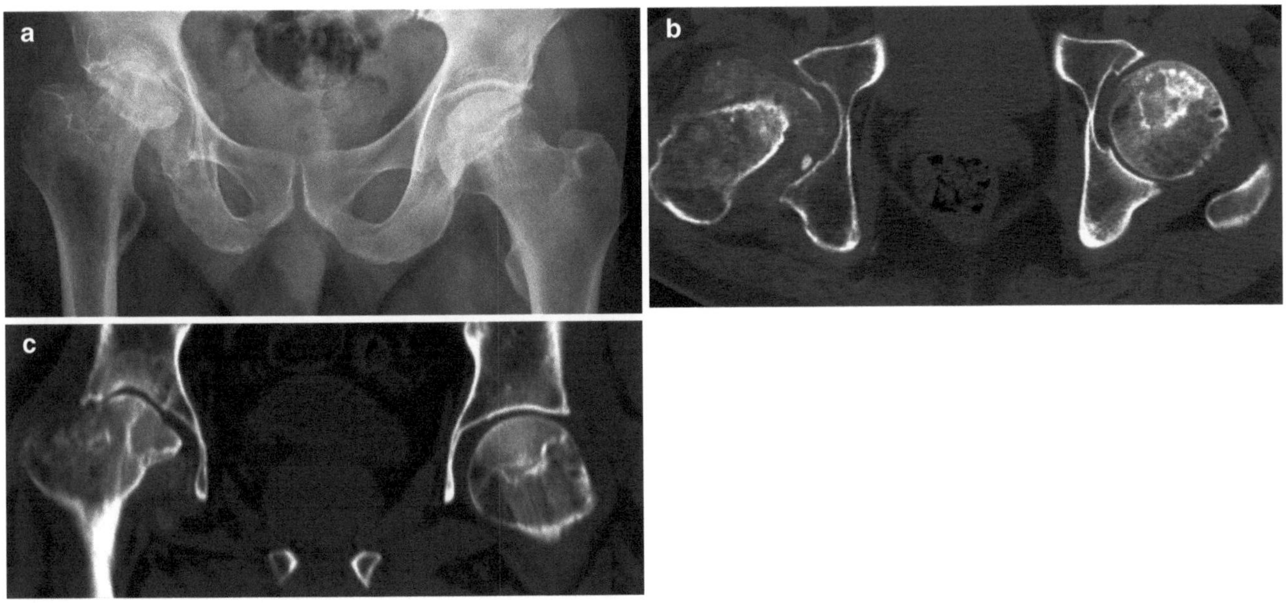

Fig. 23.13 Secondary osteoarthritis caused by ON in a 59-year-old female patient. (**a**) Plain radiograph of the hip shows advanced ON of the right femoral head with subchondral collapse and secondary osteoarthritis of the right hip. The left femoral head shows early ON with curvilinear sclerosis. (**b**) In axial CT image, bone fragments are seen within the joint space. The left femoral head shows loss of asterisk sign with irregularly margined sclerosis

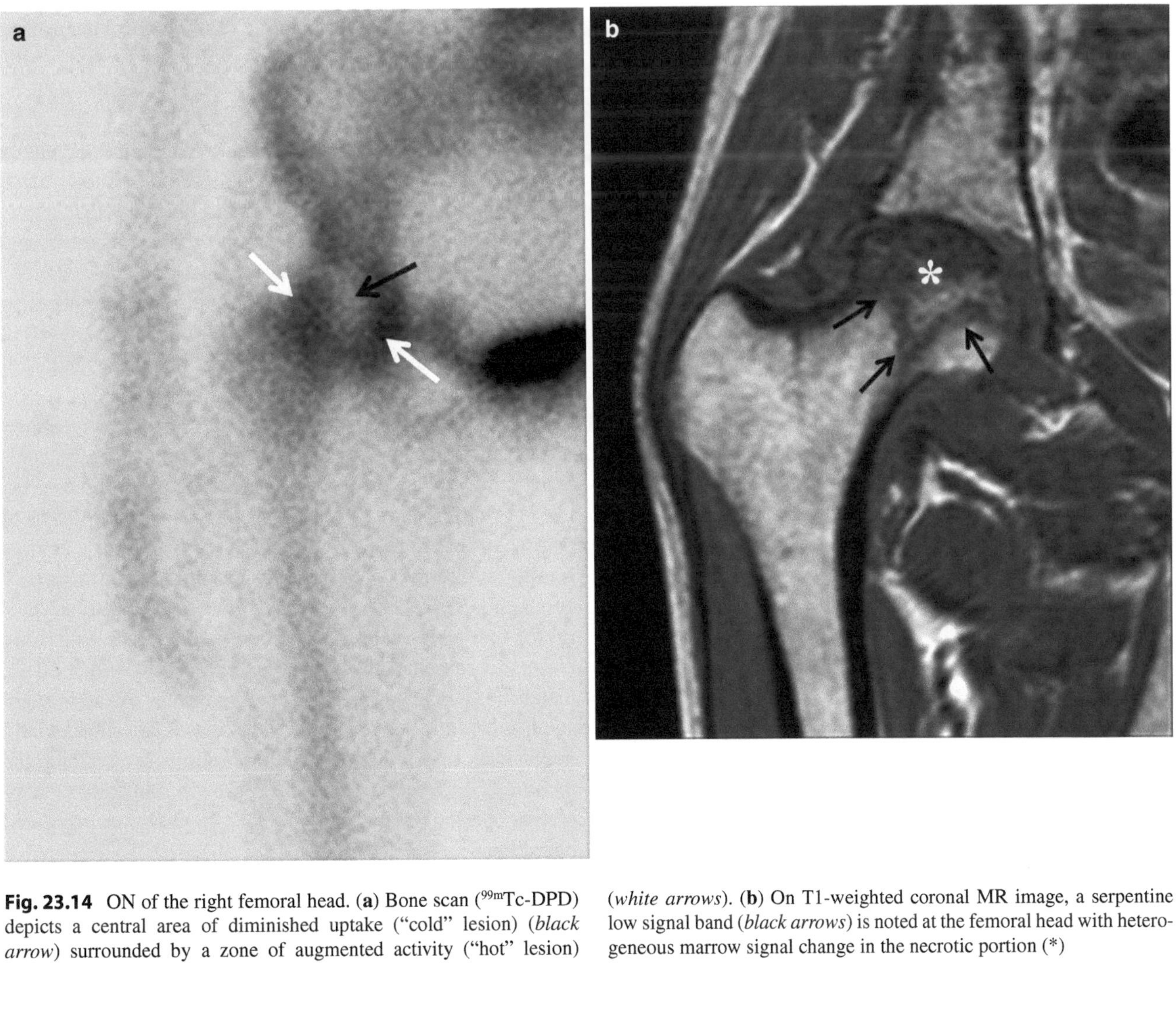

Fig. 23.14 ON of the right femoral head. (**a**) Bone scan (^{99m}Tc-DPD) depicts a central area of diminished uptake ("cold" lesion) (*black arrow*) surrounded by a zone of augmented activity ("hot" lesion) (*white arrows*). (**b**) On T1-weighted coronal MR image, a serpentine low signal band (*black arrows*) is noted at the femoral head with heterogeneous marrow signal change in the necrotic portion (*)

economic cost, and high accessibility. Cross-sectional imaging such as CT and MRI are necessary for earlier and more accurate evaluation of the lesions which may be detected on follow-up radiographs, for assessment of soft tissue lesions despite normal radiography, and for differential diagnosis of postoperative complications [47]. Meanwhile, ultrasound is useful for detecting postoperative fluid collection with or without infection and guiding a needle in aspiration procedure or injection therapy [48].

In this session, the imaging findings of the common complications after representative surgical procedures for ON, including core decompression, total hip replacement (THR), and resurfacing arthroplasty (RSA), and advantages and diagnostic pitfalls of each imaging modality, with current technical development especially in cross-sectional images, are discussed.

23.3.1 Core Decompression

The primary treatment modality for early ON is core decompression (CD), despite some argument. And sometimes bone grafting may be accompanied. The purpose of postprocedural imaging studies is the monitoring of disease progression and interval changes. During follow-up periods after CD, points of postprocedural assessment are the following: (1) whether the extent and location of ON are progressing to be more than 25 % of the articular surface [49] and (2) whether there is marrow edema along the double-line sign, which have been known to be a predictor of subchondral collapse or need for THR [50]. Plain radiographs with different views including anteroposterior, frog leg, and groin lateral views, used as a basic imaging study on postoperative follow-up, can show the progressed periodic changes such as subchondral collapse/fracture and secondary osteoarthritis (Fig. 23.15). MRI is the most feasible modality for assessing the above two findings possibly related to prognosis of ON in early postoperative follow-up period prior to disease progression. CT also may be used for the detailed evaluation of subchondral fracture and preoperative measurement before second procedures such as THR.

23.3.2 Total Hip Replacement (THR)

THR is the most common surgical treatment for advanced stage of ON involving the hip. As described in many previous literatures, the complications after THR, including loosening, osteolysis (so-called aggressive granulomatous disease, particle inclusion disease, hypersensitivity reaction), infection, periprosthetic fracture, dislocation, liner wearing/dissociation, heterotopic ossification, gluteus muscle injury, deep vein thrombosis, stress shielding, and tumor, can be developed as a solitary form or combination of two or more [47].

As for most hip surgeries, plain radiograph is used as a primary imaging tool for follow-up of THR. In relatively common complications such as loosening, osteolysis, or infection, serial plain radiographs reveal progression of periprosthetic radiolucency (more than 2 mm). Additionally, changes of bone/soft tissue densities, breakdown of surgical fixatives, joint alignment, and position of fixatives should be assessed on serial radiographs. For early diagnosis of these complications, acquisition of two and more different views and a meticulous comparison with previous serial radiographs including initial postoperative film are very important, because subtle or minimal changes may be detected only in one image among different views. Actually, cross-sectional imaging such as CT and MRI were limited by artifacts related to large metallic devices inserted in THR. These metallic artifacts (i.e., beam hardening/streak artifacts in CT, metal susceptibility artifact in MRI) contribute to imaging distortion, blurring, or signal void particularly in the area adjacent to the prosthesis. However, trials for decreasing the imaging artifacts and optimizing imaging quality have been performed and continued by many investigators even nowadays. Currently used imaging techniques for decreasing the metal artifacts are as follows: widening of bandwidth, increasing the number of excitations (NEX), increasing echo train length (ETL), use of view angle tilting (VAT), small field of view with thin section, low magnetic field strength, use of titanium hardware instead of stainless steel, metal positioning parallel to main magnetic field in MRI; use of high-voltage, high tube charge, thin section thickness, and narrow collimation during image acquisition, and extended CT scale and thick section thickness during postprocessing reconstruction in CT [46, 47, 51]. These technical developments lead to the increased use of these modalities in evaluation of postoperative hip in many orthopedic clinics.

Loosening, a main cause of painful prosthetic hip, shows progressive radiolucency of more than 2 mm along the interfaces of metal-cement-bone (Fig. 23.16). Migration of prosthesis is observed as a positional change or subsidence of prosthesis in different radiographic views, and it is a definite finding suggestive of loosening. Additionally, fracture of cement materials or wires, sclerosis adjacent to distal femoral tip, and periosteal reaction may be seen. Poor prognostic factors of radiolucency are: large area of more than 50 %, distal 2/3 part of the lateral aspect adjacent to the femoral stem, and young active patient. These cases can substantially necessitate revision THR. Stable radiolucency along the prosthesis may be due to fibrous ingrowth if in early postoperative period within less than 2 years or repeated operations.

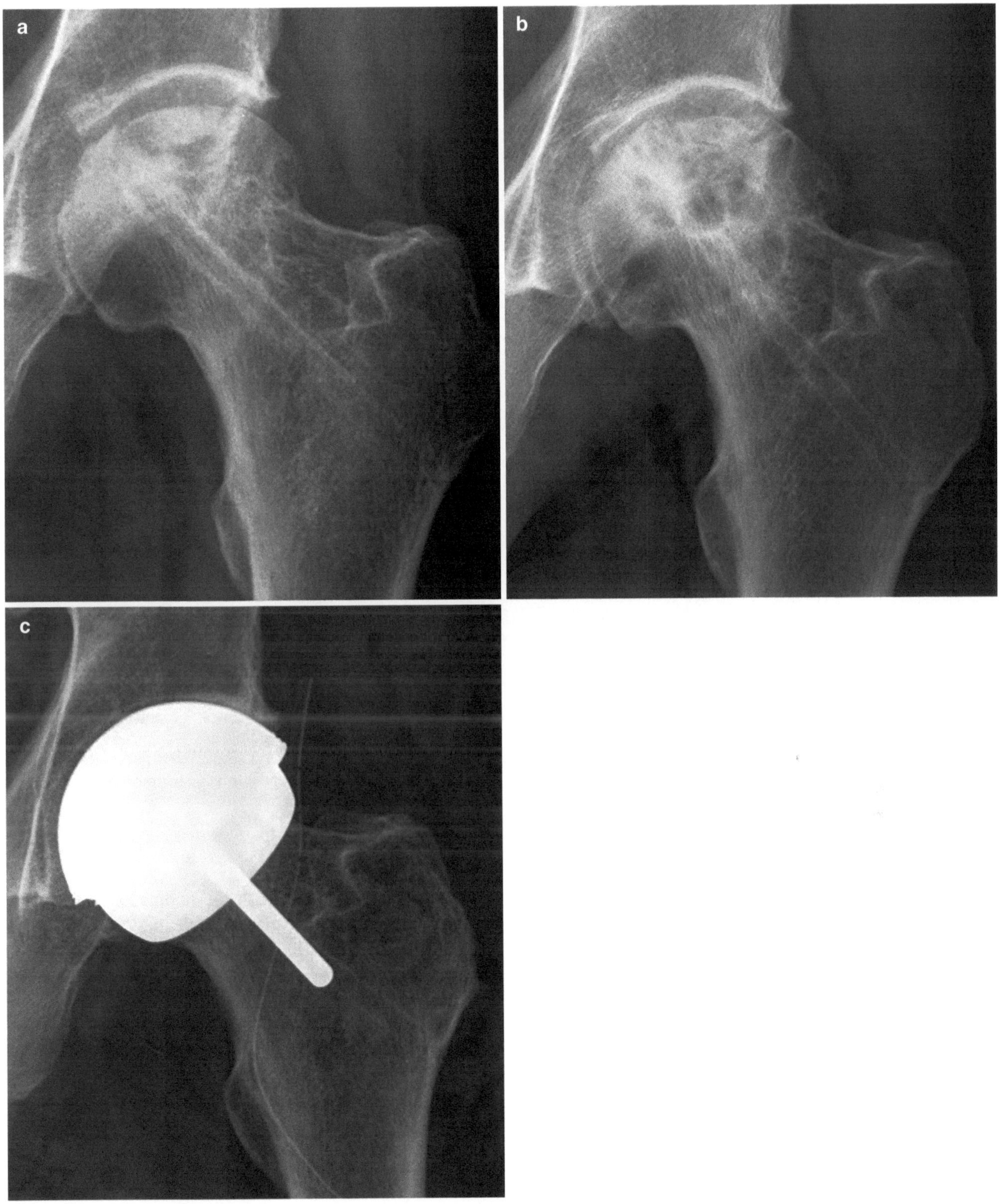

Fig. 23.15 Serial radiographs of left hip anteroposterior views in a 46-year-old man with ON initially treated by core decompression. (**a**) Left femoral head reveals heterogeneously sclerotic lesion at the superior aspect, with subchondral collapse. Narrow radiolucent tubular area with sclerotic rim crossing femoral head-neck-greater trochanter means previous core decompression. (**b**) After 5 years, the lesions involving the femoral head progressed, with increased extent of the lesions and aggravation of subchondral collapse. Secondary osteoarthritis of the left hip is also noted. (**c**) As a result of progression of ON, resurfacing arthroplasty was performed

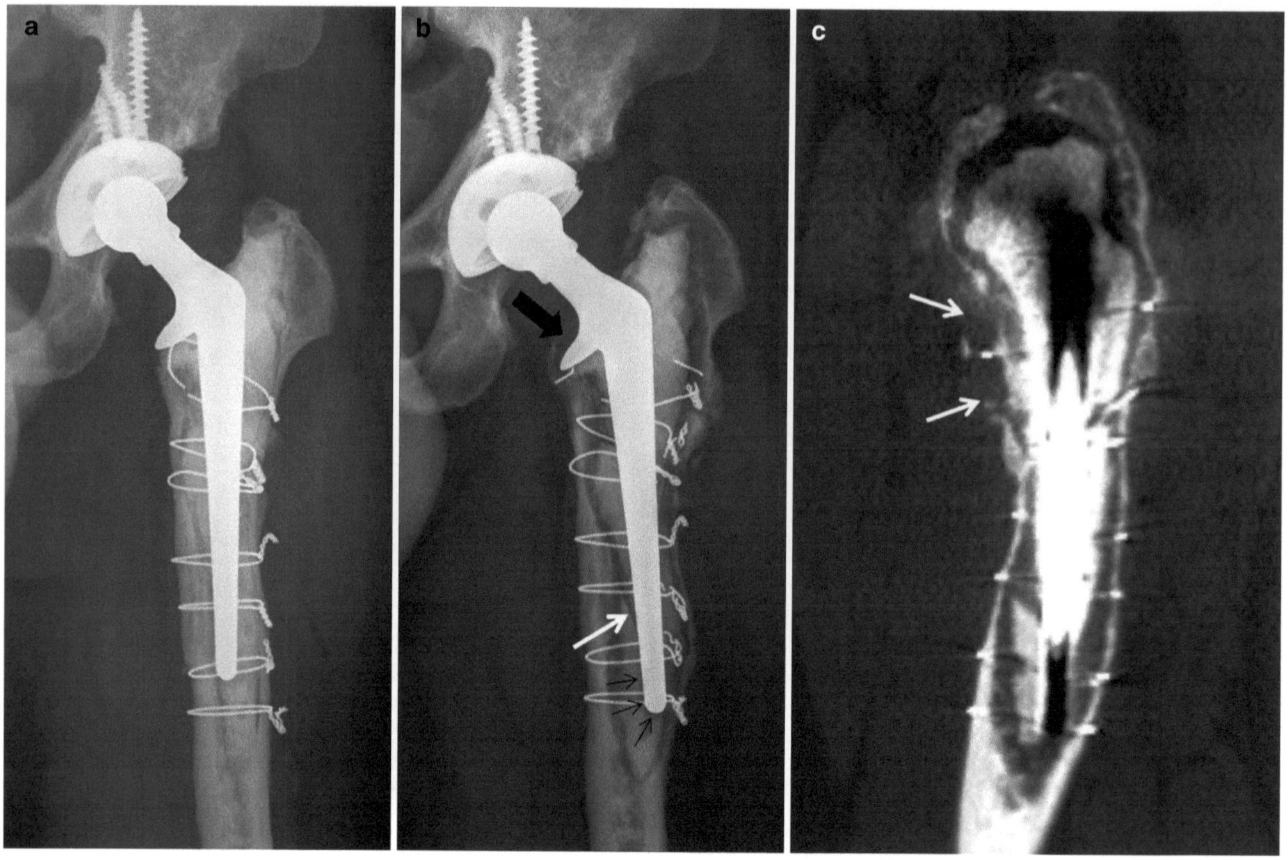

Fig. 23.16 Loosening of femoral component in left THR. (**a**) Anteroposterior radiograph taken on the 3rd postoperative year reveals thin radiolucency along the interfaces between the cement and femur. The uppermost wire is broken. (**b**) On follow-up radiograph taken on the 10th postoperative year, the thickness of periprosthetic radiolucent lesion increased more than 2 mm. Cement fracture (*white arrow*) and new periprosthetic radiolucency (*thin black arrows*) along the interfaces between the prosthesis and cement are noted at distal part of femoral component. Note the subsidence of prosthesis (*thick black arrow*). (**c**) Reformatted sagittal CT scan demonstrates cortical changes such as thinning, remodeling, and disruption (*arrows*), with bulged soft tissue

Osteolysis manifests as a not-conforming radiolucency adjacent to the prosthesis. Not-conforming radiolucency is an important differential point from a loosening, which shows conforming radiolucency along the prosthetic axis. Radiolucent lesions of osteolysis have a well-defined margin and focal or multilobular shape (Fig. 23.17). It frequently accompanies cortical remodeling with thinning and soft tissue mass through cortical disruption. And pseudobursa formation or metallosis presenting as increased radiodensity can be associated (Fig. 23.18). CT with reformatted images or MRI must be performed to evaluate the exact extent of the lesions prior to revision surgery, because the complete removal of the lesions extending to deep soft tissue layer such as pelvic cavity is important for prevention of recurrence. On MRI, osteolysis is seen as intermediate to low signal intensity on T2-weighted image [52]. Involvement of both femoral and acetabular components, well-demarcated margin of soft tissue lesion, and no fatty infiltration are differential points of infectious or tumorous condition.

Infection reveals no remarkable finding on plain radiographs in many cases because it can be diagnosed clinically based on laboratory finding in early stage. Instead, increased uptake on bone scintigraphy with ^{67}Ga-citrate or ^{111}In-WBC in combination with ^{99m}Tc-sulfur colloid and fluid collection adjacent to the prosthesis detected on US are useful. Differentiation of infection from aseptic fluid collection on US, even in conjunction with laboratory results, may be ambiguous in some cases [48]. For such cases, US-guided aspiration or synovial biopsy has an important role in diagnosing infectious condition and its causing organism by microbiologic study. Rarely, in the cases with more aggressive organisms, radiographic findings suggestive of typical osteomyelitis, such as rapidly destructive, ill-defined osteolytic lesion, periosteal reaction, and soft tissue edema, can be observed. Soft tissue abnormalities such as fluid collection or sinus tract detected on CT or US are a more feasible diagnostic points rather than periprosthetic bone abnormalities [53] (Fig. 23.19).

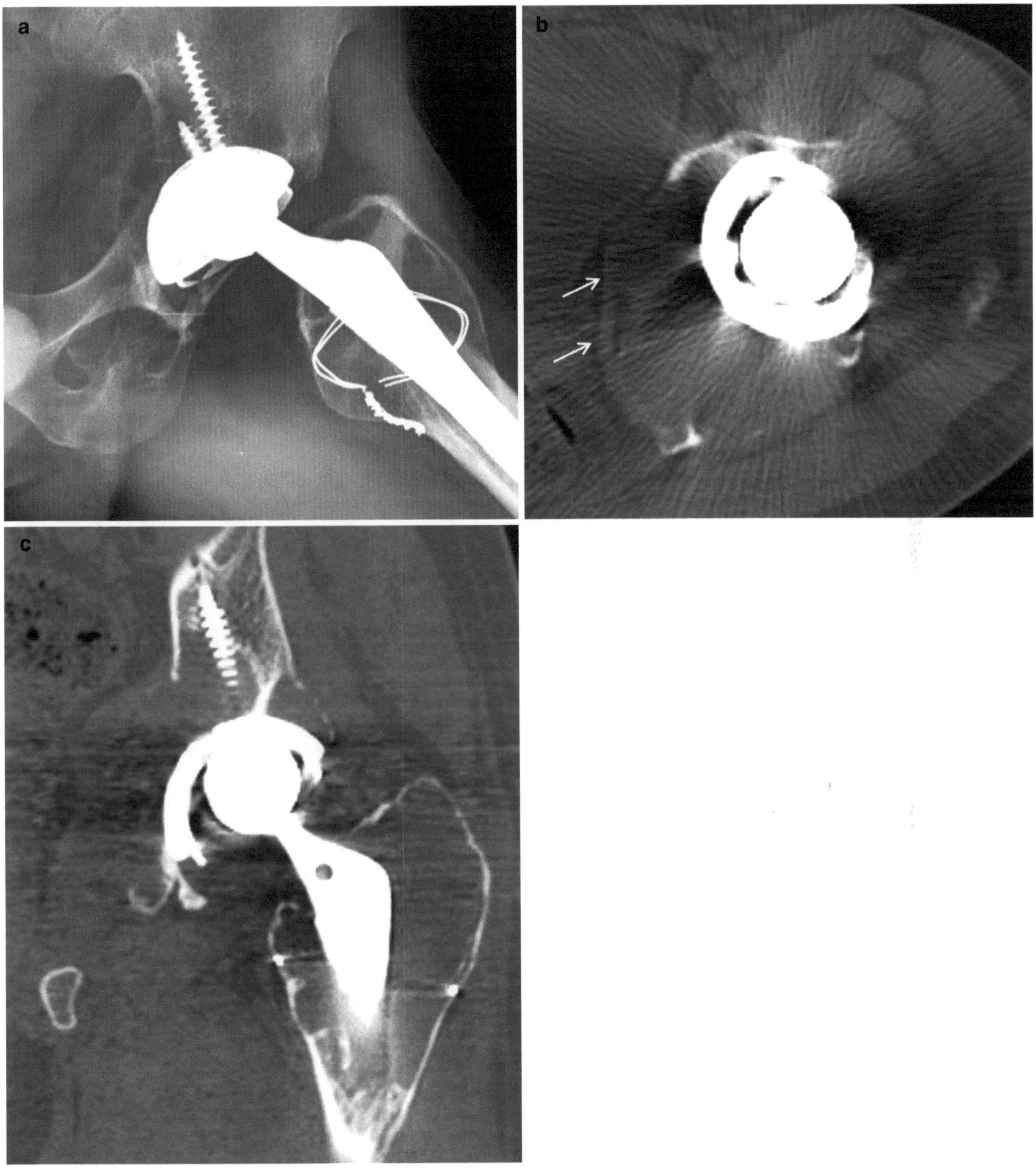

Fig. 23.17 Osteolysis in a 73-year-old male with hip arthroplasty 17 years ago. (**a**) Frog leg view of the left hip shows well-defined, multilobular, expansile, osteolytic lesions involving both femoral and acetabular components. Joint space narrowing of superior direction, suggestive of liner wear, and wire fracture of femoral component are also seen. (**b**, **c**) Axial (**b**) and reformatted coronal (**c**) CT images clearly exhibit the extent of expansile osteolytic lesions. A soft tissue mass originating from the acetabulum via cortical discontinuity displaces the obturator internus muscle (*arrows*). Endosteal scalloping of femoral lesion and loss of superior joint space due to liner wear are well visualized

Periprosthetic fracture occurs commonly in femoral shaft adjacent to the tip of the femoral stem. Dislocation may develop in trauma, imbalance of muscle tone, or infection. These complications can be diagnosed only using plain radiographs. But the associated or related lesions should be evaluated by cross-sectional images and US.

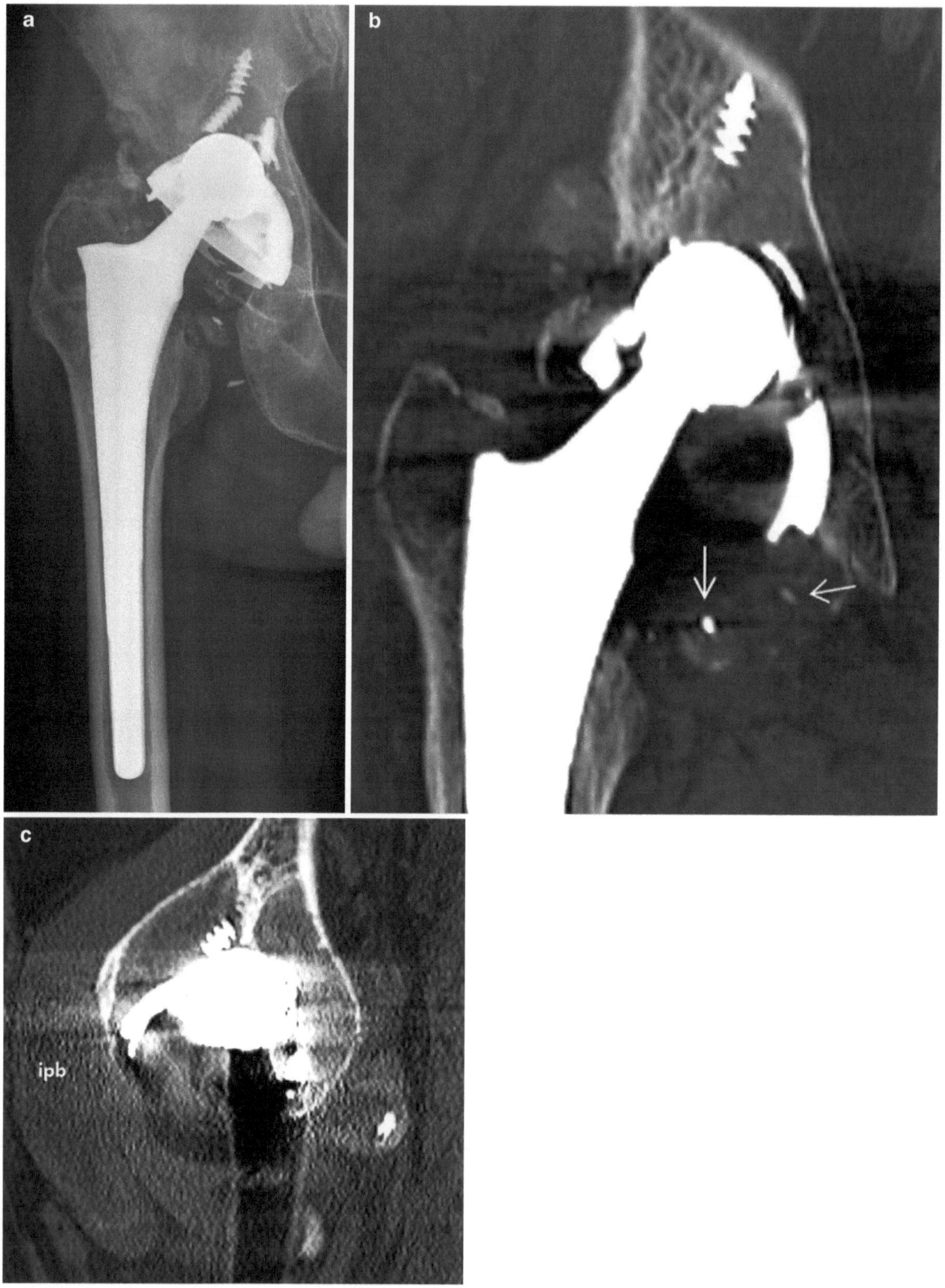

Fig. 23.18 Osteolysis and metallosis with severe wearing of polyethylene liner in a 60-year-old male who underwent hip arthroplasty 18 years ago. (**a**) Anteroposterior view of the right hip joint shows relatively well-defined, multilobular osteolytic lesions involving both the acetabular and femoral components, with internal radiodense opacities. Superior migration of the femoral head through the defect of acetabular cup and polyethylene liner is noted. (**b**) Coronal reformatted CT image demonstrates the extent of expansile osteolytic lesions and intralesional metallic radiodense opacities. Scattered liner fragments (*arrows*) are noted at inferomedial aspect of the right hip. (**c**) On sagittal reformatted CT image, iliopsoas bursitis (*IPB*) and soft tissue mass communicating with osteolysis are located at the anterior and posterior aspects of the right acetabulum and reveal radiodense peripheral rims, predictive of metallosis

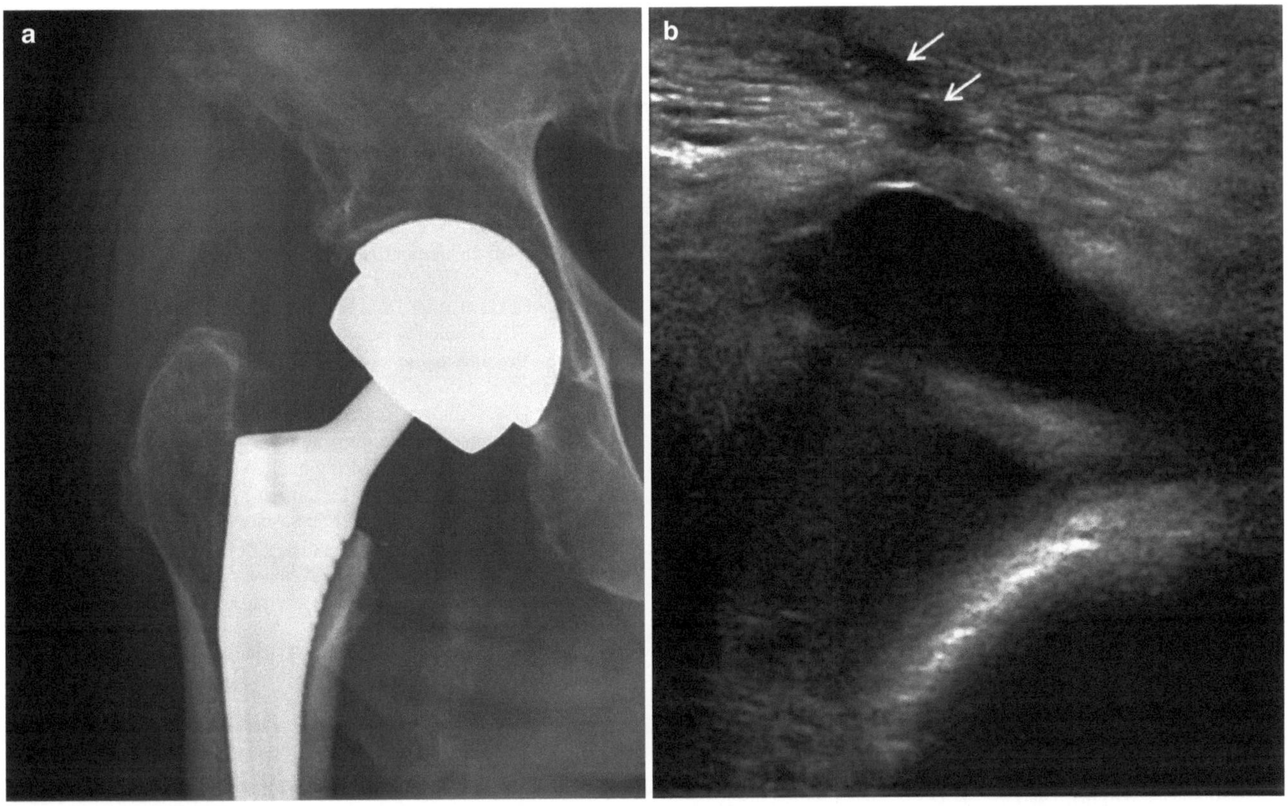

Fig. 23.19 Infected arthroplasty in an 84-year-old patient. (**a**) Hip anteroposterior view demonstrates soft tissue edema at lateral aspect of right hip without osseous abnormality. (**b**) On ultrasonography, large amount of fluid collection with echogenic debris are observed at lateral aspect of right hip. This lesion is contiguous with sinus tract (*arrows*), suggestive of infected fluid collection

Wearing or dissociation of polyethylene liner manifest as asymmetric location of the femoral head in the acetabular cup on radiographs. It is commonly accompanied by osteolysis, metallosis, and loosening (Figs. 23.17 and 23.18).

Stress shielding develops due to altered stress loading on the native bone. It shows decreased bone density with intracortical tunneling, corticocancellization, and rounding of the medial cortex in the proximal femoral component of cementless THR. Most cases stabilize within the first postoperative year, but it may progress to fracture.

Rupture of the adductor tendon, atrophy or tear of the abductor tendons such as gluteus medius/minimus, or trochanteric bursitis can result in symptomatic hips. These soft tissue lesions can be diagnosed using MRI and US [48, 54].

23.3.3 Resurfacing Arthroplasty (RSA)

RSA or metal-on-metal prosthesis is increasingly performed for the active or younger patients with limited extent of ON. Although better clinical outcome was reported compared with THR, most complications after THR can also occur after RSA, except liner wear. Particularly, synovitis is common in RSA, with similar incidence compared with THR [55]. MRI with metal artifact reducing sequences (MARS) exhibits fluid signal intensity or intermediate to low signal debris communicating with the pseudocapsule of the hip joint.

23.4 Summary

Radiological examinations of ON of the femoral head are important not only for diagnostic purposes but also for evaluation of disease progression during follow-up. Imaging modalities such as MRI, CT, radionuclide examination, PET-CT including plain radiograph show characteristic findings. However, plain radiograph and MRI are the most important modalities considering sensitivity and specificity. Radionuclide examination with unilateral osteonecrosis would show subsidiary roles when diagnosing the contralateral side. The rest of the imaging modalities are not used for diagnostic purposes. Knowledge and recognition for the imaging findings of ON involving femoral head can reduce misdiagnosis for other conditions and lead to appropriate management.

References

1. Mitchell MD, Kundel HL, Steinberg ME, Kressel HY, Alavi A, Axel L. Avascular necrosis of the hip: comparison of MR, CT, and scintigraphy. AJR Am J Roentgenol. 1986;147(1):67–71.
2. Lavernia CJ, Sierra RJ, Grieco FR. Osteonecrosis of the femoral head. J Am Acad Orthop Surg. 1999;7(4):250–61.
3. Malizos KN, Karantanas AH, Varitimidis SE, Dailiana ZH, Bargiotas K, Maris T. Osteonecrosis of the femoral head: etiology, imaging and treatment. Eur J Radiol. 2007;63(1):16–28.
4. Kokubo T, Takatori Y, Ninomiya S, Nakamura T, Kamogawa M. Magnetic resonance imaging and scintigraphy of avascular necrosis of the femoral head: prediction of subsequent. Segmental collapse. Clin Orthop. 1992;277:54–60.
5. Mitchell DG, Rao VM, Dalinka MK, Spritzer CE, Alavi A, Steinberg ME, Fallon M, Kressel HY. Femoral head avascular necrosis: correlation of MR imaging, radiographic staging, radionuclide imaging, and clinical findings. Radiology. 1987;162(3):709–15.
6. Beltran J, Herman LJ, Burk JM, Zuelzer WA, Clark RN, Lucas JG, Weiss LD, Yang A. Femoral head avascular necrosis: MR imaging with clinical-pathologic and radionuclide correlation. Radiology. 1988;166(1 Pt 1):215–20.
7. Dasa V, Adbel-Nabi H, Anders MJ, Mihalko WM. F-18 fluoride positron emission tomography of the hip for osteonecrosis. Clin Orthop Relat Res. 2008;466(5):1081–6.
8. Gayana S, Bhattacharya A, Kashyap R, Sen RK, Mittal BR. 18F-fluoride PET/CT in avascular necrosis of the femoral head. Clin Nucl Med. 2013;38(6):e265–6.
9. Ficat RP, Arlet J. Ischemia and necrosis of bone. Baltimore: Williams & Wilkins; 1980. p. 29–52.
10. Ficat RP. Idiopathic bone necrosis of the femoral head: early diagnosis and treatment. J Bone Joint Surg Br. 1985;67(1):3–9.
11. Marcus ND, Enneking WF, Massam RA. The silent hip in idiopathic aseptic necrosis: treatment by bone-grafting. J Bone Joint Surg Am. 1973;55(7):1351–66.
12. Steinberg ME, Hayken GD, Steinberg DR. A quantitative system for staging avascular necrosis. J Bone Joint Surg Br. 1995;77(1):34–41.
13. Ohzono K, Saito M, Takaoka K, Ono K, Saito S, Nishina T, Kadowaki T. Natural history of nontraumatic avascular necrosis of the femoral head. J Bone Joint Surg Br. 1991;73(1):68–72.
14. Ohzono K, Saito M, Sugano N, Takaoka K, Ono K. The fate of nontraumatic avascular necrosis of the femoral head: a radiologic classification to formulate prognosis. Clin Orthop. 1992;277:73–8.
15. Mont MA, Hungerford DS. Non-traumatic avascular necrosis of the femoral head. J Bone Joint Surg Am. 1995;77(3):459–74.
16. Sugano N, Takaoka K, Ohzono K, Matsui M, Masuhara K, Ono K. Prognostication of nontraumatic avascular necrosis of the femoral head: significance of location and size of the necrotic lesion. Clin Orthop. 1994;303:155–64.
17. Ryu KN, Kim EJ, Yoo MC, Park YG, Sartoris DJ, Resnick D. Ischemic necrosis of the entire femoral head and rapidly destructive hip disease: potential causative relationship. Skeletal Radiol. 1997;26(3):143–9.
18. Genez BM, Wilson MR, Houk RW, Weiland FL, Unger Jr HR, Shields NN, Rugh KS. Early osteonecrosis of the femoral head: detection in high-risk patients with MR imaging. Radiology. 1988;168(2):521–4.
19. Coleman BG, Kressel HY, Dalinka MK, Scheibler ML, Burk DL, Cohen EK. Radiographically negative avascular necrosis: detection with MR imaging. Radiology. 1988;168(2):525–8.
20. Fordyce MJ, Solomon L. Early detection of avascular necrosis of the femoral head by MRI. J Bone Joint Surg Br. 1993;75(3):365–7.
21. Markisz JA, Knowles RJ, Altchek DW, Schneider R, Whalen JP, Cahill PT. Segmental patterns of avascular necrosis of the femoral heads: early detection with MR imaging. Radiology. 1987;162(3):717–20.
22. Karantanas AH, Drakonaki EE. The role of MR imaging in avascular necrosis of the femoral head. Semin Musculoskelet Radiol. 2011;15(3):281–300.
23. Huang GS, Chan WP, Chang YC, Chang CY, Chen CY, Yu JS. MR imaging of bone marrow edema and joint effusion in patients with osteonecrosis of the femoral head: relationship to pain. AJR Am J Roentgenol. 2003;181(2):545–9.
24. Koo KH, Ahn IO, Kim R, Song HR, Jeong ST, Na JB, Kim YS, Cho SH. Bone marrow edema and associated pain in early stage osteonecrosis of the femoral head: prospective study with serial MR images. Radiology. 1999;213(3):715–22.
25. Tervonen O, Mueller DM, Matteson EL, Velosa JA, Ginsburg WW, Ehman RL. Clinically occult avascular necrosis of the hip: prevalence in an asymptomatic population at risk. Radiology. 1992;182(3):845–7.
26. Stoller DW, Sampson T, Bredella M. The hip. In: Stoller DW, editor. Magnetic resonance imaging in orthopaedics and sports medicine. 3rd ed. Philadelphia: Lippincott Williams & Wilkins; 2007.
27. Vande Berg BE, Malghem JJ, Labaisse MA, Noel HM, Maldague BE. MR imaging of avascular necrosis and transient marrow edema of the femoral head. Radiographics. 1993;13(3):501–20.
28. Duda SH, Laniado M, Schick F, Claussen CD. The double-line sign of osteonecrosis: evaluation on chemical shift MR images. Eur J Radiol. 1993;16(3):233–8.
29. Sugimoto H, Okubo RS, Ohsawa T. Chemical shift and the double-line sign in MRI of early femoral avascular necrosis. J Comput Assist Tomogr. 1992;16(5):727–30.
30. Mitchell DG. MR of the normal and ischemic hip. Magn Reson Annu. 1988:37–69.
31. Iida S, Harada Y, Shimizu K, Sakamoto M, Ikenoue S, Akita T, Kitahara H, Moriya H. Correlation between bone marrow edema and collapse of the femoral head in steroid-induced osteonecrosis. AJR Am J Roentgenol. 2000;174(3):735–43.
32. Ito H, Matsuno T, Minami A. Relationship between bone marrow edema and development of symptoms in patients with osteonecrosis of the femoral head. AJR Am J Roentgenol. 2006;186(6):1761–70.
33. Nadel SN, Debatin JF, Richardson WJ, Hedlund LW, Senft C, Rizk WS, Malizos KN, Stahl DL, Martinez S. Detection of acute avascular necrosis of the femoral head in dogs: dynamic contrast-enhanced MR imaging vs spin-echo and STIR sequences. AJR Am J Roentgenol. 1992;159(6):1255–61.
34. Vande Berg B, Malghem J, Labaisse MA, Noel H, Maldague B. Avascular necrosis of the hip: comparison of contrast-enhanced and nonenhanced MR imaging with Histologic correlation. Radiology. 1992;182(2):445–50.
35. Kaushik A, Sankaran B, Varghese M. To study the role of dynamic magnetic resonance imaging in assessing the femoral head vascularity in intracapsular femoral neck fractures. Eur J Radiol. 2010;75(3):364–75.
36. Kaushik A, Sankaran B, Varghese M. Prognostic value of dynamic MRI in assessing post-traumatic femoral head vascularity. Skeletal Radiol. 2009;38(6):565–9.
37. Chan WP, Liu YJ, Huang GS, Lin MF, Huang S, Chang YC, Jiang CC. Relationship idiopathic osteonecrosis of the femoral head to perfusion changes in the proximal femur by dynamic contrast-enhanced MRI. AJR Am J Roentgenol. 2011;196(3):637–43.
38. Wang YX, Griffith JF, Deng M, T Ma H, Zhang YF, Yan SX, Ahuja AT. Compromised perfusion in femoral head in normal rats: distinctive perfusion MRI evidence of contrast washout delay. Br J Radiol. 2012;85(1016):e436–41.
39. Dihlmann W. CT analysis of the upper end of the femur: the asterisk sign and ischaemic bone necrosis of the femoral head. Skeletal Radiol. 1982;8(4):251–8.
40. Mitchell DG, Kressel HY, Arger PH, Dalinka M, Spritzer CE, Steinberg ME. Avascular necrosis of the femoral head: morphologic

assessment by MR imaging with CT correlation. Radiology. 1986;161(3):739–42.

41. Conway WF, Totty WG, McEnery KW. CT and MR imaging of the hip. Radiology. 1996;198(2):297–307.
42. Resnick D, Sweet DE, Madewell JE. Osteonecrosis: pathogenesis, diagnostic techniques, specific situations, and complications. In: Resnick D, editor. Bone and joint imaging. 3rd ed. Philadelphia: Saunders; 2005.
43. Collier BD, Carrera GF, Johnson RP, Isitman AT, Hellman RS, Knobel J, Finger WA, Gonyo JE, Malloy PJ. Detection of femoral head avascular necrosis in adults by SPECT. J Nucl Med. 1985;26(9):979–87.
44. Cook GJ, Fogelman I. The role of positron emission tomography in skeletal disease. Semin Nucl Med. 2001;31(1):50–61.
45. Forrest N, Welch A, Murray AD, Schweiger L, Hutchison J, Ashcroft GP. Femoral head viability after Birmingham resurfacing hip arthroplasty: assessment with use of [18F] fluoride positron emission tomography. J Bone Joint Surg Am. 2006;88 Suppl 3:84–9.
46. Sofka CM. Optimizing techniques for musculoskeletal imaging of the postoperative patient. Radiol Clin North Am. 2006;44(3):323–9.
47. Beall DP, Martin HD, Ly JQ, Campbell SE, Anderson S, Tannast M. Postoperative imaging of the hip. Radiol Clin North Am. 2006;44(3):343–65.
48. Douis H, Dunlop DJ, Pearson AM, O'Hara JN, James SL. The role of ultrasound in the assessment of post-operative complications following hip arthroplasty. Skeletal Radiol. 2012;41(9):1035–46.
49. Beltran J, Knight CT, Zuelzer WA, Morgan JP, Shwendeman LJ, Chandnani VP, Mosure JC, Shaffer PB. Core decompression for avascular necrosis of the femoral head: correlation between long-term results and pre-operative MR staging. Radiology. 1990;175(2):533–6.
50. Radke S, Kirschner S, Seipel V, Rader C, Eulert J. Magnetic resonance imaging criteria of successful core decompression in avascular necrosis of the hip. Skeletal Radiol. 2004;33(9):519–23.
51. Lee MS, Kim SJ, Lee SA, Song HT, Huh YM, Kim DH, Han SH, Suh JS. Overcoming artifacts from metallic orthopedic implants at high-field-strength MR imaging and multidetector CT. Radiographics. 2007;27(3):791–803.
52. White LM, Kim JE, Mehta M, Merchant N, Schweitzer ME, Morrison WB, Hutchison CR, Gross AE. Complications of total hip arthroplasty: MR imaging-initial experience. Radiology. 2000;215(1):254–62.
53. Cyteval C, Hamm V, Sarrabère MP, Lopez FM, Maury P, Taourel P. Painful infection at the site of hip prosthesis: CT imaging. Radiology. 2002;224(2):477–83.
54. Pfirrmann CW, Notzli HP, Dora C, Hodler J, Zanetti M. Abductor tendons and muscles assessed at MR imaging after total hip arthroplasty in asymptomatic and symptomatic patients. Radiology. 2005;235(3):969–76.
55. Hayter CL, Gold SL, Koff MF, Perino G, Nawabi DH, Miller TT, Potter HG. MRI findings in painful metal-on-metal hip arthroplasty. AJR Am J Roentgenol. 2012;199(4):884–93.

Part VIII

Staging and Classification

24 Ficat Staging System

Kyung-Hoi Koo

24.1 Introduction

Osteonecrosis of the femoral head is progressive to collapse of the femoral head and secondary osteoarthritis of the hip in 60–80 % of the cases. However, when the necrosis is small and a considerable portion of the weight-bearing dome of the femoral head is viable, the disease is not progressive and patients are doing well for a prolonged time or during their whole life without any medical or surgical intervention. Thus, the classification of osteonecrosis should include the "stage," which expresses the status of disease progression, and the "extent," which describes the size of necrosis.

Several different systems to categorize the stage and size of the necrotic portion have been developed and used.

In terms of staging, the Ficat system [1] and ARCO system [2] have been used. For the evaluation of the necrotic extent, the Kerboul method [3] and its modification using MRI [4] and JIC (Japanese Investigation Committee) classification [5] are used.

Steinberg et al. have developed a comprehensive system including both stage and extent [6].

Ficat developed a staging system of femoral head osteonecrosis based on clinical symptoms, functional evaluation of bone, and radiologic findings [1].

Although his staging system was developed in the early 1980s and not based on MRI, it is still in use worldwide because it is simple and easy to use.

K.-H. Koo
Department of Orthopaedic Surgery,
Seoul National University College of Medicine, Seoul National University Bundang Hospital, 166 Gumi-ro,
Seongnam 463-707, South Korea
e-mail: khkoo@snu.ac.kr

24.2 Functional Exploration of Bone

Ficat's classification was based on two fundamental concepts. The first concept is that all osteonecrosis should pass through a preradiologic stage, which has no specific radiographic appearance. Thus, a radiograph cannot detect early-stage osteonecrosis and a normal radiograph does not necessarily mean a normal hip. Radiographic changes do appear after the reaction of living tissue to the ischemia. The second fundamental concept is that osteonecrosis is the end result of severe and prolonged ischemia. This again presupposes an initial stage in which vascular and medullary abnormality passes undetected by routine radiography.

Because MRI was not available in the early 1980s, he emphasized the need for a study of the hemodynamics of the medullary circulation, which he termed the functional exploration of bone (FEB) [7]. Functional exploration of bone is a method for diagnosis of early-stage osteonecrosis. It consisted of three stages: (1) measurement of bone marrow pressure, (2) intramedullary venography, and (3) core biopsy.

Measurement of bone marrow pressure can be done through a cannula placed in the intertrochanteric area under local anesthesia. The baseline pressure is usually about 20 mmHg, and 30 mmHg is regarded as the upper limit of normal.

If the baseline pressure is within normal limits, 5 ml of isotonic saline is injected into the bone and the pressure recorded 5 min after injection. This, the "stress test" pressure, is normally less than 10 mmHg above the baseline pressure. In cases of bone necrosis, the baseline pressure is above 30 mmHg, and the stress test pressure is 10 mmHg or more above the baseline after 5 min.

To obtain intramedullary venography, 10 ml of contrast medium is injected through the cannula used for the stress test. In a normal hip the medium can be injected without a

K.-H. Koo et al. (eds.), *Osteonecrosis*,
DOI 10.1007/978-3-642-35767-1_24, © Springer-Verlag Berlin Heidelberg 2014

resistance and is quickly cleared. In cases of osteonecrosis the injection is difficult and painful, with a reflux into the diaphysis and intramedullary stasis 15 min after injection.

Core biopsy establishes the diagnosis with certainty. The histological lesions have been classified by Arlet and Durroux (1973) into four types:

Type 1. Disappearance of the hemopoietic marrow, separation of the lipocytes by edema or hemorrhage, and the presence of foam cells

Type 2. Necrosis of the fatty marrow, which is largely changed to an eosinophilic reticular pattern, sometimes with oil cysts and necrosis of the hemopoietic marrow of a granular type

Type 3. Complete medullary and trabecular necrosis

Type 4. Complete necrosis with dense medullary fibrosis and new bone formation in apposition to the dead trabeculae

The histology should be interpreted cautiously. First, it should be stated that Type 1 histology is not diagnostic of osteonecrosis. Secondly, all four types may be observed in the same specimen. Thirdly, it seems logical to suppose that the ischemic process develops in three successive stages: circulatory (Type I), medullary (Type 2), and osseous (Types 3 and 4). Finally, it should be emphasized that there is little or no correlation between the histological typing and the radiographic or clinical features.

Since the wide use of MRI in the diagnosis of early-stage osteonecrosis, the functional exploration of bone is not done as a diagnostic workup.

24.3 Staging

Ficat divided the disease process into five stages. He defined asymptomatic period as stage 0 and painful period as stage I. In stage 0 and stage 1, the diagnosis of osteonecrosis cannot be made by standard radiographs. Because MRI was not available at that time, the diagnosis in the early stage can be made only through the functional exploration of bone. In his staging, an important consideration is collapse of the femoral head. He thought the collapse as the point of no return in the progression of the disease. He thought the medical or surgical treatment can aborts the progression of the disease and a complete recovery may be possible prior to collapse. However, the recovery is not possible once a collapse occurred.

Stage 0. This stage is both preclinical and preradiographic. Ficat suspected this stage in one hip when the other has definite osteonecrosis. Hungerford described this stage as "silent hip" [8–10].

Stage I. This is the earliest clinical manifestation of the hip pain before radiographic changes appear.

Stage II. Radiographs show changes in the femoral head. Curvilinear sclerosis is seen around the necrotic portion. Decalcification may also be seen in the form of small cysts in the necrotic potion.

Transition Between Stages II and III. There are a crescentic line due to a subchondral fracture and *segmental flattening* of the femoral head giving the so-called "out of round" appearance.

Stage III. This stage is characterized by the pathognomonic appearance of a sequestrum on the radiograph. The sequestrum later becomes manifest by a break in the articular margin extending from one end of the affected area to the other, followed by collapse of the sequestrated area into the femoral head. However, the joint space is preserved.

Stage IV. This is the terminal phase of the necrotic process and is characterized by progressive loss of articular cartilage and the development of acetabular osteophytes; the radiographic picture is of osteoarthritis superimposed on a deformed femoral head.

References

1. Ficat RP. Idiopathic bone necrosis of the femoral head. Early diagnosis and treatment. J Bone Joint Surg Br. 1985;67(1):3–9.
2. ARCO (Association Research Circulation Osseous): Committee on terminology and classification. ARCO News. 1992;4:41–6.
3. Kerboul M, Thomine J, Postel M, Merle d'Aubigné R. The conservative surgical treatment of idiopathic aseptic necrosis of the femoral head. J Bone Joint Surg Br. 1974;56(2):291–6.
4. Ha YC, Jung WH, Kim JR, Seong NH, Kim SY, Koo KH, et al. Prediction of collapse in femoral head osteonecrosis: a modified Kerboul method with use of magnetic resonance images. J Bone Joint Surg Am. 2006;88:35–40. doi:10.2106/JBJS.F.00535. 88/suppl_3/35 [pii].
5. Ohzono K, Saito M, Sugano N, Takaoka K, Ono K. The fate of nontraumatic avascular necrosis of the femoral head. A radiologic classification to formulate prognosis. Clin Orthop Relat Res. 1992;277:73–8.
6. Steinberg ME, Hayken GD, Steinberg DR. A quantitative system for staging avascular necrosis. J Bone Joint Surg Br. 1995;77(1):34–41.
7. Ficat RP, Arlet J. Ischemia and necrosis of bone. Baltimore/London: Williams & Wilkins; 1980. p. 196.
8. Marcus ND, Enneking WF, Massam RA. The silent hip in idiopathic aseptic necrosis. Treatment by bone-grafting. J Bone Joint Surg Am. 1973;55(7):1351–66.
9. Hungerford DS. Bone marrow pressure, venography and core decompression in ischemic necrosis of the femoral head. In: The hip: proceedings of the seventh open scientific meeting of The Hip Society. St Louis: CV Mosby; 1979. p. 218–37.
10. Hungerford DS, Zizic TM. Pathogenesis of ischemic necrosis of the femoral head. In: Hungerford DS, editor. The hip: proceedings of the eleventh open scientific meeting of The Hip Society. St Louis/Toronto: CV Mosby; 1983. p. 249–62.

The University of Pennsylvania Classification of Osteonecrosis

25

David R. Steinberg and Marvin E. Steinberg

25.1 Introduction

The management of osteonecrosis (ON) remains one of the more perplexing problems facing the orthopedic surgeon. There is still much to be learned about the etiology, pathophysiology, and management of this condition. Because prognosis and treatment are determined in large part by the stage of the disease, it is important to use a reliable and efficient method of evaluation and staging. The uniform use of such a system of classification would also enable us to compare the effectiveness of various methods of treatment and determine the best method of management for different stages of osteonecrosis.

During the 1970s we began to see a steady increase in the number of patients with osteonecrosis being treated at our institution. In attempting to evaluate these patients, we found that the classification systems in use at that time were helpful, but none was ideal [1, 2]. These included the classifications of Ficat and Arlet [3, 4]; the system of Marcus, Enneking, and Massam [5]; the use of angular measurements described by Kerboul [6]; and the radiographic staging of Sugioka [7]. We therefore felt that it would be valuable to formulate a new, comprehensive, and quantifiable system of classification and staging. Initially we set down the parameters to be included in an ideal system:

- It should correspond closely to the pathologic and radiographic changes that occur in osteonecrosis.
- It should clearly and distinctly characterize each separate stage.
- In addition to the stage, it must allow us to measure and indicate both the size of the necrotic lesion and the extent of joint involvement.
- It should be objective, simple to use, and reproducible.
- It should allow us to trace progression or resolution from the earliest to the latest stages.
- Symptoms and physical findings, although important in management, should not be part of the classification itself.
- Older, invasive techniques should be eliminated and newer diagnostic modalities such as MRI must be included.
- The system should allow for the future development of even more sensitive methods of diagnosis and evaluation.
- Its effectiveness should be established in actual clinical use and its advantages over other systems should be documented.

In 1979, in conjunction with our colleagues in the Department of Radiology, we began to develop a quantitative method for classification and staging which would include the parameters outlined above. Initially, technetium scans and computerized tomography were used to identify pre-radiographic lesions. By 1982 we had begun to use nuclear magnetic resonance (NMR) – later designated as magnetic resonance imaging (MRI) [8–10]. We examined 55 hips with biopsy-proven ON which were studied by radiographs, technetium scans, CT, and MRI. We found MRI to be the single most effective method for early diagnosis of this condition with a high degree of sensitivity and specificity. It was found to be significantly more accurate in diagnosis of pre-radiographic lesions than either technetium scans or CT. On the basis of these studies, MRI became an integral part of our staging system, and CT and technetium scans were rarely used [11, 12].

D.R. Steinberg (✉)
Department of Orthopaedic Surgery, Perelman School of Medicine, University of Pennsylvania, Philadelphia, PA, USA

Department of Orthopaedic Surgery, Penn Presbyterian Medical Center, 3900 Market Street, One Cupp Pavilion, Philadelphia, PA 19104, USA
e-mail: david.steinberg@uphs.upenn.edu

M.E. Steinberg
Department of Orthopaedic Surgery, Perelman School of Medicine, University of Pennsylvania, Philadelphia, PA, USA

Department of Orthopaedic Surgery, Hospital of the University of Pennsylvania, Silverstein 2 3400 Spruce Street, Philadelphia, PA 19104, USA
e-mail: marvin.steinberg@uphs.upenn.edu

K.-H. Koo et al. (eds.), *Osteonecrosis*,
DOI 10.1007/978-3-642-35767-1_25, © Springer-Verlag Berlin Heidelberg 2014

The classification that was developed was presented in 1982 at the Third International Symposium on Circulation in Bone in Toulouse, France, and published in 1984 [13]. Initially the type of pathologic change identified on imaging studies is used to place the hip in one of seven stages. Once the stage has been determined, the size of the necrotic segment and the extent of involvement of the femoral head and acetabulum are indicated as mild (A), moderate (B), or severe (C). For routine clinical use a simple estimate of the extent of involvement is sufficient, whereas for research projects and publications, it can be measured [11, 14] (Table 25.1).

25.1.1 Determining Stage

- Stage 0. Stage 0 indicates that a hip is suspected of having ON although radiographs and MR are normal or nondiagnostic, such as a painful hip in a patient with proven ON in the opposite hip. Stage 0 would include hips evaluated too soon after a precipitating event for changes to appear or hips with too small an area of involvement to be detected with current modalities. The diagnosis might be made some time after the original evaluation when the lesion appears on imaging studies. A definitive diagnosis in stage 0 will also most likely be possible in the future with further refinements in our diagnostic techniques. Thus, inclusion of stage 0 will extend the useful life of this classification.
- Stage I. Plain radiographs are normal, but MRI and/or technetium scans indicate the presence of ON.
- Stage II. Radiographs now show definitive abnormalities consistent with ON. These consist of radiolucent and/or sclerotic regions, at times demarcated from normal bone by a sclerotic border. Rarely, the earliest radiographic findings will include generalized osteopenia of the femoral head.
- Stage III. Stage III is diagnosed by the appearance of a radiolucent crescent line just beneath the subchondral end plate, but without flattening of the femoral head. This indicates collapse of the cancellous trabeculae beneath an intact articular surface. A crescent sign does not always appear as the head progresses from earlier to later stages and may be seen in only one radiographic projection. A relatively small percentage of hips will fit the criteria for stage III. However, we feel that they should be assigned a separate stage rather than being grouped together with hips which show gross flattening of the articular surface because clinical experience documents a better outcome for hips in stage III than for hips in stage IV, where flattening is already present [1, 15–18]. The hip is still spherical at this stage and it is theoretically possible to preserve its normal anatomy by bone grafting or other procedures.

Table 25.1 University of pennsylvania classification of osteonecrosis

Stage	Criteria	
0	Normal or nondiagnostic radiograph, bone scan, and MRI	
I	Normal radiograph; abnormal bone scan and/or MRI	
	A – Mild	(<15 % of head affected)
	B – Moderate	(15–30 %)
	C – Severe	(>30 %)
II	Lucent and sclerotic changes in femoral head	
	A – Mild	(<15 %)
	B – Moderate	(15–30 %)
	C – Severe	(>30 %)
III	Subchondral collapse (crescent sign) without flattening	
	A – Mild	(<15 % of articular surface)
	B – Moderate	(15–30 %)
	C – Severe	(>30 %)
IV	Flattening of femoral head	
	A – Mild	(<15 % of surface and <2 mm depression)
	B – Moderate	(15–30 % of surface or 2–4 mm depression)
	C – Severe	(>30 % of surface or >4 mm depression)
V	Joint narrowing and/or acetabular changes	
	A – Mild B – Moderate C – Severe	Average of femoral head involvement, as determined in stage IV, and estimated acetabular involvement
VI	Advanced degenerative changes	

- Stage IV. There is now definite flattening of the femoral head which appears in either the AP, lateral, or both views. Occasionally small areas of collapse cannot be seen on plain radiographs but can be detected with CT. The acetabulum appears radiographically normal at this stage. However, early changes in the acetabular cartilage have been identified in the majority of stage IV hip patients whose pain and disability were sufficient for them to require arthroplasty. Stage IV has serious implications, because irreversible changes have taken place and a "normal" femoral head cannot be anticipated despite appropriate treatment.
- Stage V. In addition to flattening of the femoral head, there is now clear radiographic evidence of joint line narrowing and later sclerosis and cystic changes in the acetabulum. Progressive degenerative changes follow.
- Stage VI. Degenerative changes in both the femoral head and acetabulum have progressed to the point where the joint line is virtually obliterated and marked deformity appears. Other staging systems have grouped stages V and VI together; however, a small but definite number of hips develop changes so advanced that they can be distinguished from stage V. We thus feel that they deserve a separate designation and this allows us to follow progression more accurately.

25.1.2 Determining Extent of Involvement

After the type of radiographic and pathologic changes has determined the stage, the extent of involvement is next estimated or measured. For clinical purposes it is adequate to make a simple estimate and to describe this as mild (A), moderate (B), or severe (C). However, for research purposes it is preferable to make actual measurements as described below. No attempt is made to quantify the extent of involvement in stages 0 or VI.

In stages I and II the three-dimensional size or volume of the necrotic lesion is determined and expressed as a percentage of the entire head. In stage I this is estimated or calculated from serial MRI sections. In stage II, the MRI can be used in a similar fashion if it is available. However, in many cases where the lesion is clearly seen on radiographs, MRI will not be available and several methods can be used to determine the lesion size from plain radiographs. The most accurate involve the use of computerized image analysis. However, a reasonable estimate of lesion size has been made by some investigators using different types of angular measurements or by a simple visual estimate [1, 2, 6, 19–23].

In stage III it is first determined whether the crescent sign is more prominent in the AP or the lateral view. This view is then used to measure the length of the crescent and to express it as a percent of the length of the entire articular surface of the femoral head. This can be done with modern imaging techniques. If not available, one can use a map reading planimeter, a specially designed grid, or simple angular measurements.

In stage IV, as in stage III, measurements are made on either the AP or the lateral film, whichever shows the greatest amount of collapse. The normal contour of the femoral head before collapse is reconstituted, and then the length of the collapsed segment is measured and expressed as a percentage of the entire articular surface. The maximum depression of the collapsed segment is also measured and expressed in millimeters. This can be done as described for stage III.

In stage V the length of the collapsed segment and the amount of collapse of the femoral head are determined as described above. The degree of acetabular involvement is then estimated. The average of the femoral head and acetabular involvement determines the overall grade.

More detailed information about the University of Pennsylvania Classification can be found in our earlier publications [13, 14, 21]. These include a specific description of the methods originally used to measure lesion size and the extent of joint involvement. However, a number of technological advances using image analysis software have been made since that time, making it simpler and more accurate to obtain these measurements [22, 24].

25.2 Evaluation and Comparison with Other Classifications

The two most important features of the University of Pennsylvania Classification are the incorporation of MRI and specific measurements of lesion size as integral parts of the system. Both of these are now recognized as essential for inclusion in any effective classification. MRI is the single best modality for the early diagnosis of ON, before changes appear on radiographs. Its sensitivity and specificity have been confirmed [1, 10–12, 22–25]. Its use has made invasive mechanism for diagnosis, scintigraphy, and CT no longer necessary.

It is well established that the prognosis and hence the treatment of hips with ON is directly related to the size of the necrotic region even within the same stage [1, 15, 17–20, 22, 23, 26]. It is therefore essential to include an accurate measurement of lesion size as an integral part of the classification. This allows us to establish a prognosis, follow progression or resolution, compare different methods of treatment, and determine the best management for a patient with osteonecrosis. These represent significant improvements over older methods of classification which indicated only the stage and not the extent of involvement (Fig. 25.1).

The importance of lesion size is further supported by the number of more recent publications which describe

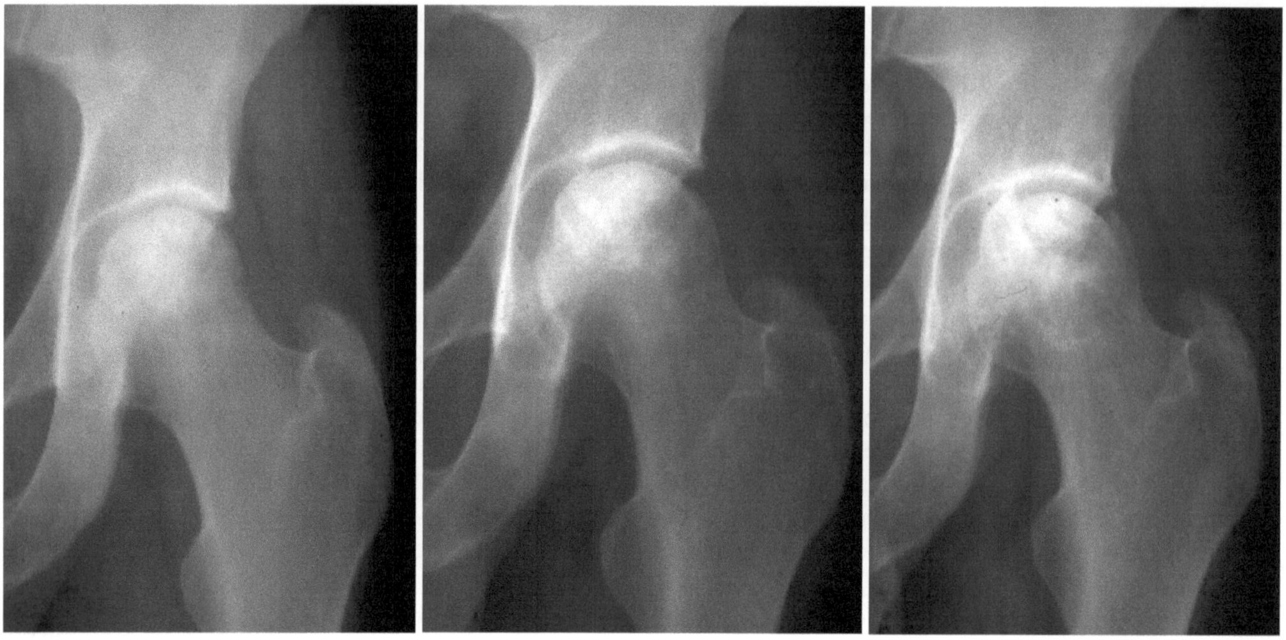

IV-A IV-B IV-C

Fig. 25.1 Anteroposterior radiographs of the left hip of a patient with stage IV osteonecrosis. In 4 months the condition progressed from stage IV-A to stage IV-B and eventually to stage IV-C. This obvious progression could not be indicated by using older non-quantitative methods of staging

alternate methods of measurement [19, 20, 23]. Several of these use angular measurements made on radiographs or MRI. Essentially all of these techniques have demonstrated some degree of correlation between lesion size and outcome. However, it is virtually impossible to determine which is more accurate because of the large number of variables involved, including the different methods of management they are used to evaluate. Although these techniques are useful and relatively simple to use, they cannot provide an accurate measurement of an irregular three-dimensional lesion. Neither are they designed to measure the extent of femoral head flattening or joint involvement. These techniques have been used to supplement an older, non-quantitative classification, such as that of Ficat and Arlet, and have not been incorporated into a comprehensive classification [2, 21].

Concern has been expressed that the University of Pennsylvania Classification may be too complex for general use. This concern has led to support for simpler methods to measure the size of the necrotic region such as the angular measurements described. It should be noted that the use of modern techniques of image analysis have simplified our ability to obtain accurate measurements compared to our original methods. In addition, both we and other investigators have found that visual estimates of lesion size made from radiographs or MRI by experienced examiners are both simple to obtain and reasonably accurate [2, 20, 21, 24].

Attempts to simplify this classification have also led some to combine our stages III and IV and eliminate stage VI. However, it has been shown that the prognosis and hence the management is different for hips with subchondral collapse alone (stage III), from hips with flattening of the articular surface (stage IV) [1, 15, 16, 18, 26]. Thus, not distinguishing between these stages has inherent disadvantages. This has also been supported by Arlet and Ficat who expanded their four-part classification to six parts to include a transition stage [3, 4, 27].

It has also been suggested that this classification be modified by adding an additional parameter of evaluation which combines the location with the size of the necrotic region [28, 29], as proposed by the Japanese Investigation Committee [30]. However, it is well established that the majority of necrotic lesions involve the anterolateral aspect of the femoral head and attempting to classify them as medial, central, or lateral does not accurately reflect the pathophysiology of ON. This modification would make the classification unnecessarily complex and provide little additional information [2, 26, 31, 32].

There are several other features of ON which are important to consider. For example, clinical evaluation of the patient with ON is, of course, essential to determine management. However, there is often little correlation between the radiographic stage and a patient's symptoms or physical findings, and therefore they are not included in this staging system. Whether the necrotic region appears primarily radiolucent or sclerotic may correlate with outcome. This should be noted, but likewise this is not part of the classification per se. We sought to include the most important factors but tried to prevent the system from becoming so complex as to be unwieldy.

The University of Pennsylvania Classification has been in use essentially unchanged since 1982. It has been used clinically to evaluate numerous patients with ON of the hip or shoulder, has been described in several publications, and specifically cited over 253 times. It was endorsed in 1991 by the ARCO Committee on Terminology and Staging [33], although it was modified in 1992 [29] and 1993 [34]. In 1992 it was also endorsed by the Committee on the Hip of the American Academy of Orthopaedic Surgeons. The essential parts of the system have been validated [14, 22, 24, 26], and it has proven itself quite useful in the evaluation and management of patients with ON. It has allowed us to develop an effective algorithm for the treatment of patients with osteonecrosis.

A recent review of articles on the treatment of ON, published in the past 25 years, showed that, although non-quantitative classifications are still frequently used and the four-part classification of Ficat and Arlet [4] is still the most often cited, there has been a steady trend towards the use of more comprehensive, quantitative systems of staging. The University of Pennsylvania Classification was cited next in frequency to that of Ficat and Arlet [32, 35].

25.3 Summary and Conclusions

The University of Pennsylvania Classification of osteonecrosis was first presented in 1982 at the Third International Symposium on Circulation in Bone and published in 1984. It was designed to identify each of the pathophysiologic changes which take place in joints afflicted by osteonecrosis, from the earliest to the most advanced. Seven specific stages were described based upon the type of change present. The extent of involvement was then identified and indicated by "A" (mild), "B" (moderate), or "C" (severe). To the best of our knowledge, this was the first classification to include both MRI and the extent of involvement as integral parts of a comprehensive method of evaluation and staging. It has withstood the test of time, has been validated, and has been described and cited in many publications. It allows us to establish a prognosis, follow progression or resolution, compare different methods of treatment, and determine the best method of management for a patient with osteonecrosis. It has proven more effective than earlier, non-quantitative methods of staging and has improved our ability to evaluate and treat patients with osteonecrosis. It is being used with increasing frequency by investigators treating and studying patients with osteonecrosis.

References

1. Steinberg ME. Diagnostic imaging and the role of stage and lesion size in determining outcome in osteonecrosis of the femoral head. Tech Orthop. 2001;16(1):6–15.
2. Steinberg ME, Steinberg DR. Classification systems for osteonecrosis: an overview. Orthop Clin North Am. 2004;35:273–83.
3. Arlet J, Ficat RP. Forage-biopsie de la tete femorale dans l'osteonecrose primitive. Observations histopathologiques portant sur huit foranes. Rev Rhum. 1964;31:257–64.
4. Ficat RP, Arlet J. Necrosis of the femoral head. In: Hungerford DS, editor. Ischemia and necrosis of bone. Baltimore: Williams and Wilkins; 1980. p. 53–74.
5. Marcus ND, Enneking WF, Massam RA. The silent hip in idiopathic aseptic necrosis: treatment by bone grafting. J Bone Joint Surg Am. 1973;55:1351–66.
6. Kerboul M, Thomine J, Postel M, Merle D'Aubigne R. The conservative surgical treatment of idiopathic aseptic necrosis of the femoral head. J Bone Joint Surg Br. 1974;56:291–6.
7. Sugioka Y, Katsuki I, Hotokebuchi T. Transtrochanteric rotational osteotomy of the femoral head for the treatment of osteonecrosis: follow-up statistics. Clin Orthop. 1982;169:115–25.
8. Axel L, Thickman D, Kressel HY, Weingrad T, Steinberg ME, Chen H, Edelstein W. NMR imaging of avascular necrosis. Magn Reson Med. 1984;1:93–4.
9. Steinberg ME, Chen HH, Thickman D, Alavi KA, Axel L, Fallon M, Kressel HY, Steinberg DR, Velchick MG. Early diagnosis of avascular necrosis by nuclear magnetic resonance. Orthop Trans. 1985;9(3):419.
10. Mitchell MD, Kundel HL, Steinberg ME, Kressel HY, Alavi A, Axel L. Avascular necrosis of the hip: comparison of MR. CT and scintigraphy. AJR Am J Roentgenol. 1986;147:67–71.
11. Steinberg ME, Brighton CT, Steinberg DR, Tooze SE, Hayken GD. Treatment of avascular necrosis of the femoral head by a combination of bone grafting, decompression, and electrical stimulation. Clin Orthop Relat Res. 1984;186:137–53.
12. Steinberg ME. Early diagnosis of avascular necrosis of the femoral head. Instructional course lectures. Published by the American Academy of Orthopaedic Surgeons. Vol 37. p. 51–7. Chapter 6; 1988.
13. Steinberg ME, Hayken GD, Steinberg DR. A new method for evaluation and staging of avascular necrosis of the femoral head. In: Arlet J, Ficat RP, Hungerford DS, editors. Bone circulation. Baltimore: Williams and Wilkins; 1984. p. 398–403.
14. Steinberg ME, Hayken GD, Steinberg DR. A quantitative system for staging avascular necrosis. J Bone Joint Surg Br. 1995;77:34–41.
15. Mont MD, Jones LC, Hungerford DS. Nontraumatic osteonecrosis of the femoral head: ten years later. J Bone Joint Surg Am. 2006;88:1117–32.
16. Hernigou P, Beaujean F. Treatment of osteonecrosis with autologous bone marrow grafting. Clin Orthop Relat Res. 2002;405:14–23.
17. Steinberg ME, Bands RE, Parry S, Hoffman E, Chan T, Hartman KM. Does lesion size affect the outcome in avascular necrosis? Clin Orthop. 1999;367:262–71.
18. Steinberg ME, Larcom PG, Strafford B, Hosick WB, Corces A, Bands RE, Hartman KE. Core decompression with bone grafting for osteonecrosis of the femoral head. Clin Orthop Relat Res. 2001;386:71–8.
19. Koo K-H, Kim R. Quantifying the extent of osteonecrosis of the femoral head: a new method using MRI. J Bone Joint Surg Br. 1995;77:875–80.
20. Cherian SF, Laorr A, Saleh KJ, et al. Quantifying the extent of femoral head involvement is osteonecrosis. J Bone Joint Surg Am. 2003;85:309–15.
21. Steinberg DR, Steinberg ME, Garino JP, Dalinka M, Udupa JK. Determining lesion size in osteonecrosis of the femoral head. J Bone Joint Surg. 2006;88-A(Supplement 3):27–34.

22. Hernigou P, Lambotte SC. Volumetric analysis of osteonecrosis of the femur: anatomical correlation using MRI. J Bone Joint Surg Br. 2001;83-B:672–5.
23. Ha YC, Jung WH, Kim JR, et al. Prediction of collapse in femoral head osteonecrosis: a modified Kerboul method with use of magnetic resonance images. J Bone Joint Surg Am. 2006;88(Supp 3):35–40.
24. Theodorou DJ, Malizos KN, Beris AE, Theodorou SF, Soucacos PN. Multimodal imaging quantitation of the lesion size in osteonecrosis of the femoral head. Clin Orthop. 2001;386: 54–63.
25. Thickman D, Axel L, Kressel HY, Steinberg M, Chen H, Velchick M, Fallon M, Dalinka M. Magnetic resonance imaging of avascular necrosis of the femoral head. Skeletal Radiol. 1986;15: 133–40.
26. Mont MA, Jones LC, Pacheo I, Hungerford DS. Radiographic predictors of outcome of core decompression for osteonecrosis stage III. Clin Orthop. 1998;354:159–68.
27. Ficat RP. Idiopathic bone necrosis of the femoral head: early diagnosis and treatment. J Bone Joint Surg Br. 1985;67:3–9.
28. ARCO Committee on Terminology and Staging. Gardeniers JWM, Chairman. The ARCO perspective for reaching one uniform staging system of osteonecrosis. In: Schoutens A, Arlet J, Gardeniers JWM, Huges SPF, editors. Bone circulation and vascularization in normal and pathological conditions. New York/London: Plenum Press and NATO Scientific Affairs Division; 1993. p. 375–80.
29. Gardeniers J. A New international classification of osteonecrosis of the ARCO committee on terminology and classification. ARCO Newsl. 1992;4:41–6.
30. Sugano J, Atsumi T, Ohzone K, et al. The 2001 revised criteria for diagnosis, classification and staging of idiopathic osteonecrosis of the femoral head. J Orthop Sci. 2002;7(5):601–5.
31. Sugano N, Takaoka K, Ohzono K, Matsui M, Masuhara K, One K. Prognostication of non-traumatic avascular necrosis of the femoral head: significance of location and size of the necrotic lesion. Clin Orthop. 1994;303:155–64.
32. Mont MA, Marulanda GA, Jones LC, Saleh KJ, Gordon N, Hungerford DS, Steinberg ME. Systematic analysis of classification systems for osteonecrosis of the femoral head. J Bone Joint Surg. 2006;88-A(Supplement 3):16–26.
33. Gardeniers J. ARCO committee on terminology and staging. A new proposition of terminology and an international classification of osteonecrosis. ARCO Newsl. 1991;3:153–9.
34. Gardeniers J. ARCO Committee on terminology and staging report on the committee meeting at Santiago de Compostela. ARCO Newsl. 1993;5:79–82.
35. Lee GC, Steinberg ME. Are we evaluating osteonecrosis adequately? Int Orthop (SICOT). 2012;36:2433–9.

26 Natural Course and the JIC Classification of Osteonecrosis of the Femoral Head

Nobuhiko Sugano and Kenji Ohzono

26.1 Introduction

To standardize clinical definitions and management of idiopathic osteonecrosis of the femoral head, criteria for the diagnosis, classification, and staging of osteonecrosis of the femoral head (ONFH) were developed in 1986 by the Japanese Investigation Committee (JIC) under the auspices of the Ministry of Health and Welfare [1]. Since then, revision was made three times and the 2001 version [2] is still used widely in Japan. We describe here the JIC diagnostic criteria and JIC classification of ONFH.

26.2 JIC Diagnostic Criteria

Although many different techniques had been used to diagnose osteonecrosis as early as possible by x-rays, venography, bone marrow pressure measurement, biopsy, computerized tomography, bone scans, and MRI, no single modality had been shown to be superior to the others for accurate diagnosis. Therefore, the JIC took an alternative method to use clinical diagnostic criteria. A revised version of the JIC diagnostic criteria was proposed in 1996, after analysis of the sensitivity and specificity of diagnosis based on the original criteria [3]. The five most effective and simple diagnostic criteria for osteonecrosis were chosen (Table 26.1): collapse of the femoral head without joint-space narrowing or acetabular abnormality on x-ray images (including crescent sign), demarcating sclerosis in the femoral head without joint-space narrowing or acetabular abnormality, "cold in hot" on bone scans, low-intensity band on T1-weighted images (band-like pattern), and trabecular and marrow necrosis on biopsy histology. It was found that for diagnosis of osteonecrosis based on any two positive criteria out of these five, the sensitivity and specificity were 91 and 99 %, respectively. The diagnostic criteria had not been changed in the 2001 version [2], and it is still used in Japan as standard diagnostic criteria for patients with ONFH to receive the public financial support of treatment.

N. Sugano (✉)
Department of Orthopaedic Medical Engineering, Osaka University Graduate School of Medicine, 2-2 Yamadaoka, Suita 565-0871, Japan
e-mail: n-sugano@umin.net

K. Ohzono
Department of Orthopaedic Surgery, Kansai Rousai Hospital, 3-1-69 Inabasou, Amagasaki 660-8511, Japan
e-mail: ozono-takuya@aist.go.jp

26.3 JIC Classification

Massive collapse of the femoral head is a crucial event that leads to the functional devastation of the hip joint with ONFH. To evaluate the susceptibility for collapse or to predict impending collapse for each case in the early stage of ONFH, the JIC proposed a classification in 1986 [1]. It consisted of three major types, based on the following specific radiographic findings (Fig. 26.1): type 1, demarcating sclerosis; type 2, flattening; and type 3, cystic radiolucency. Type 1 and type 3 are divided into subtypes 1A, 1B, 1C, 3A, and 3B, based on the location of the lesion in the weight-bearing area. A type 3A cystic lesion is located far from the weight-bearing surface. A lesion surrounded by demarcating sclerosis and located far from the weight-bearing surface is classified as type 1A. The prevalence of collapse was reported as 0 % in type 1A, 44 % in type 1B, 88 % in type

Table 26.1 Diagnostic criteria for osteonecrosis

Criteria
1. Collapse of the femoral head without joint-space narrowing or acetabular abnormality on x-rays (including crescent sign)
2. Demarcating sclerosis in the femoral head without joint-space narrowing or acetabular abnormality
3. "Cold in hot" on bone scans
4. Low-intensity band on T1-weighted images (band-like pattern)
5. Trabecular and marrow necrosis on histology

Definite diagnosis requires any two positive criteria out of the five
Bone tumors and dysplasias should be excluded

K.-H. Koo et al. (eds.), *Osteonecrosis*,
DOI 10.1007/978-3-642-35767-1_26, © Springer-Verlag Berlin Heidelberg 2014

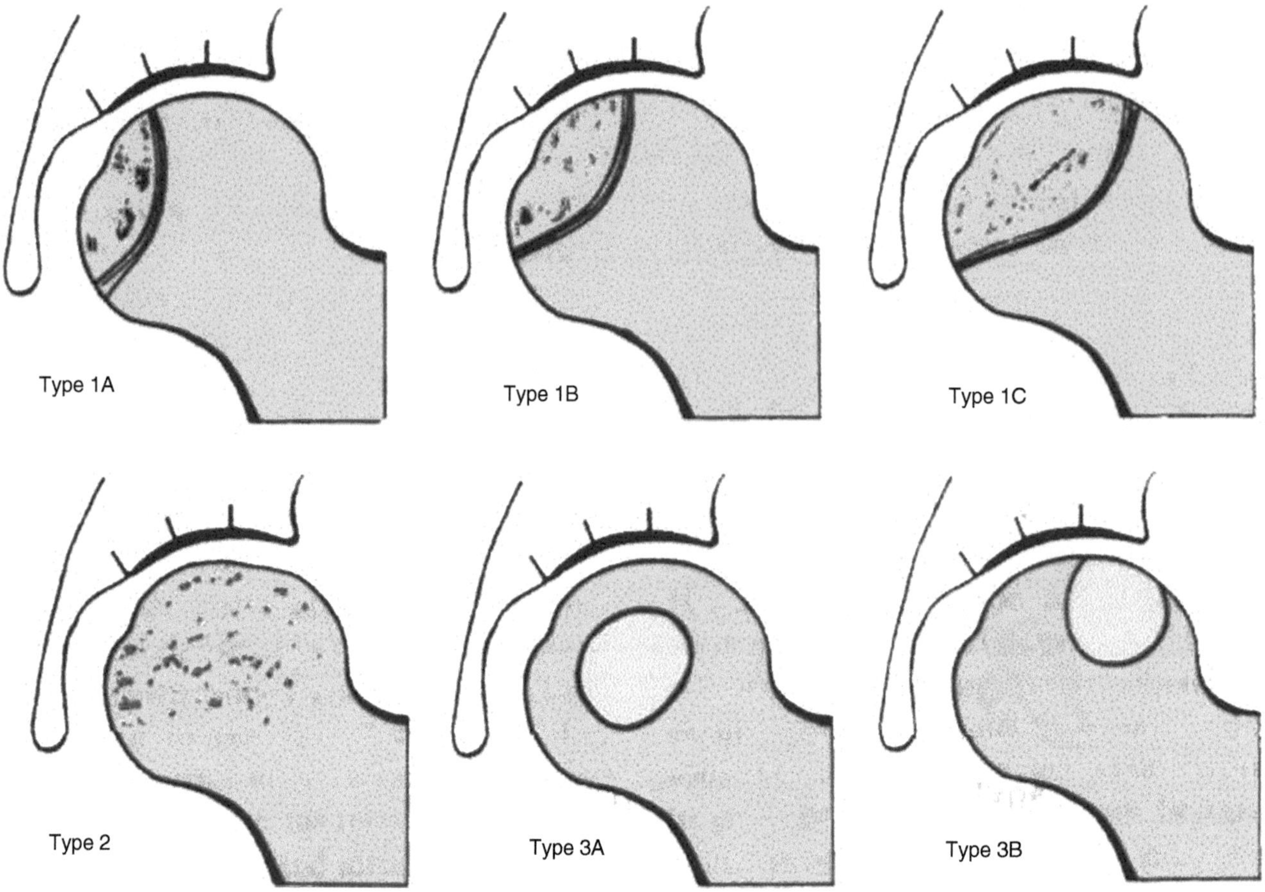

Fig. 26.1 The JIC 1986 radiographic classification of ONFH. The classification scheme consists of three types (1, 2, and 3). Type 1 is characterized by the presence of a demarcation line in the femoral head and is divided into three subtypes, 1-A, 1-B, and 1-C, according to its relationship to the weight-bearing surface. Type 2 shows early flattening of the weight-bearing surface but has no demarcation line around the necrotic area. Type 3 has cystic lesions and is divided into two subtypes according to their site in the femoral head

1C, 100 % in type 2, 0 % in type 3A, and 100 % in type 3B [4, 5]. Surgical treatment is seldom necessary in type 1A and type 3A. Varus femoral osteotomy or transtrochanteric rotational femoral osteotomy can be good indication for type 1B and 1C. The necrotic lesions were not able to be quantitatively evaluated on radiographs in type 2 and type 3 ONFH because they did not show demarcating sclerosis until the late stage. These types were often seen in patients with steroid-induced ONFH. Failure rates of osteotomies for type 2 and type 3B are high. The location of the lesion in these types was shown to occupy all weight-bearing area when MRI was used [2]. Therefore, a high prevalence of collapse in type 2 and 3B can be explained by the location of the lesion that occupied the most of the weight-bearing area of the femoral head.

As the location of lesion is an important factor to predict impending collapse, a prospective MRI study in patients with SLE was conducted to detect ONFH in the pre-radiographic stage and to prognosticate ONFH [6]. A low-intensity band in the femoral head of normal fat intensity on T1-weighted images was a specific finding of ONFH. The lesions demarcated by a low-intensity band were classified into type A, B, and C like type 1A, 1B, and 1C of the radiographic classification on the coronal image through the femoral head center. As the location of the lesion extended more weight-bearing area, the prevalence of collapse increased. Although some early lesions detected less than a year after initial steroid treatment can show size reduction, the location of lesions does not change later in most of the cases [7, 8]. The MRI classification system based on the location of the lesion surrounded by a low-intensity band on T1-weighted images was found to have the same predictive power as the radiographic classification system. Furthermore, when type C was divided into subtypes C1 and C2, the incidence of progressive collapse of the femoral head varies significantly. A type C2 lesion extends laterally to the acetabular edge, whereas a type C1 lesion does not (Fig. 26.2). The prevalence of collapse was less than 10 % in type A, 40 % in type B, 80 % in type C1, and 90 % or more in type C2. Even after collapse occurs in type A and B, subsequent cessation of collapse can be expected and improvement of symptoms with no surgical intervention required [9]. This new classification

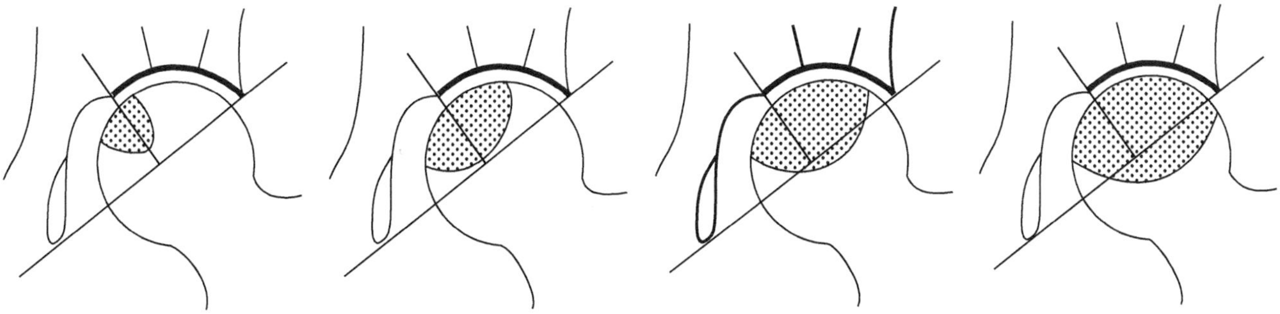

Fig. 26.2 The JIC 2001 classification of ONFH. The classification scheme consists of four types (A, B, C1, and C2) and is based on the central coronal section of the femoral head on T1-weighted MRI or the anteroposterior x-ray view

was adopted in the 2001 JIC classification and it has not changed since then.

The location and size of lesions are thought to be independently related to the prevalence of collapse. Therefore, these two parameters were analyzed by a three-dimensional quantification of lesions to clarify how these two morphological factors were related to the occurrence of collapse using 3D MR imaging [10]. Lesion volume as well as latitude and longitude of the center of gravity of the lesion within the femoral head were calculated. Multiple logistic regression analysis showed a significant relationship between lesion volume and radiological collapse. In comparison with non-collapsed hips, collapsed hips had a significantly higher combined value for latitude and longitude of the lesion, corresponding to the anterosuperior portion of the femoral head. Quantitative analysis of lesion morphology demonstrated that lesion volume is strongly correlated with risk of collapse and that lesion location is an important prognostic indicator of collapse in small necrotic lesions. None the less, the JIC classification of ONFH based on two-dimensional anteroposterior radiographs or coronal MRI can provide useful information on the prevalence of collapse easily. The outcome of total hip arthroplasty including resurfacing may not be affected by the location and size of the lesion [11]; however, the JIC classification is useful to understand how various joint-preserving treatment options can be effective to improve the natural course of ONFH in each case.

26.4 Summary

The JIC 2001 criteria for the diagnosis and classification idiopathic osteonecrosis of the femoral head (ONFH) were described. Five criteria that showed high specificity were selected for diagnosis: collapse of the femoral head (including crescent sign) without joint-space narrowing or acetabular abnormality on x-ray images, demarcating sclerosis in the femoral head without joint-space narrowing or acetabular abnormality, "cold in hot" on bone scans, low-intensity band on T1-weighted MRI (band-like pattern), and trabecular and marrow necrosis on histology. ONFH is diagnosed if the patient fulfills two of these five criteria. Necrotic lesions are classified into four types, based on their location on T1-weighted MRI or x-ray images. Type A lesions occupy the medial one-third or less of the weight-bearing portion. Type B lesions occupy the medial two-thirds or less of the weight-bearing portion. Type C1 lesions occupy more than the medial two-thirds of the weight-bearing portion but do not extend laterally to the acetabular edge. Type C2 lesions occupy more than the medial two-thirds of the weight-bearing portion and extend laterally to the acetabular edge. The prevalence of collapse was less than 10 % in type A, 40 % in type B, 80 % in type C1, and 90 % or more in type C2.

References

1. Ono K. Diagnostic criteria, staging system, and roentgenographic classification of avascular necrosis of the femoral head (steroid induced, alcohol associated, or idiopathic nature) In: Ono K, editor. Annual report of Japanese investigation committee for intractable diseases, avascular necrosis of the femoral head, under the auspices of Ministry of Health and Welfare; 1987. p. 331 (in Japanese).
2. Sugano N, Atsumi T, Ohzono K, Kubo T, Hotokebuchi T, Takaoka K. The 2001 revised criteria for diagnosis, classification, and staging of idiopathic osteonecrosis of the femoral head. J Orthop Sci. 2002;7(5):601–5.
3. Sugano N, Kubo T, Takaoka K, Ohzono K, Hotokebuchi T, Matsumoto T, Igarashi H, Ninomiya S. Diagnostic criteria for non-traumatic osteonecrosis of the femoral head. A multicentre study. J Bone Joint Surg Br. 1999;81(4):590–5.
4. Ohzono K, Saito M, Takaoka K, Ono K, Saito S, Nishina T, Kadowaki T. Natural history of nontraumatic avascular necrosis of the femoral head. J Bone Joint Surg Br. 1991;73(1):68–72.
5. Sugano N, Takaoka K, Ohzono K, Matsui M, Masuhara K, Ono K. Prognostication of nontraumatic avascular necrosis of the femoral head. Significance of location and size of the necrotic lesion. Clin Orthop Relat Res. 1994;303:155–64.

6. Sugano N, Ohzono K, Masuhara K, Takaoka K, Ono K. Prognostication of osteonecrosis of the femoral head in patients with systemic lupus erythematosus by magnetic resonance imaging. Clin Orthop Relat Res. 1994;305:190–9.
7. Takao M, Sugano N, Nishii T, Miki H, Sato Y, Tamura S, Yoshikawa H. Longitudinal quantitative evaluation of lesion size change in femoral head osteonecrosis using three-dimensional magnetic resonance imaging and image registration. J Orthop Res. 2006;24(6):1231–9.
8. Takao M, Nishii T, Sakai T, Yoshikawa H, Sugano N. Repair in osteonecrosis of the femoral head: MR imaging features at long-term follow-up. Clin Rheumatol. 2010;29(8):841–8.
9. Nishii T, Sugano N, Ohzono K, Sakai T, Haraguchi K, Yoshikawa H. Progression and cessation of collapse in osteonecrosis of the femoral head. Clin Orthop Relat Res. 2002;400:149–57.
10. Nishii T, Sugano N, Ohzono K, Sakai T, Sato Y, Yoshikawa H. Significance of lesion size and location in the prediction of collapse of osteonecrosis of the femoral head: a new three-dimensional quantification using magnetic resonance imaging. J Orthop Res. 2002;20(1):130–6.
11. Nakasone S, Takao M, Sakai T, Nishii T, Sugano N. Does the extent of osteonecrosis affect the survival of hip resurfacing? Clin Orthop Relat Res. 2013;471(6):1926–34.

Modified Kerboul Classification System of Necrotic Extent Using MRI

27

Yong-Chan Ha, Young-Kyun Lee, and Kyung-Hoi Koo

27.1 Introduction

The prognosis of osteonecrosis of the femoral head is related to the location and extent of the necrotic lesion [1–6]. Therefore, several methods have been introduced to quantify or categorize the location and extent of osteonecrosis [1, 7–11].

In 1974, Kerboul et al. developed a simple and easy method of measuring the extent of necrosis in early-stage osteonecrosis of the femoral head that involved measuring the arc of the femoral surface involved by necrosis on an anteroposterior as well as a lateral radiograph and then calculating the sum of these two angles [8].

Magnetic resonance image (MRI) is more accurate in evaluating the extent of osteonecrosis than radiographs [12, 13]. The extent of necrosis should be measured in the both coronal and sagittal planes, because the measurement in the coronal plane alone is not accurate to quantify the necrosis and, accordingly, is not accurate in predicting further collapse of the femoral head.

In this chapter, we describe the modified Kerboul method using MRI.

27.2 Modified Kerboul Method Using MRI

27.2.1 The First Modification

In 1995, the first modified method using MRI scans instead of radiographs was introduced [11]. The arc of necrotic area was measured at the subchondral portion of the femoral head on the mid-coronal image (*A*) and the midsagittal image (*B*) (Fig. 27.1).

The necrotic index was calculated by the formula: $(A/180) \times (B/180) \times 100$. In a pilot study to determine the reproducibility of this measurement, the coefficient of variation was 32 %. There was a strong correlation between this index and the risk of future collapse. If the cutoff point of 30 % is used, the predictive value of a negative test would be 100 % and that of a positive test 91 %. Likewise, a cutoff at 40 % gives a predictive value for a positive test of 100 % and for a negative test of 82 %. None of hips with necrosis less than 30 % collapsed, but all hips with more than 40 % necrosis collapsed, and half of hips with necrosis of between 30 and 40 % collapsed. Thus, hips with necrosis of less than 30 % are were classified as a low-risk group, those with necrosis of 30–40 % as a moderate-risk group, and those with more than 40 % as a high-risk group in terms of future collapse of the femoral head.

Although this method showed a strong correlation with the risk of collapse and the index was a major predictor of future collapse, a conversion table or a calculator was necessary to obtain the index.

27.2.2 The Second Modification

To simplify the method, a second modification was done in 2006 [14]. The arc of the necrotic portion on both the mid-coronal (*A*) and the midsagittal images (*B*) was measured (Fig. 27.1), and the sum of these two angles was then calculated. There was a strong correlation between the combined necrotic angle ($A+B$) and the risk of future collapse. None of hips with a combined necrotic angle of ≤190° collapsed, all hips with an angle of ≥240°collapsed, and 50 % of hips with an angle between 190° and 240° collapsed during the study period (Fig. 27.2). This would suggest that hips with a combined necrotic angle of ≤190° are in a low-risk group, those with an angle between 190° and 240° are in a moderate-risk group, and those with an angle of ≥240° are in a high-risk group.

Y.-C. Ha (✉)
Department of Orthopaedic Surgery,
Chung-Ang University College of Medicine,
224-1 Heukseok-dong, Seoul 156-755, South Korea
e-mail: hayongch@naver.com

Y.-K. Lee • K.-H. Koo
Department of Orthopaedic Surgery, Seoul National University College of Medicine, Seoul National University Bundang Hospital,
166 Gumi-ro, Seongnam 463-707, South Korea
e-mail: ykleemd@gmail.com; khkoo@snu.ac.kr

K.-H. Koo et al. (eds.), *Osteonecrosis*,
DOI 10.1007/978-3-642-35767-1_27, © Springer-Verlag Berlin Heidelberg 2014

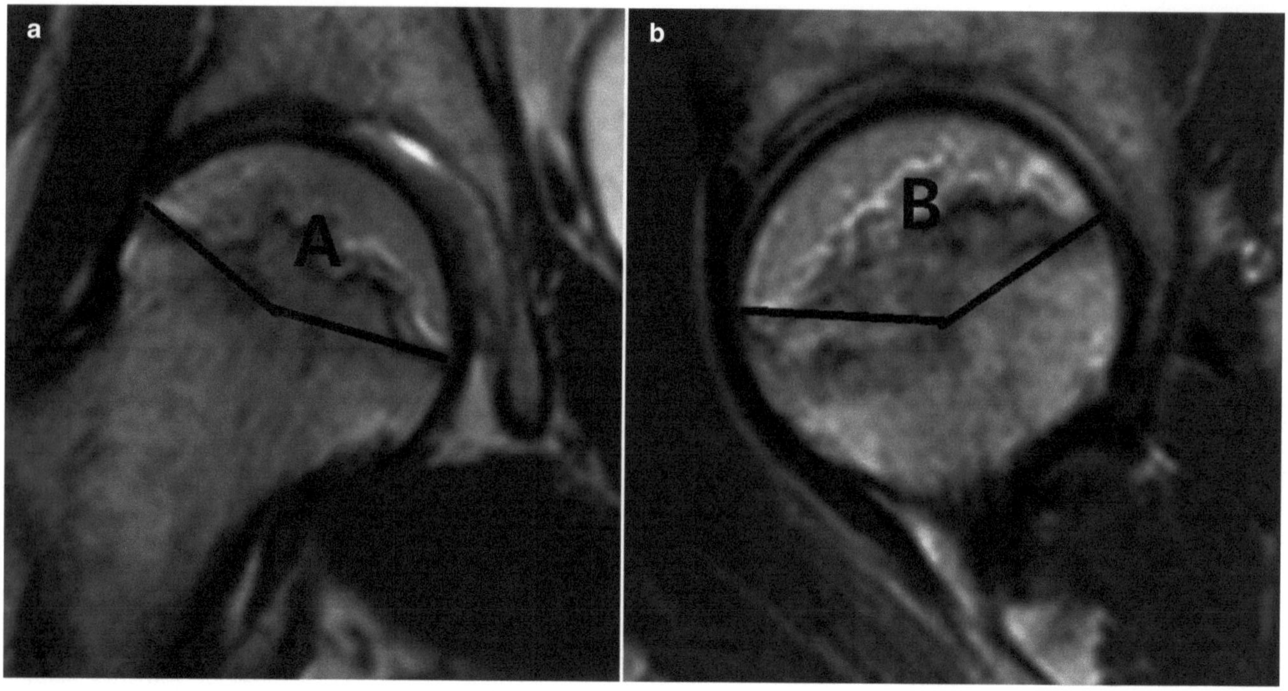

Fig. 27.1 *A* is the angle of necrotic area in mid-coronal image and *B* is the angle of necrotic area in midsagittal image. The angle is measured at the subchondral portion

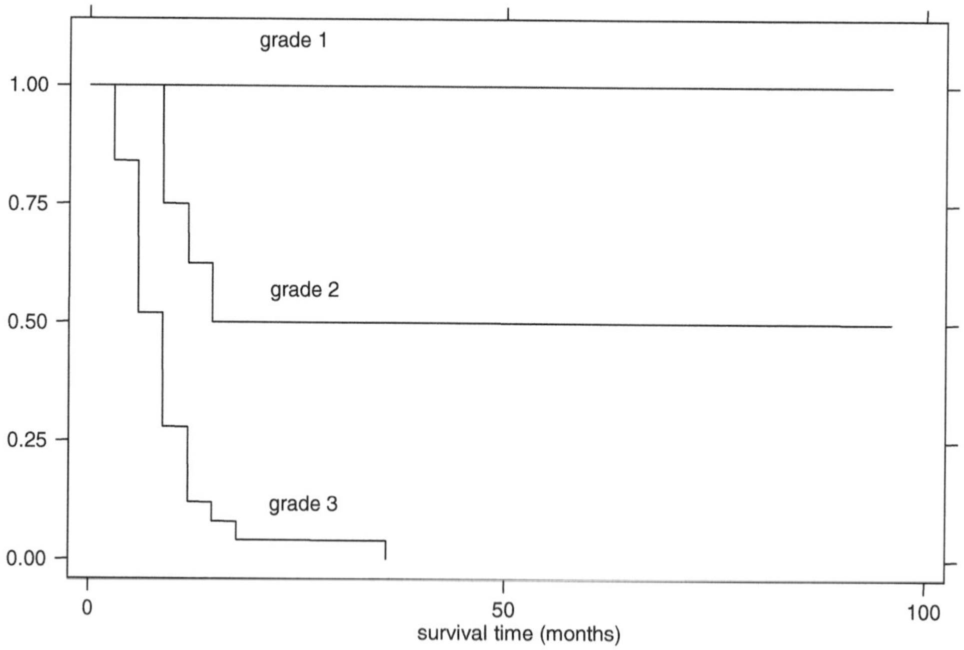

Fig. 27.2 Kaplan-Meier survival curve according to the categories of the combined necrotic angle, which were classified by cut points of 190° and 240°. Grade 1 denotes hips with combined necrotic angle ≤190°, grade 2 denotes hips with combined necrotic angle between 190° and 240°, and grade 3 denotes hips with combined necrotic angle ≥240°. Survival distributions for three grades were different by log rank test ($p<0.01$)

27.3 Summary

The measurement of necrotic arc on mid-coronal and mid-sagittal MRI scans is simple and easy and reproducible. The combined necrotic angle, the sum of the two necrotic arcs on mid-coronal and midsagittal MRI scans, is based on biplanar MRI scans and provides a three-dimensional assessment of the extent of the necrosis. The categorization of femoral head osteonecrosis according to the combined necrotic angle may accurately predict the risk of subsequent collapse of the femoral head.

Medical or surgical treatment to prevent collapse is not justified in the low-risk group. Any intervention should be limited to hips in the moderate to high-risk groups.

References

1. Ohzono K, Saito M, Takaoka K, Ono K, Saito S, Nishina T, et al. Natural history of nontraumatic avascular necrosis of the femoral head. J Bone Joint Surg Br. 1991;73(1):68–72.
2. Lieberman JR, Engstrom SM, Meneghini RM, SooHoo NF. Which factors influence preservation of the osteonecrotic femoral head? Clin Orthop Relat Res. 2012;470(2):525–34. doi:10.1007/s11999-011-2050-4.
3. Ha YC, Kim HJ, Kim SY, Kim KC, Lee YK, Koo KH. Effects of age and body mass index on the results of transtrochanteric rotational osteotomy for femoral head osteonecrosis. J Bone Joint Surg Am. 2010;92(2):314–21. doi:10.2106/JBJS.H.01020.
4. Nam KW, Kim YL, Yoo JJ, Koo KH, Yoon KS, Kim HJ. Fate of untreated asymptomatic osteonecrosis of the femoral head. J Bone Joint Surg Am. 2008;90(3):477–84. doi:10.2106/JBJS.F.01582.
5. Steinberg DR, Steinberg ME, Garino JP, Dalinka M, Udupa JK. Determining lesion size in osteonecrosis of the femoral head. J Bone Joint Surg Am. 2006;88 Suppl 3:27–34. doi:10.2106/JBJS.F.00896.
6. Nishii T, Sugano N, Ohzono K, Sakai T, Sato Y, Yoshikawa H. Significance of lesion size and location in the prediction of collapse of osteonecrosis of the femoral head: a new three-dimensional quantification using magnetic resonance imaging. J Orthop Res. 2002;20(1):130–6. doi:10.1016/S0736-0266(01)00063-8.
7. Steinberg ME, Brighton CT, Steinberg DR, Tooze SE, Hayken GD. Treatment of avascular necrosis of the femoral head by a combination of bone grafting, decompression, and electrical stimulation. Clin Orthop Relat Res. 1984;186:137–53.
8. Kerboul M, Thomine J, Postel M, Merle d'Aubigne R. The conservative surgical treatment of idiopathic aseptic necrosis of the femoral head. J Bone Joint Surg Br. 1974;56(2):291–6.
9. Steinberg ME, Hayken GD, Steinberg DR. A quantitative system for staging avascular necrosis. J Bone Joint Surg Br. 1995;77(1):34–41.
10. Kim HJ, Yoo JJ, Song WS. Quantifying the extent of femoral head involvement in osteonecrosis. J Bone Joint Surg Am. 2003;85-A(12):2481–2; author reply 2.
11. Koo KH, Kim R. Quantifying the extent of osteonecrosis of the femoral head. A new method using MRI. J Bone Joint Surg Br. 1995;77(6):875–80.
12. Gillespy 3rd T, Genant HK, Helms CA. Magnetic resonance imaging of osteonecrosis. Radiol Clin North Am. 1986;24(2):193–208.
13. Glickstein MF, Burk Jr DL, Schiebler ML, Cohen EK, Dalinka MK, Steinberg ME, et al. Avascular necrosis versus other diseases of the hip: sensitivity of MR imaging. Radiology. 1988;169(1):213–5.
14. Ha YC, Jung WH, Kim JR, Seong NH, Kim SY, Koo KH. Prediction of collapse in femoral head osteonecrosis: a modified Kerboul method with use of magnetic resonance images. J Bone Joint Surg Am. 2006;88 Suppl 3:35–40. doi:10.2106/JBJS.F.00535.

28 The ARCO Staging System: Generation and Evolution Since 1991

J.W.M. Gardeniers, A.C. Gosling-Gardeniers, and W.H.C. Rijnen

28.1 Introduction

Various classification systems have been proposed and used to distinguish the different stages and necrotic extent of femoral head osteonecrosis.

Conventional staging systems include those described by Marcus and coauthors [1], Ficat and Arlet [2], and Steinberg and associates [3], and the classification system of Ohzono and associates [4]. The necrotic extent has been evaluated with use of Steinberg system or JIC (Japanese Investigation Committee) classification.

After the widespread use of MRI for the diagnostic workup of osteonecrosis in the late 1980s, there has been an urgent need for a single unified classification, which is based on MRI, easy to understand, and valid to compare treatment results in the different reports in international literatures.

28.2 Generation of the ARCO Classification

At the time of the second General Assembly of the Association Research Circulation Osseous (ARCO), which was held on the island of Ischia, Italy, in November 1990, the "International ARCO committee on Terminology and Classification" was installed.

In May 1991, the members of the committee assembled for the first time in Nijmegen, the Netherlands. The first ARCO classification system was designed at that meeting.

The committee reported as follows:

Currently, osteonecrosis has become an increasingly significant phenomenon, especially manifest in the large joints and with the highest incidence in the younger age groups and with the vast majority of cases younger than 50 years. In 1978, John Paul Jones Jr. wrote about osteonecrosis in the femoral head that it had become a significant problem in connection with deep-diving and high-altitude operations and alcohol and corticosteroid treatment in recipients of organ transplants [5]. The precise etiology of both traumatic and nontraumatic or idiopathic osteonecrosis was unknown. This is still true today.

The assignment of the committee was to establish one uniform definition, histopathological terminology, and classification of osteonecrosis. The reason for this was that in literatures we can find various classifications on osteonecrosis based on slight or completely different definitions, terminologies, and diagnostic criteria. These will cause authors to have differences in opinions and different interpretations of each other work.

Therefore, the committee had to be "international." It should be kept in mind that the proposed classification is also a composition of all the previously or recently published scientific work and staging systems by many authors.

The members of the committee decided that the following problems had to be solved first:

- Terminology
- Diagnostic criteria
- A uniform international classification

28.2.1 Terminology

Many terms had been used to designate the necrosis of bone including avascular necrosis, osteonecrosis, aseptic necrosis, creeping substitution, necrotic bone disease, and bone infarction, which were very confusing.

The committee agreed upon that the definition of necrosis of bone had to be the following:

"Bone" is an organ that consists of mineralized and nonmineralized tissues.

Bone necrosis is a disease which causes death of bone and is called "osteonecrosis."

J.W.M. Gardeniers (✉) • A.C. Gosling-Gardeniers
W.H.C. Rijnen
Department of Orthopaedics, Radboud University Medical Centre, Geert Grooteplein zuid 10, 9101, 6500 HB Nijmegen, The Netherlands
e-mail: jeanwmgardeniers@me.com; wim.rijnen@radboudumc.nl

K.-H. Koo et al. (eds.), *Osteonecrosis*,
DOI 10.1007/978-3-642-35767-1_28, © Springer-Verlag Berlin Heidelberg 2014

28.2.2 Diagnostic Criteria

The diagnosis "true osteonecrosis" should be made as early as possible in the course of the disease.

The diagnostic criteria that are available at this moment are:

- Radiography
- Scintigraphy
- Functional bone investigation
- MRI
- Histology

The problem with radiography is that when the signs are visible on radiographs, the disease has already progressed beyond the initial stage.

This is also true for scintigraphy; and the scintigraphic sign "cold in hot" is not frequently observed. The reliability of scintigraphy is low.

"Functional bone investigation" [2] is not to be used in a staging system. It is an invasive technique and the derived data, the intraosseous pressure, and the venography are not pathognomonic for osteonecrosis. Differences from the normal values can also be seen in other circulatory bone diseases.

However, "functional bone investigation" was of great value to distinguish the so-called preradiological stage of osteonecrosis, which we now recognize as probably the onset of the disease. "Functional bone investigation" remains of great value in the research of osteonecrosis and other bone disorders.

MRI is a noninvasive method and it can visualize early changes in the bone. It is both more sensitive and more specific than all the other noninvasive diagnostic measures. It gives us an image of the existing process in the bone. Classic T1-weighted images in coronal and axial planes were recommended. This is the minimum requirement in stage 0 and 1 when there are no radiological signs. T2-weighted MRI images can give supplemental information as diagnostic tool. MRI gives us an image of a process in the bone seen as a "band-like image of low intensity" on the classic T1-weighted image and a "double-line sign" on a classic T2-weighted image. When there is a clinical suspicion of osteonecrosis, MRI should be taken immediately.

Histology remains the "golden standard" to make a definite diagnosis of osteonecrosis. Although it is an invasive method, it might be a curative procedure. A descriptive histological classification of the disease is not yet available, and for the time being a "simple descriptive histological classification" was designed as a working scheme.

Further histological data collection is of the utmost importance to be able to make a histological classification. However, it must be stated that in the very early onset of the disease, histology is not conclusive. Marrow edema, scattered lesions of necrosis, and red blood cells outside the vessels can also be seen in other bone diseases. However, when the area of necrosis with empty osteocyte lacunae is larger than 1 cm^2, the disease has already passed beyond the early ischemic stage and is no longer reversible.

28.2.3 ARCO Classification System Established in 1991

As mentioned above, the committee agreed to the necessity of one uniform classification of the various stages of osteonecrosis. The committee agreed upon that staging is a method of defining the development of the disease. Staging has to include the onset of the disease, "stage 0," and has to extend to the end stage of complete joint destruction. The committee also agreed upon that the quantification of necrotic extent was important and a descriptive histological classification was urgently needed.

In the first ARCO classification system, the progression of osteonecrosis was divided into six stages with a subdivision of location and size of the necrotic portion [6].

Stage 0 All present diagnostic techniques are normal or non-diagnostic except histology. Future diagnostic techniques will at some point enable us to make the diagnosis in this stage "0."

Diagnostic techniques are beyond the plain X-rays, the use of scintigraphy, and MRI.

Stage I Plain X-ray and CT scan are normal.

At least one of the following techniques is positive: scintigraphy and MRI.

An open biopsy will confirm the diagnosis. The classic MR image is pathognomonic.

It is important to subdivide this stage in three categories A, B, and C, according to the extension of the area of femoral head involvement. A=<15 % involvement, B=15–30 % involvement, and C=>30 % involvement.

Stage II Radiography shows areas of abnormalities: mottled aspect, sclerosis, cysts, and porosis. However, there are no signs of collapse, and the femoral head remains spherical on AP and lateral views on X-ray and CT scan. Again scintigraphy and MRI are positive. Subclassification in A, B, and C is important, as described in stage 1.

Stage III The femoral head has begun to fail mechanically.

The axial X-ray shows a fine radiolucent subchondral fracture line, usually referred to as the "crescent sign." However, there are no signs of flattening of the femoral dome. The spherical configuration remains intact.

The same subclassification as in the two previous stages described must be included. First, it is determined whether the crescent sign appears more prominent in the AP or lateral view. After selection of the most prominent view, the length of the crescent is expressed as a percentage of the entire articular surface.

Stage IV Radiographs show the articular surface of the femoral head to be flattened, but there is no evidence of joint line narrowing or acetabular involvement. CT scanning might be helpful if there is no evidence of collapse on the plain X-rays.

The same recommended subclassification in A, B, and C is added but must also be done by the amount of flattening: A=<15 % involvement or a depression of <2 mm, B = 15–30 % involvement or a depression of 2–4 mm, and C=>30 % involvement or a depression of more than 4 mm.

Stage V Radiographically the articular surface is flattened and the joint space starts narrowing. This is often associated with changes on the acetabular side of the joint and with signs of a beginning osteoarthritis with areas of sclerosis, cysts, and marginal osteophytes. Subclassification has to be done as in stage 4 and the acetabular involvement has to be estimated.

Stage VI The radiographic examinations show advanced degenerative changes and finally a complete joint destruction.

This classification was accepted by the "General Assembly of ARCO" in Basel, Switzerland, in December 1991 as a "proposal for an international classification."

The committee suggested the following requirements in reporting clinical and scientific work on osteonecrosis:

1. A clinical evaluation by means of any hip score rating
2. Staging according to this *international classification*
3. Radiographic and/or MRI quantitation of necrotic extent
4. Therapeutic results on survival of the femoral head

28.3 ARCO Classification Modified in 1994

The first ARCO classification was comprehensive but complicated. Thus, the classification was simplified for the practical use by every physician in the world. The original stages III and IV were combined into stage 3 and original stages V and VI into stage 4. This modification was discussed and approved at the General Assembly of ARCO in 1994.

Since then, this modification was accepted as the ARCO classification system.

The modified ARCO classification (Fig. 28.1):

Stage 0: All diagnostic studies are normal and diagnosis is made by histology only. A painful hip in a patient who has either one or more risk factors for osteonecrosis or who has a proven osteonecrosis on the contralateral side.

ARCO INTERNATIONAL CLASSIFICATION OF OSTEONECROSIS 2002

STAGE	0	1	2	Early 3	Late 3	4
FINDINGS	All present techniques normal or non-diagnostic	X-ray, and CT are normal at least ONE of the below mentioned is positive	NO CRESCENT SIGN! X-RAY ABNORMAL: sclerosis, osteolysis, focal porosis	CRESCENT SIGN! on the X-ray and/or flattening of articular surface of femoral head.NO COLLAPSE	COLLAPSE ! on the X-ray and/or flattening of articular surface of femoral head.	OSTEOARTHRITIS! joint space narrowing, acetabular changes, joint destruction
TECHNIQUES	X-ray, CT Scintigraph MRI	Scintigraph MRI * QUANTITATE on MRI	X-ray, CT Scintigraph MRI * QUANTITATE MRI & X-ray	X-ray, CT ONLY * QUANTITATE on X-ray	X-ray CT ONLY * QUANTITATE on X-ray	X-Ray ONLY
SUBCLASSIFICATION	NO	LOCATION: 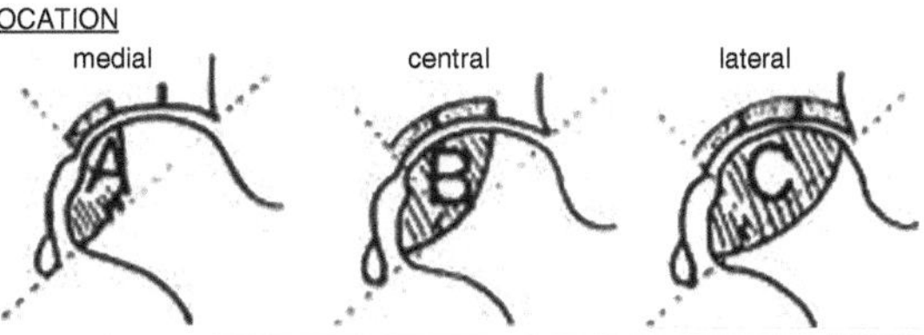				NO
QUANTITATION	NO	QUANTITATION % AREA INVOLVEMENT: minimal A < 15%, moderate B > 15% - 30%, extensive C > 30% LENGTH Of CRESCENT: A < 15%, B > 15% - 30%, C > 30% % SURFACE COLLAPSE & DOME DEPRESION 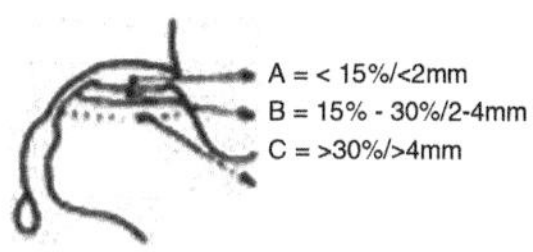				NO

Fig. 28.1 ARCO international classification of osteonecrosis

NIJMEGEN PROTOCOL: ARCO INTERNATIONAL CLASSIFICATION OF OSTEONECROSIS 2002

STAGE	0	1	2	Early 3	Late 3	4
FINDINGS	All present techniques normal or non-diagnostic	X-ray and CT are normal at least ONE of the below mentioned is positive	NO CRESCENT SIGN! X-RAY ABNORMAL: sclerosis, osteolysis, focal porosis	CRESCENT SIGN! on the X-ray and/or flattening of articular surface of femoral head. NO COLLAPSE	COLLAPSE! on the X-ray and/or flattening of articular surface of femoral head.	OSTEOARTHRITIS' joint space narrowing, acetabular changes, joint destruction
TECHNIQUES	X-ray, CT Scintigraph MRI	Scintigraph MRI *QUANTITATE on MRI	X-ray, CT Scintigraph MRI *QUANTITATE MRI & X-ray	X-ray, CT ONLY * QUANTITATE on X-ray	X-ray, CT ONLY * QUANTITATE on X-ray	X-Ray ONLY
SUBCLASS-IFICATION	NO	LOCATION medial central lateral 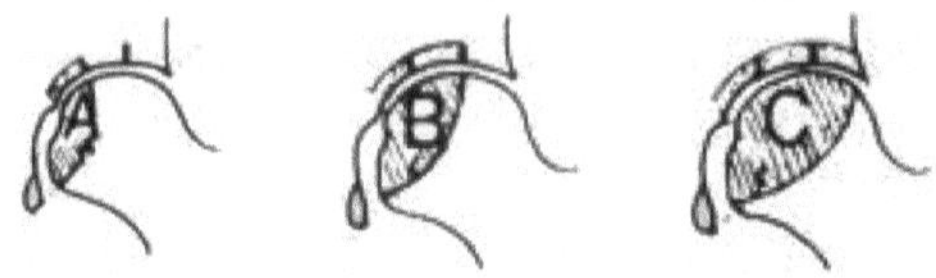				NO
QUANTITATION	NO	QUANTITATION % Area Involvement minimal A < 15% msxlcute B > 15% – 30% extensive C > 30%	Length of Crescent A < 15% B >15% – 30% C > 30%	% Surface Collapse & Dome Depression 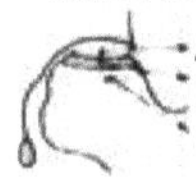 A – < 15% / < 2 mm B –15– 30% / 2–4 mm C – > 30% / > 4 mm		NO

Fig. 28.2 New Nijmegen addition to the ARCO International Classification of osteonecrosis [3]

Stage 1: A band lesion of a low signal intensity around the necrotic area is seen on MRI scans. No changes are seen on plain radiographs.

Stage 2: Subtle signs of osteosclerosis, focal osteoporosis, or cystic change can be identified in the femoral head on plain radiographs. Still there is no evidence of subchondral fracture.

Stage 3: Early fracture in the subchondral portion is seen on plain radiography or by computed tomography or tomograms.

Stage 4: There is osteoarthritis of the joint with accompanying joint space narrowing, acetabular changes, and finally destruction of the joint.

28.4 Latest Modification in Nijmegen (Fig. 28.2)

Subsequently after using this classification, there was a need to subdivide stage 3 into early and late stages. Sometimes, osteonecrosis in early collapse does not progress to further stage, and patients are doing well for a prolonged time without any intervention. The results of the joint preserving procedures such as bone grafting and osteotomies showed a clear difference between the head with and without collapse. The results in early stage 3 without definite collapse were significantly better than those in late stage 3 with definite collapse. This subdivision seems to be of crucial importance, particularly for the evaluation of outcome after treatment of osteonecrosis. Besides, other classification systems have a separation between the "early" stage before a collapse of the femoral head develops and the "late" stage when a definite collapse is already present.

References

1. Marcus ND, Enneking WF, Massam RA. The silent hip in idiopathic aseptic necrosis: treatment by bone grafting. J Bone Joint Surg Am. 1973;55:1351–66.
2. Ficat RP, Arlet J. Functional investigation of bone under normal conditions. In: Hungerford DS, editor. Ischemia and necrosis of bone. Baltimore: Williams and Wilkins; 1980. p. 29–52.
3. Steinberg ME, Hayken GD, Steinberg DR. A new method for evaluation and staging of avascular necrosis of the femoral head. In: Arlet J, Ficat RP, Hungerford DS, editors. Bone circulation. Baltimore: Williams and Wilkins; 1984. p. 398–403.
4. Ohzono K, Saito M, Sugano N, Takaoka K, Ono K. The fate of nontraumatic avascular necrosis of the femoral head: a radiologic classification to formulate prognosis. Clin Orthop Relat Res. 1992;277:73–8.
5. Jones Jr JP. Osteonecrosis. Clin Orthop Relat Res. 1978;130:2–4.
6. ARCO (Association Research Circulation Osseous): Committee on Terminology and Classification. ARCO News 1992;4:41–6.

Part IX

Differential Diagnosis

Subchondral Stress Fracture of the Femoral Head

29

Hee Joong Kim, Jeong Joon Yoo, and Pil Whan Yoon

29.1 Introduction

Subchondral stress fracture occurs most frequently in the femoral head, but it can occur in other anatomical locations such as the femoral condyle, tibial condyle, talar dome, humeral head, and acetabulum [1–8]. Although it is a recently recognized disease condition with the advent of magnetic resonance (MR) imaging [9–13], the occurrence of fatigue fractures in the subchondral trabecular bone was confirmed histologically in the early 1970s by cadaver or surgical specimen studies [14–17].

The symptoms and imaging findings of subchondral stress fracture of the femoral head (SSFFH) are similar to those of osteonecrosis of the femoral head [ONFH]. The possibility for SSFFH to be misdiagnosed as ONFH is high, as confirmed by referral to previous publications regarding cases of ONFH [18–24]. The differential diagnosis of SSFFH from ONFH is very important because its clinical course is much more benign than that of ONFH.

The clinical course and image findings of transient osteoporosis of the hip (TOH) are almost identical to those of SSFFH [25–31]. The only one difference is that no subchondral fracture line is detected in TOH. Therefore, it has been suggested that TOH might be a milder form of trabecular bone injury than SSFFH [28–31].

The first reported cases of SSFFH were insufficiency type [32]. Thereafter, the majority of reported cases were insufficiency type [2, 9–13, 33–39]. Later, the fatigue-type SSFFH was reported to occur in healthy adults with good bone quality who had suddenly increased their physical activity [8, 29, 40, 41]. In addition, SSFFH in normal healthy people without any increase of activity has been recognized [42–45].

H.J. Kim (✉) • J.J. Yoo
Department of Orthopedic Surgery,
Seoul National University College of Medicine,
101 Daehak-ro, Jongno-gu, Seoul 110-744, Korea
e-mail: oskim@snu.ac.kr; jjyos@snu.ac.kr

P.W. Yoon
Department of Orthopedic Surgery,
Seoul National University Boramae Hospital,
41 Boramae-Gil, Dongjak-Gu, Seoul 156-707, Korea
e-mail: orthoyoon@snu.ac.kr

29.2 Clinical Features

An insufficiency-type fracture occurs when normal or physiological stress is applied to abnormally weakened bone. In 1993, Grignon et al. reported 13 cases of insufficiency-type SSFFH in elderly people that were treated successfully with several weeks of nonweight bearing [9]. The authors emphasized the importance of differential diagnosis of this condition from TOH or ONFH. Since then, there have been reports of cases occurring mainly in osteoporotic elderly people and also in patients with poor bone quality such as renal transplant recipients, systemic lupus erythematosus, and osteogenesis imperfecta [2, 10–13, 33–38, 46–49]. On the contrary, fatigue-type fractures occur in people with normal bone quality after a sudden increase in activity; the first report included cases that occurred in military recruits during military drills [8, 29, 40, 41]. Later, it was recognized that SSFFH can occur in healthy adults with good bone quality without any increase in activity [42–45].

The insufficiency type is more common in women and the fatigue type is more common in men. Bilateral hip involvement is not rare and multiple site involvements have been reported (Fig. 29.1) [1–3, 29, 38, 43, 50, 51]. Fractures are usually located in the anterosuperior portion of the femoral head but can be located in the posterosuperior portion [29, 43].

In any type of fractures, common clinical findings include hip pain and limping of sudden onset without any antecedent trauma. The pain is aggravated with activity and improves with rest. Pain and limping decrease gradually as the fracture heals. In young patients, pain disappears completely 3–9 months after pain onset even in the cases with femoral head collapse [29, 41, 43]. However, in

K.-H. Koo et al. (eds.), *Osteonecrosis*,
DOI 10.1007/978-3-642-35767-1_29, © Springer-Verlag Berlin Heidelberg 2014

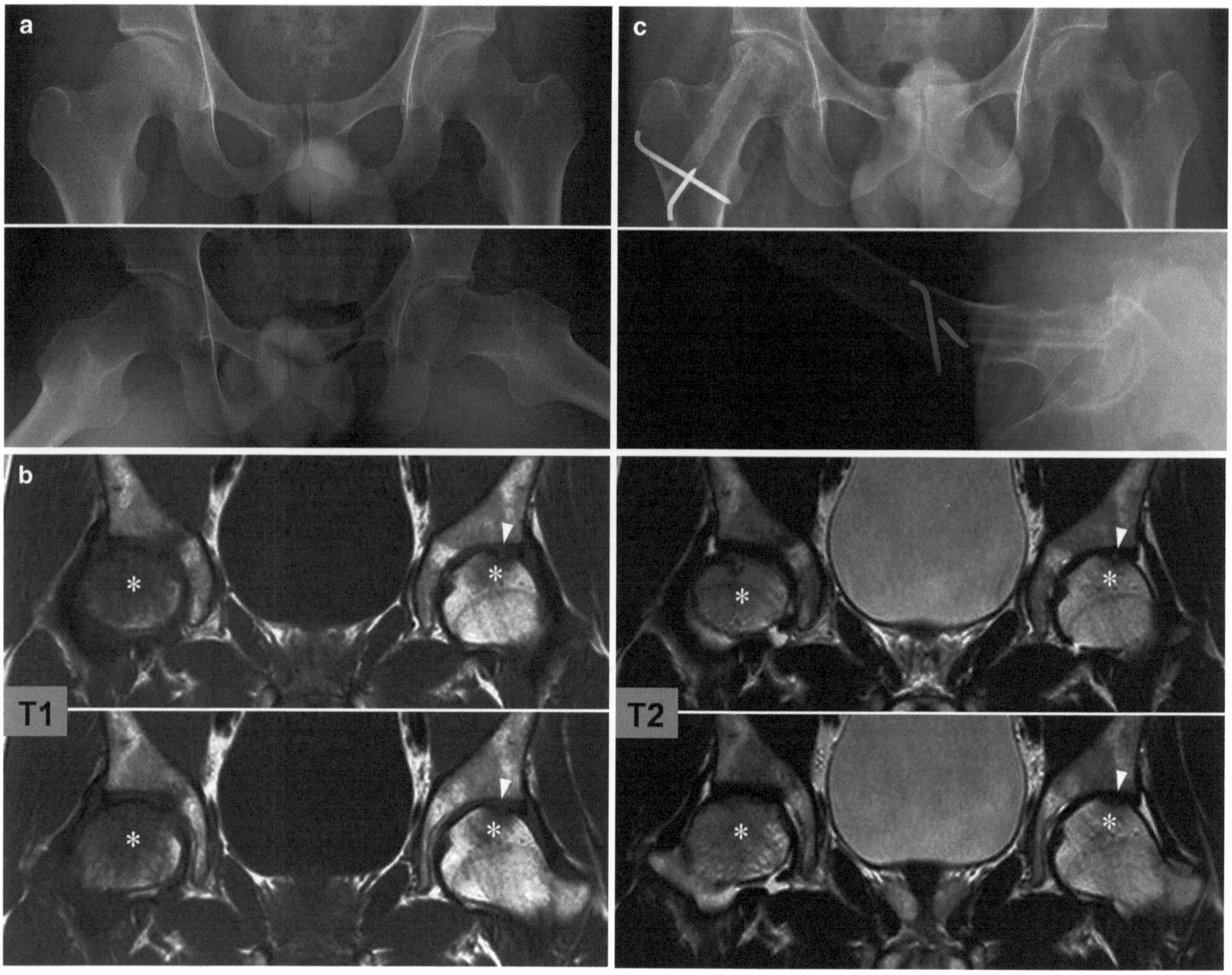

Fig. 29.1 A 27-year-old man with bilateral fatigue-type subchondral stress fracture of the femoral head. (**a**) Plain radiographs taken 2 weeks after the onset of both left and right hip pain show linear increased density lesion in both femoral heads and collapse of the right femoral head. (**b**) MR images of the hip show a subchondral fracture line (*arrow heads*) and bone marrow edema pattern (*asterisks*) extending to the subchondral area. (**c**) Radiographs taken 3 years after restoring right femoral head collapse using a fibular allograft demonstrate that the fracture is healed with partial restoration of the collapse

insufficiency-type fracture in elderly patients, incomplete resolution of pain is frequent and half of the cases need total hip arthroplasty [32, 45, 52].

29.3 Image Findings

Immediately after the onset of pain, usually no remarkable abnormal findings are detected unless collapse of the femoral head has already occurred. With time, osteopenia in the proximal femur and/or subchondral fracture line can be detected together with femoral head collapse when it occurs, but not always (Figs. 29.1, 29.3, 29.4 and 29.6c). In insufficiency-type fractures of the elderly, joint space narrowing is frequently observed, but the mechanism is not known (Fig. 29.2). The subchondral fracture line is usually more apparent on frog-leg view as in ONFH (Figs. 29.3, 29.5c and 29.6c).

Bone scintigraphy always shows focal or diffuse increased uptake in the femoral head (Fig. 29.3). It is nonspecific for the diagnosis but valuable as a screening test.

MR imaging is the most valuable and indispensible diagnostic tool (Figs. 29.1, 29.2, 29.3 and 29.4). Characteristic findings are subchondral abnormal intensity band and surrounding bone marrow edema pattern. The subchondral abnormal signal intensity band representing the fracture line is an essential finding for diagnosis. This irregular linear band is low signal intensity on T1-weighted images and variable abnormal signal intensity on T2-weighted images. The area of bone marrow edema pattern can be localized to the fracture line or diffuse in the femoral head and sometime extends to the

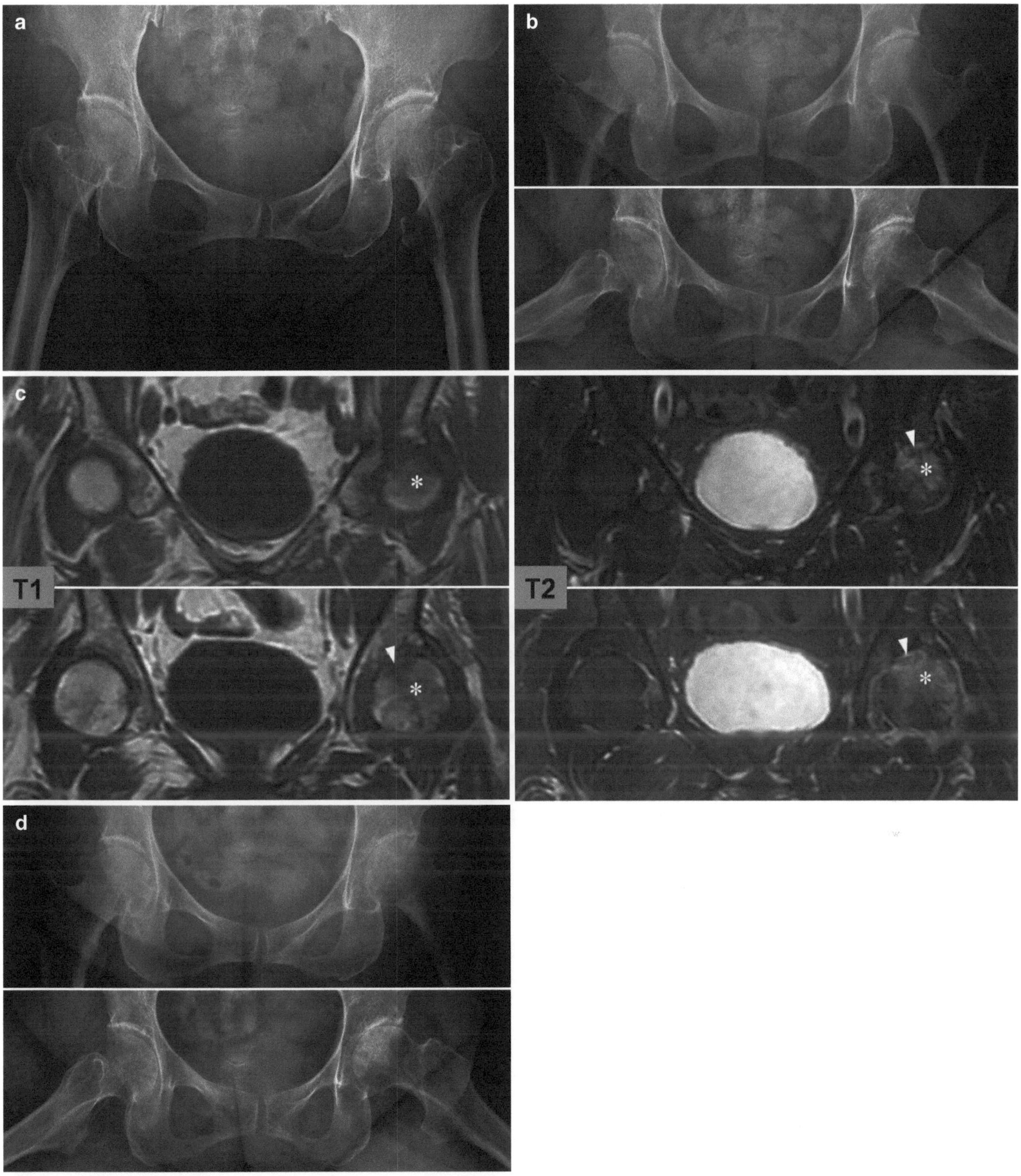

Fig. 29.2 A 65-year-old woman with insufficiency-type subchondral stress fracture of the femoral head. (**a**) Plain radiograph taken 2 months before the onset of left hip pain shows no remarkable abnormalities. (**b**) Radiographs taken 2 months after the onset of the left hip pain show joint space narrowing of the left hip without any other bony abnormality. (**c**) MR images of the hip show a subchondral fracture line (*arrow heads*) and bone marrow edema pattern (*asterisks*) extending to the subchondral area. (**d**) Radiographs taken 8 months later show slight progress of the joint space narrowing. Pain persists with some improvement

intertrochanteric area. Bone marrow edema pattern decreases gradually and disappears completely together with the symptoms as the fracture heals. The collapse of the femoral head or thinning of the articular cartilage is identifiable when existing, and joint effusion is a frequent finding.

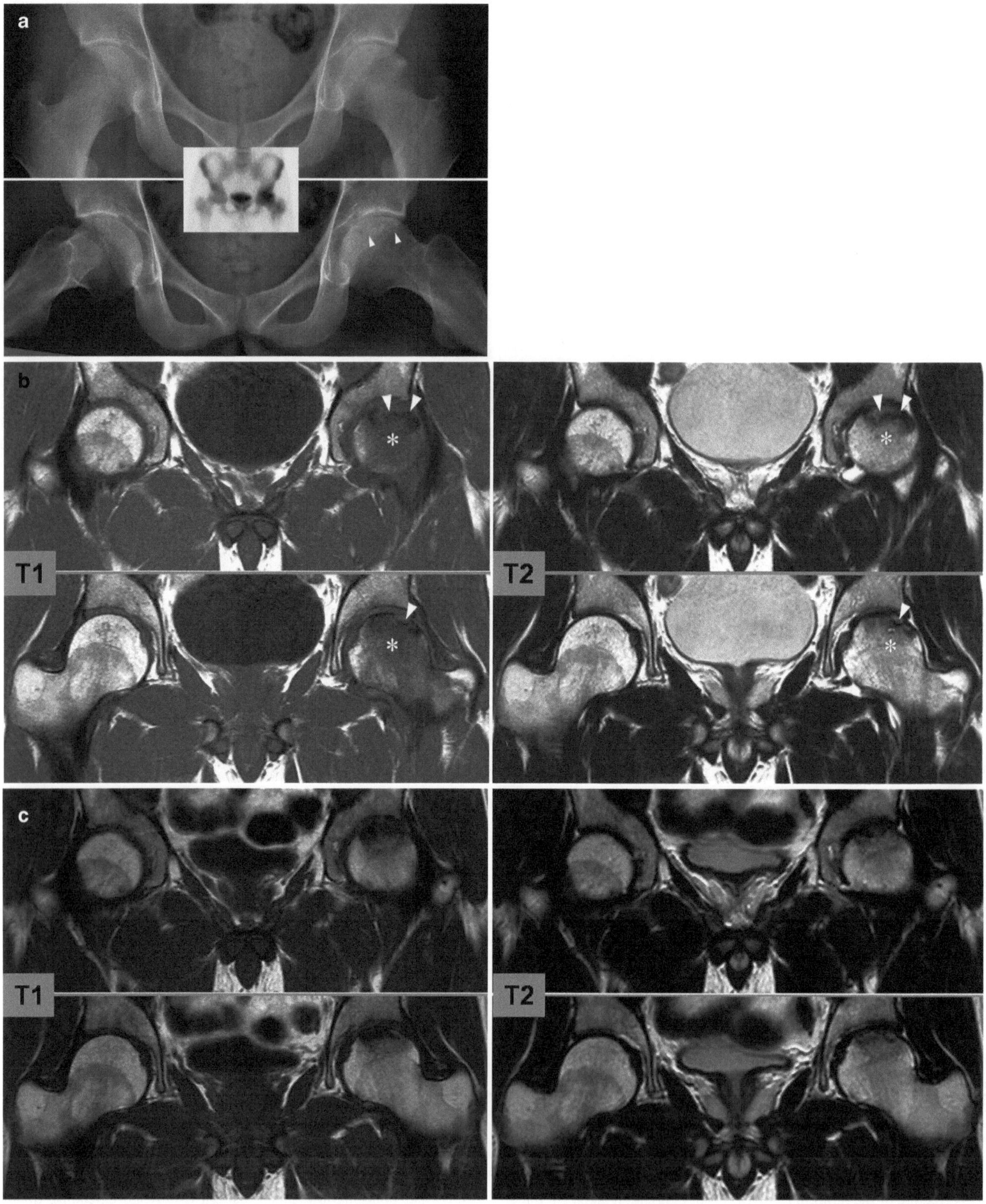

Fig. 29.3 A 20-year-old man with fatigue-type subchondral stress fracture of the femoral head.(**a**) Plain radiographs taken 1 month after the onset of the left hip pain show mild flattening of the left femoral head and a subchondral fracture line (*arrow heads*). Bone scintigraphy shows increased uptake in the left femoral head (*inset*). (**b**) MR images taken 1 month after the onset of the left hip show a subchondral fracture line (*arrow heads*) and bone marrow edema pattern (*asterisks*) extending to the subchondral area. (**c**) MR images taken 6 months later show marked decrease in the area of bone marrow edema pattern. (**d**) Radiographs taken 1.5 years after the onset of left hip pain show no further flattening of the femoral head

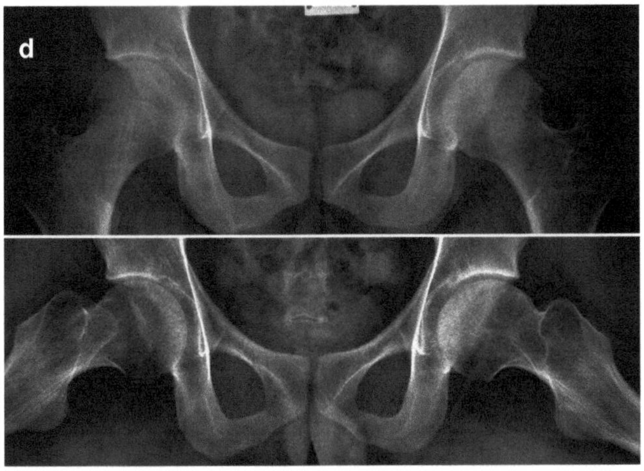

Fig. 29.3 (continued)

29.4 Treatment

No or protected weight bearing is a basic initial treatment for SSFFH with no or mild collapse of the femoral head. The duration of limitation in weight bearing has not been established.

The management for the collapsed femoral head is also not clear. When detected early, it is possible to elevate the collapsed area and maintain it until fracture healing by impaction of strut bone graft (Fig. 29.1); a few reports have described this approach [8, 29]. Recently, Yamamoto et al. reported successful short-term results of transtrochanteric rotational osteotomy for collapsed cases [44].

When symptoms persist with or without improvement with conservative treatment, usually in insufficiency-type fractures, THA is necessary.

29.5 Prognosis

Symptoms decrease gradually and disappear completely within several months. Symptoms tend to persist longer in collapsed cases, up to 9 months. When the fracture heals without collapse of the femoral head, no subsequent problems arise. In fatigue-type fractures, cases healed with moderate-to-severe collapse have been reported to do well without any significant symptom for more than 10 years (Fig. 29.4) [50].

Unlike fatigue-type fractures, conservative treatment is not successful in the large proportion of insufficiency-type fractures. Almost half of the reported cases received total hip arthroplasty because of inadequate improvement with conservative treatment [32, 45, 52]. The reason for this poorer result than fatigue-type fracture is not clear, but old age and joint space narrowing have been suggested to be associated with the poor result. Development of rapidly destructive coxopathy subsequent to insufficiency-type fractures has been reported [53–55].

29.6 Differential Diagnosis

As was pointed out in the first report of insufficiency-type SSFFH, the differentiation of ONFH and TOH from SSFFH is both necessary and important. ONFH has similar clinical and image findings, but the prognosis is very different from that of SSFFH; after the onset of pain, collapse of the femoral head and subsequent joint destruction progresses, and most cases need total hip arthroplasty.

Subchondral fracture and bone marrow edema also occur in ONFH. However ONFH differs in two aspects (Fig. 29.5). In ONFH, an additional abnormal signal intensity band is detected outside the subchondral fracture line. The outer abnormal signal intensity band is the outer margin of the necrotic lesion, the reactive interface between dead and living bones [56, 57]. The reactive interface is apparent as a low signal intensity band on T1-weighted images and the band is the first detectable abnormal MR finding of ONFH [58–60]. In the early stage of ONFH, the reactive interface appears as an inner high and outer low signal intensity band, the so-called double line sign, on T2-weighted images. The other point of difference is the extent of the bone marrow edema [8, 29, 43, 61]. In ONFH, bone marrow edema occurs only outside the reactive interface and not in the necrotic area. On the contrary, bone marrow edema extends up to or over the subchondral fracture line in SSFFH. The convexity of the subchondral fracture line was proposed as a differential point because subchondral fracture lines are usually convex to the articular surface, and reactive interface lines are usually concave to the articular surface [62, 63]. However, both the concave subchondral facture lines and the convex reactive interfaces are detected occasionally (Figs. 29.5a and 29.6) [64]. Osteonecrotic lesions without subchondral fracture are always painless, and two bands of subchondral fracture and reactive interface are usually observed in symptomatic ONFH. When the reactive interface is detected clearly as a sclerotic line on plain radiographs, a differential diagnosis can be made without MR images (Fig. 29.5c).

The clinical course and image findings of TOH, a condition of unknown etiology, are identical to those of SSFFH without femoral head collapse [25–31]. The only difference is that the subchondral fracture line is not detected in TOH. Miyanish et al. [28] detected suggestive findings of subchondral fracture in a retrospective review of MR images of cases previously diagnosed as TOH; subchondral fracture line was recognized in the MR images of many past publications of transient osteoporosis of the hip [65–76]. The differential diagnosis depends solely on the detection of the subchondral fracture line, but sometimes the fracture line can be detected

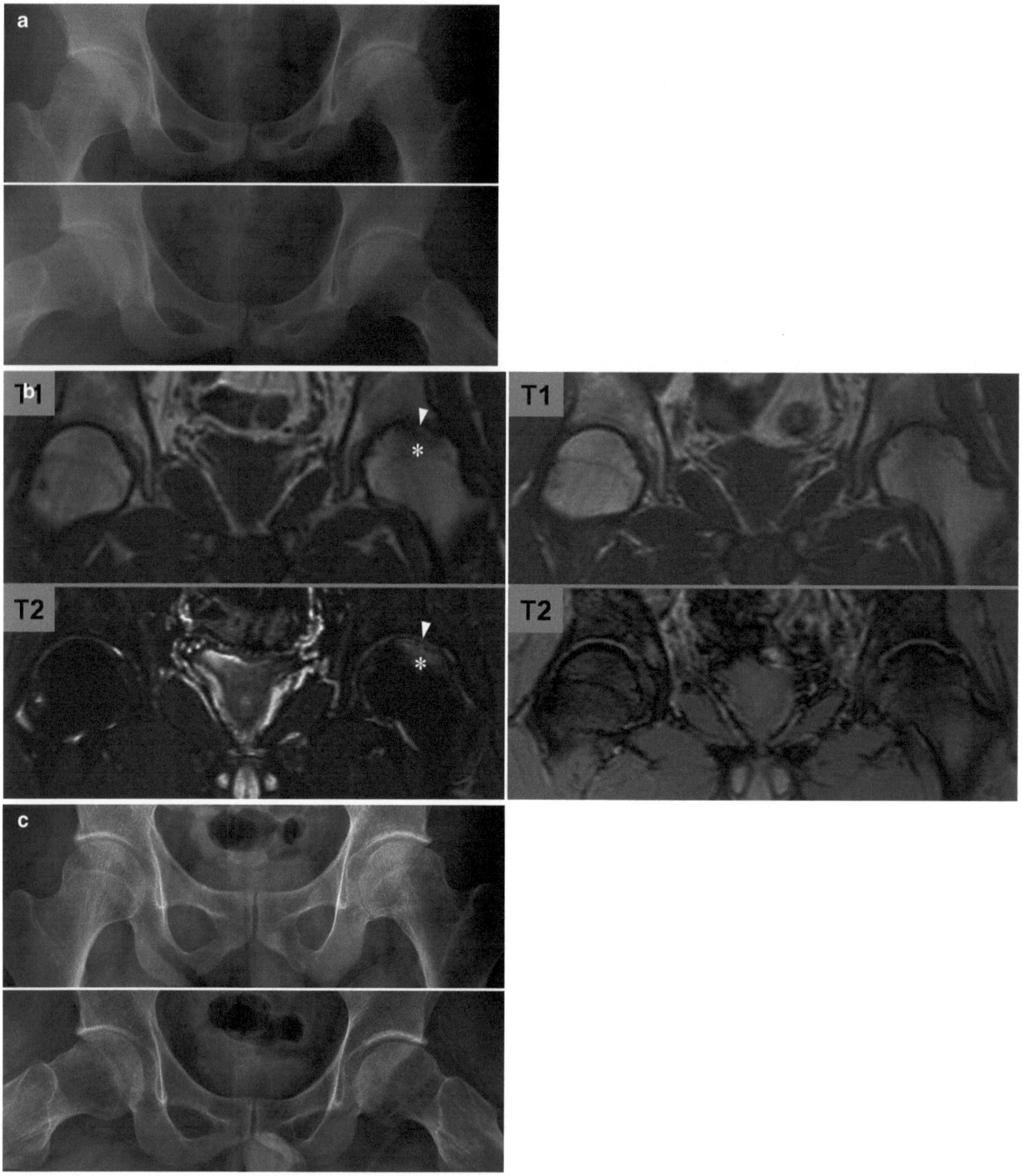

Fig. 29.4 A 20-year-old man with fatigue-type subchondral stress fracture of the femoral head. (**a**) Plain radiographs taken 4 months after the onset of left hip pain show moderate collapse of the left femoral head. (**b**) MR images taken 6 months after the onset of the left hip (*left column*) show a subchondral fracture line (*arrow heads*) and bone marrow edema pattern (*asterisks*) extending to the subchondral area. MR images taken 5 months later (*right column*) show disappearance of the bone marrow edema pattern and subchondral fracture line. (**c**) Radiographs taken 10 years after the onset of left hip pain show flattened femoral head with mild degenerative change. Patient has no pain and no limitation in daily activities

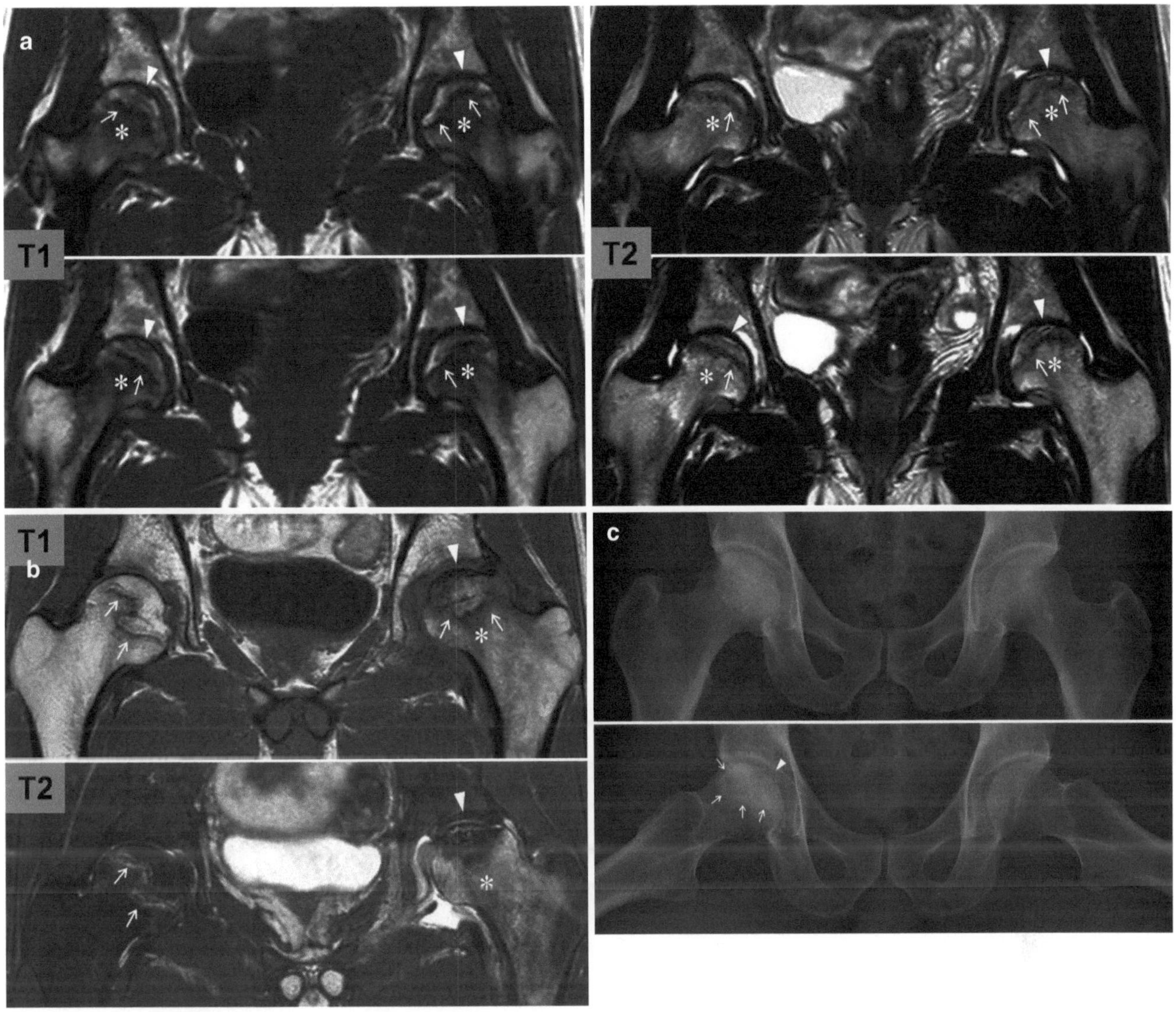

Fig. 29.5 Image findings of osteonecrosis of the femoral head. (**a**) A 31-year-old woman had both left and right hip pain for 1 month. In addition to a subchondral fracture line (*arrow heads*), an outer abnormal signal band (reactive interface, *arrows*) is detected on MR images. The bone marrow edema pattern (*asterisks*) is located distal to the reactive interface. (**b**) A 28-year-old man had left hip pain for 6 months. There has been no pain in the right hip. In the left hip, a subchondral fracture line (*arrow heads*) is observed proximal to the reactive interface band (*arrows*) and bone marrow edema pattern (*asterisks*) is found distal to the band. In the right hip, only the reactive interface (*arrows*) is observed. Neither a subchondral fracture line nor a bone marrow edema pattern is detected. (**c**) A 53-year-old man had right hip pain for 3 years. Plain radiographs show sclerotic margin (reactive interface, *arrows*) of the necrotic lesion and a subchondral fracture line (*arrow head*) in the right femoral head

only on some slices of MR images made with various techniques including gadolinium enhancement. In addition, it is likely to be more difficult or even impossible to detect the fracture line when it is incomplete. Recently, Kim et al. reported a case of bilateral TOH in which serial MPR CT findings suggested callus formation in the subchondral trabeculae followed by remodeling [31]. These propose that subchondral trabecular injury is likely the etiology of TOH.

29.7 Summary

SSFFH and ONFH are similar but definitely different diseases. The prognosis of SSFFH is much better than that of ONFH. Therefore, it is extremely important to make a differential diagnosis and it is possible with MR images. TOH may well be the milder form of subchondral trabecular bone injury.

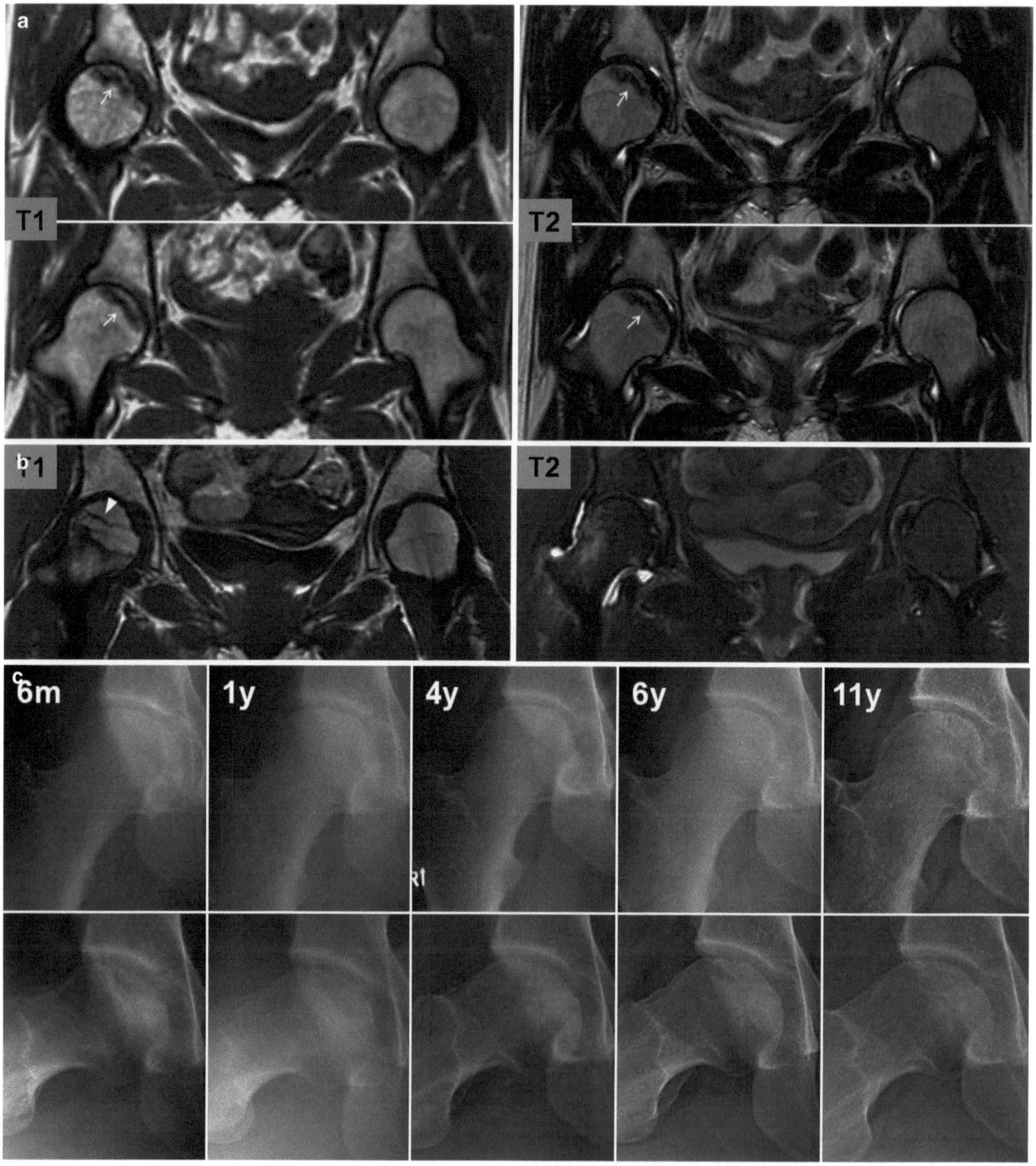

Fig. 29.6 Various convexity of the subchondral fracture line and the reactive interface. (**a**) MR images of a 17-year-old woman who had a history of steroid therapy for Hodgkin's disease show an asymptomatic osteonecrosis in the right femoral head. The abnormal signal intensity band (*arrows*) in the right femoral head is the outer margin of the necrotic lesion, the reactive interface. The band is convex to the articular surface. There is neither a subchondral fracture line nor a bone marrow edema pattern. (**b**) MR images of a 28-year-old woman with hypophosphatemic rickets show subchondral fracture findings in both femoral heads. The fracture line (*arrow heads*) in the right femoral head is concave to the articular surface. (**c**) Serial radiographs of a 21-year-old man show healing of a fatigue-type subchondral fracture of the femoral head. The fracture fragment is large and the fracture line is concave to the articular surface

References

1. Yamamoto T, Bullough PG. Subchondral insufficiency fracture of the femoral head and medial femoral condyle. Skeletal Radiol. 2000;29(1):40–4.
2. Motomura G, Yamamoto T, Miyanishi K, Shirasawa K, Noguchi Y, Iwamoto Y. Subchondral insufficiency fracture of the femoral head and acetabulum: a case report. J Bone Joint Surg Am. 2002;84(6):1205–9.
3. Narvaez JA, Narvaez J, De Lama E, Sanchez A. Spontaneous osteonecrosis of the knee associated with tibial plateau and femoral condyle insufficiency stress fracture. Eur Radiol. 2003;13(8):1843–8.
4. Tokuya S, Kusumi T, Yamamoto T, Sakurada S, Toh S. Subchondral insufficiency fracture of the humeral head and glenoid resulting in rapidly destructive arthrosis: a case report. J Shoulder Elbow Surg. 2004;13(1):86–9.
5. Pateder DB, Park HB, Chronopoulos E, Fayad LM, McFarland EG. Humeral head osteonecrosis after anterior shoulder stabilization in an adolescent: a case report. J Bone Joint Surg Am. 2004;86(10):2290–3.
6. Yamamoto T, Schneider R, Iwamoto Y, Bullough PG. Rapid acetabular osteolysis secondary to subchondral insufficiency fracture. J Rheumatol. 2007;34(3):592–5.
7. Fotiadou A, Karantanas A. Acute nontraumatic adult knee pain: the role of MR imaging. Radiol Med. 2009;114(3):437–47.
8. Yoon PW, Yoo JJ, Yoon KS, Kim HJ. Multifocal subchondral stress fracture of the femoral heads and tibial condyles in a young military recruit. Clin Orthop Relat Res. 2012;470(12):944–9.
9. Grignon B, Pere P, Regent D, Pourel J, Gaucher A. Fractures intracupitales du femur par insuffisance osseuse: une localization meconnue. Rev Im Med. 1993;5(1):83–8.
10. Vande Berg BC, Malghem J, Goffin EJ, Duprez TP, Maldague BE. Transient epiphyseal lesions in renal transplant recipients: presumed insufficiency stress fractures. Radiology. 1994;191(2):403–7.
11. Bangil M, Soubrier M, Dubost JJ, Rami S, Carcanagues Y, Ristori JM, Bussiere JL. Subchondral insufficiency fracture of the femoral head. Rev Rhum Engl Ed. 1996;63(11):859–61.
12. Rafii M, Mitnick H, Klug J, Firooznia H. Insufficiency fracture of the femoral head: MR imaging in three patients. AJR Am J Roentgenol. 1997;168(1):159–63.
13. Yamamoto T, Bullough PG. Subchondral insufficiency fracture of the femoral head: a differential diagnosis in acute onset of coxarthrosis in the elderly. Arthritis Rheum. 1999;42(10):2719–23.
14. Freeman MAR, Day WH, Swanson SA. Fatigue fracture in the subchondral bone of the human cadaver femoral head. Med Biol Eng. 1971;9(6):619–29.
15. Todd RC, Freeman MA, Pirie CJ. Isolated trabecular fatigue fractures in the femoral head. J Bone Joint Surg Br. 1972;54(4):723–8.
16. Cameron HU, Fornasier VL. Trabecular stress fractures. Clin Orthop Relat Res. 1975;111(6):266–8.
17. Fazzalari NL. Trabecular microfracture. Calcif Tissue Int. 1993;53 Suppl 1:S143–7.
18. Bassett LW, Gold RH, Reicher M, Bennett LR, Tooke SM. Magnetic resonance imaging in the early diagnosis of ischemic necrosis of the femoral head: preliminary results. Clin Orthop Relat Res. 1987;214(1):237–48.
19. Powell ET, Lanzer WL, Mankey MG. Core decompression for early osteonecrosis of the hip in high risk patients. Clin Orthop Relat Res. 1997;335(2):181–9.
20. Montella BJ, Nunley JA, Urbaniak JR. Osteonecrosis of the femoral head associated with pregnancy: a preliminary report. J Bone Joint Surg Am. 1999;81(5):790–8.
21. Aigner N, Schneider W, Eberl V, Knahr K. Core decompression in early stages of femoral head osteonecrosis: an MRI-controlled study. Int Orthop. 2002;26(1):31–5.
22. Reis ND, Schwartz O, Militianu D, Ramon Y, Levin D, Norman D, Melamed Y, Shupak A, Goldsher D, Zinman C. Hyperbaric oxygen therapy as a treatment for stage-I avascular necrosis of the femoral head. J Bone Joint Surg Br. 2003;85(2):371–5.
23. Radke S, Rader C, Kenn W, Kirschner S, Walther M, Eulert J. Transient marrow edema syndrome of the hip: results after core decompression: a prospective MRI-controlled study in 22 patients. Arch Orthop Trauma Surg. 2003;123(5):223–7.
24. Gangji V, Hauzeur JP, Matos C, De Maertelaer V, Toungouz M, Lambermont M. Treatment of osteonecrosis of the femoral head with implantation of autologous bone-marrow cells: a pilot study. J Bone Joint Surg Am. 2004;86(6):1153–60.
25. Guerra JJ, Steinberg ME. Distinguishing transient osteoporosis from avascular necrosis of the hip. J Bone Joint Surg Am. 1995;77(4):616–24.
26. Noorda RJP, van der Aa JPW, Wuisman PIJM, David EFL, Lips PTAM, van der Valk P. Transient osteoporosis and osteogenesis imperfecta: a case report. Clin Orthop Relat Res. 1997;337(4):249–55.
27. Karagkevrekis CB, Ainscow DA. Transient osteoporosis of the hip associated with osteogenesis imperfecta. J Bone Joint Surg Br. 1998;80(1):54–5.
28. Miyanishi K, Yamamoto T, Nakashima Y, Shuto T, Jingushi S, Noguchi Y, Iwamoto Y. Subchondral changes in transient osteoporosis of the hip. Skeletal Radiol. 2001;30(5):255–61.
29. Song WS, Yoo JJ, Koo K-H, Yoon KS, Kim Y-M, Kim HJ. Subchondral fatigue fracture of the femoral head in military recruits. J Bone Joint Surg Am. 2004;86(9):1917–24.
30. Miyanishi K, Kaminomachi S, Hara T, Maeda H, Watanabe H, Shimizu A, Torisu T. A subchondral fracture in transient osteoporosis of the hip. Skeletal Radiol. 2007;36(7):677–80.
31. Kim YL, Nam KW, Yoo JJ, Hong SH, Kim HJ. CT evidence for subchondral trabecular injury of the femoral head in transient osteoporosis of the hip: a case report. J Korean Med Sci. 2010;25(1):192–5.
32. Yoon PW, Yoo JJ, Koo KH, Yoon KS, Kim HJ. Subchondral insufficiency fracture of the femoral head in elderly people. J Korean Med Sci. In press.
33. Yamamoto T, Schneider R, Bullough PG. Insufficiency subchondral fracture of the femoral head. Am J Surg Pathol. 2000;24(3):464–8.
34. Yamamoto T, Schneider R, Bullough PG. Subchondral insufficiency fracture of the femoral head: histopathologic correlation with MRI. Skeletal Radiol. 2001;30(5):247–54.
35. Uetani M, Hashmi R, Ito M, Okimoto T, Kawahara Y, Hayashi K, Enomoto H, Shindo H. Subchondral insufficiency fracture of the femoral head: magnetic resonance imaging findings correlated with micro-computed tomography and histopathology. J Comput Assist Tomogr. 2003;27(2):189–93.
36. Buttaro M, Gonzalez Della Valle A, Morandi A, Sabas M, Pietrani M, Piccaluga F. Insufficiency subchondral fracture of the femoral head: report of 4 cases and review of the literature. J Arthroplasty. 2003;18(3):377–82.
37. Davies M, Cassar-Pullicino VN, Darby AJ. Subchondral insufficiency fractures of the femoral head. Eur Radiol. 2004;14(2):201–7.
38. Ikemura S, Yamamoto T, Nakashima Y, Shuto T, Jingushi S, Iwamoto Y. Bilateral subchondral insufficiency fracture of the femoral head after renal transplantation: a case report. Arthritis Rheum. 2005;52(4):1293–6.
39. Yamamoto TIY, Schneider R, Bullough PG. Histopathological prevalence of subchondral insufficiency fracture of the femoral head. Ann Rheum Dis. 2008;67(2):150–3.
40. Visuri T. Stress osteopathy of the femoral head. 10 military recruits followed for 5–11 years. Acta Orthop Scand. 1997;68(2):138–41.

41. Lee YK, Yoo JJ, Koo KH, Yoon KS, Min BW, Kim HJ. Collapsed subchondral fatigue fracture of the femoral head. Orthop Clin North Am. 2009;40(2):259–65.
42. Yamamoto T, Nakashima Y, Shuto T, Jingushi S, Iwamoto Y. Subchondral insufficiency fracture of the femoral head in younger adults. Skeletal Radiol. 2007;36 suppl 1:38–42.
43. Kim JW, Yoo JJ, Min BW, Hong SH, Kim HJ. Subchondral fracture of the femoral head in healthy adults. Clin Orthop Relat Res. 2007;464(11):196–204.
44. Yamamoto T, Iwasaki K, Iwamoto Y. Transtrochanteric rotational osteotomy for a subchondral insufficiency fracture of the femoral head in young adults. Clin Orthop Relat Res. 2010;468(12):3181–5.
45. Iwasaki K, Yamamoto T, Motomura G, et al. Prognostic factors associated with a subchondral insufficiency fracture of the femoral head. Br J Radiol. 2012;85(1011):214–8.
46. Yamamoto T, Schneider R, Iwamoto Y, Bullough PG. Subchondral insufficiency fracture of the femoral head in a patient with systemic lupus erythematosus. Ann Rheum Dis. 2006;65(6):837–8.
47. Hagino H, Okano T, Teshima R, et al. Insufficiency fracture of the femoral head in patients with severe osteoporosis—report of 2 cases. Acta Orthop Scand. 1999;70(1):87–9.
48. Yamanaka H, Goto K, Murata Y, Miyamoto K. Subchondral insufficiency fracture of the femoral head after total knee arthroplasty in a patient with rheumatoid arthritis. Mod Rheumatol. 2006;16(2):105–8.
49. Iwasaki K, Yamamoto T, Nakashima Y, Mawatari T, Motomura G, Ikemura S, Iwamoto Y. Subchondral insufficiency fracture of the femoral head after liver transplantation. Skeletal Radiol. 2009;38(9):925–8.
50. Sudo A, Hasegawa M, Kato K, Uchida A. Bilateral subchondral insufficiency fracture of the femoral head. Orthopedics. 2008;31(4):399.
51. Chouhan V, Agrawal K, Vinothkumar TK, Mathesul A. Bilateral insufficiency fracture of the femoral head and neck in a case of oncogenic osteomalacia. J Bone Joint Surg Br. 2010;92(9): 1028–31.
52. Miyanishi K, Ishihara K, Jingushi S, Torisu T. Risk factors leading to total hip arthroplasty in patients with subchondral insufficiency fractures of the femoral head. J Orthop Surg (Hong Kong). 2010;18(3):271–5.
53. Yamamoto T, Bullough PG. The role of subchondral insufficiency fracture in rapid destruction of the hip joint: a preliminary report. Arthritis Rheum. 2000;43(11):2423–7.
54. Yamamoto T, Takabatake K, Iwamoto Y. Subchondral insufficiency fracture of the femoral head resulting in rapid destruction of the hip joint: a sequential radiographic study. AJR Am J Roentgenol. 2002;178(2):435–7.
55. Niimi R, Hasegawa M, Sudo A, Uchida A. Rapidly destructive coxopathy after subchondral insufficiency fracture of the femoral head. Arch Orthop Trauma Surg. 2005;125(6):410–3.
56. Glimcher MJ, Kenzora JE. Nicolas Andry Award. The biology of osteonecrosis of the human femoral head and its clinical implications: 1. Tissue Biology. Clin Orthop Relat Res. 1979;138(1): 284–309.
57. Mitchell DG, Steinberg ME, Dalinka MK, Rao VM, Fallon M, Kressel HY. Magnetic resonance imaging of the ischemic hip. Alterations within the osteonecrotic, viable, and reactive zones. Clin Orthop Relat Res. 1989;244(7):60–77.
58. Nakamura T, Matsumoto T, Nishino M, Tomita K, Kadoya M. Early magnetic resonance imaging and histologic findings in a model of femoral head necrosis. Clin Orthop Relat Res. 1997;334(1):68–72.
59. Sakamoto M, Shimizu K, Iida S, Akita T, Moriya H, Nawata Y. Osteonecrosis of the femoral head: a prospective study with MRI. J Bone Joint Surg Br. 1997;79(2):213–9.
60. Kubo T, Yamazoe S, Sugano N, Fujioka M, Naruse S, Yoshimura N, Oka T, Hirasawa Y. Initial MRI findings of non-traumatic osteonecrosis of the femoral head in renal allograft recipients. Magn Reson Imaging. 1997;15(9):1017–23.
61. Kim YM, Oh HC, Kim HJ. The pattern of bone marrow oedema on MRI in osteonecrosis of the femoral head. J Bone Joint Surg Br. 2000;82(6):837–41.
62. Zhao G, Yamamoto T, Ikemura S, et al. A histopathological evaluation of a concave-shaped low-intensity band on T1- weighted MR images in a subchondral insufficiency fracture of the femoral head. Skeletal Radiol. 2010;39(2):185–8.
63. Ikemura S, Yamamoto T, Motomura G, Nakashima Y, Mawatari T, Iwamoto Y. MRI evaluation of collapsed femoral heads in patients 60 years old or older: differentiation of subchondral insufficiency fracture from osteonecrosis of the femoral head. AJR Am J Roentgenol. 2010;195(1):W63–8.
64. Yamaguchi R, Yamamoto T, Motomura G, Ikemura S, Iwamoto Y. MRI-detected double low-intensity bands in osteonecrosis of the femoral head. J Orthop Sci. 2011;16(4):471–5.
65. Bloem JL. Transient osteoporosis of the hip: MR imaging. Radiology. 1988;167(3):753–5.
66. Hauzeur JP, Hanquinet S, Gevenois PA, Appelboom T, Bentin J, Perlmutter N. Study of magnetic resonance imaging in transient osteoporosis of the hip. J Rheumatol. 1991;18(8):1211–7.
67. Takatori Y, Kokubo T, Ninomiya S, Nakamura T, Okutsu I, Kamogawa M. Transient osteoporosis of the hip: magnetic resonance imaging. Clin Orthop Relat Res. 1991;271(10):190–4.
68. Potter H, Moran M, Schneider R, Bansal M, Sherman C, Markisz J. Magnetic resonance imaging in diagnosis of transient osteoporosis of the hip. Clin Orthop Relat Res. 1992;280(7):223–9.
69. Hofmann S, Engel A, Neuhold A, Leder K, Kramer J, Plenk Jr H. Bone-marrow oedema syndrome and transient osteoporosis of the hip: an MRI-controlled study of treatment by core decompression. J Bone Joint Surg Br. 1993;75(2):210–6.
70. Hayes CW, Conway WF, Daniel WW. MR imaging of bone marrow edema pattern: transient osteoporosis, transient bone marrow edema syndrome, or osteonecrosis. Radiographics. 1993;13(5):1001–11.
71. Yamamoto T, Kubo T, Hirasawa Y, Noguchi Y, Iwamoto Y, Sueishi K. A clinicopathologic study of transient osteoporosis of The hip. Skeletal Radiol. 1999;28(11):621–7.
72. Andrews CL. From the RSNA Refresher Courses. Radiological Society of North America. Evaluation of the marrow space in the adult hip. Radiographics. 2000;20 Suppl 1:S27–42.
73. Uematsu N, Nakayama Y, Shirai Y, Tamai K, Hashiguchi H, Banzai Y. Transient osteoporosis of the hip during pregnancy. J Nippon Med Sch. 2000;67(6):459–63.
74. Fazekas JE, Losada R, Fruauff AA, Ortiz AO, Katz DS. Migratory transient osteoporosis of the hip occurring before and during pregnancy. J Women's Imaging. 2002;4(2):80–5.
75. Akisue T, Matsumoto K, Tsumura N, Fujita I, Yamamoto T, Yoshiya S. Bone marrow edema syndrome associated with uterine myoma: a case report. Clin Orthop Relat Res. 2003;409(4):151–7.
76. Balakrishnan A, Schemitsch EH, Pearce D, McKee MD. Distinguishing transient osteoporosis of the hip from avascular necrosis. Can J Surg. 2003;46(2):187–92.

Bone Marrow Edema Syndrome of the Hip

30

Young-Kyun Lee and Kyung-Hoi Koo

30.1 Introduction

Bone marrow edema syndrome (BMES) is an uncommon disease of the hip, which causes an acute disabling hip pain. It is a self-limiting disease, which regresses spontaneously within several months. In 1892, Hanau first described osteomalacia of the hip due to vitamin D deficiency during pregnancy [1]. In 1959, Curtiss and Kincaid reported three cases of transitory demineralization of the hip in pregnancy [2]. In 1968, Hunder and Kelly used the term "transient osteoporosis of the hip" because of the focal loss of radiodensity in the affected femoral head and its later spontaneous recovery [3].

In 1988, Bloem performed MR imaging in three patients with transient osteoporosis of the hip. MR images showed decreased signal intensity of bone marrow in the femur on T1-weighted images and increased signal intensity relative to the intensity of normal bone marrow on T2-weighted images. Joint effusions were seen on MR images of all patients on T2-weighted images [4]. Because of this, Wilson et al. proposed that the term "transient osteoporosis" be replaced by "transient marrow edema syndrome" [5].

The pathophysiology of BMES is controversial and the histology of BMES is similar to early-stage osteonecrosis (ON). Thus, there has been diagnostic confusion between these two diseases, and several authors thought BMES might be the earliest stage of ON [6]. Most authors believe that BMES is associated with an ischemia of the femoral head. It is a distinct self-limiting disease which does not progress to ON.

In this chapter, we describe the pathophysiology, clinical features, radiologic findings, and treatment of BMES. The disease is a continuous process and there is no consensus about the staging of BMES. We classified the pathological process into three stages: (1) ischemic stage, (2) hyperemic stage, and (3) recovery stage, which are useful for understanding the nature of BMES progression.

Y.-K. Lee • K.-H. Koo (✉)
Department of Orthopaedic Surgery,
Seoul National University College of Medicine, Seoul National University Bundang Hospital, 166 Gumi-ro,
Seongnam 463-707, South Korea
e-mail: ykleemd@gmail.com; khkoo@snu.ac.kr

30.2 Pathophysiology

While ON frequently occurs in people with certain risk factors such as alcohol abuse and high-dose steroid use, those risk factors are not found in patients with BMES. An association between decreased fibrinolytic potential and the subsequent development of BMES has been reported [7] and the late (third trimester) pregnancy is the only known risk factor for BMES [2].

Ischemia due to intravascular coagulation of the microcirculation seems to be the most probable cause of BMES as well as ON. However, subsequent events after the ischemia are quite different in the two diseases [8, 9]. In the absence or paucity of risk factors, intravascular coagulation is followed by a complete fibrinolysis and reactive vasodilatation [10]. Thus, there is only a brisk period of subthreshold ischemic hypoxia.

30.2.1 Ischemic Stage

The hematopoietic cells, which are most sensitive to ischemia, disappear usually within 12 h of ischemia [11]. Thus, fatty marrow conversion, which is known to correlate with the decrease in intramedullary blood flow, occurs in the proximal femur [12, 13]. Then, the marrow fat cells die from the second day of ischemia [14]. However, most osteocytes remain viable.

30.2.2 Hyperemic Stage

After a brisk ischemic stage, reactive neovascularization, arterial dilatation, and hyperemia occur in the marrow. The

K.-H. Koo et al. (eds.), *Osteonecrosis*,
DOI 10.1007/978-3-642-35767-1_30,

marrow space is filled with edematous fluid, which elevates bone marrow pressure.

The increased perfusion induces transient demineralization of the trabecular bone in the proximal femur.

30.2.3 Recovery Stage

After the hyperemic stage, a spontaneous recovery occurs within 6–12 months [1–6]. The edema is resolved, the necrotic marrow is replaced with viable fat cells, and the mineral content becomes normalized.

30.3 Histology

Histologic findings of BMES are similar to those of early-stage ON [11, 14].

In the ischemic stage, hematopoietic cells are not seen in the marrow space. Marrow fat cells are necrotic and their nucleuses are lost. Most lacunae are filled with osteocytes. Necrotic lesions are not conglomerated but scattered in the marrow space. Sequestrum, a focal lesion of completely dead marrow cells and osteocytes, is not formed, and there is no evidence of reparative processes, so-called reparative zone of osteonecrosis, at the periphery of the necrotic zone.

In the hyperemic stage, marrow space is filled with eosinophilic fluid. An active repair process is seen in this stage. Dilated vessels are observed between necrotic fat cells. Necrotic marrow is replaced by fibroblast proliferation and fibrous matrix.

The bone mass is not decreased and there is no sign of osteoporosis. Thus, the term of transient osteoporosis is a misnomer [5, 6]. Reactive bone formation is observed around the trabeculae. Extensive osteoid seams, which are covered by active osteoblasts, are formed around the trabeculae. However, the mineral content in trabecular bone is reduced [6] (Fig. 30.1).

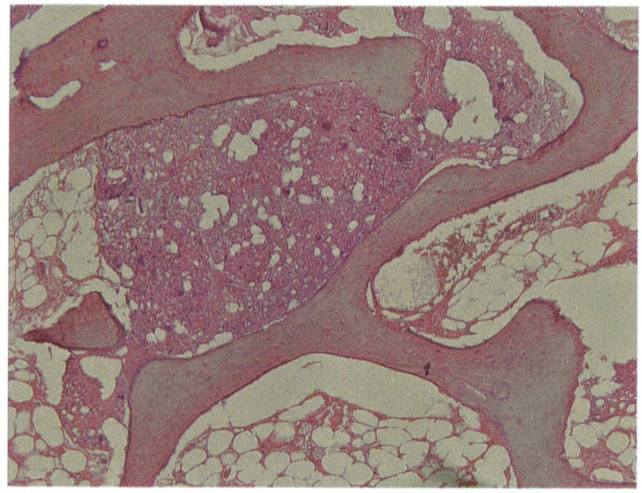

Fig. 30.1 A core biopsy specimen of bone marrow edema syndrome (stain, hematoxylin and eosin; original magnification, ×100) shows hematopoietic cells are depleted and fatty cells are necrotic in the marrow. The marrow space is filled with eosinophilic fibrinoid material and trabecular bone appears to be viable

30.4 Clinical Features, Laboratory Findings, and Natural Course

In the ischemic stage, the pain is absent or minimal. During the hyperemic stage, bone marrow pressure is elevated and patients suffer hip pain. Most patients are diagnosed in this hyperemic stage. A severe hip pain usually appears suddenly. In BMES the pressure is usually elevated to higher than 30 mmHg. The elevated bone marrow pressure is the main cause of hip pain [6, 10].

Hematological studies including erythrocyte sedimentation rate, white blood cell count, and C-reactive protein level are normal. The pain improves spontaneously within 6–12 months.

The improvement of pain parallels the normalization of findings on bone scan and MRI, which reflects the resolution of edema.

30.5 Magnetic Resonance Imaging

In the ischemic stage, the only MRI finding is the conversion of hematopoietic marrow to fatty marrow in proximal femoral metaphysis. The signal intensity of the proximal femoral metaphysis is similar to that of the greater trochanter. Otherwise, no abnormal findings are seen on MRI [15].

During this hyperemic stage, MRI shows findings of marrow edema in the proximal femur. T1-weighted images reveal a low-signal intensity in the femoral head, femoral neck, and the intertrochanteric region (Fig. 30.2), which changes to a high-signal intensity on the T2-weighted image (Fig. 30.3). No focal lesion suggestive of ON is seen on the MRI scans. Hip joint effusion, which appears as a high-signal lesion on T2-weighted image, is usually seen. The findings on MRI disappear gradually with the resolution of the edema [4–6].

30.6 Radiographs

In the initial ischemic stage, no abnormal findings are seen on radiographs. The radiographic findings become evident several weeks after the onset of pain. The radiographs show focal loss of radiodensity with blurring of the trabecular structure and cortical borders due to demineralization in the

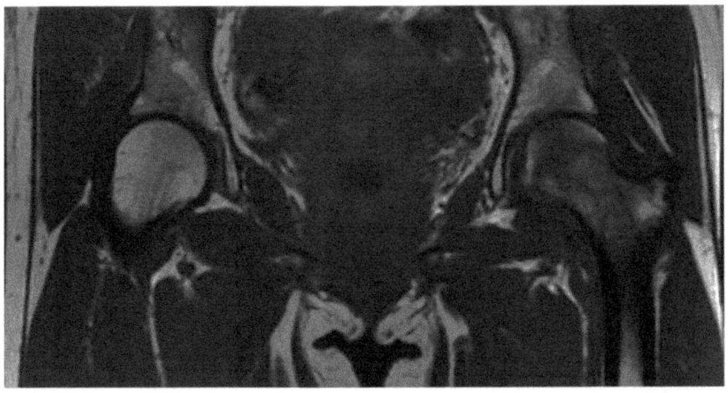

Fig. 30.2 T1-weighted spin-echo image (TR/TE: 549 ms/22 ms) reveals diffuse, low-signal intensity in the left proximal femur

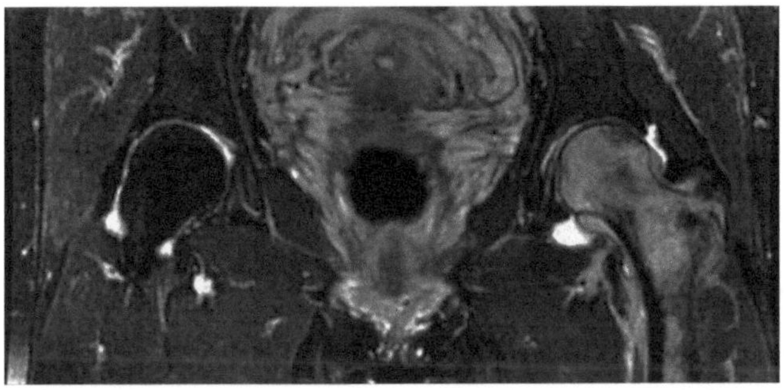

Fig. 30.3 On T2-weighted spin-echo image (TR/TE: 3,337 ms/100 ms), the lesion changes to a high-signal intensity

proximal femur. However, subchondral crescent sign (sub chondral fracture), femoral head flattening (collapse), and joint space narrowing, which are seen in ON, are not observed in BMES.

The radiolucency on radiographs gradually normalizes with the resolution of the edema.

30.7 Bone Scan

In the hyperemic stage, bone scan reveals an increased uptake involving the entire femoral head and neck often extending to the trochanteric area [4–6]. The uptake is diffuse and homogenous (Fig. 30.4). The improvement of pain parallels the normalization of findings on bone scan, which reflects the resolution of edema.

30.8 Angiography

In this ischemic stage, it is barely possible to demonstrate the arterial interruption. During the hyperemic stage, angiography shows dilatation of the medial femoral circumflex artery, superior retinacular arteries, and lateral epiphyseal artery (Fig. 30.5) [14].

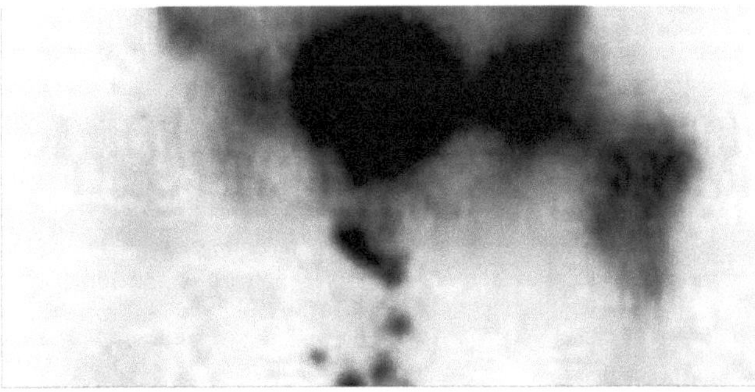

Fig. 30.4 Bone scan shows an increased uptake in the femoral head, neck, and trochanteric region (Permission from Koo et al. [10])

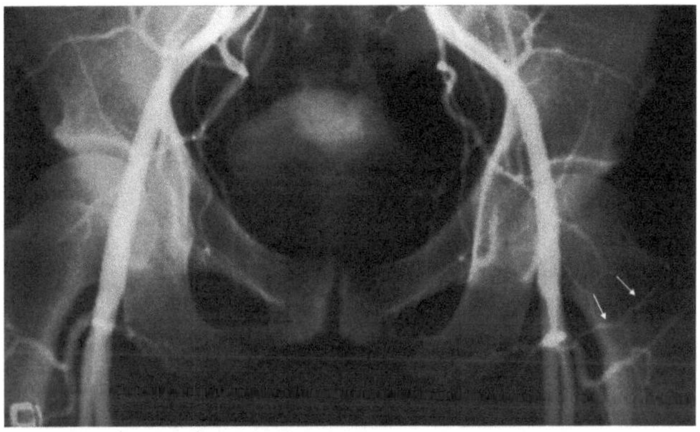

Fig. 30.5 Angiography shows dilatation of the medial femoral circumflex artery and superior retinacular arteries (*arrows*), whereas the arteries of the unaffected right hip are not dilated and barely seen (Permission from Koo et al. [10])

30.9 Treatment Strategies

Since BMES is a self-limiting disease, conservative treatments including protected weight-bearing and use of analgesics are recommended [2, 4, 5]. Some authors advocated core decompression, because it relieves the pain immediately and reduces the duration of symptoms [6]. However, it should be done cautiously in patients who have persistent and intractable pain even with conservative treatments, because of the risk of perioperative complications such as fracture and infection.

References

1. Hanau A. Ueber knochenveranderungen in der schwangerschaft und uber die bedeutung des puerperalen osteophyts. Fortschr Med Berl. 1892;10:237.
2. Curtiss Jr PH, Kincaid WE. Transitory demineralization of the hip in pregnancy. A report of three cases. J Bone Joint Surg Am. 1959;41-A:1327–33.
3. Hunder GG, Kelly PJ. Roentgenologic transient osteoporosis of the hip. Ann Intern Med. 1968;68(3):539.
4. Bloem JL. Transient osteoporosis of the hip: MR imaging. Radiology. 1988;167(3):753–5.

5. Wilson AJ, Murphy WA, Hardy DC, Totty WG. Transient osteoporosis: transient bone marrow edema? Radiology. 1988;167(3):757–60.
6. Hofmann S, Engel A, Neuhold A, Leder K, Kramer J, Plenk H. Bone-marrow oedema syndrome and transient osteoporosis of the hip: an MRI-controlled study of treatment after core decompression. J Bone Joint Surg Br. 1993;75B:210–6.
7. Van Veldhuizen PJ, Neff J, Murphey MD, Bodensteiner D, Skikne BS. Decreased fibrinolytic potential in patients with idiopathic avascular necrosis and transient osteoporosis of the hip. Am J Hematol. 1993;44(4):243–8. doi:10.1002/ajh.2830440405.
8. Jones Jr JP. Intravascular coagulation and osteonecrosis. Clin Orthop Relat Res. 1992;277:41–53.
9. Koo KH, Jeong ST, Jones Jr JP. Borderline necrosis of the femoral head. Clin Orthop Relat Res. 1999;358:158–65.
10. Koo KH, Ahn IO, Song HR, Kim SY, Jones Jr JP. Increased perfusion of the femoral head in transient bone marrow edema syndrome. Clin Orthop Relat Res. 2002;402:171–5.
11. Fondi C, Franchi A. Definition of bone necrosis by the pathologist. Clin Cases Miner Bone Metab. 2007;4(1):21–6.
12. Koo KH, Dussault R, Kaplan P, Kim R, Ahn IO, Christopher J, et al. Age-related marrow conversion in the proximal metaphysis of the femur: evaluation with T1-weighted MR imaging. Radiology. 1998;206(3):745–8.
13. Mitchell DG, Rao VM, Dalinka M, Spritzer CE, Axel L, Gefter W, et al. Hematopoietic and fatty bone marrow distribution in the normal and ischemic hip: new observations with 1.5-T MR imaging. Radiology. 1986;161(1):199–202.
14. Catto M. Pathology of aseptic bone necrosis. In: Davidson JK, editor. Aseptic necrosis of bone. Amsterdam: Excepta Medica; 1976. p. 3–100.
15. Kim SY, Koo KH, Suh KT, Kim YS, Cho YJ, Min BW, et al. Fatty marrow conversion of the proximal femoral metaphysis in transient bone marrow edema syndrome. Arch Orthop Trauma Surg. 2005;125(6):390–5. doi:10.1007/s00402-005-0824-4.

Distinguishing Bone Marrow Edema Syndrome from Osteonecrosis

31

Marc W. Hungerford and Kyung-Hoi Koo

31.1 Introduction

The histology of bone marrow edema syndrome (BMES) is similar to that of early stage osteonecrosis (ON) [1]. This similarity results in a diagnostic confusion between these two diseases. However, their natural courses are quite different from each other. While ON is frequently progressive, BMES usually recovers completely without any medical or surgical intervention. Thus, it is practically important to differentiate these two diseases.

31.2 Epidemiology

Bone marrow edema syndrome is a very uncommon disorder that affects the weight-bearing joints. Although originally described in pregnant females [2], it commonly affects middle-aged males [1, 3–5]. When women are affected, it usually occurs in the third trimester of pregnancy. Clinical presentation and clinical course do not differ from BMES in men or in nonpregnant women.

Osteonecrosis is much more common than BMES. Patients are typically in their third, fourth, or fifth decade of life [6]. In both of ON and BMES, the most frequently involved joint is the hip, followed by the knee and the shoulder. Multiple joints are occasionally involved in ON, whereas it is uncommon in BMES.

31.3 Association of Risk Factors

Risk factors, including alcohol consumption, corticosteroid use, renal transplantation, a blood clotting abnormality, radiation therapy, chemotherapy, organ transplantation, systemic lupus erythematosus, sickle cell disease, HIV infection, and Gaucher disease, can be identified in 80 % of ON patients [6]. Alcohol-related ON is frequent in males, while steroid-related ON is frequent in females. In BMES such risk factors are not associated. The only known risk factor is pregnancy at the third trimester [2].

31.4 Clinical Features and Natural Course

In both of BMES and ON, patients have an acute hip pain without any history of trauma. Hematological studies including erythrocyte sedimentation rate, white blood cell count, and C-reactive protein level are normal.

Usually, BMES completely recovers spontaneously. The clinical course is self-limiting and the pain improves within 3–18 months [1–5]. The improvement of pain parallels the resolution of edema. The extent and location of marrow edema do not affect the fate of BMES.

A spontaneous resolution of ON can occur, when the size is less than 1 cm [7]. However, once developed, ON usually persists and the size does not change. Osteonecrosis frequently leads to a collapse of the femoral head and degenerative arthritis of the hip. Size and location of a necrotic lesion are major determining factors for the collapse [8–10]. In ON, marrow edema can occur around the necrotic portion, even prior to collapse. The edema is the main cause of hip pain in early stage ON, which improves with the resolution

M.W. Hungerford
Orthopedics and Joint Replacement,
Mercy Medical Center, 301 Saint Paul Place,
Baltimore, MD 21202, USA
e-mail: mhunger@mdmercy.com

K.-H. Koo (✉)
Department of Orthopaedic Surgery,
Seoul National University College of Medicine,
Seoul National University Bundang Hospital,
166 Gumi-ro, Seongnam 463-707, South Korea
e-mail: khkoo@snu.ac.kr

K.-H. Koo et al. (eds.), *Osteonecrosis*,
DOI 10.1007/978-3-642-35767-1_31, © Springer-Verlag Berlin Heidelberg 2014

of edema [11]. As ON progresses, the femoral head collapses and subsequent osteoarthritis occurs, which is the cause of hip pain in advanced stage ON.

31.5 Magnetic Resonance Imaging

Because of its ability to image water content, MRI has become the most reliable imaging modality in the diagnosis of BMES. Abnormal findings on MRI precede abnormal radiographs by several months. The MR findings of BMES are characteristic and different from ON. The edema appears as low signal intensity on T1-weighted images and high signal intensity on STIR or fat-suppressed T2-weighted images in the proximal femur, including the femoral head, femoral neck, and the intertrochanteric region [1, 4, 5].

The defining characteristic of ON on MRI is the appearance of a band lesion. This represents the reactive zone surrounding the necrotic portion. The band lesion appears as a region of low signal intensity on T1-weighted images, which changes into a high increased signal intensity on T2-weighted spin echo (SE) or turbo-spin-echo (TSE) images [12].

The reactive band is not seen in BMES. Usually hip joint effusion, which appears as a high signal lesion on T2-weighted image, is associated in BMES. The edema resolves spontaneously within several months to a few years (Fig. 31.1).

31.6 Radiographic Findings

In the early stages of disease, plain radiographs of patients with BMES are negative. Demineralization may become evident within 3–6 weeks of onset of symptoms. A focal loss of radiodensity is seen with blurring of the trabecular structure and cortical borders in the femoral head and neck and sometimes extending down to the intertrochanteric region. The radiolucency may remain evident on plain radiographs even after full resolution of symptoms [13]. During the entire course of disease, the bony margins are preserved and no subchondral lesions are evident.

In ON patients, a radiolucent lesion surrounded by a sclerotic rim of reactive bone or a subchondral area of bone collapse or "crescent sign" is typically seen. These findings are not seen in BMES.

31.7 Bone Scan

Bone scanning using TC^{99} has been useful in detecting preradiographic lesions of BMES. Bone scan shows an increased uptake within a few days of symptoms. Generally diffuse uptake throughout the femoral head and into the neck and metaphysis is seen. Bone scan may be used to differentiate BMES from ON, as ON will typically show an area of photopenia ("cold spot") in the anterior–superior region of the femoral head [13]. The uptake normalizes in accordance with the resolution of edema.

In ON, a cold spot, which represents necrotic potion, is surrounded by a band of hot uptake, which represents the reactive zone.

Currently, bone scanning has been largely replaced by MRI in the diagnosis of BMES, due to its lack of specificity and radiation hazard.

31.8 Histology

Histological findings of BMES are similar to those of early stage ON [1, 14, 15].

Hematopoietic cells are not seen in the marrow. The marrow is filled with eosinophilic fluid and necrotic fat. Fibrosis and dilated vessels are observed in the marrow space. However, most lacunae are filled with osteocytes. Sequestrum of completely dead marrow cells and osteocytes is not formed, and there is no evidence of reparative processes, so called reparative zone of osteonecrosis.

The mineral content in the bone is reduced, which results in visible radiolucency on radiographs. Reactive bone

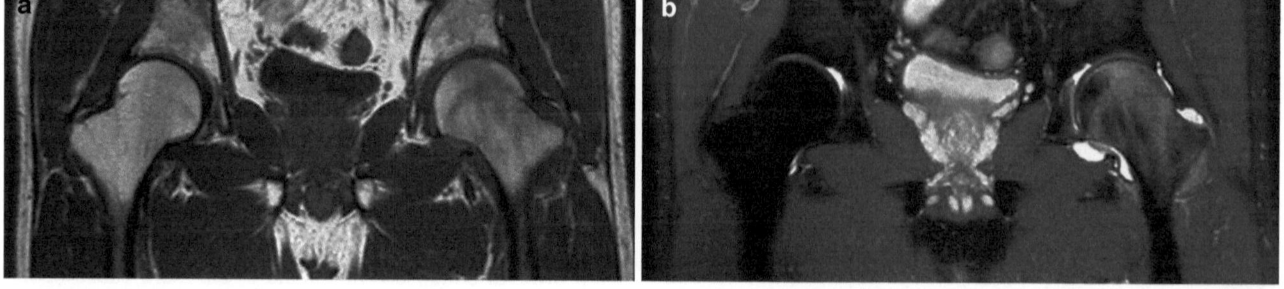

Fig. 31.1 A 44-year-old man had left hip pain for 2 weeks. (**a**) T1-weighted spin-echo image (TR/TE: 450 ms/20 ms) reveals diffuse, low signal intensity in the left proximal femur. (**b**) On proton density image (TR/TE: 4,500 ms/15 ms), the lesion changes to a high signal intensity. Hip joint effusion is associated. There is no focal lesion suggestive of osteonecrosis

formation with osteoid seams is observed around the trabeculae. Thus, bone formation is increased and there is no evidence of osteoporosis. The term of "transient osteoporosis of the hip" was a misnomer [1].

31.9 Pathophysiologic Relation of ON and BMES

The relationship between BMES and ON remains controversial. Given the self-limiting nature of BMES, some investigators hypothesize that BMES is a separate and distinct condition from ON, while others note that BMES can occasionally progress to ON and therefore suppose that BMES represents an abortive, reversible form of ON [1, 14–16].

Ischemia seems to be the common cause of both ON and BMES. Jones has theorized that intravascular coagulation of the intraosseous microcirculation may be the common pathway to both BMES and ON [14, 15]. However, subsequent events after an ischemic event are different between the two diseases. In BMES the ischemic event is subcritical and reversible. The fatty marrow in BMES specimens can be seen to undergo fibrosis, but the osteocytes remain viable and thus able to recover. In this hypothesis, the determining factor of whether an ischemic event produces BMES or ON is the speed and quality of reperfusion after thrombosis. If the reperfusion is complete, then the patient develops BMES rather than frank necrosis. Angiographic studies of patient with BMES showed arterial dilatation and hyperemia of the proximal femur [17].

Like ON, femoral heads with BMES demonstrate intraosseous hypertension [1, 17]. The bone marrow pressure is usually elevated above 30 mmHg. This intraosseous hypertension is most likely the cause of both the pain and the edema. It is this persistent hypervascularity, which probably causes the demineralization eventually detected on plain radiography. Quantitative radiography confirms a loss of hydroxyapatite without a loss of bone mass (Table 31.1) [1].

31.10 Regional Migratory Osteoporosis

Regional migratory osteoporosis (RMO) is defined as sequential arthralgia of the weight-bearing joints associated with a focal radiolucency [18, 19]. Clinical presentation, imaging results, and clinical course are identical to BMES with the exception that another joint or the same joint is affected at a different time interval. RMO most typically affects the joint nearest the previously diseased joint, although a variant with combined axial and skeletal involvement has been described. Like BMES, RMO typically affects middle-aged men. Due to its identical presentation, imaging, and clinical course, RMO should be considered a subset or recurrence of BMES, rather than a distinct clinical entity.

Table 31.1 Osteonecrosis and bone marrow edema syndrome

	ON	BMES
Risk factor	Associated in 80 %	Not associated
MRI	Band lesion in the femoral head	Diffuse lesion in the proximal femur Low signal intensity in T1-weighted image High signal intensity in T2-weighted image
Bone scan	Cold spot surrounded with band-like hot uptake	Diffuse hot uptake
Histology	Marrow necrosis and empty lacunae Reactive zone around necrosis	Marrow necrosis with interstitial edema
Natural course	Progressive to femoral head collapse in medium to large lesion	Spontaneous recovery

References

1. Hofmann S, Engel A, Neuhold A, Leder K, Kramer J, Plenk H. Bone-marrow oedema syndrome and transient osteoporosis of the hip: an MRI-controlled study of treatment after core decompression. J Bone Joint Surg Br. 1993;75B:210–6.
2. Curtiss Jr PH, Kincaid WE. Transitory demineralization of the hip in pregnancy. A report of three cases. J Bone Joint Surg Am. 1959;41-A:1327–33.
3. Hunder GG, Kelly PJ. Roentgenologic transient osteoporosis of the hip. Ann Intern Med. 1968;68(3):539.
4. Bloem JL. Transient osteoporosis of the hip: MR imaging. Radiology. 1988;167(3):753–5.
5. Wilson AJ, Murphy WA, Hardy DC, Totty WG. Transient osteoporosis: transient bone marrow edema? Radiology. 1988;167(3):757–60.
6. Mont MA, Zywiel MG, Marker DR, McGrath MS, Delanois RE. The natural history of untreated asymptomatic osteonecrosis of the femoral head: a systematic literature review. J Bone Joint Surg Am. 2010;92(12):2165–70.
7. Cheng EY, Thongtrangan I, Laorr A, Saleh KJ. Spontaneous resolution of osteonecrosis of the femoral head. J Bone Joint Surg Am. 2004;86-A(12):2594–9.
8. Steinberg ME, Hayken GD, Steinberg DR. A quantitative system for staging avascular necrosis. J Bone Joint Surg Br. 1995;77(1):34–41.
9. Koo KH, Kim R. Quantifying the extent of osteonecrosis of the femoral head. A new method using MRI. J Bone Joint Surg Br. 1995;77(6):875–80.
10. Cherian SF, Laorr A, Saleh KJ, Kuskowski MA, Bailey RF, Cheng EY. Quantifying the extent of femoral head involvement in osteonecrosis. J Bone Joint Surg Am. 2003;85-A(2):309–15.
11. Koo KH, Ahn IO, Kim R, Song HR, Jeong ST, Na JB, Kim YS, Cho SH. Bone marrow edema and associated pain in early stage osteonecrosis of the femoral head: prospective study with serial MR images. Radiology. 1999;213(3):715–22.
12. Mitchell DG, Rao VM, Dalinka MK, Spritzer CE, Alavi A, Steinberg ME, Fallon M, Kressel HY. Femoral head avascular necrosis: correlation of MR imaging, radiographic staging, radionuclide imaging, and clinical findings. Radiology. 1987;162(3):709–15.

13. Korompilias AV, Karantanas AH, Lykissas MG, Beris AE. Transient osteoporosis. J Am Acad Orthop Surg. 2008;16(8):480–9. Review.
14. Jones Jr JP. Intravascular coagulation and osteonecrosis. Clin Orthop Relat Res. 1992;277:41–53.
15. Koo KH, Jeong ST, Jones Jr JP. Borderline necrosis of the femoral head. Clin Orthop Relat Res. 1999;358:158–65.
16. Jones LC, Hungerford DS. The pathogenesis of osteonecrosis. Instr Course Lect. 2007;56:179–96. Review.
17. Koo KH, Ahn IO, Song HR, Kim SY, Jones Jr JP. Increased perfusion of the femoral head in transient bone marrow edema syndrome. Clin Orthop Relat Res. 2002;402:171–5.
18. Duncan H, Frame B, Frost H, Arnstein AR. Regional migratory osteoporosis. South Med J. 1969;62(1):41–4.
19. Malizos KN, Zibis AH, Dailiana Z, Hantes M, Karachalios T, Karantanas AH. MR imaging findings in transient osteoporosis of the hip. Eur J Radiol. 2004;50(3):238–44.

Part X

Non-surgical Treatments

Treatment of Osteonecrosis of the Hip and Knee with Enoxaparin

32

Charles J. Glueck, Richard A. Freiberg, and Ping Wang

32.1 Introduction

Osteonecrosis (ON) can be secondary to diverse risk factors including high-dose/long-term corticosteroids, alcoholism, the antiphospholipid antibody syndrome, exogenous estrogens or testosterone, pregnancy, HIV-proteases, and hip dislocation or fracture (Fig. 32.1). In men given exogenous testosterone, 40 % develop high estradiol (E2) levels as the testosterone is aromatized to E2, and they often then develop osteonecrosis when the thrombophilic E2 interacts with underlying and previously undiagnosed familial thrombophilia, particularly Factor V Leiden heterozygosity [1]. Primary (idiopathic) osteonecrosis of hips and knees [2] in adults [1, 3–14] and Legg-Calvé-Perthes disease in children [15, 16] are commonly associated with heritable thrombophilia, hypofibrinolysis, or reduction of nitric oxide (NO) production by the T-786C mutation of the endothelial nitric oxide synthase gene (eNOS), Fig. 32.1. The association of heritable thrombophilia-hypofibrinolysis with ON is important because the diagnosis provides an opportunity to decrease the frequency of total hip replacement (THR) [7, 17] by using anticoagulation with enoxaparin to stop the progression of Ficat stage I and II primary ON of the femoral head. Moreover, patients with thrombophilia-hypofibrinolysis recognized before THR should be candidates for increased intensity and duration of postoperative anticoagulation [18–22] Table 32.1.

The pathogenesis of ON probably reflects a "multiple etiology" [23–29] model, Fig. 32.1. We, and then others, have postulated a sequence for the development of ON. Osseous venous outflow obstruction is caused by venous thrombosis due to thrombophilia-hypofibrinolysis [1, 3–5, 7, 17], leading to increased intraosseous venous pressure, reduced arterial flow, ischemia, and bone death [10, 11, 13, 23–26, 30–33], Fig. 32.1. Experimental models of ON [23–26] confirm venous occlusion as a primary event. We have speculated that anticoagulation facilitates lysis of intraosseous thrombi, reducing elevated intraosseous venous pressure, improving arterial flow, reversing hypoxia, stopping bone death, and allowing bone healing (Fig. 32.1) [17].

In the current report, our focus is on intact functional hip survival 4.2–7 years after a 3-month course of enoxaparin. We have previously reported [17] a prospective pilot study of 16 primary ON patients (25 hips) with thrombophilia-hypofibrinolysis treated with enoxaparin for the same duration as used in deep venous thrombosis of leg veins [34] (60 mg/day, 3 months). This treatment stopped the progression of ischemic Ficat [35] stages I or II primary ON over ≥ 108 week follow-up. Survival of 19 of 25 hips (76 %), based on intent to treat, compared favorably with untreated historical controls (~20 % 2 year survival) [36–38]. We concluded that enoxaparin often prevents progression of primary hip ON in patients with thrombophilia-hypofibrinolysis, decreasing THR [17]. We concluded [17] that seeking a nonoperative anticoagulant route for treatment of Ficat stage I or II primary ON holds considerable promise in preserving the femoral head. However, in thrombophilic-hypofibrinolytic patients with

C.J. Glueck (✉) • P. Wang
The Cholesterol Center, Jewish Hospital of Cincinnati, ABC Building, 3200 Burnet Ave, Cincinnati, OH 45229, USA
e-mail: cjglueck@health-partners.org; pxwang@health-partners.org

R.A. Freiberg
Department of Surgery, Orthopedic Surgery Service VA Hospital, Cincinnati, OH, USA
e-mail: raf@cinci.rr.com

K.-H. Koo et al. (eds.), *Osteonecrosis*,
DOI 10.1007/978-3-642-35767-1_32, © Springer-Verlag Berlin Heidelberg 2014

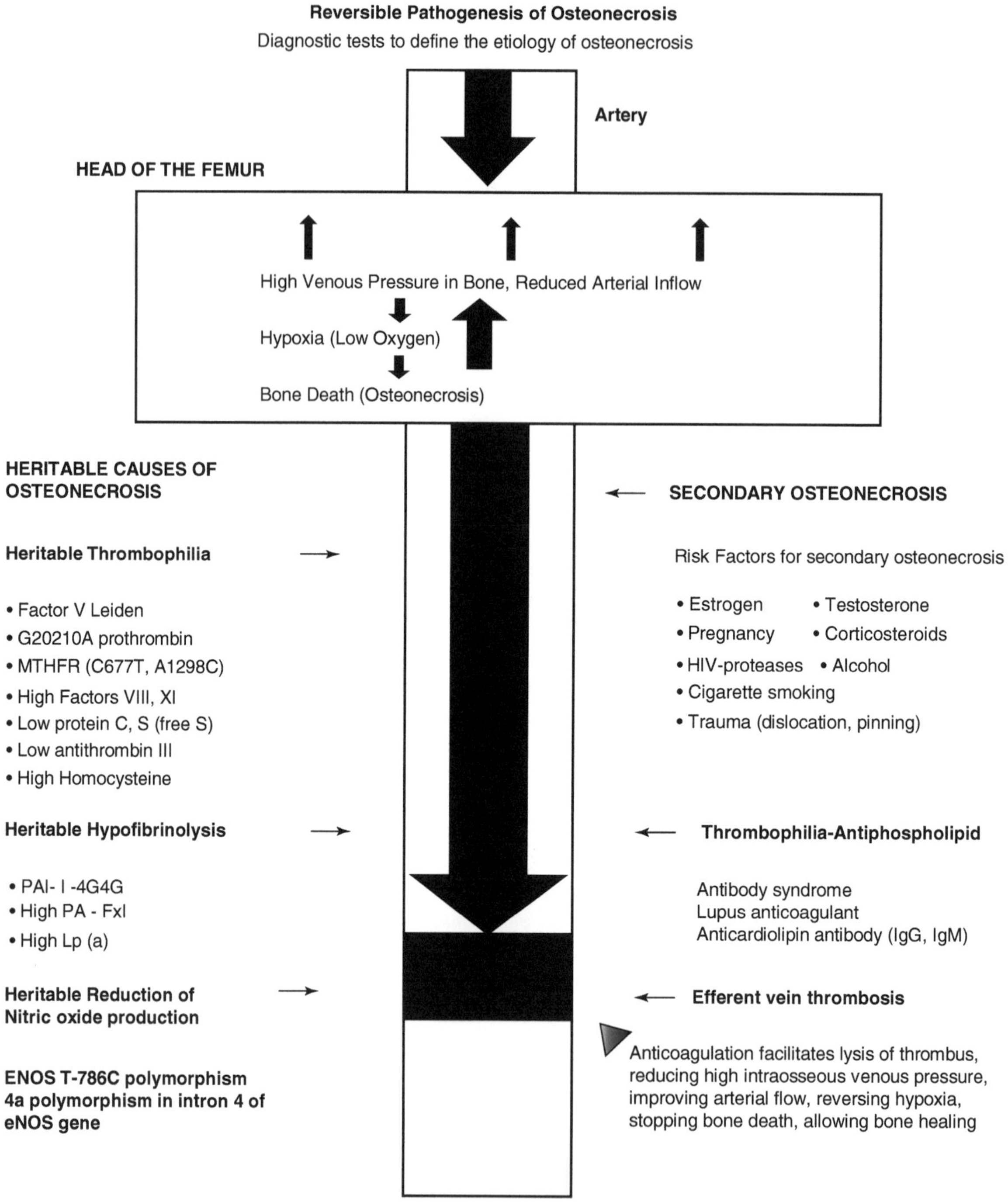

Fig. 32.1 Reversible pathogenesis of osteonecrosis

osteonecrosis secondary to corticosteroids, alcohol, etc., 3 months therapy with enoxaparin does not stop the progression of Ficat stages I or II osteonecrosis, and these patients have the same hip failure rate as untreated patients [17], requiring THR.

We are now reporting prospectively on outcomes in 20 patients (30 hips), over 4.2–7-year follow-up after initial enoxaparin treatment (60 mg/day for 3 months) [17] in preventing progression of stages I and II primary ON of the hip(s) associated with thrombophilia and/or hypofibrinolysis. We also assessed 36–40-month follow-up success of enoxaparin treatment (1.5 mg/kg/day for 3 months) in 7 patients (11 knees) in preventing progression of primary ON of the knee.

Table 32.1 Screening tests for thrombophilia, hypofibrinolysis, and impairment of nitric oxide production

Thrombophilia
PCR studies
G1691A Factor V Leiden
G20210A prothrombin
C677T/A1298C MTHFR
Serologic studies
Factor VIII
Factor XI
Antigenic protein C
Antigenic protein S (total and free)
Antigenic antithrombin III
Homocysteine
Anticardiolipin antibody IgG
Anticardiolipin antibody IgM
Beta-2-glycoprotein
Lupus anticoagulant
Hypofibrinolysis
PCR studies
Plasminogen activator inhibitor-1 gene 4G4G mutation
Serologic studies
Lipoprotein (a)
Plasminogen activator inhibitor activity
Genetic predisposition due to nitric oxide production impairment
PCR studies
Endothelial nitric oxide synthase (eNOS) gene polymorphisms (T-786C polymorphism, 4a intron 4 polymorphism)

32.2 Prospective Study of 4- to 7-Year Outcomes in 20 Patients (30 Hips) and in 7 Patients (11 Knees) After Initial Treatment with Enoxaparin

The Cincinnati studies described in this chapter were approved by the Food and Drug Administration (FDA) and by the Institutional Review Board at the Jewish Hospital; signed informed consent was obtained.

32.2.1 Hip Outcomes

Based on intent to treat, at 4-year follow-up, 22 of the original 30 hips (73 %) remained unchanged (Ficat stages I or II), as did 16 of 30 hips (53 %) at 7 years (Fig. 32.2). Those hips showing no change from Ficat stages I or II also remained asymptomatic and fully functional.

The Kaplan-Meier survival estimate (Fig. 32.3) is defined as "products of loss." The Kaplan-Meier survival estimate distinguishes between end of follow-up without hip failure (censored) and real hip failure requiring THR (uncensored). At the beginning of the study, the survival function is 1. At each time point, if there are any real failures, then the survival function will be reduced by the number of failures divided by the number of observations left just before this time point. The Kaplan-Meier hip survival (Ficat I or II) probability was 80 % at 7-year follow-up, Fig. 32.3.

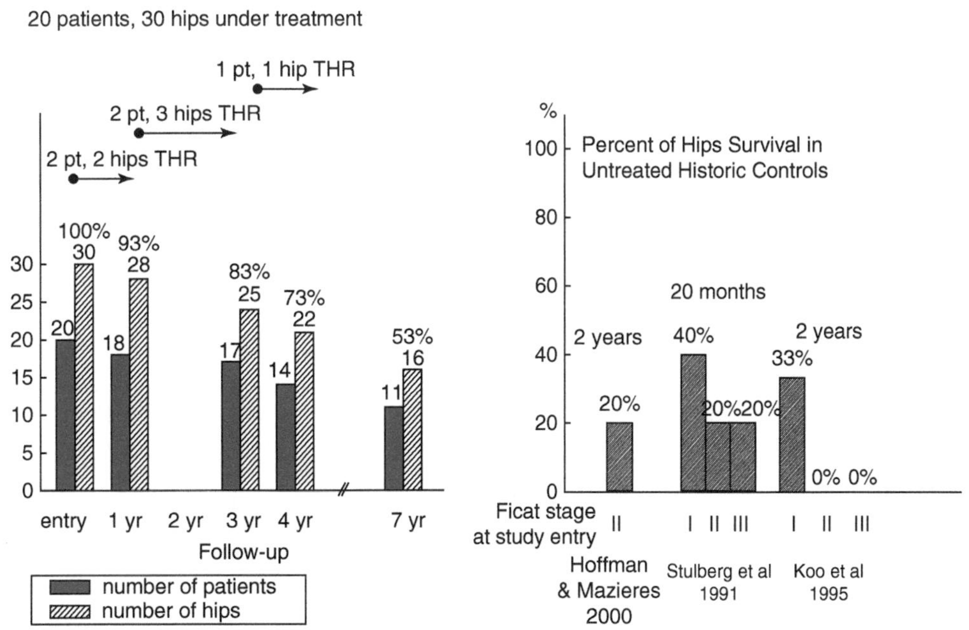

Fig. 32.2 Hip survival over 7-year prospective follow-up in 20 patients (30 hips) with primary ON (initial Ficat stage I or II), all receiving an initial 3-month therapy with enoxaparin. Hip survival in untreated historical controls and 20-month and 2-year follow-up

Two patients, both heterozygous for the Factor V Leiden mutation, required chronic anticoagulation, one with enoxaparin followed by Xarelto (6 years) and one with Warfarin (13 years), because of ≥ 2 thrombotic events. These two patients had no change from pretreatment Ficat I or II ON of ≥ 1 hip at 6 and 13 years follow-up, respectively.

Compared with untreated historical controls (approximately 20 % 2-year hip survival, Fig. 32.2), 4-year survival of 22 of 30 (73 %) hips based on intent to treat, and 80 % survival by Kaplan-Meier analysis (Fig. 32.3), suggests that the original 12-week enoxaparin thromboprophylaxis produced lasting benefit in primary ON in patients with heritable thrombophilia-hypofibrinolysis.

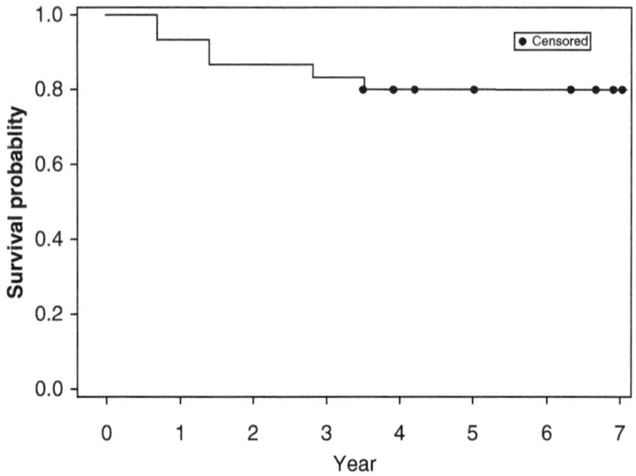

Fig. 32.3 Kaplan-Meier plot of hip survival, over 7-year prospective follow-up, starting with 30 hips in 20 patients with primary ON, all receiving an initial 3-month therapy with enoxaparin, initial Ficat stage I or II

32.2.2 Knee Outcomes

The extent of knee ON in 7 patients (11 knees) was prospectively determined by X-rays and magnetic resonance imaging (MRI). All 7 patients received enoxaparin (1.5 mg/kg/day for 3 months).

At 4 months, 2 patients (2 knees) had total knee replacement because of joint collapse, Fig. 32.4. At 20 months, 5 patients (9 knees, 82 %) had no progression by X-ray and MRI. At 36 months, 8 of the 11 knees survived (73 %) with no progression by X-ray and MRI, Fig. 32.4. At 40 months, 5 of the 11 knees survived (45 %), Fig. 32.4. Two patients (3 knees) had ≥ 8 years of follow-up, with 100 % knee survival. In 1 patient (2 knees) with 15 years follow-up, there was no progression by X-ray and MRI, with 100 % knee survival (Fig. 32.4).

In the five patients (nine knees) still undergoing follow-up, their knees were predominantly pain free and functional.

The Kaplan-Meier knee survival-probability was 82 % up to 15 year follow-up, Fig. 32.5.

Satku et al. [39] have prospectively studied 21 untreated adults with ON of the knee for at least 3 years and described three distinct patterns of outcome: (1) acute extensive collapse within 3 months of onset in 2 patients, (2) rapid progression to varying degrees of osteoarthritis in 12 knees (8 within 1 year, all 12 within 2 years), and (3) complete resolution in 4 knees. The 2 patients with acute extensive collapse and 3 who had rapid progression to severe osteoarthritis required total knee arthroplasty.

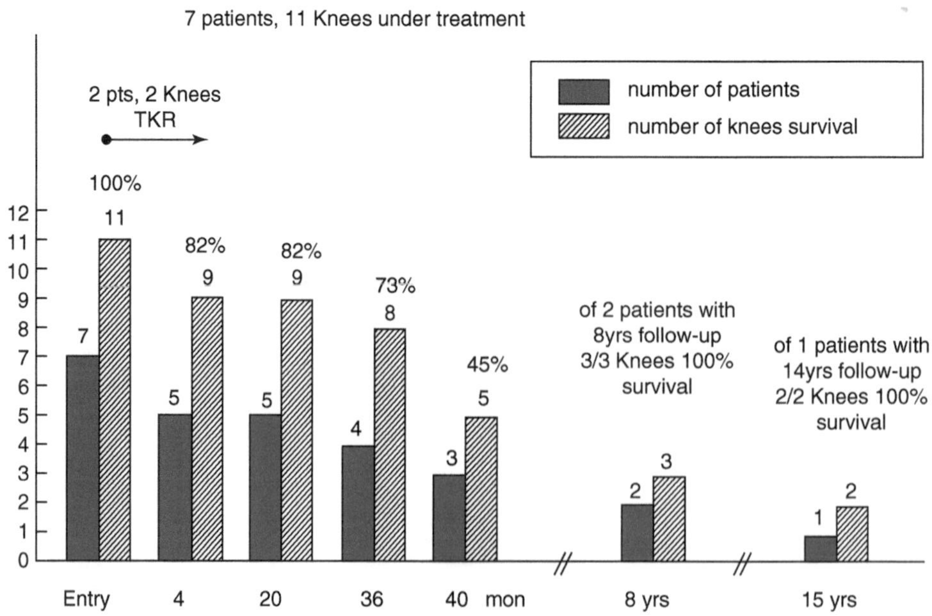

Fig. 32.4 Knee survival over prospective 15-year follow-up in 7 patients (11 knees) with primary ON, all receiving an initial 3-month therapy with enoxaparin

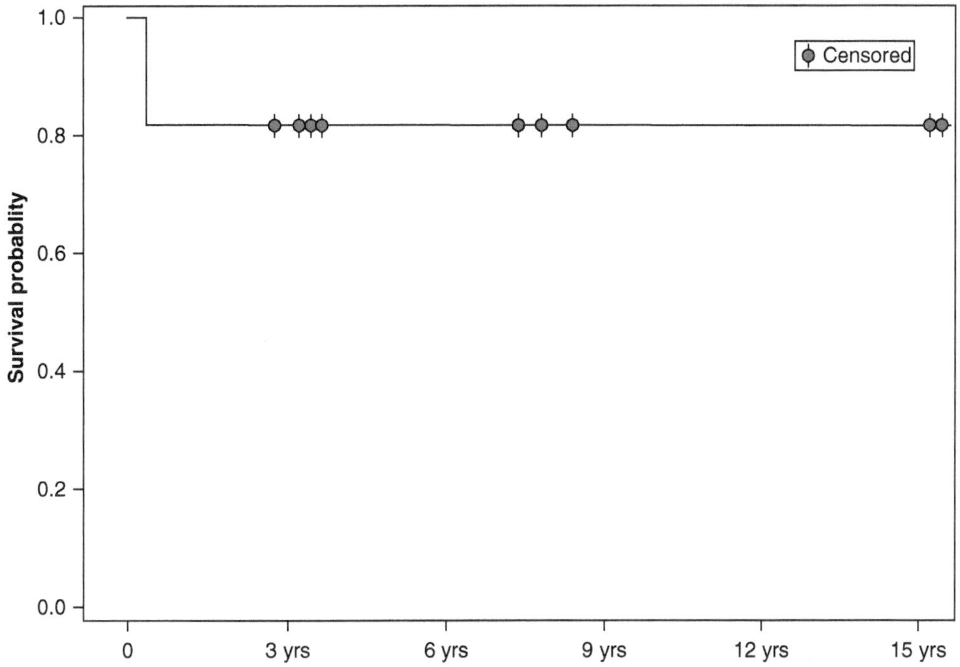

Fig. 32.5 Kaplan-Meier plot of knee survival over 15-year prospective follow-up, starting with 11 knees in 7 patients with primary ON, all receiving an initial 3-month therapy with enoxaparin

32.3 Discussion

Previous studies have suggested that all strategies for treatment of ON have certain limitations [36–38, 40–46], are difficult to develop [47], do not reverse ON's primary pathologies [48], and may not halt progression to segmental collapse [48]. Our goal is preservation of the femoral head [47] and the knee by treating ON caused by thrombophilia-hypofibrinolysis with enoxaparin, reversing a primary (coagulation) pathology of ON [48]. In our current study, compared with untreated historical controls, approximately 20 % 2-year hip survival (Fig. 32.2), 4-year survival of 22 of 30 (73 %) of hips based on intent to treat (Fig. 32.2), and 80 % survival by Kaplan-Meier analysis (Fig. 32.3), suggests that the original 12 week enoxaparin therapy produced lasting benefit in primary ON in patients with heritable thrombophilia-hypofibrinolysis. Enoxaparin may prevent progression of primary hip ON [17], allowing many patients to avoid THR. The 6- and 13-year survival of 3 hips in 2 patients heterozygous for the V Leiden mutation chronically anticoagulated with warfarin or enoxaparin and then Xarelto suggests that chronic anticoagulation might be very useful in stopping progression of primary hip ON. Except these 2 patients, however, we have not studied repeated courses of enoxaparin treatment or constant anticoagulation due to FDA restrictions when we began our initial study [17]. However, we suspect that the results would likely to be improved as new occurrences of femoral head venous thrombosis are probably likely after cessation of the 13-week initial course of enoxaparin, leading to delayed failure of the initial treatment regimen.

Because the natural history of ON of the knees is highly variable [39], any generalization about success of enoxaparin treatment for ON of the knees associated with familial thrombophilia-hypofibrinolysis is limited by our small sample size and relatively short follow-up, but our data suggests lasting benefits from the initial 3-month treatment with enoxaparin.

An optimal study of anticoagulation in patients with thrombophilia-hypofibrinolysis and Ficat [35] stage I–II primary ON of the hips or ON of the knees would be double blind, with placebo and enoxaparin injections (1.5 mg/kg for 3 months). A single 12 week enoxaparin treatment [17] also may not protect from recurrent thrombi related to underlying thrombophilia-hypofibrinolysis. A future study might evaluate whether prophylactic, continuous anticoagulant treatment might improve the lifetime results in thrombophilic-hypofibrinolytic patients with primary ON, particularly in patients heterozygous for the Factor V Leiden mutation, as in our current report.

In primary hip ON associated with thrombophilia-hypofibrinolysis [17], if enoxaparin is started during Ficat stages I or II, we postulate that ON may be safely arrested or possibly reversed over 4–7 years, potentially avoiding surgical intervention.

Acknowledgments This study followed a protocol approved by the Jewish Hospital IRB, with written informed consent.

The study was supported by the Lipoprotein Research Fund and by the Medical Research Council of the Jewish Hospital

References

1. Glueck CJ, Goldenberg N, Budhani S, Lotner D, Abuchaibe C, Gowda M, et al. Thrombotic events after starting exogenous testosterone in men with previously undiagnosed familial thrombophilia. Transl Res. 2011;158(4):225–34. doi:S1931-5244(11)00191-5 [pii] 10.1016/j.trsl.2011.06.003.
2. Bjorkman A, Burtscher IM, Svensson PJ, Hillarp A, Besjakov J, Benoni G. Factor V Leiden and the prothrombin 20210A gene mutation and osteonecrosis of the knee. Arch Orthop Trauma Surg. 2005;125(1):51–5. doi:10.1007/s00402-004-0760-8.
3. Glueck CJ, Freiberg RA, Fontaine RN, Tracy T, Wang P. Hypofibrinolysis, thrombophilia, osteonecrosis. Clin Orthop Relat Res. 2001;386:19–33.
4. Glueck CJ, Freiberg RA, Boppana S, Wang P. Thrombophilia, hypofibrinolysis, the eNOS T-786C polymorphism, and multifocal osteonecrosis. J Bone Joint Surg Am. 2008;90(10):2220–9. doi:90/10/2220 [pii] 10.2106/JBJS.G.00616.
5. Glueck CJ, Freiberg RA, Wang P. Heritable thrombophilia-hypofibrinolysis and osteonecrosis of the femoral head. Clin Orthop Relat Res. 2008;466(5):1034–40. doi:10.1007/s11999-008-0148-0.
6. Pierre-Jacques H, Glueck CJ, Mont MA, Hungerford DS. Familial heterozygous protein-S deficiency in a patient who had multifocal osteonecrosis. A case report. J Bone Joint Surg Am. 1997;79(7): 1079–84.
7. Glueck CJ, Freiberg RA, Wang P. Detecting thrombophilia, hypofibrinolysis, and reduced nitric oxide production in osteonecrosis. Semin Arthroplasty. 2007;18:184–91.
8. Zalavras C, Dailiana Z, Elisaf M, Bairaktari E, Vlachogiannopoulos P, Katsaraki A, et al. Potential aetiological factors concerning the development of osteonecrosis of the femoral head. Eur J Clin Invest. 2000;30(3):215–21.
9. Jones JJ. Activating intravascular coagulation and causing nontraumatic osteonecrosis. In: Urbaniak JR, Jones Jr JP, editors. Osteonecrosis: etiology, diagnosis, and treatment. Rosemont: American Academy of Orthopedic Surgeons; 1997. p. 89–97.
10. Jones LC, Mont MA, Le TB, Petri M, Hungerford DS, Wang P, et al. Procoagulants and osteonecrosis. J Rheumatol. 2003;30(4):783–91.
11. Koo KH, Kim R, Cho SH, Song HR, Lee G, Ko GH. Angiography, scintigraphy, intraosseous pressure, and histologic findings in high-risk osteonecrotic femoral heads with negative magnetic resonance images. Clin Orthop. 1994;308:127–38.
12. Korompilias AV, Ortel TL, Urbaniak JR. Coagulation abnormalities in patients with hip osteonecrosis. Orthop Clin North Am. 2004;35(3):265–71. vii.
13. Bjorkman A, Svensson PJ, Hillarp A, Burtscher IM, Runow A, Benoni G. Factor V leiden and prothrombin gene mutation: risk factors for osteonecrosis of the femoral head in adults. Clin Orthop Relat Res. 2004;425:168–72.
14. Nilsson IM, Krook H, Sternby NH, Soderberg E, Soderstrom N. Severe thrombotic disease in a young man with bone marrow and skeletal changes and with a high content of an inhibitor in the fibrinolytic system. Acta Med Scand. 1961;169:323–37.
15. Balasa VV, Gruppo RA, Glueck CJ, Wang P, Roy DR, Wall EJ, et al. Legg-Calve-Perthes disease and thrombophilia. J Bone Joint Surg Am. 2004;86-A(12):2642–7.
16. Vosmaer A, Pereira RR, Koenderman JS, Rosendaal FR, Cannegieter SC. Coagulation abnormalities in Legg-Calve-Perthes disease. J Bone Joint Surg Am. 2010;92(1):121–8. doi:92/1/121 [pii] 10.2106/JBJS.I.00157.
17. Glueck CJ, Freiberg RA, Sieve L, Wang P. Enoxaparin prevents progression of stages I and II osteonecrosis of the hip. Clin Orthop Relat Res. 2005;435:164–70.
18. Lindahl TL, Lundahl TH, Nilsson L, Andersson CA. APC-resistance is a risk factor for postoperative thromboembolism in elective replacement of the hip or knee–a prospective study. Thromb Haemost. 1999;81(1):18–21. doi:99010018 [pii].
19. Szucs G, Ajzner E, Muszbek L, Simon T, Szepesi K, Fulesdi B. Assessment of thrombotic risk factors predisposing to thromboembolic complications in prosthetic orthopedic surgery. J Orthop Sci. 2009;14(5):484–90. doi:10.1007/s00776-009-1368-1.
20. Wahlander K, Larson G, Lindahl TL, Andersson C, Frison L, Gustafsson D, et al. Factor V Leiden (G1691A) and prothrombin gene G20210A mutations as potential risk factors for venous thromboembolism after total hip or total knee replacement surgery. Thromb Haemost. 2002;87(4):580–5.
21. Mont MA, Jones LC, Rajadhyaksha AD, Shuler MS, Hungerford DS, Sieve-Smith L, et al. Risk factors for pulmonary emboli after total hip or knee arthroplasty. Clin Orthop Relat Res. 2004;(422):154–63. doi:00003086-200405000-00026 [pii].
22. Salvati EA, Della Valle AG, Westrich GH, Rana AJ, Specht L, Weksler BB, et al. The John Charnley Award: heritable thrombophilia and development of thromboembolic disease after total hip arthroplasty. Clin Orthop Relat Res. 2005;441:40–55. doi:00003086-200512000-00010 [pii].
23. Boss JH, Misselevich I. Osteonecrosis of the femoral head of laboratory animals: the lessons learned from a comparative study of osteonecrosis in man and experimental animals. Vet Pathol. 2003;40(4):345–54.
24. Laroche M. Intraosseous circulation from physiology to disease. Joint Bone Spine. 2002;69(3):262–9.
25. Liu SL, Ho TC. The role of venous hypertension in the pathogenesis of Legg-Perthes disease. A clinical and experimental study. J Bone Joint Surg Am. 1991;73(2):194–200.
26. Norman D, Miller Y, Sabo E, Misselevich I, Peskin B, Zinman C, et al. The effects of enoxaparin on the reparative processes in experimental osteonecrosis of the femoral head of the rat. Apmis. 2002;110(3):221–8.
27. Norman D, Reis D, Zinman C, Misselevich I, Boss JH. Vascular deprivation-induced necrosis of the femoral head of the rat. An experimental model of avascular osteonecrosis in the skeletally immature individual or Legg-Perthes disease. Int J Exp Pathol. 1998;79(3):173–81.
28. Lafforgue P. Pathophysiology and natural history of avascular necrosis of bone. Joint Bone Spine. 2006;73:500–7.
29. Ficat P. Cortisone associated necrosis of bone. In: Hungerford D, editor. Ischemia and necrosis of bone. Baltimore: Williams and Wilkins; 1980. p. 171–6.
30. Glueck CJ, Freiberg RA, Fontaine RN, Sieve-Smith L, Wang P. Anticoagulant therapy for osteonecrosis associated with heritable hypofibrinolysis and thrombophilia. Expert Opin Investig Drugs. 2001;10(7):1309–16.
31. Glueck CJ, Freiberg RA, Wang P. Role of thrombosis in osteonecrosis. Curr Hematol Rep. 2003;2(5):417–22.
32. Jones JP. Risk factors potentially activating intravascular coagulation and causing nontraumatic osteonecrosis. In: Urbaniak JR, Jones Jr JP, editors. Osteonecrosis: etiology, diagnosis, and treatment. Rosemont: American Academy of Orthopedic Surgeons; 1997. p. 89–97.
33. Zalavras CG, Vartholomatos G, Dokou E, Malizos KN. Genetic background of osteonecrosis: associated with thrombophilic mutations? Clin Orthop. 2004;422:251–5.
34. CotBTS R. Optimum duration of anticoagulation for deep-vein thrombosis and pulmonary embolism. Research Committee of the British Thoracic Society. Lancet. 1992;340(8824):873–6.
35. Arlet J, Ficat P. Diagnosis of primary femur head osteonecrosis at stage 1 (preradiologic stage). Rev Chir Orthop Reparatrice Appar Mot. 1968;54(7):637–48.

36. Hofmann S, Mazieres B. Osteonecrosis: natural course and conservative therapy. Orthopade. 2000;29(5):403–10.
37. Koo KH, Kim R, Ko GH, Song HR, Jeong ST, Cho SH. Preventing collapse in early osteonecrosis of the femoral head. A randomised clinical trial of core decompression. J Bone Joint Surg Br. 1995;77(6):870–4.
38. Stulberg BN, Davis AW, Bauer TW, Levine M, Easley K. Osteonecrosis of the femoral head. A prospective randomized treatment protocol. Clin Orthop. 1991;268:140–51.
39. Satku K, Kumar VP, Chong SM, Thambyah A. The natural history of spontaneous osteonecrosis of the medial tibial plateau. J Bone Joint Surg Br. 2003;85(7):983–8.
40. Coogan PG, Urbaniak JR. Multicenter experience with free vascularized fibular grafts for osteonecrosis of the femoral head. In: Urbaniak JR, Jones Jr JP, editors. Osteonecrosis: etiology, diagnosis, and treatment. Rosemont: American Academy of Orthopedic Surgeons; 1997. p. 327–52.
41. Garino JP, Steinberg ME. Total hip arthroplasty in patients with avascular necrosis of the femoral head: a 2- to 10-year follow-up. Clin Orthop. 1997;334:108–15.
42. Ritter MA, Helphinstine J, Keating EM, Faris PM, Meding JB. Total hip arthroplasty in patients with osteonecrosis. The effect of cement techniques. Clin Orthop. 1997;338:94–9.
43. Robinson Jr HJ. Success of core decompression in the management of early stages of avascular necrosis: a four year prospective study. In: Proceedings of the American Academy of Orthopaedic Surgeons 59th annual meeting. Washington, DC: American Academy of Orthopedic Surgeons; 1992. p. 177.
44. Steinberg M, Larcom PG, Stafford BB. Treatment of osteonecrosis of the femoral head by core decompression, bone grafting, and electrical stimulation. In: Urbaniak JR, Jones Jr JP, editors. Osteonecroiss: etiology, diagnosis, and treatment. Rosemont: American Academy of Orthopedic Surgeons; 1997. p. 293–9.
45. Stulberg BN, Singer R, Goldner J, Stulberg J. Uncemented total hip arthroplasty in osteonecrosis: a 2- to 10-year evaluation. Clin Orthop. 1997;334:116–23.
46. Yasunaga Y, Ikuta Y, Omoto O, Shigenobu T, Itoh K, Fukuoka H, et al. Transtrochanteric rotational osteotomy for osteonecrosis of the femoral head with preoperative superselective angiography. Arch Orthop Trauma Surg. 2000;120(7–8):437–40.
47. Lieberman JR. Core decompression for osteonecrosis of the hip. Clin Orthop. 2004;418:29–33.
48. Assouline-Dayan Y, Chang C, Greenspan A, Shoenfeld Y, Gershwin ME. Pathogenesis and natural history of osteonecrosis. Semin Arthritis Rheum. 2002;32(2):94–124.

The Role of Coagulopathy in the Pathogenesis and Prevention of Corticosteroid-Induced Osteonecrosis

33

Takuaki Yamamoto, Goro Motomura, Ryosuke Yamaguchi, and Yukihide Iwamoto

33.1 Corticosteroid-Induced Animal Model for ON

In nontraumatic osteonecrosis (ON) of the femoral head, several abnormalities in the coagulation-fibrinolysis system have been reported, including increase of plasminogen activator inhibitor-1 level [1], the presence of antiphospholipid antibodies [2], familial heterozygous protein S deficiency [3], and antithrombin III deficiency [4]. These abnormalities are thought to induce hypercoagulability in the blood vessels.

Based on several animal ON model experiments, the relationship between hypercoagulability and corticosteroid-induced ON was also indicated [5–7]. Corticosteroid-induced osteonecrosis was firstly developed in rabbits, in which high-dose methylprednisolone (MPSL) (20 mg/kg) can induce multifocal ON in conjunction with thrombocytopenia, hypofibrinogenemia, and hyperlipemia (Fig. 33.1). In this model, the blood platelet levels significantly decreased 1 week after the injection of MPSL ($p<0.05$) and then gradually recovered and reached almost a normal level or even a little higher after 5 weeks. Histologically, an organizing thrombus was observed in the intraosseous arteriole, indicating the presence of some degree of coagulopathy.

Based on this animal model for ON, several investigations for the prevention of ON has recently been reported [6–9].

T. Yamamoto (✉) • G. Motomura • R. Yamaguchi • Y. Iwamoto
Department of Orthopaedic Surgery, Kyushu University,
3-1-1 Maidashi, Higashi-ku, Fukuoka 812-8582, Japan
e-mail: yamataku@ortho.med.kyushu-u.ac.jp;
yamaryo@ortho.med.kyushu-u.ac.jp;
yiwamoto@ortho.med.kyushu-u.ac.jp

33.2 Combined Effects of Warfarin and Lipid-Lowering Agent [6]

In 2004, combined effects of warfarin and lipid-lowering agent (probucol) on the prevention of corticosteroid-induced ON have been proposed for the prevention of corticosteroid-induced ON [6].

Male adult Japanese white rabbits were injected once intramuscularly with 20 mg/kg of methylprednisolone acetate (MPSL) into the right gluteus medius muscle. These rabbits were divided into four groups, (1) warfarin plus probucol (WP group, $n=25$), (2) probucol alone (PA group, $n=30$), (3) warfarin alone (WA group, $n=26$), or (4) no treatment (non-prophylactic (NP) group, $n=20$). Both the femora and humeri were histopathologically examined for the presence of ON 2 weeks after the MPSL injection and hematological examinations before and after steroid injection were performed.

The incidence of ON in the WP group (5 %) was significantly lower than that observed in the NP group (70 %) ($p<0.0001$). While the incidences of ON in the PA and WA groups (37 and 33 %, respectively) were also significantly lower than that seen in the NP group ($p<0.05$), they were significantly higher than that in the WP group ($p<0.01$ and $p<0.05$, respectively) (Fig. 33.2).

The levels of PT-INR in both the WP and WA groups were significantly higher ($p<0.01$, $p<0.05$, respectively) than those observed in either the NP or PA group throughout the experimental period (Fig. 33.3a). The LDL levels in the WP group remained at significantly lower levels at all the time points tested than those seen in the NP and WA groups ($p<0.05$, Fig. 33.3b). The PA group showed significantly lower LDL levels during the study than the NP or WA groups ($p<0.05$, Fig. 33.3a). The plasma LDL/HDL cholesterol ratios were significantly lower in the WP group than those in the NP group at all of the time points tested ($p<0.05$). The LDL/HDL cholesterol ratios observed in the PA group were

K.-H. Koo et al. (eds.), *Osteonecrosis*,
DOI 10.1007/978-3-642-35767-1_33, © Springer-Verlag Berlin Heidelberg 2014

also significantly lower than those in the NP group ($p<0.05$) at every time point (Fig. 33.3c). There were no significant differences in plasma lipid levels (LDL, VLDL, triglyceride, and LDL/HDL cholesterol) between the WP and PA groups (Fig. 33.3a, b).

33.3 Effects of Antiplatelet Drug [7]

In 2010, the effects of antiplatelet drug (clopidogrel) on the prevention of corticosteroid-induced ON have been proposed [7].

Sixty-five adult male Japanese white rabbits ranging in age from 28 to 32 weeks were used. The body weight was 3,490 ± 180 g (mean ± SD). These rabbits were randomly divided into two groups. One group received 5 mg/kg of body weight of clopidogrel (Sanofi-Aventis, Paris, France) mixed with normal saline (5 ml/kg/day) which was administered intragastrically through a rubber gastric tube into the stomach (AP group; $n=35$). The other group received normal saline alone (5 ml/kg/day) intragastrically (NS group; $n=30$). All rabbits were given the drug or normal saline once daily for 3 weeks. One week after the initiation of the study, all rabbits were injected intramuscularly 20 mg/kg of body weight of

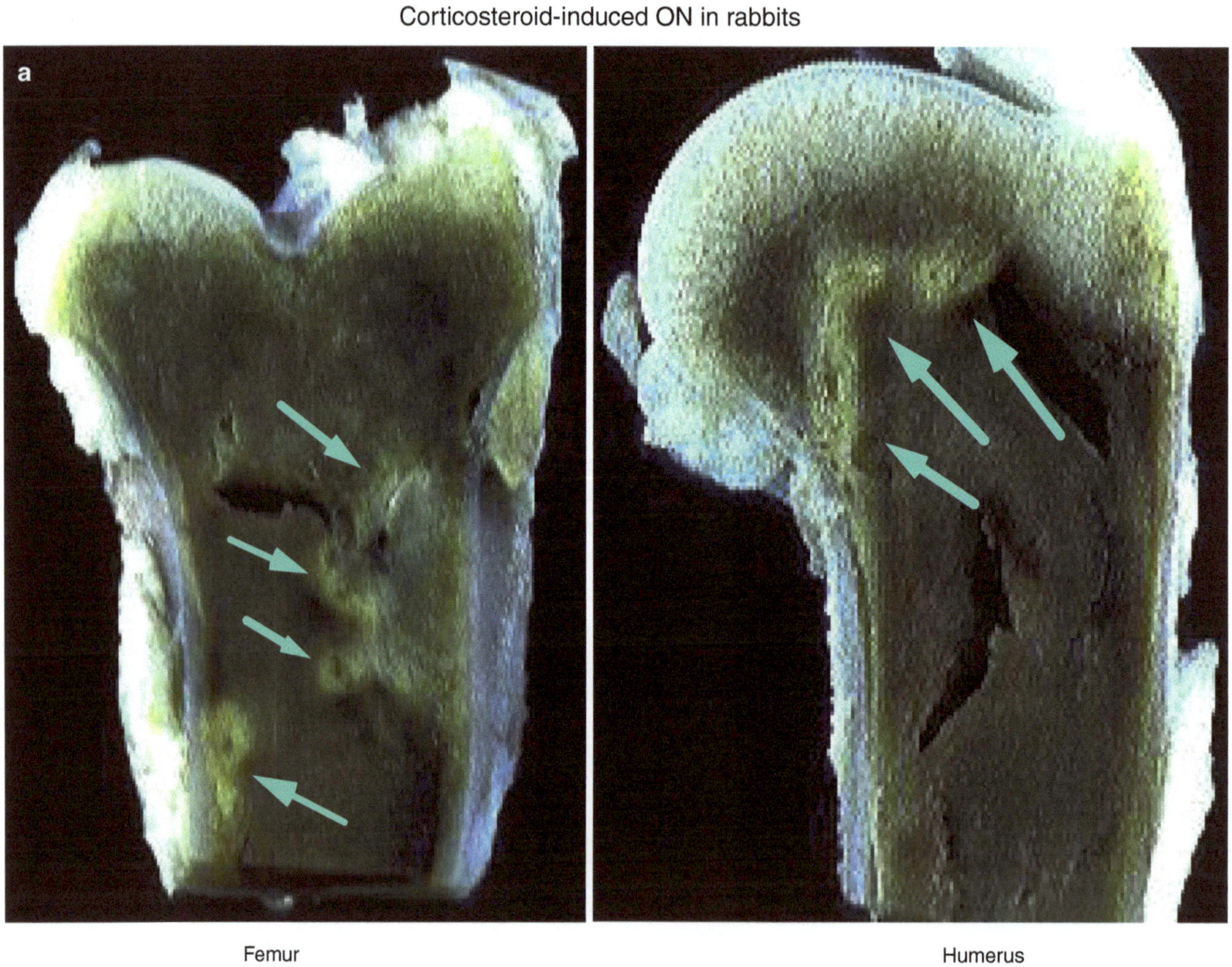

Fig. 33.1 (**a**) The macroscopical appearance of ON in the femur and humerus 4 weeks after corticosteroid injection. The yellowish-colored areas (*arrows*) mainly located in the metaphysis represent osteonecrosis area. (**b**) The sequential changes in the blood platelet levels. Although there was no significant difference between the rabbits with ON (ON+) and those without ON (ON−), the blood platelet levels significantly decreased 1 week after the injection of MPSL ($p<0.05$) and then gradually recovered and reached almost a normal level after 5 weeks. *ON* osteonecrosis. (**c**) Morphological changes in the vessels of the femur 4 weeks after corticosteroid injection. An organizing thrombus is seen in the intraosseous arteriole, which is accompanied with fibrinous exudate in its wall, just adjacent to the ON in the metaphysis (hematoxylin and eosin, ×200) (Permission from Yamamoto et al. [5])

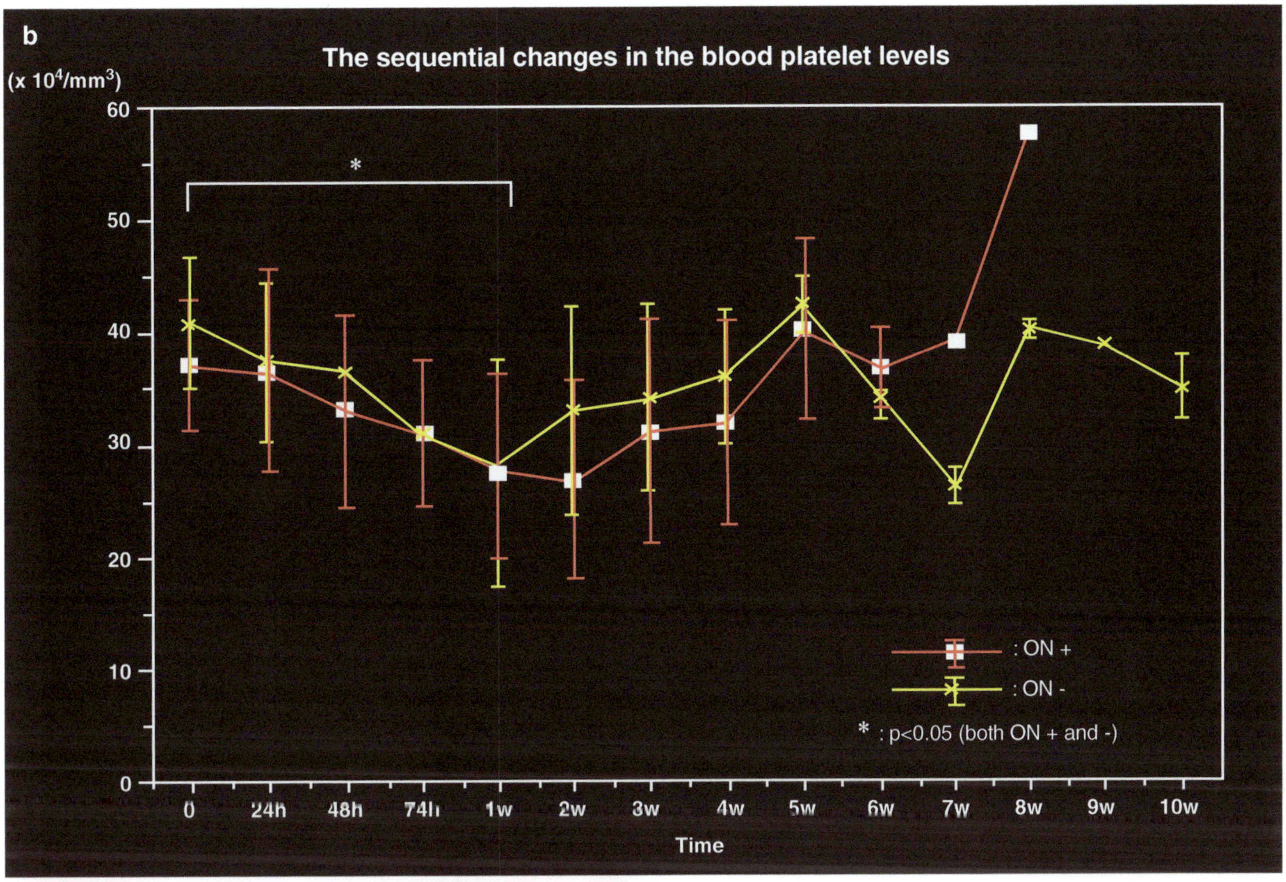

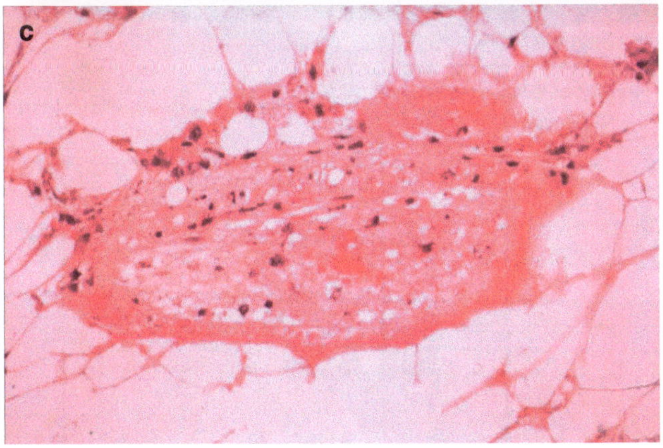

Fig. 33.1 (continued)

methylprednisolone acetate (MPSL; Pfizer, New York, USA) into the right gluteus medius muscle. Both the femora and humeri were examined histopathologically for the presence of ON 3 weeks later. Both the platelet aggregation assay and hematologic examinations were performed before and after the MPSL injection.

The incidence of ON in the AP group (48.5 %) was significantly lower than that observed in the NS group (73.3 %) (Fig. 33.4). The platelet aggregations in the AP group were significantly inhibited by the administration of clopidogrel. The levels of total cholesterol and triglycerides showed no significant differences between the AP and NS group.

Fig. 33.2 The incidence of osteonecrosis (ON) in the warfarin plus probucol treatment group (WP group, 5 %) was significantly lower than that seen in the non-prophylactic treatment group (NP group, 70 %) ($p<0.0001$). While the incidence of ON in the probucol treatment group (PA group, 37 %) and the warfarin treatment group (WA group, 33 %) was significantly lower than that observed in the NP group ($p<0.05$), these levels are significantly higher than those seen in the WP group ($p<0.01$ and $p<0.05$, respectively) (Reproduced from Motomura et al. [6])

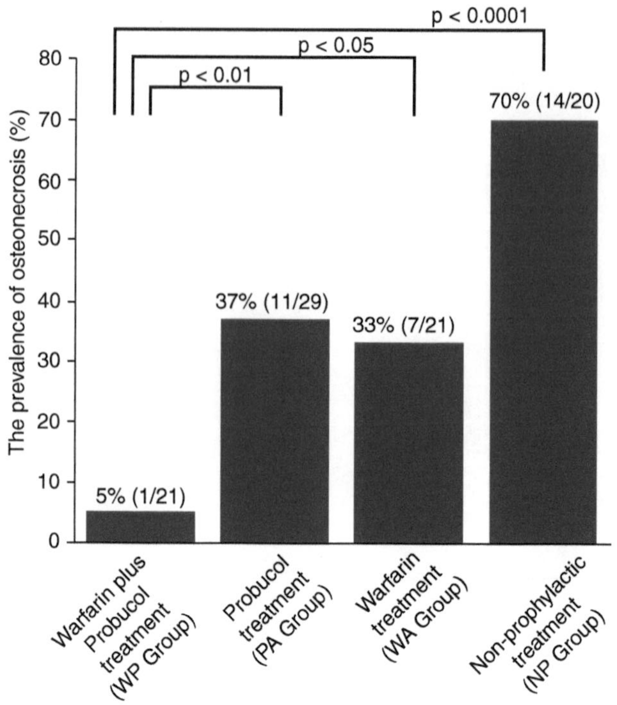

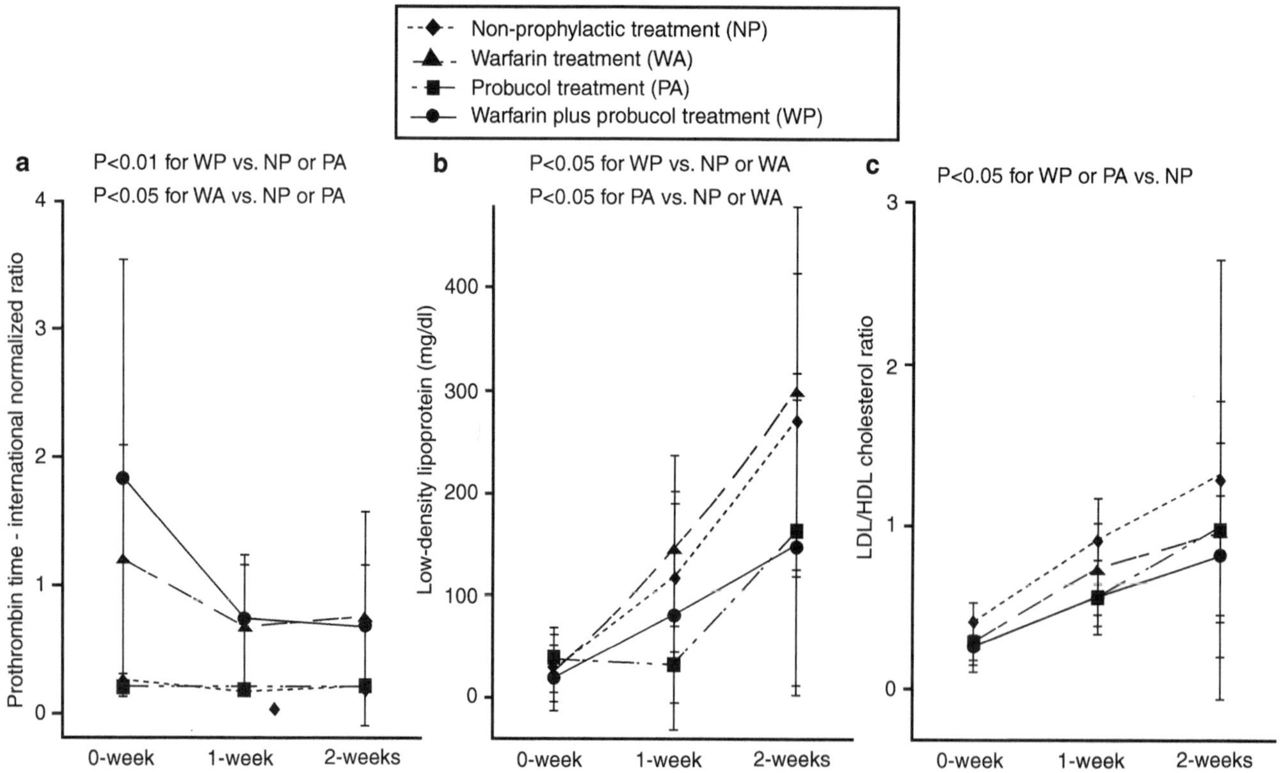

Fig. 33.3 (**a**) The levels of PT-INR in the WP group were significantly higher than those seen in either the NP or PA groups during the experimental period ($p<0.01$). The PT-INR levels in the WA group were also significantly higher than those in NP or PA groups at any of the time points tested ($p<0.05$). (**b**) The LDL levels in the WP group remained significantly lower than those seen in the NP or WA groups at all of the time points tested ($p<0.05$). The PA group also exhibited significantly lower LDL levels than the NP or WA groups throughout the study ($p<0.05$). (**c**) Plasma LDL/HDL cholesterol ratios were significantly lower in the WP group than that seen in the NP group at all of the time points tested ($p<0.05$). The LDL/HDL cholesterol ratios in the PA group were also significantly lower than those in the NP group at any time point examined ($p<0.05$) (Reproduced from Motomura et al. [6])

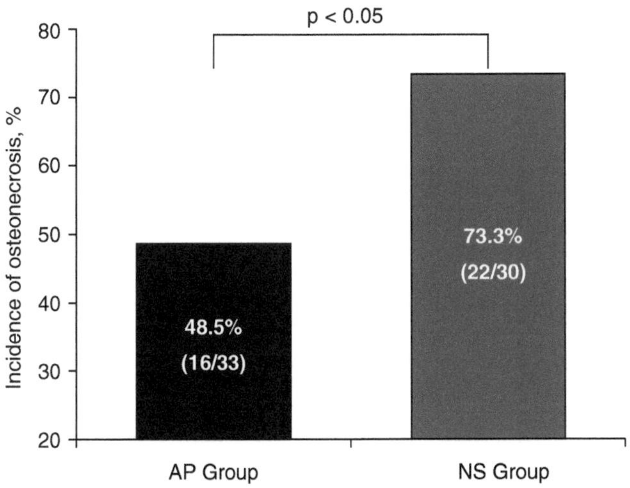

Fig. 33.4 The incidence of ON in each group. The incidence of ON in the AP group (48.5 %) was significantly lower than that observed in the NS group (73.3 %)

33.4 Perspective

Corticosteroids, a classic risk factor of ON, are known to induce hyperlipidemia as well as a hypercoagulable and hypofibrinolytic state of plasma. The pathogenesis of nontraumatic ON is generally considered to be multifactorial, and it seems that no one factor adequately accounts for the development of ON. Combination treatments, such as anti-coagulopathy drugs and lipid-lowering agents, seem to be the useful candidates for considering the prevention of corticosteroid-induced ON.

References

1. Glueck CJ, Freiberg R, Glueck HI, et al. Hypofibrinolysis: a common, major cause of osteonecrosis. Am J Hematol. 1994;45:156–66.
2. Korompilias AV, Gilkeson GS, Ortel TL, Seaber AV, Urbaniak JR. Anticardiolipin antibodies and osteonecrosis of the femoral head. Clin Orthop. 1997;345:174–80.
3. Pierre-Jacques H, Glueck CJ, Mont MA, Hungerford DS. Familial heterozygous protein-S deficiency in a patient who had multifocal osteonecrosis. A case report. J Bone Joint Surg. 1997;79A:1079–84.
4. Kubo Kubo T, Tsuji H, Yamamoto T, Nakahara H, Nakagawa M, Hirasawa Y. Antithrombin III deficiency in a patient who had multifocal osteonecrosis. Clin Orthop Relat Res. 2000;378:306–11.
5. Yamamoto AR, Yamamoto T, Irisa T, Sugioka Y, Sueishi K. Effects of pulse methylprednisolone on bone and marrow tissues. Corticosteroid-induced osteonecrosis in rabbits. Arthritis Rheum. 1997;40:2055–64.
6. Motomura Motomura G, Yamamoto T, Miyanishi K, Jingushi S, Iwamoto Y. Combined effects of an anticoagulant and a lipid-lowering agent on the prevention of steroid-induced osteonecrosis in rabbits. Arthritis Rheum. 2004;50:3387–91.
7. Yamaguchi Yamaguchi R, Yamamoto T, Motomura G, Ikemura S, Iwasaki K, Zhao G, Iwamoto Y. Effects of an anti-platelet drug on the prevention of steroid-induced osteonecrosis in rabbits. Rheumatology. 2012;51:789–93.
8. Nishida Nishida K, Yamamoto T, Motomura G, Jingushi S, Iwamoto Y. Pitavastatin may reduce risk of steroid-induced osteonecrosis in rabbits. Clin Orthop Relat Res. 2008;466:1054–8.
9. Ikemura Ikemura S, Yamamoto T, Motomura G, Yamaguchi R, Zhao G, Iwasaki K, Iwamoto Y. Preventive effects of the anti-vasospasm agent via the regulation of the Rho-kinase pathway on the development of steroid induced osteonecrosis in rabbits. Bone. 2013;53:329–35.

34 Lipid-Lowering Agents and Their Effects on Osteonecrosis: Pros and Cons

Abdurrahman Kandil and Quanjun Cui

34.1 Introduction

Osteonecrosis is a debilitating disease with many causes. It has been linked to processes that affect vascular perfusion to the bone. Systemic steroid use is a significant risk factor for the development of osteonecrosis. It is postulated that prolonged steroid use produces a hyperlipidemic state in patients and puts them at risk for osteonecrosis. The idea is that steroid use increases the fat content within the bone (most commonly the femoral head), resulting in increased intracortical pressure that may lead to sinusoidal collapse and osteonecrosis. Statins are lipid-lowering agents that dramatically reduce lipid levels in blood and tissues. They are widely used to prevent cardiovascular disease and have been shown to reduce the adverse effects of steroids on lipid metabolism as will be outlined in this chapter. As a result, the effect of lipid-lowering agents on the development and progression of osteonecrosis has been an interesting area of research.

Basic science research to understand the pathophysiology of osteonecrosis and to develop therapies that can be translated to clinical application has progressed rapidly over the past two decades, and these advances offer promise for the future treatment of osteonecrosis. One significant area and the focus of this chapter is the effect of lipid-lowering agents – primarily statins – on osteonecrosis.

A. Kandil
Department of Orthopaedic Surgery,
University of Virginia, 800159, Charlottesville,
VA 22908-0159, USA
e-mail: ak3ue@virginia.edu

Q. Cui (✉)
Department of Orthopaedic Surgery,
University of Virginia School of Medicine, 800159,
Charlottesville, VA 22908-0159, USA
e-mail: qc4q@virginia.edu

34.2 Pathogenesis

The most common area of osteonecrosis in the body is the femoral head, and it is the focus of most basic science, translational, and clinical studies on osteonecrosis. The blood supply to the femoral head originates primarily from the ascending branch of the medial femoral circumflex artery, as well as smaller secondary contributions from inferior and superior gluteal arteries and artery of the ligamentum teres [1]. The interruption of this blood supply can be multifactorial, either extravascular or intravascular. Extravascular disruption is commonly attributed to traumatic causes. The focus of this chapter is on the intravascular interruptions in blood supply that can be targeted with lipid-lowering agents. Intravascular embolic matter such as clots, lipids, or abnormal RBC morphologies occludes the terminal arterioles in the subchondral bone of the femoral head [2–4]. Adipogenesis has been shown to be a possible causal factor in steroid- and alcohol-related osteonecrosis, as it leads to compression of venous sinusoids and congestion. The venous congestion increases intraosseous pressure, preventing adequate arterial blood flow, eventually leading to bone infarction [5, 6] (see Fig. 34.1 below).

34.3 Literature Review

34.3.1 Introduction

Many studies have sought to better understand the pathophysiology of osteonecrosis and, by extension, nonoperative interventions targeting the disease process itself. Most of the early research involves basic science studies on cell/tissue or animal models, but more recently, human clinical studies have been conducted. Several animal models have been developed to evaluate various treatment strategies. Intramuscular injection of methylprednisolone has been used to develop steroid-induced osteonecrosis in primarily rabbit [7] models. However, other animal models have been

K.-H. Koo et al. (eds.), *Osteonecrosis*,
DOI 10.1007/978-3-642-35767-1_34, © Springer-Verlag Berlin Heidelberg 2014

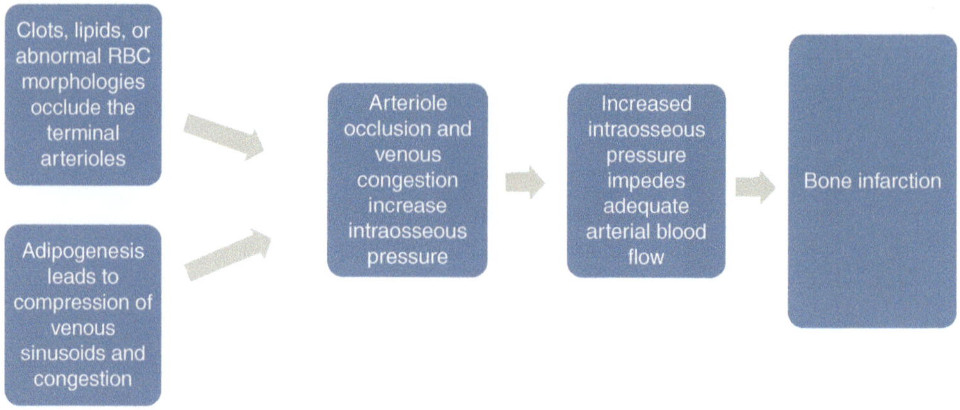

Fig. 34.1 Proposed pathogenesis of nontraumatic osteonecrosis

developed including mouse [8], rat [9], pig [10], and chicken [6] models. These animal models have been used to study the molecular mechanisms of osteonecrosis and assess the usefulness of several therapies over the last few decades.

Lipid-lowering drugs such as statins decrease the incidence of steroid-induced osteonecrosis [11, 12]. Other studies have also shown that the simultaneous use of anticoagulants along with lipid-lowering agents can decrease the prevalence of steroid-induced osteonecrosis in rabbits [13, 14].

Table 34.1 Pros and cons of statin use

Pros	Cons
Safe Lowers cholesterol Decreased risk of MI, stroke Decreased risk of arterial revascularization, hospitalization for unstable angina, or death from cardiovascular causes	Possible small increased risk of diabetes Very low risk of serious liver injury, muscle injury, and cognitive changes Increased likelihood of diagnoses of musculoskeletal conditions, arthropathies, and injuries

34.3.2 Statins: Pros and Cons

Statins are 3-hydroxy-3-methylglutaryl coenzyme A (HMG-CoA) reductase inhibitors whose mechanism of actions is competitive inhibition of HMG-CoA reductase, the rate-limiting step in cholesterol biosynthesis. They occupy a portion of the binding site of HMG-CoA, blocking access of this substrate to the active site on the enzyme [15]. They are very common lipid-lowering drugs that have a wide variety of indications. Most common among these are dyslipidemia and coronary artery disease. Despite their success and popularity, statins like most drugs provide health benefits with some degree of risk, and risk–benefit assessments require ongoing review as new data become available.

Pros: Statins are safe lipid-lowering agents that have a wide range of benefits. A large FDA clinical trial has recently been conducted to look at the safety of statins. In this JUPITER study [16], the authors found that the participants previously considered to have low cardiovascular risk had clinically important health improvements with a hazard rate 44 % lower than that of the placebo group for myocardial infarction, stroke, arterial revascularization, hospitalization for unstable angina, or death from cardiovascular causes. A meta-analysis of 13 randomized statin trials with 91,140 participants showed an odds ratio of 1.09 for a new diagnosis of diabetes [17]. These studies suggest that the net cardiovascular benefit for people at high cardiovascular risk strongly favors statin use and that even patients with lower cardiovascular risk benefit greatly from these drugs.

Cons: It has been suggested that statins may lead to an increased risk of developing diabetes. The JUPITER study [16] showed that the hazard ratio for newly diagnosed diabetes was increased 25 % in the rosuvastatin group than in the placebo group [18]. However, as mentioned in the "Pros" section, other studies have shown that effect is very modest and primarily involves patients who were prone to developing diabetes. With regard to side effects that have been reported with statins, the FDA has determined that statins appear to be associated with a very low risk of serious liver injury, muscle injury (unless lovastatin is taken at high doses with other medications), and cognitive changes [19]. Recently, Mansi et al. tried to determine whether statin use is associated with musculoskeletal conditions, including arthropathy and injury [20]. They found that statin use is associated with an increased likelihood of diagnoses of musculoskeletal conditions, arthropathies, and injuries. This study did not imply any causality but is very interesting given the context of it being considered a nonoperative modality in the management of osteonecrosis (Table 34.1).

34.3.3 Effect of Steroids on Stem Cell Morphology, Adipogenesis, and Bone Histology

The association between steroid therapy and the development of osteonecrosis has been observed since 1957 [21]. However, the pathophysiology behind this relationship has been elucidated in the past couple of decades. Stem cell studies have played an integral role in understanding the pathophysiology of steroid-induced osteonecrosis. Early studies with a cloned cell, D1, from the bone marrow have indicated that steroid-induced fatty changes in the bone marrow may be the mechanism whereby nontraumatic osteonecrosis occurs [22]. The effects of steroids on a cloned bone marrow cell showed that steroids produced adipogenesis and stimulated fat-specific gene, 422(aP2), expression which was dose dependent [23]. Other studies have shown that steroids decrease collagen synthesis and osteoblastic gene expression [24]. A study by Wang et al. developed a steroid-induced osteonecrosis model by treating pluripotential cells with dexamethasone and observing that these cells began to differentiate into adipocytes and expressed a fat-specific gene, whereas the expression of type I collagen and osteocalcin messenger ribonucleic acid decreased [25]. Kabata et al. found histological evidence of osteonecrosis first occurred 1–2 weeks after initial steroid [26]. At the same time there were significantly abnormal elevations in serum lipids, which persisted for between 1 and 2 weeks after the initial corticoid treatment. This study shows that osteonecrosis appears in rabbits shortly after steroids are first administered and that osteonecrosis in rabbits is chronologically associated with the onset of hyperlipidemia. This supports the occurrence of intraosseous fat embolism as a cause of osteonecrosis.

One can deduce from these studies that steroids increase fat accumulation in the marrow cavity leading to decreased blood inflow, increased intraosseous pressure, producing an intraosseous compartment syndrome, and leading to ischemia and nontraumatic osteonecrosis.

34.3.4 Effects of Statins on Stem Cell Morphology, Adipogenesis, and Bone Histology in Steroid-Induced Osteonecrosis Models

A landmark study by Cui et al. showed that lovastatin inhibited steroid-induced fat-specific gene expression, 422(aP2), and counteracted the inhibitory effects of steroids on osteoblastic gene expression [6]. In addition, when lovastatin was administered with steroids, less adipogenesis was observed and no bone death. Another study showed that lovastatin inhibited steroid-induced fat gene expression and counteracted the inhibitory effect of steroids on osteoblastic gene expression [26]. Li et al. helped elucidate the mechanism by which statins counteract steroid-induced osteonecrosis and osteoporosis [27]. They found that lovastatin enhanced osteoblast differentiation as assessed by a 1.8 times increase in expression of bone cell and fat cell transcription factors Cbfa1/Runx2 and by a 5 times increase in osteocalcin promoter activity. By enhancing osteoblast gene expression and inhibiting adipogenesis, the authors postulate that lovastatin may shunt uncommitted osteoprogenitor cells in the marrow from the adipocytic to the osteoblastic differentiation pathway. Iwakiri et al. found that simvastatin and pravastatin significantly reduced the incidence of steroid-induced osteonecrosis in rabbits via histological analysis of femurs [28]. Pengde et al. corroborated Iwakiri's findings by histological analysis of femora and humeri. Pathological examination showed less serious adipogenesis and bone death in the statin group. In addition the size and area of the fat cells in the bone marrow were significantly smaller in the statin and normal saline groups than in the placebo group. This study showed that in an animal model, lovastatin can inhibit adipogenesis and decrease the rate of osteonecrosis [11]. Nishida et al. also found that statins (pitavastatin) decreased the incidence of steroid-induced osteonecrosis via histological analysis in rabbits and that the size of the bone marrow fat cells was smaller in the statin-treated group [29]. The data suggest pitavastatin has the potential to lower the incidence of steroid-induced osteonecrosis in rabbits.

These results indicate that steroid-induced adipogenesis in the bone marrow may contribute to osteonecrosis and that statins (esp. lovastatin) may be helpful in preventing the development of steroid-induced osteonecrosis.

34.3.5 Effects of Statins and Anticoagulants on Osteonecrosis

Kang et al. looked at the effects of the combined treatment with an anticoagulant (enoxaparin) agent and a lipid-lowering agent (lovastatin) on prevention or decrease in the occurrence of steroid-induced osteonecrosis in rabbits [13]. Hematological examination for serum lipid levels and prothrombin time was carried out, and both femora and humeri were examined histopathologically for the presence of osteonecrosis. The incidence of osteonecrosis in the combined enoxaparin + lovastatin group (15 %) was significantly lower than that observed in the no-treatment group (68 %). The incidence in the enoxaparin-only and lovastatin-only groups was also significantly lower than that in the no-treatment group (31 and 35 %). The fat cell sizes of the bone marrow in both enoxaparin-only and lovastatin-only groups were lower than in the no-treatment group. The prothrombin time was prolonged and plasma lipid levels were reduced in the combined enoxaparin + lovastatin group during the study. This study showed that the combination treatment with an anticoagulant agent and a lipid-lowering agent can reduce the incidence of steroid-induced osteonecrosis in rabbits. Future evaluation in clinical practice is necessary, taking into account the deleterious effects of Lovenox therapy when not otherwise clinically indicated.

34.3.6 Clinical Effects of Statins on Osteonecrosis

One of the earlier clinical studies was performed by Pritchett et al. who looked at whether the use of statins affects later development of osteonecrosis in patients receiving steroids

[12]. They examined the records of 284 patients who were taking statins at the time they were started on high-dose steroids and were followed to determine whether osteonecrosis had developed. After a minimum of 5 years, only 1 % from the group had osteonecrosis develop. This 1 % incidence is much less than the 3–20 % incidence usually reported for patients receiving high-dose steroids. Although a retrospective case series, this paper suggests that statins may offer some protection against having osteonecrosis develop when steroid treatment is necessary.

Another study by Pritchett explored the effects of fish oils and statins on lipid composition in the bone marrow and joint fluid in patients having total joint replacements [30]. Statins reduced the amount of lipid by 22 % in patients with osteoporosis, 26 % in patients with osteoarthritis, and 41 % in patients with osteonecrosis compared with pretreatment lipid levels in the same patients. Interestingly, lipid profiles of disturbed marrow and joint fluid from patients who took statins or dietary fish oil showed an increase in the proportion of unsaturated fatty acids and longer-chain fatty acids relative to pretreatment profiles. This study further supported the notion that lipid-lowering agents have the ability to change the amount and character of bone and joint lipids.

Ajmal et al. analyzed their prospective renal transplant database to determine if statin usage reduces the incidence of corticosteroid-related osteonecrosis [31]. They identified 2,881 renal transplantation patients who met the entry criteria. Among 338 patients on statins, 15 (4.4 %) developed osteonecrosis, versus 180 of 2,543 (7 %) patients who were not on statins.

Over the span of two decades, numerous studies have been conducted to better understand the pathogenesis of steroid-induced osteonecrosis. In addition, studies have specifically looked at the effect of lipid-lowering agents (primarily statins) on the development, progression, and severity of osteonecrosis. The majority of these studies are cellular or animal model based with only a few studies looking at case series of human patients. These studies have helped elucidate the pathophysiology of steroid-induced osteonecrosis and have shown the beneficial role lipid-lowering agents can play in preventing or blunting the progression of osteonecrosis.

34.4 Summary

Osteonecrosis is a debilitating disease process with many causes. Systemic steroid use is a significant risk factor for the development of osteonecrosis. Statins are lipid-lowering agents that dramatically reduce lipid levels in blood and tissues. As a result, the effect of lipid-lowering agents on the development and progression of osteonecrosis has been an interesting area of research.

Most of the early research on this topic consists of basic science studies on cell/tissue or animal models, but more recently, human clinical studies have been conducted. Basic science research has helped us understand the pathophysiology of osteonecrosis and suggest therapies that can be translated to clinical application. This research has progressed rapidly over the past two decades, and these advances offer promise for the future treatment of osteonecrosis.

One of the factors that limit the systemic evaluation of the effectiveness of the treatments is the lack of an animal model that replicates the natural history and progression of osteonecrosis in humans. Moreover, since the majority of research on the use of statins in patients with osteonecrosis is either bench research or research on animal models, the need for human studies is needed before any strong recommendations are made for or against the use of statins as an adjunct therapy in the management of osteonecrosis. The few human studies in the literature are level 3 or 4 studies. There are no double-blinded randomized controlled trials looking at the preventive and therapeutic effects of statins on osteonecrosis and these studies are needed before widespread recommendations can be made.

Based on the current literature on this topic, patients on systemic steroid therapy and those with a high lipid profile are encouraged to strongly consider statin therapy. There are no recommendations for or against the use of statins in patients with a low lipid profile and those with traumatic or extravascular causes of osteonecrosis.

References

1. Grose AW, Gardner MJ, Sussmann PS, Helfet DL, Lorich DG. The surgical anatomy of the blood supply to the femoral head: description of the anastomosis between the medial femoral circumflex and inferior gluteal arteries at the hip. J Bone Joint Surg Br. 2008;90(10):1298–303.
2. Mont MA, Hungerford DS. Review non-traumatic avascular necrosis of the femoral head. J Bone Joint Surg Am. 1995;77(3):459–74.
3. Lavernia CJ, Sierra RJ, Grieco FR. Osteonecrosis of the femoral head. J Am Acad Orthop Surg. 1999;74:250–61.
4. Jones Jr JP. Fat embolism, intravascular coagulation, and osteonecrosis. Clin Orthop Relat Res. 1993;292:294–308.
5. Wang GJ, Sweet DE, Reger SI, Thompson RC. Fat-cell changes as a mechanism of avascular necrosis of the femoral head in cortisone-treated rabbits. J Bone Joint Surg Am. 1977;59(6):729–35.
6. Cui Q, Wang GJ, Su CC, Balian G. The Otto Aufranc Award. Lovastatin prevents steroid induced adipogenesis and osteonecrosis. Clin Orthop Relat Res. 1997;344:8–19.
7. Kuribayashi M, Fujioka M, Takahashi KA, Arai Y, Ishida M, Goto T, Kubo T. Vitamin E prevents steroid-induced osteonecrosis in rabbits. Acta Orthop. 2010;81(1):154–60.
8. Yang L, Boyd K, Kaste SC, Kamdem Kamdem L, Rahija RJ, Relling MV. A mouse model for glucocorticoid-induced osteonecrosis: effect of a steroid holiday. J Orthop Res. 2009;27(2):169–75.
9. Han N, Yan Z, Guo CA, Shen F, Liu J, Shi Y, Zhang Z. Effects of p-glycoprotein on steroid-induced osteonecrosis of the femoral head. Calcif Tissue Int. 2010;87(3):246–53.

10. Drescher W, Weigert KP, Bünger MH, Ingerslev J, Bünger C, Hansen ES. Femoral head blood flow reduction and hypercoagulability under 24 h megadose steroid treatment in pigs. J Orthop Res. 2004;22(3):501–8.
11. Pengde K, Fuxing P, Bin S, Jing Y, Jingqiu C. Lovastatin inhibits adipogenesis and prevents osteonecrosis in steroid-treated rabbits. Joint Bone Spine. 2008;75(6):696–701.
12. Pritchett JW. Statin therapy decreases the risk of osteonecrosis in patients receiving steroids. Clin Orthop Relat Res. 2001;386:173–8.
13. Kang P, Gao H, Pei F, Shen B, Yang J, Zhou Z. Effects of an anticoagulant and a lipid-lowering agent on the prevention of steroid-induced osteonecrosis in rabbits. Int J Exp Pathol. 2010;91:235–43.
14. Motomura G, Yamamoto T, Miyanishi K, Jingushi S, Iwamoto Y. Combined effects of an anticoagulant and a lipid-lowering agent on the prevention of steroid-induced osteonecrosis in rabbits. Arthritis Rheum. 2004;50:3387–91.
15. Istvan ES, Deisenhofer J. Structural mechanism for statin inhibition of HMG-CoA reductase. Science. 2001;292(5519):1160–4.
16. AstraZeneca; JUPITER - Crestor 20mg Versus Placebo in Prevention of Cardiovascular (CV) Events. In: ClinicalTrials.gov [Internet]. Bethesda (MD): National Library of Medicine (US). 2000 [January 22, 2014]. Available from: http://clinicaltrials.gov/show/NCT00239681. NLM Identifier: NCT00239681.
17. Sattar N, Preiss D, Murray HM, et al. Statins and risk of incident diabetes: a collaborative meta-analysis of randomised statin trials. Lancet. 2010;375:735–42.
18. Ridker PM, Danielson E, Fonseca FA, et al. Rosuvastatin to prevent vascular events in men and women with elevated C-reactive protein. N Engl J Med. 2008;359:2195–207.
19. http://www.fda.gov/drugs/drugsafety/ucm293101.htm#dose. FDA drug safety communication: important safety label changes to cholesterol-lowering statin drugs. Feb 2012.
20. Mansi I, Frei CR, Pugh MJ, et al. Statins and musculoskeletal conditions, arthropathies, and injuries. JAMA Intern Med. 2013;173:1–10.
21. Arlet J. Nontraumatic avascular necrosis of the femoral head. Past, present, and future. Clin Orthop. 1992;277:12–21.
22. Cui Q, Wang GJ, Balian G. Steroid induced fat specific gene expression and adipogenesis in cells from bone marrow stroma. J Bone Joint Surg. 1997;79A:1054–63.
23. Bernlohr JN, Bennet J, Devlin C, et al. Expression of specific mRNAs during adipose differentiation: identification of an mRNA encoding a homologue of myelin P2 protein. Proc Natl Acad Sci U S A. 1984;81:5468–72.
24. Delamy AM, Dong Y, Canalis E. Mechanisms of glucocorticoid action in bone cells. J Cell Biochem. 1994;56:295–302.
25. Wang GJ, Cui Q, Balian G. The Nicolas Andry award. The pathogenesis and prevention of steroid-induced osteonecrosis. Clin Orthop Relat Res. 2000;370:295–310.
26. Kabata T, Kubo T, Matsumoto T, Hirata T, Fujioka M, Takahashi KA, Yagishita S, Kobayashi M, Tomita K. Onset of steroid-induced osteonecrosis in rabbits and its relationship to hyperlipaemia and increased free fatty acids. Rheumatology (Oxford). 2005;44(10):1233–7. Epub 2005 Jun 21.
27. Li X, Cui Q, Kao C, Wang GJ, Balian G. Lovastatin inhibits adipogenic and stimulates osteogenic differentiation by suppressing PPARgamma2 and increasing Cbfa1/Runx2 expression in bone marrow mesenchymal cell cultures. Bone. 2003;33(4):652–9.
28. Iwakiri K, Oda Y, Kaneshiro Y, Iwaki H, Masada T, Kobayashi A, Asada A, Takaoka K. Effect of simvastatin on steroid-induced osteonecrosis evidenced by the serum lipid level and hepatic cytochrome P4503A in a rabbit model. J Orthop Sci. 2008;13(5):463–8. doi:10.1007/s00776-008-1257-z. Epub 2008 Oct 9.
29. Nishida K, Yamamoto T, Motomura G, Jingushi S, Iwamoto Y. Pitavastatin may reduce risk of steroid-induced osteonecrosis in rabbits: a preliminary histological study. Clin Orthop Relat Res. 2008;466(5):1054–8. doi:10.1007/s11999-008-0189-4. Epub 2008 Mar 19.
30. Pritchett JW. Statins and dietary fish oils improve lipid composition in bone marrow and joints. Clin Orthop Relat Res. 2007;456:233–7.
31. Ajmal M, Matas AJ, Kuskowski M, Cheng EY. Does statin usage reduce the risk of corticosteroid-related osteonecrosis in renal transplant population? Orthop Clin North Am. 2009;40(2):235–9.

Is There a Role for BMPs in the Treatment of Osteonecrosis?

35

Philipp Leucht and Stuart B. Goodman

35.1 Introduction

The cause for osteonecrosis (ON) is still largely unknown and might in fact be multifactorial [1–3]. Multiple theories exist and almost all lead to impaired osseous blood flow with subsequent bone and marrow cell death. In cases of steroid- and alcohol-induced ON, current research points towards a predominance of adipogenic over osteogenic differentiation of mesenchymal stem cells, leading to osteocyte death and impaired remodeling with fatty atrophy of the subchondral bone [4, 5]. The foundation for the vascular insult theory is thought to be either from a traumatic disruption of the vasculature, from stenosis (i.e., compression), or from occlusion (i.e., thromboembolic event) [6]. After the initial ischemic event, necrosis of the cancellous bone and adjacent bone marrow ensues. This leads to an activation of signaling pathways that cumulate in an inflammatory response. Macrophages and osteoclasts home to the site of acute necrosis and initiate a resorption phase. In cases where only a small area of bone is involved, creeping substitution will replace the necrotic bone and the process will likely resolve without any clinically significant sequelae. If, however, the area of necrosis exceeds the size that can be regenerated through creeping substitution, then osteoclastic resorption can lead to structural compromise with the detrimental result of collapse. At this final stage of osteonecrosis, regenerative treatment options are futile and replacement of the involved joint is most commonly the last option. It is estimated that about 5–12 % of total hip arthroplasties are performed for sequelae of osteonecrosis of the femoral head [7, 8]. Current research focuses on the development of regenerative strategies that could lead to an osteogenic response during the pre-collapse state. Growth factors are the main target of this research. If we understand how to control the choice between proliferation and differentiation, then theoretically we will have the ability to expand what might be a limited population of progenitor cells within the site of osteonecrosis, induce their timely differentiation, and thus restore the function of the involved bone segment.

Recent publications suggest that BMPs are among the most attractive targets for such therapeutic interventions [9]. In this chapter, we will introduce the concept of BMP-induced bone regeneration during the repair of osteonecrotic lesions and will discuss current preliminary basic science and clinical trials.

35.2 Osteonecrosis and Bone Morphogenetic Proteins

Bone morphogenetic proteins (BMPs) were discovered by Marshall Urist in 1965 [10]. Since then, seven BMPs have been identified; six of these belong to the transforming growth factor beta superfamily [11, 12]. BMPs have become the focus of recent investigations with the goal to stimulate bone formation by adding exogenous growth factors. It is now clear that BMPs achieve their dramatic effect by inducing cells to adopt a chondrogenic fate and depositing an extracellular matrix rich in proteoglycans [13]. The resulting cartilaginous callus is then slowly replaced by bone through the process of endochondral ossification, which appears to be independent from the BMP response [12]. Besides this best known and understood role, BMPs play a role in a variety of cell fate decision involving chondrocytes, osteoblasts, and osteoclasts. The latter have been the source of recent debate, as new data showed a BMP-dependent activation of osteoblast-dependent osteoclastogenesis via

P. Leucht
Department of Orthopaedic Surgery, Stanford University Medical Center Outpatient Center, 450 Broadway St. M/C 6342, Redwood City, CA 94063, USA
e-mail: pleucht@stanford.edu

S.B. Goodman (✉)
Department of Orthopaedic Surgery and Bioengineering, Stanford University Medical Center Outpatient Center, 450 Broadway St. M/C 6342, Redwood City, CA 94063, USA
e-mail: goodbone@stanford.edu

K.-H. Koo et al. (eds.), *Osteonecrosis*,
DOI 10.1007/978-3-642-35767-1_35, © Springer-Verlag Berlin Heidelberg 2014

the RANKL-OPG pathway. This increased osteoclastogenesis results in bone resorption rather than bone deposition, and therefore, a revision of the traditional understanding of the BMP pathway in clinical therapeutics may be warranted [14, 15].

Currently there are two BMP formulations (BMP-2 (Infuse, Medtronic) and BMP-7 (OP-1, Stryker)) approved by the FDA for treatment of acute open fractures of the tibial shaft, for spinal fusion procedures (BMP-2), and for treatment of recalcitrant long bone nonunions (BMP-7). The use of BMPs in orthopedic surgery otherwise is off-label. We have searched the current literature for evidence suggesting that BMPs have been used for the treatment of pre-collapse osteonecrosis.

As described above, osteonecrosis is thought to be the result of a microvascular insult, which then leads to bone and marrow necrosis. This sequence of pathologic events offers three distinct targets as therapeutic approaches: lack of (1) angiogenesis, (2) viable progenitor cells within the defect, and (3) osteogenic stimulus to the few remaining progenitor cells in the periphery of the lesion.

Cui et al. proposed an experiment in which all three deficits were targeted with a simple experimental strategy [16]. They suggest the use of genetically engineered bone marrow stromal cells, carrying VEGF and BMP-6 genes, to enhance angiogenesis and osteogenesis in necrotic bone using a chicken ON model. By delivering genetically engineered progenitor cells, they not only supply the needed growth factors but also the cellular machinery required to establish the bony regenerate. Unfortunately, the results of these proposed experiments are not yet published and therefore can only provide basis for speculations. As with all gene therapy approaches, this idea will need rigorous preclinical testing followed by extensive clinical trials prior to an approval for the common treatment of osteonecrosis.

There are, however, attempts of mimicking and simplifying the abovementioned approach by administering the purified protein into the area of osteonecrosis. Recent data suggest that BMP not only induces osteogenesis but also acts as a very potent stimulator of angiogenesis [17]. This effect is achieved through osteoblast-derived vascular endothelial growth factor A expression. Thus, addition of BMP to the site of osteonecrosis would potentially induce angiogenesis through the effect of VEGF expression, followed by increased osteogenesis, which is a direct BMP-dependent mechanism. This strategy addresses two of the three main therapeutic hurdles that we are facing in the treatment of ON. Wang et al. published their results using this approach in a murine model of ON [18]. In detail, they set out to test whether rhBMP2 was able to penetrate into the area of necrosis and, if so, could promote angiogenesis and creeping substitution of the nonviable bone. They first tested three different rhBMP-2 carriers, all containing hydroxyapatite and poly (D,L-lactide-co-glycolide)(PLGA65/35), in which the BMP protein is either contained within microspheres or tethered to the outside of spheres at different concentration. By using a murine model, in which a fragment of necrotic bone was interposed into a tibial defect, they showed that the higher concentration of rhBMP-2 (2,000 ng) tethered to the outside of the microsphere lead to a daily release of approximately 80 ng/ml per day. This release concentration resulted in a strong angiogenic response within the necrotic bone and a subsequent solid callus formation around the fragment. Despite this significant healing response in this model, there are clear differences between this model and the clinical presentation of ON. ON of the subchondral bone presents a slightly different environment than the tibial defect with intercalary necrotic segment model that is presented by the authors. There is abundant evidence that suggests that BMPs act on osteochondral progenitor cells that reside within the cambial layer of the periosteum [13, 19], but until now, there is no published evidence that BMPs activate osteoprogenitor cells within the bone marrow. Considering this caveat, other experimental designs that mimic the condition of osteonecrosis more closely will be needed.

Several animal models for osteonecrosis exist, but only a few recapitulate the various aspects of the early histopathological features combined with the late macroscopic collapse. Experimental models in goat [20], rabbit [21], and emu [22] have been published, and all have in common that osteonecrosis was created by ligation of the vascular supply to the femoral head in addition to deep-freezing of the cancellous bone of the femoral head with liquid nitrogen. In these models, ON occurs reliably and leads to subsequent collapse of the subchondral bone. This feature allows the investigators to not only investigate the early effect of BMP treatment but also to ensure that the BMP-induced bone regenerate provides a mechanically stable scaffold for maintenance of joint congruity. Tang et al. [23] employed the abovementioned goat model to evaluate if hBMP-2-gene-modified bone marrow stromal cells can be utilized for the treatment of ON of the femoral head. Three weeks after establishment of ON in the femoral head, core decompression was performed, and the defect was filled with either β-tricalcium phosphate loaded with BMP-2-gene-modified bone marrow mesenchymal stem cells or β-TCP with β-gal-gene-modified bone marrow mesenchymal stem cells. Sixteen weeks after surgery, femoral heads in both groups maintained their original shape without any signs of collapse. Histology revealed lamellar bone formation in the BMP group, compared to some fibrous tissue in the β-gal group. Biomechanical analysis revealed a significant difference between the two groups with a higher maximum compressive strength and Young's modulus in the BMP-2 group. This study provides sound evidence that BMP-2 gene therapy provides a feasible, and most importantly, successful approach in the prevention of subchondral collapse due to ON.

Ischemic necrosis of the femoral head is the cause of Legg-Calvé-Perthes disease, a condition affecting 4–31/100,000 children worldwide [24]. Since the first description by Legg, Calve, and Perthes in the early 1900s, significant research has been performed in an attempt to understand the cause and its natural history and to devise possible treatment option. Recent nonoperative treatment includes bisphosphonates, which inhibit osteoclastic resorption of the necrotic femoral head [25]. This potential delay in resorption is thought to allow osteoblasts to lay down an osteoid matrix and stabilize the necrotic area before collapse can occur. In a piglet model, both systemic and intraosseous bisphosphonates were shown to delay remodeling; however, intraosseous administration was shown to be more effective, even as a single dose [26–28]. This effect was attributed to the lower bioavailability of the IV drug in the necrotic, and therefore avascular, femoral epiphysis. Histology of these femoral heads showed a lack of osteoclastic resorption in the necrotic epiphysis, but also a lack of osteoblasts and osteoid matrix. The next logical step therefore was to add a growth factor to the bisphosphonate injection. This would theoretically inhibit remodeling of the necrotic epiphysis and at the same time induce osteogenesis and angiogenesis. Vandermeer et al. published their results on a combination therapy consisting of ibandronate and bone morphogenetic protein-2 (BMP-2) [29]. They tested if this therapy can preserve the shape of the femoral head and stimulate new bone formation in an immature pig model of ischemic osteonecrosis. Histological analysis showed increased trabecular bone in the ibandronate-BMP-2 group compared to the saline group. Trabecular volume, thickness, and osteoblast number were all significantly increased, whereas the osteoclast number was significantly reduced in response to the ibandronate-BMP-2 injection. These data provide preliminary evidence that a combination of antiresorptive and anabolic agents can not only improve bone healing but also decrease deformity following ischemic osteonecrosis. In addition, local delivery into the lesion allows for a lower dose of the bisphosphonates and restricts the growth factor to the site of interest. In this study, however, the investigators found some evidence of heterotopic ossification (HO) in the hip capsule. It is unclear if this HO formation was due to the extravasation of the BMP into the joint or from the trauma associated with the surgically induced ON of the head, which could possibly make the pericapsular tissues more receptive to the BMP. The leakage of BMP into the joint could theoretically be avoided by performing the injection through the greater trochanter into the neck and head instead of passing the needle through the joint space into the femoral head. The major advantage of the above-described bisphosphonate/BMP treatment approach is the relative ease of administration without much anticipated postsurgical pain and immobilization.

35.3 Summary

The ultimate goal of nonoperative and operative treatment of osteonecrosis is preservation of the joint space and maintenance of the bony architecture. Recent advances in basic science have opened new avenues including antiresorptive and anabolic regimens. Thus far, there is preliminary evidence, at least in animal models, that bone resorption can be delayed by administration of bisphosphonates and that regeneration of the necrotic area can be enhanced by BMP treatment. This recent research suggests new treatment options that could potentially make a significant impact on the outcome of patients with osteonecrosis.

References

1. Amanatullah DF, Strauss EJ, Di Cesare PE. Current management options for osteonecrosis of the femoral head: part 1, diagnosis and nonoperative management. Am J Orthop. 2011;40(9):E186–92.
2. Mont MA, Marker DR, Zywiel MG, Carrino JA. Osteonecrosis of the knee and related conditions. J Am Acad Orthop Surg. 2011;19(8):482–94.
3. Petrigliano FA, Lieberman JR. Osteonecrosis of the hip: novel approaches to evaluation and treatment. Clin Orthop Relat Res. 2007;465:53–62. doi:10.1097/BLO.0b013e3181591c92.
4. Wang Y, Li Y, Mao K, Li J, Cui Q, Wang GJ. Alcohol-induced adipogenesis in bone and marrow: a possible mechanism for osteonecrosis. Clin Orthop Relat Res. 2003;410:213–24. doi:10.1097/01.blo.0000063602.67412.83.
5. Asano T, Takahashi KA, Fujioka M, Inoue S, Okamoto M, Sugioka N, et al. ABCB1 C3435T and G2677T/A polymorphism decreased the risk for steroid-induced osteonecrosis of the femoral head after kidney transplantation. Pharmacogenetics. 2003;13(11):675–82. doi:10.1097/01.fpc.0000054135.14659.65.
6. Chandler FA. Coronary disease of the hip. 1949. Clin Orthop Relat Res. 2001;386:7–10.
7. Mankin HJ. Nontraumatic necrosis of bone (osteonecrosis). N Engl J Med. 1992;326(22):1473–9. doi:10.1056/NEJM199205283262206.
8. Steinberg ME, Hayken GD, Steinberg DR. A quantitative system for staging avascular necrosis. J Bone Joint Surg Br. 1995;77(1):34–41.
9. Haidar ZS, Hamdy RC, Tabrizian M. Delivery of recombinant bone morphogenetic proteins for bone regeneration and repair. Part A: current challenges in BMP delivery. Biotechnol Lett. 2009;31(12):1817–24. doi:10.1007/s10529-009-0099-x.
10. Urist MR. Bone: formation by autoinduction. Science. 1965;150:893.
11. Chen G, Deng C, Li YP. TGF-beta and BMP signaling in osteoblast differentiation and bone formation. Int J Biol Sci. 2012;8(2):272–88. doi:10.7150/ijbs.2929.

12. Chen D, Zhao M, Mundy GR. Bone morphogenetic proteins. Growth Factors. 2004;22(4):233–41. doi:10.1080/0897719041233 1279890.
13. Yu YY, Lieu S, Lu C, Colnot C. Bone morphogenetic protein 2 stimulates endochondral ossification by regulating periosteal cell fate during bone repair. Bone. 2010;47(1):65–73. doi:10.1016/j.bone.2010.03.012.
14. Tachi K, Takami M, Zhao B, Mochizuki A, Yamada A, Miyamoto Y, et al. Bone morphogenetic protein 2 enhances mouse osteoclast differentiation via increased levels of receptor activator of NF-kappaB ligand expression in osteoblasts. Cell Tissue Res. 2010;342(2):213–20. doi:10.1007/s00441-010-1052-y.
15. Toth JM, Boden SD, Burkus JK, Badura JM, Peckham SM, McKay WF. Short-term osteoclastic activity induced by locally high concentrations of recombinant human bone morphogenetic protein-2 in a cancellous bone environment. Spine (Phila Pa 1976). 2009;34(6):539–50. doi:10.1097/BRS.0b013e3181952695.
16. Cui Q, Botchwey EA. Emerging ideas: treatment of precollapse osteonecrosis using stem cells and growth factors. Clin Orthop Relat Res. 2011;469(9):2665–9. doi:10.1007/s11999-010-1738-1.
17. Deckers MM, van Bezooijen RL, van der Horst G, Hoogendam J, van Der Bent C, Papapoulos SE, et al. Bone morphogenetic proteins stimulate angiogenesis through osteoblast-derived vascular endothelial growth factor A. Endocrinology. 2002;143(4):1545–53.
18. Wang CK, Ho ML, Wang GJ, Chang JK, Chen CH, Fu YC, et al. Controlled-release of rhBMP-2 carriers in the regeneration of osteonecrotic bone. Biomaterials. 2009;30(25):4178–86. doi:10.1016/j.biomaterials.2009.04.029.
19. Minear S, Leucht P, Miller S, Helms JA. rBMP represses Wnt signaling and influences skeletal progenitor cell fate specification during bone repair. J Bone Miner Res. 2010;25(6):1196–207. doi:10.1002/jbmr.29.
20. Newton B, Crawford CJ, Powers DL, Allen Jr BL. The immature goat as an animal model for Legg-Calve-Perthes disease. J Invest Surg. 1994;7(5):417–30.
21. Boss JH. Experimental models of osteonecrosis of the femoral head. J Orthop Sci. 2004;9(5):533–4. doi:10.1007/s00776-004-0817-0.
22. Conzemius MG, Brown TD, Zhang Y, Robinson RA. A new animal model of femoral head osteonecrosis: one that progresses to human-like mechanical failure. J Orthop Res. 2002;20(2):303–9. doi:10.1016/S0736-0266(01)00108-5.
23. Tang TT, Lu B, Yue B, Xie XH, Xie YZ, Dai KR, Lu JX, Lou JR. Treatment of osteonecrosis of the femoral head with hBMP-2-gene-modified tissue-engineered bone in goats. J Bone Joint Surg Br. 2007;89(1):127–9. Erratum in J Bone Joint Surg Br. 2007;89(3):421.
24. Perry DC, Hall AJ. The epidemiology and etiology of Perthes disease. Orthop Clin North Am. 2011;42(3):279–83, v. doi:10.1016/j.ocl.2011.03.002.
25. Chen CH, Chang JK, Lai KA, Hou SM, Chang CH, Wang GJ. Alendronate in the prevention of collapse of the femoral head in nontraumatic osteonecrosis: a two-year multicenter, prospective, randomized, double-blind, placebo-controlled study. Arthritis Rheum. 2012;64(5):1572–8. doi:10.1002/art.33498.
26. Little DG, Peat RA, McEvoy A, Williams PR, Smith EJ, Baldock PA. Zoledronic acid treatment results in retention of femoral head structure after traumatic osteonecrosis in young Wistar rats. J Bone Miner Res. 2003;18(11):2016–22. doi:10.1359/jbmr.2003.18.11.2016.
27. Peled E, Bejar J, Zinman C, Reis DN, Boss JH, Ben-Noon H, et al. Alendronate preserves femoral head shape and height/length ratios in an experimental rat model: a computer-assisted analysis. Indian J Orthop. 2009;43(1):22–6. doi:10.4103/0019-5413.44630.
28. Little DG, McDonald M, Sharpe IT, Peat R, Williams P, McEvoy T. Zoledronic acid improves femoral head sphericity in a rat model of perthes disease. J Orthop Res. 2005;23(4):862–8. doi:10.1016/j.orthres.2004.11.015.
29. Vandermeer JS, Kamiya N, Aya-ay J, Garces A, Browne R, Kim HK. Local administration of ibandronate and bone morphogenetic protein-2 after ischemic osteonecrosis of the immature femoral head: a combined therapy that stimulates bone formation and decreases femoral head deformity. J Bone Joint Surg Am. 2011;93(10):905–13. doi:10.2106/JBJS.J.00716.

36 Alendronate in the Prevention of Collapse of the Femoral Head in Nontraumatic Osteonecrosis

Chung-Hwan Chen and Gwo-Jaw Wang

36.1 Introduction

Nontraumatic osteonecrosis (ON) is one of the most debilitating skeletal complications, yet the cause of the disease remains controversial. Each year, 10,000–20,000 new cases are diagnosed in the United States alone [1, 2], and about half of the total hip replacement cases in Taiwan were the result of debilitating osteoarthritis from ON [3]. Moreover, with the majority of the disease population comprising younger patients with late diagnosis, this leads to severe socioeconomic burdens and increased suffering on the part of the patient, beyond the problems of early loosening and multiple procedures [1].

Several pharmacological agents that have been used to treat ON of the hip include statins [4, 5], anticoagulants [6, 7], prostacyclin [8, 9], and bisphosphonates [10–14]. The theoretical benefit of statins is based on the association of increased fat cell size with an increased risk of the development of ON of the hip [15, 16]. Anticoagulants may inhibit the aggregation of platelets and enhance blood flow to ischemic bone areas [6]. Prostacyclin may promote bone regeneration on a cellular or systemic level [9]. Bisphosphonates, which inhibit osteoclastic activity, may decrease the incidence of femoral head collapse [10–12, 14].

At the present time, there is no efficient pharmacological treatment for ON. The reparative process at the junction between living and necrotic bone frequently leads to osteochondral sequestration. This phenomenon remains as the main reason for the collapse of the joint surface with joint destruction [11].

C.-H. Chen
Departments of Orthopedics and Orthopedic Research Center, College of Medicine, Kaohsiung Medical University, Kaohsiung, Taiwan

Department of Orthopedics, Kaohsiung Medical University Hospital, Kaohsiung Medical University, Kaohsiung, Taiwan

Medical Device Innovation Center, National Cheng-Kung University, Tainan, Taiwan

Skeleton-Joint Research Center, National Cheng-Kung University, Tainan, Taiwan

G.-J. Wang (✉)
Departments of Orthopedics and Orthopedic Research Center, College of Medicine, Kaohsiung Medical University, Kaohsiung, Taiwan

Department of Orthopedic Surgery, National Cheng-Kung University and Hospital, Tainan, Taiwan

Medical Device Innovation Center, National Cheng-Kung University, Tainan, Taiwan

Skeleton-Joint Research Center, National Cheng-Kung University, Tainan, Taiwan

Department of Orthopedic Surgery, University of Virginia, Charlottesville, VA, USA
e-mail: gwojaw2939@yahoo.com

36.2 Bisphosphonates (BPs) and Alendronate (Aln)

BPs are currently the most widely used treatment of common skeletal disorders such as osteoporosis, metastatic bone disease, and Paget's disease of bone. The P–C–P moiety is responsible for the strong affinity of the bisphosphonates for the skeleton. BPs containing a basic primary nitrogen atom in an alkyl chain (as in Aln) were found to be 10- to 100-fold more potent than those without nitrogen [17].

BPs are selective uptake in the skeleton preferentially at sites with increased bone remodeling and slow release from bone. BPs are currently administered either orally or intravenously. Oral BPs are absorbed throughout the entire gastrointestinal (GI) tract by paracellular transport with better absorption from segments of the tract with larger surface areas [18]. The absorption of BPs is very low, and the most widely used nitrogen-containing BP (N-BP), Aln, has an absorption of about 0.7 % [19]. BPs have high affinity for bone mineral and can prevent calcification both in vitro and in vivo. The main uptake of BPs in the skeleton is on the mineral surfaces in bone, taking them into close extracellular

K.-H. Koo et al. (eds.), *Osteonecrosis*,
DOI 10.1007/978-3-642-35767-1_36, © Springer-Verlag Berlin Heidelberg 2014

contact with osteoclasts [20]. BPs have been shown to interfere with osteoclast recruitment, differentiation, and action. During bone resorption by osteoclasts, the acidic pH in the resorption lacuna leads to the dissociation of BP from the bone mineral surface, followed by intracellular uptake of the BP into osteoclasts by fluid-phase endocytosis [21]. Since only osteoclasts can acidify the bone surface to release bone-bound BPs, osteoclasts are the only cell type capable of internalizing substantial amounts of these drugs in vivo [22]. Following internalization, bisphosphonates seem to act as analogs of pyrophosphate and interfere with intracellular metabolic pathways required for normal cell function. Aln disrupts the formation of the cytoskeletal actin ring in polarized, resorbing osteoclasts [23].

Nitrogen-containing bisphosphonates are inhibitors of the mevalonate pathway, a pathway for the production of cholesterol and isoprenoid lipids such as isopentenyl pyrophosphate (IPP), farnesyl pyrophosphate (FPP), and geranylgeranyl pyrophosphate (GGPP) [24]. FPP and GGPP are required for the posttranslational modification (prenylation) of small GTPases such as Ras, Rho, and Rac, which are prenylated at a cysteine residue [25]. Small GTPases are important signaling proteins that regulate a variety of cell processes important for osteoclast function, including cell morphology, membrane ruffling, trafficking of endosomes, and cell survival (i.e., prevention of apoptosis) [26]. Inhibition of the mevalonate pathway, leading to loss of prenylated proteins and/or accumulation of unprenylated proteins, could therefore account for most of the various effects of N-BPs on osteoclasts [24]. Loss of geranylgeranylated proteins causes disruption of actin rings, inhibits bone resorption, and stimulates osteoclast apoptosis [27].

36.3 The Anabolic Effect of Alendronate on Bone Metabolism

Aln is one of the most commonly used bisphosphonates for osteoporosis treatment [28]. Aln suppresses osteoclast activity by inhibiting the activity of farnesyl pyrophosphate synthetase. Some studies reveal that bisphosphonates increase proliferation, stimulate differentiation toward the osteoblastic lineage, and enhance mineralization in stem and osteoblastic lineage cells. Recent studies suggest that Aln enhances the osteogenesis of osteoblasts and bone marrow mesenchymal stem cells (BMSCs) [29–31]. Im et al. showed that Aln enhanced the expression of osteogenic marker genes and the activity of alkaline phosphatase (ALP) in human osteoblasts [31]. Von Knoch et al. [30] and Duque et al. [29] reported that Aln enhanced the proliferation and osteogenesis of human BMSCs (hBMSCs). We also found Aln acts as an osteo-inductive factor to stimulate the osteogenic differentiation of human adipose-derived stem cells (hADSCs) for bone regeneration [32]. In vivo studies showed that BPs promote early osteoblastogenesis in mice [33] and increase the expression of osteoblast differentiation markers and improve calvarial wound closure in rats [34]. Besides, Aln prevented the increase in osteoblast and osteocyte apoptosis induced by glucocorticoids in mice [35, 36]. Aln were also shown to inhibit osteocyte apoptosis induced by fatigue cyclic loading in rats [37].

36.4 Application of Aln in ON

Even though ON is the result of various conditions, the common final pathway leading to collapse of the femoral head is an uncoupling of the rates of osteoclastic bone resorption and osteoblastic bone regeneration. Lai et al. reasoned that by inhibiting the activity of the osteoclasts, collapse of the femoral head might be delayed or even prevented. They evaluated the effect of Aln in preventing early collapse of the femoral head in patients with nontraumatic ON. Forty patients with Steinberg stage II or III ON and a necrotic area of >30 % (class C) were randomly divided into Aln and control groups of 20 patients each. Placebo or 70 mg of Aln orally per week for 25 weeks was prescribed. Two years later, only 2 of 29 femoral heads in the Aln group collapsed, whereas 19 of 25 femoral heads in the control group collapsed ($p<0.001$). One hip in the Aln group underwent total hip arthroplasty (THA), whereas 16 hips in the control group underwent total hip arthroplasty ($p<0.001$). The result was promising because Aln appeared to prevent early collapse of the femoral head in the hips with Steinberg stage II or IIIC nontraumatic ON [11]. Nishii et al. reported Aln group had a lower incidence of collapse and worsening of hip pain than patients in the control group. On serial radiographs, collapse was observed in 6 of 13 hips in the control group and in 1 of 20 hips in the Aln group. They concluded Aln has the potential to prevent collapse of the femoral head, even with extensive necrosis, presumably by inhibiting bone resorption in the necrotic region [12]. Agarwala et al. reported the result of clinicoradiological analysis of 395 hips with ON treated with oral Aln for 3 years with a mean follow-up of 4 years (1–8). They found patients treated with Aln had an improvement in the clinical function, a reduction in the rate of collapse, and a decrease in the requirement for total hip replacement, compared with those with no treatment given. This improvement was particularly marked if the treatment is begun in the pre-collapse stages of the disease [13].

36.5 The Randomized, Double-Blind, Placebo-Controlled Trial of Aln on ON

Because the anti-catabolic and potential anabolic effect of Aln in the previous clinical studies, we hypothesized that Aln can delay or prevent the progression of the reparative process and then reduce the need of THA in patients who have ON. We conducted a multicenter, randomized, double-blind, placebo-controlled trial to prove or disprove Aln's ability to delay or prevent the progression of the reparative process. The primary object of this study was to determine the cumulative incidence of THA and time to event after treatment with Aln or placebo during the study period. The secondary objects were to determine the cumulative incidence of progression of femoral head collapse and time to event; to assess the change in the stage using X-ray and the necrotic area as assessed by MRI after a 2-year treatment period or before THA with Aln or placebo; and to assess the change in HHS and Short Form-36 after treatment with Aln or placebo during the study period. The primary endpoint was prosthetic arthroplasty as the end of survival. When the patients still had intractable pain more than 1 month after treatment with analgesia after the collapse of femoral head, THA was suggested. The primary goal was to evaluate whether Aln can decrease the need for THA in patients with nontraumatic ON of the femoral head. The secondary goal was to evaluate whether Aln can decrease the progression of ON. The tertiary goal was to evaluate whether Aln can improve quality of life [38].

All the patients presented with University of Pennsylvania System stage IIC and IIIC ON of the femoral head. Exclusion criteria were as follows: (1) being under 20 years of age; (2) prior bisphosphonate use; (3) having contraindications to the use of Aln; (4) unwillingness or inability to provide informed consent, (5) a history or evidence of metabolic bone disease (other than postmenopausal bone loss) including but not limited to hyper- or hypoparathyroidism, Paget's disease, osteomalacia, renal osteodystrophy, or osteogenesis imperfecta; (6) having received anabolic steroids and glucocorticoids for more than 2 weeks within the 6 months prior to the start of the study; (7) pregnant or lactating women; (8) severe cardiac disease and a history of recent (within 1 year) major upper gastrointestinal disease; (9) the presence of cancer(s) with known metastasis of the bone; (10) bilateral hip replacements; and (11) those with a serum creatinine level > 1.6 mg/dL. When the patients who had bilateral hip replacements met the inclusion criteria, two hips were counted in the statistics. Each treatment group of patients received oral Aln (70 mg) [Fosamax® 70 mg tablets, MSD] or a placebo weekly for 104 weeks. In addition, all patients received daily oral calcium (500 mg) and vitamin D (400 IU), as a supplement. In the end, there were 52 patients whose data were assessed for the study results. There was no statistical significance between the two groups in terms of demographics and the distribution of baseline severity of bilateral hip collapse in the radiographic evaluation [38].

At the end of this study, 4 of 32 hips in the treatment group, i.e., 13.06 % (95 % C.I. of cumulative incidence, 1.1–25.0 %), received THA, while 5 of 33 hips in the placebo group, i.e., 15.6 % (95 % C.I. of cumulative incidence, 3.0–28.2 %), underwent THA ($p = 0.837$) (Fig. 36.1). At the end of the study, 21 of 32 hips in the treatment group and 20 of 33 hips in the placebo group had progressed ($p = 0.636$) (Table 36.1). In the MRI evaluation, there was no difference between the groups (Table 36.2). There was no difference in the HHS between the groups at the beginning and the end of this study. In addition, the difference in the HHS between the groups during the study was not significant. There was no difference between the groups at the beginning and the end of the study, and the difference during the study in all dimensions of the Short Form-36 except the decrease in the dimension of vitality which was obvious in the Aln group

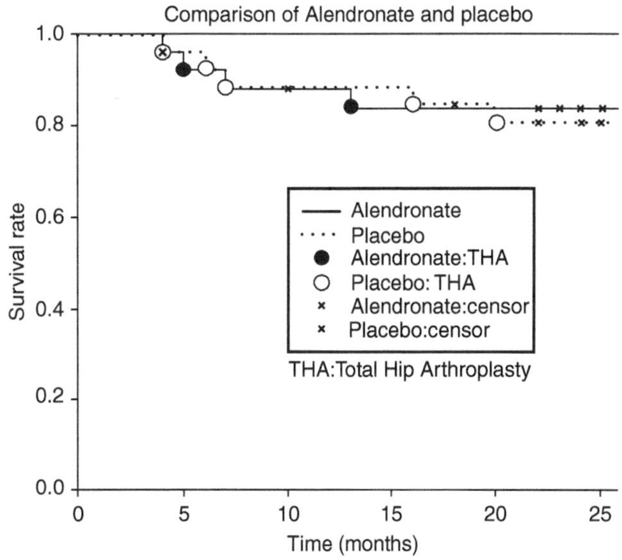

Censored: no event during the observational period 24 hips in alendronate group and 23 hips in placebo group were censored at the end of study
1 hip at 3 months and 3 hips at 12 months in the alendronate group lost follow-up
1 hip at 15 months, 2 hip at 18 months and 2 hips at 21 months lost follow-up in the placebo group lost follow-up

Fig. 36.1 Comparison of alendronate and placebo

Table 36.1 Radiographic evaluation (University of Pennsylvania System)

Fosamax							
Stage	0	I	IIC	IIIC	IV	V and VI	THA
Baseline	–	–	20	12	–	–	–
Follow-up	0	0	11	11	9	1	4
Placebo							
Stage	0	I	IIC	IIIC	IV	V and VI	THA
Baseline	–	–	25	8	–	–	–
Follow-up	1	0	14	9	9	0	5

Table 36.2 MRI evaluation and Harris Hip Score

% of the area of osteonecrosis in femoral head	Alendronate (*N*)	Placebo (*N*)	*p*-value[a]
Baseline	47.0±19.4 (32)	45.8±19.4 (30)	0.6262
End of study/THA/withdrew	37.9±19.9 (26)	38.8±16.6 (22)	0.8920
Difference	−6.6±11.9 (26)	−6.6±13.9 (19)	0.5170
95 % C.I.	−11.4 to −1.8	−13.3–0.1	
Harris Hip Score (subject no.)	26	26	
Baseline	78.1±12.5	76.6±15.2	0.6804
Follow-up	79.3±14.2	83.8±12.8	0.2435

[a]There is no statistical significance in any item between two groups

at the end of the study ($p=0.029$) (Table 36.3). Our results overthrew the null hypothesis in the primary, secondary, and tertiary goals [38].

Our primary goal was to evaluate whether Aln can decrease the need for THA. Both surgical and nonsurgical approaches have been developed to preserve the joint and are used in an attempt to arrest the progression of disease, as well as to offer pain relief [39, 40]. Maintenance of the femoral head shape and articular surface, and halting the progression of the disease, appears to be one of the preferred methods of avoiding arthrosis of the hip joint. Surgical treatments with osteotomies and/or bone grafts that restore and revive the femoral head provide excellent long-term

Table 36.3 Short Form-36

Dimension	Alendronate		Placebo		*p*-value[a]
N	31		28		
Baseline	Mean±SD	Medium	Mean±SD	Medium	
Physical functioning	60.3±24.8	60.0	58.0±28.1	55.0	0.7388
Role limitation due to physical problem	46.0±40.4	50.0	50.9±44.9	62.5	0.6588
Bodily pain	58.5±20.5	57.5	56.6±24.2	62.5	0.7401
General health	56.0±17.8	55.0	53.4±20.5	55.0	0.6074
Vitality	60.5±20.3	55.0	52.3±23.7	52.5	0.1598
Social functioning	70.2±24.7	75.0	65.6±26.3	68.8	0.4972
Role limitation due to emotional problem	58.1±44.7	66.7	60.7±43.6	83.3	0.8188
Mental health	65.5±17.0	68.0	61.6±21.5	64.0	0.4310
Total score	59.2±18.6	55.9	57.0±21.9	60.1	0.6788
N	30		28		
The end of study/THA/withdrew	Mean±SD	Medium	Mean±SD	Medium	
Physical functioning	55.0±26.2	52.0	56.1±27.2	55.0	0.8742
Role limitation due to physical problem	37.5±43.4	0.0	38.4±42.7	12.5	0.9374
Bodily pain	58.1±20.4	57.5	63.3±18.6	67.5	0.3140
General health	51.0±20.4	45.0	50.8±23.8	50.0	0.9731
Vitality	53.5±18.1	50.0	54.8±20.1	52.5	0.7931
Social functioning	64.2±20.2	68.8	63.8±24.4	50.0	0.9556
Role limitation due to emotional problem	50.0±47.7	50.0	53.6±46.6	62.5	0.7743
Mental health	60.7±15.9	60.0	61.1±19.5	60.0	0.9189
Total score	53.3±20.2	53.7	54.7±21.9	61.3	0.8011

Difference of dimension	Alendronate	Placebo	*p*-value[a]
N	30	28	
	Mean±SD	Mean±SD	
Physical functioning	−5.8±26.3	−1.9±30.8	0.6024
Role limitation due to physical problem	−10.0±43.8	−12.5±45.4	0.8318
Bodily pain	−1.3±21.2	6.7±22.4	0.1656
General health	−5.8±19.8	−2.6±22.6	0.5621
Vitality	**−8.5±18.9***	2.5±18.2	0.0288
Social functioning	−7.9±21.4	−1.7±20.6	0.2718
Role limitation due to emotional problem	−10.0±51.9	−7.1±39.9	0.8160
Mental health	−5.8±17.4	−0.42±14.4	0.2027
Total score	**−6.9±19.3***	−2.2±15.4	0.3137

*$p<0.05$, tested by Signed Rank test
[a]Tested by Wilcoxon Rank sums test

results [1, 39, 41–43]. Medication that prevents the early collapse of the osteonecrotic femoral head is an attractive treatment. Using Aln in an attempt to slow down the bone remodeling process had been reported by Lai et al. [11]. In a randomized, control, prospective study, they showed the effectiveness of Aln in delaying or even avoiding THA in pre-collapse femoral heads. In the study by Agarwala et al., THA was circumvented with early use of Aln in pre-collapse femoral heads [10, 13]. In terms of our primary goal, the result was different from the above studies [11, 13]. We did not find any obvious effect of Aln in decreasing the possibility of receiving THA. Hip arthroplasty for ON is dependent on the patient's pain severity and functional needs; therefore, the disease status and the functional demand of the patient are very important factors in terms of treatment options. It is important that any decision to perform arthroplasty should be supported by robust clinical information. A double-blind design is very important because the disease course sometimes involves subjective judgment by the investigator and the expectations of individual patients when making decisions concerning undergoing surgical treatment. No standard criteria for the timing of surgical treatment have been defined. A meta-analysis of the outcomes of protected weight bearing in 819 patients demonstrated a failure rate of >80 % at a mean of 34 months [44]. Even though all patients had a large lesion (>30 %) in our study, we found a very low incidence of THA (13.06 % in the Aln group and 15.60 % in the placebo group) due to the collapse of the femoral head, as compared with the previous literature [1, 40, 44–48]. In our study, all patients received daily oral calcium (500 mg) and vitamin D (400 IU). There is no report about the therapeutic effects of calcium and vitamin D. We are not certain of the reasons for the low incidence of THA and progression of disease in the placebo group. Because there is no data about the natural course of ON in the Taiwanese population, we are not certain as to whether there might be a racial difference in the natural course of ON. As such, there was a numerical reduction in the rate of THA in the Aln group compared with placebo that did not achieve statistical significance; this was likely because the study was originally designed to detect a between-group difference based on event rates of 35.7 % (10/28) and 3.4 % (1/29) in the placebo and Aln groups, respectively.

Our secondary goal was to evaluate whether Aln can decrease the progression of ON in image studies. Early studies showed overall clinical progression rates of 77–98 % and radiographic progression rates of 68–75 %, with an average of 3 years of follow-up [47, 48]. Our results are somewhat different from the above studies, with a low stage progression rate (37 % in the Aln group and 42 % in the placebo group). On the other hand, when the size and location of the lesion are large enough (>30 %), there is concern about potential collapse [49], and preventive surgery would provide a better chance of reviving the necrotic head and preserving hip function. Nam et al. reported excellent results (near 100 % survival) for small lesions (<30 %) followed more than 5 years, among asymptomatic lesions in ON of the femoral head [50]. According to their survival analysis, about 90 % of median (30–50 %) and more than 85 % of large (>50 %) asymptomatic lesions survived at the second year of follow-up [50]. Their results are somewhat similar to ours, but in our study, all lesions were symptomatic. The prognosis may be different for asymptomatic versus symptomatic lesions.

There were some limitations in our study. First, the sample size was not large, and this may have led to inadequate power to detect differences. The number of patients who have not been exposed to Aln is less than before after some studies found that Aln was effective in the treatment of ON; therefore, it is not easy to perform a trial with a very large sample size of patients who did not use Aln in the past 2 years. Besides, the events of THA are much less than we expect from the result of the previous study [11]. The less events of THA further decrease the power of this study. In addition, not all patients received an MRI evaluation, and this may have led to a smaller sample size in terms of MRI evaluation and thus less discrimination power. Finally, although surgeons may have a consensus at the time of THA, it is not easy to standardize practice in every situation, and this may lead to some differences in decisions concerning THA.

36.6 Summary

In conclusion, in this study we used randomized, double-blind, placebo-controlled treatment for ON. There was no significant pharmacological function of Aln in terms of the need for THA, disease progression, and life quality. The esophageal or gastric irritation caused by the oral preparations is an established adverse effect. Other adverse events like osteonecrosis of the jaw (ONJ) and subtrochanteric fractures have attracted attention mainly because of their unclear pathophysiology [51]. Because of the potent inhibitory effect of Aln on osteoclast and subsequently on bone remodeling, we do not suggest the use of Aln in young patients with ON. Further study for the medical treatment of ON is still required.

References

1. Mont MA, Hungerford DS. Non-traumatic avascular necrosis of the femoral head. J Bone Joint Surg Am. 1995;77(3):459–74.
2. Mankin HJ. Nontraumatic necrosis of bone (osteonecrosis). N Engl J Med. 1992;326(22):1473–9.
3. Lai YS, Wei HW, Cheng CK. An analysis of hip replacements data of Taiwan. Read at the Northern Region Congress of the Asia Pacific Orthopaedic Association in conjunction with the third annual meeting of the Pacific Asian Society of Minimally Invasive Spine Surgery, Taipei, 5–6 Dec 2003.
4. Wang GJ, Cui Q, Balian G. The Nicolas Andry award. The pathogenesis and prevention of steroid-induced osteonecrosis. Clin Orthop Relat Res. 2000;370:295–310.
5. Pritchett JW. Statin therapy decreases the risk of osteonecrosis in patients receiving steroids. Clin Orthop. 2001;386:173–8.
6. Glueck CJ, Freiberg RA, Sieve L, Wang P. Enoxaparin prevents progression of stages I and II osteonecrosis of the hip. Clin Orthop Relat Res. 2005;435:164–70.
7. Wang Y, Yin L, Li Y, Liu P, Cui Q. Preventive effects of puerarin on alcohol-induced osteonecrosis. Clin Orthop Relat Res. 2008;466(5):1059–67.
8. Disch AC, Matziolis G, Perka C. The management of necrosis-associated and idiopathic bone-marrow oedema of the proximal femur by intravenous iloprost. J Bone Joint Surg Br. 2005;87(4):560–4.
9. Jager M, Tillmann FP, Thornhill TS, Mahmoudi M, Blondin D, Hetzel GR, Zilkens C, Krauspe R. Rationale for prostaglandin I2 in bone marrow oedema–from theory to application. Arthritis Res Ther. 2008;10(5):R120.
10. Agarwala S, Jain D, Joshi VR, Sule A. Efficacy of alendronate, a bisphosphonate, in the treatment of AVN of the hip. A prospective open-label study. Rheumatology (Oxford). 2005;44(3):352–9.
11. Lai KA, Shen WJ, Yang CY, Shao CJ, Hsu JT, Lin RM. The use of alendronate to prevent early collapse of the femoral head in patients with nontraumatic osteonecrosis. A randomized clinical study. J Bone Joint Surg Am. 2005;87(10):2155–9.
12. Nishii T, Sugano N, Miki H, Hashimoto J, Yoshikawa H. Does alendronate prevent collapse in osteonecrosis of the femoral head? Clin Orthop Relat Res. 2006;443:273–9.
13. Agarwala S, Shah S, Joshi VR. The use of alendronate in the treatment of avascular necrosis of the femoral head: follow-up to eight years. J Bone Joint Surg Br. 2009;91(8):1013–8.
14. Agarwala S, Sule A, Pai BU, Joshi VR. Alendronate in the treatment of avascular necrosis of the hip. Rheumatology (Oxford). 2002;41(3):346–7.
15. Wang GJ, Sweet DE, Reger SI, Thompson RC. Fat-cell changes as a mechanism of avascular necrosis of the femoral head in cortisone-treated rabbits. J Bone Joint Surg Am. 1977;59(6):729–35.
16. Wang GJ, Moga DB, Richemer WG, Sweet DE, Reger SI, Thompson RC. Cortisone induced bone changes and its response to lipid clearing agents. Clin Orthop Relat Res. 1978;130:81–5.
17. Shinoda H, Adamek G, Felix R, Fleisch H, Schenk R, Hagan P. Structure-activity relationships of various bisphosphonates. Calcif Tissue Int. 1983;35(1):87–99.
18. Porras AG, Holland SD, Gertz BJ. Pharmacokinetics of alendronate. Clin Pharmacokinet. 1999;36(5):315–28.
19. Cremers SC, Pillai G, Papapoulos SE. Pharmacokinetics/pharmacodynamics of bisphosphonates: use for optimisation of intermittent therapy for osteoporosis. Clin Pharmacokinet. 2005;44(6):551–70.
20. Roelofs AJ, Coxon FP, Ebetino FH, Lundy MW, Henneman ZJ, Nancollas GH, Sun S, Blazewska KM, Bala JL, Kashemirov BA, Khalid AB, McKenna CE, Rogers MJ. Fluorescent risedronate analogues reveal bisphosphonate uptake by bone marrow monocytes and localization around osteocytes in vivo. J Bone Miner Res. 2010;25(3):606–16.
21. Coxon FP, Thompson K, Roelofs AJ, Ebetino FH, Rogers MJ. Visualizing mineral binding and uptake of bisphosphonate by osteoclasts and non-resorbing cells. Bone. 2008;42(5):848–60.
22. Roelofs AJ, Thompson K, Ebetino FH, Rogers MJ, Coxon FP. Bisphosphonates: molecular mechanisms of action and effects on bone cells, monocytes and macrophages. Curr Pharm Des. 2010;16(27):2950–60.
23. Sato M, Grasser W, Endo N, Akins R, Simmons H, Thompson DD, Golub E, Rodan GA. Bisphosphonate action. Alendronate localization in rat bone and effects on osteoclast ultrastructure. J Clin Invest. 1991;88(6):2095–105.
24. Luckman SP, Hughes DE, Coxon FP, Graham R, Russell G, Rogers MJ. Nitrogen-containing bisphosphonates inhibit the mevalonate pathway and prevent post-translational prenylation of GTP-binding proteins, including Ras. J Bone Miner Res. 1998;13(4):581–9.
25. Zhang FL, Casey PJ. Protein prenylation: molecular mechanisms and functional consequences. Annu Rev Biochem. 1996;65:241–69.
26. Ridley AJ, Paterson HF, Johnston CL, Diekmann D, Hall A. The small GTP-binding protein rac regulates growth factor-induced membrane ruffling. Cell. 1992;70(3):401–10.
27. Coxon FP, Helfrich MH, Van't Hof R, Sebti S, Ralston SH, Hamilton A, Rogers MJ. Protein geranylgeranylation is required for osteoclast formation, function, and survival: inhibition by bisphosphonates and GGTI-298. J Bone Miner Res. 2000; 15(8):1467–76.
28. Kanis JA, Burlet N, Cooper C, Delmas PD, Reginster JY, Borgstrom F, Rizzoli R. European guidance for the diagnosis and management of osteoporosis in postmenopausal women. Osteoporos Int. 2008;19(4):399–428.
29. Duque G, Rivas D. Alendronate has an anabolic effect on bone through the differentiation of mesenchymal stem cells. J Bone Miner Res. 2007;22(10):1603–11.
30. von Knoch F, Jaquiery C, Kowalsky M, Schaeren S, Alabre C, Martin I, Rubash HE, Shanbhag AS. Effects of bisphosphonates on proliferation and osteoblast differentiation of human bone marrow stromal cells. Biomaterials. 2005;26(34):6941–9.
31. Im GI, Qureshi SA, Kenney J, Rubash HE, Shanbhag AS. Osteoblast proliferation and maturation by bisphosphonates. Biomaterials. 2004;25(18):4105–15.
32. Wang CZ, Chen SM, Chen CH, Wang CK, Wang GJ, Chang JK, Ho ML. The effect of the local delivery of alendronate on human adipose-derived stem cell-based bone regeneration. Biomaterials. 2010;31(33):8674–83.
33. Giuliani N, Pedrazzoni M, Negri G, Passeri G, Impicciatore M, Girasole G. Bisphosphonates stimulate formation of osteoblast precursors and mineralized nodules in murine and human bone marrow cultures in vitro and promote early osteoblastogenesis in young and aged mice in vivo. Bone. 1998;22(5):455–61.
34. D'Aoust P, McCulloch CA, Tenenbaum HC, Lekic PC. Etidronate (HEBP) promotes osteoblast differentiation and wound closure in rat calvaria. Cell Tissue Res. 2000;302(3):353–63.
35. Plotkin LI, Weinstein RS, Parfitt AM, Roberson PK, Manolagas SC, Bellido T. Prevention of osteocyte and osteoblast apoptosis by bisphosphonates and calcitonin. J Clin Invest. 1999;104(10): 1363–74.
36. Plotkin LI, Lezcano V, Thostenson J, Weinstein RS, Manolagas SC, Bellido T. Connexin 43 is required for the anti-apoptotic effect of bisphosphonates on osteocytes and osteoblasts in vivo. J Bone Miner Res. 2008;23(11):1712–21.

37. Follet H, Li J, Phipps RJ, Hui S, Condon K, Burr DB. Risedronate and alendronate suppress osteocyte apoptosis following cyclic fatigue loading. Bone. 2007;40(4):1172–7.
38. Chen CH, Chang JK, Lai KA, Hou SM, Chang CH, Wang GJ. Alendronate in the prevention of collapse of the femoral head in nontraumatic osteonecrosis: a two-year multicenter, prospective, randomized, double-blind, placebo-controlled study. Arthritis Rheum. 2012;64(5):1572–8.
39. Mont MA, Jones LC, Hungerford DS. Nontraumatic osteonecrosis of the femoral head: ten years later. J Bone Joint Surg Am. 2006;88(5):1117–32.
40. Lieberman JR, Berry DJ, Mont MA, Aaron RK, Callaghan JJ, Rajadhyaksha AD, Urbaniak JR. Osteonecrosis of the hip: management in the 21st century. Instr Course Lect. 2003;52:337–55.
41. Yoo MC, Kim KI, Hahn CS, Parvizi J. Long-term followup of vascularized fibular grafting for femoral head necrosis. Clin Orthop Relat Res. 2008;466(5):1133–40.
42. Sugioka Y, Yamamoto T. Transtrochanteric posterior rotational osteotomy for osteonecrosis. Clin Orthop Relat Res. 2008;466(5):1104–9.
43. Seyler TM, Marker DR, Ulrich SD, Fatscher T, Mont MA. Nonvascularized bone grafting defers joint arthroplasty in hip osteonecrosis. Clin Orthop Relat Res. 2008;466(5):1125–32.
44. Mont MA, Carbone JJ, Fairbank AC. Core decompression versus nonoperative management for osteonecrosis of the hip. Clin Orthop Relat Res. 1996;324:169–78.
45. Ohzono K, Saito M, Sugano N, Takaoka K, Ono K. The fate of nontraumatic avascular necrosis of the femoral head. A radiologic classification to formulate prognosis. Clin Orthop. 1992;277:73–8.
46. Arlet J. Nontraumatic avascular necrosis of the femoral head. Past, present, and future. Clin Orthop Relat Res. 1992;277:12–21.
47. Patterson RJ, Bickel WH, Dahlin DC. Idiopathic avascular necrosis of the head of the femur. A study of fifty-two cases. J Bone Joint Surg Am. 1964;46:267–82.
48. Merle D'Aubigne R, Postel M, Mazabraud A, Massias P, Gueguen J, France P. Idiopathic necrosis of the femoral head in adults. J Bone Joint Surg Br. 1965;47(4):612–33.
49. Min BW, Song KS, Cho CH, Lee SM, Lee KJ. Untreated asymptomatic hips in patients with osteonecrosis of the femoral head. Clin Orthop Relat Res. 2008;466(5):1087–92.
50. Nam KW, Kim YL, Yoo JJ, Koo KH, Yoon KS, Kim HJ. Fate of untreated asymptomatic osteonecrosis of the femoral head. J Bone Joint Surg Am. 2008;90(3):477–84.
51. Pazianas M, Abrahamsen B. Safety of bisphosphonates. Bone. 2011;49(1):103–10.

37 New Therapies of Bone Necrosis

Wolf Drescher, Matthias Knobe, Wolfgang Wagner, and Thomas Pufe

37.1 Introduction

Femoral head osteonecrosis is an ischemic necrosis of subchondral bone and bone marrow due to posttraumatic or nontraumatic causes. Nontraumatic femoral head necrosis affects mainly young people and leads to early destruction of the hip joint. However, the orthopedic surgeon is facing the challenge of treating the hip joint of a young person. Arthroplasty in young age has the risk of many future revisions, so that diagnosis should be made in the very early stage of FHN, preferably ARCO stage 1.

37.2 The Different New Therapies

37.2.1 Stem Cell Therapy

In the scientific literature, there are growing indications that the additive application of bone marrow aspirate concentrate (BMAC) as a part of core decompression increases the local osseous potency within the femur head necrotic area [1]. In this disease, it is suggested that not only the affected femoral head osteonecrosis range but the entire proximal femur of patients with osteonecrosis contains significantly less mesenchymal progenitor cells [2]. However, it is unclear whether this observation is the result of disturbed femoral head blood perfusion or if the primary reduction of progenitor cells in the femoral head is an independent risk factor for the development of femoral head osteonecrosis. With the use of BMAC on over 100 patients with local bone healing disorders, they have high osteogenic potential of this cell therapy [3]. Eighteen hips in ARCO stage 1 and 2 were part of a controlled double-blind study on core decompression only compared with additional implantation of autologous mononuclear bone marrow stem cells from the anterior iliac crest [3]. In this pilot study, they reported clinical and MRI results after 24 months. 5 of 8 hips developed to ARCO stage 3 after treatment with pure core decompression, whereas only 1 of 10 hips with additional stem cell transplantation progressed to ARCO stage 3. In addition to the direct cell application via a cannula or a hollow drill bit, this form of therapy can be combined with autologous spongiosa graft. Here too, the transplanted autologous spongiosa graft is incubated for a defined period of time with suspension mononuclear cells. To what extent this technique, especially medium and long term in ARCO stage 2, would improve the prognosis of affected patients still needs to be investigated in prospective clinical trials. Due to the lack of long-term results from such studies, and even sparser data, stem cell therapy is promising, but still classified as experimental therapy of femoral head osteonecrosis.

37.2.2 Intravenous Iloprost

In early FHN stages, pain relief and improvement of the Harris hip score were reported after application of intravenous iloprost administration, a prostacyclin analogue [4]. MRI findings during follow-up showed a decrease in the extent of bone marrow edema. However, this clinical study in 95 patients also stated that there is no benefit from iloprost treatment in advanced stages of FHN.

W. Drescher (✉)
Department of Orthopaedic Surgery,
RWTH University Hospital Aachen, Aachen, Germany

Department of Orthopaedic and Spine Surgery,
Agaplesion Ev. Bathildis-Hospital, Bad Pyrmont, Germany
e-mail: wdrescher@ukaachen.de

M. Knobe
Department of Traumatology,
RWTH University Hospital, Aachen, Germany

W. Wagner
Division for Stem Cell Biology and Cellular Engineering,
Helmholtz Institute for Biomedical Engineering,
RWTH University Hospital, Aachen, Germany

T. Pufe
Institute of Anatomy and Cell Biology,
RWTH University, Aachen, Germany

K.-H. Koo et al. (eds.), *Osteonecrosis*,
DOI 10.1007/978-3-642-35767-1_37,

37.2.3 Extracorporeal Shock Wave Therapy

We rarely find valid studies on the benefits of extracorporeal shock wave therapy (ESWT) in the treatment of femoral head necrosis. Wang et al. found, at a mean follow-up of 25 months, that 79 % of the hips examined clinically and on MRI improved, 10 % unchanged, and 10 % were worse [5]. They found a superiority of ESWT versus combined core decompression and non-vascularized fibular grafting at an average follow-up of 25 months. Heller and Niethard advised in their meta-analysis on the application of ESWT for musculoskeletal indications to use a differentiated application of the energy density [6]. Because of only few studies of higher levels of EBM, application of ESWT in the treatment of osteonecrosis is not proven.

37.2.4 Bisphosphonates

In a clinical-radiological follow-up of 395 femoral head necrosis in Ficat stages 1–3 on an average of 4 years, good results have been reported after alendronate administration [7]. All patients in this study were given 10 mg alendronate daily combined with 500–1,000 mg of calcium and 400–800 IU of vitamin D3. In 92 % of patients, a satisfactory clinical result was achieved. They needed no total hip replacement. In 2 % of Ficat-1, 8 % of Ficat-2, and 33 % of Ficat-3-hips total hip replacement was implanted. Radiologically, 12.6 % of Ficat-1-hips and 55.8 % of Ficat-2-hips collapsed on average of 4 years. Jaw necrosis has been reported as a complication of bisphosphonate therapy [8].

37.2.5 Future Therapy Methods: Vasodilatation

We could show that steroids have a vasoconstrictive effect on lateral epiphyseal arteries of the femoral head which could lead to ischemia and subsequent necrosis [9]. In an experimental study we investigated the preventive effect of a nitrate patch on steroid-related bone necrosis in the Yamamoto rabbit model [10]. New Zealand White Rabbits (male; 3–4.5 kg bodyweight) were injected with 20 mg/kg bodyweight methylprednisolone (GC group; $n=6$). Control animals ($n=6$) were treated with phosphate-buffered saline. A third group (GC+N; $n=6$) additionally received a nitrate patch (0.675 mg/day). Four weeks after i.m. methylprednisolone injection, the animals were sacrificed. For histology and immunohistochemistry, tissue samples were fixed in 3 % paraformaldehyde, embedded in paraffin, sectioned, dewaxed, and stained with Ladewig. For quantification of empty lacunae, a histologic sign of FHN, histomorphometry was performed. Histomorphometry revealed a significant increase of empty lacunae in glucocorticoid-treated animals compared to controls and GC+N-treated animals. No significant difference in empty lacunae count was detected between the GC+N group and controls. HE staining revealed the different osteocyte amount in the GC versus GC and nitrate patch-treated groups. This study demonstrates an increased number of empty osteocyte lacunae representing a pathologic feature of osteonecrosis, in the GC group. Less empty lacunae were counted in the GC animals after additional treatment with a nitrate patch. This finding suggests that nitrate co-treatment has the potential to prevent steroid-associated FHN.

Conclusion

Considering the variety of today's existing treatment methods, the damage of the chosen technique should, in our opinion, be weighed up against the patient's age and the supportive therapy method afterwards. Flexion osteotomy, e.g., makes future hip arthroplasty difficult.

Nontraumatic osteonecrosis can lead to secondary arthritis and cause destruction of the hip joint. Often, young patients are affected. The etiologic risk factors are steroids, alcohol abuse, sickle cell anemia, lupus erythematosus, inflammatory bowel disease, Caisson disease, Gaucher disease, chemotherapy, and contralateral femoral head. Doctors should make an early diagnosis FHN, and the patients need to be referred much earlier to the orthopedic surgeon knowledgeable about FHN and its early stages. ARCO stage 1 is detectable by MRI, is still reversible, and can be treated by a core decompression. As for the other stages, there are various treatment methods available which should be discussed in detail with the patient.

References

1. Hernigou P, Beaujean F. Treatment of osteonecrosis with autologous bone marrow grafting. Clin Orthop Relat Res. 2002;405:14–23.
2. Hernigou P, Poignard A, Manicom O, et al. The use of percutaneous autologous bone marrow transplantation in nonunion and avascular necrosis of bone. J Bone Joint Surg Br. 2005;87:896–902.
3. Gangji V, Hauzeur JP, Matos C, et al. Treatment of osteonecrosis of the femoral head with implantation of autologous bone-marrow cells. A pilot study. J Bone Joint Surg Am. 2004;86:1153–60.
4. Jäger M, Zilkens C, Bittersohl B, et al. Efficiency of iloprost treatment for osseous malperfusion. Int Orthop (SICOT). 2011;35(5):761–5.
5. Wang CJ, Wang FS, Huang CC, et al. Treatment for osteonecrosis of the femoral head: comparison of extracorporeal shock waves with core decompression and bone-grafting. J Bone Joint Surg Am. 2005;87:2380–7.

6. Heller KD, Niethard FU. Using extracorporeal shockwave therapy in orthopedics – a meta-analysis. Z Orthop Ihre Grenzgeb. 1998; 136:390–401.
7. Agarwala S, Shah S, Joshi VR. The use of alendronate in the treatment of avascular necrosis of the femoral head: follow-up to eight years. J Bone Joint Surg Br. 2009;91:1013–8.
8. Wirth SM, Lawson AP, Sutphin SD, et al. Osteonecrosis of the jaw associated with bisphosphonate therapy. Orthopedics. 2009;32:900–3.
9. Drescher W, Li H, Lundgaard A, et al. Endothelin-1-induced femoral head epiphyseal artery constriction is enhanced by long-term corticosteroid treatment. J Bone Joint Surg Am. 2006;88 Suppl 3:173–9.
10. Drescher W, Beckmann R, Kasch R, et al. Nitrate patch prevents steroid-related bone necrosis. J Orthop Res. 2011;29(10):1517–20.

Part XI

Surgical Treatments

Principles of Core Decompression for Osteonecrosis of the Hip

38

Bhaveen H. Kapadia, Samik Banerjee, Jeffrey J. Cherian, Julio J. Jauregui, and Michael A. Mont

38.1 Introduction

Osteonecrosis of the femoral head is a poorly understood disease with a wide range of etiologies. It has been shown to affect mostly patients in the third and fourth decades of life [1–3]. Some of the known risk factors include corticosteroid use, excessive alcohol intake, radiation therapy, chemotherapy, renal transplant recipients, systemic lupus erythematosus, human immunodeficiency virus infection, and sickle cell disease (Table 38.1) [4–9]. The most commonly used classification systems used for staging are the Ficat and Arlet, the Association Research Circulation Osseous classification (ARCO), and the Japanese Orthopaedic Association (Table 38.2).

The goal of management is early diagnosis in the precollapse stage and to prevent progression to collapse. Although various pharmacological and biophysical treatment strategies have been suggested for the prevention and treatment of disease progression, the management of osteonecrosis continues to be challenging [2]. Additionally, bone-preserving procedures such as bone grafting, osteotomies, and core decompression have been proposed to avoid the need for total joint arthroplasty.

Core decompression has been used commonly for the treatment of smaller-sized precollapse lesions [10–12]. This technique was initially developed by Ficat and Arlet [13]. The procedure was postulated to be effective because it was believed that the pathogenetic mechanism of osteonecrosis was an elevated intraosseous pressure causing extravascular compression of the blood vessels within the femoral head.

Table 38.1 Osteonecrosis risk factors

Direct risk factors
Trauma – fracture, dislocation
Sickle cell disease
Human immunodeficiency virus infection
Chemotherapy
Radiation
Indirect risk factors
Corticosteroids
Alcohol abuse
Tobacco use
Systemic lupus erythematosus
Myeloproliferative disorders
Gaucher's disease
Organ transplant
Renal failure
Coagulation abnormalities
Pregnancy
Genetic factors

It was therefore postulated that early treatment with decompression would relieve intraosseous pressure of the femoral head, thereby restoring normal vascular flow [14]. The general pathophysiology of osteonecrosis of the hip is proposed to be disruption of the microcirculation to the femoral head. The additional mechanisms leading to vascular disruption are postulated to be due to direct vascular interruption from trauma or from intravascular occlusion by thromboembolic events or fat emboli [15–17]. The following sections address preoperative planning, indications, surgical techniques, rehabilitation, and the outcomes reported in literature for core decompression.

38.2 Preoperative Planning and Indications for Core Decompression

Formulating a treatment plan should be based on clinical factors. Patients generally present with groin pain, trochanteric symptoms, or nonspecific hip pain. The treatment plan

B.H. Kapadia • S. Banerjee • J.J. Cherian
J.J. Jauregui • M.A. Mont (✉)
Department of Orthopaedic Surgery, Rubin Institute for Advanced Orthopedics, Center for Joint Preservation and Replacement, Sinai Hospital of Baltimore, 2401 West Belvedere Avenue, Baltimore, MD 21215, USA
e-mail: bhaveen.k@gmail.com; bashb02@gmail.com; jjaicherian@gmail.com; juljau@gmail.com; mmont@lifebridgehealth.org; rhondamont@aol.com

K.-H. Koo et al. (eds.), *Osteonecrosis*,
DOI 10.1007/978-3-642-35767-1_38, © Springer-Verlag Berlin Heidelberg 2014

Table 38.2 Ficat and Arlet staging

Ficat and Arlet		Association Research Circulation Osseous (ARCO)		Japanese Orthopaedic Association	
Stage	Findings	Stage	Findings	Stage	Findings
I	Normal X-ray	0	Normal hip	1	Demarcation line
II	Diffuse cystic/sclerotic lesions	1	MRI findings only	2	Early femoral head flattening
III	Crescent sign (subchondral fracture)	2	Focal osteoporosis, cystic lesions, sclerosis	3	Cystic lesions
IV	Femoral head collapse, acetabular involvement	3	Crescent sign (subchondral fracture)		
		4	Acetabular involvement		

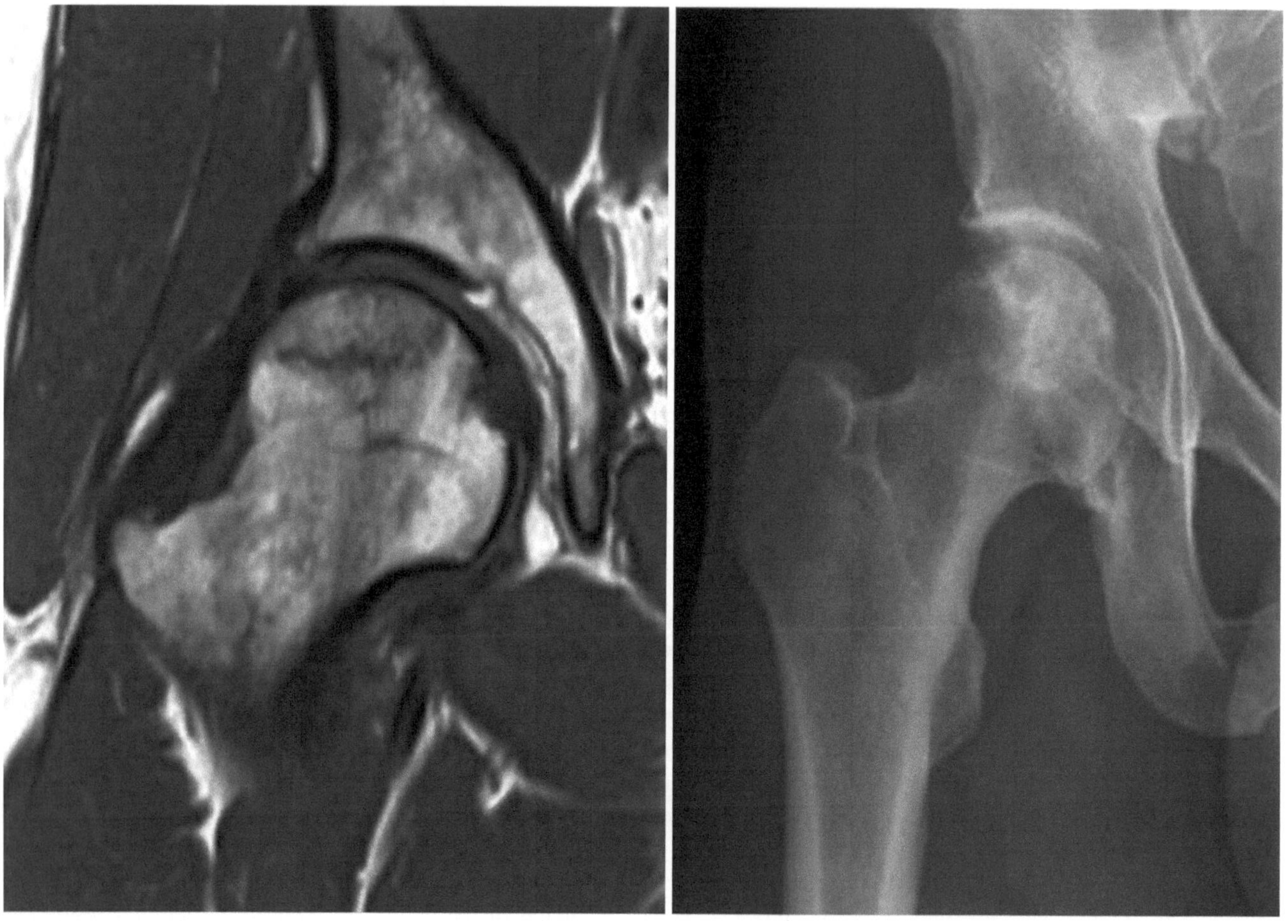

Fig. 38.1 MRI and X-ray features of osteonecrosis

should be tailored to the patients' age, the presence of medical comorbidities, and the activity level.

Radiographic factors should also be taken into consideration, as core decompression is generally recommended for patients without advanced arthritis or subchondral collapse. Early stage (Ficat and Arlet Stage I and II), smaller-sized lesions with a combined necrotic angle of less than 200° have been demonstrated to have more favorable results with this procedure [18–20]. Since the disease is often bilateral, a thorough evaluation for contralateral joint involvement should be conducted as well [14, 21–23] (Fig. 38.1).

38.3 Surgical Technique (Authors' Experience)

Currently, all of these procedures are performed using fluoroscopic guidance. The conventional core decompression involves one to three large diameter drilling. The area of the lesion should be identified on radiographs or magnetic resonance imaging (MRI) scans to identify stage 1 Ficat and Arlet disease. The position of the femoral head should be identified prior to preparing and draping the hip. The initial tract made for the core decompression should be above the superior level of the lesser trochanter, which minimizes the

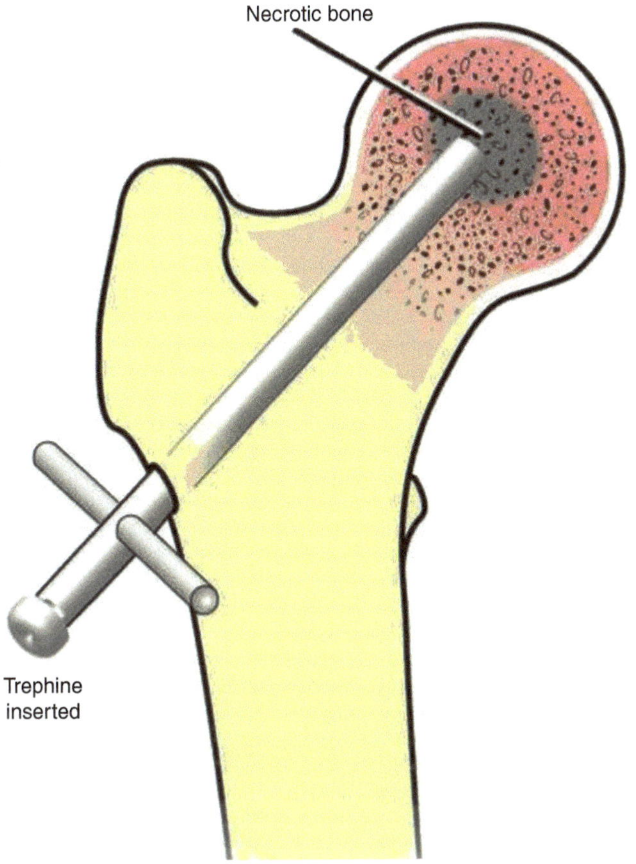

Fig. 38.2 Core decompression

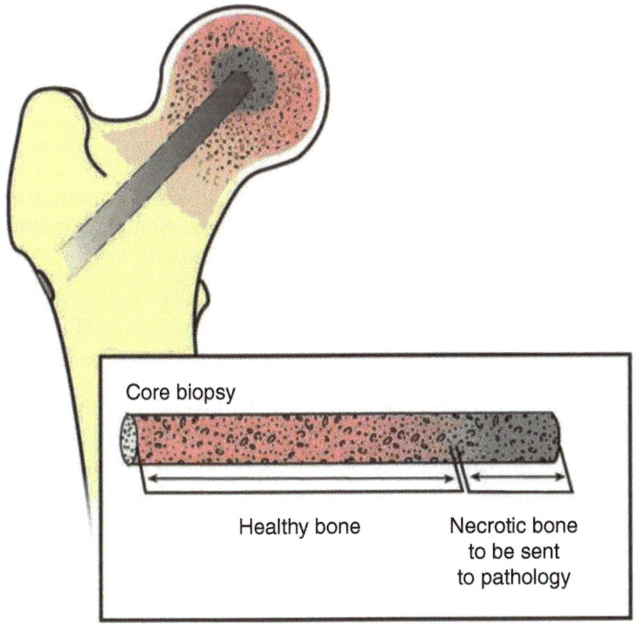

Fig. 38.3 Eight to ten millimeter of tissue removed after core

risk of developing a stress fracture of the femur. With the guide wire in place, an 8–10-mm wide cannulated trephine is generally used (Fig. 38.2). Subsequently, the necrotic bone is removed with a burr (Fig. 38.3). The Steinberg modification to the traditional core decompression involves the removal of three bone cores from the single initial hole made for the procedure. Through a lateral approach a trephine is used to remove an 8-mm core of bone from the center of the lesion. Subsequently, two 6-mm bone cores are removed from the lesion's periphery through the same entry site. Then, viable bone is grafted into the central core region of the femur.

An alternative to the conventional core decompression is multiple drilling, which consists of small diameter core tracts. Under fluoroscopic guidance the pin is slowly advanced until it comes in contact with the lateral cortex above the lesser trochanter and is subsequently passed through the femoral neck and into the femoral head to the site of the lesion.

38.4 Rehabilitation

Protective 50 % weight-bearing is recommended for 4–6 weeks postoperatively with the use of a cane or other ambulatory aids. After this period, the patient can be advanced to full weight-bearing without the use of aids as tolerated. Standard rehabilitation should include hip abductor strengthening and range of motion exercises. Patients are discouraged from engaging in high impact activities for a minimum of 10–12 months postoperatively. However, if after this time there is no radiographic evidence of collapse, the patients are allowed to resume all prior activities.

38.5 Outcomes of Core Decompression

38.5.1 Core Decompression

In 1985 Ficat et al. reported favorable outcomes in 133 patients who were treated with core decompression for early stage lesions. The survivorship was 94 % for patients who had stage I disease and 82 % for patients who had stage II disease [24]. Fairbank et al. reported similar outcomes in 128 hips (90 patients) undergoing core decompression for Ficat and Arlet stage I, II, and III disease. At a mean follow-up of 11 years, the survivorship was reported to be 88 % for stage I, 72 % for stage II, and 26 % for stage III disease [25]. A study by Steinberg et al. reviewed the outcomes of core decompression with bone grafting in 406 hips for osteonecrosis of the femoral head. At a mean follow-up of 29 months, 18 of 65 hips (28 %) with stage I disease, 45 of 133 hips (34 %) with stage II disease, 3 of 13 hips (23 %) with stage III disease, and 45 of 92 hips (49 %) with stage IV disease required a hip replacement [26]. However, a study by Markel et al. reported poorer outcomes in 53 hips with the use of core decompression. At a mean follow-up of 4 years, the survivorship was reported to be 45 % for stage I, 38 % for stage IIa, 14 % for stage IIb, and 25 % for stage III disease [22]. See Table 38.3 for a summary of results.

Table 38.3 Outcomes of core decompression

Author (year)	Level of evidence	Hips Stage 1	Stage 2a	Stage 2b	Stage 3	Mean age (years)	Follow-up (years)	Survivorship (%) Stage 1	Stage 2a	Stage 2b	Stage 3
Al Omran (2013) [23]	III	13	25	23	–	26	6.1	100	80	52	–
Lieberman et al. (2004) [27]	IV	–	15	1	1	47	4.4	–	93	0	0
Aigner et al. (2002) [28]	IV	30	9	–	6	41	5.7	97	44	–	33
Steinberg et al. (2001)[a] [26]	III	65	45[b]	–	13	37	48	72	66[b]	–	77
Lavernia and Sierra (2000) [29]	IV	15	30[b]	–	22	40.2	3.4	100	83[b]	–	44
Maniwa et al. (2000) [30]	IV	10	16[b]	–	–	46	7.8	100	56.4[b]	–	–
Bozic et al. (1999) [31]	IV	12	12	2	0	38	10	92	52	20	0
Iorio et al. (1998) [32]	IV	7	20	6	–	41	5	71	45	33	–
Powell et al. (1997) [33]	IV	18	8[b]	–	–	35	4	80	37[b]	–	–
Markel et al. (1996) [22]	IV	10	32	7	4	38	4	45	38	14	25
Fairbank et al. (1995) [25]	IV	25	51	–	52	40	11	88	72	–	26
Saito et al. (1988) [34]	III	17	–	–	–	33	4	100	–	–	–

[a]Patients also underwent bone grafting
[b]Stage 2 hips

Table 38.4 Outcomes of multiple drilling

Author (year)	Level of evidence	Hips Stage 1	Stage 2a	Stage 2b	Stage 3	Mean age (years)	Follow-up (years)	Survivorship (%) Stage 1	Stage 2a	Stage 2b	Stage 3
Al Omran (2013) [23]	III	6	14	13	–	26	6.1	100	78	53.8	–
Song et al. (2007) [35]	IV	39	64	17	43	36.1	7.2	80	77	77	35
Mont et al. (2004) [1]	IV	30	15[a]	–	–	42	2	80	57[a]	–	–

[a]Stage 2 hips

A review by Mont et al. compared the outcomes of core decompression versus nonoperative management for osteonecrosis of the hip. This study of 42 reports found that of the 1,206 hips treated with core decompression, satisfactory results were reported in 63.5 % of hips when compared to 22.7 % in the nonoperative management group of 819 hips [20]. A more recent systematic literature review by Marker et al. [36] demonstrated that techniques for core decompression prior to 1992 led to significantly inferior outcomes when compared to those after 1992. Modern techniques yielded significantly lower rates of additional surgery (mean 30 %; range, 39–100 %) when compared to older techniques (mean 41 %; range, 29–85 %; $p<0.05$). However, this analysis revealed that it may not be due solely to better surgical techniques, but rather to more careful patient selection. The review demonstrated that studies after 1992 included fewer patients with Ficat and Arlet stage III disease ($p<0.001$), which could have contributed to better clinical outcomes. Core decompression in patients with Ficat and Arlet stage III disease is more likely to lead to higher rates of failures and additional surgeries. Therefore, careful patient selection could result in more favorable results following core decompression.

38.5.2 Multiple Drilling

The conventional core decompression can lead to complications, due to the large canal that is formed, such as subtrochanteric fractures and inadvertent penetration of the femoral head. The risks associated with this technique have led surgeons to develop multiple drilling as an alternative method to relieve intraosseous pressure, venous congestion, and restoring normal vascular flow in the necrotic region [35].

A study by Mont et al. [1] in 2004 found that a multiple drilling procedure using 2–3 core tracts with a 3-mm pin led to successful results in 71 % (32 of 45) of hips with Ficat and Arlet stage I or II disease at a mean follow-up of 2 years (range, 1.7–3.3 years). When these results were substratified by disease stage, they found that patients who have stage I disease have a higher success rate than patients who have stage II disease (80 %; 24 of 30 hips versus 52 %; 8 of 15 hips, respectively).

In 2007, Song et al. reported similar successful outcomes of multiple drilling in 163 hips with Ficat and Arlet stage I to III osteonecrosis. Their results that at a mean follow-up of 7.2 years (range, 5–11.2 years), 88 % (52 of 59) of hips with small- to medium-sized lesions required no further surgery. See Table 38.4 for a summary on multiple drilling.

Multiple drilling has the potential to decrease intraosseous pressure as much as a conventional core decompression, but has the added benefit of increased accuracy in reaching osteonecrotic lesions. Factors which contributed to unsuccessful outcomes of multiple drilling were a combined necrotic angle of greater than 200° and a markedly higher intertrochanteric intraosseous pressure.

38.6 Summary

Osteonecrosis of the femoral head has been attributed to increased intraosseous hypertension and venous congestion. It is believed that core decompression may result to a decrease in intraosseous pressure within the femoral head and therefore relieve venous congestion. Patients who have successful outcomes generally have Ficat and Arlet stage I and II disease, smaller-sized lesions (<30 % femoral head involvement), and patients with poorer outcomes are those who have post-collapse or large lesions. The conventional core decompression has been demonstrated to have positive clinical outcomes; however, multiple drilling has also been reported to be equally efficacious. Additionally, multiple drilling has been associated with a low risk of stress fractures and inadvertent head penetration. The studies on core decompression are varied in their patient populations, in terms of age, gender, and disease stage, which makes it difficult to derive a statement of the efficacy of this procedure. Further prospective, randomized studies are needed to compare the long-term outcomes of the various core decompression techniques.

References

1. Mont MA, Ragland PS, Etienne G. Core decompression of the femoral head for osteonecrosis using percutaneous multiple small-diameter drilling. Clin Orthop Relat Res. 2004;429:131–8.
2. Etienne G, Mont MA, Ragland PS. The diagnosis and treatment of nontraumatic osteonecrosis of the femoral head. Instr Course Lect. 2004;53:67–85.
3. Wei BF, Ge XH. Treatment of osteonecrosis of the femoral head with core decompression and bone grafting. Hip Int. 2011;21(2):206–10. doi:10.5301/HIP.2011.6525.
4. Shim K, MacKenzie MJ, Winquist E. Chemotherapy-associated osteonecrosis in cancer patients with solid tumours: a systematic review. Drug Saf. 2008;31(5):359–71. doi:3151 [pii].
5. Powell C, Chang C, Naguwa SM, Cheema G, Gershwin ME. Steroid induced osteonecrosis: an analysis of steroid dosing risk. Autoimmun Rev. 2010;9(11):721–43. doi:10.1016/j.autrev.2010.06.007. S1568-9972(10)00125-4 [pii].
6. Milner PF, Kraus AP, Sebes JI, Sleeper LA, Dukes KA, Embury SH, et al. Sickle cell disease as a cause of osteonecrosis of the femoral head. N Engl J Med. 1991;325(21):1476–81. doi:10.1056/NEJM199111213252104.
7. Rodrigue SW, Rosenthal DI, Barton NW, Zurakowski D, Mankin HJ. Risk factors for osteonecrosis in patients with type 1 Gaucher's disease. Clin Orthop Relat Res. 1999;362:201–7.
8. Zhang LD, Kang JF, Xue HL. Distribution of lesions in the head and neck of the humerus and the femur in dysbaric osteonecrosis. Undersea Biomed Res. 1990;17(4):353–8.
9. Hedri H, Cherif M, Zouaghi K, Abderrahim E, Goucha R, Ben Hamida F, et al. Avascular osteonecrosis after renal transplantation. Transplant Proc. 2007;39(4):1036–8. doi:10.1016/j.transproceed.2007.02.031. S0041-1345(07)00202-3 [pii].
10. Learmonth ID, Maloon S, Dall G. Core decompression for early atraumatic osteonecrosis of the femoral head. J Bone Joint Surg Br. 1990;72(3):387–90.
11. Richards RR. Bone grafting with microvascular anastomosis in osteonecrosis of the femoral head. Semin Arthroplasty. 1991;2(3):198–207.
12. Tooke SM, Nugent PJ, Bassett LW, Nottingham P, Mirra J, Jinnah R. Results of core decompression for femoral head osteonecrosis. Clin Orthop Relat Res. 1988;228:99–104.
13. Arlet J, Ficat P, Lartigue G, Tran MA. Clinical research on intraosseous pressure in the upper femoral metaphysis and epiphysis in humans. Application to the diagnosis of ischemia and necrosis. Revue du rhumatisme et des maladies osteo-articulaires. 1972;39(11):717–23.
14. Mulliken BD. Osteonecrosis of the femoral head: current concepts and controversies. Iowa Orthop J. 1993;13:160–6.
15. Kenzora JE, Glimcher MJ. Pathogenesis of idiopathic osteonecrosis: the ubiquitous crescent sign. Orthop Clin North Am. 1985;16(4):681–96.
16. Jones Jr JP. Intravascular coagulation and osteonecrosis. Clin Orthop Relat Res. 1992;277:41–53.
17. Jones Jr JP. Fat embolism and osteonecrosis. Orthop Clin North Am. 1985;16(4):595–633.
18. Rajagopal M, Balch Samora J, Ellis TJ. Efficacy of core decompression as treatment for osteonecrosis of the hip: a systematic review. Hip Int. 2012;22(5):489–93. doi:10.5301/HIP.2012.9748.
19. Yoon TR, Song EK, Rowe SM, Park CH. Failure after core decompression in osteonecrosis of the femoral head. Int Orthop. 2001;24(6):316–8.
20. Mont MA, Carbone JJ, Fairbank AC. Core decompression versus nonoperative management for osteonecrosis of the hip. Clin Orthop Relat Res. 1996;324:169–78.
21. Israelite C, Nelson CL, Ziarani CF, Abboud JA, Landa J, Steinberg ME. Bilateral core decompression for osteonecrosis of the femoral head. Clin Orthop Relat Res. 2005;441:285–90.
22. Markel DC, Miskovsky C, Sculco TP, Pellicci PM, Salvati EA. Core decompression for osteonecrosis of the femoral head. Clin Orthop Relat Res. 1996;323:226–33.
23. Al Omran A. Multiple drilling compared with standard core decompression for avascular necrosis of the femoral head in sickle cell disease patients. Arch Orthop Trauma Surg. 2013;133(5):609–13. doi:10.1007/s00402-013-1714-9.
24. Ficat RP. Idiopathic bone necrosis of the femoral head. Early diagnosis and treatment. J Bone Joint Surg Br. 1985;67(1):3–9.
25. Fairbank AC, Bhatia D, Jinnah RH, Hungerford DS. Long-term results of core decompression for ischaemic necrosis of the femoral head. J Bone Joint Surg Br. 1995;77(1):42–9.
26. Steinberg ME, Larcom PG, Strafford B, Hosick WB, Corces A, Bands RE, et al. Core decompression with bone grafting for osteonecrosis of the femoral head. Clin Orthop Relat Res. 2001;386:71–8.
27. Lieberman JR, Conduah A, Urist MR. Treatment of osteonecrosis of the femoral head with core decompression and human

bone morphogenetic protein. Clin Orthop Relat Res. 2004;429: 139–45.
28. Aigner N, Schneider W, Eberl V, Knahr K. Core decompression in early stages of femoral head osteonecrosis – an MRI-controlled study. Int Orthop. 2002;26(1):31–5.
29. Lavernia CJ, Sierra RJ. Core decompression in atraumatic osteonecrosis of the hip. J Arthroplasty. 2000;15(2):171–8.
30. Maniwa S, Nishikori T, Furukawa S, Kajitani K, Iwata A, Nishikawa U, et al. Evaluation of core decompression for early osteonecrosis of the femoral head. Arch Orthop Trauma Surg. 2000;120(5–6):241–4.
31. Bozic KJ, Zurakowski D, Thornhill TS. Survivorship analysis of hips treated with core decompression for nontraumatic osteonecrosis of the femoral head. J Bone Joint Surg Am. 1999;81(2):200–9.
32. Iorio R, Healy WL, Abramowitz AJ, Pfeifer BA. Clinical outcome and survivorship analysis of core decompression for early osteonecrosis of the femoral head. J Arthroplasty. 1998;13(1):34–41.
33. Powell ET, Lanzer WL, Mankey MG. Core decompression for early osteonecrosis of the hip in high risk patients. Clin Orthop Relat Res. 1997;335:181–9.
34. Saito S, Ohzono K, Ono K. Joint-preserving operations for idiopathic avascular necrosis of the femoral head. Results of core decompression, grafting and osteotomy. J Bone Joint Surg Br. 1988;70(1):78–84.
35. Song WS, Yoo JJ, Kim YM, Kim HJ. Results of multiple drilling compared with those of conventional methods of core decompression. Clin Orthop Relat Res. 2007;454:139–46.
36. Marker DR, Seyler TM, Ulrich SD, Srivastava S, Mont MA. Do modern techniques improve core decompression outcomes for hip osteonecrosis? Clin Orthop Relat Res. 2008;466(5):1093–103. doi:10.1007/s11999-008-0184-9. Epub 2008 Apr 8. Review.

Stem Cells in Osteonecrosis: Cons

39

Anjan P. Kaushik, Anusuya Das, and Quanjun Cui

39.1 Introduction

Mesenchymal stem cells (MSCs) are progenitor cells from various tissues with the potential for self-renewal and differentiation into multiple cell lineages. The multipotency, paracrine effects, and immunomodulatory properties of these cells make them useful for the research of cell therapy modalities in bone and joint diseases, particularly osteonecrosis (ON). In addition to proliferation and differentiation, implanted MSCs also secrete angiogenic cytokines that may be significant for remodeling in osteonecrosis [1, 2].

Over the past decade, several researchers have started to evaluate the role of MSCs in osteonecrosis treatment. Gangji et al. [3] and Hernigou et al. [4] have successfully used autologous bone marrow concentrate for treatment of early stage ON. Both investigators have reported mid- to long-term favorable results. However, many questions are yet unanswered, and only limited information is available in the literature in terms of clinical trials and surgical techniques in humans using MSCs as adjunct therapies. This chapter will review literature related to MSC-utilizing surgical techniques and explore some of the limitations of using stem cell therapies in osteonecrosis.

39.2 Treatments of Osteonecrosis with MSCs

39.2.1 Animal Studies

Advancements in the techniques of obtaining MSCs efficiently from multiple tissues have prompted interest in the application of these cells into surgical techniques for treating osteonecrosis. However, the quality of the MSCs may be affected by underlying diseases in the host. Wang et al. [5] demonstrated that MSC proliferation is limited in steroid-induced ON of the femoral head. Bone marrow obtained from the proximal femur of patients with steroid-induced ON was compared to marrow from unaffected patients with femoral neck fractures, and assays demonstrated significantly decreased mitotic proliferation of MSCs in ON patients. This partially explains the limited repair capacity in the pathogenesis of ON. Similar findings were also reported by Hernigou and Beaujean [4].

Canine [6–8] and other animal models such as mice [9], rabbits [10], and sheep [11] have been used to study MSC-based treatments that transplant MSCs systemically or locally. One study examined the survival of labeled autologous MSCs after surgical transplantation into dogs that have undergone traumatic ON of the femoral head [6]. The researchers demonstrated that the number of labeled MSCs and volume of trabecular bone increased significantly from week 2 to week 12, suggesting that the implanted stem cells could survive and differentiate successfully into osteoblasts in vivo. Li et al. [10] also demonstrated the directional migration of GFP-labeled MSCs to defect sites in heat-induced femoral head necrosis in rabbits.

Evaluating surgical techniques, a recent study evaluated the value of using biphasic calcium phosphate ceramic scaffolds seeded with MSCs on inducing new bone formation in a canine model [7]. These scaffolds were created using a 3D gel-lamination technique and seeded with autologous bone marrow-derived MSCs in vitro, then implanted in vivo using a trapdoor surgical technique into the canine femoral head. Micro-CT scan analysis demonstrated that there was better osteointegration and greater compressive strength in animals that received the scaffolds containing MSCs. Another animal study evaluated the treatment of ON through a different surgical method: arterial perfusion of marrow MSCs [8]. Dogs had ON induced by surgical hip dislocation, and autologous MSCs were obtained and cultured. Arterial perfusion was completed, and tissues were examined with digital subtraction angiography 4–8 weeks afterward. Results demonstrated

A.P. Kaushik • A. Das • Q. Cui (✉)
Department of Orthopaedic Surgery, University of Virginia School of Medicine, Charlottesville, VA 22903, USA
e-mail: qc4q@hscmail.mcc.virginia.edu

K.-H. Koo et al. (eds.), *Osteonecrosis*,
DOI 10.1007/978-3-642-35767-1_39, © Springer-Verlag Berlin Heidelberg 2014

higher quantity and diameter of femoral head arteries in the MSC group than controls, and higher VEGF expression was also seen.

Other surgical techniques implementing MSCs are also currently in progress. Results from the studies above suggest improvements in properties such as osteointegration and angiogenesis in the femoral head. They do not, however, demonstrate outcomes such as functional improvement or pain relief, which would be better studied in human populations. Some animal studies also fail to show any substantial benefits of using MSCs. Cuomo et al. [12] used human bone marrow aspirate mixed with MSCs to treat critical size defects in a rat femoral head and observed no significant differences compared to the controls. This study outlines many reasons why the bench-to-bedside translation of stem cell therapy will be difficult.

39.2.2 Limitations of Animal Studies

The preclinical animal research above and other similar studies demonstrate generally favorable results for MSC-based surgical treatments for ON, and there is some promise for translational application to humans. However, at this point in time, that is the primary limitation: there are very few human studies regarding these therapies. For example, the scaffolds containing MSCs and the MSC arterial perfusion techniques have not yet been applied to humans to become clinically useful. We will explore the human research in the next section, but it is important to remember one disadvantage of stem cell research: some of the techniques used in animals, such as control group sham surgery or animal sacrifice for histology and microimaging, cannot be ethically applied to human research. Therefore, studying osteonecrosis treatment in humans will require advanced in vivo imaging techniques such as functional MRI, microangiography, and other newer methods. The availability and costs of such techniques may be a limitation to the study of ON treatments in the future.

There also exists significant controversy in parts of the world regarding the ethics of using stem cells for research, not only for animals, but also especially for human research. Each nation may have laws restricting stem cell research, or there may exist differences in institutional review board (IRB) guidelines that may inhibit the growth of meaningful clinical research. Although these ethical aspects are beyond the scope of this chapter, discussions on these topics at both the regional and international levels will have a profound impact on the progress of stem cell research.

39.2.3 Human Studies

Gangji et al. [3] studied 19 patients (24 hips) with early stage femoral head ON prospectively. The hips were allocated to either core decompression only or core decompression with bone marrow cell implantation. The treatment outcomes, including clinical symptoms and disease progression, were evaluated with a minimum of 5 years follow-up. They found that bone marrow implantation resulted in significant reduction in pain and disease progression. At 5-year follow-up, 8 of the 11 hips in the control group had progressed to collapse of the femoral head, whereas only 3 of the 13 hips in the bone marrow graft group had progressed to a similar stage.

Hernigou has pioneered bone marrow stem cell therapy for osteonecrosis in the last two decades [4]. In his 2009 case series [13], 342 patients (534 hips) ages 16–61 with early stage ON (Steinberg Stages I and II) were treated between 1990 and 2000 with core decompression and autologous iliac crest bone marrow grafting. Marrow aspirate was concentrated and injected into the femoral head after core decompression. Outcomes included Harris Hip Score, radiographic progression, changes in femoral head necrotic volume as seen on digitized MRI, and need for hip replacement. Patient follow-up was 8–18 years. Ninety-four out of 534 (18 %) hips required total hip arthroplasty, but 69 (13 %) hips with stage I ON demonstrated total resolution of osteonecrosis. The remaining 371 (69 %) hips without collapse demonstrated reductions in mean volume of femoral head necrosis from 26 to 12 cm^3. The study demonstrates that the best indication for this procedure is a symptomatic patient with pre-collapse femoral head ON.

Three additional clinical trials from China and India describe surgical treatment with core decompression (CD) combined with bone marrow-derived MSCs. Two separate research groups from China performed randomized clinical trials containing 8 [14] and 100 [15] patients. Control groups received CD only, and matched treatment groups received CD with *ex vivo* expanded autologous bone marrow MSCs. They found significant differences between the groups for volume of necrotic area in femoral head, Harris hip score, and visual analog pain scores with follow-up times of 42 and 60 months, respectively. There were no complications, and fewer patients required vascularized bone grafting or total hip arthroplasty in the MSC treatment group. Sen et al. [16] performed a similar study with 51 hips and found similar radiographic and clinical results in their patients, though they had a shorter follow-up of 24 months. Although these studies offer promising results and point toward bone marrow-derived MSCs as a safe, feasible surgical option for pre-collapse ON, they still have small sample sizes and no long-term follow-up beyond 5 years. Further studies with longer follow-up and larger sample sizes are required to draw definitive conclusions regarding the usefulness of stem cell therapy in ON.

A few other case reports and series outside of the United States have also utilized MSC-based treatments in humans and show favorable preliminary results. One study from Korea describes the percutaneous injection of autologous adipose-derived MSCs with platelet-rich plasma and hyaluronic acid in two patients with femoral head ON [17]. MRI evaluation demonstrated mild improvement of ON, and patient pain scores and physical therapy progress improved. Pak also reported in 2012 on two additional patients with femoral head ON who were treated with adipose MSCs, and they also reported improvement in Harris Hip Scores (HHS), physical therapy, and pain scores postoperatively [18]. MRI scans suggested regeneration of medullary bone-like tissue. However, these are uncontrolled clinical case series with a small number of subjects, so further study is needed to draw meaningful conclusions. No histopathological assessment can be made, and more detailed objective clinical data is required.

39.2.4 Limitations of Human Studies

Though a few human clinical studies have been done with stem cells to treat ON, certain concerns remain. It has been difficult to create and validate an animal model for ON that reflects all the symptoms and indications of ON in humans. Moreover, there is no evidence that stem cell therapy is effective on higher stage ON and femoral head collapse. A literature review [19] suggests that the reconstructive repair is a slow process, taking at least 8 years to improve the HHS to a mean of 88 points and to decrease the percent volume of necrosis involvement to a mean of 20 % of the femoral head. Though Gangji et al. showed in a 5-year study that autologous bone marrow cells transplanted into the necrotic lesion might help patients with early stages of osteonecrosis of the femoral head [3], substantial long-term data on the efficacy of transplanted stem cells is still lacking. Various studies have shown that bone marrow stem cell aspirates result in substantial reduction of necrosis and reduction of collapse, but randomized, controlled, prospective studies are needed to prove their absolute efficacy [20]. Additionally, most of the promising stem cell therapy research in humans is being done in Europe and Asia, as getting federal approval for such therapies is difficult in the United States.

39.3 Concerns with Stem Cell Transplantation

39.3.1 Autologous Stem Cells

Although autologous stem cells are the best sources for such therapy, they pose some challenges.

Morbidity: The morbidity associated with harvesting autologous MSCs makes it an operational challenge. Harvesting MSCs from iliac crest and then transplanting them prolongs the anesthesia time a patient experiences. In order to obtain adequate volume of bone marrow MSCs, multiple aspirations through different sites may be needed, which increases the surgical time, additional anesthesia risk, and expense. These factors could have unwanted consequences.

Availability: Another major hurdle to autologous stem cell transplantation is the available quantity. Regarding the issue of available technology, immediate intraoperative processing via density gradient centrifugation to get a higher concentration of cells could be utilized to overcome this [21]. However, the efficacy of this procedure is not completely proven. As another option, the cells can be harvested and allowed to expand *ex vivo* prior to implantation, but the patient would need to return for a second surgery at another time. While such efforts require concerted laboratory work, the effect of cell propagation on the biological properties of the MSCs is yet to be ascertained. The efficacy of using stem cells immediately isolated prior to transplantation compared to those that have been expanded *ex vivo* needs to be extensively evaluated. This could have repercussions on patient safety, treatment efficacy, and medical costs.

39.3.2 Allogeneic Stem Cells

Allogeneic stem cells are an alternate source for such therapy. MSCs have been successfully isolated from adipose tissue, and their use could negate the limitations of using autologous stem cells. However, allogeneic MSCs have their own set of concerning issues.

Disease Transmission: The most limiting factor is disease transmission. Transmission of disease from the donor to the host is well established in many cases of solid organ transplantation, and the same holds true for cell transplantation. Though efforts are made to screen for disease transmission, the possibility still poses an impediment toward widespread acceptance of this therapy.

Immunoprivileged Status: There is still debate about the viability of cells being transplanted and about their contribution to the formation of new vasculature in bone. The results of various in vitro and in vivo studies support the immunoprivileged status of MSCs. However, some in vivo studies in MHC-mismatched animal models contradict the theory that MSCs do not succumb to the host immune response. Murine allogeneic MSCs were rejected by MHC class I and class II mismatched hosts, and analysis of these allogeneic cell implants revealed increased proportions of host-derived CD8+ T-cells, NKT-cells, and NK cells by comparison to syngeneic controls [22]. Moreover, in a rabbit critical-sized fracture defect model, rabbit autologous MSCs but not human xenogeneic MSCs enhanced fracture healing [23].

Furthermore, the administration of immunosuppressive drugs in vivo significantly improved bone formation induced by MSCs when compared to non-immunosuppressed groups [24]. Many of the preclinical studies that evaluate the efficacy of stem cells are conducted in immunocompromised animals. Efforts to intensify the immunosuppression capability of the MSCs by co-delivering them with appropriate drugs might alleviate this concern. Additionally, there is some evidence that suggests that the viability of human MSCs in such immunocompromised animals is a function of the immaturity of the cell preparation being transplanted [25].

MSCs evoked significant cellular and humoral responses when implanted in vivo, though they were found to elicit no lymphocyte proliferation in vitro [26, 27]. In previous studies, researchers observed a significantly higher number of T-cells, B-cells, macrophages, and significantly higher expression of T-cell-derived interferon gamma (IFN-γ) in Bl/6 allogeneic implants [28]. Since MHC-mismatched allogeneic MSC implantation animal studies have shown evidence for both bone formation as well as rejection, a systematic analysis to determine if MSCs are capable of evading MHC barriers in different mouse immune models and to produce a clinically relevant bone forming response is imperative prior to widespread clinical use.

39.3.3 Other Concerns

In addition to the fact that most of the clinical trials involving stem cell therapies are still being validated, certain logistic challenges remain. These include but are not limited to the following:

1. *State of cell being transplanted* – The appropriate age of the stem cell donor is still being examined, and depending on the application, the passage of the cells being transplanted needs to be optimized. Using Brdu staining, Arthur et al. [29] showed that stem cells after 8 weeks did not have much proliferation capability. Using such mature stem cells as a therapy will likely not have positive results.
2. *Optimizing delivery* – Various scaffolds have been designed to deliver these cells to treat injuries such as large defects in long bones and craniofacial bones, fractures of long bones, vertebral disc defects, and ON of the femoral head. The treatment site dictates the design of the scaffold. However, the scaffolds used for stem cell delivery have been shown to affect the outcome of such therapies. In order to establish a scaffold-stem cell combination as a therapy, appropriate toxicity and cell dosage studies will need to be done. These studies will likely have different results in preclinical models and human trials.
3. *Cost* – The advanced laboratory and technical effort necessary undermines fast clinical translation of this technology, even if all the efficacy and safety concerns are adequately addressed. Stem cell isolation, expansion, and its subsequent transplantation require substantial investment in both the laboratory and operational front.
4. *Legal implications* – Establishing safe manufacturing practices for isolating and expanding stem cells prior to implantation is critical. Legal and bureaucratic hurdles to make such practices mainstream exist, the details of which are beyond the scope of this chapter.

References

1. Noel D, Djouad F, Jorgense C. Regenerative medicine through mesenchymal stem cells for bone and cartilage repair. Curr Opin Investig Drugs. 2002;3:1000–4. PMID: 12186258.
2. Kuo TK, Ho JH, Lee OK. Mesenchymal stem cell therapy for nonmusculoskeletal diseases: emerging applications. Cell Transplant. 2009;18:1013–28. PMID: 19523328.
3. Gangji V, De Maertelaer V, Hauzeur JP. Autologous bone marrow cell implantation in the treatment of non-traumatic osteonecrosis of the femoral head: Five year follow-up of a prospective controlled study. Bone. 2011;49(5):1005–9. PMID: 21821156.
4. Hernigou P, Beaujean F. Treatment of osteonecrosis with autologous bone marrow grafting. Clin Orthop Relat Res. 2002;405: 14–23.
5. Wang BL, Sun W, Shi ZC, et al. Decreased proliferation of mesenchymal stem cells in corticosteroid-induced osteonecrosis of femoral head. Orthopedics. 2008;31(5):444. PMID: 19292322.
6. Yan Z, Hang D, Guo C, Chen Z. Fate of mesenchymal stem cells transplanted to osteonecrosis of femoral head. J Orthop Res. 2009;27(4):442–6. PMID: 18925660.
7. Peng J, Wen C, Wang A, et al. Micro-CT-based bone ceramic scaffolding and its performance after seeding with mesenchymal stem cells for repair of load-bearing bone defect in canine femoral head. J Biomed Mater Res B Appl Biomater. 2011;96(2):316–25. PMID: 21210512.
8. Jin H, Xia B, Yu N, et al. The effects of autologous bone marrow mesenchymal stem cell arterial perfusion on vascular repair and angiogenesis in osteonecrosis of the femoral head in dogs. Int Orthop. 2012;36(12):2589–96. PMID: 23064553.
9. Cui Q, Xiao Z, Li X, Saleh KJ, Balian G. Use of genetically engineered bone-marrow stem cells to treat femoral defects: an experimental study. J Bone Joint Surg Am. 2006;88 Suppl 3:167–72. PMID: 17079384.
10. Li ZH, Liao W, Cui XL, et al. Intravenous transplantation of allogeneic bone marrow mesenchymal stem cells and its directional migration to the necrotic femoral head. Int J Med Sci. 2011;8(1):74–83. PMID: 21234272.
11. Feitosa ML, Fadel L, Beltrão-Braga PC, Wenceslau CV, Kerkis I, Kerkis A, Birgel Júnior EH, Martins JF, Martins Ddos S, Miglino MA, Ambrósio CE. Successful transplant of mesenchymal stem cells in induced osteonecrosis of the ovine femoral head: preliminary results. Acta Cir Bras. 2010;25(5):416–22.
12. Cuomo AV, Virk M, Petrigliano F, Morgan EF, Lieberman JR. Mesenchymal stem cell concentration and bone repair: potential pitfalls from bench to bedside. J Bone Joint Surg Am. 2009;91(5):1073–83. PMID: 19411455.
13. Hernigou P, Poignard A, Zilber S, Rouard H. Cell therapy of hip osteonecrosis with autologous bone marrow grafting. Indian J Orthop. 2009;43(1):40–5. doi:10.4103/0019-5413.45322.
14. Chang T, Tang K, Tao X, et al. Treatment of early avascular necrosis of femoral head by core decompression combined with autologous bone marrow mesenchymal stem cells transplantation.

Zhongguo Xiu Fu Chong Jian Wai Ke Za Zhi. 2010;24:739–43. PMID: 20632513.

15. Zhao D, Cui D, Wang B, et al. Treatment of early stage osteonecrosis of the femoral head with autologous implantation of bone marrow-derived and cultured mesenchymal stem cells. Bone. 2012;50:325–30. PMID: 22094904.
16. Sen RK, Tripathy SK, Aggarwal S, Marwaha N, Sharma RR, Khandelwal N. Early results of core decompression and autologous bone marrow mononuclear cells instillation in femoral head osteonecrosis: a randomized control study. J Arthroplasty. 2012;27(5):679–86. PMID: 22000577.
17. Pak J. Regeneration of human bones in hip osteonecrosis and human cartilage in knee osteoarthritis with autologous adipose-tissue-derived stem cells: a case series. J Med Case Rep. 2011;5(1):296. PMID: 21736710.
18. Pak J. Autologous adipose tissue-derived stem cells induce persistent bone-like tissue in osteonecrotic femoral heads. Pain Physician. 2012;15:75–85. PMID: 22270740.
19. Sen RK. Management of avascular necrosis of femoral head at pre-collapse stage. Indian J Orthop. 2009;43(1):6–16.
20. Hauzeur JP, Gangji V. Phases 1–3 clinical trials using adult stem cells in osteonecrosis and nonunion fractures. Stem Cells Int. 2010;2010:410170. PMID: 21048847.
21. Hendrich C, Franz E, Waertel G, Krebs R, Jäger M. Safety of autologous bone marrow aspiration concentrate transplantation: initial experiences in 101 patients. Orthop Rev (Pavia). 2009;1(2):e32. PMID: 21808691.
22. Eliopolous N, Stagg J, Lejeune L, Pommey S, Galipeau J. Allogeneic marrow stromal cells are immune rejected by MHC class I- and class II-mismatched recipient mice. Blood. 2005;106:4057–65. PMID: 16118325.
23. Niemeyer P, Szalay K, Luginbühl R, Südkamp NP, Kasten P. Transplantation of human mesenchymal stem cells in a non-autogenous setting for bone regeneration in a rabbit critical-size defect model. Acta Biomater. 2010;6(3):900–8. PMID: 19766744.
24. Tsuchida H, Hashimoto J, Crawford E, Manske P, Lou J. Engineered allogeneic mesenchymal stem cells repair femoral segmental defect in rats. J Orthop Res. 2003;21(1):44–53. PMID: 12507579.
25. Gronthos S, Chen S, Wang CY, Robey PG, Shi S. Telomerase accelerates osteogenesis of bone marrow stromal stem cells by upregulation of CBFA1, osterix, and osteocalcin. J Bone Miner Res. 2003;18:716–22. PMID: 12674332.
26. Poncelet AJ, Vercruysse J, Saliez A, Gianello P. Although pig allogeneic mesenchymal stem cells are not immunogenic in vitro, intracardiac injection elicits an immune response in vivo. Transplantation. 2007;83(6):783–90. PMID: 17414713.
27. Badillo AT, Beggs KJ, Javazon EH, Tebbets JC, Flake AW. Murine bone marrow stromal progenitor cells elicit an in vivo cellular and humoral alloimmune response. Biol Blood Marrow Transplant. 2007;13(4):412–22.
28. Dighe AS, Yang S, Madhu V, Balian G, Cui Q. Interferon gamma and T cells inhibit osteogenesis induced by allogeneic mesenchymal stromal cells. J Orthop Res. 2013;31(2):227–34. PMID: 17382248.
29. Arthur A, Zannettino A, Gronthos S. The therapeutic applications of multipotential mesenchymal/stromal stem cells in skeletal tissue repair. J Cell Physiol. 2009;218(2):237–45. PMID: 18792913.

Cement Techniques in Hip Osteonecrosis with Collapse: From Traditional Methyl Methacrylate to Bone Substitutes and Stem Cells

40

Philippe Hernigou and Gildasio Daltro

40.1 Introduction

Osteonecrosis of the femoral head (ONFH) is a bone disease which can affect young patients [1, 2]. Its late stages are characterized by a collapse of the femoral head due to subchondral fracture. The collapsed hip usually progresses to secondary osteoarthritis and requires total hip replacement. Therefore, in the treatment of osteonecrosis the goal should be to prevent collapse. Osteotomies and bone grafts [3–6] were proposed to resolve this problem. However, the results are irregular and need to avoid full weight bearing for a long time. The use of cement to restore and maintain the sphericity of the femoral head avoids this inconvenience of delaying full weight bearing. The first patient that we treated for osteonecrosis by injecting cement was operated in 1986 in the Henri Mondor Hospital and remained without arthroplasty until 2009. In the beginning [7], we injected low viscosity cement into the femoral heads of 16 patients with osteonecrosis secondary to sickle cell disease. In subsequent report, we [8] reported treatment of 61 patients treated for other causes of osteonecrosis. The dominant feature observed was the postoperative pain-killing effect thought to be secondary to immobilization of the sequestrum and intraosseous pressure decompression. We noted that the more depressed the fracture, the more likely the chance of repeated fracture, even if initial cement technique was able to reestablish the sphericity. This technique was used from 1986 to 2000 with methyl methacrylate for more than 300 patients and was modified to prevent late osteoarthritis in 2000 by using phosphocalcic cement loaded mixed with stem cells instead of methyl methacrylate in young people, according to the results obtained with autologous bone marrow injection in patients with stage I and stage II osteonecrosis [9].

This paper describes the different surgical techniques that can be used to restore the sphericity of the femoral head in hip osteonecrosis associated with collapse, the rational for moving from traditional methyl methacrylate to bone substitutes and stem cells, and discuss the results obtained by different series.

40.2 Techniques Used to Restore the Sphericity of the Femoral Head

40.2.1 Operative Technique with the Intra-articular Approach

The patient is placed in a supine position and the anterior capsule of the hip is exposed by a Smith-Peterson approach, using a skin incision from about 7 cm behind the anterior superior iliac spine, along the outer lip of the iliac crest and down over the groove between the sartorius and tensor of fascia lata, as described previously [7]. A capsulotomy is performed to expose the anterior part of the femoral head. Dislocation is not necessary; the exposition of the osteonecrosis is performed by moving the hip with the orthopedic Table. A pin is then driven at the junction of the living bone and the necrotic segment. The leverage on this pin elevates the necrotic bone and reduces the collapse. The pin is removed and replaced by a needle, through which low viscosity cement is injected with a cement gun. The injection is completed when the shape of the femoral head is restored. After the operation, weight bearing is immediately permitted after 3 weeks. This technique is available in patients with a crescent line without a large collapse because the technique uses only a needle or a small trocar. The advantages of this technique relate to the exposure that allows for a direct evaluation of the cartilage surface and underlying diseased

P. Hernigou (✉)
Department of Orthopaedic Surgery, University Paris East, 51 avenue du Maréchal de Lattre de Tassigny, Créteil 94010, France
e-mail: philippe.hernigou@wanadoo.fr

G. Daltro
Department of Orthopaedic Surgery, Hospital Edgar Santos, University Federal of Bahia, Salvador, Brazil
e-mail: gildasio.daltro@yahoo.com.br

K.-H. Koo et al. (eds.), *Osteonecrosis*,
DOI 10.1007/978-3-642-35767-1_40, © Springer-Verlag Berlin Heidelberg 2014

femoral head segment and allows for precise bone cement injection. There is no risk of intertrochanteric fracture. The disadvantages include the demanding technical nature of the procedure to perform it without dislocation. Another advantage is that it can be performed with arthroscopic technique.

40.2.2 Operative Technique with Core Decompression

Patients are placed on a table with two image intensifiers with a C arm. The method involves the placement of a channel through the lateral cortex of the proximal femur. A small skin incision is used and a guide wire is advanced under fluoroscopic guidance from the lateral cortex, through the femoral neck, and into the necrotic lesion within the femoral head. A drill is used over the guide wire to introduce an opening in the lateral cortex and a trephine of 8 mm is then advanced through the opening, past the femoral neck, and into the necrotic segment of the femoral head. Depending on the size and location of the lesion, trephines and curettes of various sizes can be used to remove necrotic bone. This approach can also be used to perform a wider debridement of the diseased bone and can address to patients with a more important collapse. The reduction of the collapse is performed by pushing the subchondral bone from the core track. Then the volume of bone removed (debridement) and the core track are filled with cement. The advantages of this approach include a simple and well-known technique and the absence of surgical dislocation of the hip. The disadvantages include the risk of postoperative fracture and the inability to directly visualize the joint surfaces and the inexact nature of removing diseased bone and replacing it with bone cement under fluoroscopic guidance. The principal risk of the technique is unrecognized joint penetration with cement going inside the joint. That may occur because radiograph beam projects an equatorial dimension of the femoral head on fluoroscopy as described in detail in a previous paper [10]. This problem of projection is compounded in the clinical setting by the difficulty in obtaining clear radiographs with an image intensifier.

40.2.3 Cementing Technique Through a Femoral Neck Window

The technique is done through an anterolateral approach. Hueter, Watson-Jones, or Smith- Peterson approaches can be used to expose the anterior femoral neck where a burr hole (like a window) is created at the level of the junction of the femoral head and neck. The necrotic segment is identified and removed with curettes and burrs through the window. The collapsed segment is reduced from below under direct visualization, and the cement injected through the window restores the femoral head sphericity and support the region of collapse. The advantages of this approach include the improved access to the necrotic segment and the avoidance of direct iatrogenic cartilage damage. The disadvantages of the approach include the inability to fully visualize the joint surfaces and the cartilage, the creation of a window defect in the femoral neck (with a risk of fracture), and the relative invasiveness of the surgical approach which is quite the same as for an arthroplasty.

40.3 The Rational for Moving from Methyl Methacrylate to Phosphocalcic Cement Loaded with Stem Cells

From a historical point of view, methyl methacrylate was first used to replace the cartilage with the acrylic arthroplasty of Judet. Secondary methyl methacrylate was used in giant cell tumors by Vidal; these tumors present an analogous situation to osteonecrosis because they also usually present with involvement to the subchondral bone and may be treated successfully by curettage of the lesion (to subchondral bone) followed by packing of the cavity with methyl methacrylate. The published clinical and basic science success rates using methyl methacrylate to support cartilage are encouraging [11–14]; however, there are three concerns with potential adverse affects related to cement [15, 16]. Heat generated by the exothermic polymerization of the monomer can injure the overlying cartilage [17]. Indeed, a thinner cement layer may be better for thermal bone necrosis; but correspondingly worse for the strength of the cement fixation, other reasons such as a local cytotoxic effect of the cement monomer may damage to the natural structures above (cartilage) or under (trabecular bone); there is no incorporation with time. There may be alterations in the forces on the subchondral bone and overlying cartilage after cementation that can be the cause of osteoarthritis observed later in patients.

Mesenchymal stem cells (MSCs) are multipotent stem cells that can differentiate into a variety of cell types. In the field of cell transplantation, MSCs have many advantages over other cell types such as easy isolation and culture, rapid in vitro amplification, differentiation potential, and easy collection. MSCs were proposed first in 1990 for the treatment of femoral head necrosis for stage I and stage II, by injection as the same time of core decompression [9]. The clinical data demonstrated that the implanted MSCs can not only survive but proliferate in the necrotic femoral head after transplantation, promoting the repair of injured femoral head [9, 18–20]. So we mixed MSCs to phosphocalcic cement to improve repair of osteonecrosis.

The natural bone consists of an extracellular matrix with nano-sized apatitic minerals and collagen fibers that support bone cell functions. It is advantageous for a synthetic biomimetic scaffold to contain nano-apatite crystals similar to those in bone, together with fibers to form a matrix that supports cell attachment, have mechanical properties similar to those of bone, and support cells for osteogenic differentiation and bone regeneration. Bioactive calcium phosphates such as hydroxyapatite (HA) $Ca_{10}(PO_4)_6(OH)_2$, tricalcium phosphate (TCP) $Ca_3(PO_4)_2$, tetracalcium phosphate ($Ca_4P_2O_9$), and dicalcium phosphate (DCP) $CaHPO_4$ have been widely applied for hard tissue substitute materials, due to their good biocompatibility and bioactivity [21–28]. Many studies have evidenced the excellent biocompatibility of calcium phosphates (CaPs) and their favorable interaction with hard tissue [25, 26]. One of the major improvements in CaPs in recent years is the development of an injectable system. The injectable bone graft substitutes can mold to the shape of the bone cavity and set in situ when injected. Such systems shorten the surgical operation time, reduce the damaging effects of large muscle retraction, decrease the size of the scars, and diminish postoperative pain.

The stem cell-bone substitute construct may be promising for orthopedic applications. Major reconstructions can greatly benefit from a paste that can be molded to the desired with fracture resistance and stem cell encapsulation for rapid bone regeneration. Xiao et al. [29] evaluated the effect of autologous BMSC seeded bio-derived bone materials combined with recombinant human bone morphologic protein-2 (rhBMP-2) in repairing the defect of ONFH in the rabbit. They found that collapse could be prevented and new bone formation could be generated. These novel treatment protocols conform well to the concept of in vivo tissue engineering, which is also based on three essential factors: seed cells, various scaffolds, and cytokines in an intracorporeal environment. Ito et al. [30] demonstrated bone formation using novel interconnected porous calcium hydroxyapatite ceramic hybridized with cultured marrow stromal stem cells derived from Green rat.

40.4 Results Obtained by Different Series

40.4.1 Acrylic Cement

We used low viscosity cement injected into the femoral heads [7] with a Smith-Petersen approach. The collapsed segment was reduced with a pin, then cement injected into the junction of the living and necrotic bone until the collapse of the articular cartilage has been corrected. The dominant feature observed was the postoperative pain thought to be secondary to immobilization of the sequestrum and intraosseous pressure decompression. Fourteen of 16 patients were improved clinically (some reported slight pain) at a mean follow-up of 5 years. Two patients required revision to total hip arthroplasty, both within 2 years. In subsequent follow-up, we [8] reported treatment of 61 patients and noted early failures (6 months to 1 year) in 10 patients with kidney transplant or need for hemodialysis or corticosteroids. Among 38 hips with success for greater than 5 years, five required total hip arthroplasty due to functional and radiographic arthritis. We noted that the more depressed the fracture, the more likely the chance of repeated fracture, even if initial cement technique was able to reestablish the sphericity. Furthermore, in the long term osteoarthritis occurred, probably due to degradation of the cartilage in contact with the cement. So, this technique, used from 1986 to 2000 with methyl methacrylate for more than 300 patients, was modified in 2000 to use phosphocalcic cement loaded with stem cells instead of methyl methacrylate for osteonecrosis with collapse in young people, according to the results obtained with autologous bone marrow injection in patients with stage I and stage II osteonecrosis.

Other centers have used cementation for femoral head osteonecrosis. Bresler et al. [31] reported the results of 27 cementations with 10 failures at 1–3 years are presented. He used a technique using a 12 mm trephine put in place under arthroscopic control with injection of cement through a syringe. He noted the immediate pain-killing action was distinctly superior to classic core decompression, which they related to stabilization of the sequestrum. Cheng et al. [32] describes injecting the proximal half of the tract after core decompression. A prospective randomized study comparing core decompression alone with and without cement augmentation for precollapse disease is ongoing. A prospective report of stage III hips with greater than 1 mm collapse showed 87 % conversion to total hip arthroplasty at 2-year follow-up. Wood et al. [33] reported a series of 20 cementations. Three patients had a conversion to total hip arthroplasty at follow-up from 6 months to 2 years (average = 8.7 months).

40.4.2 Stem Cell-Bone Substitute Construct

The first implantation of MSCs mixed with beta-tricalcium phosphate was used in 2000 at the Henri Mondor Hospital to treat patients with collapse. At this moment 50 patients have been treated using concentrate bone marrow and granular types (diameter, 1–3 mm) of pure porous beta-tricalcium phosphate ceramics (β-TCP). The technique was done through an anterolateral approach using a Smith-Peterson approach to expose the anterior femoral neck where a window was created at the level of the junction of the femoral head and neck. The necrotic segment was removed with curettes through the window. The collapsed segment was reduced from below under direct visualization, and the granules that had been soaked in bone marrow concentrate were packed in the femoral head to restore sphericity and support the region of collapse. We found greater clinical improvement in patients treated with core decompression and implantation of porous beta-tricalcium phosphate scaffold with stem cells versus patients treated with methyl methacrylate.

Kawate et al. [34] used in 2006 autologous mesenchymal stem cells (MSCs) cultured with beta-tricalcium phosphate (β-TCP) ceramics and with a free vascularized fibula were transplanted into three patients with steroid-induced osteonecrosis of the femoral head. About 400 mL of blood was obtained from the patients for serum separation 4 weeks before the surgery, and this serum was used for cell culture. At the same time, about 15 mL of bone marrow was obtained from the anterior iliac crest. Following 2 days of culture, nonadherent cells were removed and 13 mL culture medium was added. The medium was changed three times per week. After 10–11 days, β-TCP porous ceramic granules were immersed in the MSC cell suspension and were cultured for 2 weeks to induce osteogenic differentiation. Cultured MSCs/β-TCP composite granules were implanted into the cavity that remained after curettage of necrotic bone, and finally, a free vascularized fibula was grafted.

Sun et al. [35] reported the effect of bone marrow mononuclear cells on vascularization and bone regeneration in steroid-induced osteonecrosis of the femoral head.

Yamasaki et al. [36, 37] used BMMNCs that were transplanted into the affected area of one hip using interconnected porous calcium hydroxyapatite (IP-CHA) in two patients, while the other hip was simultaneously treated with transtrochanteric rotational osteotomy. This case report documents the potential of BMMNCs with IP-CHA for bone repair at the lesion of osteonecrosis of the femoral head.

Liu et al. [38] recently reported a study where patients with ONFH underwent core decompression and implantation of nano-hydroxyapatite/polyamide bone filler with or without BMMNCs. Granular porous medical nano-hydroxyapatite/polyamide composite bone filling material (nano-apatite composite, Sichuan National Nano Technology Co., Ltd, Chengdu, China) was soaked in the concentrated BMMNC solution for 2 min. After the BMMNC solution was completely absorbed, the bone filling particles/BMMNCs were implanted in the bone tunnel. Repeated filling and compacting of the particles was performed using a pushing bar. All patients with stage IIIA ONFH underwent reduction of the collapsed femoral head.

References

1. Jones LC, Hungerford DS. The pathogenesis of osteonecrosis. Instr Course Lect. 2007;56:179–96.
2. Mont MA, Hungerford DS. Non-traumatic avascular necrosis of the femoral head. J Bone Joint Surg Am. 1995;77:459–74.
3. Baksi DP. Treatment of osteonecrosis of the femoral head by drilling and muscle-pedicle bone grafting. J Bone Joint Surg Br. 1991; 73:241–5.
4. Steinberg ME, Brighton CT, Steinberg DR, et al. Treatment of avascular necrosis of the femoral head by a combination of bone grafting, decompression, and electrical stimulation. Clin Orthop. 1984;186:137–53.
5. Steinberg ME, Larcom PG, Strafford B, et al. Core decompression with bone grafting for osteonecrosis of the femoral head. Clin Orthop. 2001;386:71–8.
6. Urbaniak JR, Coogan PG, Gunneson EB, et al. Treatment of osteonecrosis of the femoral head with free vascularized fibular grafting. A long-term follow-up study of one hundred and three hips. J Bone Joint Surg Am. 1995;77:681–94.
7. Hernigou P, Bachir D, Galacteros F. Avascular necrosis of the femoral head in sickle-cell disease. Treatment of collapse by the injection of acrylic cement. J Bone Joint Surg Br. 1993;75:875–80.
8. Hernigou P. Treatment of hip necrosis by sequestrectomy and replacement with bone cement. Acta Orthop Belg. 1999;65 Suppl 1:89–94.
9. Hernigou P, Beaujean F. Treatment of osteonecrosis with autologous bone marrow grafting. Clin Orthop Relat Res. 2002;405: 14–23.
10. Hernigou P, Manicom O, Poignard A, Nogier A, Filippini P, De abreu L. Core decompression with marrow stem cells. Oper Tech Orthop. 2004;14(2):68–74.
11. Ewald FC, Poss R, Pugh J, et al. Hip cartilage supported by methacrylate in canine arthroplasty. Clin Orthop. 1982;171:273–9.
12. Malawer MM, Dunham W. Cryosurgery and acrylic cementation as surgical adjuncts in the treatment of aggressive (benign) bone tumors. Analysis of 25 patients below the age of 21. Clin Orthop. 1991;262:42–57.
13. Pals SD, Wilkins RM. Giant cell tumor of bone treated by curettage, cementation, and bone grafting. Orthopedics. 1992;15: 703–8.
14. Persson BM, Wouters HW. Curettage and acrylic cementation in surgery of giant cell tumors of bone. Clin Orthop. 1976;120: 125–33.
15. Fukushima H, Hashimoto Y, Yoshiya S, et al. Conduction analysis of cement interface temperature in total knee arthroplasty. Cent Jpn J Orthop Surg Trauma. 2001;44:993–1003.
16. Huiskes R. Heat-generation and conduction analyses of acrylic bone cement in situ. Acta Orthop Scand Suppl. 1980;185:43–108.
17. Schatzker J, Horne JG, Sumner-Smith G, et al. Methylmethacrylate cement: its curing temperature and effect on articular cartilage. Can J Surg. 1975;18:172–5, 178.
18. Gangji V, Hauzeur JP, Matos C, De Maertelaer V, Toungouz M, Lambermont M. Treatment of osteonecrosis of the femoral head with implantation of autologous bone-marrow cells. A pilot study. J Bone Joint Surg Am. 2004;86-A:1153–60.
19. Gangji V, De Maertelaer V, Hauzeur JP. Autologous bone marrow cell implantation in the treatment of non-traumatic osteonecrosis of the femoral head: five year follow-up of a prospective controlled study. Bone. 2011;49:1005–9.
20. Wang BL, Sun W, Shi ZC, et al. Treatment of nontraumatic osteonecrosis of the femoral head with the implantation of core decompression and concentrated autologous bone marrow containing mononuclear cells. Arch Orthop Trauma Surg. 2010;130:859–65.
21. Brown WE, Chow LC. A new calcium phosphate water setting cement. In: Brown PW, editor. Cements research progress. Westerville: American Ceramic Society; 1986. p. 352–79.
22. Drissens F, Bolton M, Bermudez O, Planell J, Ginebra M, Fernandez E. Effective formulation for the preparation of calcium phosphate hone cements. J Mater Sci. 1994;5(3):164–70.
23. LeGeros RZ. Calcium phosphate-based osteoinductive materials. Chem Rev. 2008;108(11):4742–53.
24. Rabiee SM, Mortazavi SMJ, Moztarzadeh F, et al. Mechanical behavior of a new biphasic calcium phosphate bone graft. Biotechnol Bioprocess Eng. 2008;13(2):204–9.

25. Sarkar MR, Wachter N, Patka P, Kinzl L. First histological observations on the incorporation of a novel calcium phosphate bone substitute material in human cancellous bone. J Biomed Mater Res. 2001;58:329–34.
26. Theiss F, Apelt D, Brand B, Kutter A, Zlinszky K, Bohner M. Biocompatibility and resorption of a brushite calcium phosphate cement. Biomaterials. 2005;26(21):4383–94.
27. Vallet-Regí M, González-Calbet JM. Calcium phosphates as substitution of bone tissues. Prog Solid State Chem. 2004;32(1–2):1–31.
28. Weiss P, Layrolle P, Clergeau LP, et al. The safety and efficacy of an injectable bone substitute in dental sockets demonstrated in a human clinical trial. Biomaterials. 2007;28(22):3295–305.
29. Xiao ZM, Jiang H, Zhan XL, Wu ZG, Zhang XL. Treatment of osteonecrosis of femoral head with BMSCs-seeded bio-derived bone materials combined with rhBMP-2 in rabbits. Chin J Traumatol. 2008;11:165–70.
30. Ito Y, Tanaka N, Fujimoto Y, et al. Bone formation using novel interconnected porous calcium hydroxyapatite ceramic hybridized with cultured marrow stromal stem cells derived from Green rat. J Biomed Mater Res A. 2004;69:454–61.
31. Bresler F, Roche O, Chary-Valckenaire I, Blum A, Mole D, Schmitt D. Femoral head osteonecrosis: original extra-articular cementoplasty technique. A series of 20 cases. Acta Orthop Belg. 1999;65 Suppl 1:95–6.
32. Cheng E, et al. Osteonecrosis of the femoral head: the North American perspective. In: Bulstrode CBJ, Carr A, editors. Oxford textbook of orthopedics and trauma. New York: Oxford University Press; 2002. p. 981–91.
33. Wood ML, McDowell CM, Kerstetter TL, et al. Open reduction and cementation for femoral head fracture secondary to avascular necrosis: preliminary report. Iowa Orthop J. 2000;20:17–23.
34. Kawate K, et al. Tissue-engineered approach for the treatment of steroid-induced osteonecrosis of the femoral head: transplantation of autologous mesenchymal stem cells cultured with beta-tricalcium phosphate ceramics and free vascularized fibula. Artif Organs. 2006;30(12):960–2.
35. Sun Y, Feng Y, Zhang C. The effect of bone marrow mononuclear cells on vascularization and bone regeneration in steroid-induced osteonecrosis of the femoral head. Joint Bone Spine. 2009;76:685–90.
36. Yamasaki T, Yasunaga Y, Ishikawa M, Hamaki T, Ochi M. Bone-marrow-derived mononuclear cells with a porous hydroxyapatite scaffold for the treatment of osteonecrosis of the femoral head: a preliminary study. J Bone Joint Surg Br. 2010;92:337–41.
37. Yamasaki T, Yasunaga Y, Terayama H, Ito Y, Ishikawa M, Adachi N, Ochi M. Transplantation of bone marrow mononuclear cells enables simultaneous treatment with osteotomy for osteonecrosis of the bilateral femoral head. Med Sci Monit. 2008;14(4):CS23–30.
38. Liu Y, Liu S, Su X. Core decompression and implantation of bone marrow mononuclear cells with porous hydroxylapatite composite filler for the treatment of osteonecrosis of the femoral head. Arch Orthop Trauma Surg. 2013;133:125.

Impaction Bone Grafting

41

Seung-Hoon Baek and Shin-Yoon Kim

41.1 Introduction

Osteonecrosis of the femoral head (ONFH) is a disease that commonly affects young adults progressing to collapse and osteoarthritis. Joint-preserving procedures are preferred treatments to prevent the progression to collapse and subsequent osteoarthritis [1]. Since core decompression was first described by Ficat and Arlet [2], several head-preserving procedures combined with core decompression including vascularized [3, 4] or nonvascularized bone graft [5, 6] from the fibula, iliac crest, or tibia have been performed to provide mechanical support and biological augmentation aiding bone healing [7, 8]. Most of these procedures, however, demonstrated limited successful outcomes for treating ONFH in early stage [6, 9, 10]. Some of them are technically demanding with extensive surgical time and showed donor site morbidity [11]. The residual graft can prevent optimal positioning and canal fit of the stem in later possible total hip arthroplasty (THA) after failed nonvascularized or vascularized fibular or tibial grafting [12, 13]. On the contrary, bone impaction grafting is relatively simple and does not take extensive surgical time. It does not produce donor site morbidity and does not disturb the procedure in future THA [14].

In this chapter, we are going to provide historical background of bone impaction grafting as the treatment for ONFH. Next, technical aspects of bone impaction grafting will be discussed. Third, we are going to provide results of bone impaction grafting in the treatment of ONFH according to disease stage, quantification, and location of the lesion, summarizing them as a table. Finally, we are going to suggest an opinion on the future solution and application of the bone impaction grafting combined with additives to augment mechanical and biological characteristics of the graft.

S.-H. Baek
Department of Orthopedic Surgery, School of Medicine, Kyungpook National University, 130 Dongdeok-ro, Jung-gu, Daegu 700-721, South Korea
e-mail: sbaek@knu.ac.kr

S.-Y. Kim (✉)
Department of Orthopedic Surgery, Musculoskeletal Genome Research Center, School of Medicine, Kyungpook National University, 130 Dongdeok-ro, Jung-gu, Daegu 700-721, Korea (South)
e-mail: syukim@knu.ac.kr

41.2 Background

Impaction bone grafting as the treatment for ONFH, first introduced by Gardeniers et al., has been originally developed from the technique of using morselized fresh-frozen allograft to reconstruct bone defects in revision arthroplasties [14, 15]. The construct using this technique has shown sufficient initial stability and demonstrated satisfactory long-term results in revision THA [16, 17]. The histologic evaluation retrieved from 21 revision or re-revision THAs showed rapid revascularization of the graft, directly followed by osteoclastic resorption and woven bone formation on the graft remnant; 30 % of the graft incorporated by 6 months and 90 % by 10 years [18]. Although the biological environment in ONFH and composition of the construct are different from those in revision THA, this incorporation process can be augmented by using cancellous autograft which contains osteoprogenitor cells as well as local growth factors to induce the mesenchymal cells to differentiate into mature osteoblasts.

41.3 Surgical Technique (Modified from Rijnen et al. [14]) (Fig. 41.1)

A patient is placed in the supine on the fracture table with 20° internal rotation of the leg. Gentle compression instead of traction is applied to press the femoral head against the chondral surface of the acetabulum so as to regain the sphericity and prevent the possible perforation of the femoral

K.-H. Koo et al. (eds.), *Osteonecrosis*,
DOI 10.1007/978-3-642-35767-1_41, © Springer-Verlag Berlin Heidelberg 2014

head. Five- to seven-cm-sized lateral skin incision is made centered over 1 cm distal to the vastus lateralis ridge. The fascia lata is split in the direction of the skin incision, and the vastus lateralis muscle is lifted off from the lateral cortex of the femur following L-shaped incision of the muscle. After making a small cortical window 1 cm distal to the vastus ridge, a guide pin is inserted to the direction of the center of necrosis (usually superolateral) under the guidance of the image intensifier and preoperative MRI (Fig. 41.1a, b). An intraosseous tunnel reaching the margin of necrotic area is created with the use of a 9–15 mm trephine drill (Fig. 41.1c), and the cancellous bone from the proximal femur is saved for

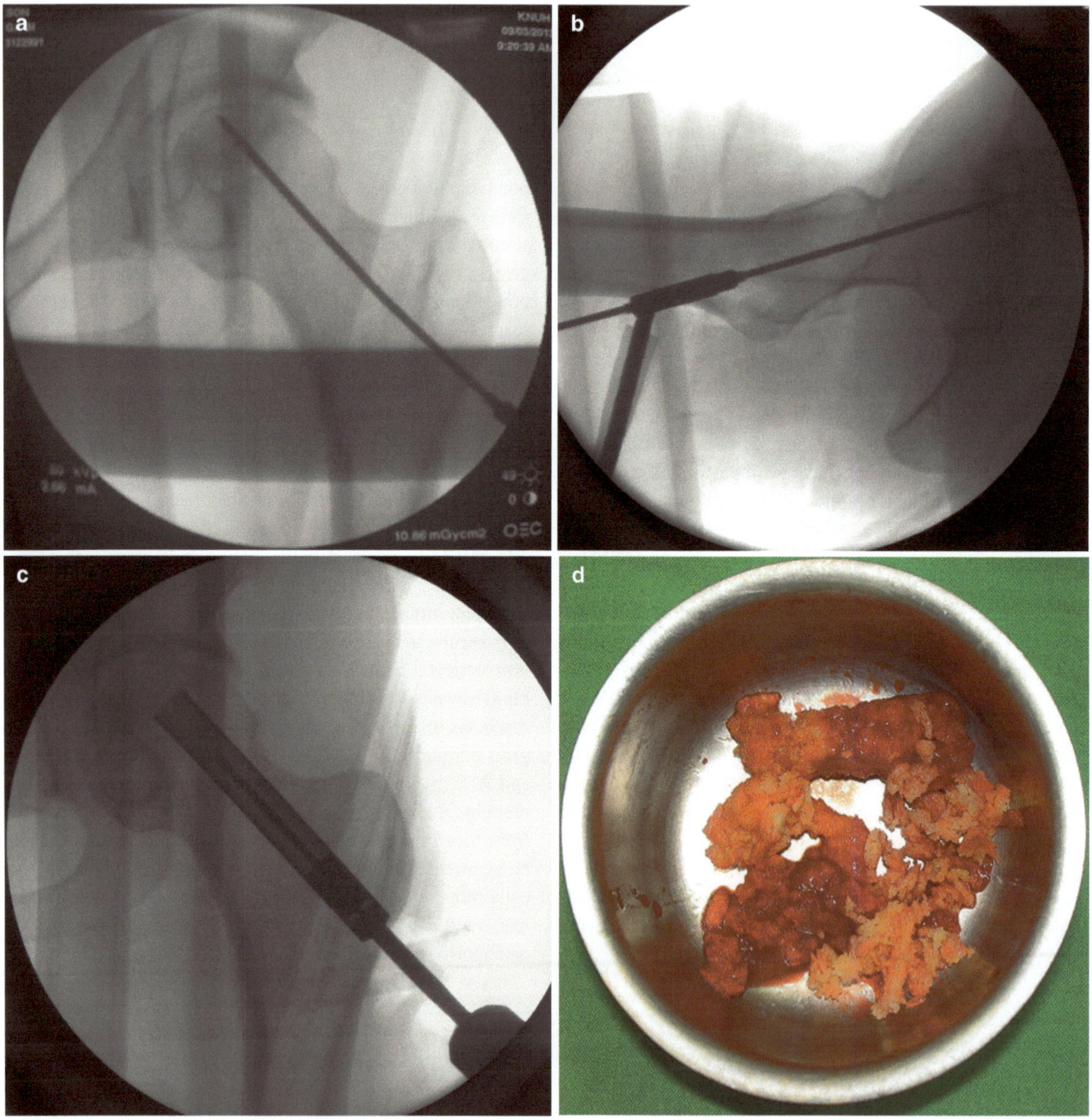

Fig. 41.1 At 1 cm distal to the vastus ridge, a guide pin is inserted to the direction of the center of necrosis under the guidance of the image intensifier in the anteroposterior (**a**) and axial direction (**b**). A tunnel reaching the margin of necrotic area is established with the use of 11 mm trephine drill (**c**) and the cancellous bone block from the proximal femur is reserved for impaction grafting (**d**). After central core biopsy, the remaining necrotic bone is completely curetted under the image intensifier in two directions (**e, f**) followed by thorough irrigation of debris (**g**). The photograph demonstrates washed and squeezed fresh-frozen allograft chips with a size of 7–10 mm (**h**), and they are impacted into the remaining void following impaction of the cancellous bone block from the proximal femur (**i**)

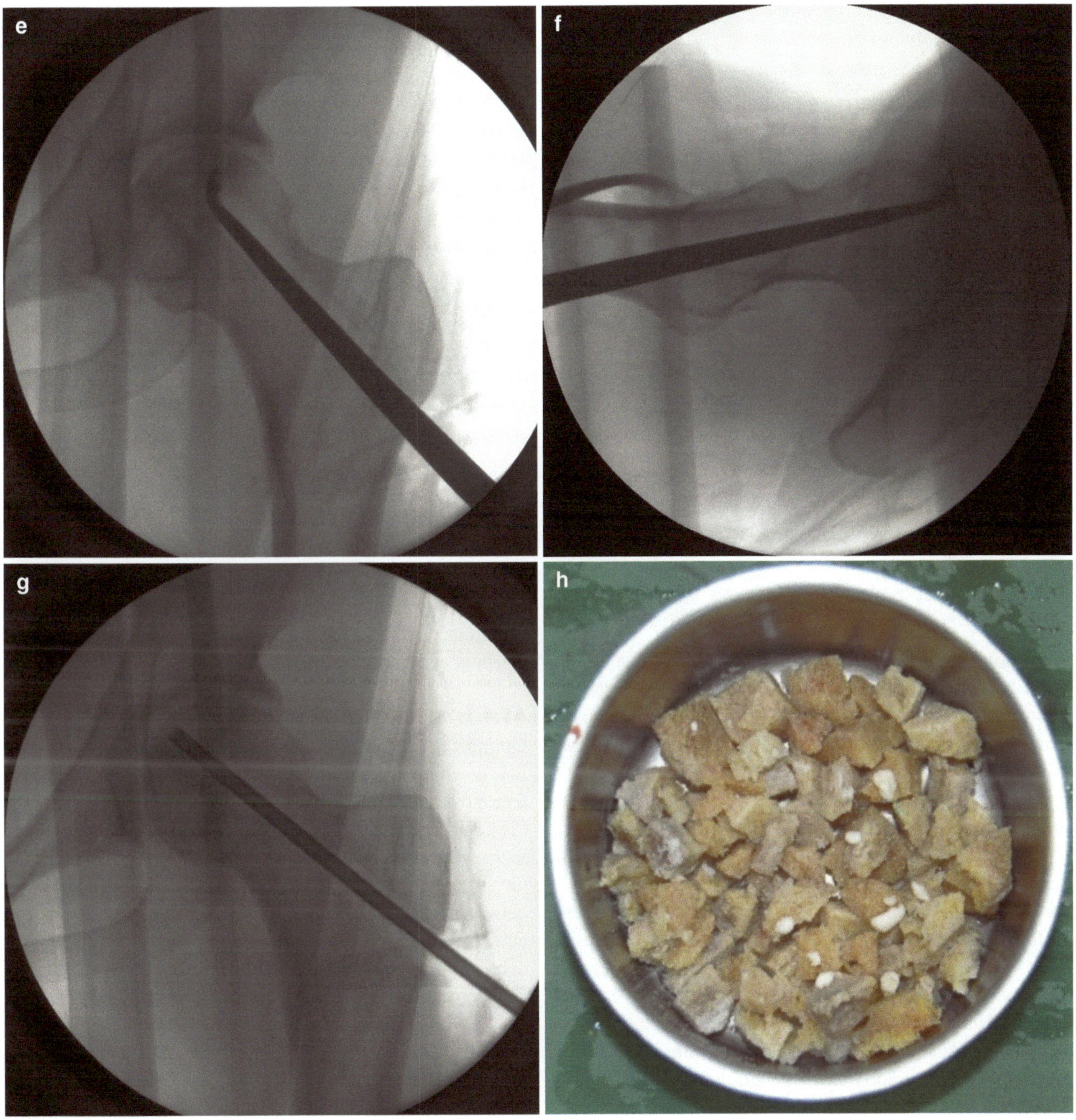

Fig. 41.1 (continued)

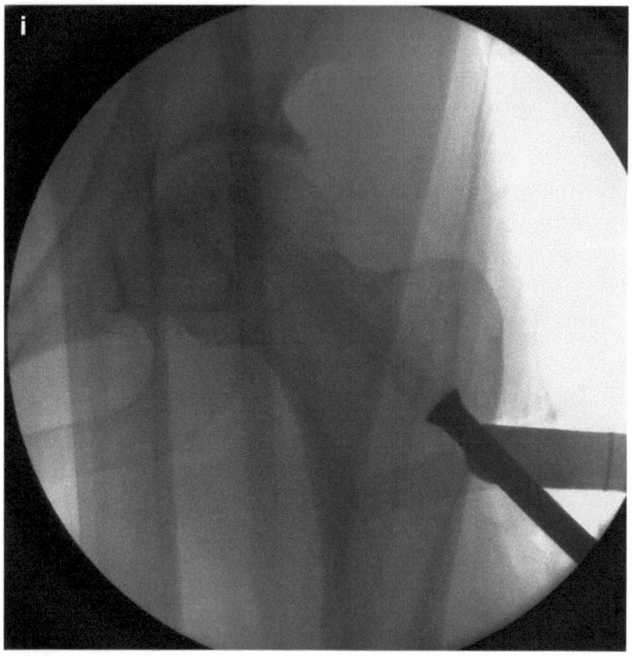

Fig. 41.1 (continued)

impaction grafting (Fig. 41.1d). For histologic evaluation, central core biopsy is taken from the necrotic bone, and the remnant necrotic bone is completely curetted or removed using high-speed burrs under the image intensifier in two directions (Fig. 41.1e, f). Following irrigation of debris, a normal cancellous bone taken during tunneling is shaped into bone chips with a size of 7–10 mm (Fig. 41.1g). The empty space in the femoral head is filled with these bone chips, and solid impaction is applied layer by layer to cover the subchondral bone thoroughly. The remaining tunnel can be filled with fresh-frozen allograft [14] or autogenous iliac bone graft with or without additional allograft [19] depending on the surgeon's preference in the same manner (Fig. 41.1h, i). Care should be taken not to put the cortical window inside the lateral cortex of the femur for possible arthroplasty. Lastly, soft tissues including the vastus lateralis and fascia lata are repaired layer by layer. During 6 weeks after surgery, touch weight-bearing with two crutches is allowed followed by weight-bearing up to a maximum of 50 % body weight in the next 6 weeks. Full weight-bearing is permitted using one crutch to slow down from 3 months after surgery [14].

41.4 Technical Considerations

In addition to head-preserving procedure for ONFH, bone impaction grafting is now widely applied to a variety of orthopedic procedures such as management of osteonecrosis in other joints [20, 21], osteosynthesis for complicated fracture [22] or nonunion with large segmental defects [23], ACL reconstruction [24], and primary arthroplasty [25]. Their results of bone impaction grafting are encouraging, but there are still much room for improvements in surgical techniques and need for standardization for optimal treatment. Long-term results after bone impaction grafting for treating ONFH would be determined by proper patient selection, progression of the disease, and graft incorporation, but initial mechanical stability of the graft by optimal surgical technique will allow for long-term incorporation into the host bone without joint destruction. The understandings of the mechanical properties of impacted bone have recently increased, and despite most of these have originated from bench research for revision arthroplasties, some technical improvement can be applied to bone impaction grafting in the treatment of ONFH as well.

41.4.1 Graft Preparation

The technique of graft preparation in bone impaction grafting has been shown to be of both mechanical and biological importance. This technique includes graft selection and washing and particle size and grading.

41.4.1.1 Choice of Allograft and Washing

Optimizing the fat and water content produces a stronger graft that is more resistant to compressive stresses, preventing the femoral head from collapsing until bone growth will occur [26]. When fresh-frozen allograft is impacted, fat, fluid, and marrow particles in the marrow are either exuded or trapped in the space between particles. Their presence acts as lubricants between particles, reducing the interlocking of particles and allowing the graft to move more freely. Furthermore, the presence of this incompressible fluid damps and resists compressive forces during impaction, preventing the graft particles from moving into a compact bone [26]. Washed graft reducing fat content, however, has little lubricating fluid and better contact between the particles. On mechanical testing, washed graft demonstrated significantly more resistance than those without washing regardless of different particle size, and thus, washing allowed the production of stronger impacted graft [27]. On the contrary, Fosse et al. compared the effect of impaction force, number of impaction strokes, and bone liquid contents on mechanical behavior and demonstrated that the overall major contributor on load stiffness was liquid content [28]. High water content decreased load stiffness during load because liquid filled up more of the pore volume surrounding the bone particles, while low fat content increased stiffness significantly only during the initial phase of loading. Thus, they concluded that the preparation and impaction should be performed under dry conditions to improve the initial stability [29]. Recently, McKenna et al. performed mechanical shear testing in vitro on morselized human femoral heads, varying the amount of fat and water to determine their optimum concentrations [26]. They found that reducing the fat and eliminating water greatly improved the strength of bone graft. They concluded that the most effective means of producing a stable graft was first washing the graft with pulsed lavage reducing the level of fat and subsequent squeezing the graft of its remaining liquid content further reducing the total volume of fluid in an operative setting although it did not reach the ideal concentration of fat and water.

While washing appears to improve the mechanical properties of fresh-frozen allograft, the effect of washing on the biological properties is less clear. Washing the trabecular allografts may enhance graft incorporation by washing out immunological inflammatory factors existing in blood, marrow, and fat, while it can also diminish the incorporation process by washing out biologically active factors stimulating new bone formation [30]. Van der Donk et al. performed animal experiments using autograft and allograft and divided them into three treatment groups as those with impacted, rinsed and impacted, and rinsed, impacted, rinsed, and impacted again. After histologic analyses at 6 weeks, they found that new bone and total tissue ingrowth were higher in autograft than in allografts, especially in the nonrinsed group. With rinsing, total tissue ingrowth increased in the allograft group to approach that of autograft, while rinsing after impaction did not additionally alter bone ingrowth. Thus, they concluded that incorporation of allografts could be improved by rinsing the grafts before impaction [30]. Because autograft contains osteoprogenitor cells and local growth factors to induce the mesenchymal cells to differentiate into mature osteoblasts, rinsing removes beneficial factors from the autograft and leads to poorer incorporation [30].

On the other hand, some authors reported that freeze-dried irradiated grafts showed higher stiffness than fresh-frozen grafts whatever the size of the particles [31, 32]. The brittleness of freeze-dried irradiated bone, caused by loss of the capacity to absorb energy in a plastic way, has been demonstrated to be superior to a fresh-frozen one in a femoral impaction model [31]. Also, Cornu et al. explained improved results with freeze-dried irradiated bone due to incomplete rehydration and increase in the interlocking effect by increasing their water content during later progressive rehydration because rehydration could last for longer than 1 day [32]. Although both fresh-frozen and freeze-dried allograft have demonstrated successful outcome after revision THA [16, 17, 33], there is clearly a lack of quality data in this area, and well-designed clinical trials are required to help inform and guide practice [34].

41.4.1.2 Particle Size

The impacted layer of large particles has been reported to be superior, as a greater magnitude of force would be required to deform the large particles compared to smaller particles [35–37]. Xu et al. compared the mechanical properties of impacted graft with a size of 7–10 mm bone and a small slurry bone with a size of 2 mm [38]. They found that 7–10 mm bone grafts showed higher height, elastic modulus, and massive extrusion strength than those of the small slurry bone grafts. Also, the bone mineral density of the 7–10 mm grafts continued to increase during impaction and became higher than that of the small slurry bone grafts after ten impactions. Bolder et al. performed a gradually increasing dynamic loading experiment with radiostereometric analysis [39]. They found that large bone grafts with an average size of 9 mm produced by hand with a rongeur did provide more initial stability than those with a mean size of 2 mm produced by a bone mill. Therefore, considering these biomechanical studies, the use of large bone chips of between 8 and 10 mm appears to be rational to provide adequate initial stability.

Larger particles have a more porous bone bed between the graft particles, and microvascularity may depend on the graft porosity. Therefore, this use of the larger chips might encourage bone ingrowth and seems to be of benefit not only biomechanically but also biologically [40].

41.4.1.3 Particle Grading

The behavior of impacted graft has been investigated largely using the principles of soil mechanics, and according to them, the mechanical properties of impacted particles are dependent on the particle size distribution (grading) as well as the mechanical properties of the individual particle [27]. Fosse et al. examined the relative influence of different bone particle size, impaction energy, and liquid content on impacted bone stiffness and found that pellets with a wider range of particle sizes had better mechanical properties than those with unisized particles [28]. During impaction, large particles in a well-graded pellet slide in between each other, and with better grading, smaller granules fill the voids resulting in more compaction and less deformation. Dunlop et al. performed mechanical shear testing using fresh-frozen allograft with differing particle size distributions. They demonstrated that a well-graded particle size of allograft was more resistant to shear force. Although these results are encouraging, the effects of a well-graded particle size may be less important than surgical technique, and the impaction may compensate the advantages of a well-graded chip size [40]. Biologically, idealized grading of particle size can make the graft more impacted but bring a detrimental effect on subsequent bone ingrowth due to decreased microcirculation [41, 42].

41.4.2 Impaction Technique

One of the fundamental difficulties of bone impaction grafting wherever it is applied is the intraoperative decision regarding how "vigorous" it should be applied and when the graft can be adequately impacted. The degree of impaction is determined by the impaction force and the number of impaction strikes [43]. No specific guideline, however, exists to standardize the amount of energy transmitted to the bone graft and enable the surgeon to determine when the graft is adequately impacted. This is of clinical importance because subchondral perforation during surgery and progression of collapse was a concern in a previous study (7 %) [14]. Also this concern regarding fracture may lead to under-impaction of the graft and subsequent collapse of femoral head. Thus, in the absence of methods for establishing when the graft is adequately impacted, there should be a significant learning curve between over-impaction causing subchondral perforation and under-impaction leading to collapse of femoral head.

Although experimental model is different from clinical situation and the clinical setting of impaction grafting for ONFH is also different from those for revision THA, Flannery et al. examined the threshold force using adult sow femurs in revision THA [44], and the threshold force before fracture was found to be 4 kN. This force was similar to the maximum force obtained from direct impaction of a slap hammer on the load cell, which was 3.5 kN. Fosse et al. also performed the same experiment using embalmed human femurs. The threshold force was found to be 0.5 kN and four-fifths of the femurs fractured above 1.6 kN. Thus, there is limited information regarding adequate force in bone impaction grafting. Further studies should be performed to determine the threshold force of bone impaction grafting in the treatment of ONFH and monitor this force in the clinical setting as well.

Increased number of strikes can bring the particles to slide in between each other and induce plastic deformation. Obviously, stiffness in impacted morselized bone to a certain extent would increase by number of impactions [45]. This rearrangement, however, would reach plateau above which further strokes fail to impact for increasing stiffness of the graft [28]. Fosse et al. measured graft stiffness stroke-by-stroke [29]. They found that no significant increase in stiffness was achieved after five strokes at the highest drop level, while drop level of the impaction slap hammer increased bone stiffness on each layer of morselized bone during impaction. They also compared factors affecting stiffness properties in impacted morselized bone one by one while keeping all other involved factors constant [28]. Graft with low water content had a major effect, while increasing the number of impaction strokes beyond five per layer had a minor effect. Thus, optimal stability was achieved with dried and well-graded particle, but the number of heavy impaction strokes could be restricted.

Because bone graft is impacted manually with a hammer, the concept of "vigorous impaction" is always subjective [40]. Even if the optimal magnitude of the impaction force as well as the number of strikes would be identified, there always exists a risk of over- or under-impaction. Hostner et al. compared conventional impaction technique with an impaction technique using polished and rotating impactors [46]. They found that this new impaction technique obtained a more reproducible procedure and less risk for fracture and resulted in stability equal to that obtained with the conventional technique. Recently, Putzer et al. compared two different methods of bone impaction grafting [47]. The pneumatic method reduced the risk of fracture in vivo, as force peaks were smaller and applied for a shorter period, while results from manual impaction demonstrated higher variability and depended much on the experience of the surgeon. Thus, they concluded that pneumatic hammer was a suitable tool to standardize the impaction process.

41.5 Results

To date, there have been limited outcomes available after bone impaction grafting in the treatment for ONFH. Rijnen et al. reported the first clinical and radiographic outcomes in English after bone impaction grafting in 28 hips with ONFH (10 steroid induced, 4 alcoholic, 1 hereditary hyperlipidemia, 5 trauma related, 1 SCFE, and 7 idiopathic) (Table 41.1) [14]. Fourteen hips (50 %) already had preoperative collapse of the femoral head. The overall clinical success rate was 64 %, whereas 15 hips (54 %) demonstrated radiographic success at an average follow-up of 43 months. Patients older than 30 years had a significantly higher chance of a radiographic failure (hazard ratio, 6.075). Thus, three patients with an average age of 21 years in stage 4 showed remarkable recoveries and had good clinical results with improvement of Harris hip score (HHS) from 45 points preoperative to 89 points postoperative, while those older than 30 years had a preoperative HHS of 60 points, increasing to 71 points postoperative. They also reported that patients with preoperative collapse and use of corticosteroids had worse results. Park et al. reported the outcome in 42 hips (15 alcoholic, 8 steroid induced, 3 posttraumatic, and 6 idiopathic) according to ARCO classification including stage, quantification, and location [48]. They evaluated radiographic results using MRI after the procedure in 25 hips in which THA was not performed at an average follow-up of 15 months (range 11–23). They demonstrated overall clinical and radiographic success rate to be 74 and 50 %, respectively. They reported that lesions with large involvement (>30 %) or lateral location were significantly associated with clinical and radiographic failure in spite of short period of follow-up (average, 29 months) emphasizing the importance of the location as well as the size of involvement. Jung et al. reported outcomes in 95 hips with ONFH (41 alcoholic, 42 steroid induced, and

Table 41.1 Clinical and radiographic results after bone impaction grafting

	Hips (patients)	F-U (range), *months*	Age (range), *years*	Stage (hips)	Quantification	Location (hips)	Clinical success (%)	Radiographic success (%)			THA conversion (hips)	Complication (hips)
								Stage	Quantification	Location		
Rijnen et al. [14][a]	28 (27)	43 (24–119)	33 (15–55)	2 (11)	Combined angle >200° in all hips	NA	2 (73)	2 (73)	NA	NA	2 (2)	Perforation of cartilage (2)
				3 early (3)			3 early (67)	3 early (33)			3 early (6)	
				3 late (11)			3 late (45)	3 late (36)			3 late (5)	
				4 (3)			4 (100)	4 (67)			4 (0)	
Park et al. [48][a,b]	42 (32)	29 (12–41)	38.2 (15–69)	1B(1)/C(8)	A(1)	M(8)	1B(100)/C(100)	1(78)	A(100)	M(88)	2C(8)	None
				2A(1)/B(6)/C(22)	B(7)	C(8)	2A(100)/B(100)/C(64)	2(45)	B(86)	C(100)	3C(3)	
				3C(4)	C(34)	L(26)	3C(75)	3(25)	C(41)	L(23)		
							M(100)					
							C(100)					
							L(58)					
Jung et al. [19][b,c,d]	95 (64)	43.3 (24–95)	36.6 (16–53)	I(18)	A(24)	M(0)	A(92)	NA	A(79)	C(92)	A(2)	Subtrochanter fracture (1)
				IIA(45)/B(27)	B(40)	C(12)	B(95)		B(55)	L(40)	B(1)	
				III(5)	C(24)	L(33)	C(50)		C(8)		C(9)	
					D(7)		D(29)		D(14)		D(4)	
							C(100)					
							L(75)					
Aarvold et al. [49][c,e]	5(4)	NA (22–44)	35.4 (31–42)	II(5)	NA	NA	60 %	II(60)	NA	NA	2 hips	None

NA not available, *F-U* follow-up, *M* medial, *C* central, *L* lateral
[a]ARCO classification [50]
[b]THA was performed only in hips with lateral involvement of the head
[c]Modified Ficat classification [51]
[d]Koo classification [52]
[e]Skeletal stem cells and milled allograft were impacted

12 idiopathic). The overall clinical success rate was 78 %, whereas 44 hips (46 %) demonstrated radiographic success at an average follow-up of 43 months. They also concluded that lesions with large involvement or lateral location were significantly associated with radiographic failure.

41.6 Future Solution and Application of Bone Impaction Grafting

41.6.1 Future Solution

In the literatures, there still is much discussion regarding the optimal treatment for the disease according to different stage, size, and location. Although the short-term outcome is encouraging, few reports using bone impaction grafting as a treatment for ONFH are available in English literatures [14]. For appropriate patient selection, more longer-term reports analyzing outcomes according to the disease stage, size, and location of the lesion will be necessary. Neither has been a report comparing with natural history or other type of head-preserving procedures such as core decompression alone, nonvascularized or vascularized bone graft, osteotomy, and electrical stimulation. Therefore, when long-term reports comparing with these procedures become available, the value of this procedure and its place in the treatment for ONFH will be determined.

Influence of packing density and thickness of cancellous graft on the graft incorporation is another concern. It still remains unclear whether or how these impacted grafts used in the femoral head for treating osteonecrosis will incorporate. Impaction can decrease the graft porosity and subsequent revascularization, and bone conduction may depend on the microporosity of the grafted impacted bone as well. Tagil et al. measured the mean distance which the ingrown bone had reached into the graft after impaction on histology [42]. With pressures of either 25 or 2,500 MPa, the ingrowth distance of the impacted bone decreased to 30 % of the unimpacted controls. They concluded that impaction itself did not have a favorable effect on the osteoconductive properties of bone graft. Therefore, more investigation regarding biological fate after bone impaction grafting in the femoral head with ONFH will be necessary.

41.6.2 Future Application

Because bone impaction grafting can provide mechanical support and has biological advantages of bone graft, interest has been shown in combining this procedure with additives such as calcium phosphate cement [53], synthetic hydroxyapatite [54], demineralized bone matrix (DBM) [55], bone morphogenetic proteins [56], and skeletal stem cell (SSC) [49] to augment mechanical and biological characteristics of the graft. To date, two literatures have been reported after bone impaction grafting combined with these additives in the clinical setting of treating ONFH. Rijnen et al. [53] created a critically sized subchondral defect model in 15 goats following the trapdoor procedure. Defects filled with morselized cancellous bone demonstrated complete incorporation and remodeling to a normal trabecular structure, while in those filled with morselized cancellous bone/calcium phosphate cement, most of the calcium phosphate cement was resorbed by 12 weeks and the mixture was largely replaced by fibrous or fatty marrow. They concluded that the addition of calcium phosphate cement to cancellous bone grafts did not improve the process of incorporation and remodeling into new bone and was not suitable to use in critically sized animal model. Recently, Aarvold et al. impacted a concentrated pool of pluripotent SSCs from the posterior iliac crest and milled allograft into necrotic bone in 5 femoral heads with osteonecrosis (1 alcoholic, 3 steroid induced, and 1 idiopathic) [49]. They found that three patients remained asymptomatic at the follow-up of 22–44 months (Table 41.1). Two hips underwent THA and retrieved femoral heads at 13 and 19 months demonstrated mature trabecular microarchitecture on histology and on micro-CT, and bone density and axial compression strength were comparable to the trabecular bone. Although clinical works at present are limited to case reports and small clinical series, the results of these combinations to improve graft incorporation and regeneration appear to be promising [57].

Conclusion

Impaction bone grafting has been originally developed from the technique for reconstruction of bone defects in revision THA. It does not produce donor site morbidity and does not disturb the procedure in future THA. Although it is relatively simple in technique, there still remained a few considerations to improve initial mechanical stability and biological incorporation simultaneously. To date, there have been limited short-term outcomes available after bone impaction grafting in the treatment for ONFH. It seems to be effective in small- or medium-sized lesion with medial or central location in early-stage ONFH. However, it does not appear to be effective for large-sized and laterally located lesion in early-stage ONFH. Additives such as calcium phosphate cement and skeletal stem cell to augment mechanical and biological characteristics of the impaction graft did not improve the outcomes. Also, there is no report comparing with natural history or other joint-preserving procedures. Appropriate selection of patients with specific lesion size and location and stage of disease should be determined for this procedure in the future.

References

1. Mont MA, Jones LC, Einhorn TA, Hungerford DS, Reddi AH. Osteonecrosis of the femoral head. Potential treatment with growth and differentiation factors. Clin Orthop Relat Res. 1998;(355 suppl):S314–35.
2. Arlet J, Ficat R. Forage-biopsie de la tete femorale dans l' osteonecrose primative. Obs ervations histopathologiques portant sur huit foranes. Rev Rhum Ed Fr. 1964;31:257–64.
3. Eisenschenk A, Lautenbach M, Schwetlick G, Weber U. Treatment of femoral head necrosis with vascularized iliac crest transplants. Clin Orthop Relat Res. 2001;386:100–5.
4. Judet H, Gilbert A. Long-term results of free vascularized fibular grafting for femoral head necrosis. Clin Orthop Relat Res. 2001;386:114–9.
5. Phemister DB. Treatment of the necrotic head of the femur in adults. J Bone Joint Surg Am. 1949;31A:55–66.
6. Smith KR, Bonfiglio M, Montgomery WJ. Non-traumatic necrosis of the femoral head treated with tibial bone-grafting. A follow-up note. J Bone Joint Surg Am. 1980;62:845–7.
7. Koo KH, Kim R, Ko GH, Song HR, Jeong ST, Cho SH. Preventing collapse in early osteonecrosis of the femoral head. A randomised clinical trial of core decompression. J Bone Joint Surg Br. 1995;77:870–4.
8. Penix AR, Cook SD, Skinner HB, Weinstein AM, Haddad Jr RJ. Femoral head stresses following cortical bone grafting for aseptic necrosis. A finite element study. Clin Orthop Relat Res. 1983;173:159–65.
9. Bakx PA, van Biezen FC, van Linge B. Failure of tibial bone grafting for femoral head necrosis. Acta Orthop Scand. 1991;62:230–1.
10. Mont MA, Hungerford DS. Non-traumatic avascular necrosis of the femoral head. J Bone Joint Surg Am. 1995;77:459–74.
11. Vail TP, Urbaniak JR. Donor-site morbidity with use of vascularized autogenous fibular grafts. J Bone Joint Surg Am. 1996; 78:204–11.
12. Fehrle MJ, Callaghan JJ, Clark CR, Peterson KK. Uncemented total hip arthroplasty in patients with aseptic necrosis of the femoral head and previous bone grafting. J Arthroplasty. 1993;8:1–6.
13. Berend KR, Gunneson E, Urbaniak JR, Vail TP. Hip arthroplasty after failed free vascularized fibular grafting for osteonecrosis in young patients. J Arthroplasty. 2003;18:411–9.
14. Rijnen WH, Gardeniers JW, Buma P, Yamano K, Slooff TJ, Schreurs BW. Treatment of femoral head osteonecrosis using bone impaction grafting. Clin Orthop Relat Res. 2003;417:74–83.
15. Slooff TJ, Huiskes R, van Horn J, Lemmens AJ. Bone grafting in total hip replacement for acetabular protrusion. Acta Orthop Scand. 1984;55:593–6.
16. te Stroet MA, Gardeniers JW, Verdonschot N, Rijnen WH, Slooff TJ, Schreurs BW. Femoral component revision with use of impaction bone-grafting and a cemented polished stem: a concise follow-up, at fifteen to twenty years, of a previous report. J Bone Joint Surg Am. 2012;94:e1731–4.
17. Schreurs BW, Bolder SB, Gardeniers JW, Verdonschot N, Slooff TJ, Veth RP. Acetabular revision with impacted morsellised cancellous bone grafting and a cemented cup. A 15- to 20-year follow-up. J Bone Joint Surg Br. 2004;86:492–7.
18. van der Donk S, Buma P, Slooff TJ, Gardeniers JW, Schreurs BW. Incorporation of morselized bone grafts: a study of 24 acetabular biopsy specimens. Clin Orthop Relat Res. 2002;396:131–41.
19. Jung K-H, Jang J-S, Choi Y-R. Core decompression and impaction bone graft in osteonecrosis of the femoral head. J Korean Hip Soc. 2005;17:223–9.
20. Rijnen WH, Luttjeboer JS, Schreurs BW, Gardeniers JW. Bone impaction grafting for corticosteroid-associated osteonecrosis of the knee. J Bone Joint Surg Am. 2006;88 Suppl 3:62–8.
21. Jiang JJ, Hussain WM, Bielski RJ. Bone impaction grafting of the lateral femoral condyle in a pediatric patient. Orthopedics. 2012;35:e1533–6.
22. Kim SH, Lee YH, Chung SW, Shin SH, Jang WY, Gong HS, Baek GH. Outcomes for four-part proximal humerus fractures treated with a locking compression plate and an autologous iliac bone impaction graft. Injury. 2012;43:1724–31.
23. Solomon LB, Callary SA, Boopalan PR, Chakrabarty A, Costi JJ, Howie DW. Impaction bone grafting of segmental bone defects in femoral non-unions. Acta Orthop Belg. 2013;79:64–70.
24. Gokce A, Beyzadeoglu T, Ozyer F, Bekler H, Erdogan F. Does bone impaction technique reduce tunnel enlargement in ACL reconstruction? Int Orthop. 2009;33:407–12.
25. Li H, Wang L, Dai K, Zhu Z. Autogenous impaction grafting in total hip arthroplasty with developmental dysplasia of the hip. J Arthroplasty. 2013;28:637–43.
26. McKenna PB, Leahy JJ, Masterson EL, McGloughlin TM. Optimizing the fat and water content of impaction bone allograft. J Orthop Res. 2013;31:243–8.
27. Dunlop DG, Brewster NT, Madabhushi SP, Usmani AS, Pankaj P, Howie CR. Techniques to improve the shear strength of impacted bone graft: the effect of particle size and washing of the graft. J Bone Joint Surg Am. 2003;85-A:639–46.
28. Fosse L, Ronningen H, Benum P, Lydersen S, Sandven RB. Factors affecting stiffness properties in impacted morsellized bone used in revision hip surgery: an experimental in vitro study. J Biomed Mater Res A. 2006;78:423–31.
29. Fosse L, Ronningen H, Benum P, Sandven RB. Influence of water and fat content on compressive stiffness properties of impacted morsellized bone: an experimental ex vivo study on bone pellets. Acta Orthop. 2006;77:15–22.
30. van der Donk S, Weernink T, Buma P, Aspenberg P, Slooff TJ, Schreurs BW. Rinsing morselized allografts improves bone and tissue ingrowth. Clin Orthop Relat Res. 2003;408:302–10.
31. Cornu O, Libouton X, Naets B, Godts B, Van Tomme J, Delloye C, Banse X. Freeze-dried irradiated bone brittleness improves compactness in an impaction bone grafting model. Acta Orthop Scand. 2004;75:309–14.
32. Cornu O, Schubert T, Libouton X, Manil O, Godts B, Van Tomme J, Banse X, Delloye C. Particle size influence in an impaction bone grafting model. Comparison of fresh-frozen and freeze-dried allografts. J Biomech. 2009;42:2238–42.
33. de Roeck NJ, Drabu KJ. Impaction bone grafting using freeze-dried allograft in revision hip arthroplasty. J Arthroplasty. 2001;16: 201–6.
34. Board TN, Brunskill S, Doree C, Hyde C, Kay PR, Meek RD, Webster R, Galea G. Processed versus fresh frozen bone for impaction bone grafting in revision hip arthroplasty. Cochrane Database Syst Rev. 2009;7141:CD006351.
35. Giesen EB, Lamerigts NM, Verdonschot N, Buma P, Schreurs BW, Huiskes R. Mechanical characteristics of impacted morsellised bone grafts used in revision of total hip arthroplasty. J Bone Joint Surg Br. 1999;81:1052–7.
36. Ullmark G. Bigger size and defatting of bone chips will increase cup stability. Arch Orthop Trauma Surg. 2000;120:445–7.
37. Arts JJ, Verdonschot N, Buma P, Schreurs BW. Larger bone graft size and washing of bone grafts prior to impaction enhances the initial stability of cemented cups: experiments using a synthetic acetabular model. Acta Orthop. 2006;77:227–33.
38. Xu ZJ, Chen LY, Zhong C, Tan YB, He RX. Mechanical properties of 7-10mm bone grafts and small slurry grafts in impaction bone grafting. J Orthop Res. 2011;29:1491–5.
39. Bolder SB, Schreurs BW, Verdonschot N, van Unen JM, Gardeniers JW, Slooff TJ. Particle size of bone graft and method of impaction affect initial stability of cemented cups: human cadaveric and synthetic pelvic specimen studies. Acta Orthop Scand. 2003;74: 652–7.
40. McNamara IR. Impaction bone grafting in revision hip surgery: past, present and future. Cell Tissue Bank. 2010;11:57–73.

41. Pratt JN, Griffon DJ, Dunlop DG, Smith N, Howie CR. Impaction grafting with morsellised allograft and tricalcium phosphate-hydroxyapatite: incorporation within ovine metaphyseal bone defects. Biomaterials. 2002;23:3309–17.
42. Tagil M, Aspenberg P. Impaction of cancellous bone grafts impairs osteoconduction in titanium chambers. Clin Orthop Relat Res. 1998;352:231–8.
43. Fosse L, Ronningen H, Lund-Larsen J, Benum P, Grande L. Impacted bone stiffness measured during construction of morsellised bone samples. J Biomech. 2004;37:1757–66.
44. Flannery OM, Britton JR, O'Reilly P, Mahony N, Prendergast PJ, Kenny PJ. The threshold force required for femoral impaction grafting in revision hip surgery. Acta Orthop. 2010;81:303–7.
45. Bavadekar A, Cornu O, Godts B, Delloye C, Van Tomme J, Banse X. Stiffness and compactness of morselized grafts during impaction: an in vitro study with human femoral heads. Acta Orthop Scand. 2001;72:470–6.
46. Hostner J, Hultmark P, Karrholm J, Malchau H, Tveit M. Impaction technique and graft treatment in revisions of the femoral component: laboratory studies and clinical validation. J Arthroplasty. 2001;16:76–82.
47. Putzer D, Mayr E, Haid C, Reinthaler A, Nogler M. Impaction bone grafting: a laboratory comparison of two methods. J Bone Joint Surg Br. 2011;93:1049–53.
48. Park YS, Rim YS, Park YK, Yun SH. Core decompression and impaction bone graft in avascular necrosis of the femoral head. J Korean Orthop Assoc. 1999;34:425–30.
49. Aarvold A, Smith JO, Tayton ER, Jones AM, Dawson JI, Lanham S, Briscoe A, Dunlop DG, Oreffo RO. From bench to clinic and back: skeletal stem cells and impaction bone grafting for regeneration of bone defects. J Tissue Eng Regen Med. 2007;459:216–21.
50. Gardeniers JWM. Report of the committee of staging and nomenclature. ARCO News Letter. 1993;2:79–82.
51. Ficat RP. Idiopathic bone necrosis of the femoral head. Early diagnosis and treatment. J Bone Joint Surg Br. 1985;67:3–9.
52. Koo KH, Kim R. Quantifying the extent of osteonecrosis of the femoral head. A new method using mri. J Bone Joint Surg Br. 1995;77:875–80.
53. Rijnen WH, Gardeniers JW, Schreurs BW, Buma P. Impacted bone and calcium phosphate cement for repair of femoral head defects: a pilot study. Clin Orthop Relat Res. 2007;459:216–21.
54. Aulakh TS, Jayasekera N, Kuiper JH, Richardson JB. Long-term clinical outcomes following the use of synthetic hydroxyapatite and bone graft in impaction in revision hip arthroplasty. Biomaterials. 2009;30:1732–8.
55. Wang BL, Sun W, Shi ZC, Zhang NF, Yue DB, Guo WS, Shi SH, Li ZR. Treatment of nontraumatic osteonecrosis of the femoral head using bone impaction grafting through a femoral neck window. Int Orthop. 2010;34:635–9.
56. Tagil M, Jeppsson C, Aspenberg P. Bone graft incorporation. Effects of osteogenic protein-1 and impaction. Clin Orthop Relat Res. 1985;67:3–9.
57. Bolland BJ, Tilley S, New AM, Dunlop DG, Oreffo RO. Adult mesenchymal stem cells and impaction grafting: a new clinical paradigm shift. Expert Rev Med Devices. 2007;4:393–404.

42 Principles of Bone Grafting for Osteonecrosis of the Hip

Julio J. Jauregui, Samik Banerjee, Bhaveen H. Kapadia, Jeffrey J. Cherian, Kimona Issa, and Michael A. Mont

42.1 Introduction

Osteonecrosis of the femoral head (ONFH) is a disease that mainly affects patients in the third and fourth decades of life, which often leads to femoral head collapse and subsequent destruction of the hip joint [1, 2]. Depending on the time of insult and the stage of osteonecrosis, many therapeutic options are available such as core decompression, rotational osteotomy, bone grafting, resurfacing of the femoral head, and total hip arthroplasty [3].

The use of a nonvascularized tibial graft to treat ONFH was described by Phemister in 1949 [4]. Subsequently, in 1958 Bonfiglio and Bardenstein described nonvascularized fibular grafting [5]. Vascularized bone grafting for ONFH was first described in 1978 by Meyers et al. who described the use of a vascularized muscle pedicle bone graft combined with fresh iliac bone chips [6]. In 1980 free fibular vascularized grafting was described by Judet et al. [7] and subsequently popularized by Urbaniak et al. in 1995 [8]. Since then, many studies have been published using vascularized and nonvascularized bone grafting for ONFH with varying success rates [9].

42.2 Bone Grafting

The results achieved with bone grafting have been shown to vary depending on the stage of osteonecrosis [1]. Furthermore, although it has been shown to be more successful in pre-collapse and early post-collapse lesions, it has not been demonstrated to be effective in advanced stages [10]. Although the decision for bone grafting is based on preoperative radiographic staging, occasionally, more advanced stage disease may be found intraoperatively, necessitating a conversion to a resurfacing arthroplasty or a total hip arthroplasty [11]. Some of the advantages of bone grafting include stimulation of repair following removal of weak necrotic bone and decompression of the femoral head [1]. Bone grafts also work as a scaffold for new bone to grow and may give structural stability to the weakened necrotic femoral head [12]. Bone grafts can be divided into two broad categories such as vascularized and nonvascularized grafts. Vascularized bone grafts have many variations, but can be broadly divided into three categories, which are vascularized free fibular grafts, vascularized iliac bone grafts, and muscle pedicle grafting. Various techniques described for nonvascularized bone grafting of the femoral head include grafting through the femoral neck or the head–neck junction (light bulb procedure) [13], cortical strut grafting through a core in the femoral head (Phemister) [5], and grafting through the articular cartilage (trapdoor procedure) [3].

42.2.1 Vascularized Bone Grafting

Vascularized bone grafting can be broadly divided into three types: The first type is muscle pedicle grafting, which uses the muscles vasculature for blood supply [2]; second, vascularized fibular grafting, which uses the vascular pedicle of the fibula anastomosed to the lateral circumflex femoral artery as blood supply [14]; and, third, an iliac bone pedicle, which gets its blood supply from the deep circumflex iliac vessels [8]. Vascularized grafting has been shown to be more efficacious than nonvascularized bone grafting due to a higher amount of osteocytes having adequate vascularity. Furthermore, it is believed that vascularized grafting maintains osteoconductive and osteoinductive properties.

J.J. Jauregui • S. Banerjee • B.H. Kapadia • J.J. Cherian • K. Issa
M.A. Mont (✉)
Department of Orthopaedic Surgery, Rubin Institute for Advanced Orthopedics, Center for Joint Preservation and Replacement, Sinai Hospital of Baltimore, 2401 West Belvedere Avenue, Baltimore, MD 21215, USA
e-mail: juljau@gmail.com; bashb02@gmail.com; bhaveen.k@gmail.com; jjaicherian@gmail.com; kissa@buffalo.edu; mmont@lifebridgehealth.org, rhondamont@aol.com

K.-H. Koo et al. (eds.), *Osteonecrosis*,
DOI 10.1007/978-3-642-35767-1_42, © Springer-Verlag Berlin Heidelberg 2014

42.2.2 Muscle Pedicle Grafting

This procedure entails the use of four muscles and their pedicles, namely, the quadratus femoris graft (posterolateral approach), the sartorius graft (anterolateral approach), the tensor fascia lata, and the gluteus medius graft (lateral approach) [2, 6, 15]. The decision on whether to use one or more muscle pedicle bone grafts (MPBG) depends mainly on the localization of the necrotic area in the femoral head. Even though the tensor fascia lata graft appears to be better vascularized than the sartorius graft, these two can be used if the anterosuperior part of the femoral head is affected. However, if the necrotic area is posterior, the quadratus femoris or the gluteus medius muscle pedicle may be used [16].

42.2.2.1 Surgical Technique

Depending on the location of the osteonecrotic segment, the muscle pedicle is chosen as described previously. The muscle pedicle bone graft is elevated from its bed, maintaining its vascular supply. Next, through an appropriate approach, an arthrotomy is made to expose the femoral neck. Using curettes or a power-assisted burr, the necrotic bone found in the femoral head should be excised through a window in the head–neck junction. Subsequently, the MPBG can be inserted into the defect previously created in the femoral neck. During mobilization of the muscle pedicle, care should be taken to avoid axial torsion of the vascular pedicle, so that the blood supply is not jeopardized [2, 6, 15].

42.2.3 Free Fibular Vascularized Grafting

Free vascularized fibular grafting is usually performed after a core is made to relieve pressure and remove the necrotic bone from the femoral head. A vascularized fibular graft provides a nascent vascular source to aid healing of the osteonecrotic region as well as providing structural support that may prevent collapse of the articular cartilage [9].

42.2.3.1 Surgical Technique

Separate teams ideally should perform this operation simultaneously. The proximal femur is exposed through the interval between the gluteus medius and tensor fascia lata muscles. The lateral circumflex artery and vein are isolated as well as their ascending cervical branches. Under fluoroscopic guidance, a guide pin is used to localize the center of the osteonecrotic lesion. Following this, cannulated reamers of increasing diameters between 16 and 21 mm are used to create a core that starts at the lateral femoral cortex (distal to the vastus ridge) and extends to within 3–5 mm of the articular cartilage of the femoral head [8, 14].

The fibular graft should be obtained from the ipsilateral leg and usually measures approximately 13 cm. It is important to leave at least 10 cm of fibula unharvested at each end. The vascular pedicle of the peroneal vessels should be left as long as possible and left attached to the graft. The graft can, however, be trimmed to obtain the desired length. The periosteum is then peeled off 3–4 mm from the insertion end of the graft and is fixed to the bone to avoid stripping of the vascular pedicle during the procedure. Care should be taken to ensure that the core diameter exceeds the graft diameter by at least 2 mm to avoid compressing the vascular supply of the fibula [17].

A gap is created by releasing the vastus intermedius and lateralis, so that the lateral circumflex and peroneal vessels can be anastomosed without any tension. The graft is then stabilized to the proximal femur with a Kirschner wire. Following completion of the procedure, back bleeding from the base of the fibular graft should be obtained to confirm viability of the graft. See Fig. 42.1.

42.2.4 Vascularized Iliac Bone Grafting

Vascularized iliac crest bone grafts is one of the many vascularized procedures used in osteonecrosis of the femoral head for restoration of blood supply [18, 19].

42.2.4.1 Surgical Technique

After an incision made along the iliac crest and downward, it is important to identify, dissect, and ligate the first few tributaries of the deep circumflex iliac artery. A tricortical iliac bone graft is harvested, keeping its vascular pedicle intact. In addition, cortico-cancellous chips are also harvested from the iliac crest [20]. The joint capsule is then exposed by separating the interval between the sartorius and tensor fascia lata superficially, and the interval between the gluteus medius and the rectus femoralis underneath. An arthrotomy is made to expose the femoral neck. With a high-speed burr, under direct vision, the necrotic bone is excised from the anterior aspect of the head–neck junction. The vascularized graft with its pedicle is then mobilized and fixed to the femoral neck after the defect is packed with cancellous bone graft.

42.3 Nonvascularized Bone Grafting

Nonvascularized bone grafting has been used because cancellous bone graft provides an osteoconductive and osteoinductive substrate for filling of voids left after decompressive procedures in the treatment of osteonecrosis of the femoral head. One of the limitations with nonvascularized bone grafting is that it fails to improve the vascularity of the recipient femoral head [12]. The three basic types of nonvascularized grafts used in ONFH are femoral neck grafting, cortical strut grafting, and grafting through the articular cartilage.

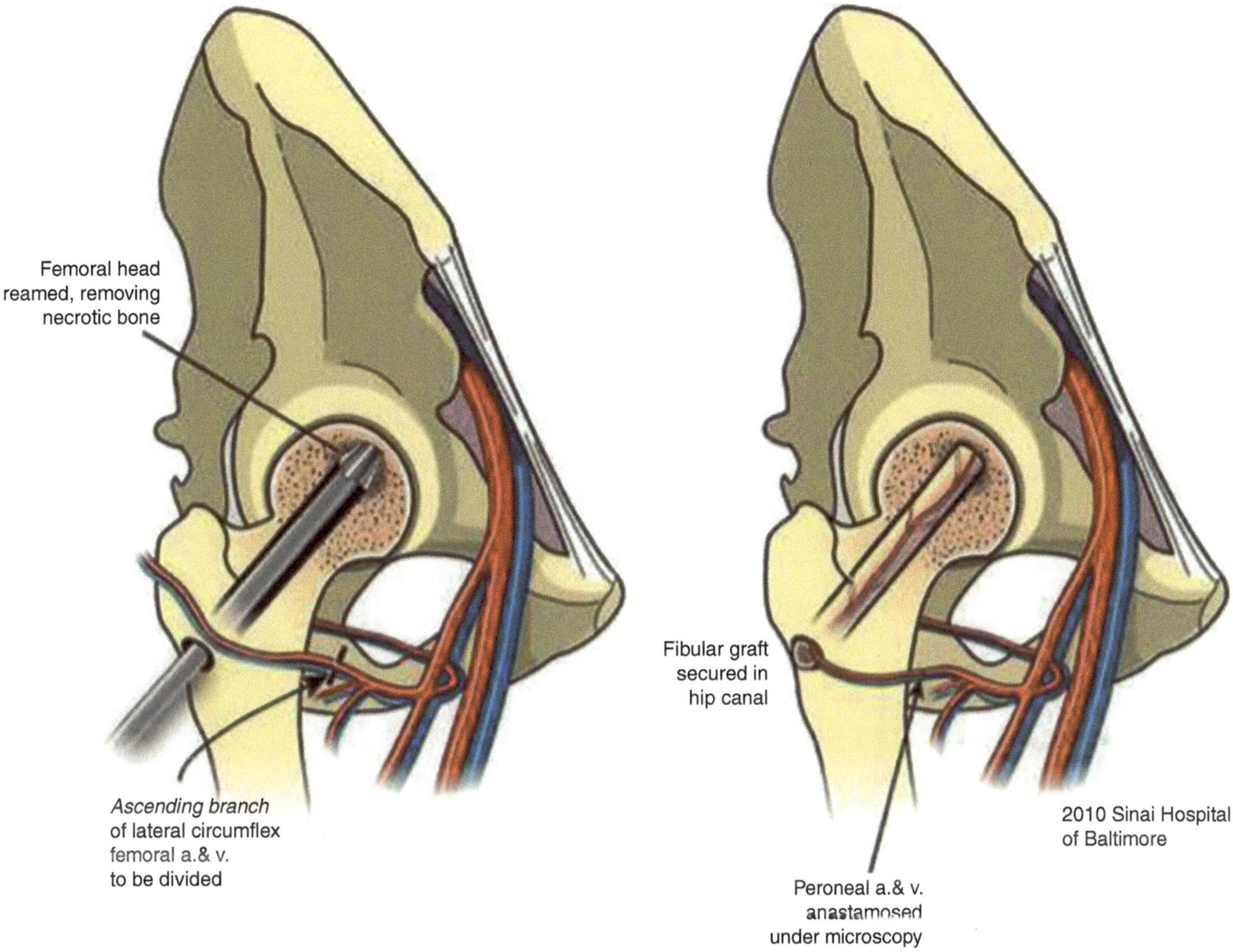

Fig. 42.1 Vascularized fibula grafting

42.3.1 Femoral Neck Grafting (Light Bulb Procedure)

In the early pre-collapse stages of the disease, the necrotic region of the femoral head can be replaced with cancellous bone graft in an effort to aid healing of the lesion.

42.3.1.1 Surgical Technique

After the proximal femur is exposed, an approximate 1.0 by 1.5 cm bone window should be made at the femoral head–neck junction using osteotomes. Through the window previously created, a curette is used to create a cavity inside the femoral head and remove all of the necrotic bone found up to the sub-cartilage bone lamellae. Then measure the volume of the light bulb-shaped cavity using saline solution. The sclerotic bone should then be perforated using a power-assisted drill until bleeding bone is found. The next would be to obtain the bone graft which can typically be an auto-iliac-harvested bone (cortical and cancellous bone) combined with demineralized bone matrix. Subsequently, bone graft should be packed into layers to fill the light bulb-shaped cavity. At last the cortical segment previously removed should be replaced and fixed with one 3-mm absorbable pin [13]. See Figs. 42.2 and 42.3.

42.3.2 Cortical Strut Grafting (Phemister)

Cortical strut grafting was first described by Phemister in 1949 [4] and is therefore commonly known as the Phemister procedure. It consists of drilling two cores of bone that will decompress the femoral head. The large surface area is presumed to act as conduit for blood vessels to grow and perfuse the femoral head. In addition, the bone grafts provide mechanical stability to prevent articular surface collapse [4].

42.3.2.1 Surgical Technique

After exposure of the greater trochanter and femoral neck, two 2-mm guide pins are inserted under fluoroscopic guidance with a power-assisted drill. The first pin is inserted

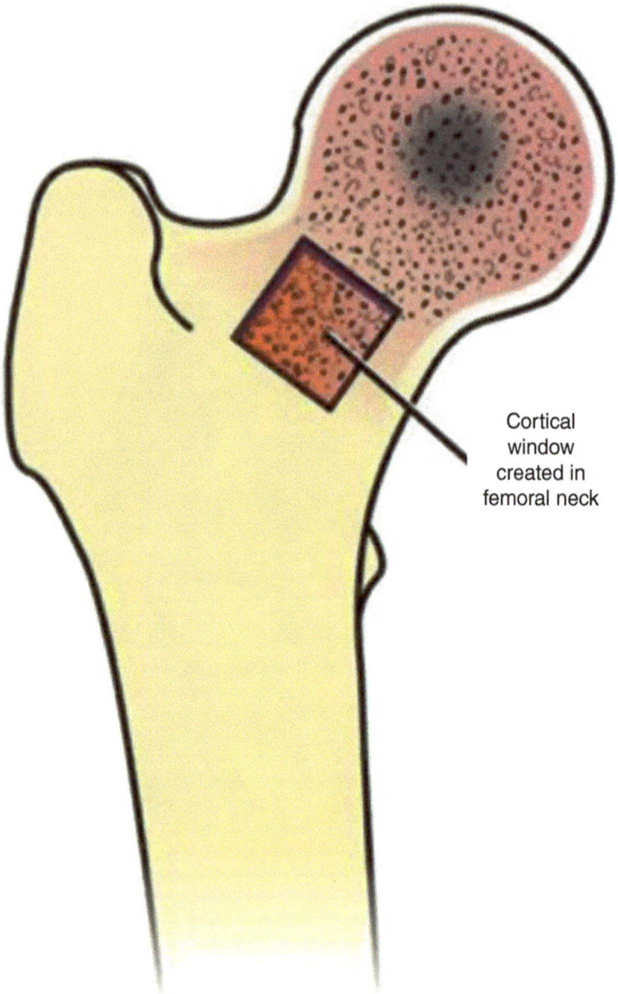

Fig. 42.2 Light bulb procedure

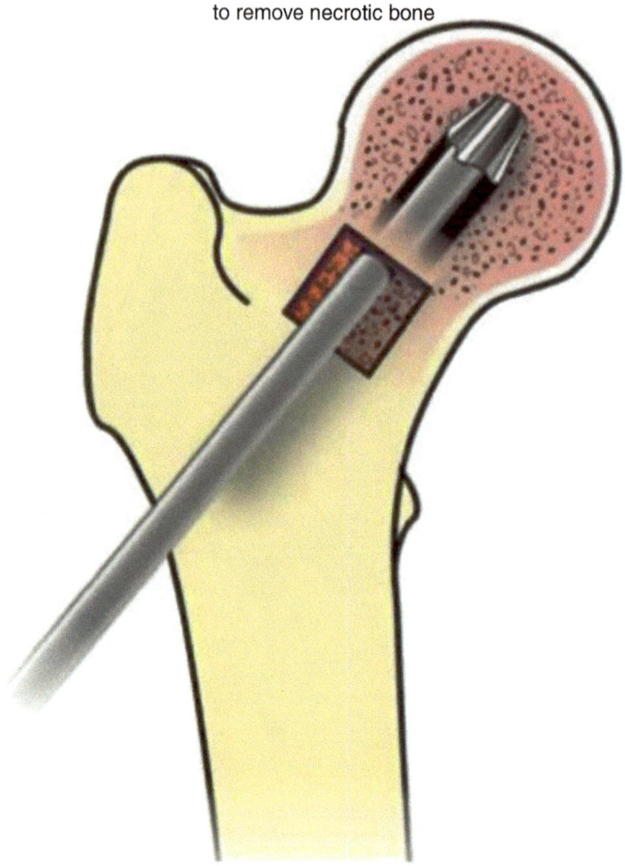

Fig. 42.3 Removal of necrotic bone during the light bulb procedure

below the vastus tubercle of the greater trochanter and directed toward the anterior superior half of the femoral head until it is placed in the subchondral bone. The second pin should be inserted 1.5–2 cm below the previous pin and should aim 1 cm below the level of the subchondral cortex. These pins are used as a guide to drill 4–5 cm with a 7- and then a 9-mm cannulated drill. This will prepare the outer portion of the channel. Subsequently, drilling is performed without the pins at low speeds with a Phemister trephine (using saline to avoid overheating) through the previous channels until the necrotic bone is taken out. The core tissue which is removed during the procedure should be sent for histopathological examination. The procedure should then be repeated in the inferior channel.

To obtain the graft, there should be an adequate exposure of the anteromedial part of the tibia, and the periosteum should be vertically stripped (approximately 13 mm wide). With a twin-oscillating saw, a 10-mm wide graft (kept cool with saline), which is long enough for both channels, should be used. The tibial bone grafts should be trimmed to remove excess cancellous bone from the posterior surface and to achieve the desired length. The exact length of the channels should be measured, and the graft should be cut to accurately fit the channel. The grafts are then inserted (so that the broad surface is in the coronal plane) and tapped until it gets to the subchondral plane [5, 21].

42.3.3 Grafting Through the Articular Cartilage (Trapdoor Procedure)

In advanced cases, or when the articular cartilage is compromised, bone grafting through a so-called trapdoor in the femoral head may be considered as an alternative procedure. The nonvascularized cortical and cancellous autografts, which replace the necrotic bone, may act as support for the subchondral bone and cartilage, as well as stimulating bone formation [3].

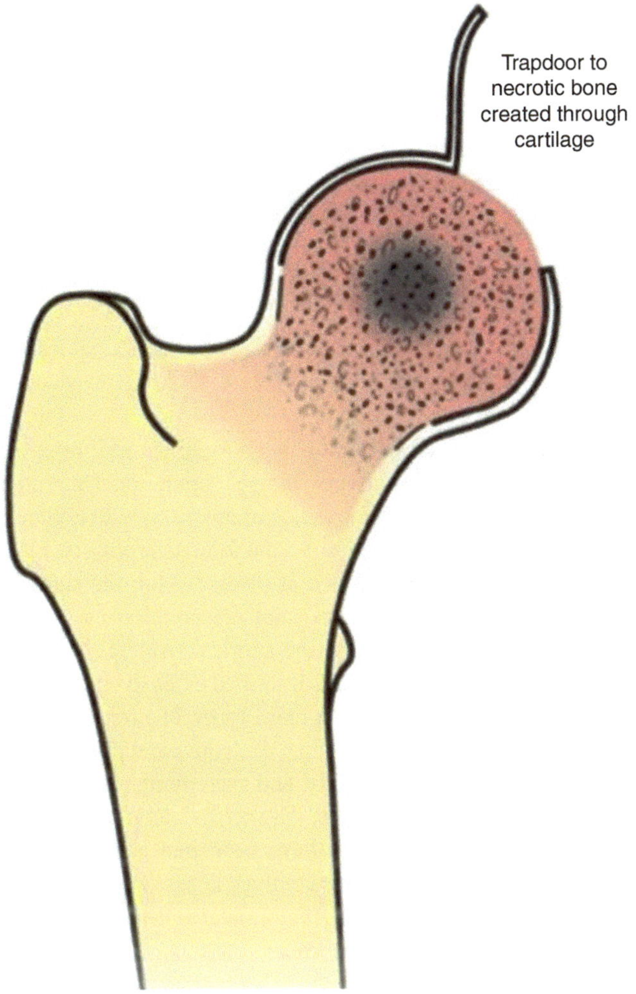

Fig. 42.4 Trapdoor procedure

42.3.3.1 Surgical Technique

After an adequate exposure of the hip's capsule is obtained, it is incised at the superior rim of the acetabulum and peeled back posteriorly and anteriorly, maintaining its blood supply. Then, dislocate the hip and expose the area of the segmental collapse. Using a scalpel and an osteotome, the edges of the necrotic segment are defined. The necrotic segment is then removed using osteotomes, curettage, and power burrs, until a bleeding surface and viable bone is encountered at the base of the cavity.

An iliac (the tibia can also be used) bone graft should be harvested consisting of cortico-cancellous struts and cancellous bone. Depending on the size of the lesion, two to three cortical struts should be placed (perpendicular) in the troughs previously made. The remaining space in the femoral head should be packed with cancellous bone graft which was previously harvested. After replacing the trapdoor, it should be fixed with two or three absorbable pins. The hip joint should then be reduced and the capsule should be sutured loosely [3]. See Figs. 42.4, 42.5, and 42.6.

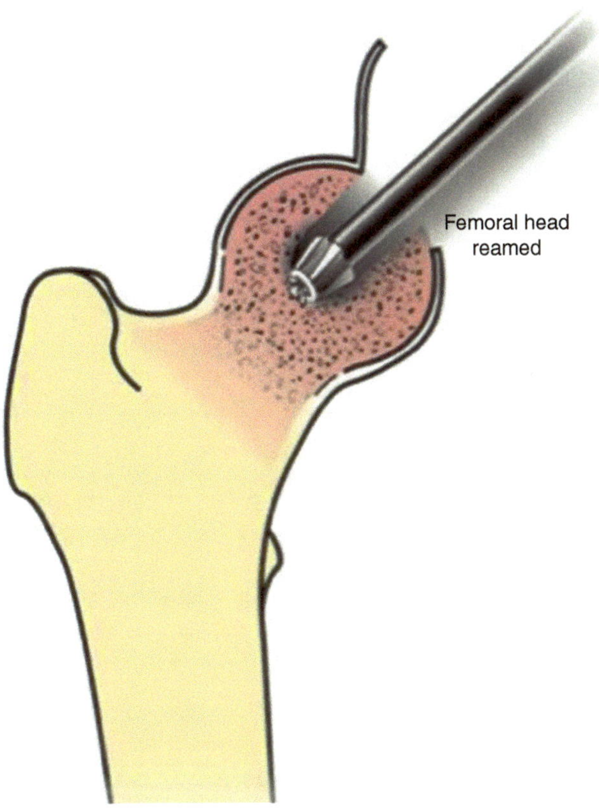

Fig. 42.5 Removal of necrotic tissue through the trapdoor

42.4 Results of Vascularized Bone Grafting

Yoo et al. reported 89 % survivorship at a mean follow-up of 13.9 years (range, 10–23.7 years) in 124 hips with Ficat and Arlet stage II or III disease [22]. Similar results were reported in a study of 103 hips at a mean of 5 year follow-up by Urbanik et al. who observed 91 and 77 % survivorship in stage II and stage III hips, respectively [8]. Results by Edward et al. were in agreement with those reported by Urbanik and Yoo [23]. Following 65 pre-collapse osteonecrotic hips treated with vascularized bone grafting for a mean of 14.4 years (range, 10.5–26 years), the results demonstrated that 75 % of the hips did not require total hip arthroplasty after 10 years. See Table 42.1 for a summary of studies on vascularized bone grafting procedures.

42.5 Results of Nonvascularized Bone Grafting

Nonvascularized bone grafting is typically limited to small- and medium-sized lesions (Ficat and Arlet stage I or II and ARCO stages I to IIIA) and is not indicated when decompression without grafting has failed. Poor results have been

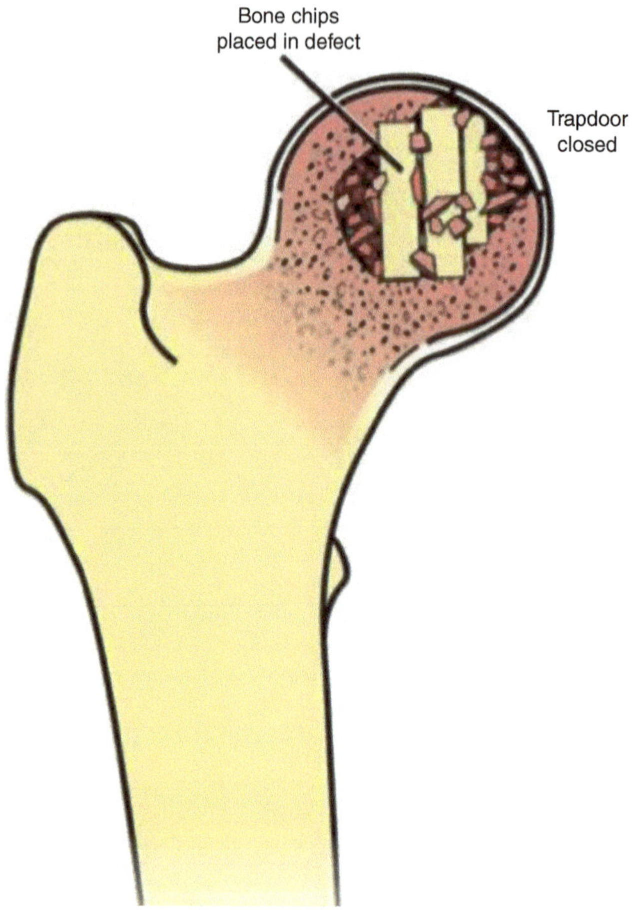

Fig. 42.6 Packing of the defect with bone grafts

noted when there is a collapse of more than 2 mm, acetabular osteonecrosis, or cartilage delamination.

Several techniques have been described, with the major difference being in the method of inserting the graft. The Phemister technique inserts the graft directly through the bored canal and has led to mixed results, with studies reporting success in 36–90 % of patients after 2–7 years [30–32]. See Table 42.2 for a summary of studies on nonvascularized bone grafting procedures.

42.6 Summary

Osteonecrosis of the femoral head is multifactorial in etiology and predominantly affects younger population. Untreated osteonecrosis has a high incidence of progression to collapse and end stage disease requiring total joint arthroplasty, once there is radiographic evidence of disease. Multiple surgical and nonsurgical strategies for joint preservation have been used over the years. One of the surgical strategies used is bone grafting, which has been described extensively over the past 60 years. There are two main types of bone grafting: vascularized and nonvascularized. Nonvascularized bone grafting was described initially, and even though some cases presented favorable outcomes, long-term outcomes were not always favorable. This may have been partly because the etiopathogenetic mechanisms involved in osteonecrosis were never adequately addressed. This stimulated the development

Table 42.1 Vascularized bone grafting

Author (year)	Level of evidence	Stage	Number of hips	Mean age (years)	Mean follow-up (years)	Survivorship
Eward et al. (2012) [23]	IV	Ficat stages I and II	65	32.1	14.4	75
Yin et al. (2011) [24]	IV	Steinberg stages II to IV	14	34	3.3	100
Chen et al. (2009) [19]	IV	ARCO stages IIIA and IIIB	33	37	6.2	24
Sun et al. (2009) [25]	IV	Steinberg stages II to V	80	31	4.3	100
Babhulkar et al. (2009) [26]	IV	ARCO stages IIB and IIIC	31	32	8	96.7
Bakshi et al. (2009) [27]	IV	Ficat stages I to III	187	35.5	16.5	71
Kawate et al. (2007) [28]	IV	Steinberg stages IB to V	71	39	7	83
Marciniak et al. (2005) [29]	IV	Marcus-Enneking stages II to IV	101	37	8	42
Hasegawa et al. (1997) [18]	IV	Inoue and Ono stages I and II	31	38.3	8	70

Table 42.2 Nonvascularized bone grafting

Author (year)	Level of evidence	Stage	Number of hips	Mean age (years)	Mean follow-up (years)	Survivorship
Zhang et al. (2012) [33]	IV	Steinberg stages II to IV	85	31.4	2.3	85.4
Wei and Ge (2011) [34]	IV	ARCO stages II to III	223	33.5	2	81
Wang et al. (2010) [13]	IV	ARCO stages IIA to IIIA	138	32.3	2	68
Yuhan et al. (2009) [35]	IV	ARCO stages IIC to III A	11	37	5	73
Seyler et al. (2008) [36]	IV	Ficat stages II and III	39	35	3	67
Mont et al. (2003) [10]	IV	Ficat stages II and III	19	31	4	86
Mont et al. (1998) [3]	IV	Ficat stages III and IV	30	26	56	80

and use of multiple vascularized bone grafting techniques, which in addition to providing mechanical support, were proposed to restore the blood supply for the femoral head. Various studies have reported improved outcomes with vascularized bone grafting procedures utilizing modern microvascular techniques. Further studies are required to determine which of the techniques has better outcomes and can be more broadly and safely used.

References

1. Dailiana ZH, Toth AP, Gunneson E, Berend KR, Urbaniak JR. Free vascularized fibular grafting following failed core decompression for femoral head osteonecrosis. J Arthroplasty. 2007;22:679–88.
2. Stein H, Volpin G, Horer D. Vascularized muscle pedicle flap for osteonecrosis of the femoral head. Orthopedics. 2002;25:485–8.
3. Mont MA, Einhorn TA, Sponseller PD, Hungerford DS. The trapdoor procedure using autogenous cortical and cancellous bone grafts for osteonecrosis of the femoral head. J Bone Joint Surg Br. 1998;80:56–62.
4. Phemister DB. Treatment of the necrotic head of the femur in adults. J Bone Joint Surg Am. 1949;31A:55–66.
5. Bonfiglio M, Bardenstein MB. Treatment by bone-grafting of aseptic necrosis of the femoral head and non-union of the femoral neck (Phemister technique). J Bone Joint Surg Am. 1958;40-A:1329–46.
6. Meyers MH. The treatment of osteonecrosis of the hip with fresh osteochondral allografts and with the muscle pedicle graft technique. Clin Orthop Relat Res. 1978;130:202–9.
7. Judet J, Judet H, Gilbert A. Trial revascularization of the femur head with a pediculed fibular transplant. Rev Chir Orthop Reparatrice Appar Mot. 1980;66 Suppl 2:65.
8. Urbaniak JR, Coogan PG, Gunneson EB, Nunley JA. Treatment of osteonecrosis of the femoral head with free vascularized fibular grafting. A long-term follow-up study of one hundred and three hips. J Bone Joint Surg Am. 1995;77:681–94.
9. Gaskill TR, Urbaniak JR, Aldridge 3rd JM. Free vascularized fibular transfer for femoral head osteonecrosis: donor and graft site morbidity. J Bone Joint Surg Am. 2009;91:1861–7.
10. Mont MA, Etienne G, Ragland PS. Outcome of nonvascularized bone grafting for osteonecrosis of the femoral head. Clin Orthop Relat Res. 2003;417:84–92.
11. Lieberman JR, Berry DJ, Mont MA, et al. Osteonecrosis of the hip: management in the 21st century. Instr Course Lect. 2003;52:337–55.
12. Myeroff C, Archdeacon M. Autogenous bone graft: donor sites and techniques. J Bone Joint Surg Am. 2011;93:2227–36.
13. Wang BL, Sun W, Shi ZC, et al. Treatment of nontraumatic osteonecrosis of the femoral head using bone impaction grafting through a femoral neck window. Int Orthop. 2010;34:635–9.
14. Garrigues GE, Aldridge 3rd JM, Friend JK, Urbaniak JR. Free Vascularized Fibular Grafting for treatment of osteonecrosis of the femoral head secondary to hip dislocation. Microsurgery. 2009;29:342–5.
15. Meyers MH. Osteonecrosis of the femoral head treated with the muscle pedicle graft. Orthop Clin North Am. 1985;16:741–5.
16. Baksi DP. Treatment of osteonecrosis of the femoral head by drilling and muscle-pedicle bone grafting. J Bone Joint Surg Br. 1991;73:241–5.
17. Aldridge 3rd JM, Berend KR, Gunneson EE, Urbaniak JR. Free vascularized fibular grafting for the treatment of postcollapse osteonecrosis of the femoral head. Surgical technique. J Bone Joint Surg Am. 2004;86(A Suppl 1):87–101.
18. Hasegawa Y, Iwata H, Torii S, Iwase T, Kawamoto K, Iwasada S. Vascularized pedicle bone-grafting for nontraumatic avascular necrosis of the femoral head. A 5- to 11-year follow-up. Arch Orthop Trauma Surg. 1997;116:251–8.
19. Chen CC, Lin CL, Chen WC, Shih HN, Ueng SW, Lee MS. Vascularized iliac bone-grafting for osteonecrosis with segmental collapse of the femoral head. J Bone Joint Surg Am. 2009;91:2390–4.
20. Matsusaki H, Noguchi M, Kawakami T, Tani T. Use of vascularized pedicle iliac bone graft combined with transtrochanteric rotational osteotomy in the treatment of avascular necrosis of the femoral head. Arch Orthop Trauma Surg. 2005;125:95–101.
21. Wang YS, Yin L, Lu ZD, Wu XJ, Liu HJ. Analysis of long-term outcomes of double-strut bone graft for osteonecrosis of the femoral head. Orthop Surg. 2009;1:22–7.
22. Yoo MC, Kim KI, Hahn CS, Parvizi J. Long-term followup of vascularized fibular grafting for femoral head necrosis. Clin Orthop Relat Res. 2008;466:1133–40.
23. Eward WC, Rineer CA, Urbaniak JR, Richard MJ, Ruch DS. The vascularized fibular graft in precollapse osteonecrosis: is long-term hip preservation possible? Clin Orthop Relat Res. 2012;470:2819–26.
24. Yin S, Zhang C, Jin D, Chen S, Sun Y, Sheng J. Treatment of osteonecrosis of the femoral head in lymphoma patients by free vascularised fibular grafting. Int Orthop. 2011;35:1125–30.
25. Sun Y, Zhang CQ, Chen SB, Sheng JG, Jin DX, Zeng BF. Treatment of femoral head osteonecrosis in patients with systemic lupus erythematosus by free vascularised fibular grafting. Lupus. 2009;18:1061–5.
26. Babhulkar S. Osteonecrosis of femoral head: treatment by core decompression and vascular pedicle grafting. Indian J Orthop. 2009;43:27–35.
27. Baksi DP, Pal AK, Baksi DD. Long-term results of decompression and muscle-pedicle bone grafting for osteonecrosis of the femoral head. Int Orthop. 2009;33:41–7.
28. Kawate K, Yajima H, Sugimoto K, et al. Indications for free vascularized fibular grafting for the treatment of osteonecrosis of the femoral head. BMC Musculoskelet Disord. 2007;8:78.
29. Marciniak D, Furey C, Shaffer JW. Osteonecrosis of the femoral head. A study of 101 hips treated with vascularized fibular grafting. J Bone Joint Surg Am. 2005;87:742–7.
30. Buckley PD, Gearen PF, Petty RW. Structural bone-grafting for early atraumatic avascular necrosis of the femoral head. J Bone Joint Surg Am. 1991;73:1357–64.
31. Israelite C, Nelson CL, Ziarani CF, Abboud JA, Landa J, Steinberg ME. Bilateral core decompression for osteonecrosis of the femoral head. Clin Orthop Relat Res. 2005;441:285–90.
32. Plakseychuk AY, Kim SY, Park BC, Varitimidis SE, Rubash HE, Sotereanos DG. Vascularized compared with nonvascularized fibular grafting for the treatment of osteonecrosis of the femoral head. J Bone Joint Surg Am. 2003;85-A:589–96.
33. Zhang HJ, Liu YW, Du ZQ, et al. Therapeutic effect of minimally invasive decompression combined with impaction bone grafting on osteonecrosis of the femoral head. Eur J Orthop Surg Traumatol. 2013;23(8):913–9.
34. Wei BF, Ge XH. Treatment of osteonecrosis of the femoral head with core decompression and bone grafting. Hip Int. 2011;21:206–10.
35. Yuhan C, Hu CC, Chen DW, Ueng SW, Shih CH, Lee MS. Local cancellous bone grafting for osteonecrosis of the femoral head. Surg Innov. 2009;16:63–7.
36. Seyler TM, Marker DR, Ulrich SD, Fatscher T, Mont MA. Nonvascularized bone grafting defers joint arthroplasty in hip osteonecrosis. Clin Orthop Relat Res. 2008;466:1125–32.

43 Vascularized Pedicle Iliac Bone Grafting for Osteonecrosis of the Femoral Head

Mel S. Lee

43.1 Introduction

Osteonecrosis of the femoral head (ONFH) is a debilitating disease and eventually leads to collapse if left untreated. This condition is estimated to account for more than 10 % of the total hip arthroplasties (THAs) performed each year in the United States and more than 50 % in many Asian countries [1–4]. ONFH often affects young active patients and the incidence of bilateral hip involvement is around 50–80 % [3, 4]. Even though the success rate and the intermediate term of prosthesis survival by using newer bearing surface are improving as compared to the conventional THA, preservation of the femoral head is still the goal in those young active patients.

Since ONFH is frequently found in patients between the ages of 20 and 50 years, many techniques to salvage the ONFH in young patients have been reported. Among them, the use of vascularized iliac bone grafting based on a pedicle of the circumflex iliac artery has become popular because it is in vicinity to the lesion and needs no microsurgical anastomosis. It has also been successfully used for nonunion of the femoral neck fracture or large defects of the proximal femur.

In addition to the vascularized iliac pedicle bone grafts, there are other alternative grafts around the hip that can be used to repair the necrotic femoral head. The quadratus femoris muscle pedicle graft is supplied by the muscular branch of the lateral femoral circumflex artery and is commonly used for the repair of femoral neck fracture nonunion (Meyer procedure). It has been successful in femoral neck fracture nonunion, but it is seldom used in the ONFH repair. The reason is because the graft is a posterior-based muscle pedicle graft, whereas the osteonecrotic lesion is usually located in the anterosuperior quadrant of the femoral head. Furthermore, there is limitation in the graft size that the mechanical strength of the proximal femur will be compromised if the donor site is too big. The gluteus minimus pedicle graft has also been used in the repair of ONFH [5]. It is a relatively simple procedure because the surgical approach is identical to the direct lateral approach to the hip. The graft is supplied by the muscular branch of the superior gluteal artery. Care should be taken in the dissection of the gluteal muscles to avoid inadvertent injury to the vessel. By gently elevating the insertion of the gluteus medius muscle, the vascular pedicle can be found in the fat pad between the gluteus medius and minimus about 2–3 cm from the greater trochanter tip. By using oscillating saw, the entire insertion of the gluteus minimus on the greater trochanter can be harvested as a corticocancellous graft. The potential drawbacks of the graft are (1) the osteonecrosis is sometimes extended to the trochanteric area that the graft itself is also necrotic; (2) the harvest of the graft may weaken the femoral neck that additional fixation may be needed; and (3) part of the hip abductor muscles are sacrificed that is less favorable for the hip function.

Vascularized iliac bone graft (VIBG) has been used for the repair of femoral neck fracture nonunion or proximal femoral deficiency [6, 7]. As compared with the free vascularized fibular grafting, the VIBG has been less reported in the literature. We and others have used VIBG for the salvage of the ONFH. This chapter will review the anatomy, the surgical technique, the indication, the clinical results, and other combined technique of the VIBG.

43.2 Anatomy

The blood supply to the iliac crest is majorly contributed by the deep circumflex iliac artery (DCIA) which is arisen from the lateral or posterolateral aspect of the external iliac artery just above the inguinal ligament and opposite to the inferior epigastric artery (Fig. 43.1). Other arteries such as

M.S. Lee
Department of Orthopaedic Surgery,
Chia-Yi Chang Gung Memorial Hospital,
College of Medicine, Chang Gung University,
6, Sec. West, Chia-Pu Road,
Putzu City, Chia-Yi 613, Taiwan
e-mail: bone@doctor.com

K.-H. Koo et al. (eds.), *Osteonecrosis*,
DOI 10.1007/978-3-642-35767-1_43, © Springer-Verlag Berlin Heidelberg 2014

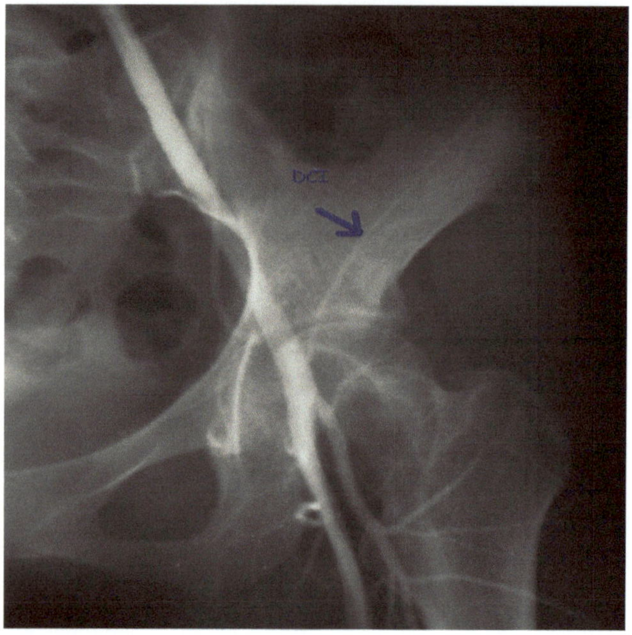

Fig. 43.1 Superselective angiography. The deep circumflex iliac (*DCI*) artery is shown

the superior gluteal, lateral circumflex femoral, and superficial circumflex iliac artery also contribute, but the tributaries are smaller in diameter. The DCIA runs upward and laterally between the transversalis fascia and the extraperitoneal fat. It gives out a number of branches in the course and pierces through the abdominal muscle layers to the inner surface of the iliac crest in the insertion of iliacus and transversus muscles [8].

The external diameter of the DCIA is usually around 2–2.5 mm and can be easily handled without microscopic magnification. The artery runs along the inner lip of the iliac crest and diverts away from the upmost point of the iliac crest to give off multiple intramuscular branches to the iliacus and anastomoses with the iliolumbar and superior gluteal artery. From the origin of the external iliac artery to the iliac crest, the vascular pedicle can be 8–10 cm in length which provides a versatile radius to swing around the proximal femur. All along its course, the DCIA is accompanied by its venae commitantes that drain into the external iliac vein or femoral vein.

Most of the surgeries use the DCIA as the vascular pedicle because the constant position and diameter of the vessels make it very suitable for harvest and transplantation. In addition to the DCIA, some surgeons used the superficial circumflex iliac artery that travels between the fatty tissue and fascia in the inguinal region [9, 10]. It is noted that the vessels of the superficial circumflex iliac artery are smaller in size and more difficult to harvest.

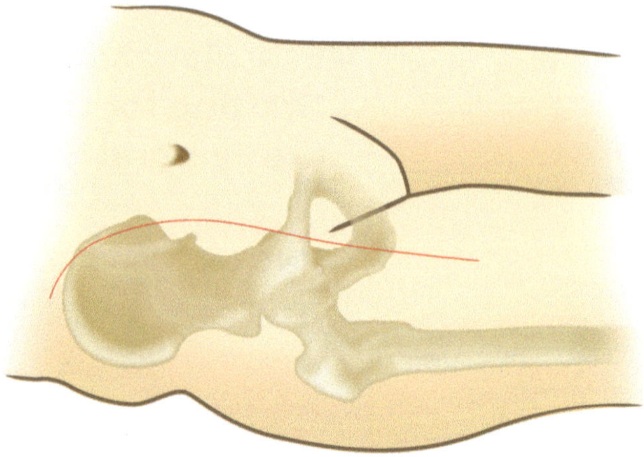

Fig. 43.2 Skin incision for VIBG surgery

43.3 Surgical Technique

Under general anesthesia, patient is put in the supine position with a sandbag behind the operated side of the pelvis. A long and curve skin incision is made on the iliac crest 8 cm pass the anterior superior iliac spine (ASIS), along the inguinal ligament, with the distal limb extended medially to the hip joint (Fig. 43.2). The femoral artery and the vein are looped to identify the external iliac artery. By gentle traction on the external iliac artery, tributaries of the external iliac artery can be exposed. The superficial circumflex iliac vessels and the deep circumflex iliac vessels are usually arising from the external iliac vessels just opposite to the origin of the inferior epigastric artery and could be easily traced to the inner lip of the iliac crest, into which feeding branches were sent (Fig. 43.3a). The external and internal oblique abdominal muscles are cut from its insertion on iliac crest. Dissection of the vascular pedicle should be carefully performed after opening the inguinal ligament and the transversalis fascia. The first few tributaries behind the inguinal ligament can be ligated. Beyond the point of ASIA, a sleeve of iliacus muscles should be left on the inner lip of the iliac bone that encases the vascular pedicle to avoid overzealous dissection and inadvertent tear of the feeding vessels. A suitable-size bone graft is harvested with its attached vascular bundle and muscle sleeve (Fig. 43.3b).

The hip joint is exposed by using the inferior limb of the skin incision. Between the sartorius muscle and the tensor fascia latae (Smith-Petersen's interval), the anterior hip joint capsule is exposed by retracting the rectus femoris medially and the hip abductors laterally. The anterior joint capsule is incised in an H-shape manner to expose the head-neck junction of the hip joint. Rotation and manipulation of the hip

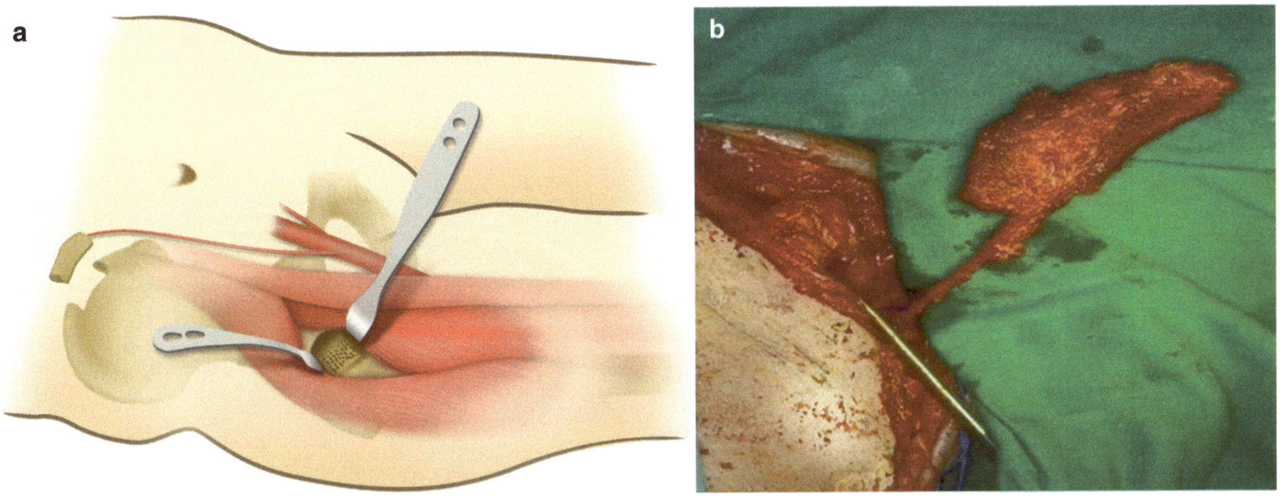

Fig. 43.3 Deep dissection. (**a**) The DCIA can be found opposite to the inferior epigastric artery. Two Hohmann retractors are put intra-articularly for exposure. A bone trough is made on the femoral neck. (**b**) VIBG with vascular pedicle

will bring the femoral head into view. A bone trough about 1.5 cm × 3 cm is made in the femoral neck leading into the head using sharp narrow osteotomies (Fig. 43.3a). Repeated sharp cuts along the top end of the trough open into the ischemia area of the femoral head. The hard and sclerotic avascular bone is removed using high-speed burrs as thoroughly as possible. If the cartilage is cracked that can been seen directly from the inside, careful out-pushing of the cartilage shell from inside the femoral head can correct the indentation and make it more congruent with the acetabulum.

The void and cavity after debridement is filled with bone chips by gentle impaction of a layer of cancellous bone to the subchondral level. The remaining space is to be filled in with a tailored piece of iliac crest bone with its intact blood supply of DCIA. A tunnel below the iliopsoas is made by blunt dissection with the hip in flexion. A large-size Penrose drain is passed beneath the inguinal ligament along the tunnel as a channel to transfer the graft to the anterior aspect of the femoral neck. The entire graft is slid into the Penrose drain and wrapped by it. By carefully pushing of the graft from the inside of the iliopsoas, the graft can be transferred to the anterior hip with intact pedicle. The Penrose drain is then incised completely with scissor to bring out the graft. As long as the graft is transferred to the anterior hip joint, it can be trimmed to a suitable size to be inserted through the bone trough into the femoral head. The graft can be pushed into the trough to produce a locked-in position and additional holding implant is unnecessary.

Postoperatively, the surgically treated hip is put in a position with 30° flexion and neutral rotation. This posture is advised for approximately 1 week to relax the tension of the vascular pedicle. Hip motion is encouraged as tolerated. The patients are instructed to use double crutches to avoid full weight bearing on the involved limb for 6 weeks. During the following weeks, the amount of weight bearing can be gradually increased by using a single crutch and progresses to a fully unassisted weight bearing by 6 months.

43.4 Indication

The indications for VIBG have not been well established in the literature. The factors affecting treatment results include staging (demonstration of the lesion by radiograph or magnetic resonance imaging, size of the necrotic segment, location of lesion relative to the weight-bearing area, the amount of femoral head depression, and the acetabular involvement), risk factors (use of steroid, medical comorbidities, or systemic disease), and patient-specific factors (age, activity level, or body mass).

In a survey of treatment modalities in the North America, total hip replacement is the most commonly selected treatment of postcollapse ONFH, and core decompression is the most frequently offered treatment for symptomatic precollapse ONFH [11]. Vascularized bone grafting is suggested by only 3–10 % of the responders who are active members of the professional society. It is generally agreed that a symptomatic case with the lesion size more than 30 % of the femoral head needs operative treatment to prevent early collapse of the femoral head. For asymptomatic necrotic lesions with an area smaller than 30 % of the femoral head, close follow-up without treatment appears to be adequate in most of the cases [3, 4, 12].

Table 43.1 Summary of success rate

Authors	Case no.	Success rate		Follow-up (years)
		Precollapse	Postcollapse	
Iwata et al. [9]	23	17/20	0/3	1–6
Leung [19]	21	4/5	4/16	5–12
Wassenaar et al. [20]	12	3/5	2/7	4.1
Ishizaka [21]	31	9/18	7/13	2–11
Hasegawa et al. [10]	31	12/27	2/4	8
Feng et al. [22]	17	7/12	3/5	5.7
Kern et al. [23]	80	Clinical 50 %; radiographic 47.5 %		5.6
Pavlovcic et al. [14]	24	7/7	3/17	12
Yen et al. [17]	39	16/23	6/16	2–6
Eisenschenk et al. [18]	102	Clinical 87 %; radiographic 56.1 %		5
Nagoya et al. [15]	35	12/28	0/7	8.5
Babhulkar [16]	31	9/9	21/22	5–8
Chen et al. [13]	33		8/33	7.1

In the literature, most of the studies of VIBG reported a mix group of hips ranging from precollapse stage to early postcollapse stage. In a study of 33 segmental collapse hips, 26 ARCO stage IIIA and 7 ARCO stage IIIB, only 24 % of the hips treated with VIBG survived without converting to total hip replacement with a mean survival of 74 months. The authors concluded that VIBG is not indicated for the treatment of ONFH with segmental collapse [13]. Other studies also reported similar results in postcollapse hips with a relatively low successful rates [9, 10, 14, 15]. As a contrast, Babhulkar reported a clinical success rate of 95 % in 22 ARCO III hips with a follow-up period of 5–8 years by using vascularized iliac pedicle grafting [16]. However, by looking at the illustrated cases in that report, many of the clinically successful cases showed radiographic collapse of the femoral head. Based on the findings, the rational indication for VIBG should be ONFH without collapse in a young active patient with the lesion more than 30 % of the femoral head. Contraindications include a segmental collapse hip, preexisting thromboembolic disease, a risk of bleeding or thrombocytopenia, a questionable vascular supply to the iliac graft due to factors such as surgery or trauma, multifocal osteonecrosis involving the ilium, untreated inguinal or femoral hernia, and asymptomatic hips [13].

43.5 Clinical Results

Between 1994 and 1999, the author had performed 100 cases of VIBG in 86 patients at the author's institute. Thirty-nine hips in 33 patients with a minimal follow-up of 2 years were reported [17]. The overall clinical success rate was 82 % and the radiographic success rate was 56 %. The rate of conversion to replacement arthroplasty was 10.3 %. We had further followed up 33 hips with preoperative segmental collapse lesions for 7.1 years. VIBG by using the technique described in this chapter had delayed the conversion to total hip arthroplasty by an average of 7 years in ARCO stage IIIA hips and by 2.9 years in ARCO stage IIIB hips [13].

Eisenschenk et al. had performed VIBG in 102 hips and achieved 87 % clinical success rate and 56.1 % radiographic success rate [18]. Many other reports have been published by using similar technique as described in this chapter [14–23]. The clinical success rate in precollapse hips ranged from 43 to 100 % with an average success rate around 72 % (Table 43.1). Iwata and Hasegawa had used superficial circumflex iliac vessels as the pedicle in their patients and had achieved a 52–74 % success rate [9, 10].

In postcollapse hips, the success rate differed between reports with 0 % in some reports and 95 % in one report [16]. The majority of the reports had a success rate less than 50 %. In view of these, some surgeons had developed combined surgical procedures to improve the clinical results and to salvage the segmental collapsed hips.

43.6 Combined Technique

Transtrochanteric osteotomy has been successful in hips where the intact articular surface is larger than 36 % of the femoral head and the extent of necrosis is limited [24]. For extensive or widely collapsed lesions, it is challenging to salvage the hip by one surgical procedure. Combined technique of proximal femur osteotomy and vascularized iliac bone grafting are intended to move the necrosis away from weight-bearing zone and provide mechanical support with viable bone at the same time. It is an appealing procedure in extensive and widely collapsed lesion in young patients. However, the combined surgical technique and procedure is more complex than either technique alone.

Two types of transtrochanteric osteotomy combined with vascularized iliac grafting were reported in the literature. One is the combination of transtrochanteric rotational osteotomy and vascularized iliac grafting. In 12 hips with extensive and widely collapsed necrotic lesion, the combined procedure was effective to prevent endoprosthesis replacement in 11 hips with a mean follow-up of 81 months [25]. In 17 hips with the necrosis more than two-thirds of the weight-bearing zone of the femoral head, the combined rotational osteotomy and vascularized iliac grafting prevented disease progression in 12 hips with a mean follow-up of 51 months [26]. When combining the rotational osteotomy with the vascularized iliac grafting, care must be taken to plan the direction of rotation and the position of the vascularized graft [27, 28]. A trough in the femoral neck to the necrotic femoral head needs to be designed properly for debridement and grafting in accordance to the degrees of rotation. The vascularized graft should be put immediately below the weight-bearing zone after rotation. Temporary fixation of the rotational osteotomy can facilitate the procedure. Definite fixation of the rotated femoral head can be done after trimming and transferring the graft through the bone tunnel.

The other type of transtrochanteric osteotomy combined with vascularized iliac grafting is a valgus/varus and/or flexion/extension osteotomy. It is simpler than the rotational osteotomy. In a series of 44 hips followed for 13.5 years, 34 % were converted to total hip arthroplasty while 90 % had progressive arthritis demonstrated by radiographs [29]. The authors suggested that this combination technique should be considered only in young symptomatic patients with good preoperative clinical function and Ficat stage II disease.

43.7 Graft Viability and Assessment Tools

The graft viability can be assessed postoperatively by several methods. Eisenschenk et al. had followed 82 patients for 5 years. In 42 patients, a superselective angiography was performed. Those angiographies showed perfusion of the grafts in 35 hips (83.3 %) [18]. The overall clinical success was achieved in 86.6 % of the patients. Although an angiography is a reliable tool to demonstrate the vascular pedicle after transplant, it is difficult to assess the viability of the necrotic femoral head and the revascularization of the necrotic lesion. In addition, an angiography is more invasive than other studies. Duchow et al. had used Doppler ultrasound to detect the blood flow of the VIBG [30]. However, it needs more experienced hands and is more technical demanding.

Nuclear medicine bone scintigraphy can also be used to evaluate the graft viability [31]. We had used single-photon emission computed tomography (SPECT) in 9 hips treated by VIBG [13]. The graft viability could be confirmed in 8 hips (89 %). However, a SPECT can only demonstrate the perfusion of the graft and the femoral head. Detailed information such as the extent of revascularization and the graft incorporation is difficult to assess by SPECT. Other nuclear medicine scan, such as positron emission tomography, theoretically can be used to evaluate the graft viability, healing, revascularization, and hemodynamic changes in the femoral head [32]. It has, however, not been reported in the literature.

In the literature, the most feasible noninvasive method to assess the graft viability and reparative process in the femoral head is a MRI study [13, 20, 33]. It is useful in most cases that the VIBG could be pushed into the bone trough without additional metal screw fixation. The signal intensity characteristics of the grafts can be compared with the normal fat marrow signals. An iso- or hyperintense signal in the graft is considered viable. Contrast enhancement by Gadolinium can be used to further evaluate the enhancement of the graft and the surrounding environment. The graft viability had been demonstrated by MRI in 82–100 % of hips treated by vascularized iliac grafting [10, 13, 18].

43.8 Summary

To preserve the femoral head and not to replace with prosthesis remains to be a challenge for the treatment of ONFH. VIBG with the feeding vessel of DCIA is a reliable graft with high rates of graft viability. The graft is corticocancellous and contains red marrow to provide osteogenic and revascularization potentials. No microsurgical anastomoses are required in the operation. The clinical results in precollapse ONFH are promising and can prevent or delay the total hip arthroplasties in most of the cases. Its use in segmental collapse ONFH remains controversial. To simultaneously transpose the intact articular surface and transfer a vascularized graft to weight-bearing zone of the necrotic femoral head has been tried. However, the combined procedure is difficult and complex to perform. Since the prognosis and long-term survival of ONFH rely on early diagnosis and intervention, the mainstay of treatment goals should emphasize on screening of patients with high risks, educate medical professions about the disease, and use of highly sensitive and accurate diagnostic tools such as MRI or PET scan to make early diagnosis.

References

1. Lee MS, Hsieh PH, Shih CH, Wang CJ. Non-traumatic osteonecrosis of the femoral head – from clinical to bench. Chang Gung Med J. 2010;33:351–60.
2. Lee MS, Chang YH, Chao EK, Shih CH. Conditions before collapse of the contralateral hip in osteonecrosis of the femoral head. Chang Gung Med J. 2002;25:228–37.
3. Lieberman JR, Berry DJ, Mont MA, Aaron RK, Callaghan JJ, Rayadhyaksha A, Urbaniak JR. Osteonecrosis of the hip: management in the twenty-first century. J Bone Joint Surg. 2002;84A: 834–53.

4. Mont MA, Jones LC, Hungerford DS. Nontraumatic osteonecrosis of the femoral head: ten years later. J Bone Joint Surg. 2006;88A: 1117–32.
5. Forgon M, Montskó P. Muscle-pedicle grafts or muscle-pedicle-bone grafts in the treatment of avascular necrotic femoral heads. Arch Orthop Trauma Surg. 1996;115:223–6.
6. Hou SM, Hang YS, Liu TK. Ununited femoral neck fractures by open reduction and vascularized iliac bone graft. Clin Orthop. 1993;294:176–80.
7. Lee SS, Ueng SWN, Shih CH. Aneurysm-induced intertrochanteric bone loss reconstructed by a vascularized iliac graft. A case report. J Trauma. 1999;46:944–7.
8. Swenson TM, Urbaniak JR, Sotereanos DG. A surgical guide for identifying the lateral femoral circumflex vessels during free vascularized fibular transfer for avascular necrosis of the femoral head. J Reconstr Microsurg. 1996;12:1–4.
9. Iwata H, Torii S, Hasegawa Y, Itoh H, Mizuno M, Genda E, Kataoka Y. Indications and results of vascularized pedicle iliac bone graft in avascular necrosis of the femoral head. Clin Orthop. 1993;295:281–8.
10. Hasegawa Y, Iwata H, Torii S, Iwase T, Kawamoto K, Iwasada S. Vascularized pedicle bone-grafting for nontraumatic avascular necrosis of the femoral head. A 5- to 11-year follow-up. Arch Orthop Trauma Surg. 1997;116:251–8.
11. McGrory BJ, York SC, Iorio R, Macaulay W, Pelker RR, Parsley BS, Teeny SM. Current practices of AAHKS members in the treatment of adult osteonecrosis of the femoral head. J Bone Joint Surg. 2007;89A:1194–204.
12. Nam KW, Kim YL, Yoo JJ, Koo KH, Yoon KS, Kim HJ. Fate of untreated asymptomatic osteonecrosis of the femoral head. J Bone Joint Surg. 2008;90A:477–84.
13. Chen CC, Lin CL, Chen WC, Shih HN, Ueng SWN, Lee MS. Vascularized iliac bone-grafting for osteonecrosis with segmental collapse of the femoral head. J Bone Joint Surg. 2009;91A:2390–4.
14. Pavlovcic V, Dolinar D, Arnez Z. Femoral head necrosis treated with vascularized iliac crest graft. Int Orthop. 1999;23:150–3.
15. Nagoya S, Nagao M, Takada J, Kuwabara H, Wada T, Kukita Y, Yamashita T. Predictive factors for vascularized iliac bone graft for nontraumatic osteonecrosis of the femoral head. J Orthop Sci. 2004;9:566–70.
16. Babhulkar S. Osteonecrosis of femoral head: treatment by core decompression and vascular pedicle grafting. Indian J Orthop. 2009;43:27–35.
17. Yen CY, Lee SS, Yuan LJ, Fu TS, Chan YS, Chen CY, Tu YK, Ueng SWN. Vascularized island pedicle iliac bone grafting for avascular necrosis of the femoral head. Chang Gung Med J. 2000;23:536–41.
18. Eisenschenk A, Lautenbach M, Schwetlick G, Weber U. Treatment of femoral head necrosis with vascularized iliac crest transplants. Clin Orthop. 2001;386:100–5.
19. Leung PC. Femoral head reconstruction and revascularization. Treatment for ischemic necrosis. Clin Orthop. 1996;323:139–45.
20. Wassenaar RP, Verburg H, Taconis WK, van der Eijken JW. Avascular osteonecrosis of the femoral head treated with a vascularized iliac bone graft: preliminary results and follow-up with radiography and MR imaging. Radiographics. 1996;16:585–94.
21. Ishizaka M, Sofue M, Dohmae Y, Endo N, Takahashi HE. Vascularized iliac bone graft for avascular necrosis of the femoral head. Clin Orthop. 1997;337:140–8.
22. Feng CK, Yu JK, Chang MC, Chen TH, Lo WH. Vascularized iliac bone graft for treating avascular necrosis of the femoral head. Zhonghua Yi Xue Za Zhi. 1998;61:463–9.
23. Kern O, Klöckner C, Weber U. Femur head preserving therapy, using vascular pedicled iliac bone graft, in segmental femoral head necrosis. Orthopade. 1998;27:482–90.
24. Sugioka Y, Hotokebuchi T, Tsutsui H. Transtrochanteric anterior rotational osteotomy for idiopathic and steroid-induced necrosis of the femoral head. Indications and long-term results. Clin Orthop. 1992;277:111–20.
25. Nakamura Y, Kumazawa Y, Mitsui H, Toh S, Katano H. Combined rotational osteotomy and vascularized iliac bone graft for advanced osteonecrosis of the femoral head. J Reconstr Microsurg. 2005;21:101–5.
26. Matsusaki H, Noguchi M, Kawakami T, Tani T. Use of vascularized pedicle iliac bone graft combined with transtrochanteric rotational osteotomy in the treatment of avascular necrosis of the femoral head. Arch Orthop Trauma Surg. 2005;125:95–101.
27. Noguchi M, Kawakami T, Yamamoto H. Use of vascularized pedicle iliac bone graft in the treatment of avascular necrosis of the femoral head. Arch Orthop Trauma Surg. 2001;121:437–42.
28. Kubo T, Kobayashi M, Ishida T, Yamazoe S, Fujioka M, Inoue S, Hirasawa Y. Non-traumatic osteonecrosis of the femoral head treated with transtrochanteric anterior rotational osteotomy combined with vascularized iliac bone grafting. J Orthop Sci. 2000;5:610–3.
29. Fuchs B, Knothe U, Hertel R, Ganz R. Femoral osteotomy and iliac graft vascularization for femoral head osteonecrosis. Clin Orthop. 2003;412:84–93.
30. Duchow J, Kubale R, Hopf T. Color Doppler imaging assessment of blood flow in vascularized pedicle grafts for avascular necrosis of the femoral head: angiographic correlation. J Ultrasound Med. 1998;17:509–12.
31. Cheung HS, Stewart IE, Ho KC, Leung PC, Metreweli C. Vascularized iliac crest grafts: evaluation of viability status with marrow scintigraphy. Radiology. 1993;186:241–5.
32. Huang MJ, Hsieh PH, Ueng SWN, Ho KC, Yen TZ, Lee MS. Use of positron emission tomography to detect infection around antibiotic-loaded cement spacers in patients with high C-reactive protein levels. Orthopedics. 2011;34:605–9.
33. Tan CF, Ng KK, Yem PS, Ng SH, Cheung YC, Wan YL. Viability of vascularized bone grafts; perfusion studies by dynamic enhanced MRI and bone scan. Transplant Proc. 2001;33:623–4.

44 The Vascularized Fibular Graft in the Treatment of Osteonecrosis: Data, Dogma, and Controversies

Will Eward

44.1 Introduction

In the debate about surgical treatment for osteonecrosis of the femoral head (ONFH), no topic is more frequently debated than the use of the free vascularized fibular graft (FVFG) as a standard treatment. Pioneered by Urbaniak in 1979, the FVFG represents a durable, biologic means of reconstructing the femoral head after removal of the osteonecrotic bone [1]. However, this technique has been criticized for its complexity and is only widely performed at several centers throughout the world. Small numbers of cases treated operatively, difficulty comparing uniform cases of ONFH, and the proclivity of many surgeons to utilize one particular operation preferentially have rendered direct comparison of FVFG to other techniques an unwieldy prospect [2]. What is agreed upon is that the goal of therapy should be to delay the progression of osteonecrosis as well as repair it. This chapter will focus upon how the FVFG addresses these goals, how it performs, and how it compares – indirectly at least – with other options such as core decompression, tantalum rod instrumentation, nonvascularized bone grafting, and corrective osteotomies.

44.2 Rationale

Although physicians have been treating osteonecrosis for over a century, the exact pathogenetic mechanisms associated with the development of this condition have not yet been thoroughly described. This places the treatment of the disease in an unfortunate position: whereas targeted therapy of diseases has become commonplace, those treating osteonecrosis are left reacting to the disease as it progresses and treating the effects of the condition on the bone rather than the fundamental underlying causes. In the case of ONFH, Korompilias et al. have described a "heterogeneous group of disorders leading to a common pathway of necrosis of the femoral head" [3]. This common pathway involves acute pain from the osteonecrosis itself and is followed by structural failure of the subchondral bone leading to femoral head collapse and chronic pain [1]. Most surgical therapies decompress and remove the area of osteonecrosis. FVFG purports to directly restore stability to the femoral head by providing a vascularized bone graft that does not depend on creeping substitution (as is the case with nonvascularized bone grafting). This direct and biologic reconstruction of the femoral head sets it apart from other operative treatments.

44.3 Efficacy

The first questions one might ask are "Does FVFG work?" and "How well does it work?" The answer to these questions should be cautiously divided between treatment of precollapse ONFH and treatment of postcollapse ONFH. For most operative interventions, the progression of ONFH can be interrupted if treatment is initiated prior to subchondral collapse [4]. Treatment with the FVFG is no exception – the results are excellent [5]. Rates of FVFG survivorship reflect successful hip preservation. When the FVFG is used to treat precollapse ONFH, rates of overall survivorship range from 61 to 96 % [5–8]. In general, survivorship decreases with time. Studies evaluating outcomes with final follow-up times of less than 5 years typically report survivorship rates in excess of 90 % [5]. Although survivorship following core decompression is similar in many studies, some authors have reported lower rates of hip preservation with this technique. Bozic, for instance, reported a 44 % rate of salvage among precollapse ONFH patients treated by core decompression with a mean follow-up time of 10 years [9]. However, it is interesting to note that half of the failures in that study occurred in patients with cystic changes in the femoral head, suggesting that core decompression alone is not ideal for this subset of patients [9]. A simple solution to treat patients with

W. Eward
Department of Orthopaedic Surgery, Duke University Medical Center, Box 3312, DUMC, Durham, NC 27710, USA
e-mail: w.eward@alumni.duke.edu

K.-H. Koo et al. (eds.), *Osteonecrosis*,
DOI 10.1007/978-3-642-35767-1_44, © Springer-Verlag Berlin Heidelberg 2014

cystic changes was nonvascularized fibular grafting. However, survivorship with this technique is generally poorer than the FVFG, ranging from 30 to 59 % with reported follow-up times between 5 and 7 years postoperatively [10, 11]. As far as "how well it works," Harris Hip Scores (HHS) are excellent following FVFG. For patients with long-term surviving FVFG (survivorship greater than 10 years), HHS are generally in excess of 80 and are comparable to HHS in patients treated with total hip arthroplasty (THA) [5, 12, 13]. Long-term functional outcomes such as HHS are not well described for nonoperative management, core decompression, nonvascularized fibular grafting, or instrumentation with a trabecular metal implant. These relatively high levels of graft survival and excellent functional outcomes do not hold true when performed in patients with postcollapse ONFH [14–16].

44.4 Technique

The second inquiry about FVFG is typically a variant of the question "Is it worth all of the effort?" While people often emphasize the highly technical nature of the case, the use of two surgical teams (one for harvest and one for the inset), and the relative paucity of patients, at our institution – where this procedure is performed multiple times weekly – we have found the process to be straightforward. A multidisciplinary, multisurgeon "FVFG team" meets weekly to screen all patients presenting for consideration for FVFG. Dedicated teams in the operating room, the postoperative orthopedic floor of the hospital, and the physical therapy department facilitate smooth transitions through the various stages of treatment. The procedure itself is broken down into several different and discrete steps [14]: first, under tourniquet, the ipsilateral fibula is harvested through a 15-cm longitudinal incision beginning 10 cm distal to the fibular head and ending 10 cm proximal to the lateral malleolus. The peroneal vessels are identified, protected, and divided after the application of vascular clips. While this is occurring, the second operative team is exposing the proximal femur. This is accomplished through a 10–15-cm, convex-anterior, curved anterolateral skin incision. One-third of the incision is superior to the tip of the greater trochanter, while two-thirds are inferior to the tip of the greater trochanter. As the vasti are reflected from their origins, the falx or aponeurotic bridge spanning from the femur to the rectus femoris can be seen. Within the adjacent fat pad, the ascending branch of the lateral circumflex femoral artery, and its two venae comitantes are identified and preserved for utilization as donor vessels. Next, under fluoroscopic guidance, a 3-mm guide pin is inserted into the center of the necrotic area within the femoral head. Sequential reaming starting with a 10-mm reamer and increasing to up to 21 mm (based on the diameter of the harvested fibula) is performed. A ball reamer is then used to further remove necrotic bone. Locally harvested autograft is impacted into the reaped areas using a custom-made bone impactor. After these steps are complete, the fibula is placed within the femoral core and secured within the core using a single 0.062-mm Kirschner wire. A standard microvascular anastomosis is performed. We typically use a coupling device (Microvascular Anastomotic Coupler System; Medical Companies Alliance, Homewood, Alabama) under loupe magnification for the venous anastomosis. The arterial anastomosis is performed under an operating microscope using 8-0 or 9-0 Nylon monofilament suture.

44.5 Why Choose FVFG?

The last question one might ask is "Why FVFG?" There are three advantages that have contributed to the FVFG being our choice for managing symptomatic Ficat Stage I and II hips that have not responded to nonoperative measures. First, the long-term results after this operation are excellent. In patients with a mean follow-up of 14.5 years, we found long-term hip preservation (defined as greater than 10 years) was achieved in 60 % of patients [5]. Second, even in patients who "fail" long-term hip preservation and convert to total hip arthroplasty within a decade of their FVFG operation, the mean duration of hip preservation is 8.3 years. With a mean patient age of 32 years at the time of vascularized fibular grafting, this means that the average "failure" still experiences an extension of the life of the femoral head and hip joint from the fourth decade of life to the fifth decade of life [5]. Third, patients undergoing FVFG can expect levels of hip function comparable to that experienced after THA but without the lifestyle restrictions that often accompany arthroplasty. Patients with successful hip preservation following FVFG are significantly more likely to participate in impact sports or active events than those patients treated with arthroplasty. Although investigation of athletic capacity after core decompression, nonvascularized bone grafting, tantalum instrumentation, and corrective osteotomy has not been well elucidated, we believe that the vascularized fibular graft offers an excellent solution for large or cystic ONFH lesions in patients who wish to return to sport in a relatively short amount of time.

44.6 Pitfalls and Risk Factors for Failure

There has been considerable debate and disagreement about what features of a patient's ONFH should be regarded as poor prognostic indicators for any particular treatment. What is widely accepted is that patients with Ficat Stage I disease do very well, regardless of the treatment chosen [17]. Similarly, patients with advanced stage disease (Ficat Stage III and above) consistently experience poorer outcomes across a variety of treatment choices [3, 4, 7, 12, 16, 18]. While most hips that have been successfully preserved for a decade do not require conversion to THA in later years, we have reported a progressive decline in survivorship beyond the 10-year mark in patients with ONFH [5]. We speculate that this is because idiopathic cases of ONFH may result from an underlying progressive disorder such as intraosseous hypertension that can progress even after treatment. Some authors have reported advanced age to be predictive of poor outcome following FVFG [12, 18]. Our experience and reports of other authors have not found this to be the case [5, 6, 9]. Berend et al. have also reported alcoholic and posttraumatic etiologies to be strongly associated with failures; however, this phenomenon is largely specific to postcollapse hips [16]. In other words, there are not specific and definite contraindications to FVFG. However, surgeons should be careful neither to have high expectations for patients with advanced disease nor to treat Ficat Stage I patients aggressively unless they have already failed conservative management.

44.7 Summary

In conclusion, we continue to regard FVFG as the treatment of choice at our institution for patients younger than 50 years with symptomatic, precollapse ONFH and especially in those patients – regardless of age – who wish to maintain a high level of athletic activity. Over half of patients with precollapse ONFH treated with FVFG can expect preservation of the hip for greater than 10 years. Those who do not have successful long-term preservation still typically experience an average of 8 years of hip preservation prior to conversion to arthroplasty. Functional outcomes that are equivalent to hip arthroplasty can be expected following this operation. Although technically more demanding than other operative treatments, this durable biologic reconstructive procedure can be an excellent option for treating patients with precollapse ONFH.

References

1. Urbaniak JR. Aseptic necrosis of the femoral head treated by vascularized fibular graft. In: Urbaniak JR, editor. Microsurgery for major limb reconstruction. St. Louis: CV Mosby; 1987. p. 178–84.
2. Korompilias AV, Beris AE, Lykissas MG, et al. Femoral head osteonecrosis: why choose vascularized fibula grafting. Microsurgery. 2001;31(3):223–8.
3. Korompilias AV, Lykissas MG, Beris AE, et al. Vascularized fibular graft in the management of femoral head osteonecrosis. Twenty years later. J Bone Joint Surg Br. 2009;91-B:287–93.
4. Soucacos PN, Beris AE, Malizos K, et al. Treatment of avascular necrosis of the femoral head with vascularized fibular transplant. Clin Orthop. 2001;386:120–30.
5. Eward WC, Rineer CA, Urbaniak JR, Richard MJ, Ruch DS. The vascularized fibular graft in precollapse osteonecrosis: is long-term hip preservation possible? Clin Orthop Relat Res. 2012;470:2819–26.
6. Cho BC, Kim SY, Lee JH, et al. Treatment of osteonecrosis of the femoral head with free vascularized fibular transfer. Ann Plast Surg. 1998;40:586–93.
7. Louie BE, McKee MD, Richards RR, et al. Treatment of osteonecrosis of the femoral head by free vascularized fibular grafting: an analysis of surgical outcome and patient health status. Can J Surg. 1999;42:274–83.
8. Scully SP, Aaron RK, Urbaniak JR. Survival analysis of hips treated with core decompression or vascularized fibular grafting because of avascular necrosis. J Bone Joint Surg Am. 1998;80:1270–5.
9. Bozic KJ, Zurakowski D, Thornhill TS. Survivorship analysis of hips treated with core decompression for nontraumatic osteonecrosis of the femoral head. J Bone Joint Surg Am. 1999;812:200–9.
10. Keizer SB, Kock NB, Dijkstra PD, et al. Treatment of avascular necrosis of the hip by a non-vascularized cortical graft. J Bone Joint Surg Br. 2006;88:460–6.
11. Plakseychuk AY, Kim SY, Park BC, et al. Vascularized compared with nonvascularized fibular grafting for the treatment of osteonecrosis of the femoral head. J Bone Joint Surg Am. 2003;85:589–96.
12. Judet H, Gilbert A. Long-term results of free vascularized fibular grafting for femoral head necrosis. Clin Orthop Relat Res. 2001;386:114–9.
13. Urbaniak JR, Coogan PG, Gunneson EB, Nunley JA. Treatment of osteonecrosis of the femoral head with free vascularized fibular grafting: a long-term follow-up study of one hundred and three hips. J Bone Joint Surg Am. 1995;77:681–94.
14. Aldridge JM, Berend KR, Gunneson EE, Urbaniak JR. Free vascularized fibular grafting for the treatment of postcollapse osteonecrosis of the femoral head. Surgical technique. J Bone Joint Surg Am. 2004;86:87–101.
15. Aldridge JM, Urbaniak JR. Avascular necrosis of the femoral head: role of vascularized bone grafts. Orthop Clin North Am. 2007;38:13–22.
16. Berend KR, Gunneson EE, Urbaniak JR. Free vascularized fibular grafting for the treatment of post collapse osteonecrosis of the femoral head. J Bone Joint Surg Am. 2003;85:987–93.
17. Fairbank AC, Bhatia D, Jinnah RH, Hungerford DS. Long-term results of core decompression for ischaemic necrosis of the femoral head. J Bone Joint Surg Br. 1995;77:42–9.
18. Yoo M, Kim K, Hahn C, Parvizi J. Long-term followup of vascularized fibular grafting for femoral head necrosis. Clin Orthop Relat Res. 2008;466:1133–40.

45 Transtrochanteric Rotational Osteotomy for Femoral Head Osteonecrosis

Yong-Chan Ha, Jae-Hwi Nho, and Kyung-Hoi Koo

45.1 Introduction

Osteonecrosis of the femoral head occurs in young adults. Total hip arthroplasty is not life-long durable in most patients with osteonecrosis. It is associated with high rates of failure due to excessive wear, osteolysis, and aseptic loosening [1–4]. This may eventually lead to a revision surgery which is usually much more difficult than a primary hip replacement. Moreover, the revision surgery is associated with high rate of failure, compromised results, and poor quality of life. Although contemporary articulations have been introduced [5–7], their long-term results are not known yet. Thus, joint-preserving procedures is desirable to avoid or delay total hip arthroplasty in patients with osteonecrosis. Transtrochanteric anterior rotational osteotomy, which was introduced by Sugioka in 1972, is one of the joint-preserving procedures, which moves the necrotic portion of the femoral head from the weight-bearing dome to the non-weight-bearing region [8].

In this chapter, we describe indications, surgical techniques, and reported results of the osteotomy.

Y.-C. Ha (✉)
Department of Orthopaedic Surgery,
Chung-Ang University College of Medicine,
102, Heukseok-ro, Seoul 156-755, South Korea
e-mail: hayongch@naver.com

J.-H. Nho
Department of Orthopaedic Surgery,
Soonchunhyang University Hospital Cheonan,
31 Soonchunhyang 6-gil, Cheonan,
330-721, South Korea

K.-H. Koo
Department of Orthopaedic Surgery,
Seoul National University College of Medicine,
Seoul National University Bundang Hospital,
82 Gumi-ro, 173 Beon-gil, Seongnam
463-707, South Korea
e-mail: khkoo@snu.ac.kr

45.2 Indications

The rotational osteotomy is indicated in patients who have painful early-collapse osteonecrosis without narrowing of the joint space or acetabular involvement (Ficat stage IIB and III). Patients should be younger than 40 years and their body mass index should be less than 24. There should have an enough viable area in the posterior aspect of the femoral head as seen on midsagittal MRI scan (arc of more than 120° between the central vertical line of the femoral head and the posterior margin of the necrotic portion) (Fig. 45.1) [9]. This osteotomy is also indicated for the treatment of Perthes' disease, insufficiency fracture of femoral head with a large extent and collapse, slipped capital femoral epiphysis, and primary osteoarthritis of the hip with localized erosion in the weight-bearing area.

45.3 Surgical Technique

We describe a modified surgical technique by Ha et al. [10], which uses a Y-shaped skin incision instead of the original U-shaped incision and a compression hip screw instead of cancellous screws. The Y-shaped incision enables a better exposure of the anterior capsule. Sugioka recommended fixing the osteotomy with two or three large cancellous screws. However, we have used a 120°-angled compression hip screw since 1999. The angled hip screw has several advantages compared to the cancellous screw. It prevents loss of fixation and nonunion at the osteotomy site. It also shortens the hospital stay and allows an early ambulation.

45.3.1 Surgical Pitfalls

A complete understanding of the anatomy of the medial femoral circumflex artery is of critical importance for the safe performance of this procedure.

K.-H. Koo et al. (eds.), *Osteonecrosis*,
DOI 10.1007/978-3-642-35767-1_45, © Springer-Verlag Berlin Heidelberg 2014

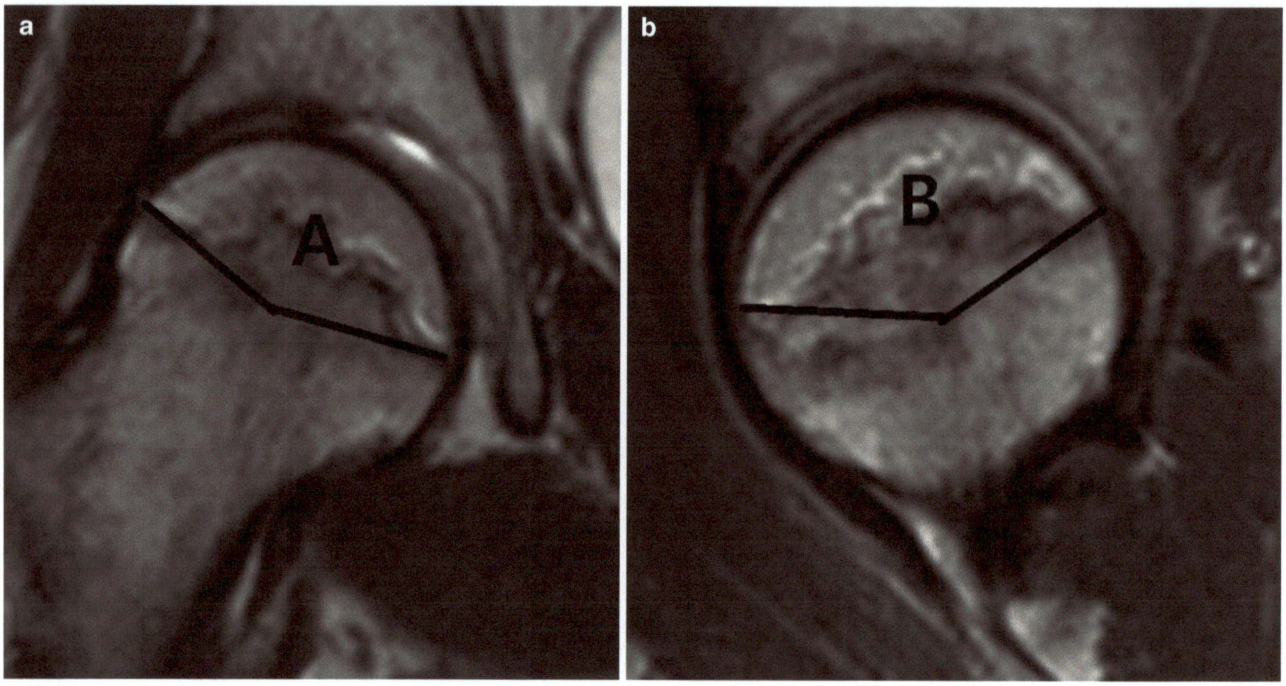

Fig. 45.1 The calculation of the combined necrotic angle from magnetic resonance imaging scans. *A* The angle of necrotic area in the midcoronal image. *B* The angle of necrotic area in the midsagittal image. The combined necrotic angle = $A+B$

The artery is located in the space between the quadratus femoris and obturator externus. During capsulotomy and osteotomy, extreme care should be taken not to damage this artery.

45.3.2 Patient Positioning

The patient is placed in the lateral decubitus position on a standard operating room table with the pelvis stabilized in the neutral position. Intraoperative fluoroscopy is used to confirm the appropriate osteotomy line and the position of compression hip screw (Fig. 45.2).

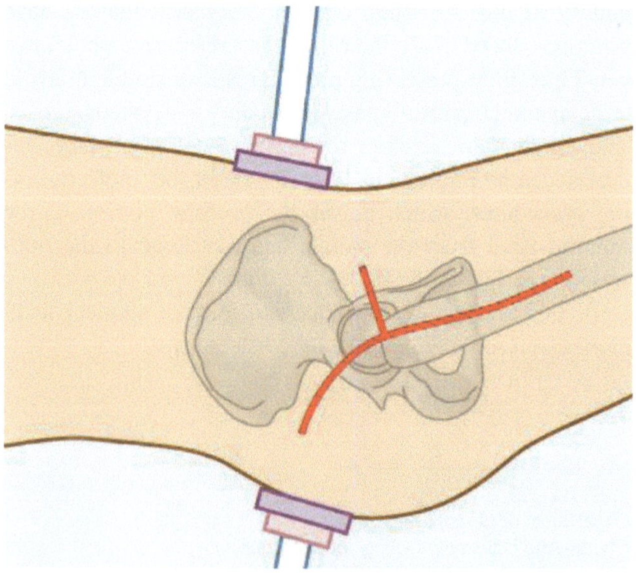

Fig. 45.2 The patient is placed in the lateral decubitus position and the pelvis is secured with holding devices and pads. The Y-shaped skin incision is centered at the greater trochanter. The posterior portion of the incision is started at a point that is level with the posterior superior iliac spine and along a line parallel to the posterior edge of the greater trochanter. The incision is extended distally to the center of the greater trochanter and then to a point 10–15 cm distal to the greater trochanter, in line with the femoral shaft. The anterior portion of the incision is made from the greater trochanter to the anterior superior iliac spine

45.3.3 Skin Incision

A Y-shaped skin incision is made. The posterior limb of the incision starts at the posterior superior iliac spine and proceeds to the greater trochanter and then extends to 10–15 cm distally in line with the axis of the femur. The anterior limb of the incision starts from the center of the greater trochanter to the anterior iliac spine by a length of 5–8 cm (Fig. 45.3). The length of the incision is adjusted according to the size and obesity of the patient.

45.3.4 Fascia Incision

The fascia lata and the gluteus maximus fascia are incised in line with the skin incision. Then gluteus maximus muscle fibers are bluntly divided, giving an access to the gluteus medius and the external rotators of the hip (Fig. 45.3).

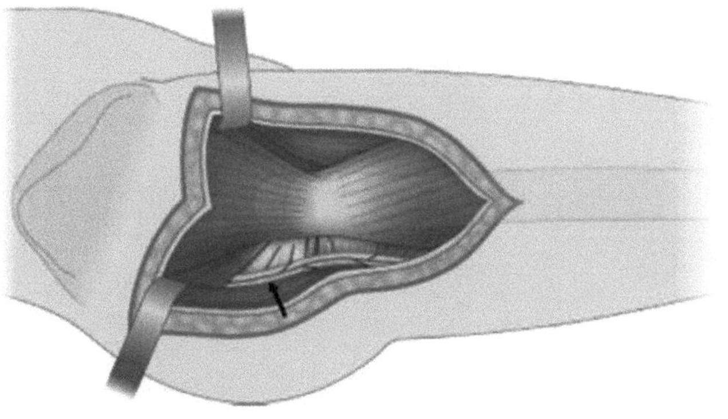

Fig. 45.3 The gluteus maximus fascia is incised in line with the posterior portion of the skin incision, and the muscle fibers of the gluteus maximus are bluntly divided. Fibers of the fascia lata are divided in line with the anterior portion of the skin incision. The fat tissues covering the external rotators and the trochanteric bursa are removed to expose the sciatic nerve (*arrow*) along its course beneath the piriformis muscle and over the short external rotators distally

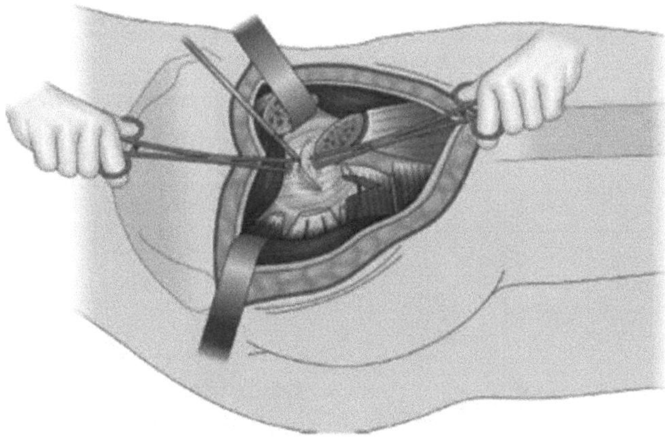

Fig. 45.4 After the complete exposure of the hip joint capsule, the joint capsule is incised circumferentially. The capsulotomy line is 1 cm away from the acetabular rim to protect the acetabular labrum and to obtain adequate rotation of the femoral head

45.3.5 Exposure of the External Rotators and Sciatic Nerve

Remove the fat tissue covering the external rotators, divide the trochanteric bursa, and bluntly sweep it posteriorly to expose the sciatic nerve along its course beneath the piriformis muscle and over the short external rotators distally. The nerve is protected during the operation (Fig. 45.3).

45.3.6 Osteotomy of the Greater Trochanter

The greater trochanter is osteotomized between the gluteus medius and piriformis posteriorly and between the gluteus medius and vastus lateralis anteriorly with an oscillating saw.

45.3.7 Exposure of the Hip Joint Capsule and Capsulotomy

Expose the superior portion of the hip joint capsule by dissecting the gluteus minimus from the capsule. Expose the posterior capsule by cutting the tendons of the piriformis and obturator internus at the trochanteric insertion. Expose the inferior capsule by cutting the quadratus femoris, superior gemellus, and inferior gemellus. To avoid damage to the medial femoral circumflex artery, cut the quadratus femoris, superior gemellus, and inferior gemellus at their muscle fibers 2 cm apart from their femoral insertions. Expose the anterior capsule by developing the interval between the gluteus medius and vastus lateralis.

Once the complete exposure of the hip joint capsule is obtained, a circumferential capsulotomy is performed. The capsulotomy line should be about 1 cm apart from the acetabular rim to avoid the injury of the acetabular labrum. During the capsulotomy hold the capsule using forceps and separate it from the underlying femoral head to avoid the injury of the femoral head cartilage (Fig. 45.4).

45.3.8 Transtrochanteric Osteotomies

Make two transtrochateric osteotomies. The first osteotomy is made about 10 mm distal to the intertrochanteric crest. The osteotomy line should be inclined at 20° from the line perpendicular to the femoral neck to place the femoral head in a varus angulation. The second osteotomy is made near the upper one-third of the lesser trochanter at 90° to the first osteotomy line (Fig. 45.5).

45.3.9 Rotation of the Proximal Segment

The proximal fragment is rotated anteriorly by 90° with a care to avoid excessive stretching or damage of the medial femoral circumflex vessels (Fig. 45.6).

45.3.10 Fixation of Transtrochanteric Osteotomy

After rotating the proximal fragment, the guide pin is positioned with the use of a 120° fixed-angle guide midway on the lateral cortex. The appropriate lag screw length and reaming distance are determined with the aid of fluoroscopy.

After verifying the position and depth of the screw with image intensification in both planes, the osteotomy is fixed

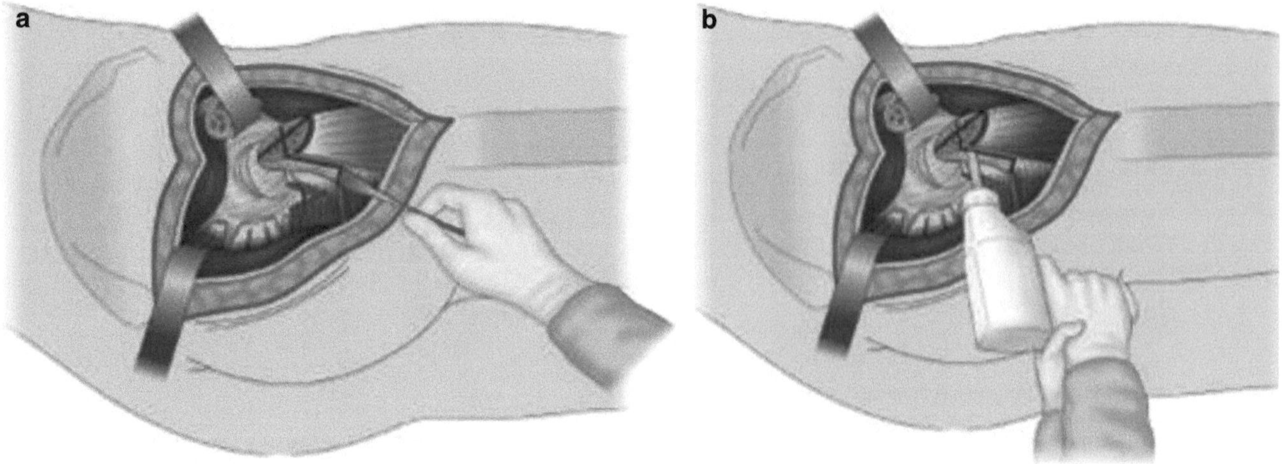

Fig. 45.5 The two osteotomy lines are marked with a broad straight osteotome (**a**), and the osteotomy is performed with the use of a reciprocating saw (**b**)

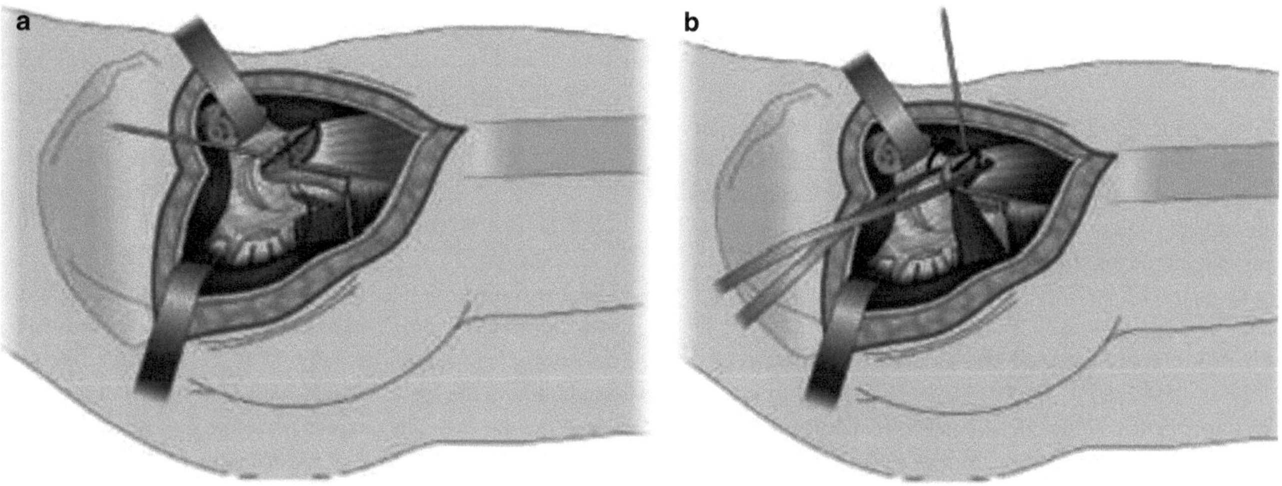

Fig. 45.6 A Kirschner wire is placed in the proximal segment (**a**). The proximal fragment is rotated anteriorly 90° (*arrow* in **b**), with care taken to avoid excessive stretching of or damage to the medial femoral circumflex vessels. The rotated proximal segment is temporarily fixed with use of clamps or Kirschner wires (**b**)

using a 120° compression hip screw and plate (Solco, Seoul, South Korea) (Fig. 45.7).

45.3.11 Reattachment of the Greater Trochanter

For reattachment of the trochanteric fragment, a folding vertical number 16 stainless steel wire is used. One side of the folding vertical wire is inserted in the hole drilled in the lateral cortex below the abductor tubercle and the hole in the osteotomized trochanter, and the other side of folding end makes a loop at the lateral cortex. Each of the two ends is crossed loop in different directions, tightening the wires and tying the knots with Kirschner wire bow. And then the transverse wire that is inserted in the hole drilled in the anteroposterior cortex and the two holes in the osteotomized trochanter is tightened and twisted (Fig. 45.8). After inserting a closed suction drainage, close the wound.

45.3.12 Postoperative Care

The suction drain is removed when the amount of daily drainage was less than 50 ml, usually 2 or 3 days after the operation. After then, patients are allowed to walk with protected weight bearing. Patients continue to use crutches for 3–6 months until there is a radiological evidence of bony union of the osteotomy.

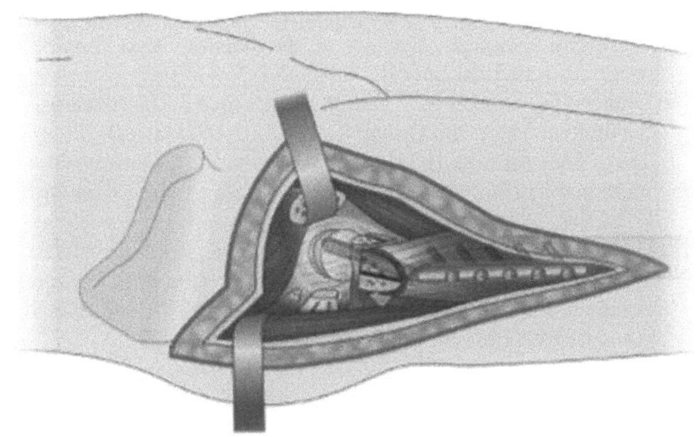

Fig. 45.7 After rotating the proximal fragment, the guide pin is positioned with the use of a 120° fixed-angle guide that is anchored on the midportion of the lateral femoral cortex. After verifying the position and depth of the lag screw in both the anteroposterior and mediolateral planes, the osteotomy is fixed with the use of a 120° compression hip screw and plate

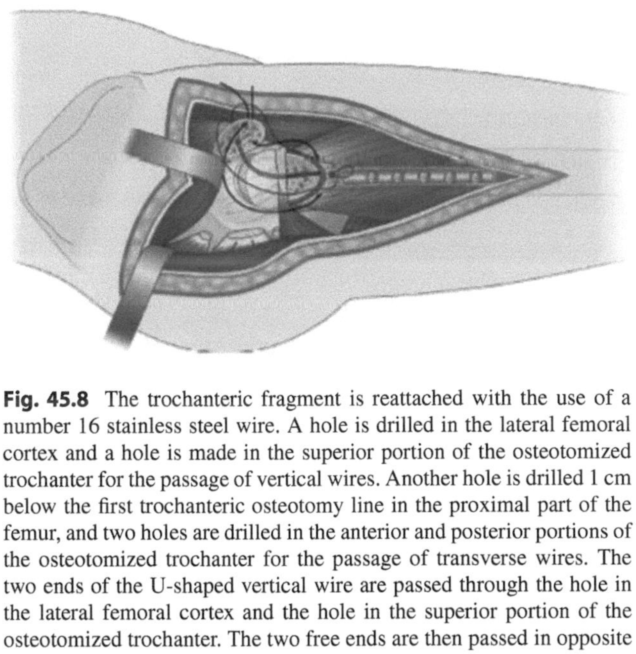

Fig. 45.8 The trochanteric fragment is reattached with the use of a number 16 stainless steel wire. A hole is drilled in the lateral femoral cortex and a hole is made in the superior portion of the osteotomized trochanter for the passage of vertical wires. Another hole is drilled 1 cm below the first trochanteric osteotomy line in the proximal part of the femur, and two holes are drilled in the anterior and posterior portions of the osteotomized trochanter for the passage of transverse wires. The two ends of the U-shaped vertical wire are passed through the hole in the lateral femoral cortex and the hole in the superior portion of the osteotomized trochanter. The two free ends are then passed in opposite directions through the loop in the lateral cortex. The two transverse wires are passed through the hole below the trochanteric osteotomy and then through the two holes in the anterior and posterior portions of the osteotomized trochanter

45.4 Reported Results

The reported results have been quite different [11–17]. Studies from Japan and Korea reported satisfactory results [8, 11–14]. However, such favorable results have not been reproduced in Western countries [15–17]. The striking difference of results was thought to be mainly related to differences in body weight and body mass index between East Asians and Caucasians [15, 18]. Other contributing factors are the preoperative stage, size of necrosis, surgical technique, method of fixation, and postoperative management.

Conclusion

Transtrochanteric osteotomy is an effective joint-preserving procedure in young patients with osteonecrosis. The success rate of the osteotomy is improved by more efficient selection of patients and improved surgical technique. The procedure should be performed in early stages before marked collapse of the head. Viable portion of the femoral head should be of such a size that restoration of adequate weight-bearing articular surface is possible after the operation. Patients should be younger than 40 years and should have a body mass index of less than 24. We recommend a Y-shaped skin incision and fixation of the osteotomy using a compression hip screw.

References

1. Cornell CN, Salvati EA, Pellicci PM. Long-term follow-up of total hip replacement in patients with osteonecrosis. Orthop Clin North Am. 1985;16(4):757–69.
2. Saito S, Saito M, Nishina T, Ohzono K, Ono K. Long-term results of total hip arthroplasty for osteonecrosis of the femoral head. A comparison with osteoarthritis. Clin Orthop Relat Res. 1989;244:198–207.
3. Kim YH, Oh JH, Oh SH. Cementless total hip arthroplasty in patients with osteonecrosis of the femoral head. Clin Orthop Relat Res. 1995;320:73–84.
4. Katz RL, Bourne RB, Rorabeck CH, McGee H. Total hip arthroplasty in patients with avascular necrosis of the hip. Follow-up observations on cementless and cemented operations. Clin Orthop Relat Res. 1992;281:145–51.
5. Daniel J, Pynsent PB, McMinn DJ. Metal-on-metal resurfacing of the hip in patients under the age of 55 years with osteoarthritis. J Bone Joint Surg Br. 2004;86(2):177–84.
6. Kearns SR, Jamal B, Rorabeck CH, Bourne RB. Factors affecting survival of uncemented total hip arthroplasty in patients 50 years or younger. Clin Orthop Relat Res. 2006;453:103–9. doi:10.1097/01.blo.0000238868.22852.dd.
7. Yoo JJ, Kim YM, Yoon KS, Koo KH, Kim JW, Nam KW, et al. Contemporary alumina-on-alumina total hip arthroplasty performed in patients younger than forty years: a 5-year minimum follow-up study. J Biomed Mater Res B Appl Biomater. 2006;78(1):70–5. doi:10.1002/jbm.b.30457.
8. Sugioka Y. Transtrochanteric anterior rotational osteotomy of the femoral head in the treatment of osteonecrosis affecting the hip: a new osteotomy operation. Clin Orthop Relat Res. 1978;130:191–201.
9. Ha YC, Jung WH, Kim JR, Seong NH, Kim SY, Koo KH. Prediction of collapse in femoral head osteonecrosis: a modified Kerboul method with use of magnetic resonance images. J Bone Joint Surg Am. 2006;88 Suppl 3:35–40. doi:10.2106/JBJS.F.00535.
10. Ha YC, Kim HJ, Kim SY, Kim KC, Lee YK, Koo KH. Effects of age and body mass index on the results of transtrochanteric rotational osteotomy for femoral head osteonecrosis: surgical technique. J Bone Joint Surg Am. 2011;93 Suppl 1:75–84. doi:10.2106/JBJS.J.01215.

11. Sugioka Y, Hotokebuchi T, Tsutsui H. Transtrochanteric anterior rotational osteotomy for idiopathic and steroid-induced necrosis of the femoral head. Indications and long-term results. Clin Orthop Relat Res. 1992;277:111–20.
12. Sugano N, Takaoka K, Ohzono K, Matsui M, Saito M, Saito S. Rotational osteotomy for non-traumatic avascular necrosis of the femoral head. J Bone Joint Surg Br. 1992;74(5):734–9.
13. Inao S, Ando M, Gotoh E, Matsuno T. Minimum 10-year results of Sugioka's osteotomy for femoral head osteonecrosis. Clin Orthop Relat Res. 1999;368:141–8.
14. Koo KH, Song HR, Yang JW, Yang P, Kim JR, Kim YM. Trochanteric rotational osteotomy for osteonecrosis of the femoral head. J Bone Joint Surg Br. 2001;83(1):83–9.
15. Dean MT, Cabanela ME. Transtrochanteric anterior rotational osteotomy for avascular necrosis of the femoral head. Long-term results. J Bone Joint Surg Br. 1993;75(4):597–601.
16. Langlais F, Fourastier J. Rotation osteotomies for osteonecrosis of the femoral head. Clin Orthop Relat Res. 1997;343:110–23.
17. Tooke SM, Amstutz HC, Hedley AK. Results of transtrochanteric rotational osteotomy for femoral head osteonecrosis. Clin Orthop Relat Res. 1987;224:150–7.
18. Ha YC, Kim HJ, Kim SY, Kim KC, Lee YK, Koo KH. Effects of age and body mass index on the results of transtrochanteric rotational osteotomy for femoral head osteonecrosis. J Bone Joint Surg Am. 2010;92(2):314–21. doi:10.2106/JBJS.H.01020.

Posterior Rotational Osteotomy for Severe Femoral Head Osteonecrosis

46

Takashi Atsumi

46.1 Introduction

Nontraumatic and post-traumatic osteonecrosis involving the femoral head related with steroid administration, alcoholic abuse, and neck fracture frequently occurs in young patients [1].

The necrotic focus is predominantly located in the loaded portion of the femoral head resulting in progressive collapse [2]. Preservation of the joint of the femoral head necrosis is important in young patients to avoid some kind of joint replacement [3–5]. The joint-preserving procedures are usually effective to cases with small or medium sized lesions in early stage of the disease [6, 7]. However, if lesion size is extensive in the weight-bearing area, the femoral head will usually progress to collapse in many cases [2]. Some kind of osteotomies [7] and vascularized fibular grafts [6] are usually not effective in extensive collapsed cases. Sugioka has reported his technique of transtrochanteric anterior rotational osteotomies for femoral head osteonecrosis with extensive lesion which might be an ideal treatment with extensive lesion and described favorable results [9]. However, in case of apparent collapse, collapsed anterior lesions are moved to the loaded portion below the acetabular roof in flexed positions after anterior rotation resulting anteroposterior instability [8] and osteoarthritic change. In contrast, by means of high posterior rotational osteotomy [10–14] for markedly collapsed cases, uncollapsed anterior viable areas are transferred to the loaded portion below the acetabular roof in flexed position receiving the load as possible advantage.

T. Atsumi
Department of Orthopaedic Surgery, Showa University Fujigaoka Hospital, Showa University School of Medicine, 1-30 Fujigaoka Aobaku, Yokohama 227-8501, Japan
e-mail: t.atsumi@mx6.ttcn.ne.jp

The author mentioned the concept, effectiveness, surgical technique, remodeling, and the results of high-degree posterior rotational osteotomy for the treatment of extensive collapsed necrotic lesions.

46.2 Concepts and Advantage

The primary concept of femoral osteotomy for the treatment of osteonecrosis is to move collapsed necrotic lesions from the major weight bearing portion. Weight bearing forces are received by transferred viable area [1]. Most necrotic portions are located in the anterior superior portion of the femoral head. Anterior rotational osteotomy developed by Sugioka [9, 15] for osteonecrosis of the femoral head with extensive lesion is that a posterior healthy portion is moved to superior area on loaded portion of the femoral head. The limitation of anterior rotational angle according to Sugioka is less than 100°. There remain many patients have large necrotic lesion that exceeds the indication of Sugioka. From the angiographic study of anterior rotational osteotomy, the posterior column artery branching off from the medial circumflex artery was demonstrated to be markedly stretched laterally, which may impair blood supply of the femoral head [16]. In contrast, the posterior column artery was moved and relaxed medially after posterior rotational osteotomy [10]. After anterior rotation, collapsed necrotic lesion is remained on anterior portion of the femoral head and moved to weight-bearing area below the acetabular roof in flexion positions. Posterior rotational osteotomy including high-degree rotation might be indicated in cases without indication of conventional anterior rotational osteotomy and with advanced collapsed lesion and had advantages comparing with anterior rotation.

K.-H. Koo et al. (eds.), *Osteonecrosis*,
DOI 10.1007/978-3-642-35767-1_46,

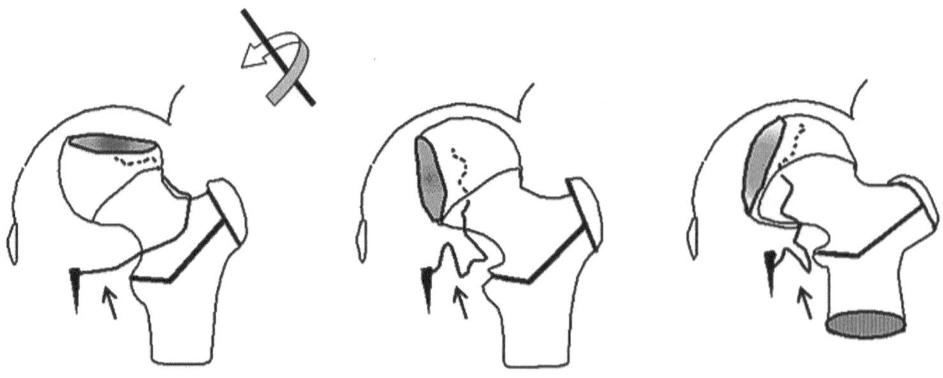

Fig. 46.1 Concept and advantage of high-degree posterior rotational osteotomy. The necrotic lesion is moved to the medial to posteromedial non-weight-bearing portion of the joint by high-degree posterior rotational osteotomy. Postoperative uncollapsed anterior viable areas are moved to the loaded portion below the acetabular roof in neutral and flexed positions. After posterior rotation, congruency can be expected in a flexed position of daily life, especially in advanced stages with apparent collapse. The posterior column artery (*arrow*) is shifted medially and is not under tension without vascular impairment by posterior rotation

46.2.1 Location of Necrotic and Viable Area After Posterior Rotation

The possible advantages of posterior rotational osteotomies are as follows [10–14]:

1. The necrotic lesion is transferred to the medial or posteromedial non-weight-bearing portion of the joint far away from high-pressure area. Postoperative uncollapsed anterior viable areas are moved to the loaded portion below the acetabular roof in flexed positions. After posterior rotation, congruency can be expected in a flexed position of daily life, especially in advanced stages with apparent collapse. These conditions are opposite to those for the traditional anterior rotational osteotomy for collapsed femoral heads.
2. The posterior column artery branched off from the femoral medial circumflex artery is shifted medially and is not under tension and without vascular impairment by posterior rotation. This has been confirmed by angiographic studies [10, 16].

Thus, a high degree of posterior rotation can be performed even when the patients have extensive lesions which are beyond the scope of Sugioka's indication for traditional anterior rotation (Fig. 46.1).

46.3 Indications

Indications of posterior rotational osteotomy are as follows: (1) Cases with the necrotic lesion are too far advanced for conservative treatment, or most other joint-preserving operations are not effective. (2) Cases with less than one-third of the viable posterior portion of the femoral head which are out of indication for conventional anterior rotational osteotomy. (3) In young patients with extensive collapsed lesion where less than one-third of anterior and posterior portion remain viable area, "high-degree" posterior rotational osteotomy might be required even if joint space narrowing already occurred [10–14].

46.3.1 Preoperative Assessment

The posterior rotational angle and intentional varus angle necessary for this procedure were determined by preoperative assessment, mainly on radiographic findings and magnetic resonance imaging (Fig. 46.2). Lateral radiographs should be taken in all hips by the method described by Sugioka [9] to observe the location and extent of necrotic region. The patients are laid in supine position; radiographs of hips were taken in 90° of flexion, 45° of abduction, and neutral rotation. This radiograph was available for decision of indications in 90° anterior or posterior rotational osteotomy. In addition, anterior-posterior radiographs in a flexed position were obtained. The patients are laid in supine position, and the affected hip was flexed with 45° of abduction with varying degrees of flexion [13, 14] (Fig. 46.3a). Location of the necrotic lesion was carefully confirmed on radiographs in various flexion positions. At that time, flexion angle could reveal the posterior rotational angle. By the use of this radiograph, the varus angle was decided by drawing a figure.

Magnetic resonance imaging can be available if the demarcation area between living and necrotic bone is not clearly visualized on radiographs. Radial MRI (Fig. 46.3b, c) was developed for decision of location of viable

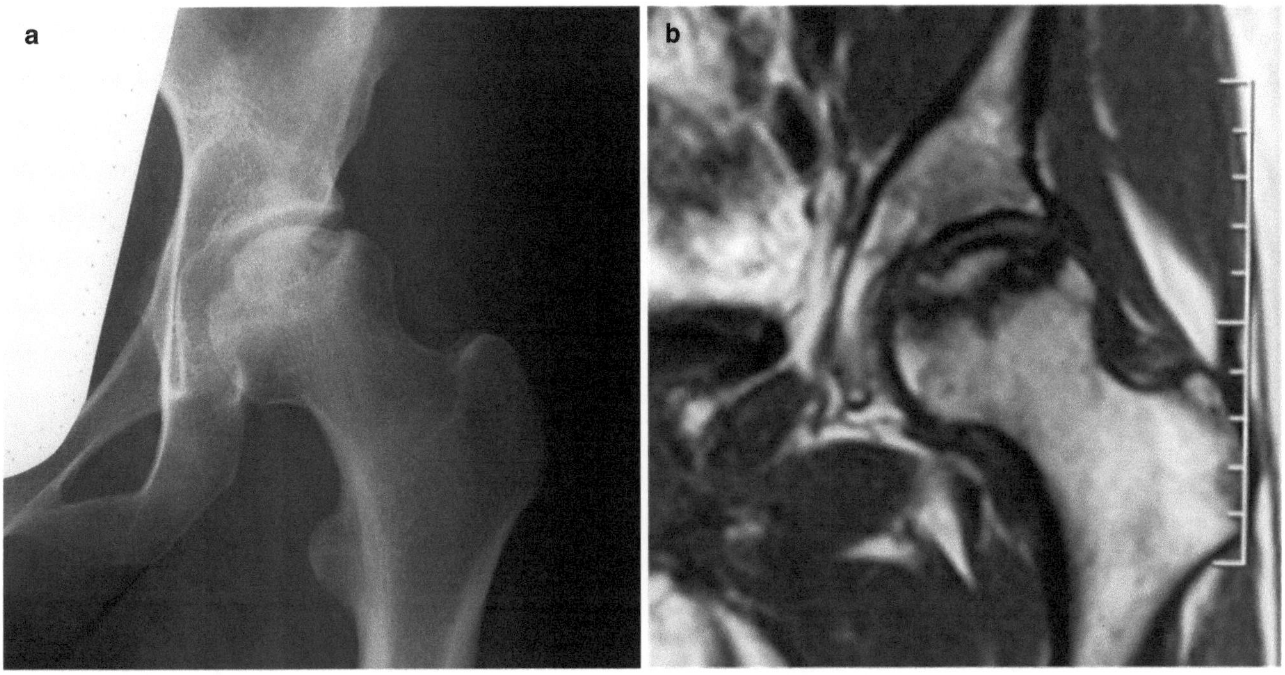

Fig. 46.2 A 27-year-old woman having high dose of corticosteroids due to treatment of sclerotic lupus erythematosus. (**a**) Preoperative anteroposterior radiograph of her left hip showed large collapsed extensive lesion. (**b**) Magnetic resonance imaging (T1-weighted image) coronal slice showed extensive low-intensity area below acetabular roof

necrotic area, and rotational angle, T1-weighted image, and T2 fat suppression image were taken perpendicular to the axis of the femoral neck 10° each (Fig. 46.3b). MRI findings were compared with radiographic findings; then, posterior rotational angle and intentional varus angle were decided.

46.4 Operative Technique

A modified Southern approach [10–14] was used with the patients in the lateral position. Skin incision was performed from distal to the anterior superior iliac spine and extended distally and posteriorly, passing through the distal portion of the greater trochanter. The fascia is incised in line with the skin incision. With the hip rotated internally, the short external rotators are incised at the acetabular margin. The location of the posterior column vessels should be carefully confirmed. The obturator externus is elevated and incised, protecting nutrient vessels. The posterior column vessels are situated along the obturator externus. The greater trochanter is osteomized and is reflected proximally with the gluteus medius and minimus. The complete incision of the iliopsoas tendon is necessary in area attached to the lesser trochanter. The capsule was exposed widely; then, the capsule is incised circumferentially except the anteroinferior portion.

Method of Decision for Osteotomy Plane: The hip is rotated internally; position with maximum lengths of femoral neck is confirmed under image intensifier, and then, one K-wire is placed into the center of the femoral neck through the trochanteric osteotomy [13]. Two additional K-wires are inserted into the intertrochanteric area, perpendicular to the axis of the femoral neck to decide the correct osteotomy plane. This technique is different from original technique described by Sugioka [9] (Fig. 46.4). A Steinman pin is inserted into anterior portion of the femoral neck. The femoral head and neck is rotated manually to posterior direction. Then, the remained anteroinferior capsular ligament (mainly the iliofemoral ligament) is detached from the femoral neck [13].

The image intensifier is used for the final determination of the correct position [10, 12, 13]. Bleeding from the osteomized area of proximal portion should be confirmed. Fixation of the transtrochanteric osteotomy is performed by screws and plate system designed by Atsumi [10, 12, 13]. For postoperative management, early motion exercises and isometric exercises of the quadriceps muscle were performed immediately after the patients became free from postoperative pain. The patients were in bed for one week and then used a wheel chair. Partial weight bearing was initiated 5–6 weeks after operation using 2 crutches. Walking with 1 crutch should be continued 6 months after operation.

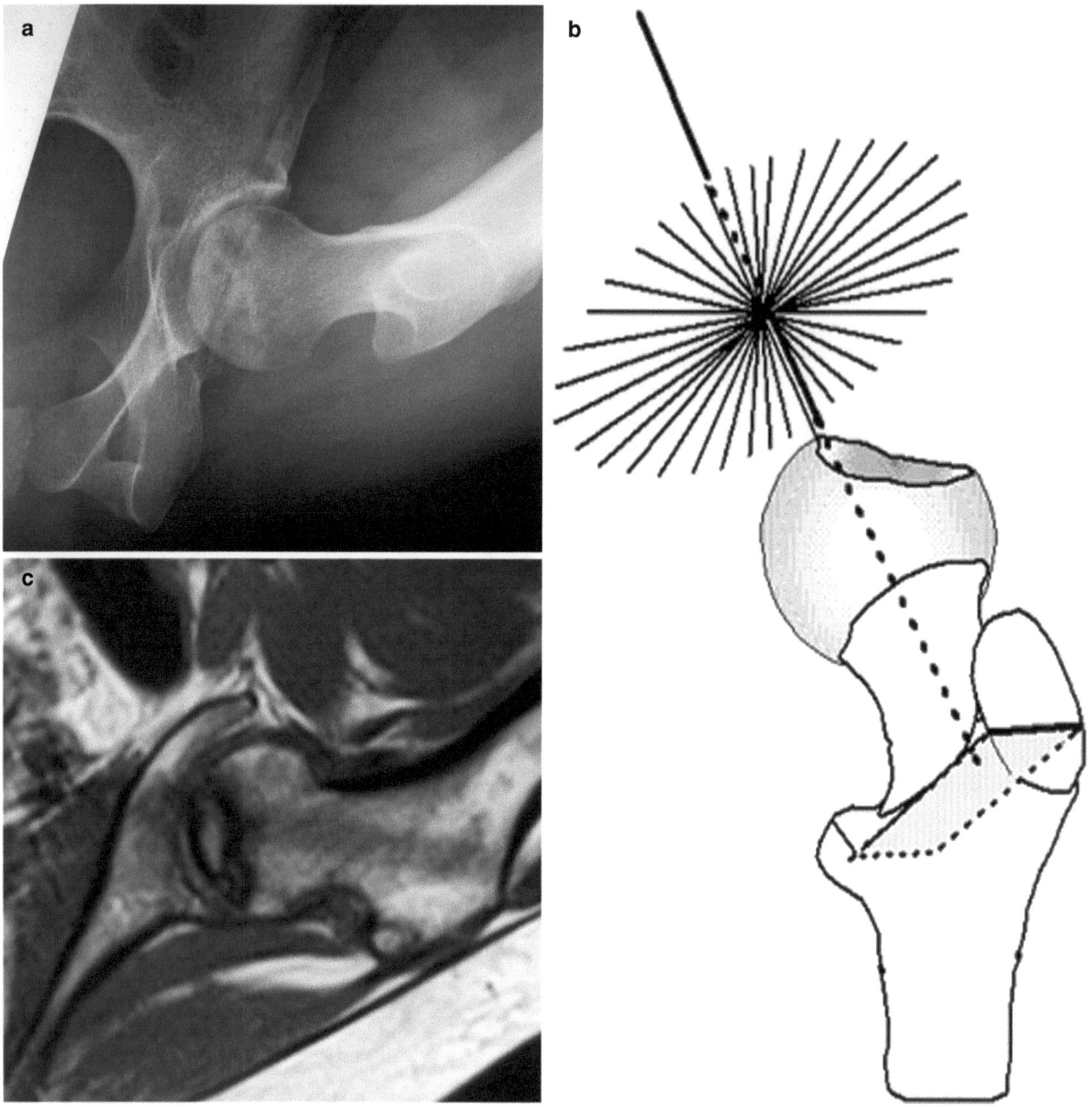

Fig. 46.3 Radial MRI and AP radiographs in a flexed position in the patient of Fig. 46.2. (**a**) AP radiograph in 120° flexion with 45° of abduction showed anterior viable area that is moved to loaded portion. (**b**) Radial MRI was developed for decision of location of viable, necrotic area, and rotational angle was taken perpendicular to the axis of the femoral neck 10° each. (**c**) Radial MRI equivalent of 120° posterior rotation indicated the anteroinferior viable portion implied by normal intensity

46.5 Calcar Remodeling

After high-degree posterior rotational osteotomy, anterolateral porotic portion is moved to medial neck. Atsumi and Kuroki described calcar remodeling after this procedure by AP radiographs. Calcar remodeling was partially observed in 61 % 1 year after operation. The entire calcar remodeled in 56 % 2 years after operation. Three years after operation, the calcar remodeling was completed [10] (Figs. 46.5a and 46.6).

46.6 Prevention of Re-collapse

Atsumi et al. reviewed the results of 35 hips affected by nontraumatic osteonecrosis with apparent extensive collapsed lesions of the femoral head in 28 young patients (mean age: 28 years) with 8-year follow-up [12]. All hips were not indicated for Sugioka's anterior rotational osteotomy.

Collapse was progressed in all hips showing greater than 3 mm of collapse on AP radiographs. Joint space narrowing

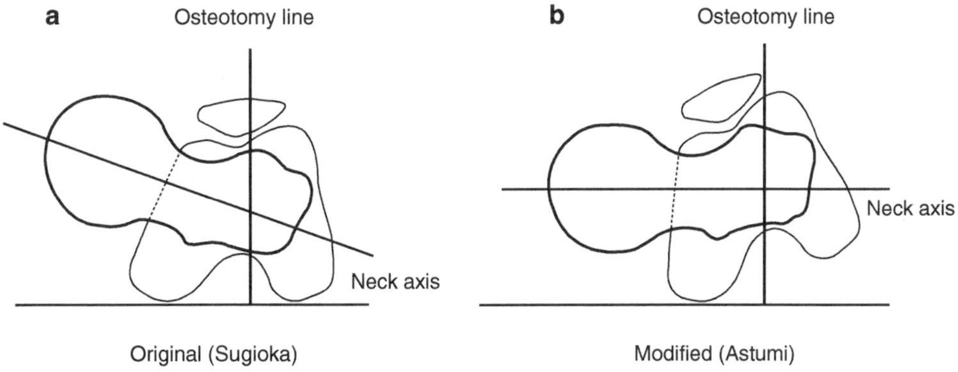

Fig. 46.4 Method of decision for osteotomy plane. The hip is rotated internally; position with maximum lengths of the femoral neck is confirmed under image intensifier; then, one K-wire is placed into the center of the femoral neck through the trochanteric osteotomy. Two additional K-wires are inserted into the intertrochanteric area, perpendicular to the axis of the femoral neck to decide the correct osteotomy plane (**b**). This technique is different form original technique described by Sugioka. The osteotomy plane described by Sugioka (**a**) is oblique to the femoral neck axis

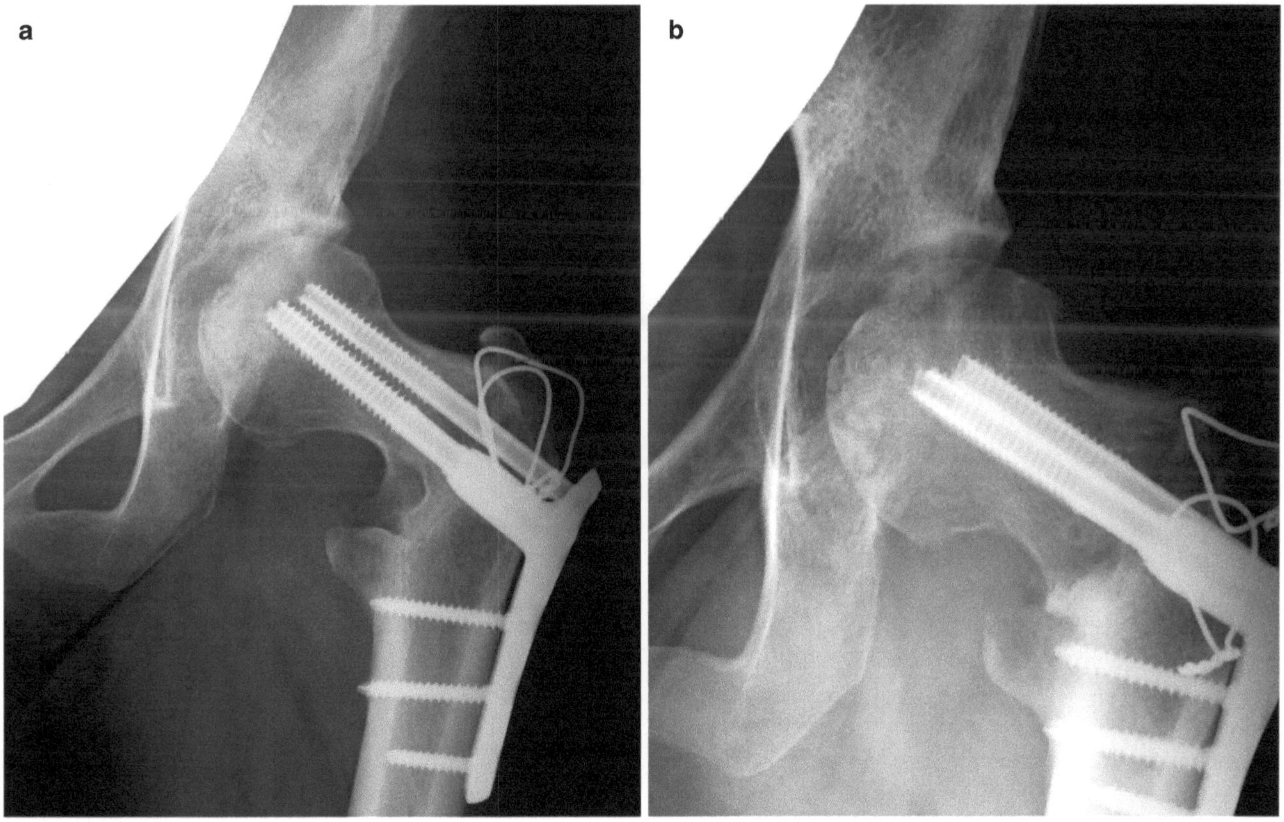

Fig. 46.5 Following radiographs of Figs. 46.2 and 46.3. (**a**). 120° posterior rotation was performed. AP radiograph taken 6 months after operation showed that collapsed lesion with subchondral fracture was moved to the medial portion. Note the spherical viable area was placed on the loaded portion below the acetabulum. Calcar was remodeled in part. (**b**) 45° flexion AP radiograph taken at the same time. Anterior viable area was seen below the acetabulum

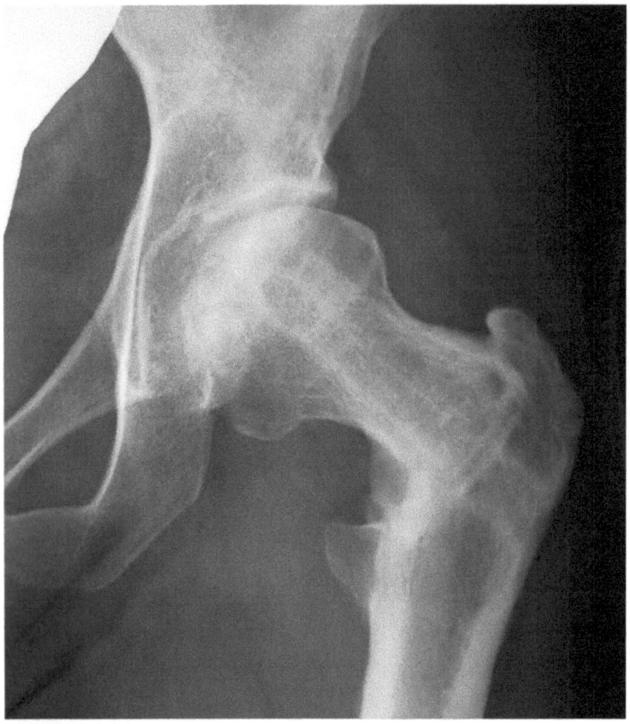

Fig. 46.6 3 years after operation of a case of Figs. 46.2 and 46.3. AP radiograph disclosed spherical contour of the medial femoral head and disappearance of medial subchondral fracture. Secondary collapse was prevented; calcar remodeling was complete. She is free from pain and has good range of motion (flexion was 140°; abduction was 30°)

was already observed on seven hips. All hips were treated by posterior rotational osteotomy (mean posterior rotational angle: 131°).

The anterior non-collapsed viable area was moved to the weight-bearing area below the acetabular roof after posterior rotation. This was confirmed by using 45° flexion position anterior-posterior radiographs showing anterior spherical portion (Figs. 46.5a, b). The extent of the viable area corresponding to the weight-bearing portion below the acetabular roof on conventional anterior-posterior radiographs was almost equivalent to the extent on the 45° flexion anteroposterior radiographs. On the final follow-up AP radiographs, re-collapse were prevented in 94 % with adequate viable area.

46.7 Remodeling

The necrotic lesion is transferred to the medial or posteromedial non-weight-bearing portion.

Respherical contour with medial collapsed portion and disappearance of subchondral fracture moved by high-degree posterior rotational osteotomy is one of the characteristic remodeling (Figs. 46.5 and 46.6). Measurement was performed that showed the greatest collapse area of the medial femoral head in 28 hips treated by high-degree posterior rotational osteotomy. The methods of Steinburg et al. [17] were used in part. The mean ratio of medial collapse of the femoral head was 18.4 % less than 6 months after operation and 8.3 % 3 years 3.4 % at final follow-up (mean, 8.5 years) after operation [14]. The ratios were equivalent between nontraumatic and traumatic cases.

Subchondral fracture disappeared on 68 % 3 years after operation and on 92 % at final follow-up [14]. Of the improvement of the acetabular subchondral roof for the seven hips with apparent joint space narrowing before operation, the shape of the acetabular roof was reformed by 2 years after the procedure in all seven hips. At final follow-up anterior-posterior radiographs, the joint space was increased, when comparing it before the procedure, and maintained [12]. These results showed apparent remodeling occurred after high-degree posterior rotational osteotomy.

46.8 Discussion

Joint preservation of femoral head osteonecrosis in young patients is widely recognized for orthopedic surgeons. However, if the patients have the extensive lesion in the weight-bearing area, collapse usually occurs within a short period [2].

In cases with extensive collapsed necrotic lesions, various types of prosthetic replacement should be performed even if patients are young although the results of prosthetic replacement for young patients are controversial [3–5]. In cases of no apparent collapse, Sugioka's conventional anterior rotational osteotomy may be effective if the posterior large viable area still remains [9, 15]. However, if the patients have apparent collapse, anterior instability occurs after anterior rotation. Anterior collapsed lesion is moved to the loaded portion below acetabular roof on flexion producing instability [8]. In contrast, the anterior viable area transferred by high-degree posterior rotation can be moved to the loaded portion below acetabular roof. The authors demonstrated using 45° flexion AP radiograph that anterior viable was placed in the weight-bearing area below the acetabular roof [12]. Collapsed necrotic lesion was moved to the medial or posteromedial portion implying low-pressure area. After high-degree posterior rotational osteotomy, containment and congruency between the femoral head and the acetabulum were improved not only in the neutral position but also in flexion of daily activities. With these reasons, the prominent remodeling might be able to occur after high-degree posterior rotational osteotomy resulting in joint preservation for young patients.

46.9 Summary

The author believes that this operation may delay the progression of degeneration if adequate viable area can be placed under the loaded portion of the acetabulum. Remodeling of the collapsed lesion and the degenerative acetabular subchondral roof might be one of the important factors for preserving the joints. High-degree posterior rotational osteotomy might be effective in young patients with extensive collapsed necrotic lesion of the femoral head.

References

1. Mont MA, Hungerford DS. Non-traumatic avascular necrosis of the femoral head. J Bone Joint Surg Am. 1995;77:459–74.
2. Ohzono K, Saito M, Takaoka K, et al. Natural history of nontraumatic avascular necrosis of the femoral head. J Bone Joint Surg Br. 1991;73-B:68–72.
3. Adili A, Trousdale T. Femoral head resurfacing for the treatment of osteonecrosis in the young patient. Clin Orthop Relat Res. 2003;417:93–101.
4. Piston RW, Engh CA. Osteonecrosis of the femoral head treated with total hip arthroplasty without cement. J Bone Joint Surg Am. 1994;76:202–14.
5. Sayeed SA, Johnson AJ, Stroh DA, Gross TP, Mont MA. Hip resurfacing in patients who have osteonecrosis and are 25 years or under. Clin Orthop Relat Res. 2011;469:1582–8.
6. Urbaniak JR, Coogan PG, Gunneson EB, Nunley JA. Treatment of osteonecrosis of the femoral head with free vascularized fibular grafting. A long-term follow-up study of one hundred and three hips. J Bone Joint Surg Am. 1995;77:681–94.
7. Mont MA, Fairbank AC, Krackow KA, Hungerford DS. Corrective osteotomy for osteonecrosis of the femoral head. J Bone Joint Surg Am. 1996;78:1032–8.
8. Hiranuma Y, Atsumi T, Kajiwara T, Tamaoki S, Asakura Y. Evaluation of instability after transtrochanteric anterior rotational osteotomy for nontraumatic osteonecrosis of the femoral head. J Orthop Sci. 2009;14:535–42.
9. Sugioka Y. Transtrochanteric anterior rotational osteotomy of the femoral head in the treatment of osteonecrosis affecting the hip. A new osteotomy operation. Clin Orthop Relat Res. 1978;130:191–201.
10. Atsumi T, Kuroki Y. Modified Sugioka's osteotomy. More than 130° posterior rotation for osteonecrosis of the femoral head with large lesion. Clin Orthop Relat Res. 1997;334:98–107.
11. Atsumi T, Muraki M, Yoshihara S, Kjiwara T. Posterior rotational osteotomy for the treatment of femoral head osteonecrosis. Arch Orthop Trauma Surg. 1999;119:388–93.
12. Atsumi T, Kajiwara T, Hiranuma Y, Tamaoki S, Asakura Y. Posterior rotational osteotomy for nontraumatic osteonecrosis with extensive collapsed lesions in young patients. J Bone Joint Surg Am. 2006;88:42–7.
13. Atsumi T, Hosalkar H. Proximal femoral osteotomies. In: Steinberg ME, editor. Osteonecrosis of the hip, Tech Orthop 2008;23:54–64.
14. Atsumi T, Kajiwara T, Tamaoki S, Maeda A, Nakanishi R. Re-spherical contour with medial collapsed femoral head necrosis after high degree posterior rotational osteotomy in young patients with extensive necrosis. Orthop Clin North Am. 2009;40:267–74.
15. Sugioka Y, Hotokebuti T, Tsutsui H. Transtrochanteric anterior rotational osteotomy for idiopathic and steroid-induced necrosis of the femoral head. Indications and long-term results. Clin Orthop Relat Res. 1992;277:111–20.
16. Atsumi T, Yamano K. Superselective angiography in osteonecrosis of the femoral head. In: Urbaniak JR, Jones JP, editors. Osteonecrosis: etiology, diagnosis, and treatment. The American Orthopaedic Association, Rosemont: American Academy of Orthopaedic Surgeons; 1997. p. 247–52.
17. Steinburg ME, Heyken GD, Steinburg DR. A quantitative system for staging avascular necrosis. J Bone Joint Surg Br. 1995;77:34–41.

47 Transtrochanteric Curved Varus Osteotomy for the Treatment of Osteonecrosis of the Femoral Head

Takuaki Yamamoto, Satoshi Ikemura, and Yukihide Iwamoto

47.1 Background of the Transtrochanteric Curved Varus Osteotomy

Osteonecrosis (ON) of the femoral head often occurs in adolescents and in middle-aged patients. Accordingly, joint preservation may be one of the ideal options, when a surgical treatment is considered. We believe the principles of the treatment of ON are (1) to eliminate the shear stress from the necrotic region and to prevent a progression of collapse and (2) to obtain joint realignment of the femoral head subluxated due to collapse. To satisfy these principles, we have performed transtrochanteric curved varus osteotomy for ON patients who have an intact non-collapsed lesion in the lateral part of the femoral head. The purpose of this curved varus osteotomy is to move the necrotic lesion medially and then to bring the intact lateral articular surface into a weight-bearing position.

Originally, the varus wedge osteotomy was developed for the treatment of hip osteoarthritis [1], which later was adapted for the treatment of osteonecrosis by Merle d'Aubigne et al. [2] and Kerboul et al. [3]. This varus wedge osteotomy, however, has some disadvantages, such as causing elevation or lateral displacement of the greater trochanter, potential possibility of nonunion or delayed union, and leg length discrepancy (ranging from 29 to 38 mm) [4–6].

In order to overcome these problems, Nishio developed a transtrochanteric curved varus osteotomy, which is performed between the greater and the lesser trochanters (Fig. 47.1) [7]. In this transtrochanteric curved varus osteotomy, the leg length discrepancy has been reported to range from around 0.5–20 mm [8–11], and good clinical and radiological outcomes have been reported (success rate is around 90 %) [8–11].

T. Yamamoto (✉) • S. Ikemura • Y. Iwamoto
Department of Orthopaedic Surgery, Kyushu University, 3-1-1 Maidashi, Higashi-ku, Fukuoka 812-8582, Japan
e-mail: yamataku@ortho.med.kyushu-u.ac.jp; sikemura@ortho.med.kyushu-u.ac.jp; yiwamoto@ortho.med.kyushu-u.ac.jp

47.2 Indication of the Curved Varus Osteotomy

This procedure is indicated in cases with a residual intact area in the lateral part of the femoral head with an intact area ratio to the acetabular weight-bearing area of 33.6 % or more in a maximum abduction position (Fig. 47.2), since patients who had more than 33.6 % of the intact articular surface of the femoral head postoperatively had been reported to have a good clinical outcome (Figs. 47.3 and 47.4) [11]. Therefore, patients who had the prospect of obtaining more than 34 % intact articular surface on preoperative AP hip radiograph in maximum abduction were indicated for this operation. To prevent adduction contracture, cases in which the hip joints could not be abducted more than 20° are not indicated.

47.3 Operative Procedures

47.3.1 Operative Position

Osteotomy is performed in a complete lateral decubitus position. Since an image will be used during the operation, secure fixation should be achieved so as to obtain an accurate anteroposterior radiograph of the pelvis.

47.3.2 Skin Incision

A 15–20-cm lateral longitudinal incision is made from the proximal end of the greater trochanter to the distal end.

47.3.3 Expansion of the Hip

An incision is made on the deep fascia of the thigh and on the iliotibial band as well. The thin membranes or synovial capsules around the greater trochanter are incised with the lower extremities in a medial rotation position so that the

K.-H. Koo et al. (eds.), *Osteonecrosis*,
DOI 10.1007/978-3-642-35767-1_47, © Springer-Verlag Berlin Heidelberg 2014

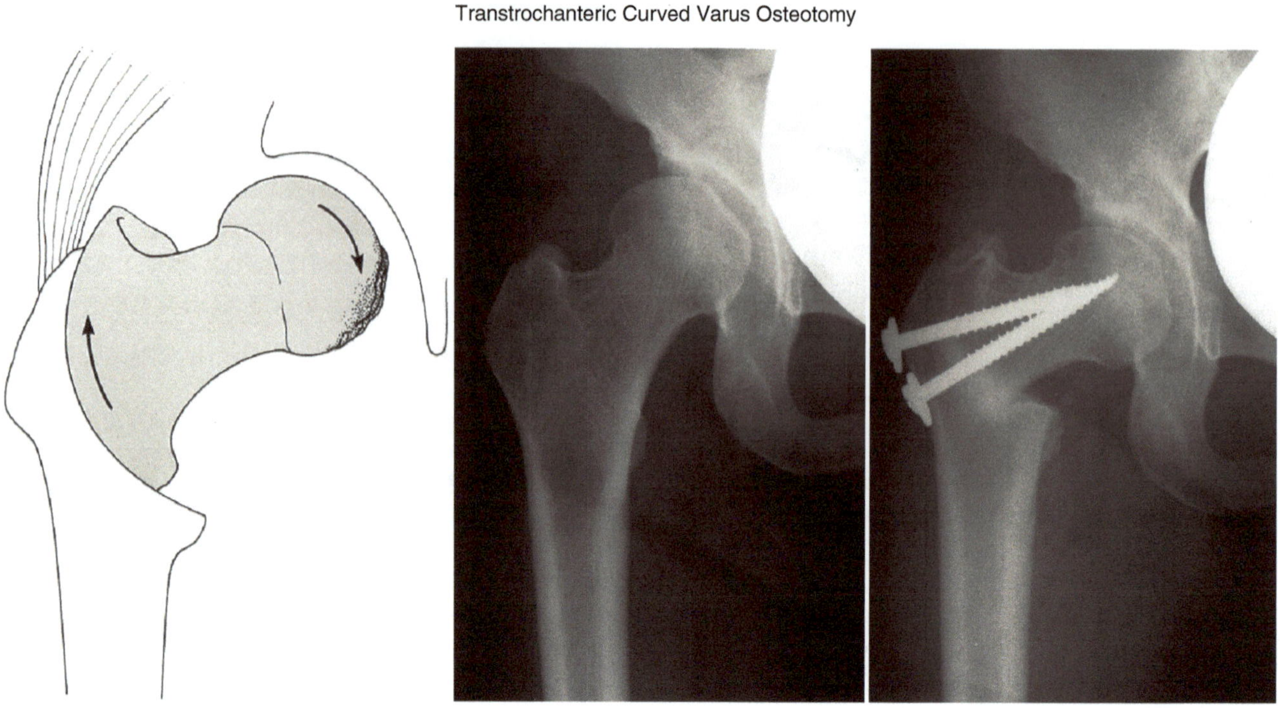

Fig. 47.1 Transtrochanteric curved varus osteotomy is performed between the greater and the lesser trochanters, which has a merit to prevent elevation of the greater trochanter, lateral displacement of the femoral shaft which causes gluteus medius and minimus muscle disorders, delayed union or nonunion at the site of osteotomies, and leg length discrepancy, which has been commonly observed after wedge varus osteotomies

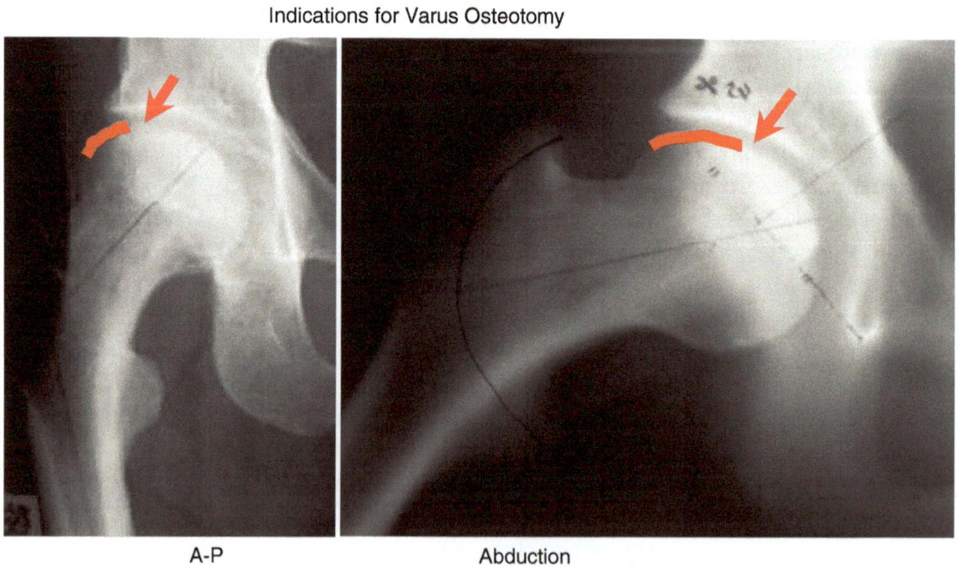

Fig. 47.2 Cases who have a residual intact area in the lateral part of the femoral head with an intact area ratio to the acetabular weight-bearing area of 33.6 % or more in a maximum abduction position (*red arrow*: borderline between necrotic and intact area)

intertrochanteric crest is exposed. The lesser trochanter is exposed subperiosteally, and the intertrochanteric crest is also elevated along the planned osteotomy line. During this process, care should be taken not to damage the nutrient vessels supplying the femoral head in the medial intertrochanteric crest. Since osteotomy is performed from the posterior side, forward expansion is not required.

47.3.4 Osteotomy Guide Setting

The varus osteotomy guide is posteriorly applied to the lateral intertrochanteric crest slightly distal end to the center of the lesser trochanter. Care should be taken to ensure that the central part of the guide is inserted 5 mm away from the intertrochanteric crest to be fixed with two pieces of cortex screw

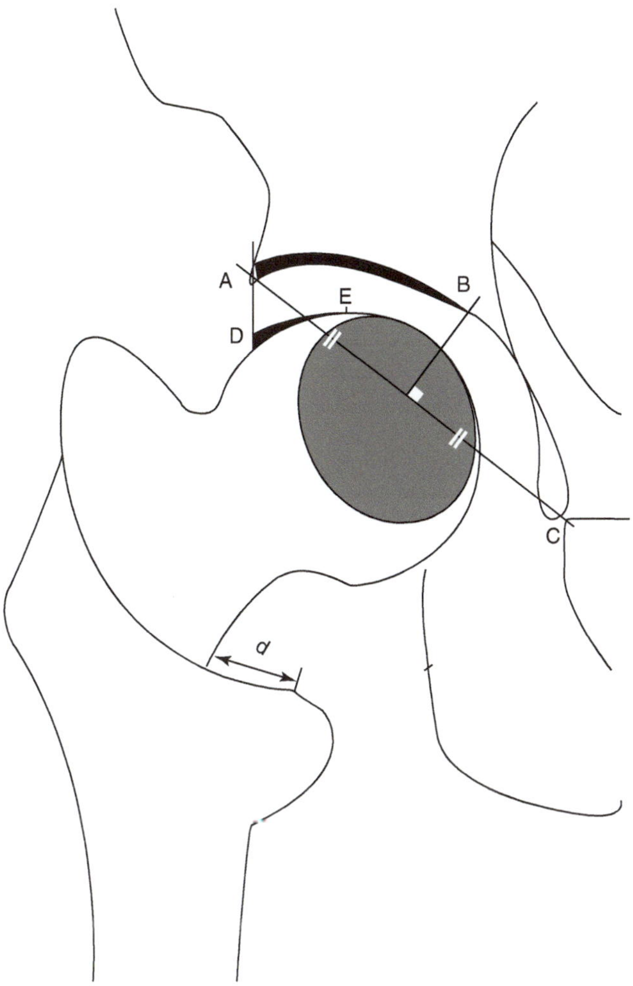

Fig. 47.3 The postoperative intact area ratio of the articular surface of the femoral head to the weight-bearing area of the acetabulum on postoperative anteroposterior (*AP*) radiographs. Point *B* is determined by drawing a perpendicular line from the midpoint of *A* (the edge of the acetabulum) and *C* (the lowest point of the teardrop) to the acetabular roof. Point *D* represents the lateral edge of the load-bearing portion. Point *E* represents the medial edge of the intact articular surface of the femoral head. The postoperative intact area ratio is expressed as *D*–*E*/*A*–*B*. The planned varus angle is confirmed during surgery by measuring the moving distance of proximal femur (*d*), which was calculated preoperatively (Reproduced with permission and copyright© of the British Society of Bone and Joint Surgery [11])

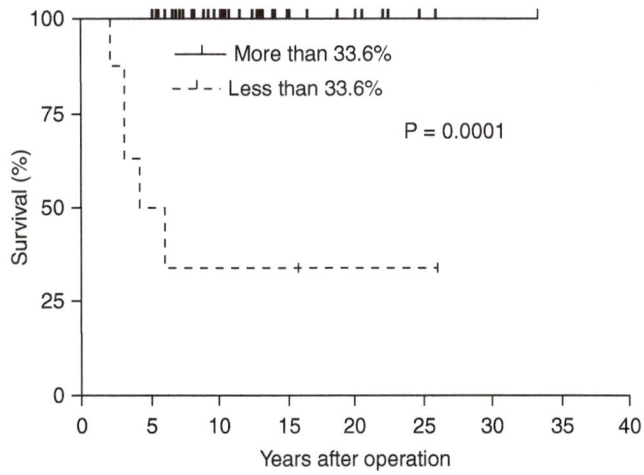

Fig. 47.4 Kaplan-Meier survival curve shows the radiological survival rate based on the postoperative intact area ratio of 33.6 %. The endpoint is the time when the progression of collapse was observed (Reproduced with permission and copyright© of the British Society of Bone and Joint Surgery [11])

Posterior View of the left hip

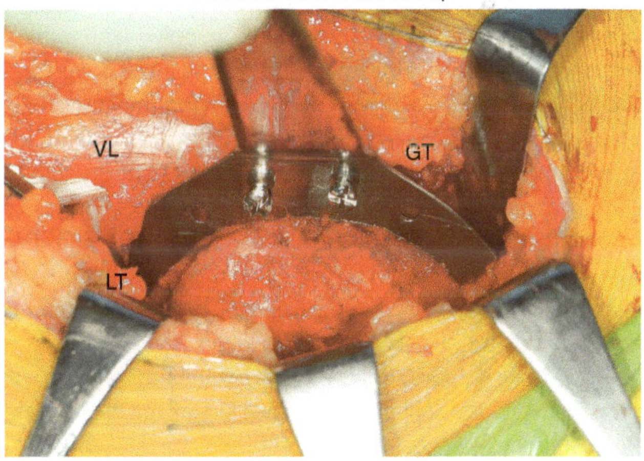

Fig. 47.5 The varus osteotomy guide is posteriorly applied to the lateral intertrochanteric crest slightly distal end to the center of the lesser trochanter. Care should be taken to ensure that the central part of the guide is inserted 5 mm away from the intertrochanteric crest to be fixed with two pieces of cortex screw. *GT* greater trochanter, *LT* lesser trochanter, *VL* vastus lateralis

(Fig. 47.5). Also, the greater trochanter and its base should be sufficiently thick. The position should be reconfirmed on an image, and it should be adjusted as needed; the knee joint flexed to 90° and the lower leg parallel to the X-ray incident direction is the accurate median position (Fig. 47.6).

47.3.5 Osteotomy

After partially removing the adhesion of the gluteus medius, osteotomy is performed with a reciprocator in a curved fashion from the tip of the greater trochanter along the guide with careful attention to the depth and direction. When osteotomy is performed from the lesser trochanter side, the relatively soft bone of the greater trochanter side remains, and there is a risk that this bone may break.

47.3.6 Varus Control by Moving the Proximal Fragment

The moving distance determined during preoperative planning should be marked on the distal and the proximal bone fragments by using a chisel. The lower extremity is set in a medial rotation–adduction position by towing it so that the

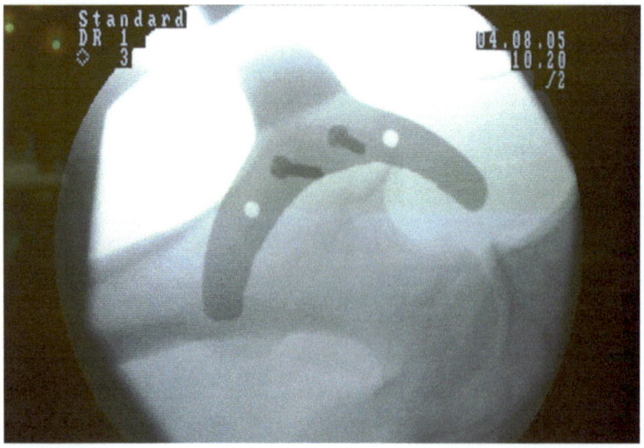

Fig. 47.6 The guide position should be reconfirmed on an image, and it should be adjusted as needed; the knee joint flexed to 90°and the lower leg parallel to the X-ray incident direction is the accurate median position

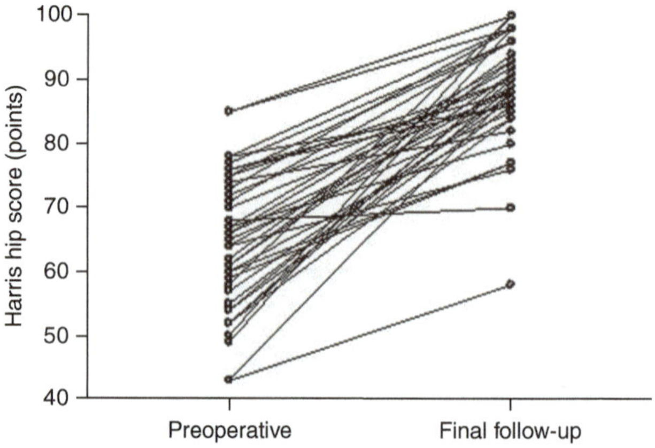

Fig. 47.7 Preoperative and final follow-up Harris hip score. The mean preoperative Harris hip score was 64.0 ± 10.7 points, which improved to 88.7 ± 8.5 points at the final follow-up examination (Wilcoxon signed-rank test; $n = 42$, $p < 0.0001$) (Reproduced with permission and copyright© of the British Society of Bone and Joint Surgery [10])

osteotomy site is expanded and then the osteotomy section of the lesser trochanter, which is located at the inferomedial margin of the central bone fragment, is grappled with a sharp retractor to be towed toward the head so that the bone fragment is in a varus position. The gluteus minimus muscle is isolated from the joint capsule at the proximal end of the greater trochanter, and a part of the anterior joint capsule of the proximal bone fragment and the adhesion of the lesser trochanter of the iliopsoas muscle are resected to facilitate translation. The proximal bone fragment is translated till the points marked on the proximal and distal bone fragments meet, and then the extremity in a medial rotation position is relieved to be reduced. Since the sharp retractor is slippery at this moment, care should be taken not to damage the nutrient vessels in the intertrochanteric crest.

47.3.7 Fixation of Bone Fragments

A longitudinal incision is made on the lateral great muscle and expanded so that a plate can be inserted. A Steinmann pin and guide pins for fixing different plates are inserted into the proximal and the distal fragments, respectively, and they are provisionally fixed there. Confirmation is made on the basis of the varus angle, the position of pins, and the direction and length of the pins on an image. First, the proximal side is fixed with a large lag screw to prevent rotation. Subsequently, fixation is achieved with a plate. Following these procedures, reconfirmation is made on the basis of the planned varus angle, the length of screws, and their position on an image.

47.3.8 Wound Closure

A drain is left, and then layer-by-layer suturing is performed.

47.4 Clinical Results [10]

Between January 1993 and March 2004, a transtrochanteric curved varus osteotomy was performed on 42 hips in 36 ON patients (6 patients had operation on both hips). The patients included 15 men and 21 women with a mean age at the time of surgery of 34 years (range 15–68 years). All patients were followed up at least 1-year intervals, and the mean duration of follow-up was 5.9 years (range 2.0–12.5 years).

Thirty-two hips were classified as steroid-related diseases, 4 were secondary to excessive alcohol consumption, 2 were post-traumatic, and 4 were idiopathic.

According to the classification of the Japanese Investigation Committee of Health and Welfare [12], 37 hips were classified as stage 3A, 4 as stage 3B, and one as stage 4. The localization of the affected necrotic lesion [12] was type B in one hip, type C1 in 36, and type C2 in 5.

The mean preoperative Harris hip score was 64.0±10.7 (mean ± standard deviation) points, which improved to 88.7 ± 8.5 points at the final follow-up (Fig. 47.7). More than 34 % of the postoperative intact area ratio was obtained in 41 of the 42 hips (Fig. 47.8), and the mean postoperative intact area ratio was 53.0 % (range 30–81 %). Only 2 of the 42 hips developed osteoarthritic changes during the follow-up period. One case is a 27-year-old female, who had only 30 % postoperative intact area ratio. The hip pain recurred 2 years after the operation, followed by progressive collapse, which resulted in undergoing total hip arthroplasty (THA). The other case is a 37-year-old male, who had 45 % postoperative intact articular surface. However, 2 years after the operation, mild osteoarthritic changes occurred but neither hip pain nor progression of a collapse on radiographs was noted, and this patient is being followed up [10].

A mean varus angulation of 25.0°(range 12–38°) was obtained (10–15° in 2 cases, 16–20° in 11 cases, 21–25° in 10 cases, 26–30° in 11 cases, 31–35° in 6 cases, and 36–40° in 2 cases, respectively). No increase in the varus angulations was

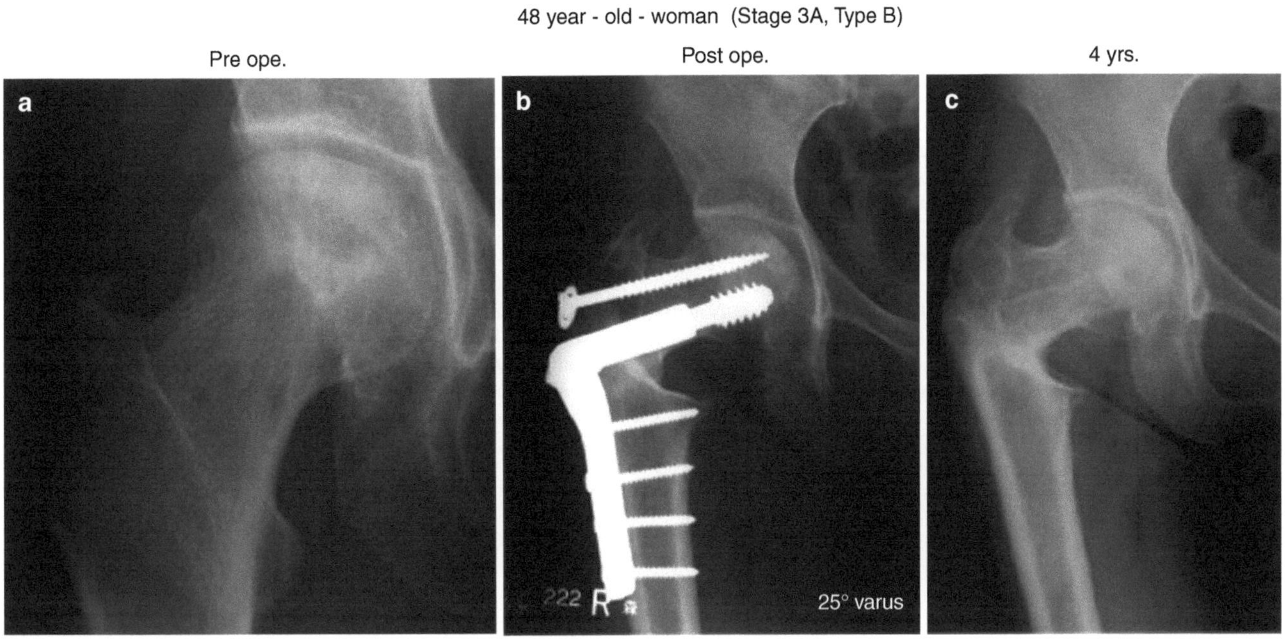

Fig. 47.8 Osteonecrosis in a 48-year-old male. (**a**) Preoperative radiograph. The right hip was classified as stage 3A and type B. (**b**) Postoperative radiograph. After 25° of varus osteotomy, an 80 % postoperative intact ratio was obtained. (**c**) Radiographs 4 years after the operation. Neither the progression of collapse nor any joint-space narrowing was observed. The size of the necrotic area, which is surrounded by a sclerotic line, was observed to have decreased, thus indicating that a sufficient repair was obtained by the varus osteotomy

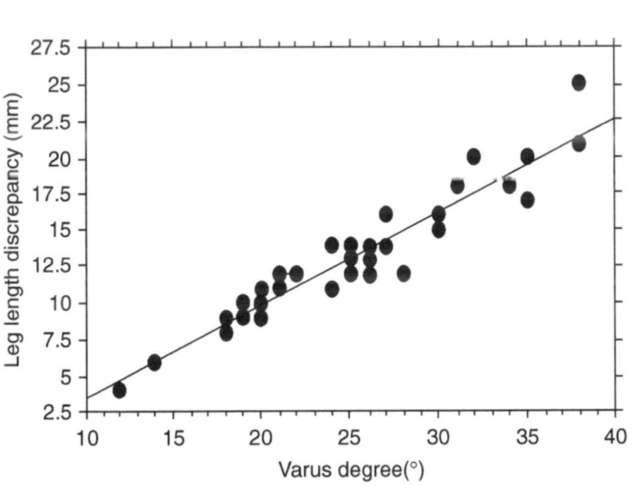

Fig. 47.9 The varus degree and postoperative leg length discrepancy. The postoperative leg length discrepancy showed a very strong correlation with the ratio of varus angulation (Pearson's correlation coefficient; $n=42$, $r=0.9530$, $p<0.0001$) (Reproduced with permission and copyright© of the Britsh Society of Bone and Joint Surgery [10])

observed in any cases during the follow-up period [10]. The postoperative leg length discrepancy showed a very strong correlation with the ratio of varus angulation (Pearson's correlation coefficient; $n=42$, $r=0.9530$, $p<0.0001$) (Fig. 47.9).

47.5 Discussion

A curved varus osteotomy is performed in patients with an intact area ratio of approximately 34 % in a maximum abduction position. During curved varus osteotomy, collapsed necrotic areas can be moved medially so that the intact area, which remains in the lateral portion, supports load. This procedure is considered to be an effective joint-preserving modality with a relatively low surgical stress for patients with an intact area ratio to the weight-bearing area of 1/3 or higher in a preoperative maximum abduction position.

This curved varus osteotomy has been designed to prevent elevation of the greater trochanter (Trendelenburg limp), lateral displacement of the femoral shaft which causes gluteus medius and minimus muscle disorders, delayed union or nonunion at the site of osteotomies, and leg length discrepancy, which has been commonly observed after wedge varus osteotomies [4–6]. There have been several reports which investigated the good clinical results of a transtrochanteric curved varus osteotomy [9–11, 13]. Leg length discrepancy has been reported to range from 0.5 to 20 mm in transtrochanteric curved varus osteotomy [8, 9] compared with 29–38 mm in varus wedge osteotomy [6]. Recently, Ikemura first reported the correlation between the varus degree and the leg length discrepancy (Fig. 47.9) [10]. This paper seems to be a useful preoperative information for the ON patients who are scheduled to undergo transtrochanteric curved varus osteotomy and have some concerns regarding the postoperative leg length discrepancies.

References

1. Pauwels F. The place of osteotomy in the operative management of osteoarthritis of the hip. Triangle. 1968;8:196–210.
2. Merle d'Aubigne R, Postel M, Mazabraud A, Massias P, Gueguen J, France P. Idiopathic necrosis of the femoral head in adults. J Bone Joint Surg [Br]. 1965;47-B:612–33.

3. Kerboul M, Thomine J, Postel M, Merle d'Aubigne R. The conservative surgical treatment of idiopathic aseptic necrosis of the femoral head. J Bone Joint Surg [Br]. 1974;56-B:291–6.
4. Mont MA, Fairbank AC, Krackow KA, Hungerford DS. Corrective osteotomy for osteonecrosis of the femoral head: the results of a long-term follow-up study. J Bone Joint Surg Am. 1996;78-A:1032–8.
5. Ito H, Kaneda K, Matsuno T. Osteonecrosis of the femoral head: simple varus intertrochanteric osteotomy. J Bone Joint Surg [Br]. 1999;81-B:969–74.
6. Bombelli R. Osteoarthritis of the hip: pathogenesis and consequent therapy. Berlin: Springer; 1976.
7. Nishio A, Sugioka Y. A new technique of the varus osteotomy at the upper end of the femur. Orthop Trauma. 1971;20:381–6.
8. Sugioka Y, Ogata K, Kitajima T, Nishio A. Transtrochanteric curved varus osteotomy in the treatment of dysplastic hip. In: The hip: proceedings of the eighth open scientific meeting of The Hip Society. St. Louis: Mosby; 1980. p. 227–44.
9. Sakano S, Hasegawa Y, Torii Y, Kawasaki M, Ishiguro N. Curved intertrochanteric varus osteotomy for osteonecrosis of the femoral head. J Bone Joint Surg [Br]. 2004;86-B:359–65.
10. Ikemura S, Yamamoto T, Jingushi S, Nakashima Y, Mawatari T, Iwamoto Y. Leg length discrepancy after transtrochanteric curved varus osteotomy for osteonecrosis of the femoral head. J Bone Joint Surg Br. 2007;89B:725–9.
11. Zhao G, Yamamoto T, Ikemura S, Motomura G, Mawatari T, Nakashima Y, Iwamoto Y. Radiological outcome analysis of transtrochanteric curved varus osteotomy for osteonecrosis of the femoral head at a mean follow-up of 12.4 years. J Bone Joint Surg Br. 2010;92B:781–6.
12. Sugano N, Atsumi T, Ohzono K, Kubo T, Hotokebuchi T, Takaoka K. The 2001 revised criteria for diagnosis, classification, and staging of idiopathic osteonecrosis of the femoral head. J Orthop Sci. 2002;7:601–5.
13. Saito S, Ohzono K, Ono K. Joint-preserving operations for idiopathic avascular necrosis of the femoral head: results of core decompression, grafting and osteotomy. J Bone Joint Surg [Br]. 1988;70-B:78–84.

Total Hip Arthroplasty Using Ceramic-on-Ceramic Articulation

48

Young-Kyun Lee, Ki-Choul Kim, Bun Jung Kang, and Kyung-Hoi Koo

48.1 Introduction

Severely collapsed or advanced osteonecrosis requires total hip arthroplasty (THA). When a THA is performed for osteonecrosis (ON), problems with polyethylene wear can arise in the medium and long term [1–3]. Furthermore, the wear rate of conventional polyethylene and the prevalence of osteolysis associated with THA in younger patients with osteonecrosis of femoral head are unacceptably high at the midterm follow-up [1–3]. The factors that contribute to high failure rates include a relatively young age, long life expectancy, higher activity, increased body weight, and poor quality of the femoral bone. Therefore, the minimization of wear is essential for improving the results of THA in these populations. More durable articulations have been introduced, such as highly cross-linked polyethylene-on-metal articulation [4], metal-on-metal articulation [5], and ceramic-on-ceramic articulation [6].

48.2 Main Text

Ceramic-on-ceramic articulation was developed and introduced by Boutin in the 1970s [7] and later was popularized worldwide by Mittelmeier [8]. The advantages of a ceramic bearing surface in THA are hardness, wettability, fluid film lubrication, inertness, and a high oxidation level, which theoretically should provide scratch resistance, increased implant longevity, and biocompatibility. However, as was experienced for first-generation metal-on-metal articulations, early experiences of early generation alumina ceramic bearings were disappointing, because of design issue and inadequate material properties, such as low density and a coarse microstructure [6, 9]. Poor designs, such as conically threaded "monobloc" or spherical press-fit cups, were problematic with respect to prosthesis-bone integration [6, 9]. Furthermore, because of inadequate material properties, early generation ceramic bearings showed higher rates of acetabular component loosening, and ceramic component fracture, and isolated examples of accelerated bearing surface wear [6, 9].

These early designs are now being replaced by modular systems with taper fixation of metal-backed alumina components, and these newer designs have shown better midterm outcomes [10, 11]. In addition, since 1990, many improvements have been adopted to produce third-generation ceramics, such as hot isostatic pressing, laser marking, and nondestructive proof-testing [12]. Furthermore, grain size has been reduced from 4.2 to 1.8 μm, and burst strength improved from 46 to 65 kN. Furthermore, ceramic is biocompatible, which precludes concerns regarding metal ion release. For these reasons, it is hoped that advanced high-quality alumina ceramic bearings with excellent tribological properties are a durable option for THA in young active patients [6, 13–18].

Although few studies on ceramic-on-ceramic THA have been conducted in patients with osteonecrosis, results may be similar to those of young active patients.

Nich et al. reported the long-term results of ceramic-on-ceramic THA in patients with ON. Fifty-two ceramic-on-ceramic THAs were performed in 41 patients with ON (mean age, 41 years; age range, 22–79 years). At an average follow-up of 16 years (range 11–24 years), no osteolysis was observed and no wear was detected. With revision for aseptic loosening as the end point, the survival rates of acetabular and femoral components were 88.5 and 100 % at 10 years, respectively [19].

Y.-K. Lee (✉) • K.-H. Koo
Department of Orthopaedic Surgery, Seoul National University College of Medicine, Seoul National University Bundang Hospital, 82 Gumi-ro, 173 Beon-gil, Seongnam 463-707, South Korea
e-mail: ykleemd@gmail.com; khkoo@snu.ac.kr

K.-C. Kim
Department of Orthopaedic Surgery, Dankook University college of Medicine, 119, Dandae-ro, Dongnam-gu, Cheonan, 330-714, South Korea
e-mail: puhoo73@hanmail.net

B.J. Kang
Department of Orthopaedic Surgery, Gyeongsang National University School of Medicine, 79, Gangnam-ro, Jinju-si, Jinju 660-702, South Korea
e-mail: bunjung0111@hanmail.net

K.-H. Koo et al. (eds.), *Osteonecrosis*,
DOI 10.1007/978-3-642-35767-1_48,

Kim et al. used plain radiography and computed tomography (CT) to investigate 93 cementless THAs performed using alumina-on-alumina ceramic bearings in 64 young patients with femoral head osteonecrosis. At follow-up visits conducted at least 10 years after surgery, no hip required revision or showed aseptic loosening, and CT demonstrated no acetabular or femoral osteolysis [20].

Although no case of ceramic fracture occurred in these series, ceramic fracture is a well-recognized problem [16, 21]. Recent studies have described that third-generation ceramic bearing can be also fractured [10, 22, 23].

Ha et al. reported that ceramic liner fracture can occur after third-generation alumina-on-alumina cementless THA [24]. One hundred and forty-four cementless alumina-on-alumina THAs were performed in 17–78-year-old patients, 69 % of whom had AVN. The acetabular component consisted of an alumina liner (BIOLOX forte, CeramTec AG, Plochingen, Germany) housed in a polyethylene shell (Lima, Udine, Italy), which was housed in a porous titanium-coated hemispheric cup (SPH CONTACT, Lima). This sandwich-type acetabular component was designed to reduce the rigidity of the ceramic-on-ceramic bearing by inserting a layer of polyethylene between the ceramic liner and metal shell. Ceramic liner fractures occurred in five hips (3.5 %) at a mean of 35 months (range, 24–48 months) postoperatively. These five patients were fitted with a more anteverted cup than the remainder. Furthermore, in three patients fracture apparently occurred during squatting, resulting in hyperflexion and wide hip abduction. Thus, early ceramic liner fracture was associated with impingement associated with excessive anteversion of the acetabular cup in patients who habitually squat. For this design of acetabular component, fracture problems were attributed to impingement between the metal neck and the ceramic liner during squatting.

Koo et al. also reported that ceramic head fracture can occur after third-generation alumina-on-alumina THA [25]. Three hundred and five patients (359 hips), who had undergone cementless alumina-on-alumina THA at four participating centers using the 28-mm BIOLOX forte femoral head and a BIOLOX forte liner, were evaluated at a mean of 45 months postoperatively. It was found that 5 (1.4 %) ceramic head fractures occurred during normal daily activities at a mean of 22.6 months postoperatively and were associated with one design of a short-neck modular alumina femoral head in this study. On the other hand, the following causative factors have been suggested by others, such as component design, material properties of ceramic components, and manufacturing defects, including cone-trunnion mismatch and ceramic material deterioration [13, 26, 27].

Lee et al. evaluated 16 patients that underwent reoperation more than 1 year after previous third-generation ceramic-on-ceramic THA, with respect to impingement [28]. In this study, 4 (25 %) of the 16 revision cases showed impingement. Retrieved alumina liners showing evidence of impingement were examined visually and by scanning electron microscopy (SEM). One of the 4 retrieved liners exhibited multiple microcracks, and cross-sectional SEM revealed a microcrack propagating deep into the ceramic liner. These findings suggest that metal neck-to-ceramic impingement in ceramic-on-ceramic THA can cause microcracking of the ceramic liner.

Baek et al. reported noise after third-generation ceramic-on-ceramic THA in patients with ON. These authors prospectively evaluated 71 ceramic-on-ceramic THAs in 60 patients with ON (mean age, 39.1 years; age range, 18–49 years). After average follow-up of 7.1 years (range, 6–9 years), 13 patients (14 hips, 20 %) reported noise in the hip. However, no osteolysis was observed, no revision was required, and no ceramic fracture occurred during follow-up [29].

Lee et al. reported long-term outcomes for third-generation alumina-on-alumina bearings in 88 consecutive cementless alumina-on-alumina THAs performed in 18–65-year-old patients, 50 % of whom had AVN [17]. At last follow-up evaluations, mean WOMAC score was 12.9 points (range, 0–44 points). Twelve (14 %) of the 88 hips produced an intermittent clicking sound and one squeaking. Another patient that reported an audible squeak during swaying sideward could not reproduce the noise during the outpatient evaluation. The remaining total hip prostheses were completely problem-free. At an average follow-up of 11 years (range, 10–11.8 years), no osteolysis was observed and no wear was detectable. Two hips required a bearing change because of ceramic head fracture. The cumulative survival rate at 10 years was 99.0 % (95 % confidence interval, 97.0–100 %) when implant revision for any reason was considered as the end point.

Byun et al. reported the results of third-generation ceramic-on-ceramic THA in active young patients with ON. They evaluated 56 ceramic-on-ceramic THAs in 41 patients of mean age 25.6 years (range 16–29 years). At an average follow-up of 7.7 years (range, 6–8.5 years), no osteolysis was observed and no revision was required. Furthermore, no ceramic fracture occurred during follow-up [30].

Solarino et al. reported the long-term results of third-generation ceramic-on-ceramic THA in patients with ON. These authors used a large ceramic head ball (32 mm) for 68 ceramic-on-ceramic THAs in 61 patients with ON (mean age, 49.9 years; range, 29–72 years). At an average follow-up of 12.9 years (range, 11–15 years), two revisions have been performed for one periprosthetic infection and one excessive abduction of acetabular component, respectively. No ceramic fracture or osteolysis was observed [31].

The possibility of ceramic failure, noise, and impingement between the metal neck and the ceramic liner remains to be major concerns when ceramic bearing surfaces are used in THA [24, 25], despite advancement made in the quality of third-generation alumina ceramic bearings [12, 14]. Nevertheless, these studies show that the results of third-generation alumina-on-alumina THA are satisfactory for long-term follow-up in ON patients [19, 20, 28–43].

At present, research and design efforts are targeted toward the developments of alumina-zirconia composite implants [44, 45]. Zirconia toughened alumina designs could improve fracture resistance, while maximizing biocompatibility and minimizing particulate wear debris [32].

Better implant designs and new ceramic materials and advanced surgical techniques have produced promising long-term results that may minimize the negative impact of high activity in patients with ON.

References

1. Dunkley AB, Eldridge JD, Lee MB, Smith EJ, Learmonth ID. Cementless acetabular replacement in the young. A 5- to 10-year prospective study. Clin Orthop Relat Res. 2000;376:149.
2. Beaule PE, Dorey FJ. Survivorship analysis of cementless total hip arthroplasty in younger patients. J Bone Joint Surg Am. 2001;10:1590.
3. Fye MA, Huo MH, Zatorski LE, Keggi KJ. Total hip arthroplasty performed without cement in patients with femoral head osteonecrosis who are less than 50 years old. J Arthroplasty. 1998;8:876.
4. D'Antonio JA, Manley MT, Capello WN, Bierbaum BE, Ramakrishnan R, Naughton M, Sutton K. Five-year experience with crossfire highly cross-linked polyethylene. Clin Orthop Relat Res. 2005;441:143.
5. Schmalzried TP, Peters PC, Maurer BT, Bragdon CR, Harris WH. Long-duration metal-on-metal total hip arthroplasties with low wear of the articulating surfaces. J Arthroplasty. 1996;3:322.
6. Hamadouche M, Boutin P, Daussange J, Bolander ME, Sedel L. Alumina-on-alumina total hip arthroplasty: a minimum 18.5-year follow-up study. J Bone Joint Surg Am. 2002;1:69.
7. Boutin P. Total arthroplasty of the hip by fritted aluminum prosthesis. Experimental study and 1st clinical applications. Rev Chir Orthop Reparatrice Appar Mot. 1972;3:229.
8. Mittelmeier H, Heisel J. Sixteen-years' experience with ceramic hip prostheses. Clin Orthop Relat Res. 1992;282:64.
9. Mahoney OM, Dimon 3rd JH. Unsatisfactory results with a ceramic total hip prosthesis. J Bone Joint Surg Am. 1990;5:663.
10. Yoo JJ, Kim YM, Yoon KS, Koo KH, Song WS, Kim HJ. Alumina-on-alumina total hip arthroplasty. A five-year minimum follow-up study. J Bone Joint Surg Am. 2005;3:530.
11. Ha YC, Koo KH, Jeong ST, Joon Yoo J, Kim YM, Joong Kim H. Cementless alumina-on-alumina total hip arthroplasty in patients younger than 50 years: a 5-year minimum follow-up study. J Arthroplasty. 2007;2:184.
12. Skinner HB. Ceramic bearing surfaces. Clin Orthop Relat Res. 1999;369:83.
13. Willmann G. Ceramic femoral head retrieval data. Clin Orthop. 2000;379:22.
14. Bierbaum BE, Nairus J, Kuesis D, Morrison JC, Ward D. Ceramic-on-ceramic bearings in total hip arthroplasty. Clin Orthop Relat Res. 2002;405:158.
15. Bizot P, Hannouche D, Nizard R, Witvoet J, Sedel L. Hybrid alumina total hip arthroplasty using a press-fit metal-backed socket in patients younger than 55 years. A six- to 11-year evaluation. J Bone Joint Surg Br. 2004;2:190.
16. D'Antonio J, Capello W, Manley M, Bierbaum B. New experience with alumina-on-alumina ceramic bearings for total hip arthroplasty. J Arthroplasty. 2002;4:390.
17. Lee YK, Ha YC, Yoo JJ, Koo KH, Yoon KS, Kim HJ. Alumina-on-alumina total hip arthroplasty: a concise follow-up, at a minimum of ten years, of a previous report. J Bone Joint Surg Am. 2010;8:1715.
18. Sedel L. Evolution of alumina-on-alumina implants: a review. Clin Orthop Relat Res. 2000;379:48.
19. Nich C, Sariali el H, Hannouche D, Nizard R, Witvoet J, Sedel L, Bizot P. Long-term results of alumina-on-alumina hip arthroplasty for osteonecrosis. Clin Orthop Relat Res. 2003;417:102.
20. Kim YH, Choi Y, Kim JS. Cementless total hip arthroplasty with ceramic-on-ceramic bearing in patients younger than 45 years with femoral-head osteonecrosis. International Orthopaedics. 2010;8:1123.
21. Garino JP. Modern ceramic-on-ceramic total hip systems in the United States: early results. Clin Orthop Relat Res. 2000;379:41.
22. Hannouche D, Nich C, Bizot P, Meunier A, Nizard R, Sedel L. Fractures of ceramic bearings: history and present status. Clin Orthop Relat Res. 2003;417:19.
23. Hasegawa M, Sudo A, Uchida A. Alumina ceramic-on-ceramic total hip replacement with a layered acetabular component. J Bone Joint Surg Br. 2006;7:877.
24. Ha YC, Kim SY, Kim HJ, Yoo JJ, Koo KH. Ceramic liner fracture after cementless alumina-on-alumina total hip arthroplasty. Clin Orthop Relat Res. 2007;458:106.
25. Koo KH, Ha YC, Jung WH, Kim SR, Yoo JJ, Kim HJ. Isolated fracture of the ceramic head after third-generation alumina-on-alumina total hip arthroplasty. J Bone Joint Surg Am. 2008;2:329.
26. Callaway GH, Flynn W, Ranawat CS, Sculco TP. Fracture of the femoral head after ceramic-on-polyethylene total hip arthroplasty. J Arthroplasty. 1995;6:855.
27. Masonis JL, Bourne RB, Ries MD, McCalden RW, Salehi A, Kelman DC. Zirconia femoral head fractures: a clinical and retrieval analysis. J Arthroplasty. 2004;7:898.
28. Lee YK, Yoo JJ, Koo KH, Yoon KS, Kim HJ. Metal neck and liner impingement in ceramic bearing total hip arthroplasty. J Orthop Res. 2011;2:218.
29. Baek SH, Kim SY. Cementless total hip arthroplasty with alumina bearings in patients younger than fifty with femoral head osteonecrosis. J Bone Joint Surg Am. 2008;6:1314.
30. Byun JW, Yoon TR, Park KS, Seon JK. Third-generation ceramic-on-ceramic total hip arthroplasty in patients younger than 30 years with osteonecrosis of femoral head. J Arthroplasty. 2012;7:1337.
31. Solarino G, Piazzolla A, Notarnicola A, Moretti L, Tafuri S, De Giorgi S, Moretti B. Long-term results of 32-mm alumina-on-alumina THA for avascular necrosis of the femoral head. J Orthop Traumatol. 2012;1:21.
32. Affatato S, Testoni M, Cacciari GL, Toni A. Mixed-oxides prosthetic ceramic ball heads. Part 2: effect of the ZrO2 fraction on the wear of ceramic on ceramic joints. Biomaterials. 1999;20:1925.
33. Beaule PE, Amstutz HC. Management of ficat stage III and IV osteonecrosis of the hip. J Am Acad Orthop Surg. 2004;2:96.
34. Schneider W, Knahr K. Total hip replacement in younger patients: survival rate after avascular necrosis of the femoral head. Acta Orthop Scand. 2004;2:142.
35. Hungerford DS. Treatment of osteonecrosis of the femoral head: everything's new. J Arthroplasty. 2007;22(4 Suppl 1):91.
36. Panagiotopoulos EC, Kallivokas AG, Koulioumpas I, Mouzakis DE. Early failure of a zirconia femoral head prosthesis: fracture or fatigue? Clin Biomech (Bristol, Avon). 2007;7:856.
37. Seyler TM, Cui Q, Mihalko WM, Mont MA, Saleh KJ. Advances in hip arthroplasty in the treatment of osteonecrosis. Instr Course Lect. 2007;56:221.
38. Nizard R, Pourreyron D, Raould A, Hannouche D, Sedel L. Alumina-on-alumina hip arthroplasty in patients younger than 30 years old. Clin Orthop Relat Res. 2008;2:317.

39. Regis D, Sandri A, Bartolozzi P. Delayed diagnosis of low-symptomatic ceramic acetabular liner fracture in ceramic-on-ceramic total hip arthroplasty. Orthopedics. 2008;31:10.
40. Amstutz HC, Esposito C, Campbell P. Long term preservation of femoral bone following hemiresurfacing. Hip Int. 2010;2:236.
41. Millar NL, Halai M, McKenna R, McGraw IW, Millar LL, Hadidi M. Uncemented ceramic-on-ceramic THA in adults with osteonecrosis of the femoral head. Orthopedics. 2010;11:795.
42. Finkbone PR, Severson EP, Cabanela ME, Trousdale RT. Ceramic-on-ceramic total hip arthroplasty in patients younger than 20 years. J Arthroplasty. 2012;2:213.
43. Kim YH, Park JW, Kim JS. Cementless metaphyseal fitting anatomic total hip arthroplasty with a ceramic-on-ceramic bearing in patients thirty years of age or younger. J Bone Joint Surg Am. 2012;17:1570.
44. Lombardi Jr AV, Berend KR, Seng BE, Clarke IC, Adams JB. Delta ceramic-on-alumina ceramic articulation in primary THA: prospective, randomized FDA-IDE study and retrieval analysis. Clin Orthop Relat Res. 2010;2:367.
45. Hamilton WG, McAuley JP, Dennis DA, Murphy JA, Blumenfeld TJ, Politi J. THA with delta ceramic on ceramic: results of a multicenter investigational device exemption trial. Clin Orthop Relat Res. 2010;2:358.

Highly Crosslinked Polyethylene Liners in Patients with Osteonecrosis of the Femoral Head in the United States and Europe

49

Patrick O'Toole and Javad Parvizi

49.1 Introduction

The treatment of patients with osteonecrosis (ON) of the femoral head has changed over the last 30 years from the concept of saving the femoral head at all costs to the more recent concept of treating symptomatic femoral head collapse, in the setting of ON, with total hip arthroplasty. Approximately 20,000 patients are diagnosed in the United States with ON of the femoral head every year [1] with the average age at presentation being 38 years. Although femoral head core decompression, with or without bone grafting, for the early stages of ON is still performed with reasonable success, it plays no role in the patient with collapse. Free vascularized bone grafting of the femoral head and neck has been shown to have marginally superior results to core decompression in the treatment of pre-collapse lesions [2]; however, results are much better when used for lesions with early collapse, but subsequent THA can be less successful as a result [3]. Proximal femoral redirectional osteotomies are described in the treatment of ON of the femoral head; however, these are technically demanding surgeries with significant associated complications and can make any subsequent THA more difficult [4]. These osteotomies should be reserved for the much younger patient with modest-sized lesions [5].

Younger patients with end-stage hip arthritis secondary to ON were traditionally offered a range of surgical options including resection arthroplasty, resurfacing arthroplasty, and arthrodesis; however, there were multiple limitations and complications related to these options. The average age of a patient undergoing THA as a result of ON is approximately 40 years. These patients are typically more active and have a higher demand on their hip prosthesis. This high level of activity with repetitive loading especially in the adolescent and young adult patient group has previously lead to mixed results post-THA [6]. Overall improvement in bearing surfaces and prosthetic design as well as operative techniques and better instrumentation has made THA a more favorable option in the treatment of those patients with ON of the femoral head.

49.2 Total Hip Arthroplasty in the Young Patient: Alternative Bearings

Surgical techniques, cementless fixation methods, and bearing surfaces have all improved greatly in the area of total hip arthroplasty. Osteolysis as a result of polyethylene wear particles resulting in premature failure of the prosthesis with associated bone loss has led to the consideration of alternative articulating or bearing surfaces in the younger patient population.

The development of severe and painful hip arthritis in the younger patient can occur as a result of ON, infection, Legg-Calvé-Perthes disease, slipped capital femoral epiphysis, or femoroacetabular impingement. THA is performed in patients with ON when conservative measures have been exhausted. Traditionally the demand placed on the hip prosthesis by the younger patient has led to accelerated failure [7] making this surgical option less attractive. Higher loading cycles and increased requirements on the longevity of the implants in younger patients have traditionally led the orthopedic surgeon away from THA as a treatment option for ON of the femoral head [8, 9]. High wear rates and subsequent osteolysis associated with conventional ultrahigh-molecular-weight polyethylene (UHMWPE) have prompted the need to search for alternative bearing surfaces in younger patients [10]. Alternative bearing surfaces include ceramic on ceramic (COC), metal on metal (MOM), ceramic on metal (COM), and highly cross-linked polyethylene.

P. O'Toole • J. Parvizi (✉)
The Rothman Institute at Thomas Jefferson University, 925 Chestnut Street, Philadelphia, PA 19107, USA
e-mail: parvj@aol.com

K.-H. Koo et al. (eds.), *Osteonecrosis*,
DOI 10.1007/978-3-642-35767-1_49, © Springer-Verlag Berlin Heidelberg 2014

49.2.1 Ceramic on Ceramic

COC bearing surfaces in THA were approved by the Food and Drug Administration for use in the United States in 2003 and were available in Europe since the 1970s [11]. Ceramic bearings have low surface roughness and as a result have a low coefficient of friction, which lends itself to exceedingly low wear rates. However, there are complications specifically associated with the use of COC articulations with head fracture and liner fracture rates at 0.004–1.4 % and 0.01–2.0 %, respectively. Squeaking, which can be early or late [12], is deemed to be a multifactorial problem that occurs in 0.48–7.0 % and may be improved using more recently developed alumina matrix composite ceramics [13].

49.2.2 Metal on Metal

MOM bearing surfaces have been used with some success in younger patients in the treatment of end-stage arthritis secondary to ON [14]; however, some authors would advise against this practice due to increase stress placed on the bone cement interface on the femoral side [15]. A MOM bearing can also be facilitated in these patients by way of a stemmed femoral component. Advantages of MOM bearings include initial postoperative joint stability, as a result of the bigger head sizes, and in resurfacing the femoral bone stock can be preserved. The use of MOM articulations are currently proving divisive among orthopedic surgeons with concerns over adverse soft tissue reactions, metal ion release, and carcinogenic risk [16, 17].

49.2.3 Ceramic on Metal

COM articulations represent an alternative hard bearing in the treatment of young patients with ON; however, there may be a concern regarding the level of metal ions produced [11].

49.3 Highly X-Linked Polyethylene

Aseptic loosening and acetabular component wear are the leading causes of late revision in THA. The revision burden in THA is predicted to increase by 137 % (97,000 revisions) in the United States by the year 2030. Newer cementless THA fixation techniques have allowed hip replacement surgery to be more successful in the treatment of young patients with ON [18, 19]. However, the success of the procedure has been limited by the use of conventional polyethylene (UHMWPE) as part of the bearing surface [20] due to the high wear rates and subsequent osteolysis requiring revision.

Highly cross-linked UHMWPE has rapidly become the polyethylene of choice for use in THA as it has enhanced wear-resistant properties over its conventional counterparts. Ionizing radiation is used to increase the number of cross-links in the manufacturing process thereby reducing the amount of polyethylene wear debris created during cyclical loading of the prosthetic joint [21]. Reduction in wear rates have been as great as 80 % when compared to conventional polyethylene for the 28 and 32 mm head sizes [22].

Increased cross-linking of polyethylene was initially achieved either by chemical means or more reliably by using high doses of radiation; however, these first-generation techniques did not use any post-treatment to prevent later oxidation. Second-generation cross-linking uses thermal techniques to reduce the number of free radicals and demonstrate excellent wear characteristics [23]; however, there have been isolated reports regarding fracture of the polyethylene liner. Current third-generation techniques were introduced around 2006/2007 and use gamma-rays in place of electron beam irradiation. Subsequent annealing of the polyethylene is used by all of the current manufacturers; however, there are different techniques described to "quench" the free radicals in order to prevent post-manufacture oxidation. Some highly cross-linked polyethylene has shown a dramatic decrease in wear rates when compared to a conventional polyethylene from the same company (Table 49.1). The Zimmer longevity liner (Zimmer, Warsaw, Indiana) showed a steady-state wear rate that was eight times lower than the conventional Zimmer UHMWPE [24].

Table 49.1 Comparison of highly cross-linked polyethylene liners with their conventional (UHMWPE) liners

Study	UHMWPE[a] (mm/year)	Highly x-linked (mm/year)	*P* value
Thomas et al.[b] [24]	0.037	0.025	0.007
Geerdink et al.[c] [25]	0.142	0.088	0.007
McCalden et al.[d] [26]	0.051	0.003	0.006
Mutimer et al.[e] [27]	0.26	0.05	<0.001

Although different wear measurement parameters were used in the different studies, the important comparison is between the conventional polyethylene and its highly cross-linked counterpart

[a]UHMWPE: conventional ultrahigh-molecular-weight polyethylene

[b]Thomas et al. (Zimmer, Warsaw, Indiana). Zimmer longevity vs conventional Zimmer poly liner. Measurement: steady-state linear wear rate

[c]Geerdink et al. (Stryker Orthopaedics, Mahwah, NJ). Duration vs conventional Stryker poly liner. Measurement: linear wear rate

[d]McCalden et al. (Zimmer, Warsaw, Indiana). Zimmer longevity vs conventional Zimmer poly liner. Measurement: femoral head penetration in years 1–5 post implantation

[e]Mutimer et al. (DePuy, Warsaw, IN). Highly cross-linked Marathon vs conventional Enduron poly liner. Measurement: linear wear rate

49.4 Current Performance of Highly X-Linked Polyethylene in Younger Patient Population

Highly cross-linked polyethylene liners can be coupled with either cobalt chromium or ceramic femoral head prostheses to form a "hard on soft" bearing. Over the last decade or so, there has been a huge interest in the use of highly cross-linked polyethylene liners to help decrease and prevent wear particles and their sequelae. This is particularly true in patients suffering from ON of the femoral head, who tend to be younger and more active at the time of THA. Highly cross-linked polyethylene liners are an obvious choice for the younger patient as osteolysis has been reported in up to 60 % of young patients, at 5 years, treated with conventional UHMWPE [28, 29]; however, there is little clinical or in vivo evidence supporting the use of highly cross-linked polyethylene in younger patients.

Osteolysis is one of the most important factors affecting the longevity of a total hip replacement. Osteolysis is uncommon with wear rates of <0.1 mm/year [30]; however, wear rates of >0.2 mm/year can cause 100 % failure of THAs, with wear rates of >0.15 mm/year putting the hip at risk over time [31]. Initial early and midterm results of highly cross-linked polyethylene are promising, showing excellent wear rates and low levels of osteolysis. Nikolaou et al., in a prospective study, randomized patients to three groups with different bearing surfaces in each group, cobalt chrome on UHMWPE, cobalt chrome on highly cross-linked polyethylene, and COC bearings. They concluded that there were no significant differences in radiological outcomes or hip outcome scores at 5 years, but did show a significant difference in wear rates between the UHMWPE and the highly cross-linked version [32]. All patients were <65 years of age with a mean age of 53 years, while the majority of these patients were diagnosed with primary osteoarthritis, ON represented the next largest group.

Younger patients are more active post-THA and may also participate in manual labor postoperatively. As THA techniques are improving and prosthetic design as well as cementless fixation technology is becoming more robust, the indications for THA are expanding to include younger and more active patients. A ceramic on highly cross-linked polyethylene bearing was used in patients under the age of 30 years with results showing no osteolysis or aseptic loosening at a mean follow-up time of 10.8 years [33], using a Marathon liner (DePuy, Warsaw, Indiana). The range of wear rates for highly cross-linked polyethylene in the literature varies from 0.002 to 0.15 mm/year [34, 35]; however, the majority of studies do not specifically look at the younger patient. Trousdale et al. [36] investigated the relatively long-term outcome in 54 hips in patients <50 years of age. Although the patient numbers were low, survivorship was 100 % using highly cross-linked polyethylene liners.

While the average age of the ON patient undergoing THA is approximately 40 years, the majority of studies dealing with the midterm results of highly cross-linked polyethylene in younger patients have primary osteoarthritis as the most common pathology requiring THA. However, despite this, as younger patients will cyclically load their hip prosthesis and will be more active, it is fair to draw comparisons from these studies for young patients requiring THA for ON.

Patients with ON requiring THA have always been a challenging group to treat. The main reason for this is that the outcome post-THA in this group has been poor owing to the high demands placed on the prosthesis. Cementless fixation has continued to develop and now offers an excellent form of fixation for both the femoral and acetabular components in this group. The durability of a cementless THA in a patient with ON has been shown to be excellent and comparable to that of the general population and may even surpass its cemented counterpart [37].

The long-term effects, in patients with ON, of the altered mechanical properties of the highly cross-linked polyethylene liners remain unknown, but there is short-term 5-year follow-up data to suggest that the clinical and radiological results are promising for this patient population [38]. Kim et al. showed a polyethylene linear penetration rate of 0.05+/−0.02 mm/year with no aseptic loosening or osteolysis in 73 hips treated with THA for ON in a population with an average age of 45.5 years and a mean follow-up of 8.5 years [39].

49.5 Complications of Highly Cross-Linked Polyethylene

Highly cross-linked polyethylene is only in use long enough to show early to midterm results; however, these initial results are so promising that if they are to continue, the longevity of a cementless THA may increase dramatically. For the same reason there is a question mark over the mechanical properties of these liners with time. The wear characteristics and the risk of liner fracture and failure are different for the different manufacturing techniques. Although it is presumed that there is a minimum liner thickness that should be adhered to, this measurement may be different for different highly cross-linked polyethylene liners. Keeping the liner thickness >6 mm to prevent fracture has been advocated by some authors [33].

When the in vivo studies cannot be relied upon, during the recent introduction of these new polyethylene liners, in vitro studies can be used to simulate long-term loading of a prosthesis; however, these studies can result in catastrophe when there is a mismatch between the in vitro and in vivo wear characteristics [40, 41].

Retrieval analyses of highly cross-linked polyethylene liners have also revealed that cracks may exist especially near notches in the unsupported rims of some particular liners [42]. The majority of modern liners have a similar design, and it is not yet known whether these cracks may propagate to cause catastrophic liner failure.

49.6 Summary

ON of the femoral head is a relatively common condition. The pre-collapse or early stages can be treated successfully with core decompression. Once collapse is present, and the patient's symptoms are significant, then a modern cementless THA with a highly cross-linked polyethylene liner is an excellent choice. Initial and midterm results with these liners are encouraging, and the longevity of a THA in this high-demand group may increase. Recent reports of trunnion-related pathology may be decreased or eliminated by using a modern ceramic femoral head prosthesis.

References

1. Mont MA, Hungerford DS. Non-traumatic avascular necrosis of the femoral head. J Bone Joint Surg Am. 1995;77(3):459–74.
2. Berend KR, Gunneson EE, Urbaniak JR. Free vascularized fibular grafting for the treatment of postcollapse osteonecrosis of the femoral head. J Bone Joint Surg Am. 2003;85-A(6):987–93.
3. Davis ET, McKee MD, Waddell JP, Hupel T, Schemitsch EH. Total hip arthroplasty following failure of free vascularized fibular graft. J Bone Joint Surg Am. 2006;88 Suppl 3:110–5.
4. Shinar AA, Harris WH. Cemented total hip arthroplasty following previous femoral osteotomy: an average 16-year follow-up study. J Arthroplasty. 1998;13(3):243–53.
5. Hungerford DS. Treatment of osteonecrosis of the femoral head: everything's new. J Arthroplasty. 2007;22(4 Suppl 1):91–4.
6. Kamath AF, Sheth NP, Hosalkar HH, Babatunde OM, Lee GC, Nelson CL. Modern total hip arthroplasty in patients younger than 21 years. J Arthroplasty. 2012;27(3):402–8.
7. Puolakka TJ, Pajamaki KJ, Halonen PJ, Pulkkinen PO, Paavolainen P, Nevalainen JK. The Finnish arthroplasty register: report of the hip register. Acta Orthop Scand. 2001;72(5):433–41.
8. Bessette BJ, Fassier F, Tanzer M, Brooks CE. Total hip arthroplasty in patients younger than 21 years: a minimum, 10-year follow-up. Can J Surg. 2003;46(4):257–62.
9. Cage DJ, Granberry WM, Tullos HS. Long-term results of total arthroplasty in adolescents with debilitating polyarthropathy. Clin Orthop Relat Res. 1992;283:156–62.
10. Kim SM, Lim SJ, Moon YW, Kim YT, Ko KR, Park YS. Cementless modular total hip arthroplasty in patients younger than fifty with femoral head osteonecrosis: minimum fifteen-year follow-up. J Arthroplasty. 2013;28(3):504–9.
11. Kamath AF, Prieto H, Lewallen DG. Alternative bearings in total hip arthroplasty in the young patient. Orthop Clin North Am. 2013;44(4):451–62.
12. Restrepo C, Matar WY, Parvizi J, Rothman RH, Hozack WJ. Natural history of squeaking after total hip arthroplasty. Clin Orthop Relat Res. 2010;468(9):2340–5.
13. Hamilton WG, McAuley JP, Dennis DA, Murphy JA, Blumenfeld TJ, Politi J. THA with delta ceramic on ceramic: results of a multicenter investigational device exemption trial. Clin Orthop Relat Res. 2010;468(2):358–66.
14. Amstutz HC, Le Duff MJ. Hip resurfacing results for osteonecrosis are as good as for other etiologies at 2 to 12 years. Clin Orthop Relat Res. 2010;468(2):375–81.
15. McMinn DJ, Daniel J, Ziaee H, Pradhan C. Indications and results of hip resurfacing. Int Orthop. 2011;35(2):231–7.
16. Daniel J, Ziaee H, Pradhan C, Pynsent PB, McMinn DJ. Blood and urine metal ion levels in young and active patients after Birmingham hip resurfacing arthroplasty: four-year results of a prospective longitudinal study. J Bone Joint Surg Br. 2007;89(2):169–73.
17. Migaud H, Putman S, Combes A, Berton C, Bocquet D, Vasseur L, et al. Metal-on-metal bearing: is this the end of the line? We do not think so. HSS J. 2012;8(3):262–9.
18. Xenakis TA, Gelalis J, Koukoubis TA, Zaharis KC, Soucacos PN. Cementless hip arthroplasty in the treatment of patients with femoral head necrosis. Clin Orthop Relat Res. 2001;386:93–9.
19. Babis GC, Soucacos PN. Effectiveness of total hip arthroplasty in the management of hip osteonecrosis. Orthop Clin North Am. 2004;35(3):359–64, x.
20. Min BW, Song KS, Bae KC, Cho CH, Lee KJ, Kim HJ. Second-generation cementless total hip arthroplasty in patients with osteonecrosis of the femoral head. J Arthroplasty. 2008;23(6):902–10.
21. Muratoglu OK, Bragdon CR, O'Connor DO, Jasty M, Harris WH. A novel method of cross-linking ultra-high-molecular-weight polyethylene to improve wear, reduce oxidation, and retain mechanical properties. Recipient of the 1999 HAP Paul Award. J Arthroplasty. 2001;16(2):149–60.
22. Hermida JC, Bergula A, Chen P, Colwell Jr CW, D'Lima DD. Comparison of the wear rates of twenty-eight and thirty-two-millimeter femoral heads on cross-linked polyethylene acetabular cups in a wear simulator. J Bone Joint Surg Am. 2003;85-A(12): 2325–31.
23. Rohrl SM, Li MG, Nilsson KG, Nivbrant B. Very low wear of non-remelted highly cross-linked polyethylene cups: an RSA study lasting up to 6 years. Acta Orthop. 2007;78(6):739–45.
24. Thomas GE, Simpson DJ, Mehmood S, Taylor A, McLardy-Smith P, Gill HS, et al. The seven-year wear of highly cross-linked polyethylene in total hip arthroplasty: a double-blind, randomized controlled trial using radiostereometric analysis. J Bone Joint Surg Am. 2011;93(8):716–22.
25. Geerdink CH, Grimm B, Vencken W, Heyligers IC, Tonino AJ. Cross-linked compared with historical polyethylene in THA: an 8-year clinical study. Clin Orthop Relat Res. 2009;467(4):979–84.
26. McCalden RW, MacDonald SJ, Rorabeck CH, Bourne RB, Chess DG, Charron KD. Wear rate of highly cross-linked polyethylene in total hip arthroplasty. A randomized controlled trial. J Bone Joint Surg Am. 2009;91(4):773–82.
27. Mutimer J, Devane PA, Adams K, Horne JG. Highly crosslinked polyethylene reduces wear in total hip arthroplasty at 5 years. Clin Orthop Relat Res. 2010;468(12):3228–33.
28. Wangen H, Lereim P, Holm I, Gunderson R, Reikeras O. Hip arthroplasty in patients younger than 30 years: excellent ten to 16-year follow-up results with a HA-coated stem. Int Orthop. 2008;32(2):203–8.
29. Schmalzried TP, Kwong LM, Jasty M, Sedlacek RC, Haire TC, O'Connor DO, et al. The mechanism of loosening of cemented acetabular components in total hip arthroplasty. Analysis of specimens retrieved at autopsy. Clin Orthop Relat Res. 1992;274: 60–78.
30. Dumbleton JH, Manley MT, Edidin AA. A literature review of the association between wear rate and osteolysis in total hip arthroplasty. J Arthroplasty. 2002;17(5):649–61.
31. Sochart DH. Relationship of acetabular wear to osteolysis and loosening in total hip arthroplasty. Clin Orthop Relat Res. 1999;363:135–50.
32. Nikolaou VS, Edwards MR, Bogoch E, Schemitsch EH, Waddell JP. A prospective randomised controlled trial comparing three

alternative bearing surfaces in primary total hip replacement. J Bone Joint Surg Br. 2012;94(4):459–65.
33. Kim YH, Park JW, Patel C, Kim DY. Polyethylene wear and osteolysis after cementless total hip arthroplasty with alumina-on-highly cross-linked polyethylene bearings in patients younger than thirty years of age. J Bone Joint Surg Am. 2013;95(12):1088–93.
34. Reynolds SE, Malkani AL, Ramakrishnan R, Yakkanti MR. Wear analysis of first-generation highly cross-linked polyethylene in primary total hip arthroplasty: an average 9-year follow-up. J Arthroplasty. 2012;27(6):1064–8.
35. Capello WN, D'Antonio JA, Ramakrishnan R, Naughton M. Continued improved wear with an annealed highly cross-linked polyethylene. Clin Orthop Relat Res. 2011;469(3):825–30.
36. Babovic N, Trousdale RT. Total hip arthroplasty using highly cross-linked polyethylene in patients younger than 50 years with minimum 10-year follow-up. J Arthroplasty. 2013;28(5):815–7.
37. Bedard NA, Callaghan JJ, Liu SS, Greiner JJ, Klaassen AL, Johnston RC. Cementless THA for the treatment of osteonecrosis at 10-year follow-up: have we improved compared to cemented THA? J Arthroplasty. 2013;28(7):1192–9.
38. Min BW, Lee KJ, Song KS, Bae KC, Cho CH. Highly cross-linked polyethylene in total hip arthroplasty for osteonecrosis of the femoral head: a minimum 5-year follow-up study. J Arthroplasty. 2013;28(3):526–30.
39. Kim YH, Choi Y, Kim JS. Cementless total hip arthroplasty with alumina-on-highly cross-linked polyethylene bearing in young patients with femoral head osteonecrosis. J Arthroplasty. 2011;26(2):218–23.
40. Livingston BJ, Chmell MJ, Spector M, Poss R. Complications of total hip arthroplasty associated with the use of an acetabular component with a hylamer liner. J Bone Joint Surg Am. 1997;79(10):1529–38.
41. Scott DL, Campbell PA, McClung CD, Schmalzried TP. Factors contributing to rapid wear and osteolysis in hips with modular acetabular bearings made of hylamer. J Arthroplasty. 2000;15(1):35–46.
42. Furmanski J, Kraay MJ, Rimnac CM. Crack initiation in retrieved cross-linked highly cross-linked ultrahigh-molecular-weight polyethylene acetabular liners: an investigation of 9 cases. J Arthroplasty. 2011;26(5):796–801.

50 Alumina Ceramic-on-Highly Cross-Linked Polyethylene Bearing in Cementless Total Hip Arthroplasty in Young Patients with Osteonecrosis of Femoral Head

Young-Hoo Kim

50.1 Introduction

Although total hip arthroplasties (THAs) have been extremely successful, survivorship of THAs in young patients with osteonecrosis of femoral head has been limited by aseptic loosening and osteolysis secondary to wear and particulate polyethylene debris [1–4]. Highly cross-linked polyethylene (HXLPE) has been introduced to decrease osteolysis secondary to polyethylene wear debris generation, thereby increasing long-term survivorship of the THAs [5–7]. There are a variety of types of HXLPE sold worldwide today.

Three versions of intentionally HXLPE have been historically used in THA; one of those types have been chemically cross-linked, while the other two were cross-linked using high doses of irradiation. Retrospective wear measurements and anecdotal results of more than 10 years are available; Wroblewski [7] reports in his 10-year data a wear rate of 0.037 mm/year, a reduction of 75 % versus conventionally sterilized PE. Oohnishi [8] and Grobbelaar [9] report 20-year results with similar reduction in wear rate. Nevertheless, the historical cross-linking methods used the standard sterilization technology of those days and, therefore, were suboptimal. Gamma irradiation sterilization in inert gas was introduced in 1986 [10], and since the late 1990s, the second generation of HXLPE has been used successfully as bearing surfaces using two thermal methods to reduce the free radicals generated during the cross-linking process. Despite a dramatic reduction in wear and positive clinical results with the second-generation HXLPE [11], it was necessary to compromise between oxidation resistance and preservation of toughness, which has been addressed by various manufactures in different ways. Second-generation HXLPE have been used on a limited basis as bearing surfaces for total knee replacement (TKR), and there is limited clinical information on their success but no reports of failures of tibial inserts. Nevertheless, isolated reports of fracture of remelted HXLPE hip liners have been reported [12, 13], and degradation due to oxidation remains a long-term concern.

The newest third generation of HXLPE has been introduced in 2005/2007 to address the deficiencies of the previous generation by usage of enhanced technologies to minimize the compromise made with second-generation materials. All new-generation HXLPE are now irradiated by gamma rays instead of electron beam. To retain the mechanical properties, the annealing procedures are used for all materials on the market, while for the quenching of the free radicals, two different methods are used. One uses a sequential irradiation/annealing process repeated three times (×3), others incorporate vitamin E as radical scavenger in various amounts and process into the HXLPE.

Alumina ceramic bearings offer the advantage of improved lubrication, smoother surface finish, and improved resistance to scratching and are biologically inert compounds. Ceramic femoral heads therefore have substantial tribologic advantages over metal femoral heads and result in much lower wear and osteolysis [14]. Furthermore, alumina ceramic-on-highly cross-linked polyethylene bearing in total hip arthroplasty would reduce more polyethylene wear and osteolysis.

Y.-H. Kim
The Joint Replacement Center, Ewha Womans University School of Medicine, Seoul, Republic of Korea

The Joint Replacement Center, Ewha Womans University MokDong Hospital, 911-1, MokDong, YangChun-Gu, Seoul 158-710, Korea
e-mail: younghookim@ewha.ac.kr

K.-H. Koo et al. (eds.), *Osteonecrosis*,
DOI 10.1007/978-3-642-35767-1_50, © Springer-Verlag Berlin Heidelberg 2014

We investigated whether cementless total hip arthroplasties using alumina ceramic-on-second generation of highly cross-linked polyethylene bearings would improve hip score and functional activity and reduce the incidence of polyethylene wear, osteolysis, and aseptic loosening.

50.2 Materials and Methods

From February 2000 to April 2002, the senior author performed 146 consecutive total hip arthroplasties using alumina ceramic-on-highly cross-linked polyethylene (Marathon, DePuy, Warsaw, Indiana) in 133 patients. The study was approved by our institutional review board, and all patients provided informed consent. Twelve patients were lost to follow-up (before 2 years), leaving 121 patients (133 hips) in this study.

There were 82 men and 39 women. The average age at the time of the index arthroplasty was 36.9 years (range, 20–50 years). The average weight of the patients was 67.8 kg (range, 47–98 kg). The average height was 164.8 kg (range, 147–189 kg), and the average body mass index was 24.9 kg/m^2 (range, 18.8–30.5 kg/m^2). The preoperative diagnosis was osteonecrosis of femoral head in all hips. All hips with osteonecrosis of femoral head had Ficat and Arlet stage III or IV [15]. The presumed cause of osteonecrosis was ethanol abuse in 85 patients (70 %), idiopathic in 31 patients (26 %), and steroid use in five patients (4 %). The average follow-up was 11.6 years (range, 10.5–12.8 years).

All operations were performed through a posterolateral approach. A cementless Duraloc 100 or 1,200 series acetabular component with a highly cross-linked polyethylene liner of 28 mm inner diameter was used in all hips. The solid acetabular component was fixed with a press fit only in 122 hips (92 %), and one or two screws were inserted for supplemental fixation of the cups with screw holes in the remaining 11 hips (8 %). All patients received an Immediate Postoperative Stability (IPS; DePuy, Leeds, United Kingdom) femoral component with a 28 mm alumina forte ceramic femoral head. The femoral component was inserted with a press-fit technique. The largest broach that would fit the metaphysis was used. The IPS femoral component is an anatomical metaphyseal-fitting titanium stem with a polished and tapered distal stem, designed to provide fixation in the metaphysis only, thereby avoiding metal-to-bone contact below this point. The proximal 30 % of stem was porous coated with sintered titanium beads, with a mean pore size of 250 μm to which a hydroxyapatite coating was applied to a thickness of 30 μm.

The patients were allowed to stand on the second postoperative day, and they progressed to full weight bearing with crutches as tolerated. They were advised to use a pair of crutches for 4 weeks and walk with a cane thereafter if required.

Clinical follow-up was performed at 3 months and 1 year and yearly thereafter. Harris hip score [16] and Western Ontario and McMaster Universities Osteoarthritis (WOMAC) [17] score were determined before surgery and at each follow-up examination. Patients subjectively evaluated thigh pain on a 10-point visual analog scale (0 = no pain; 10 = severe pain). The level of activity of the patients after the total hip arthroplasty was assessed with the activity score of the University of California, Los Angeles (UCLA) [18].

Radiographic follow-up was performed at 3 months and 1 year and yearly thereafter. A supine anteroposterior radiograph of the pelvis with both hips in neutral rotation and 0° of abduction was made for every patient. Consistent patient positioning was ensured with the use of x-ray frame. Cross-table lateral radiographs were also made of each hip.

Femoral bone type was determined in preoperative radiographs using Dorr's classification [19]. Definite loosening of the femoral component was defined if there was a progressive axial subsidence of >2 mm or varus or valgus shift of >2° [20]. A femoral component was considered to be possibly loose when there was a complete radiolucent line surrounding the entire porous-coated surface on both the anteroposterior and lateral radiographs [20]. Definite loosening of the acetabular component was diagnosed when there was a change in the position of the component (>2 mm vertically and/or medially or laterally) or a continuous radiolucent line wider than 2 mm on both the anteroposterior and the lateral radiographs [20].

Penetration of the polyethylene liner was measured with AutoCAD 2013 (Autodesk, Inc., Sauslito, California [21]), by three observers who was blinded to the clinical results. The observers made three measurements in each radiograph. A ScanMaker 9600XL flat-bed imaging scanner (Microtek, Carson, California) digitized the anteroposterior radiograph of the pelvis as two-dimensional grayscale arrays of 12-bit (256-gray-level) integers. The scanning resolution was 600 pixels per square inch (psi). Penetration of the head into the polyethylene liner was determined annually from anteroposterior pelvic radiographs. The amount of head penetration into the polyethylene liner on radiographs made 3 months postoperatively was considered to be the "zero position."

The presence and location of areas of osteolysis in the acetabulum and in the femur were recorded in the anteroposterior and lateral radiographs according to the system of DeLee and Charnley [22] and Gruen et al. [23], respectively. The length and width of osteolytic lesions were measured, and the area was expressed in square centimeters.

Computed tomography of one or both hips was performed at 1 week after the operation and at final follow-up to determine osteolysis. We developed an algorithm to address the beam hardening artifacts, as well as to measure the volume of osteolytic lesions. We then developed a segmentation algorithm to segment the lytic lesions from image data and to measure their volumes. Computed tomographic images were acquired using Siemens AG (Munich, Germany) with 1 mm collimation, a pitch of 1.5, and a 14–22 cm field of view. The raw data was reconstructed for 1 mm slices. The area within 5 cm from the prosthesis-bone interface in all directions was evaluated. The volume of osteolysis was calculated by VirtualScopics (Rochester, New York).

Survivorship analysis was performed with the Kaplan-Meier method [24] with revision for any reason as one end point and revision due to mechanical failure (clinical and radiographic evidence of aseptic loosening) at the time of follow-up as the other end point. We determined differences in continuous variances (Harris hip score and range of motion) between preoperative and postoperative results using Student's paired *t*-test and in categorical variances (details of functional evaluation and deformity according to the Harris hip score) and limb length between preoperative and postoperative evaluations using chi-square test. Univariate regression analysis was used to evaluate the relationship, if any, between osteolysis and the variables of age, gender, weight, diagnosis, the duration of follow-up, and acetabular inclination and anteversion. The level of significance was set at $p<0.05$.

50.3 Results

Preoperative Harris hip score was improved significantly ($p=0.005$). The mean preoperative Harris hip score was 44.3 points (range, 6–55 points), which was improved to 96 points (range, 85–100 points) at 11.6-year follow-up. Preoperative functional activity was improved significantly ($p=0.001$) at 11.6-year follow-up. The ability to put on footwear and to cut toenails and to use stairs and public transportation was improved markedly at 11.6-year follow-up. Preoperative WOMAC score was 65.3 points (range, 52–82 points), and it was improved to 13 points (range, 9–14 points) at 11.6-year follow-up.

Activity level of patients was improved very much after the operation. Many patients were quite active despite our admonitions to avoid activities involving high impact, following the total hip arthroplasty. The preoperative UCLA activity score was 2 points (range, 1–3 points), which was improved to 6.5 points (range, 5–10 points) at 11.6-year follow-up.

No hip had aseptic loosening of any acetabular or femoral component. All hips had Dorr type A or type B bones. The mean inclination and anteversion of acetabular component was 43.2° (range, 35–45°) and 21° (range, 19–25°), respectively. All acetabular and femoral components were fixed by bone ingrowth. Calcar rounding off was observed in all hips, but no hip had stress-shielding-related proximal femoral bone resorption. No hip had ceramic femoral head or acetabular liner fracture.

The mean total amount of HXLPE linear penetration was 0.381 ± 0.298 mm (range, 0.000–1.296 mm), and mean annual penetration rate was 0.033 ± 0.002 mm per year (range, 0.000–0.111 mm per year). Normal accuracy of measurement of this system was 0.001 mm. The chance-corrected kappa coefficient that was calculated to determine interobserver agreement of hip scoring and wear measurement was between 0.81 and 0.87. We noted that increased head penetration into polyethylene during the first postoperative year suggested the bedding-in period. At 11.6-year follow-up, four hips were an outlier for the so-called osteolysis threshold of 0.10 mm per year [26–29], with remaining 129 polyethylene liners having a penetration rate below this level. In the four hips with an outlier for the osteolysis threshold, there was no evidence of acetabular or femoral osteolysis. With the numbers available, univariate regression analysis did not demonstrate that age, gender weight, activity, cup inclination, or cup anteversion had any influence on polyethylene linear penetration.

Radiographs and computer tomographic scans demonstrated that no acetabular or femoral osteolysis was detected in any hip at 11.6-year follow-up (Fig. 50.1).

Two hips (1.5 %) were dislocated 3 and 5 days, respectively, after the operation and were treated successfully with a closed reduction and an abduction brace for 3 months. No further dislocation was observed in these hips until 11.6-year follow-up. No hip had a revision or aseptic loosening of acetabular and/or femoral component. Kaplan-Meier survival analysis, with revision as the end point for failure, showed that the rates of survival of both acetabular and femoral components at 11.6 years were 100 % (95 % confidence interval, 98–100).

50.4 Discussion

Survivorship of total hip arthroplasty in young patients is poorer than in older patients. Young patients may have acquired hip disease from a multitude of different causes and have different activity levels. The majority of patients in our series continue to participate in high-demand activities, including moderate to heavy manual labor. These disease entities (osteonecrosis) and the level of activity did not seem to affect the longevity of fixation of acetabular and femoral components in these young cohorts. We believe that several factors were responsible for our good results: improved design (the proximal canal-fitting design of the femoral stem including pronounced lateral flare, anteroposterior buildup, and short and narrow polished distal stem) and surgical technique for implantation of the cementless stem, the strong trabecular bone in young patients, utilization of an alumina ceramic femoral head with HXLPE liner, and small and light patients.

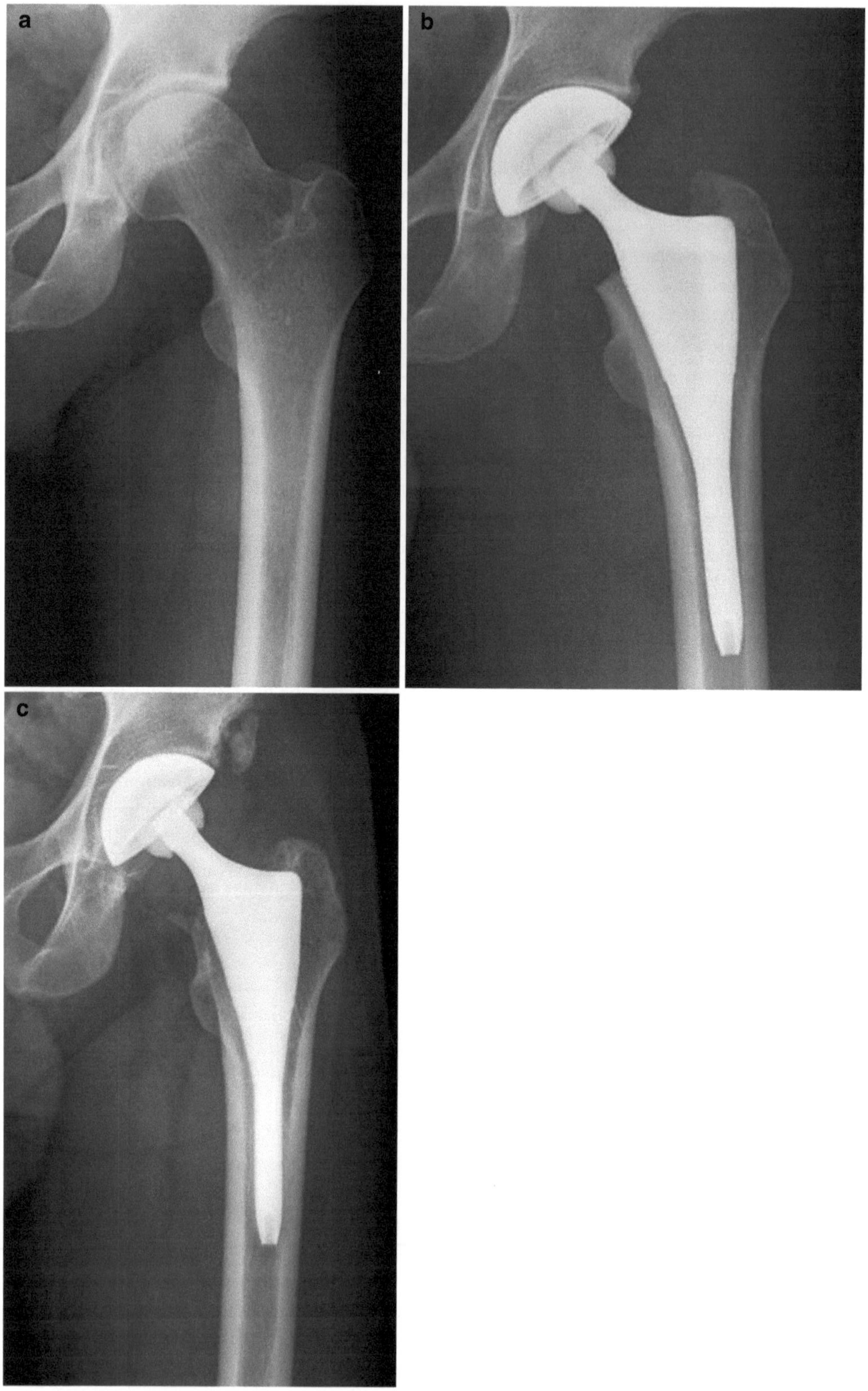

Fig. 50.1 Radiographic and computed tomographic evaluation of osteolysis of left hip of a 46-year-old man with osteonecrosis of femoral head. (**a**) An anteroposterior view of left hip before the operation shows sclerotic lesion in the femoral head. (**b**) An anteroposterior view of the left hip made 7 days after surgery reveals that Duraloc 100 series cementless acetabular component and IPS femoral component are fixed in a satisfactory position. (**c**) An anteroposterior view of the left hip made 12 years after surgery shows that acetabular and femoral component are fixed in a satisfactory position. Calcar round off is observed. There is no evidence of radiolucent line, polyethylene wear, or osteolysis around the acetabular or femoral component. (**d**) Computed tomographic scanning of left hip taken 12 years after the surgery reveals no evidence of osteolysis around the acetabular or femoral components

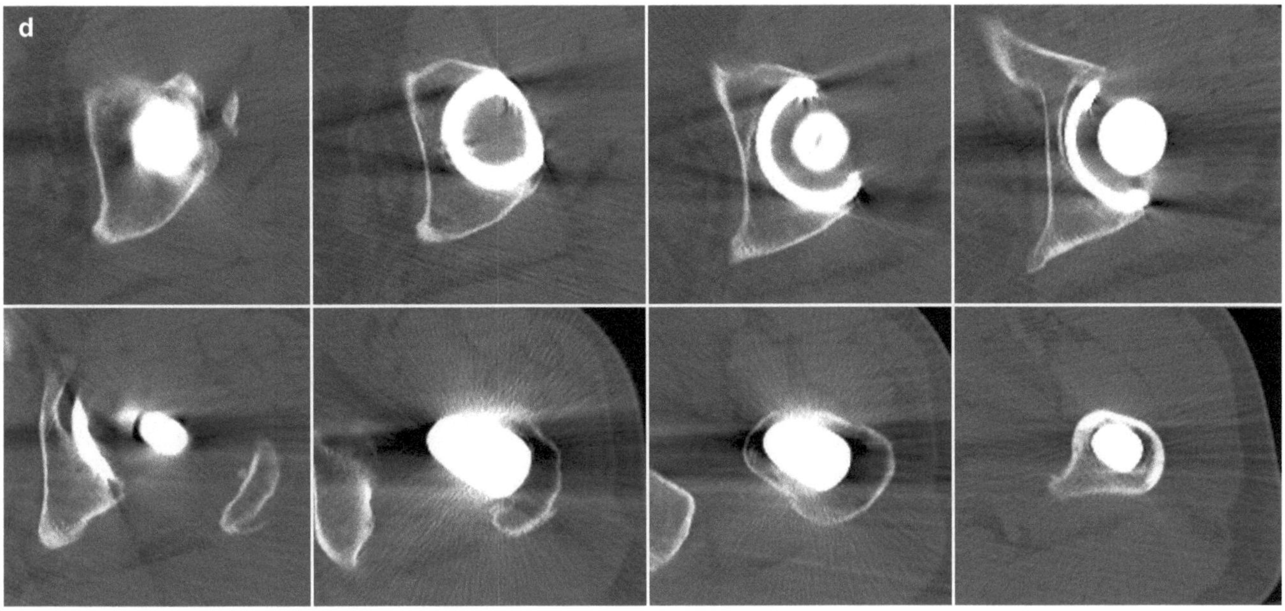

Fig. 50.1 (continued)

Our results are consistent with other studies [20, 25, 28–36]. In one study with a minimum 5-year follow-up, the wear rate of the HXLPE liner was 0.029 mm per year and 0.065 mm per year for conventional polyethylene [29]. In another study with a minimum 7-year follow-up, the mean steady-state wear rate of highly cross-lined polyethylene was 0.005 mm per year (95 % confidence interval, ±0.15 mm per year) [35]. McCalden et al. [36] reported that the mean femoral head penetration rate in the first through fifth years in patients treated with the HXLPE was 0.003 mm per year (95 % confidence interval, ±0.027 mm per year). Using edge-detection techniques at 4 years, the rate for HXLPE wear was 0.007 mm per year and 0.174 mm per year for conventional polyethylene [31, 32].

Bitsch et al. [32] reported, after a mean follow-up of 5.8 years (range, 5.0–7.7 years), that the mean femoral head penetration was 0.031 mm per year (range, 0.04–0.196 mm per year) in hips with a Marathon HXLPE (DePuy, Warsaw, Indiana) and 0.104 mm per year (range 0.04–0.196 mm per year) in hips with an Enduron polyethylene liner (DePuy). Osteolysis was not observed in any of hips with a Marathon HXLPE. Engh et al. [33] reported a reduction in the mean wear rate for Marathon HXLPE of 95 % (0.01 ± 0.12 mm per year) compared with Enduron liners (0.19 ± 0.12 mm per year). Kim et al. [35] observed that the mean Marathon HXLPE penetration rate was 0.05 ± 0.02 mm per year and no hip had aseptic loosening or osteolysis in young patients with femoral head osteonecrosis. In all but four patients in our study, the penetration rate of Marathon HXLPE was below the osteolysis threshold (0.1 mm per year). No detectable osteolysis using plain x-ray and computed tomography was observed in any hip in our study, which is consistent with other studies [29, 32, 33].

The first generation of HXLPE had documented reductions in fatigue, tensile, and toughness properties [30]. In the current series, no hip had polyethylene liner fracture. We believe that the use of adequate thickness of acetabular polyethylene liner (thicker than 6 mm) and satisfactory position of acetabular component led to absence of polyethylene liner fracture.

There has been some concern that smaller wear particles are produced with HXLPE than with conventional polyethylene, leading to a higher functional biologic activity [37, 38]. However, in our 11.6-year follow-up data, no evidence of acetabular or femoral osteolysis was observed. A longer follow-up is necessary to make conclusions about the biologic activity of HXLPE.

While there is a risk of ceramic femoral head fracture, the risk was low enough to go undetected in our small series and was outweighed by the excellent 11.6-year outcomes in a highly active, young group of patients.

There are some limitations of this study. First, the hip scoring system and the measurement of polyethylene wear are prone to interobserver variability. However, the chance-corrected kappa coefficient that was calculated to determine interobserver agreement of hip scoring and wear measurement was between 0.78 and 0.85. Second, there is some potential for bias as this is one technique and does not have a control or comparison group. Finally, the follow-up was not long enough to make conclusions regarding the theoretical advantage of alumina ceramic-on-HXLPE bearing. Strengths of this study are completeness and length of follow-up as well as consistency of clinical and radiographic examinations.

Our data suggest that the current generation of cementless acetabular and femoral components with alumina ceramic-on-HXLPE bearing has been functioning well, with no osteolysis at a 10.5-year minimum and average of 11.6-year follow-up in young patients with osteonecrosis of femoral head. While the long-term survival of implants and prevalence of HXLPE wear and osteolysis remain unknown, the midterm data are promising.

References

1. Kim Y-H, Kook H-K, Kim J-S. Total hip replacement with a cementless acetabular component and a cemented femoral component in patients younger than fifty years of age. J Bone Joint Surg Am. 2002;84(5):770–4.
2. Kim Y-H, Oh S-H, Kim J-S, Koo K-H. Contemporary total hip arthroplasty with and without cement in patients with osteonecrosis of the femoral head. J Bone Joint Surg Am. 2003;85(4):675–81.
3. Kim Y-H, Oh S-H, Kim J-S. Primary total hip arthroplasty with a second-generation cementless total hip prosthesis in patients younger than fifty years of age. J Bone Joint Surg Am. 2003; 85(1):109–14.
4. Kim Y-H. Cementless total hip arthroplasty with a close proximal fit and short tapered distal stem (third-generation) prosthesis. J Arthroplasty. 2002;17(7):841–50.
5. Jasty M, Haire T, Tanzer M. Femoral osteolysis: a generic problem with cementless and cemented femoral components. Orthop Trans. 1991;15:758–9.
6. Willert HG, Bertram H, Buchhorn GH. Osteolysis in alloarthroplasty of the hip. The role of ultra-high molecular weight polyethylene wear particle. Clin Orthop Relat Res. 1990;258:95–107.
7. Wroblewski BM, Siney PD, Fleming PA. Low-friction arthroplasty of the hip using alumina ceramic and cross-linked polyethylene. J Bone Joint Surg Br. 1990;81(1):54–5.
8. Oonishi H. Long term clinical results of THR. Clinical results of THR of an alumina head with a cross-linked UHMWPE cup. Orthop Surg Traumatol. 1995;38:1255–64.
9. Grobbelaar CJ. Long term results with cross linked PE. Abstr, 4th EFORT. 1999:158.
10. Streicher RM. Investigation on sterilization and modification of high molecular weight polyethylenes by ionizing radiation. Beta Gamma. 1989;89(1):34–43.
11. Röhrl SM, Li MG, Nilsson KG, Nivbrant B. Very low wear of non-remelted highly cross-linked polyethylene cups: an RSA study lasting up to 6 years. Acta Orthop. 2007;78(6):739–45.
12. Harris W. Three revolutions in acetabular revision surgery. Abstr. 2003 16th ISTA:24–8.
13. Rowell SL, Duffy G, Wannomae KK. Failure of a MarathonTM UHMWPE acetabular liner: a case study. Trans 53rd ORS. 2007:1646.
14. Urban JA, Garvin KL, Boese CK, Bryson L, Pedersen DR, Callaghan JJ, Miller RK. Ceramic-on-polyethylene bearing surfaces in total hip arthroplasty. Seventeen to twenty-one-year results. J Bone Joint Surg Am. 2001;83(11):1688–94.
15. Ficat RP, Arlet J. Treatment of bone ischemia and necrosis. In: Hungerford DS, editor. Ischemia and necrosis of bone. Baltimore: Williams & Wilkins; 1980. p. 171.
16. Harris WH. Traumatic arthritis of the hip after dislocation and acetabular fractures: treatment by mold arthroplasty. An end-result study using a new method of result evaluation. J Bone Joint Surg Am. 1969;51(4):737–55.
17. Bellamy N, Buchanan WW, Goldsmith CH, Campbell J, Stitt LW. Validation study of WOMAC: a health status instrument for measuring clinically important patient relevant outcomes to antirheumatic drug therapy in patients with osteoarthritis of the hip or knee. J Rheumatol. 1988;15(12):1833–40.
18. Zahiri CA, Schmalzried TP, Szuszczewicz ES, Amstutz HC. Assessing activity in joint replacement patients. J Arthroplasty. 1998;13(8):890–5.
19. Dorr LD. Total hip replacement using APR system. Tech Orthop. 1986;1(3):22–34.
20. Kim Y-H, Kim J-S, Oh S-H, Kim J-M. Comparison of porous-coated titanium femoral stem with and without hydroxyapatite coating. J Bone Joint Surg Am. 2003;85(9):1682–8.
21. Kim Y-H, Kim J-S, Chi S-H. A comparison of polyethylene wear in hips with cobalt-chrome or zirconia heads. A prospective, randomized study. J Bone Joint Surg Br. 2001;83(5):742–50.
22. DeLee JG, Gharnley J. Radiological demarcation of cemented sockets in total hip replacement. Clin Orthop Relat Res. 1976;121:20–32.
23. Gruen TA, McNeice GM, Amstutz HC. "Modes of failure" of cemented stem-type femoral components: a radiographic analysis of loosening. Clin Orthop Relat Res. 1979;141:17–27.
24. Kaplan EL, Meier P. Nonparametric estimation from incomplete observation. J Am Stat Assoc. 1958;53:457–81.
25. Dumbleton JH, Manley MT, Edidin AA. A literature review of the association between wear rate and osteolysis in total hip arthroplasty. J Arthroplasty. 2002;17(5):649–61.
26. Leung SB, Egawa H, Stepniewski A, Beykirch S, Engh Jr CA, Engh Sr CA. Incidence and volume of pelvic osteolysis at early follow-up with highly cross-linked and noncross-linked polyethylene. J Arthroplasty. 2007;22(6 suppl 2):134–9.
27. Garvin KL, Hartman CW, Mangla J, Murdoch N, Martell JM. Wear analysis in THA utilizing oxidized zirconium and crosslinked polyethylene. Clin Orthop Relat Res. 2009;467(1):141–5.
28. Kim Y-H, Kim J-S, Choi Y-W, Kwon O-R. Intermediate results of simultaneous alumina-on-alumina bearing and alumina-on-highly cross-linked polyethylene bearing total hip arthroplasties. J Arthroplasty. 2009;24(6):885–91.
29. Dorr LD, Wan Z, Shahrdar C, Sirianni L, Boutary M, Yun A. Clinical performance of a Durasul highly cross-linked polyethylene acetabular liner for total hip arthroplasty at five years. J Bone Joint Surg Am. 2005;87(8):1816–21.
30. Bradford L, Baker D, Ries MD, Pruitt LA. Fatigue crack propagation resistance of highly crosslinked polyethylene. Clin Orthop Relat Res. 2004;429:68–72.
31. Manning DW, Chiang PP, Martell JM, Galante JO, Harris WH. In vivo comparative wear study of traditional and highly cross-linked polyethylene in total hip arthroplasty. J Arthroplasty. 2005;20(7): 880–6.
32. Bitsch RG, Loidolt T, Heisel C, Ball S, Schmalzried TP. Reduction of osteolysis with use of Marathon cross-linked polyethylene. A concise follow-up, at a minimum of five years, of a previous report. J Bone Joint Surg Am. 2008;90(7):1487–91.
33. Engh Jr CA, Stepniewski AS, Ginn SD, Beykirch SE, Sychterz-Terefenko CJ, Hopper Jr RH, Engh CA. A randomized prospective evaluation of outcomes after total hip arthroplasty using cross-linked marathon and non-cross-linked Enduron polyethylene liners. J Arthroplasty. 2006;21(6 suppl 2):17–25.
34. Dowd JE, Sychterz CJ, Young AM, Engh CA. Characterization of long-term femoral-head-penetration rates. Association with and prediction of osteolysis. J Bone Joint Surg Am. 2000;82(8): 1102–7.
35. Kim Y-H, Choi Y-W, Kim J-S. Cementless total hip arthroplasty with alumina-on-highly cross-linked polyethylene bearing in young patients with femoral head osteonecrosis. J Arthroplasty. 2011;26(2):218–23.

36. McCalden RW, MacDonald SJ, Rorabeck CH, Bourne RB, Chess DG, Charron KD. Wear rate of highly cross-linked polyethylene in total hip arthroplasty. A randomized controlled trial. J Bone Joint Surg Am. 2009;91(4):773–82.
37. Endo M, Tipper JL, Barton DC, Stone MH, Ingham E, Fisher J. Comparison of wear, wear debris and functional biological activity of moderately crosslinked and non-crosslinked polyethylenes in hip prostheses. Proc Inst Mech Eng H. 2002;216(2):111–22.
38. Fisher J, McEwen HM, Tipper JL, Galvin AL, Ingram J, Kamali A, Stone MH, Ingham E. Wear, debris, and biologic activity of cross-linked polyethylene in the knee: benefits and potential concerns. Clin Orthop Relat Res. 2004;428:114–9.

51 Hip Arthroplasty for Osteonecrosis of the Femoral Head

Harlan C. Amstutz, Michel J. Le Duff, and Mariam Al-Hamad

51.1 Introduction

The typical patient affected by osteonecrosis (ON) of the hip joint ranges in age from 20 to 50 years [1], and men are usually more prone to idiopathic ON than women [2]. Also, bilateral involvement is quite frequent [3–5]. Acute discomfort is felt by the patient when necrotic bone no longer performs its support function and a subchondral fracture or collapse occurs [6]. Accurate staging of the disease is essential to select the appropriate treatment option, and many surgical procedures exist for the treatment of ON of the femoral head. A treatment algorithm can be defined, which will take into consideration (1) the age of the patient, (2) the development stage of the disease, and (3) the clinical and survivorship results of various procedures available to the treating physician. Here, we can see that this treatment algorithm is not set in stone as the evolution of surgical techniques can alter outcomes, possibly reducing the usefulness of a procedure while expanding the indications for another. Several staging systems exist [7–10] and some may be preferred in the description of the early stages of the disease, but we believe that the Ficat and Arlet classification provides the essential information to treat patients who may be best treated with one type of hip arthroplasty [7].

In this chapter, an overview of popular treatment options for hip ON will be given, and the senior author's clinical results with hemiresurfacing, full resurfacing, and THR will be presented.

H.C. Amstutz (✉) • M.J. Le Duff • M. Al-Hamad
Joint Replacement Institute at St Vincent Medical Center, 2200 West Third Street, Suite 400, Los Angeles, CA 90057, USA
e-mail: harlanamstutz@dochs.org; michelleduff@dochs.org; mariam.alhamad@gmail.com

51.2 Non-prosthetic Operative Treatments

All the operative treatments commonly elected for ON of the hip joint aim to (1) relieve pain and (2) restore the congruence of the articular surfaces whether natural or artificial. Generally speaking, as long as the femoral head has not collapsed, there is a chance that a conservative non-prosthetic solution might be sufficient to achieve both these objectives by reestablishing blood flow to the femoral head.

Core decompressions have been performed since the 1960s, but there is still a paucity of studies reporting long term results of this procedure [11]. However, it is clear that the efficacy of core decompression is limited to Ficat stage I and II ON [12] in consideration of the high rates of progression of the disease leading to the need for arthroplasty in hips with Ficat grade III or higher [13]. The surgical technique used for core decompression has evolved including using smaller, multiple drill holes or using bone grafts, but the improvement observed in the last 15 years may to some extent be a factor of patient selection by the surgeons performing the procedures [14].

Free vascularized fibular grafting (FVFG) was initially utilized for all stages of disease but most would now agree that the procedure's morbidity and quality of results do not justify the procedure in Ficat stage III or IV because restoration of the sphericity of the head and damaged cartilage repair are not possible and prosthetic solutions are preferable. The probability for conversion to THA within 5 years is lower for precollapsed hips (Ficat stages I and II) with increasing likelihood up to ~30 % in Ficat stages III and IV [15–17]. The indications for FVFG are even controversial for stages 1 and II because of safety and efficacy issues. Complications include ankle pain, motor weakness, sensory abnormalities, and a 2.5 % rate of subtrochanteric fractures [18, 19]. It has also been shown that patients who undergo FVFG can have diminished success with THA and THR later in life when needed because the grafted bone hinders

K.-H. Koo et al. (eds.), *Osteonecrosis*,
DOI 10.1007/978-3-642-35767-1_51, © Springer-Verlag Berlin Heidelberg 2014

optimal placement of the femoral component [20]. Therefore, it is important to carry out a careful preoperative staging with attention to age, duration of symptoms, and radiographs to ensure good outcomes in these patients [21]. Eward et al. [22], however, reported hip preservation lasting greater than 10 years in the majority of 65 hips, and those who were eventually revised had hip preservation at a mean duration of 8 years. The results in other series have been less favorable.

Circa 2005, a new procedure was introduced that had for objective to restore blood flow and femoral head structural support by insertion of a threaded rod featuring trabecular tantalum porous coating (Osteonecrosis Intervention Implant, Zimmer, Warsaw, IN). Several preliminary studies reported encouraging results [23–25]. However, the latest clinical report showed a high (44 %) conversion rate to total hip arthroplasty 4 years after the procedure [26], and several cases of femoral neck fracture have been reported [27, 28]. In addition, the main characteristic of this procedure is the implantation of a device that is difficult to remove when comes the time to proceed with hip arthroplasty, in the event of a collapse of the femoral head. The need to resect the femoral neck to extract the device [29] precludes performing any type of resurfacing arthroplasty (even though the patients are usually still young when this happens) and can complicate the implantation of a conventional total hip device [30].

Our belief is that stage one requires no immediate treatment other than periodical follow-up. The results of simple bone grafting seem to be equivalent to those of FVFG and may even be preferable considering the high morbidity associated with FVFG. Nonetheless, our preference goes to low morbidity procedures for symptomatic patients such as hemi- or full resurfacing which remains bone conserving in anticipation of a possible revision in these young patients. The results of cancellous head grafting are also unpredictable with insufficient midterm success [31–33] even with the adjunction of bone morphogenetic protein [34].

51.3 Prosthetic Solutions

Unfortunately, the currently dominant prosthetic solution for ON is conventional total hip arthroplasty, despite the success of more bone-conserving and better bone-preserving alternatives.

51.3.1 Hemiresurfacing: The Forgotten Procedure

51.3.1.1 Rationale for Hemiresurfacing

In the 1980s, the high failure rates of metal-on-polyethylene resurfacings [35] and THR [36] in young patients with Ficat stage III or early stage IV ON prompted the use of hemiresurfacing (resurfacing of the femoral head only) in cases where the acetabular cartilage damage was not severe. The absence of bearing material in hemiresurfacing eliminates failures associated with wear products [37]. Consequently, loosening of the device is extremely rare, and the only anticipated adverse outcome is the inevitable acetabular cartilage wear over time.

51.3.1.2 Indications for Hemiresurfacing

Hemiresurfacing is a bone-preserving and "time-buying" alternative to THA particularly suited for very young patients with Ficat stage II or III osteonecrosis of the femoral head and occasionally for a very young patient with early stage IV (but minimal acetabular cartilage changes). This method should be considered as part of a lifetime treatment plan for young patients despite the potentially better initial performance of full resurfacing or conventional total hip arthroplasty. Very young patients are likely to need revision surgery no matter what prosthetic solution is opted for, but hemiresurfacing is the only one to delay the insertion of an acetabular component and an artificial bearing susceptible to release wear particles.

The indications include young patients (now generally less than 25 year) with Ficat II or III who have normal, grade I or no more than grade II cartilage changes (absence of any full thickness cartilage loss) [38]. We do include hips with "whole head" lesions, which, after subsequent debridement, retain at least some circumferential cylindrically reamed portion of the head. Bone preparation and cement technique (including cementing the metaphyseal stem in components that feature one) are critical. From our experience, hemiresurfacing is not indicated in heavy patients (BMI>30), workman's compensation cases, or those who must work standing and walking on hard cement floors. Our early unsatisfactory results with these patients are the justification for such exclusion criteria.

51.3.1.3 Methods and Materials

Patient Demographics

Our first 54 hips in 46 patients underwent hemiresurfacing for osteonecrosis of the femoral head between 1981 and 2004 and have been followed a minimum of 8 years. Risk factors for the development of ON were diverse in this group and distributed as follows:

Steroids 24 (45 %)
Alcohol 11 (20 %)
Trauma 13 (24 %)
No dominant risk factor (idiopathic ON) 4 (7 %)
Gaucher's disease 2 (4 %)

There were 4 hips rated Ficat stage II, 44 hips rated Ficat stage III, and 4 hips rated early Ficat stage IV. The average age of the patients was 34.2 (range, 18–51). Thirty-four patients were male (74 %) and 12 were female (26 %).

Table 51.1 Demographics of the patients operated with hemiresurfacing secondary to osteonecrosis

	Male and female combined
Age (years)	34.2 (18–51)
Weight (kg)	74.6 (40–120)
Femoral component size (mm)	49.2 (40–54)
Charnley class	
A	17 (37 %)
B	22 (48 %)
C	7 (15 %)

Twenty-three patients had bilateral disease (50 %), among which 8 were treated with bilateral hemiresurfacing (5 one-stage and 3 two-stage procedures). Six hips (11 %) had undergone at least one previous surgery including 3 core decompressions, 1 Bonfiglio graft, and 2 free vascularized fibular grafts (in one patient) [21]. At last follow-up, 6 patients had died of causes unrelated to the surgery. The demographics of our cohort of patients treated with hemiresurfacing are summarized in Table 51.1.

In our series, three different materials were used to replace the femoral head: titanium (11 hips), alumina ceramic (11 hips), and cobalt-chromium (32 hips). The titanium and alumina components were custom-made by Zimmer Inc. (Warsaw, IN) and Kinamed Inc. (Newbury Park, CA), respectively. Two of the CoCr components were femoral shells from THARIES hip resurfacing systems (Zimmer Inc., Warsaw, IN), while the remaining 30 were Conserve® femoral resurfacing components (Wright Medical Technology Inc., Arlington, TN). All components were cemented with the exception of one alumina component that was press fit. A posterior approach was used in the last 37 hips, while the first 17 were resurfaced through a posterolateral approach with a trochanteric osteotomy. The details of the surgical technique used have been previously described [39–41], but it is useful to emphasize the need to completely remove the necrotic bone from the reamed femoral head in order to limit the bone-cement interface to vascularized bone only.

51.3.1.4 Results of Hemiresurfacing

Clinical Scores

The average UCLA hip scores all improved significantly ($p<0.001$) between preoperative and last follow-up visits. The pain score increased from 4.8 ± 1.8 to 8.4 ± 1.7, the walking score from 5.8 ± 1.8 to 8.9 ± 1.4, the function score from 5.2 ± 1.6 to 7.9 ± 2.0, and the activity score from 4.2 ± 1.3 to 5.9 ± 1.3. The mean postoperative Harris hip score was 82.3 ± 12.4 (range, 54–100). In this series 13 patients (13 hips, 24 %) reported incomplete pain relief (highest UCLA pain score of 7 or less). We found a weak but significant negative correlation in male patients between weight at the time of surgery and the maximum UCLA pain score reported during the follow-up period ($r=-0.38$, $p=0.022$). Patients weighing 77 kg or less had a mean pain score of 9.0 (range, 5–10) while patients heavier than 77 kg had a mean score of 7.4 (range 5–10). This difference was significant ($p=0.006$).

Conversions and Survivorship

Twenty-nine hips have now been revised in this series at a mean time of 100.8 months (range, 3–278 months) most for cartilage wear [27]. There was one each revised for sepsis and enigmatic pain at 3 and 12 months. Most failed hemiresurfacing procedures were revised to conventional stem-type total hip replacements with 4 exceptions: Two hips (2 patients) with ceramic hemiresurfacing components received a metal-on-metal hip resurfacing devices (Conserve®Plus, Wright Medical technology Inc., Arlington, TN) after removal of the alumina femoral component, one hip with a CoCr femoral component had a custom cross-linked PE liner cemented on the acetabular side now 10 years post-op, and one hip with a super finished CoCr component (the current Conserve®Plus device, available in 2 mm increments) was converted to a metal-on-metal resurfacing by inserting the Conserve®Plus porous-coated monoblock acetabular component of the corresponding size. The overall Kaplan-Meier survivorship of this series was 79.3 % (95 % confidence interval 65–88 %) at 5 years, 56.4 % (95 % CI 39–70 %) at 10 years, and 26.3 % (95 % CI 12–43 %) at 15 years. The comparative survivorship curves generated by type of material used revealed no significant difference in favor of any of the materials (logrank test $p=0.6628$) as shown in Fig. 51.1. We found no association between survivorship and the following variables: gender, age at surgery, Ficat stage, acetabular cartilage grading, component size, and patient weight at the time of surgery.

51.3.1.5 Discussion

The clinical scores showed considerable variability, and this result has also been observed by others [42]. Some patients often report incomplete pain relief during the first few months after the procedure but this typically abates over time due to "accommodation" although these patients rarely become as pain free as those receiving a full replacement. When the acetabular cartilage finally wears out, pain may reappear. However, the longest survivor is a woman with SLE who is now 31 years post-op with no increase in symptoms. Although her joint space has somewhat narrowed, the patient's UCLA hip scores remain high with 9, 7, 8, and 6 for pain, walking, function and activity, respectively. Weight appears to be related to the magnitude of pain relief, and this was observed particularly in our male patients. Our current recommendation is to reserve this procedure to lighter patients, in particular if the acetabular cartilage has already been somewhat compromised. However, the difficulty to predict the postoperative clinical scores requires that the

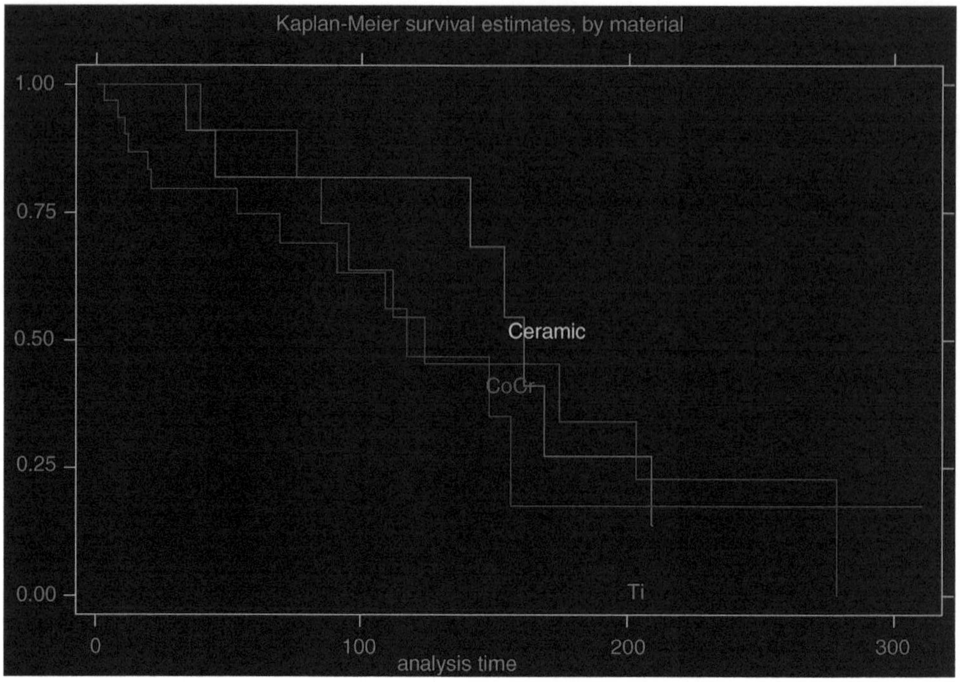

Fig. 51.1 Comparative Kaplan-Meier survivorship curve by femoral head material used in hemiresurfacing procedures between 1981 and 2004. There was no significant superiority of any material (logrank test $p=0.6628$)

patient understands the benefit of delaying the implantation of an artificial bearing material. Seven of our patients have been implanted with a hemiresurfacing on one side and a full resurfacing on the contralateral side. Five of these hemiresurfacing have been revised at a mean follow-up time of 59.6 months (range, 11–109) which is less than the mean 100 months of all the revised hips. A possible explanation is that the patients who can compare the hemiresurfacing side with another prosthetic joint are more likely to request a revision because the pain relief is not as good on the hemiresurfacing side.

The survivorship of hemiresurfacing does not match that of other prosthetic treatments (i.e., full resurfacing or conventional THA) but fits within acceptable ranges for a "time-buying" procedure with extremely low morbidity destined to restore the patient's lifestyle without compromising bone stock in anticipation of an inevitable revision surgery. It was our belief that hard bearing surfaces such as cobalt-chromium or alumina would reduce the friction against the acetabular cartilage and eliminate the metallic debris possibly generated by the relatively soft titanium alloy component (our first hemiresurfacing device). Our comparative survivorship results show that femoral head material has no effect on the durability of the procedure. The advantage of the ceramic is that it can be cracked and removed without loss of bone, and full resurfacing has been successful in 2 patients for over 15 years after such revision. Unfortunately, ceramic components are not now available but would be my choice if still available. With our relatively small series, there has not been an association between survivorship gender, age, or Ficat stage, acetabular cartilage grading, component size, or patient weight, and this illustrates the difficulty to profile the ideal candidate for the procedure. We do believe that the long-term survival of some of these prostheses had to do with how precisely these implants were fitted to the acetabular cartilage in patients with relatively low activity levels.

When reoperation was needed, revision to either full surface or total hip replacement was easy and much like a primary replacement because of bone stock preservation, because of intact intramedullary canals, and because there was no debris-induced granuloma. It is important to note that a regular radiographic follow-up of the patients with hemiresurfacing devices is needed because once the acetabular cartilage is worn, a rapid migration of the femoral head through the acetabulum can occur, leading to bone loss and therefore negating one of the main advantages of hemiresurfacing. The histological response has been very benign with a few macrophages and some metallic debris scattered throughout a predominantly loose connective tissue despite significant burnishing of some titanium alloy components.

At the beginning of the series, in 1981, our indications for hemiresurfacing included patients in their 40s or even 50s or with advanced cartilage defects because there was no alternate conservative prosthetic solution available with demonstrated potential for durability. However, because of the recent success of our metal-on-metal resurfacing series for osteonecrosis [43–45], our indications for hemiresurfacing have narrowed to very young with a well-preserved joint space. We do not include heavy patients anymore, considering that the results of full hip resurfacing are excellent in this patient population [46]. In addition, hemiresurfacing components once available in 1 mm increments for

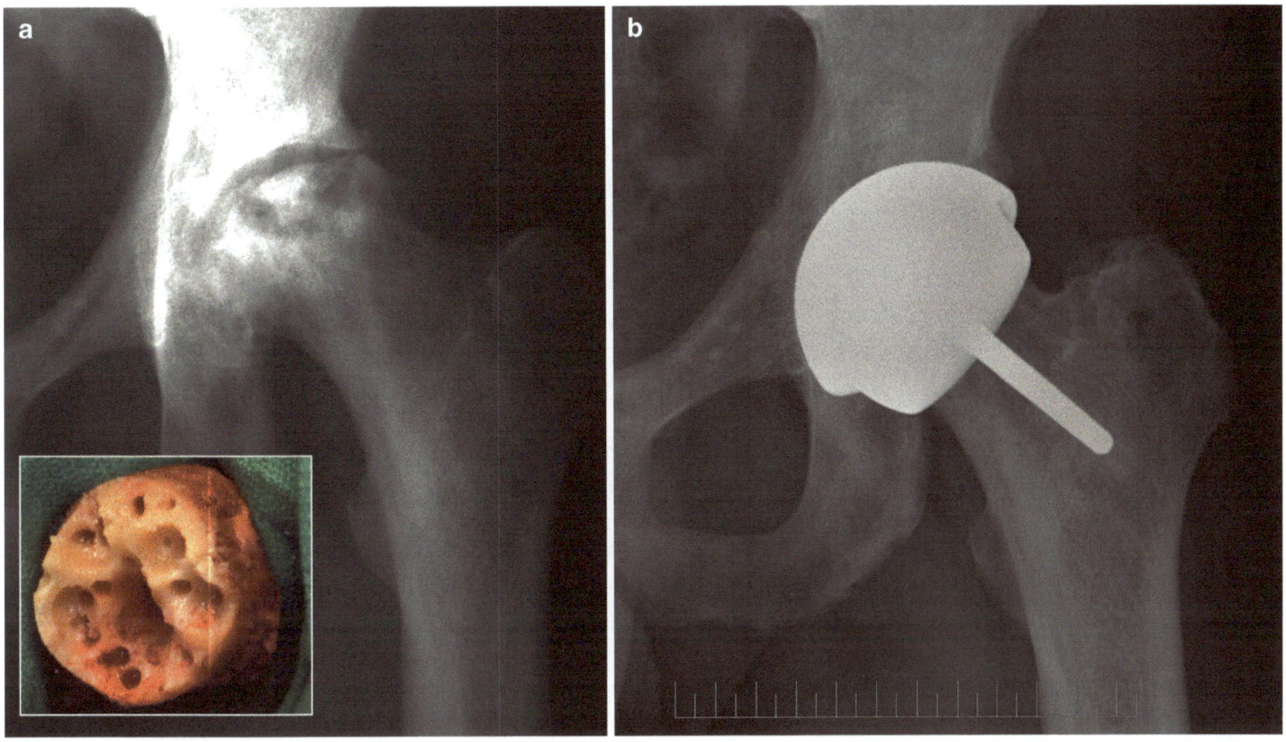

Fig. 51.2 (**a**) Anteroposterior radiograph of a 46-year-old bus driver with a history of sickle cell disease and Ficat stage IV osteonecrosis of the left hip. The femoral head defects were extensive as shown on the intraoperative photograph of the femoral head after preparation (inset). (**b**) Twelve years after surgery, the components show perfect interfaces with the bone, and the patient's UCLA hip scores are 10, 10, 10, and 8 for pain, walking, function, and activity, respectively

optimal precision fitting to the acetabulum are now only manufactured in 2 mm increments because of cost-efficiency concerns. However, they are finished so that an acetabular component can be inserted, provided there is enough acetabular bone stock.

51.3.1.6 Summary for Hemiresurfacing

From our experience and that of others, we can conclude that it is unrealistic to expect a pain relief and survivorship results comparable to that of full resurfacing or conventional THA in every case. The patients who could benefit from hemiresurfacing are very young and should be fully informed and accept the "time-buying" objectives before undergoing surgery. A surprisingly long durability has been demonstrated in some patients, which may have been favored by low activity levels without participation in sports.

51.3.2 Full Hip Resurfacing

51.3.2.1 Rationale for Full Hip Resurfacing

Primary hip replacement surgery is such a successful procedure that the percent of young patients seeking this type of treatment is increasing every year worldwide [47]. Although the durability has been impressive for some patients, conversion to THR may still be necessary for others. However, full hip resurfacing is a bone-conserving procedure that will provide complete pain relief and preserve both bone quality [48, 49] and quantity [50] for an eventual revision surgery.

51.3.2.2 Indications for Full Hip Resurfacing

Full hip resurfacing should be considered in patients about 25 years of age or over with Ficat III ON or younger with advanced Ficat III or IV ON with extensive cartilage damage. A recent publication showed that the size of the lesion does not alter the survivorship results of hip resurfacing [51] even though previous work with finite element analysis predicted adverse biomechanical effects after resurfacing in presence of large femoral defects [52]. In our series, decision was made from the beginning to include very large lesions as long as most of the cylindrically reamed bone was intact circumferentially. Figure 51.2 shows an example of large defects associated with longstanding osteonecrosis of the femoral head in a patient who received a Conserve®Plus hip resurfacing device.

51.3.2.3 Methods and Materials

Patient Demographics

From our series of 1,366 hips (1,097 patients), 100 hips (82 patients) received a Conserve®Plus hip resurfacing system

Table 51.2a Demographics of the patients operated with full resurfacing for arthritis secondary to osteonecrosis

	Male and female combined
Age (years)	41.2 (14–64)
Weight (kg)	81.9 (46–116)
Femoral component size (mm)	46.7 (36–54)
Cysts >1 cm	85 (85 %)
Charnley class	
A	42 (51 %)
B	33 (40 %)
C	7 (9 %)

Table 51.2b Distribution of hip bone quality by femoral defect size

	n	% of hips
Good bone – no defect	6	6 %
Defects 0–1 cm	9	9 %
Defects 1–2 cm	42	42 %
Defects 2–3 cm	43	43 %

(Wright medical Technology, Inc.) for a diagnosis of arthritis secondary to osteonecrosis of the femoral head. The risk factors for the development of ON were distributed as follows:

Steroids 34 (34 %)
Trauma 23 (23 %)
Alcohol 7 (7 %)
Sickle cell disease 1 (1 %)
No dominant risk factor (idiopathic ON) 35 (35 %)

There were 22 hips rated ON Ficat stage III and 78 rated Ficat stage IV.

The average age of the patients was 41.2 (range, 14–64). Most of the patients were male (67/82, 81.2 %).

From this cohort, 36 patients had bilateral disease (44 %). However, excluding the 23 patients with post-trauma (all unilateral), the incidence of bilaterality was 61 %. There were 4 patients with a contralateral hemiresurfacing, 18 with bilateral full metal-on-metal resurfacing (one of them with one device from another manufacturer), 3 with a contralateral conventional THR, and 7 with a contralateral core decompression. Thirty-six hips (36 %) had undergone at least one previous surgery: 21 had a core decompression, 3 had a hemiresurfacing, 9 had been pinned, 2 had previous free vascularized fibula graft, and 1 had a Judet graft.

The demographics of this group of patients are shown in Tables 51.2a and 51.2b.

The percentage of large defects was the highest of any etiologic group undergoing metal-on-metal hip resurfacing with only 15 % having none or a defect size of 1 cm or less.

51.3.2.4 Surgical Technique

The surgical technique used in this series for preparation of the femoral head is quite similar to our current technique for hemiresurfacing and has been described in detail in a previous publication [45]. In this series, 55 hips (55 %) were implanted with the femoral metaphyseal stem cemented [53].

51.3.2.5 Results of Full Hip Resurfacing

Clinical Scores

The average UCLA hip scores all improved significantly ($p<0.0001$) between preoperative and last follow-up visits. The pain score increased from 3.6 ± 1.5 to 9.3 ± 1.1, the walking score from 5.8 ± 1.6 to 9.5 ± 1.1, the function score from 5.3 ± 1.6 to 9.3 ± 1.4, and the activity score from 4.2 ± 1.4 to 7.0 ± 1.6. The postoperative Harris hip score was 91.9 ± 11.3.

51.3.2.6 Conversions to THR and Survivorship

There were four conversions to THR in this series. Three were consecutive to a loosening of the femoral component at 23, 61, and 85 months (hips #6, #25, and #455) and one secondary to a loosening of the acetabular component at 56 months.

In addition, one patient with poor bone quality who underwent one-stage bilateral procedures required a revision of the acetabular component after this one protruded through the acetabular wall 3 days after surgery. This complication was attributed to over-reaming with new very sharp "bear claw" reamers on the first side of a bilateral simultaneous hip resurfacing.

Using any cause for revision as end point, the Kaplan-Meier survivorship results for this group of patients were the following (Fig. 51.3):

5 years: 96.6 % (95 % confidence interval 90–99 %)
10 years: 93.6 % (95 % CI 85–97 %)

We also computed the Kaplan-Meier survivorship results for this group of patients using femoral failure only as end point. This analysis yielded a 98.9 % survivorship at 5 years (95 % CI 92–100 %) and a 95.8 % survivorship at 10 years (95 % CI 87–99 %).

51.3.2.7 Discussion

From the results shown above, it is safe to say that the etiology of osteonecrosis is a good indication for hip resurfacing when performed with optimal technique. Both survivorship and clinical scores match those obtained with idiopathic osteoarthritis [43, 54] and other etiologies [45]. Our survivorship results even surpass those of conventional THR for osteonecrosis listed in the 2012 Australian National registry report (AOANJRR) which shows a 91.8 % survival at 10 years [55]. Two aseptic femoral component loosenings occurred in hips that were implanted with our early surgical technique, before the use of suction, and additional drill holes was implemented [56]. Two hips show radiolucencies around the metaphyseal stem but these have been stable and asymptomatic for over 11 years. There has been no femoral component loosening in the 55 hips with a cemented metaphyseal stem. Since 2005, several studies have suggested that

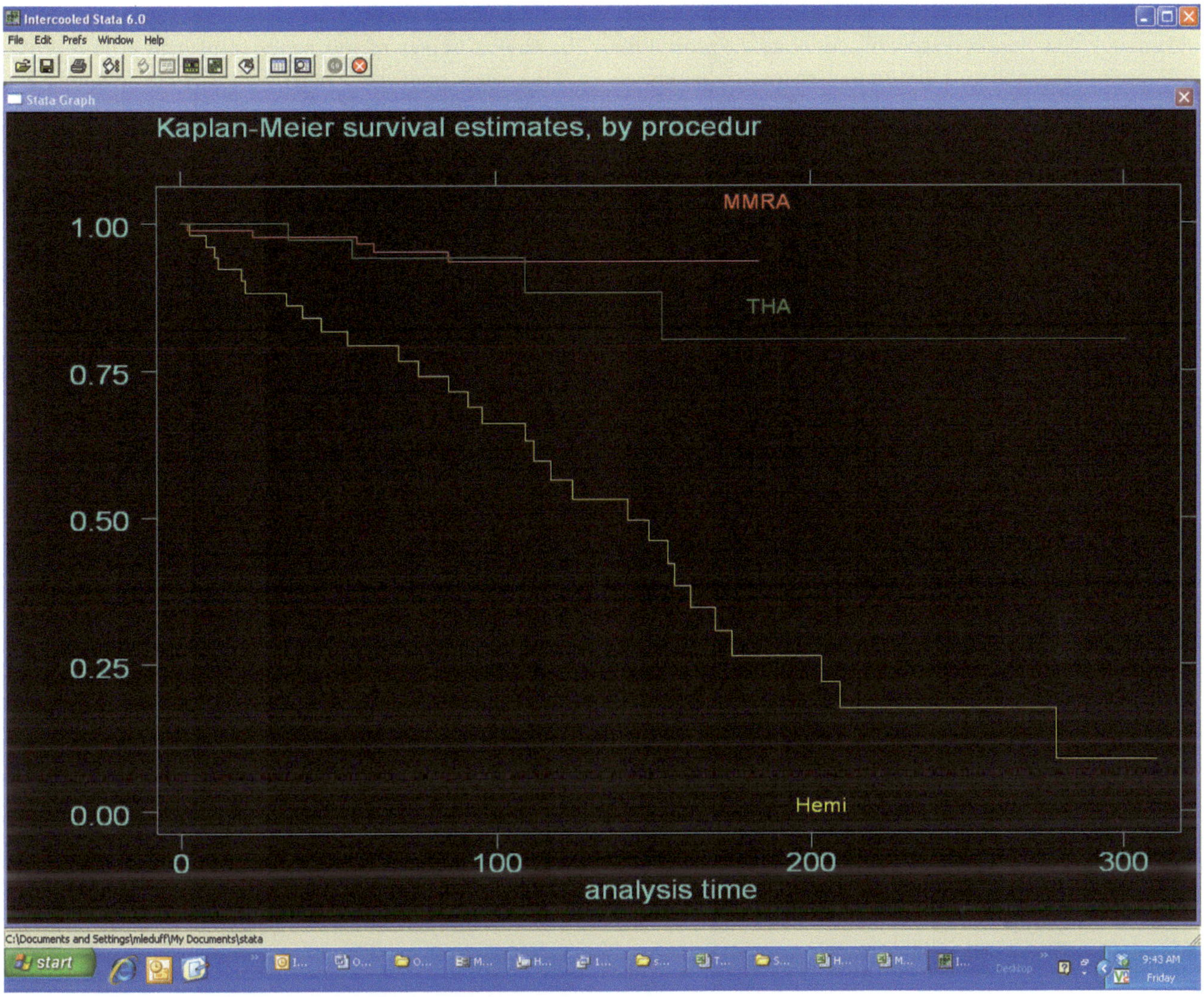

Fig. 51.3 Comparative Kaplan-Meier survivorship curve by procedure used in the treatment of patients with hip osteonecrosis between 1981 and 2012. There was no significant difference between MMRA and THA (logrank test $p = 0.3707$) while both MMRA and THA were more durable than hemiresurfacing (logrank test $p = 0.0001$)

hip resurfacing may be a viable option for patients with femoral head osteonecrosis but none has offered long-term results to this day [43, 44, 57–59]. In the present report, follow-up time ranged from 1 month to 16 years, providing meaningful Kaplan-Meier survival estimates at 10 years.

The question of how much femoral head involvement can be accepted for a resurfacing procedure remains, and both Mont and Revell suggested <33 % of the head as a guideline. Our results confirm with long-term follow-up those of Nakasone [51] and suggest that the extent of femoral head defects should not be a limitation as long as the procedure remains technically possible and the biomechanics of the reconstructed hip are sound.

Summary

Osteonecrosis of the hip presents specific challenges when performing hip resurfacing because of the large defects often present and filled with yellowish, friable necrotic bone. This necrotic bone must be completely removed down to the underlying white hard reparative bone to ensure proper component fixation and durability. Cementing the metaphyseal stem maximizes the fixation area. Our results with the Conserve®Plus device highlight that hip resurfacing should be the treatment of choice for young patients up to the age of 65 with Ficat stage III and IV osteonecrosis.

51.3.3 Conventional Total Hip Arthroplasty

51.3.3.1 Rationale for THA

Conventional (stem type) THA has been the gold standard for the treatment of hip osteonecrosis because of an established reliability in pain relief and longevity. However, we believe that THA should only be performed in patients old enough that there is reasonable certainty the procedure will outlast the patient's lifetime. Because revisions of conventional THA are often technically difficult, have poor survivorship (83.8 % at 5 years) [55], and are associated with an increased complication rate compared with primary surgeries, it is our strong belief that THA is better reserved as the last element of a lifetime treatment plan.

51.3.3.2 Indications for THA

In our center, recommendations for a primary THA have been made to patients with hip ON when hip resurfacing was not an option (either for technical reasons or limited insurance coverage) or when the patient was old enough that a conventional THA was likely to outlive the patient.

51.3.3.3 Methods and Materials

Patient Demographics

Between 1981 and 2004, 42 patients (47 hips) received a primary THA for the treatment of hip ON. The mean patient age at the time of surgery was 58.4 years (range, 20–83). The cohort consisted of 22 men and 20 women. At the time of review, 21 patients (25 hips) had died of causes unrelated to the surgery. The hips were reconstructed with a variety of implants combining 15 cementless and 32 cemented stems. The bearing materials used included high-density polyethylene (36 hips), cross-linked polyethylene (4 hips), and metal-on-metal (7 hips). The mean femoral head size was 31.2 mm (range, 28–54).

51.3.3.4 Results of THA

Clinical Scores

At last follow-up, the mean UCLA activity scores were 9.0 ± 1.5 for pain, 8.4 ± 1.9 for walking, 7.3 ± 2.4 for function, and 5.2 ± 1.4 for activity.

51.3.3.5 Conversions and Survivorship

Four hips (4 patients) underwent revision surgery at a mean time of 87.8 months (range, 34–152) in this cohort. The reasons for revisions included sepsis (1 hip – 34 months after surgery), wear of the polyethylene liner (1 hip – 109 months after surgery), and aseptic loosening (2 hips – one acetabular at 55 months and one femoral at 152 months).

The Kaplan-Meier survivorship was 94.2 % (95 % confidence interval 79–98 %) at 5 years, 88.3 % (95 % CI 66–96 %) at 10 years, and 80.3 % (95 % CI 52–93 %) at 15 years. These figures are certainly on the conservative side because of the large number of patients who died before 10 years of follow-up (15 hips in 13 patients), therefore lowering the survivorship value and increasing the width of the 95 % confidence interval.

51.3.3.6 Discussion

The clinical scores of this series of patients who received a THA show good pain relief and walking, function, and activity scores consistent with those of an older population. There is no doubt that the procedure was beneficial to all, especially considering that this group of patients was overall less demanding of the reconstruction than the typical young patient with Ficat II or IV ON. However, in this group, 4 patients (4 hips) underwent revision surgery, among which 2 had a subsequent re-revision. Considering that these 2 patients were relatively young (46 and 57 years of age at the time of primary surgery), one would wonder if these patients would not have better benefitted from a resurfacing as a primary operation.

51.4 Comparative Evaluation of the Three Prosthetic Solutions

This comparison is certainly limited in its applications because the three populations in which hemiresurfacing, full resurfacing, and THA were used differ significantly in terms of age and activity levels, reflecting the senior author's approach to the treatment of ON. However, we believe that it still presents some value for the surgeon trying to establish a treatment algorithm for the wide range of patients presenting with ON.

51.4.1 Clinical Scores

Pain scores were greater for MMRA compared with hemiresurfacing ($p=0.0003$) while we found no significant difference between MMRA and THA ($p=0.2288$) or hemiresurfacing and THA ($p=0.1119$).

Walking scores were greater for MMRA compared with both hemiresurfacing ($p=0.005$) and THA ($p=0.0001$) while there was no significant difference between hemiresurfacing and THA ($p=0.1516$).

Similarly, function scores were greater for MMRA compared with both hemiresurfacing ($p=0.0001$) and THA ($p=0.0001$) while there was no significant difference between hemiresurfacing and THA ($p=0.2081$).

Finally, activity scores were greater for MMRA compared with both hemiresurfacing ($p=0.0001$) and THA ($p=0.0001$) but also greater for hemiresurfacing compared with THA ($p=0.0175$).

Pain relief is clearly better for MMRA and THA as compared with hemiresurfacing, and this is unlikely to be the reflection of differences between the patient population. However, if walking, function, and activity scores were better in the MMRA group compared with the hemiresurfacing group, this could be interpreted as a consequence of the difference in pain relief while the difference in walking function and activity between MMRA and THA is likely an effect of the normal aging process.

51.4.2 Survivorship (Fig. 51.3)

The survivorship curve for hemiresurfacing showed significantly shorter times to revision compared with both MMRA (logrank test $p=0.0001$) and THA (logrank test $p=0.0001$). However, this is to be expected for this time-buying procedure which we now restrict to lighter patients in the under 25-year age group.

We found no significant difference in survivorship between MMRA and THA (logrank test $p=0.3707$).

51.4.3 Current Treatment Recommendations

Stage I: Observation if the hip is asymptomatic.
Stage II: If asymptomatic, continue with observation.
If symptomatic, the practical options are:
Core decompression. Multiple small core tracks [14] are less likely to weaken the head and lead to collapse.
Hemiresurfacing if patient <25 years of age and perfect fit can be achieved.
Stages III and IV:
Hemiresurfacing if patient <25 years of age with good cartilage and close to or perfect fit can be achieved (<1 mm difference in roundness of the prosthetic ball size to the acetabular cavity).
Full hip resurfacing.
Total hip arthroplasty for patients >65 years of age or in case of a total head necrosis that precludes performing hip resurfacing.

51.5 Surgical Technique for Hip Resurfacing Arthroplasty

The success of hip resurfacing arthroplasty in patients with advanced Ficat stages (III or IV) ON heavily relies on a careful application of surgical techniques. The challenge is essentially to utilize as much viable bone from the femoral head as possible instead of just resecting the entire problem area as in the implantation of a THR.

51.5.1 Templating

We use 20 % magnified templates which are placed over both the AP and Johnson lateral radiographs which have an approximate magnification comparable to an analog X-ray taken at a tube to cassette of 40 in. The template is oriented so that the metaphyseal stem forms approximately anatomical 135–140° angle with the femoral shaft on the AP radiograph. The 5-mm dotted lines help determine the optimal point of entry for the pin with respect to the ligamentum teres. The dotted lines which are parallel to the neck indicate how much bone the reamer will take away and how close the reamer will come to the external surface of the femoral neck. For patients with ON, careful templating allows to anticipate how much of the femoral head and neck will be available for component fixation after all the necrotic lesion has been removed.

51.5.2 Centering the Pin: A Key Step

The Conserve®Plus instrumentation provides two methods of insertion for the pin: one uses the pin-centering guide and the other the "lollipop." With the pin-centering guide, the angle finder is positioned so that the pin forms an angle which follows approximately the main axis of the femoral neck, and the entry point of the pin is consistent with the location determined by templating. A Steinman pin (3.2 mm) is then inserted 3–5 cm deep, using the guide to keep the determined alignment during insertion. With the lollipop guide pin system, a measurement of the neck width is made using a caliper or notch guide and the lollipop of appropriate size is selected. The device is then aligned and the head is marked with the electrocautery. The hip is then rotated 90° in the other plane and a similar mark is made.

After pin insertion, the cylindrical reamer gauge for the anticipated final femoral head size is used to check the positioning of the pin and that there is sufficient clearance around the neck to ensure that the femoral neck will not be notched during cylindrical reaming. Repositioning of the pin can be achieved if needed using the relocator guide. In patients with ON, relocating the pin is often necessary because preserving the viable bone takes precedence over following the predetermined orientation suggested by the template. To more accurately assess the final size the femoral component, use the ring gauge internal dimension. This will establish the final size of the component for hemiresurfacing, while in general the size may be smaller for the full resurfacing in order to save acetabular bone stock.

51.5.3 Cylindrical Reaming

An oversized reamer (2–3 sizes larger than the final anticipated size) is selected to debulk the femoral head, irrigating copiously to avoid seizing. Smaller reamers are then used similarly down to ~1 size greater than the final anticipated size from the template and verified size by the ring gauge measurement. Carefully avoid notching the superior neck. After this initial reaming, the remaining anterior capsule can be more easily excised which will facilitate the positioning of the femoral head into a muscle pocket superiorly and anteriorly (which is smaller than if the head had not been debulked) to provide wide access to the acetabulum (the leg is then extended and slightly internally rotated). If a full hip resurfacing is performed, then the acetabular cavity is prepared and the socket inserted.

51.5.3.1 Final Femoral Preparation

After implantation of the acetabular component, the femoral head is delivered again, the neck elevator repositioned, and the pin reinserted through the last cylindrical reamer used. A final check is useful before reaming to the final size. The location of the pin may be changed to optimize the final reaming and maximize surface area for fixation and offset. To minimize impingement, the pin may be moved superiorly to produce more lateral offset. After final reaming, the saw cutoff guide is positioned covering all the reamed bone at the head-neck junction and the resection of the dome performed with a saber or oscillating saw. The tower alignment guide is positioned flush with the top of the cutoff guide. A starter drill is selected to make the final hole for the tapered metaphyseal stem based on the chosen method of stem fixation: one or two sizes deeper if the stem is to be cemented and one size under if press fit. A chamfer guide of the corresponding size is then inserted into the drilled hole and the final shape of the femoral head obtained with the chamfer reamer. An "eye" vidrape can be placed over the head prior to chamfer reaming to collect bone debris.

The femoral head trial is used for a final check of the femoral head shape and should rotate freely to leave room for a 1 mm cement mantle. All cystic material and soft tissue should be curetted out and burred, and additional fixation holes made in both the dome and the nonporous chamfered areas. This is the most important phase for patients with ON of the femoral head because ALL yellowish necrotic bone needs to be removed to provide a sound and vascular basis for the cementing of the femoral component. Multiple drill 1/8 in. (~3 mm) holes are placed in the dome and chamfered areas. For the hard and relatively avascular areas, the holes should be drilled into areas of bleeding bone. Short 2–3 mm holes should be drilled into the base of cystic areas.

51.5.4 Femoral Head Cementation

After jet lavage and irrigation with duo-biotic, a suction tip is then inserted through the stem hole. A second suction is inserted in the lesser trochanter. The bone-cement interface needs to be clean and dry at the time the cement is applied, until it has cured. A CO_2 blow-dry carbo-jet™ (Kinamed Inc., Camarillo, CA) is useful to dry the field and to identify any tissue which would prevent intimate contact of the cement to bone. A small amount of bone cement (Surgical Simplex P, Howmedica Inc., Rutherford, NJ) in the liquid state is poured into the femoral component and smeared to provide a thin layer to cover all of the metal. When the acrylic reaches the doughy stage, it is hand-pressurized into the cylindrical portion of the head. Additional cement is hand-pressurized down the central hole if the stem is to be cemented. The femoral component is inserted until complete seating and pressure maintained until the cement has set. Excess cement should be trimmed carefully so that acrylic is not pulled out from the interface.

2,000–3,000 cc of saline and 1,000 cc of antibiotic solution are used for a final irrigation. This phase is important as it contributes to maintain the temperature low under the femoral component and prevent possible thermal necrosis.

Currently, our recommendation for the acetabular component is the new Biofoam® socket (Wright Medical Technology Inc., Arlington, TN) which features a uniform head coverage >166° across all sizes to avoid any wear issues so long as they are implanted with an angle of abduction of 42° ± 10° and anteversion of 15° ± 10°. The technique of reaming and impaction should be followed carefully to provide enough stability to ensure long-lasting durability [60].

References

1. Hungerford D. Treatment of ischemic necrosis of the femoral head. In: Evarts C, editor. Surgery of the musculoskeletal system. New York: Churchill Livingstone; 1983. p. 5.
2. Taylor L. Multifocal avascular necrosis after short-term high-dose steroid therapy. A report of three cases. J Bone Joint Surg Br. 1984;66(3):431–3.
3. Ficat R. Treatment of avascular necrosis of the femoral head. Hip. 1983:279–95.
4. Hauzeur J, Pasteels J, Orloff S. Bilateral non-traumatic aseptic osteonecrosis in the femoral head. An experimental study of incidence. J Bone Joint Surg Am. 1987;69(8):1221–5.
5. Merle D'Aubigné R, Postel M, Mazabraud A, Massias P, Gueguen J, France P. Idiopathic necrosis of the femoral head in adults. J Bone Joint Surg Br. 1965;47(4):612–33.
6. Hedley A, Kim W. Prosthetic replacement in osteonecrosis of the hip. Instr Course Lect. 1983;32:265–71.
7. Ficat R, Arlet J. Ischaemia and necrosis of bone. Baltimore: Williams & Watkins; 1980.
8. Ficat RP. Idiopathic bone necrosis of the femoral head. Early diagnosis and treatment. J Bone Joint Surg Br. 1985;67(1):3–9.
9. Marcus N, Enneking W, Massam R. The silent hip in idiopathic aseptic necrosis. Treatment by bone-grafting. J Bone Joint Surg Am. 1973;55(7):1351–66.
10. Steinberg M, Hayken G, Steinberg D. A new method for evaluating and staging of avascular necrosis of the femoral head. In: Arlet J, Ficat R, Hungerford D, editors. Proceedings of the third international symposium on circulation in bone, Toulouse, France. Baltimore: Williams & Watkins; 1982.

11. Rajagopal M, Balch Samora J, Ellis T. Efficacy of core decompression as treatment for osteonecrosis of the hip: a systematic review. Hip Int. 2012;22(5):489–93.
12. Bozic K, Zurakowski D, Thornhill T. Survivorship analysis of hips treated with core decompression for nontraumatic osteonecrosis of the femoral head. J Bone Joint Surg Am. 1999;81(2):200–9.
13. Lavernia C, Sierra R. Core decompression in atraumatic osteonecrosis of the hip. J Arthroplasty. 2000;15(2):171–8.
14. Marker D, Seyler T, Ulrich S, Srivastava S, Mont M. Do modern techniques improve core decompression outcomes for hip osteonecrosis? Clin Orthop Relat Res. 2008;466(5):1093–103.
15. Urbaniak JR, Coogan PG, Gunneson EB, Nunley JA. Treatment of osteonecrosis of the femoral head with free vascularized fibular grafting. J Bone Joint Surg Am. 1995;77A(5):681–94.
16. Sotereanos D, Plakseychuk A, Rubash H. Free vascularized fibula grafting for the treatment of osteonecrosis of the femoral head. Clin Orthop Relat Res. 1997;344:243–56.
17. Beaulé PE, Amstutz HC. Management of ficat stage III and IV osteonecrosis of the hip. J Am Acad Orthop Surg. 2004;12:96–105.
18. Marciniak D, Furey C, Shaffer J. Osteonecrosis of the femoral head. A study of 101 hips treated with vascularized fibular grafting. J Bone Joint Surg Am. 2005;87(4):742–7.
19. Aluisio F, Urbaniak J. Proximal femur fractures after free vascularized fibular grafting to the hip. Clin Orthop Relat Res. 1998;356:192–201.
20. Davis E, McKee M, Waddell J, Hupel T, Schemitsch E. Total hip arthroplasty following failure of free vascularized fibular graft. J Bone Joint Surg Am. 2006;88 Suppl 3:110–5.
21. Beaulé P, Le Duff M, Amstutz H. Hemiresurfacing arthroplasty of the hip for failed free-vascularized fibular graft. J Arthroplasty. 2003;18(6):519–23.
22. Eward W, Rineer C, Urbaniak J, Richard M, Ruch D. The vascularized fibular graft in precollapse osteonecrosis: is long-term hip preservation possible? Clin Orthop Relat Res. 2012;470(10):2819–26.
23. Veillette C, Mehdian H, Schemitsch E, McKee M. Survivorship analysis and radiographic outcome following tantalum rod insertion for osteonecrosis of the femoral head. J Bone Joint Surg Am. 2006;88 Suppl 3:48–55.
24. Shuler M, Rooks M, Roberson J. Porous tantalum implant in early osteonecrosis of the hip: preliminary report on operative, survival, and outcomes results. J Arthroplasty. 2007;22(1):26–31.
25. Tsao A, Roberson J, Christie M, Dore D, Heck D, Robertson D, et al. Biomechanical and clinical evaluations of a porous tantalum implant for the treatment of early-stage osteonecrosis. J Bone Joint Surg Am. 2005;87 Suppl 2:22–7.
26. Floerkemeier T, Thorey F, Daentzer D, Lerch M, Klages P, Windhagen H, et al. Clinical and radiological outcome of the treatment of osteonecrosis of the femoral head using the osteonecrosis intervention implant. Int Orthop. 2011;35(4):489–95.
27. Fung D, Frey S, Menkowitz M, Mark A. Subtrochanteric fracture in a patient with trabecular metal osteonecrosis intervention implant. Orthopedics. 2008;31(6):614.
28. Stronach B, Duke J, Rozensweig S, Stewart R. Subtrochanteric femur fracture after core decompression and placement of a tantalum strut for osteonecrosis of the femoral head. J Arthroplasty. 2010;25(7):1168.e5–7.
29. Zimmer I. Trabecular metal osteonecrosis intervention implant-removal instruments – surgical technique. 2007. Accessed 31 Jan 13.
30. Owens J, Ely E, Guilliani N, Suarez J, Patel P. Removal of trabecular metal osteonecrosis intervention implant and conversion to primary total hip arthroplasty. J Arthroplasty. 2012;27(6):1251–3.
31. Mont M, Einhorn T, Sponseller P, Hungerford D. The trapdoor procedure using autogenous cortical and cancellous bone grafts for osteonecrosis of the femoral head. J Bone Joint Surg Br. 1998;80-B(1):56–62.
32. Rosenwasser M, Garino J, Kiernan H, Michelsen C. Long term followup of thorough debridement and cancellous bone grafting of the femoral head for avascular necrosis. Clin Orthop Relat Res. 1994;306:17–27.
33. Yuhan C, Hu C, Chen D, Ueng S, Shih C, Lee M. Local cancellous bone grafting for osteonecrosis of the femoral head. Surg Innov. 2009;16(1):63–7.
34. Mont M, Etienne G, Ragland P. Outcome of nonvascularized bone grafting for osteonecrosis of the femoral head. Clin Orthop Relat Res. 2003;417:84–92.
35. Amstutz HC, Dorey F, O'Carroll PF. THARIES resurfacing arthroplasty. Evolution and long-term results. Clin Orthop. 1986;213:92–114.
36. Ortiguera C, Pulliam I, Cabanela M. Total hip arthroplasty for osteonecrosis. Matched-pair analysis of 188 hips with long-term follow-up. J Arthroplasty. 1999;14(1):21–8.
37. Schmalzried TP, Noordin S, Zahiri CA, Sarkany A, Campbell PA, Amstutz HC, editors. The critical difference in hemi-surface replacement vs. total hip resurfacing: absence of a polyethylene acetabular component. 44th annual meeting of the Orthopaedic Research Society, New Orleans, 16–19 Mar 1998.
38. Beaulé P, Schmalzried T, Campbell P, Dorey F, Amstutz H. Duration of symptoms and outcome of hemiresurfacing for hip osteonecrosis. Clin Orthop. 2001;385:104–17.
39. Amstutz H, Le Duff M. Current status of hemi-resurfacing arthroplasty for osteonecrosis of the hip. A 27-year experience. Orthop Clin North Am. 2009;40(2):275–82.
40. Beaulé P, Amstutz H. Hemiresurfacing arthroplasty for osteonecrosis of the hip. Oper Tech Orthop. 2000;10(2):123–32.
41. Tooke SM, Amstutz HC, Delaunay C. Hemiresurfacing for femoral head osteonecrosis. J Arthroplasty. 1987;2(2):125–33.
42. Cuckler J, Moore K, Estrada L. Outcome of hemiresurfacing in osteonecrosis of the femoral head. Clin Orthop Relat Res. 2004;429:146–50.
43. Mont M, Seyler T, Marker D, Marulanda G, Delanois R. Use of metal-on-metal total hip resurfacing for the treatment of osteonecrosis of the femoral head. J Bone Joint Surg Am. 2006;88 Suppl 3:90–7.
44. Revell M, McBryde C, Bhatnagar S, Pynsent P, Treacy R. Metal-on-metal hip resurfacing in osteonecrosis of the femoral head. J Bone Joint Surg Am. 2006;88 Suppl 3:98–103.
45. Amstutz H, Le Duff M. Hip resurfacing results for osteonecrosis are as good as for other etiologies at 2- to 12-years. Clin Orthop. 2009;468(2):375–81.
46. Le Duff M, Amstutz H, Dorey F. Metal-on-metal hip resurfacing for obese patients. J Bone Joint Surg Am. 2007;89(12):2705–11.
47. Sahlgrenska University Hospital DoO. The Swedish National Hip Arthroplasty Register – annual report 2010. http://www.shpr.se/en/Publications/DocumentsReportsaspx. 2010. p. 1–107.
48. Cordingley R, Kohan L, Ben-Nissan B. What happens to femoral neck bone mineral density after hip resurfacing surgery? J Bone Joint Surg Br. 2010;92(12):1648–53.
49. Kishida Y, Sugano N, Nishii T, Miki H, Yamaguchi K, Yoshikawa H. Preservation of the bone mineral density of the femur after surface replacement of the hip. J Bone Joint Surg. 2004;86 B(3):185–9.
50. Su E, Sheehan M, Su S. Comparison of bone removed during total hip arthroplasty with a resurfacing or conventional femoral component a cadaveric study. J Arthroplasty Suppl. 2010;25(2):325–9.
51. Nakasone S, Takao M, Sakai T, Nishii T, Sugano N. Does the extent of osteonecrosis affect the survival of hip resurfacing? Clin Orthop Relat Res. 2013;471(6):1926–34.
52. Sakagoshi D, Kabata T, Umemoto Y, Sakamoto J, Tomita K. A mechanical analysis of femoral resurfacing implantation for osteonecrosis of the femoral head. J Arthroplasty. 2010;25(8):1282–9.

53. Amstutz H, Le Duff M. Cementing the metaphyseal stem in metal-on-metal resurfacing: when and why. Clin Orthop. 2009;467(1):79–83.
54. Madadi F, Eajazi A, Kazemi S, Aalami Harandi A, Madadi F, Sharifzadeh S. Total hip arthroplasty in advanced osteonecrosis: the short-term results by metal-on-metal hip resurfacing. Med Sci Monit. 2011;17(2):78–82.
55. Australian Orthopaedic Association National Joint Replacement Registry [database on the Internet]. 2012. Available from: http://www.dmac.adelaide.edu.au/aoanjrr/documents/AnnualReports2011/AnnualReport_2011_WebVersion.pdf. Accessed 14 Feb 2013.
56. Amstutz H, Le Duff M, Campbell P, Dorey F. The effects of technique changes on aseptic loosening of the femoral component in hip resurfacing. Results of 600 conserve plus with a 3–9 year follow-up. J Arthroplasty. 2007;22(4):481–9.
57. Aulakh T, Rao C, Kuiper J, Richardson J. Hip resurfacing and osteonecrosis: results from an independent hip resurfacing register. Arch Orthop Trauma Surg. 2010;130(7):841–5.
58. McMinn D, Daniel J, Pradhan C, Ziaee H. Avascular necrosis in the young patient: a trilogy of arthroplasty options. Orthopedics. 2005;28(9):945–7.
59. Sayeed S, Johnson A, Stroh D, Gross T, Mont M. Hip resurfacing in patients who have osteonecrosis and are 25 years or under. Clin Orthop Relat Res. 2011;469(6):1582–8.
60. Amstutz H, Le Duff M, Johnson A. Socket position determines hip resurfacing 10-year survivorship. Clin Orthop Relat Res. 2012;470(11):3127–33.

Resurfacing Arthroplasty for Osteonecrosis of the Femoral Head

52

Bernard N. Stulberg and Jayson D. Zadzilka

52.1 Introduction

Patients with osteonecrosis of the femoral head (ONFH) are often in their third to fifth decade of life. If their collapse is sufficiently advanced, or if they have failed preservative treatment, they become candidates for arthroplasty approaches to management. In our practice, if this is radiographically an obvious stage IV or V disease (University of Pennsylvania Classification) or have collapse demonstrated on CT (not MRI), they would fit into this category. As these patients are young, may be very active, and are likely to face more than one surgical intervention for the involved hip in their lifetime, less aggressive approaches to bone removal in arthroplasty, such as modern day resurfacing arthroplasty (RSTHA), may be appealing. This chapter will combine the literature's and authors' experience in evaluating the use of RSTHA for ONFH and provide guidance as to when this approach is likely to work predictably and when other options might prove more predictable. The authors will show this and other alternative approaches as a strategy for addressing long-term success in the young patient with ONFH.

52.2 Indications

ONFH is found in up to 14 % of those that undergo total hip arthroplasty (THA) for end-stage disease of the hip joint. This number includes those who experience ONFH late in life (where the etiology is often related to arteriolar compromise) and those who experience ONFH related to inflammatory arthropathy and corticosteroid usage. The patient population affected is likely to have diminished bone density and perhaps smaller head sizes, both characteristics that put them at greater risk for failure of RSTHA. As a general rule, both of these groups are best treated with standard THA approaches, whether cemented, hybrid, or uncemented arthroplasty. Thus, the majority of the population of ONFH patients who might be considered candidates for RSTHA will be young males with either alcohol-related (ETOH) or idiopathic ONFH. In addition, the current understanding of RSTHA in general suggests that males under age 65 with femoral head diameters ≥50 mm are likely to have the best outcomes of RSTHA [1] and are the preferred group of patients for whom this arthroplasty approach should be considered.

The above criteria represent the general indications for consideration for RSTHA as applied to the patient population that experiences ONFH. In addition, there will be disease-specific indications. For these indications, the etiology of the disease may play a role (as above) and the quantitative involvement and location of the lesion might play a role. Therefore, it is our belief that the surgeon should be selective about the population of the ONFH patient who becomes a candidate for RSTHA and should carefully classify the patients' femoral head involvement (using the modified Ficat, ARCO, or University of Pennsylvania classification system and consider adding the Japanese Orthopaedic Association's (JOA) classification of surface involvement), before choosing to use RSTHA as an arthroplasty choice. As a general rule, any lesion over 1 cm^3 suggests a level of involvement that is too large to provide sufficient bone support for the femoral head component. The surgeon should also be aware of the likelihood of periarticular osteopenia related to the inflammatory component of the hip with ONFH. This could affect acetabular component stabilization and perhaps the femoral head resurfacing component as well.

We do not believe there is a role for isolated resurfacing of the femoral head in early collapse disease, where the acetabulum has a normal radiographic appearance and perhaps a normal clinical appearance intraoperatively. There is sufficient literature (see below) to suggest that the histological

B.N. Stulberg (✉) • J.D. Zadzilka
Department of Orthopaedic Surgery, Orthopaedic and Rheumatologic Institute, Cleveland Clinic,
1730 W. 25th Street, Suite 4E, Cleveland, OH 44113, USA
e-mail: stulbeb@ccf.org; zadzilj@ccf.org

K.-H. Koo et al. (eds.), *Osteonecrosis*,
DOI 10.1007/978-3-642-35767-1_52, © Springer-Verlag Berlin Heidelberg 2014

abnormality of the acetabular cartilage is suspected [2, 3] and that the clinical performance of isolated femoral head resurfacing and hemiarthroplasty is less satisfactory than THA as it relates to short- and long-term outcomes.

52.3 Technical Aspects of Implantation

The technique for predictable resurfacing arthroplasty has been well documented in the literature, and the reader is referred to the references listed. It is appropriate to follow the guidelines of implantation of the device chosen and to be certain of the appropriate technical steps to ensure proper placement of the device. In addition, the surgical approach may influence the potential for damage to the blood supply of the femoral neck, and use of modified posterolateral approaches or an anterior approach is recommended [4–7].

Acetabular reaming and positioning must take into account the possibility of significant osteopenia of the acetabular bone bed, as well as the desire to be conservative in the removal of bone. On the femoral side, in addition to being careful to preserve the blood supply to the remaining femoral head and neck, reaming of the upper femur must be precise, and cysts or necrotic areas must be debrided. In a suitable candidate for resurfacing, the reaming process will likely remove most of the necrotic segment, and a small defect, less than 1 cm^3, may require particulate grafting, if any. If the lesion size remains greater than 1 cm^3, it is best to consider abandoning the procedure and proceed with THA. Amstutz however has had good success with his device in this subpopulation of patients with ONFH, with a technique that involves cementing the femoral stem [8]. Other devices might not perform well with this approach. He is an expert in this technique with a broad experience in performing it.

52.4 Results

52.4.1 General Comment

The published results of RSTHA for ONFH are mixed, with some experts suggesting that the failure rate in patients with ONFH is sufficiently greater than the OA patient of similar characteristics that an alternative approach should be used, while others remain enthusiastic about its role for this subpopulation of patients. Femoral head resurfacing, in isolation, has shown unsatisfactory results and has been abandoned as an alternative for the osteonecrosis (ON) patient in the USA.

52.4.2 Results of Resurfacing for ON

We have reported an initial and early experience with RSTHA for ONFH as a subset of the population initially studied as a requirement of premarket approval (PMA) process for a specific resurfacing device introduced in to the USA in 2007 [9]. One thousand one hundred and forty-eight patients were implanted with a third-generation metal-on-metal (MOM) hip resurfacing system as part of this US multicenter investigational device exemption (IDE) study. Of these, 116 subjects had a preoperative diagnosis of ON. As we had seen differences in component survival between those patients with a diagnosis of OA and those with a diagnosis "other than OA," we were concerned that the ON patient population might represent a very specific group with a high risk – despite the appeal of applying this treatment approach to the young male patient that is a portion of the population that experiences ON. It was our hypothesis that by comparing the OA group to the ON group (a subset of the non-OA group) the Kaplan-Meier survival estimates would be significantly lower for the ON group. That was not what we encountered, however, as the survival estimates were not significantly different (95.9 and 95.8 % at 24 months for OA and ON, respectively, $p=0.46$). Comparing the Ficat stages III and IV to the OA population (there were a few Ficat stage II hips) also did not show a significant difference in implant survival (95.9 % OA and 96.1 % ON III/IV at 24 months, $p=0.57$). We concluded that, at least in the short term, resurfacing arthroplasty appeared to be a reasonable option for patients with ON *if* judgments of implant size, patient gender, and size of femoral deficiency were taken into consideration. That population is not available to study at longer term. Required postmarket surveillance is available for only a limited number of this group, although we personally have experienced 3 late failures of RSTHA in 2 patients with bilateral hips: 1 due to femoral loosening and 2 late acetabular loosening (Figs. 52.1 and 52.2).

Several new reports have shed more light on the long-term behavior of RSTHA in the ON patient, although the results are conflicting. Gross and Liu [10] reviewed their findings in 122 hips with ON, matching them for surgical date, gender, size, and component type with 122 OA hips in

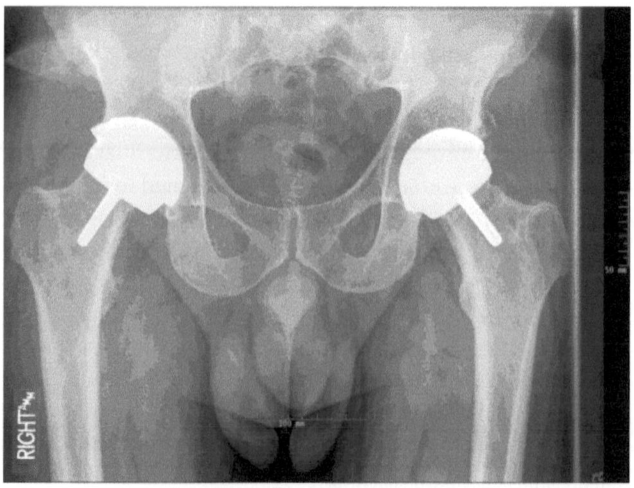

Fig. 52.1 Ten years post-RSTHA for ON on the *right side* (pre-revision)

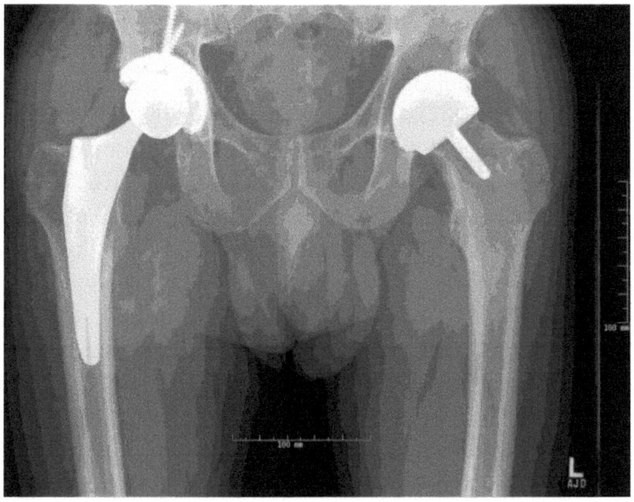

Fig. 52.2 Post-revision RSTHA for acetabular loosening on *right side*; 8 years post-RSTHA for ON on the *left side* doing well

their extensive database. Using revision for any reason as an endpoint, their survivorship rate at 10 years was 88 % for the ON hips and 100 % for the OA hips. They noted no failures when uncemented femoral components were used in the ON patients ($N=47$). They concluded that the ON patient might not be a suitable candidate for RSTHA.

Woon et al. [11] evaluated RSTHA in patients with diagnosis posttraumatic OA (PTOA) versus patients with posttraumatic ON (PTON – an ON population that may behave slightly differently than idiopathic ON, but of interest nonetheless). They report on 63 patients, 43 of whom had PTOA and 19 with PTON. At an average of 87.2 months follow-up, survival rates were 95 % at 8 years for the PTOA group and 91 % for the PTON group, not a statistically significant difference.

Several shorter-term follow-up reports from outside the USA report satisfactory outcomes for their patients using RSTHA for ON. Madadi et al. [12] retrospectively assessed outcomes for "end-stage ON" in 28 patients and compared them to 24 patients using RSTHA for OA. While there were differences in mean age between the populations (47.9 for OA population versus 30.9 for ON population), they found no differences in clinical and functional results as measured by Harris Hip Scores between the two groups at an average of 41 months follow-up. Bose and Baruah [13] reported on 96 RSTHA in 71 patients at mean follow-up of 5.4 years (4.0–8.1), with cumulative survival rate of 95.4 %. They do not provide a comparative study group, but do report the importance of optimum positioning and describe their neck-capsule-preserving modification of the posterolateral approach, raising the issue of surgical approach and technique to the discussion of success of RSTHA. He et al. [14] provide their experience in 37 patients (43 hips) for ARCO stage 3A, 3B, 3C, and 4 ON, with the ability to follow the results in 40/43 hips with mean follow-up of 32.4 months. They have no revisions at that time point (survival 100 %) with 37 excellent and 3 good results (Harris Hip Scores).

Large database assessments through joint registries have also been used to comment on the appropriateness of RSTHA for the ON patient. Corten and Macdonald [1] note that overall cumulative revision rates are higher at 5 years for RSTHA than THA (3.7 % versus 2.7 %) pointing out that the diagnoses "other than primary OA" bear a higher risk of early revision of RSTHA versus THA. Cuckler [15] notes a 7.2 % cumulative 9-year revision rate in the Australian registry, argues that rate, as well as other concerns of femoral neck erosion and metal-on-metal articulation complications, should encourage surgeons to use RSTHA with caution, and notes that "hip resurfacing is contraindicated in cases of avascular necrosis especially with cysts >1 cm in diameter."

In a unique article focusing on RSTHA for ONFH in patients under 25 years of age, Sayeed et al. [16] identified 17 patients with 20 RSTHA, with a mean follow-up of 62 months (range 32–103 months). They compared this group to a matched population of 16 patients (20 hips) with THA (mean follow-up 61 months) and 78 patients (87 hips) with RSTHA who were over the age of 25. They noted 100 % survivorship for the study population at 7.5 years, with a 93.3 % for the THA population at that same time interval, and a 94 % survival for the group of RSTHA over 25 years of age. They concluded that the results were similar for all three groups.

52.5 Revision of Resurfacing for ON

There are several issues of concern that relate to revision of RSTHA: the size of the necrotic defect, how it is addressed, and its effect on implant support; the blood supply to the femoral neck and the influence of surgical approach; the incidence of post-implantation ON and perhaps cementation approaches; and the results of revision of failed resurfacing.

52.5.1 Size of the Necrotic Defect

There are few studies that have predictably quantified the size of lesions in the series of patients studied. Most discussions refer to ">1 cm^3" as the defect size that is the limit beyond which RSTHA becomes inappropriate. Only 1 study has examined actual defect size before and after preparation of the femoral head for resurfacing [17]. In 33 patients with 39 hips they used three-dimensional MRI templating to estimate lesion size before and after machining and followed their patients for a mean of 8 years. According to their estimates, the mean percentage of ON in the bony bed was 5 % smaller after machining, and they found no difference in implant survival between small and large lesions. This led them to conclude that "neither the residual osteonecrosis volume… after femoral head machining nor the total amount of osteonecrosis before femoral head machining had significant influence on the survival of hip resurfacing." Similarly,

He et al. [14] noted no difference in short-term results when using a quantifiable staging system. Gross and Liu [18] evaluated 117/939 RSTHA that demonstrated femoral head cysts >1 cm at time of surgery. These were bone grafted using shavings from acetabular reamings (as opposed to filling with bone cement). They used a computer algorithm to compare results at a minimum of 24 months with those with no cysts identified at surgery. Early femoral failure was identified in 3/117 (2.6 %) versus 0/117 (0 %) in the control group, which was not statistically different. Two of three (2/3) failures were femoral neck fractures and 1/3 was a femoral component loosening. They suggest bone grafting as a possible approach to those femoral heads with cysts >1 cm^3. Amstutz [8] has recommended cementing the stem in patients with significant cyst formation/bone deficiency and has shown reasonable results of RSTHA using his device.

52.5.2 Femoral Head Blood Flow/ON

In the broader literature of RSTHA, there is concern regarding the influence of the surgical approach on the viability of the proximal femoral blood flow, and those would be pertinent to discussions relative to RSTHA for ON. However, histological evaluation of retrieved femoral heads at time of revision RSTHA suggests that ON itself is minimally involved in the loosening or failure process and that necrosis that is seen is most likely the result of upper femoral remodeling and accompanying loosening. This may not be the case for femoral neck fracture after RSTHA, as a recent report of 19 hips retrieved after fracture of the femoral head was compared with femoral heads retrieved at THA for OA and ON (controls) and for 13 retrieved RSTHA for other reasons. In the THA controls, 9 % of OA hips had empty osteocyte lacunae versus 85 % for ON hips, and the retrieved implants following fracture showed 71 % empty lacunae versus 21 % empty lacunae in those retrieved for other reasons ($p<0.001$). The authors believe that these findings indicate established ON related to compromised blood supply to the femoral neck, which they attribute to surgical trauma (surgical approach).

A recent article from Falez et al. [19] is an in vitro study suggesting that cement technique and cement type (high versus low viscosity) may be critical to failure – with polar concentration of cement – most commonly seen with low viscosity cement, being particularly harmful. Similar concerns regarding cementation are reported by Krause et al. [20].

52.5.3 Revision RSTHA

One of the arguments used to justify RSTHA is that the revision is straightforward and results in a successful arthroplasty that does not differ from a primary THA. There are two concerns that question the validity of that argument. The first is that many proponents of RSTHA have felt that the revision would be conversion to THA, leaving the MOM acetabular component in place and revising to a large diameter THA with MOM bearings. Recent increased concerns regarding failure of those devices and concerns for taper corrosion now make that a less desirable alternative for the young active patient. Although many current patients with large head MOM THA are doing very well without complication, enthusiasm for this approach to THA has diminished significantly.

The second is the result of the revision RSTHA itself. De Smet and colleagues [21] reviewed their single surgeon experience with revision RSTHA over the period of 2001–2010. In 113 revisions evaluated at "midterm," 11 patients (9.7 %) suffered complications, of which 6 have required a subsequent revision. Most of these revisions were done for malpositioning of components with associated wear-induced metallosis.

52.6 Results of Isolated Femoral Head Resurfacing

Femoral head resurfacing (FSR) without acetabular component placement would have some appeal in the young patient population that often is afflicted with ON and indeed is still used in the very young patients by one of the lead proponents of RSTHA (Amstutz HC, 2011, personal communication). Its success has been variable, however, and for most US surgeons, this approach has been abandoned. Adili and Trousdale [22] reported the Mayo Clinic results in 2003 (before RSTHA was available in the USA other than through IDE assessment). They reported 29 FHR in 28 patients implanted from February 1997 to April 2000. In patients with mean age of 31.6 (range 12–48), they showed clinical improvement to a mean Harris hip score of 79.3. Overall survivorship was 75.9 % at 3 years. They note that "the majority of patients were satisfied with the procedure but outcomes are unpredictable."

Squire et al. [2] reported their results in 37 FSR implanted between 1997 and 2003. They judged failure as Harris hip pain scores of ≤20, or revision to THA. Their overall failure rate was 64.8 % (24/37 hips), with 15/24 failed because of revision surgery and 9/24 failed because of poor pain relief. They concluded that FSR "for ON is an unpredictable procedure" and no longer includes this approach in the treatment of the ON patient at their institution.

52.7 Summary

Hip arthroplasty for the young patient with ON represents a viable alternative for the patient with femoral head collapse when all other nonoperative strategies have been exhausted. Given that these patients are young and may have a life expectancy well beyond the expected life span of the device implanted, it is natural that the surgeon treating these patients will look for alternatives that are somewhat more conservative in approach and provide failure mechanisms that provide predictable approaches to revision treatment with substantially positive outcomes.

The senior author has taken care of young patients with ON of the femoral head for more than 30 years. He has long believed that arthroplasty approaches for ON behave similarly to those done for comparable young patients with OA, either primary or secondary, and he has become familiar with the failure patterns of all devices in these patients. He believes that it is important to have a philosophy about arthroplasty management in the young patient, and he believes it very important to include the patient and, if appropriate, family members, thoroughly in the discussion of available treatment options. He believes that none of the currently available arthroplasty approaches can be expected to last the lifetime of a patient with a life expectancy of 30 years or more, and while it may, both the patient and surgeon should recognize that a subsequent operation is likely. This then requires both surgeon and patient to understand the failure potentials and revision needs of all arthroplasty approaches and work with the patient to determine which approach is most reasonable for that patient. Figures 52.3 and 52.4 demonstrate this approach for a patient now 20+ years since initial arthroplasty and show one of the many possible approaches. Resurfacing THA for the properly selected patient can represent one form of this type of approach.

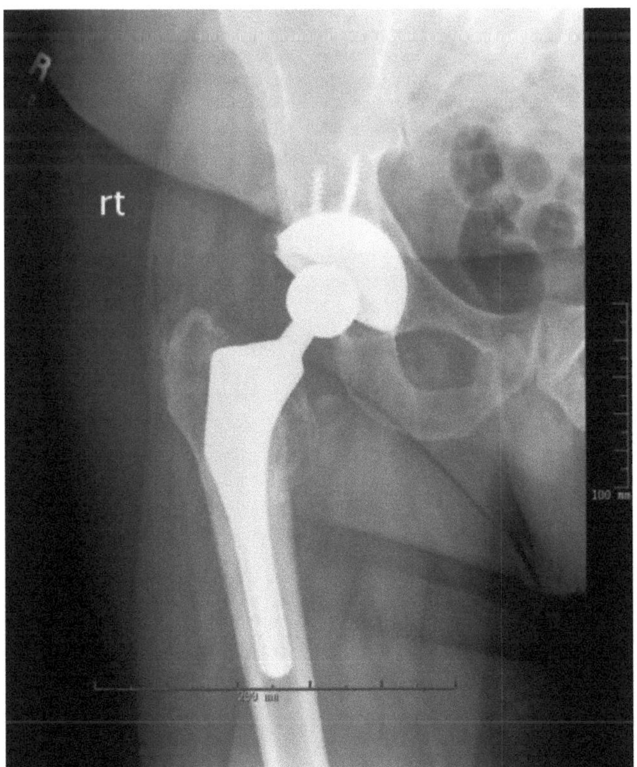

Fig. 52.3 20+ years post-primary THA for ON on the *right* (required acetabular revision in 2002)

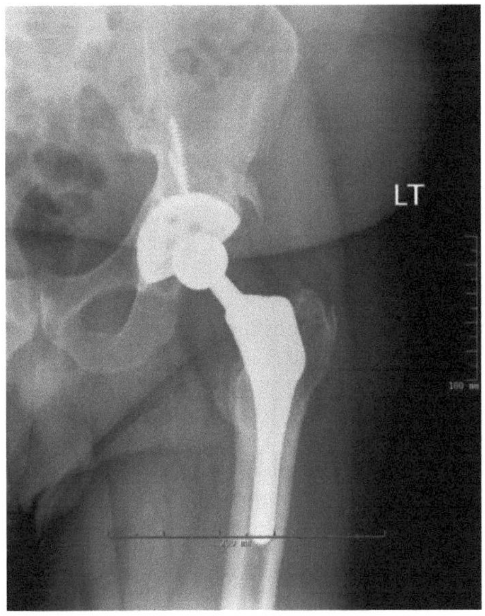

Fig. 52.4 20+ years post-primary THA for ON on the *left* (required acetabular revision in 2004)

References

1. Corten K, MacDonald SJ. Hip resurfacing data from national joint registries: what do they tell us? what do they not tell us? Clin Orthop Relat Res. 2010;468(2):351–7.
2. Squire M, Fehring TK, Odum S, Griffin WL, Bohannon Mason J. Failure of femoral surface replacement for femoral head avascular necrosis. J Arthroplasty. 2005;20(7 Suppl 3):108–14.
3. Steinberg ME, Corces A, Fallon M. Acetabular involvement in osteonecrosis of the femoral head. J Bone Joint Surg Am. 1999;81(1):60–5.
4. Amarasekera HW, Roberts P, Costa ML, Parsons N, Achten J, Griffin DR, et al. Scintigraphic assessment of bone status at one year following hip resurfacing: comparison of two surgical approaches using SPECT-CT scan. Bone Joint Res. 2012;1(5):86–92.
5. Gross TP, Liu F. Risk factor analysis for early femoral failure in metal-on-metal hip resurfacing arthroplasty: the effect of bone density and body mass index. J Orthop Surg Res. 2012;7:1, 799X–7–1.
6. Steffen RT, De Smet KA, Murray DW, Gill HS. A modified posterior approach preserves femoral head oxygenation during hip resurfacing. J Arthroplasty. 2011;26(3):404–8.
7. Kreuzer S, Leffers K, Kumar S. Direct anterior approach for hip resurfacing: surgical technique and complications. Clin Orthop Relat Res. 2011;469(6):1574–81.
8. Amstutz HC, Le Duff MJ. Cementing the metaphyseal stem in metal-on-metal resurfacing: when and why. Clin Orthop Relat Res. 2009;467(1):79–83.
9. Stulberg BN, Fitts SM, Zadzilka JD, Trier K. Resurfacing arthroplasty for patients with osteonecrosis. Bull NYU Hosp Jt Dis. 2009;67(2):138–41.
10. Gross TP, Liu F. Comparative study between patients with osteonecrosis and osteoarthritis after hip resurfacing arthroplasty. Acta Orthop Belg. 2012;78(6):735–44.

11. Woon RP, Johnson AJ, Amstutz HC. Results of conserve plus(R) metal-on-metal hip resurfacing for post-traumatic arthritis and osteonecrosis. Hip Int. 2012;22(2):195–202.
12. Madadi F, Eajazi A, Kazemi SM, Aalami Harandi A, Madadi F, Sharifzadeh SR. Total hip arthroplasty in advanced osteonecrosis: the short-term results by metal-on-metal hip resurfacing. Med Sci Monit. 2011;17(2):CR78–82.
13. Bose VC, Baruah BD. Resurfacing arthroplasty of the hip for avascular necrosis of the femoral head: a minimum follow-up of four years. J Bone Joint Surg Br. 2010;92(7):922–8.
14. He ZY, Di ZL, Tao K, Zhang JH, Feng JX, Wu HS. Short-term result of hip resurfacing arthroplasty in the treatment of patients with femoral head necrosis. Zhongguo Gu Shang. 2011;24(12):997–1000.
15. Cuckler JM. Metal-on-metal surface replacement: a triumph of hope over reason: affirms. Orthopedics. 2011;34(9):e439–41.
16. Sayeed SA, Johnson AJ, Stroh DA, Gross TP, Mont MA. Hip resurfacing in patients who have osteonecrosis and are 25 years or under. Clin Orthop Relat Res. 2011;469(6):1582–8.
17. Nakasone S, Takao M, Sakai T, Nishii T, Sugano N. Does the extent of osteonecrosis affect the survival of hip resurfacing? Clin Orthop Relat Res. 2013;471(6):1926–34.
18. Gross TP, Liu F. Is there added risk in resurfacing a femoral head with cysts? J Orthop Surg Res. 2011;6:55, 799X–6–55.
19. Falez F, Favetti F, Casella F, Papalia M, Panegrossi G. Results of hip resurfacing. Int Orthop. 2011;35(2):239–43.
20. Krause M, Breer S, Hahn M, Ruther W, Morlock MM, Amling M, et al. Cementation and interface analysis of early failure cases after hip-resurfacing arthroplasty. Int Orthop. 2012;36(7): 1333–40.
21. De Smet KA, Van Der Straeten C, Van Orsouw M, Doubi R, Backers K, Grammatopoulos G. Revisions of metal-on-metal hip resurfacing: lessons learned and improved outcome. Orthop Clin North Am. 2011;42(2):259–69, ix.
22. Adili A, Trousdale RT. Femoral head resurfacing for the treatment of osteonecrosis in the young patient. Clin Orthop Relat Res. 2003;(417):93–101.

Part XII

Osteonecrosis in Bones Other than the Hip

53 Multifocal Osteonecrosis

Samik Banerjee, Bhaveen H. Kapadia, Jeffrey J. Cherian, Julio J. Jauregui, and Michael A. Mont

53.1 Introduction

Osteonecrosis of the hip is an incapacitating condition that often affects patients in their second to fifth decades of their lives. It is estimated that about 10,000–20,000 patients are diagnosed with this condition every year in the United States. When this condition affects multiple skeletal structures, the debilitation is even more magnified.

53.2 Definition and Etiopathogenesis

Multifocal osteonecrosis is defined by simultaneous or sequential involvement of three or more separate anatomic sites [1, 2]. For example, involvement of the hip, knee, and shoulder or disease involving the shoulder, knee, or ankle would qualify as multifocal osteonecrosis. However, affection of both hips and knee joints should not be classified as multifocal osteonecrosis as it involves only two separate anatomic regions. It is a rare clinical condition, which is found to occur in approximately 3 % of patients with osteonecrosis [1, 2]. Typically, most patients have about six joints involved. However, recent reports suggest higher incidence of multifocal involvement than have been previously reported because many of these lesions were clinically silent [3, 4]. Several risk factors are known to be associated with the development of osteonecrotic lesions at multiple sites (see Table 53.1).

Although corticosteroid use is often reported as the most common risk factor in 90 % of patients with multifocal osteonecrosis, other associated conditions include renal failure, alcohol abuse, inflammatory bowel disease, systemic lupus erythematosus, human immunodeficiency virus infection, coagulation abnormalities (e.g., antithrombin III deficiency, protein S deficiency, factor V Leiden mutation, or increased activity of plasminogen activator), multiple sclerosis, Sjogren's syndrome, sickle-cell disease, leukemia, and lymphoma. However, due to paucity of reports and a high incidence of asymptomatic lesions, our understanding of the true incidence of multifocal osteonecrosis in various individual disease conditions is limited. Nevertheless, one study on 200 patients with sickle-cell disease reported that multifocal involvement occurred in 44 % of patients (87 out 200 patients) [4]. While the underlying pathoetiology in the development appears to be multifactorial (e.g., venous hypertension, altered fat metabolism, mechanical stress, and primary cell death), recent reports suggest that familial thrombophilia, hypofibrinolysis, and genetic polymorphisms of the endothelial nitric oxide synthetase (e.g., 4a and T-786C) causing reduction in nitric oxide production may play a role [3].

Osteonecrosis is considered a well-recognized complication during the maintenance phase following treatment of acute lymphoblastic leukemia (ALL) and non-Hodgkin's lymphoma. A higher incidence of lesions in the lower

Table 53.1 Risk factors associated with multifocal osteonecrosis

Risk factors for multifocal osteonecrosis
1. Corticosteroid use
2. SLE
3. Sickle-cell disease
4. HIV infection
5. Alcohol abuse
6. Multiple sclerosis
7. Coagulation disorders
8. Inflammatory bowel disease
9. Organ transplant recipients, e.g., renal, liver
10. Malignancy/chemotherapy
11. Sjogren's syndrome/inflammatory arthritis

S. Banerjee • B.H. Kapadia • J.J. Cherian • J.J. Jauregui
M.A. Mont (✉)
Department of Orthopaedic Surgery, Rubin Institute for Advanced Orthopedics, Center for Joint Preservation and Replacement, Sinai Hospital of Baltimore, 2401 West Belvedere Avenue, Baltimore, MD 21215, USA
e-mail: bashb02@gmail.com; bhaveen.k@gmail.com; jjaicherian@gmail.com; juljau@gmail.com; mmont@lifebridgehealth.org, rhondamont@aol.com

K.-H. Koo et al. (eds.), *Osteonecrosis*,
DOI 10.1007/978-3-642-35767-1_53, © Springer-Verlag Berlin Heidelberg 2014

extremities compared to upper extremities with a predilection towards bilateral involvement. Multifocal involvement is also found to be more common in this population than previously reported, with 82 % of patients affected in one series who had undergone whole-body screening MRI following chemotherapy for acute lymphoblastic leukemia [5, 6]. This increase in incidence is potentially related to prolonged use of high-dose dexamethasone in the recent chemotherapeutic regimens and low threshold for ordering MRI scans in chemotherapy patients complaining of musculoskeletal symptoms. A complex interplay of pathogenetic factors such as suppression of bone formation, expansion of intramedullary adipocytes causing elevated intraosseous pressure, and secondary marrow ischemia has been postulated to predispose these patients to develop osteonecrosis. In a large retrospective study on 111 patients, Mattano et al. reported that a higher incidence of osteonecrosis was found in the age group between 10 and 20 years compared to younger children who were below 10 years of age [5]. This was potentially related to the improved buffering of the intraosseous pressure by the immature bone prior to the epiphyseal closure. In contrast to more recent reports, they found a 6 % incidence of multifocal osteonecrosis in their patients.

53.3 Location of Involvement and Clinical Features

Typically, when long bones are involved, it affects the epiphyseal region, although less commonly it can involve the metaphysis and the diaphysis [7]. In multifocal osteonecrosis, femoral head involvement is found to occur most commonly, followed by the knee, shoulder, and talus. Less common sites of involvement include the elbow (the trochlea and the capitellum), wrist (distal radius and other carpal metacarpal heads), and tarsal bones such as the cuboid, cuneiform, and the navicular bone. In two large reports on multifocal osteonecrosis, it was found that the mean number of skeletal sites involved was found to vary between 5.2 and 6.3 [2, 4]. Majority of the patients with multifocal disease present in the early pre-collapse stage of the disease (Ficat-Arlet stages 1 and 2), with either hip symptoms or multiple joint pain (Table 53.2).

Flouzat-Lachaniete et al., in a study on 200 patients with osteonecrosis at multiple skeletal sites, due to sickle-cell disease, reported that 25 % of patients ($n=49$) had multifocal disease [4]. Multifocal disease was found to occur more commonly in sickle-cell SS genotype followed by SC and Sβ^+ genotypes. The high incidence of multifocal involvement found in this series was attributed to the routine use of MRI scans for screening. The authors also reported that 90 % of patients with shoulder and 95 % with knee involvement had evidence of multifocal disease. When patients present initially with osteonecrotic involvement of joints other than the hip (e.g., shoulder, ankle, or knee), a high index of suspicion for multifocal disease should be suspected, and routine imaging of the hips is advised. In this situation, the incidence of multifocal involvement was reported to be approximately 50 %, in one study [2]. Similarly, Orlic et al., in a study of 62 patients, who had alcohol-related osteonecrosis found that 6 % (5 out of 62 patients) had multifocal involvement [13]. However, the dose and the duration of alcohol intake that predisposed patients to multifocal involvement were not adequately defined.

Patients typically present with insidious onset and slowly progressive joint pain which increase with activity and weight bearing. The time period from onset of symptoms and the loss of joint function varies considerably and can range from months to years. In the later stages of the disease, rest pain and reduction in the range of motion often occurs, leading to substantial loss of function. The severity of pain varies from initially mild to severe when substantial joint destruction has taken place.

53.4 Diagnosis

53.4.1 Radiographs

Initial radiographic investigations should always include standard plain film radiographs of the affected site, in two or more orthogonal planes. In the early stages of the disease, radiographs can either be normal or show signs of mixed sclerosis and lysis. Occasionally, bone infarction is present in the meta-diaphyseal region as evidenced by multiple, incomplete, linear, sclerotic lines.

53.4.2 Bone Scan

Typically, in the early stages, due to increased vascularity in the region surrounding the osteonecrotic region, a bone scan shows reactive increase in the uptake of the tracer. The avascular region itself shows a cold spot (photopenic defect). However, the ability to detect a cold spot by planar scintigraphy decreases within a few weeks as a result of increased background activity. This prevents the differentiation between osteonecrosis and other causes of increased activity [14]. Historically, studies evaluating the efficacy of bone scans over radiographs found that bone scans were more sensitive than plain films [15]. In a study of 36 patients with systemic lupus erythematosus, Conklin et al. evaluated the sensitivity of bone scans and radiographs for the detection of steroid-induced osteonecrosis [15]. The authors found that 24 out of 27 joints (89 %) with elevated pressures had

Table 53.2 Patient demographics reported in studies on multifocal osteonecrosis

Author/study	No. of patients	Age/gender	Follow-up	Location in long bones	Diagnosis	Bones involved	Risk factors	Treatment
Fajardo-Hermosillo et al. [8]	1	24/W	3.3	Meta-diaphyseal	Multifocal ON	Tibia, fibula, talus	SLE associated with corticosteroids	NS
Gonzalez-Garcia et al. [9]	1	49/M	NS	Epiphyseal, meta-diaphyseal	Multifocal ON	Hip, knee, tibia, calcaneus, navicular, cuboid, metatarsals	HIV	NS
Miettunen et al. [6]	11	5.4	NS	Epiphyseal, meta-diaphyseal	Multifocal ON	Distal femur, proximal tibia, ankle, proximal femur	ALL; post-chemotherapy	
Sinclair et al. [7]	1	42/F	NS	Meta-diaphyseal	Multifocal ON	Femur, tibia, talus	MS associated with corticosteroids	IM reaming
Flouzat-Lachaniete et al. [4]	49	46	15	Epiphyseal, meta-diaphyseal	Multifocal ON	Hip, knee shoulder, and ankle	Sickle-cell disease	NS
Solarino et al. [10]	1	14	5.3	Epiphyseal	Multifocal ON	Hip, knee, and shoulders	ALL, post-chemotherapy	Bilateral THA
Gutierrez et al. [11]	3	NS	NS	Epiphyseal, meta-diaphyseal	Multifocal ON	Shoulder, hip, and knee	HIV	NS
Mullan et al. [12]	1	42/M	NS	Epiphyseal, meta-diaphyseal	Multifocal ON	Hip, talus, knee, shoulder	HIV	NS
Collaborative study group [1]	101	36	NS	Epiphyseal, meta-diaphyseal	Multifocal ON	6.2 lesions/patient hip, knee, shoulder, ankles, foot	Multiple factors	NS
LaPorte et al. [2]	32	34(24 women/8 men)	NS	Epiphyseal, meta-diaphyseal	Multifocal ON	Hip, knee, ankle, shoulder	Multiple factors	NS

ON osteonecrosis, *HIV* human immunodeficiency virus, *NS* not specified, *M* male, *W* women, *MS* multiple sclerosis abnormal scans, while 11 out of 27 joints (41 %) with elevated bone marrow pressures had abnormal radiographs [15]. However, most recent literature do not support the use of bone scanning as a diagnostic imaging modality for the diagnosis of osteonecrosis over magnetic resonance imaging due to its slower sensitivity. The current authors do not recommend using this imaging for screening of osteonecrosis.

53.4.3 Single-Photon Emission Computerized Tomography

These scans provide three-dimensional imaging of radioactivity in the target tissues. Sequential imaging can separate out overlying and underlying areas of radioactivity, thereby providing better image contrast, superior lesion detection, and localization. Collier et al. in a study of 20 hips compared the efficacy of single-photon emission tomography (SPECT) bone scintigraphy, radionuclide angiography, and planar bone scintigraphy in diagnosing osteonecrosis [16]. The authors found higher sensitivity with SPECT (85 %) compared to the planar imaging (55 %). However, artifacts from the bladder can obscure the images of the femoral head resulting in lower sensitivity compared to magnetic resonance imaging. With the advent of multi-head cameras that lead to shorter acquisition times and improved image resolution, the sensitivity of this modality in diagnosing multifocal osteonecrosis has improved.

More recently SPECT has been combined with bone scintigraphy for improved accuracy in detecting osteonecrotic lesions in the hip region. Ryu et al. compared the diagnostic sensitivity of MRI (1.5 T scanner) and bone scan with SPECT in a study of 24 renal transplant patients with osteonecrosis of the hip [17]. The authors reported that combining bone scan with SPECT improved the sensitivity of this imaging modality to 100 % compared to 66 % with MRI in this selected group of patients. This may be related to the increased skeletal uptake of Tc-99 m methylene diphosphonate in the bone surrounding the osteonecrotic region providing a better contrast leading to an earlier diagnosis compared to magnetic resonance scans. Nevertheless, despite these improvements, magnetic resonance imaging has currently superseded SPECT as the initial diagnostic imaging for osteonecrosis due to advantages of lack of radiation and detection of other concurrent hip pathologies.

53.4.4 Magnetic Resonance Imaging

MRI is the most sensitive and specific imaging modality currently available for the diagnosis of osteonecrosis. Initial studies also found that low-field MRI and bone scans were equally sensitive in diagnosing osteonecrotic lesions. However, recent evidence suggests that the specificity, sensitivity, and accuracy of high-strength (1.5–3 T) MRI in diagnosing osteonecrosis are considerably higher. Mont et al. in a comparative study evaluated the sensitivity of bone scans and MRI in multifocal disease. The authors found that the sensitivity of diagnosing multifocal disease was 100 % with MRI compared to 45 % with bone scan. The sensitivity with bone scans were higher for hip and knee lesions and later stages of the disease compared to the shoulder and ankle lesions and early-stage disease.

Despite the advantages, the time taken for scanning and the high costs were the main deterrents against its use for screening of multifocal osteonecrosis. Khanna et al. evaluated the effectiveness of a rapid sequence imaging protocol for the diagnosis of osteonecrotic lesions in 172 hips in 92 patients [18]. The authors found marked agreements between limited and full sequence MRI in 98.8 % cases (177 out of 179 hips; $k=0.97$) for detecting and determining the extent of osteonecrosis [18]. Since then multiple authors have reported that rapid sequence imaging with improved protocols of whole-body STIR sequences are effective in the screening of multifocal disease. Recently, Miettunen et al. evaluated the incidence of osteonecrosis using whole-body MRI in 11 pediatric patients who complained of musculoskeletal pain following chemotherapy for acute lymphoblastic leukemia [6]. The authors found that 9 out of 11 patients (82 %) had multifocal involvement. A high incidence of osteonecrotic lesions were found in proximity to the knee, with 89 % (8 out of 9 patients) of patients having lesions in the distal femur, while 78 % had disease affecting the proximal tibia. However, only 22 % (2 out of 9 patients) of patients had osteonecrotic lesions in the hip. Similarly, Tania et al. in their report of a 13-year-old patient with chemotherapy-induced multifocal osteonecrosis found that whole-body MRI STIR sequences provided excellent quality images and were an effective screening tool for detection of multifocal disease. However, further studies are needed to evaluate whole-body MRI STIR sequences as a screening tool for multifocal osteonecrosis.

Early lesions show an area of hypointense signal intensity in both T1and T2W images. Various patterns of signals have been reported with these early lesions such as homogenous (well-defined lesions), inhomogeneous (large irregular areas of decreased signal intensity), and ring patterns (area of decreased intensity surrounded by relatively normal intensity). The double-line sign on T2W images has been reported by many authors as the most consistent MRI feature of osteonecrotic lesions. This consists of an outer rim of low signal intensity (sclerotic bone) with an adjacent inner rim of high signal intensity (vascularized granulation tissue) with serpentine borders.

The optimal method of screening for both symptomatic and asymptomatic multifocal lesions has been debated in

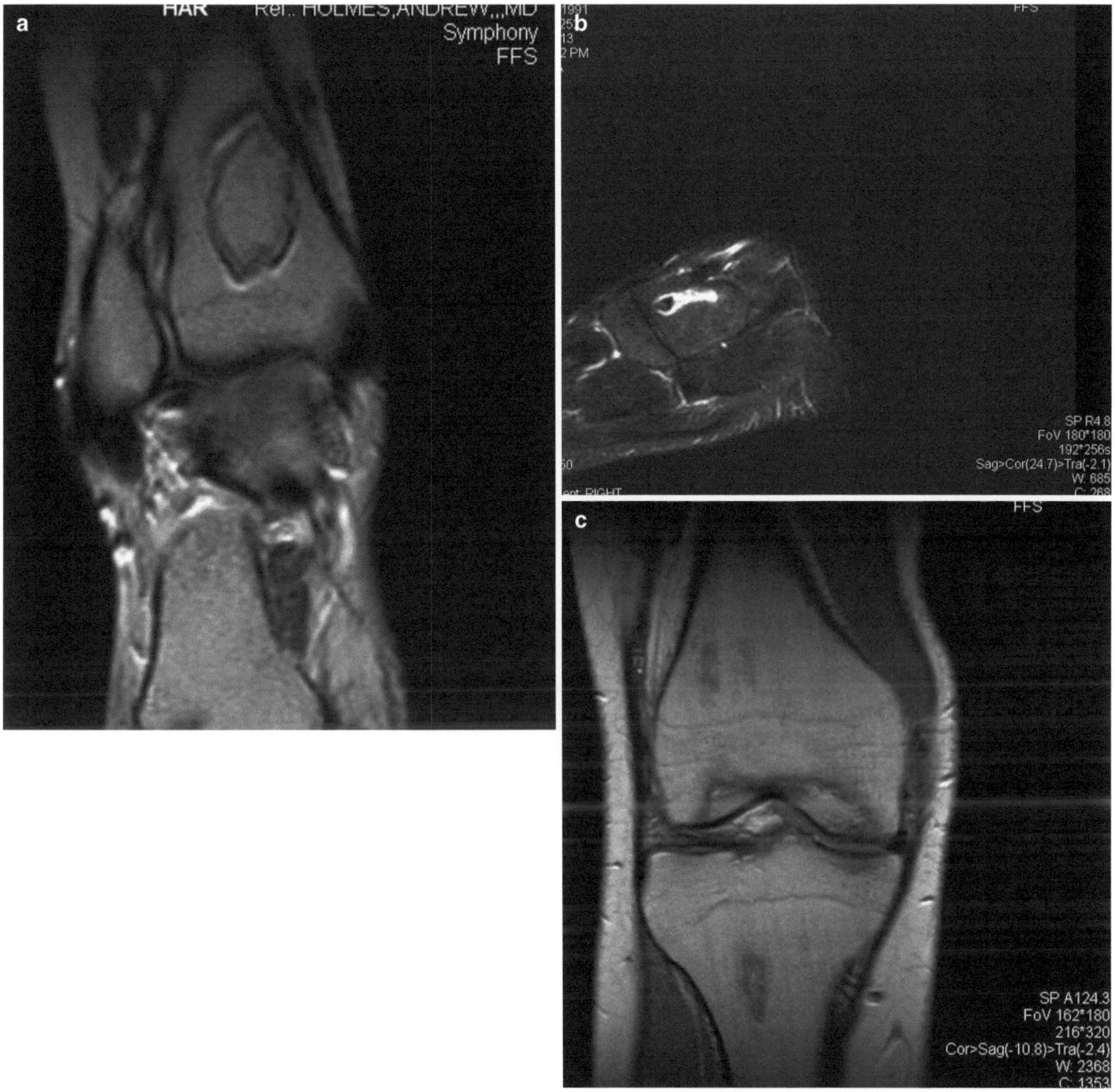

Fig. 53.1 (**a**) T1W sagittal image showing osteonecrotic lesion in the distal tibia of a 25-year-old lady with corticosteroid-induced multifocal osteonecrosis. (**b**) Involvement of the medial cuneiform in the same patient in T2W MRI. (**c**) T1W coronal images showing osteonecrosis in the subchondral region of the distal femur in the same patient

literature. Plain radiographs are considered nonsensitive tests for diagnosis of asymptomatic multifocal disease. Despite this, one approach could be obtaining a focused skeletal survey of the painful joints as the initial investigation followed by joint-specific MRI of the symptomatic joints if plain radiographs were found to be inconclusive. The other approach could be a whole-body MRI with STIR sequences followed by focused joint-specific MRI or bone scintigraphy. However, the superiority of one approach over another in the early detection of lesions remains to be proven. Nevertheless, further imaging of the contralateral side is recommended when osteonecrosis is diagnosed on one side due to the high incidence of bilaterality (70–100 %) reported with this condition [2, 4] (Fig. 53.1).

53.5 Management

The goal of management of multifocal disease is early diagnosis and treatment of the osteonecrotic lesions to prevent progression to collapse and end-stage arthritis. Regular follow-up of high-risk patients with low thresholds for cross-sectional imaging may detect asymptomatic lesions at an earlier stage of the disease. The treatment varies according to the stage of the disease for each joint. For early-stage (Ficat-Arlet stages 1 and 2) symptomatic disease, joint-preserving procedures such as core decompression, multiple drilling, vascularized, and nonvascularized bone grafting are usually advised. Less optimal outcomes are reported with joint-conserving procedures when substantial collapse (>2 mm) of more than 50 % involvement of the joint surface has occurred. Late-stage disease (Ficat stages 3 and 4) often requires a total joint arthroplasty for relief of symptoms. For meta-diaphyseal involvement, intramedullary reaming has been advised to stimulate a healing response [7].

Conclusion

Recent evidence suggests that a higher incidence of multifocal involvement can occur with known risk factors like corticosteroid use, alcohol abuse, HIV infection, and sickle-cell disease. A low threshold for whole-body planar imaging with magnetic resonance scanning may be necessary for early diagnosis and follow-up evaluations, when clinical suspicion remains high. The goal of treatment should be to diagnose these lesions at an early stage to avoid progression to collapse. Management of individual lesions should be based on the stage of the disease, with total joint arthroplasty reserved for end-stage disease.

References

1. Symptomatic multifocal osteonecrosis. A multicenter study. Collaborative Osteonecrosis Group. Clin Orthop Relat Res. 1999;(369):312–26.
2. LaPorte DM, Mont MA, Mohan V, Jones LC, Hungerford DS. Multifocal osteonecrosis. J Rheumatol. 1998;25(10):1968–74.
3. Glueck CJ, Freiberg RA, Boppana S, Wang P. Thrombophilia, hypofibrinolysis, the eNOS T-786C polymorphism, and multifocal osteonecrosis. J Bone Joint Surg Am. 2008;90(10):2220–9. doi:10.2106/JBJS.G.00616. 90/10/2220 [pii].
4. Flouzat-Lachaniete CH, Roussignol X, Poignard A, Mukasa MM, Manicom O, Hernigou P. Multifocal joint osteonecrosis in sickle cell disease. Open Orthop J. 2009;3:32–5. doi:10.2174/187432500 0903010032.
5. Mattano Jr LA, Sather HN, Trigg ME, Nachman JB. Osteonecrosis as a complication of treating acute lymphoblastic leukemia in children: a report from the Children's Cancer Group. J Clin Oncol. 2000;18(18):3262–72.
6. Miettunen PM, Lafay-Cousin L, Guilcher GM, Nettel-Aguirre A, Moorjani V. Widespread osteonecrosis in children with leukemia revealed by whole-body MRI. Clin Orthop Relat Res. 2012;470(12):3587–95. doi:10.1007/s11999-012-2579-x.
7. Sinclair V, Shepard G. Symptomatic, steroid-induced, multifocal diaphyseal osteonecrosis in a patient with multiple sclerosis. Mult Scler. 2010;16(3):370–2. doi:10.1177/1352458509358091. 1352458509358091 [pii].
8. Fajardo-Hermosillo LD, Lopez-Lopez L, Nadal A, Vila LM. Multifocal osteonecrosis in systemic lupus erythematosus: case report and review of the literature. BMJ Case Rep. 2013. doi:10.1136/bcr-2013-008980. bcr2013008980 [pii].
9. Gonzalez Garcia A, Sifuentes Giraldo WA, Blazquez Canamero MA, Ahijon Lana M, Navas Elorza E, Vazquez Diaz M. Multifocal osteonecrosis associated with human immunodeficiency virus infection. Reumatol Clin. 2012;8(6):361–4. doi:10.1016/j.reuma.2012.01.008. S1699-258X(12)00055-1 [pii].
10. Solarino G, Scialpi L, Bruno M, De Cillis B. On a case of multifocal osteonecrosis in a patient suffering from acute lymphoblastic leukemia. Chir Organi Mov. 2008;92(2):119–22. doi:10.1007/s12306-008-0047-2.
11. Gutierrez F, Padilla S, Masia M, Flores J, Boix V, Merino E, et al. Osteonecrosis in patients infected with HIV: clinical epidemiology and natural history in a large case series from Spain. J Acquir Immune Defic Syndr. 2006;42(3):286–92. doi:10.1097/01.qai.0000225012.53568.20.
12. Mullan RH, Ryan PF. Multiple site osteonecrosis in HIV infection. Rheumatology (Oxford). 2002;41(10):1200–2.
13. Orlic D, Jovanovic S, Anticevic D, Zecevic J. Frequency of idiopathic aseptic necrosis in medically treated alcoholics. Int Orthop. 1990;14(4):383–6.
14. Maillefert JF, Toubeau M, Piroth C, Piroth L, Brunotte F, Tavernier C. Bone scintigraphy equipped with a pinhole collimator for diagnosis of avascular necrosis of the femoral head. Clin Rheumatol. 1997;16(4):372–7.
15. Alavi A, McCloskey JR, Steinberg ME. Early detection of avascular necrosis of the femoral head by 99m technetium diphosphonate bone scan: a preliminary report. Clin Orthop Relat Res. 1977;127:137–41.
16. Collier BD, Carrera GF, Johnson RP, Isitman AT, Hellman RS, Knobel J, et al. Detection of femoral head avascular necrosis in adults by SPECT. J Nucl Med. 1985;26(9):979–87.
17. Ryu JS, Kim JS, Moon DH, Kim SM, Shin MJ, Chang JS, et al. Bone SPECT is more sensitive than MRI in the detection of early osteonecrosis of the femoral head after renal transplantation. J Nucl Med. 2002;43(8):1006–11.
18. Khanna AJ, Yoon TR, Mont MA, Hungerford DS, Bluemke DA. Femoral head osteonecrosis: detection and grading by using a rapid MR imaging protocol. Radiology. 2000;217(1):188–92.

54 Osteonecrosis of the Humeral Head

Nobuhiko Sugano

54.1 Introduction

Osteonecrosis of the humeral head (ONHH) is thought to occur when the vascularity of the proximal part of the humerus is impaired. An ascending branch of the anterior circumflex artery on the anterolateral aspect of the humeral head is a principal blood supply to the humeral head (Fig. 54.1). The ascending branch of the anterior circumflex (the arcuate artery) enters the proximal humerus at the superior end of the bicipital groove or by way of its branches into the adjacent greater and lesser tuberosities [1, 2]. Once the arcuate artery becomes intraosseous, it pursues a tortuous posteromedial course just below the epiphysis. Although a posterior circumflex artery branch can be the second supply, few anastomoses exist once the artery becomes intraosseous. The existence of only one principal artery and the tortuousness of the subchondral arterioles are the reasons for the vulnerability of the vascularity of the humeral head to impairment due to trauma and thromboembolic events. Traumatic ONHH can be seen after humeral neck fractures, shoulder dislocations, or surgery of the shoulder [3–5]. However, the majority of ONHH related to humeral neck fractures is quickly revascularized with creeping substitution without collapse, and the clinical impact of ONHH in fracture cases is relatively small compared to the fracture itself. Therefore, this chapter focuses on nontraumatic ONHH.

54.2 Etiology and Pathogenesis of Nontraumatic ONHH

Nontraumatic ONHH is an uncommon disease. Before steroid-induced osteonecrosis had been recognized, nontraumatic osteonecrosis was thought to be caused by vascular occlusion due to systemic diseases such as Gaucher's disease, sickle-cell disease, caisson disease, and collagen vascular diseases [6–9]. In 1960, Heimann and Freiberger [10] first reported in the English literature two

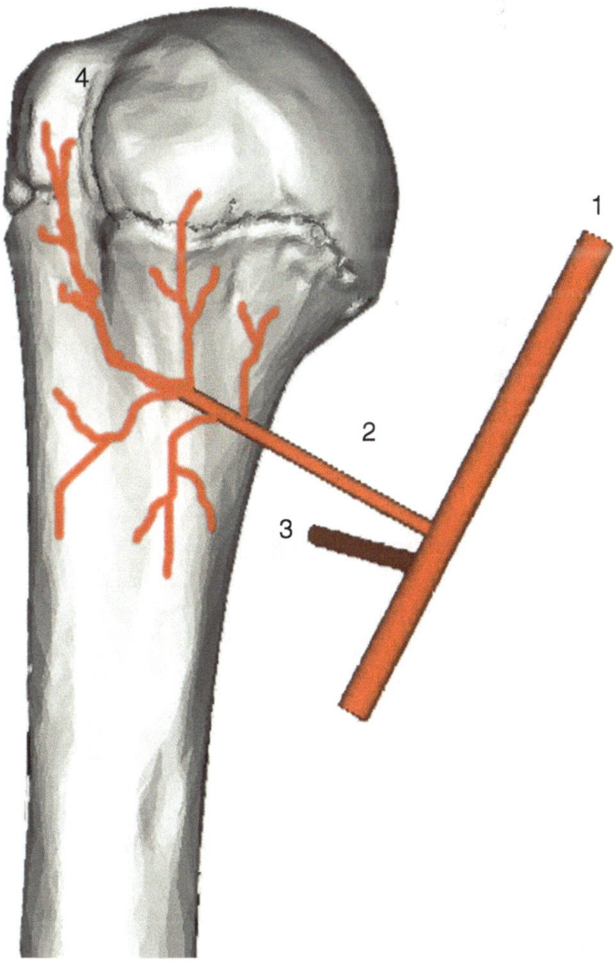

Fig. 54.1 Principal blood supply to the humeral head. The drawing of the anterior aspect of the humeral head shows the axillary artery (*1*), anterior humeral circumflex artery (*2*), posterior circumflex artery (*3*), andintertubercular groove (*4*)

N. Sugano
Department of Orthopaedic Medical Engineering, Osaka University Graduate School of Medicine, 2-2 Yamadaoka, Suita 565-0871, Japan
e-mail: n-sugano@umin.net

K.-H. Koo et al. (eds.), *Osteonecrosis*,
DOI 10.1007/978-3-642-35767-1_54, © Springer-Verlag Berlin Heidelberg 2014

cases with nontraumatic ONHH that occurred in four patients with osteonecrosis of the femoral head (ONFH) after high-dosage corticosteroid therapy for pemphigus and thrombotic thrombocytopenic purpura. Cruess et al. reported three cases of ONHH after steroid treatment for renal transplantation in 1968 [11]. Two of the three cases also had ONFH, while the third had no other site of osteonecrosis. After that, the number of reports about steroid-induced ONHH increased [12, 13], and steroid is the most frequently observed etiology of nontraumatic ONHH nowadays. Steroid-induced ONHH often manifests itself as multiple or multifocal osteonecrosis with an incidence of 3 % in osteonecrosis patients [14]. The shoulder is one of the major affected sites of osteonecrosis, secondary to the hip and knee [15]. Although the correlation between corticosteroids and osteonecrosis has been well described, the pathogenesis remains unclear. Corticosteroid administration may induce a fatty liver with possible systemic fat embolism [16, 17]. It may also increase the size of intraosseous adipocytes leading to an increase in the intraosseous pressure [18], which in turn may lead to ischemia causing osteonecrosis. The interval between corticosteroid administration and the onset of shoulder symptoms is variable, ranging from 6 to 18 months [19].

Excessive alcohol intake may cause osteonecrosis in a pathomechanism similar to steroid-induced osteonecrosis [20, 21]. In patients who had medical treatment for excessive consumption of alcohol, the incidence of osteonecrosis was reported to be 5.3 %. Eighty-nine percent of lesions developed in the femoral head, while 11 % of lesions developed in the humeral head [22]. Multiple foci of osteonecrosis were found in 6.1 % of the patients. When excessive alcohol intake was combined with steroid administration, more bone sites including femoral heads and humeral heads can be involved with osteonecrosis [23].

Increased blood coagulability is another etiology of osteonecrosis, and there is a report of ONHH associated with multi-foci osteonecrosis in a patient with type I congenital antithrombin III deficiency [24]. Idiopathic ONHH is extremely rare, and it has been recently reported in an adolescent amateur swimming athlete [25].

54.3 Diagnosis and Staging

The maximum weight-bearing of the shoulder during daily activities is generally smaller than that of the hip. In addition, the glenoid can withstand greater deformity than the acetabulum because of its less conforming morphology. Furthermore, compensatory motion at adjacent joints preserves considerable shoulder motion and function despite glenohumeral joint destruction and stiffness. Therefore, patients with ONHH frequently do not show symptoms until collapse of the humeral head [26]. The usual complaint

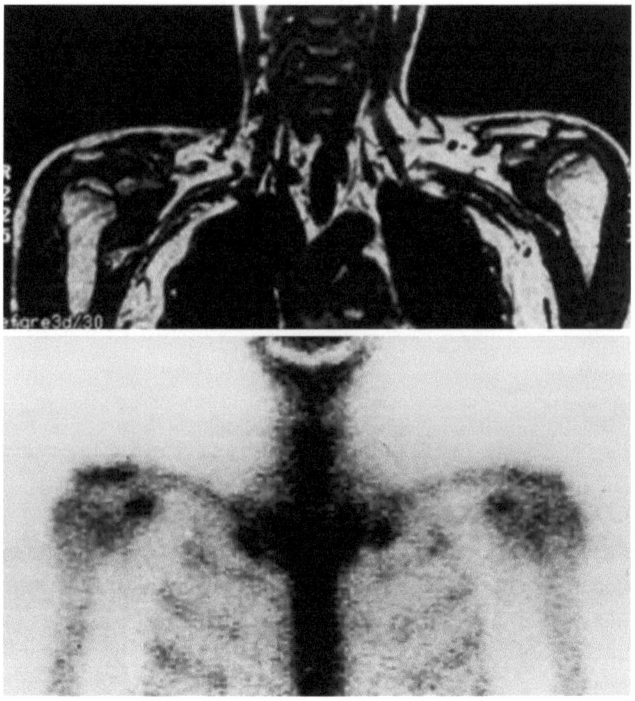

Fig. 54.2 Stage I ONHH. A coronal MR image on a spoiled gradient-recalled echo pulse sequence (SPGR; TR/TE = 14/2.3 ms) of bilateral shoulders (*top*) shows a low-intensity band in the humeral heads. Anteroposterior bone scintigrams of bilateral shoulders (*bottom*) show increased bone uptake in the coracoid process and the acromioclavicular joint and marginal increased bone uptake in the bilateral humeral heads

is a gradual onset of pain during joint movement. There is usually no pain at rest, and night pain is not a prominent complaint early in the course of ONHH. Later, a click during joint movement may be heard, which is usually painful [27]. This results from joint incongruity, a cartilage flap, or a large loose body. Passive range of motion is preserved until relatively late.

Plain radiographs are essential for the diagnosis of ONHH and its staging. True anteroposterior and axillary radiographs are usually obtained, and 40° posterior oblique radiographs in internal and external rotation may also be helpful. Experience with ONFH has shown the value of a staging system based upon the radiographic appearance of bony changes, and ARCO staging can be applied to ONHH. However, adaptation of Ficat-Arlet classification to the humeral head by Cruess [27] is the most widely used.

The preradiologic stage (stage I) shows no abnormality on radiographs. Magnetic resonance imaging (MRI) or radionuclide imaging [28] is required for diagnosis (Fig. 54.2). The diagnostic MRI signs of osteonecrosis are similar to those observed in femoral head osteonecrosis. Stage I osteonecrosis appears on MRI as linear bands of low signal on both T1- and T2-weighted images that

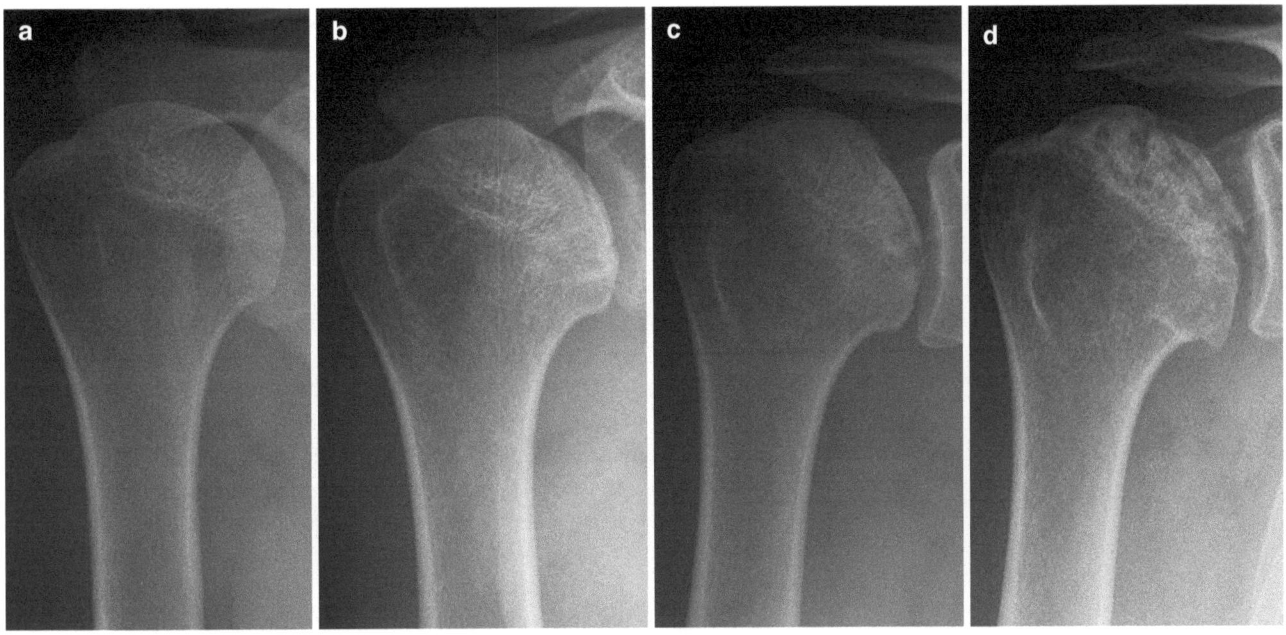

Fig. 54.3 Plain radiographs of ONHH. No radiologic abnormality is seen in stage I (**a**). An early sign of subchondral fracture is seen in stage III (**b**). Flattening of the humeral head follows (**c**), and fragmentation of the necrotic lesion may be seen later (**d**)

represent reactive bone at the margins of the infarct. A double-line sign representing bands of alternating high and low signal intensity can be observed in some patients on T2-weighted images. The scintigraphic appearance of early osteonecrosis is a photopenic zone corresponding to the necrotic segment. Increased radionuclide uptake accompanies revascularization and repair, producing a "cold in hot" pattern in ONFH [28]. However, the cold area is not always apparent because the necrotic lesions in ONHH are shallower than the lesions commonly seen in ONFH. A marginal increase in bone uptake in the humeral head is a sign of ONHH.

The early radiologic stage (stage II) may show an osteolytic area in the portion of the humeral head that articulates with the glenoid at 90° of abduction. Sclerosis can be also seen, and it may be wedge shaped or mottled and diffuse. However, these radiologic changes are not often apparent before collapse of the humeral head. The differential diagnosis of a lucent lesion includes bone cyst, benign or malignant bone tumor, and infection. Extensive resorption of the subchondral bone can lead to a subchondral fracture seen as a "crescent" sign even under ordinary forces transmitted across the shoulder joint (stage III). Massive collapse of the humeral head then develops (Fig. 54.3). The articular cartilage may separate from the underlying bone after collapse and, occasionally, may become detached and turn into a loose body. With extensive collapse, humeral head incongruity can lead to early degenerative changes (stage IV). Advanced collapse of the humeral head and arthritic changes of the glenoid then reveal a humeral head with a totally distorted shape, subchondral sclerosis of the glenoid, osteophytes, loss of joint space, and cystic changes in the entire glenohumeral joint (stage V).

54.4 Extent of Lesions and Natural Course

Large lesions in ONHH and collapsed-stage cases on plain radiographs tend to have poor prognoses. Several studies suggest the extent of a necrotic lesion on radiographs correlates with the prognosis and with the results of surgical treatment in patients with corticosteroid-related ONHH or traumatic ONHH [29–31]. The necrotic angle which was originally described for the hip adapted to ONHH to quantify the size of the lesion. Outlines of the lesions on AP and lateral radiographs were traced and the arc of the surface involving the necrosis was measured using a goniometer. These two angles were added to derive a combined necrotic angle. These studies reported that large lesions in ONHH and patients with collapse on plain radiographs tend to have poor prognoses. However, accurate evaluation of a lesion on radiographs is difficult at best and impossible at stage I. MRI is superior to radiographs in the early detection of necrotic lesions as well as in evaluating the extent and location of lesions [32, 33]. Early diagnosis and understanding of the natural history are important for joint-preserving treatment planning. When the necrotic angles are evaluated on MRI (Fig. 54.4), lesions with a necrotic angle of 90° or less both on the mid-oblique-coronal and mid-oblique-sagittal planes have a very small risk of collapse. In the case of lesions with

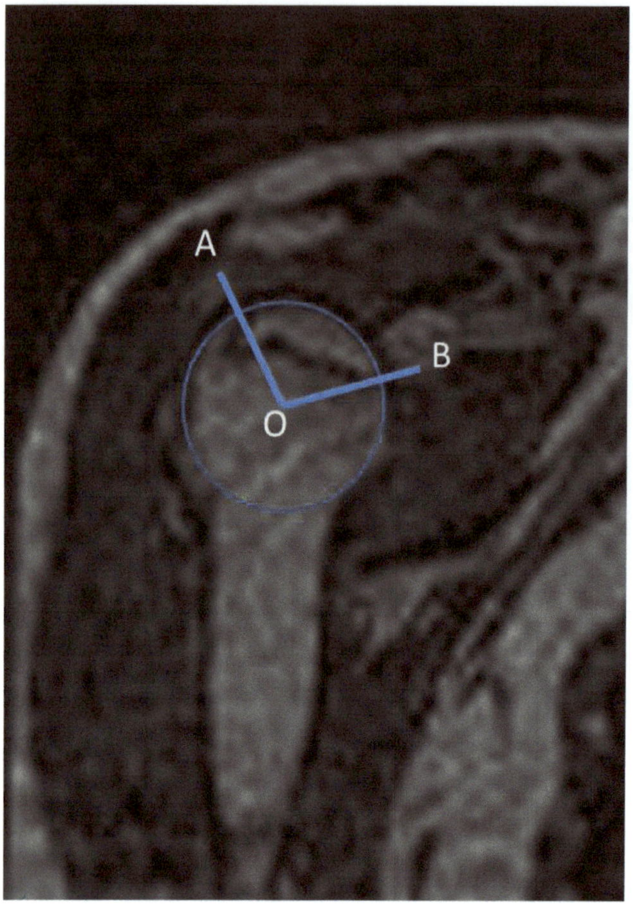

Fig. 54.4 The necrotic angles of ONHH on MRI. The center of the humeral head was defined as point *O*, and two end points of the necrotic lesion on the joint surface were defined as points *A* and *B* on mid-oblique-coronal and mid-oblique-sagittal SPGR images of the humeral head. The necrotic angle was calculated as the angle AOB

necrotic angles between 90° and 100°, collapse will occur but will not progress to osteoarthritis, followed by reparative reaction on plain radiographs. In the case of larger lesions with necrotic angles of more than 100° on mid-oblique-coronal and mid-oblique-sagittal planes, collapse seems inevitable followed by degenerative arthritis of the shoulder [32]. Another MRI study shows that the stage at initial visit, occurrence of pain, and continuation of peak doses of corticosteroids predicted progression of the disease in asymptomatic shoulders, whereas in symptomatic shoulders, extent and location of lesions were the main risk factors for progression [33].

54.5 Treatment

Although clinical symptoms and etiology of ONHH play a critical role in the treatment of each patient, staging is the most objective criterion in determining the most appropriate treatment. Conservative treatment can be effective in stages I and II (precollapse stages), when patients' symptoms are relatively mild. This is also considered for patients with minimal collapse and symptoms or for patients with limited physical demands. To prevent joint stiffness from disuse, physical therapy should include full passive range of motion and pendulum exercises without active overhead exercises. Administration of analgesics and nonsteroidal anti-inflammatory drugs may ease patient pain and increase comfort in everyday activities. Overall, the goal of conservative treatment is to relieve pain, restore normal range of motion, and delay the progression of the disease. When symptoms persist, and collapse progresses despite conservative treatment, surgical interventions including core decompression, vascularized bone grafting, arthroscopic debridement, and shoulder arthroplasty are considered.

Mont et al. first described the surgical technique for core decompression of the humeral head [34]. They made a small incision in the anterior axillary fold just above the pectoralis major tendon, reaching the proximal humerus with blunt dissection in the deltopectoral groove. A cannulated reamer was then inserted into the lesion lateral to the bicipital groove over a guide-wire pin under fluoroscopic guidance. The latest study by Mont et al. includes 63 shoulders in 43 patients with an average follow-up of 10 years. Preoperative Ficat-Arlet stage I disease had 15 of 16 (94 %) successful outcomes, and stage II had 15 of 17 (88 %) successful outcomes. Stage III had 16 of 23 (70 %) successful results, and stage IV had one of seven (14 %) successful results. They recommend core decompression for stages I, II, and III when conservative treatment fails. In contrast, L'Insalata et al. reported that humeral head drilling was not effective in preventing clinical or radiographic progression in stage III ONHH. The effectiveness of core decompression versus conservative treatment for humeral head necrosis stages I and II is not clear in the literature, although patients with stage I or stage II ONHH and intolerable pain are possible candidates for core decompression.

There are a few case studies of arthroscopic treatment for ONHH. Removal of loose bodies and joint debridement for steroid-induced ONHH successfully improved the patient's functional status through relief of pain, improved range of motion, and elimination of locking [35]. Repositioning of the joint cartilage and bone engraftment from an iliac crest through her humeral head from under the greater tuberosity with shoulder arthroscopy was tried for stage IV ONHH, and the patient wore an abduction brace for 8 weeks after the operation to hold the joint surface in its new position. Considerable improvement of the functional status of the shoulder by relieving pain and increasing range of motion was obtained at 2 years' follow-up [36]. Another study of arthroscopic debridement for ONHH revealed that relief of pain and improved range of motion were obtained in stage III

ONHH with episodes of locking [37]. A recent paper presented the case of endoscopically guided thorough debridement of the humeral head combined with nonvascularized bone grafting of the residual cavity and stabilization and concomitant arthroscopy [38].

The indications for shoulder arthroplasty in ONHH are similar to those for degenerative shoulder diseases with severe pain and dysfunction for which conservative treatment is unsatisfactory. Shoulder arthroplasty that is either hemiarthroplasty (humeral head replacement) or total shoulder arthroplasty (TSA) seems to be the most reliable surgical treatment for ONHH. Age is a major concern in shoulder arthroplasty, and several surgeons have questioned the durability of prosthetic implants, stressing the necessity for multiple shoulder revisions in young patients. In patients aged 50 years and younger, Sperling et al. have reported success rates of 84 and 73 % for TSA and hemiarthroplasty, respectively, in a 15-year follow-up period [39]. In this study, however, the indications of shoulder arthroplasty were mostly the sequelae of trauma and rheumatoid arthritis. The number of patients with ONHH in the series was small (5 %). Only small series are available in the literature regarding shoulder arthroplasty for ONHH. Little difference was noted between hemiarthroplasty and TSA in terms of pain relief and range of motion in the early studies [40–42]. In recent studies with shoulder arthroplasty for ONHH, progressive glenoid erosion or preoperative glenoid destruction is one of the main causes of failure when hemiarthroplasty is used [43, 44]. On the other hand, Feeley et al. showed that TSA had a higher complication rate and decreased mobility compared to hemiarthroplasty [45]. The authors recommended that TSA should be reserved for patients with stage V ONHH. Therefore, further studies are needed to clarify the indications for TSA and hemiarthroplasty and design and material improvements for the glenoid component may be necessary to provide longevity and good shoulder function for young patients with ONHH.

54.6 Summary

Osteonecrosis of the humeral head (ONHH) is thought to occur when the vascularity of the proximal part of the humerus is impaired. Traumatic ONHH can be seen after humeral neck fractures, shoulder dislocations, or surgery of the shoulder. However, the majority of ONHH related to humeral neck fractures is quickly revascularized with creeping substitution without collapse, and the clinical impact of ONHH in fracture cases is relatively small compared to the fracture itself. Nontraumatic ONHH is an uncommon disease. Before steroid-induced osteonecrosis had been recognized, nontraumatic osteonecrosis was thought to be caused by vascular occlusion due to systemic diseases such as Gaucher's disease, sickle-cell disease, caisson disease, and collagen vascular diseases. Since Heimann and Freiberger first reported two cases with steroid-induced ONHH, the number of reports about it increased, and steroid is the most frequently observed etiology of nontraumatic ONHH nowadays. Steroid-induced ONHH often manifests itself as multiple or multifocal osteonecrosis with an incidence of 3 % in osteonecrosis patients. The shoulder is one of the major affected sites of osteonecrosis secondary to the hip and knee. Plain radiographs are essential for the diagnosis of ONHH and staging. However, MRI is useful for the early diagnosis of ONHH and evaluation of the extent of the necrotic lesion. Staging is the most objective criterion in determining the treatment methods. Conservative treatment can be effective in stages I and II (precollapse stages), when patients' symptoms are relatively mild. When symptoms persist and collapse progresses despite conservative treatment, surgical interventions including core decompression, vascularized bone grafting, arthroscopic debridement, and shoulder arthroplasty are considered.

References

1. Laing PG. The arterial supply of the adult humerus. J Bone Joint Surg Am. 1956;38:1105–16.
2. Gerber C, Schneeberger AG, Vinh TS. The arterial vascularization of the humeral head. J Bone Joint Surg Am. 1990;72:1486–94.
3. Lee CK, Hansen HR. Post-traumatic avascular necrosis of the humeral head in displaced proximal humeral fractures. J Trauma. 1981;21(9):788–91.
4. Pateder DB, Park HB, Chronopoulos E, et al. Humeral head osteonecrosis after anterior shoulder stabilization in an adolescent. A case report. J Bone Joint Surg Am. 2004;86:2290–3.
5. Wang Jr P, Koval KJ, Lehman W, et al. Salter-Harris type III fracture-dislocation of the proximal humerus. J Pediatr Orthop B. 1997;6:219–22.
6. Dubois EL, Cozen L. Avascular (aseptic) bone necrosis associated with systemic lupus erythematosus. JAMA. 1960;174:966–71.
7. Amstutz HC, Carey EJ. Skeletal manifestations and treatment of Gaucher's disease. Review of twenty cases. J Bone Joint Surg Am. 1966;48(4):670–701.
8. McCallum RI, Walder DN. Bone lesions in compressed air workers, with special reference to men who worked on the Clyde Tunnels 1958 to 1963. Report of Decompression Sickness Panel Medical Research Council. J Bone Joint Surg Br. 1966;48(2):207–35.
9. Chung SM, Ralston EL. Necrosis of the femoral head associated with sickle-cell anemia and its genetic variants. A review of the literature and study of thirteen cases. J Bone Joint Surg Am. 1969;51(1):33–58.
10. Heimann WG, Freiberger RH. Avascular necrosis of the femoral and humeral heads after high-dosage corticosteroid therapy. N Engl J Med. 1960;263:672–5.
11. Cruess RL, Blennerhassett J, MacDonald FR, MacLean LD, Dossetor J. Aseptic necrosis following renal transplantation. J Bone Joint Surg Am. 1968;50:1577–90.
12. Fisher DE, Bickel WH. Corticosteroid-induced avascular necrosis. A clinical study of seventy-seven patients. J Bone Joint Surg Am. 1971;53(5):859–73.
13. Cruess RL. Steroid-induced avascular necrosis of the head of the humerus. J Bone Joint Surg Br. 1976;58:313–7.

14. LaPorte DM, Mont MA, Mohan V, Jones LC, Hungerford DS. Multifocal osteonecrosis. J Rheumatol. 1998;25:1968–74.
15. Mont MA, Jones LC, LaPorte DM, Collaborative Osteonecrosis Group. Symptomatic multifocal osteonecrosis. A multicenter study. Clin Orthop. 1999;369:312–26.
16. Jones Jr JP, Engleman EP, Najarian JS. Systemic fat embolism after renal homotransplantation and treatment with corticosteroids. N Engl J Med. 1965;273(27):1453–8.
17. Jones Jr JP, Sakovich L. Fat embolism of bone. A roentgenographic and histological investigation, with use of intra-arterial lipiodol, in rabbits. J Bone Joint Surg Am. 1966;48(1):149–64.
18. Hungerford DS, Lennox DW. The importance of increased intraosseous pressure in the development of osteonecrosis of the femoral head: implications for treatment. Orthop Clin North Am. 1985;16(4):635–54.
19. Cruess RL. Experience with steroid-induced avascular necrosis of the shoulder and etiologic considerations regarding osteonecrosis of the hip. Clin Orthop. 1978;130:86–93.
20. Hungerford DS, Zizic TM. Alcoholism associated ischemic necrosis of the femoral head. Early diagnosis and treatment. Clin Orthop Relat Res. 1978;130:144–53.
21. Mielants H, Veys EM, DeBussere A, van der Jeught J. Avascular necrosis and its relation to lipid and purine metabolism. J Rheumatol. 1975;2(4):430–6.
22. Orlić D, Jovanović S, Anticević D, Zecević J. Frequency of idiopathic aseptic necrosis in medically treated alcoholics. Int Orthop. 1990;14(4):383–6.
23. Nishii T, Sugano N, Ohzono K, Takaoka K. Multiple lesions of osteonecrosis depicted by magnetic resonance imaging. Am J Knee Surg. 1995;8(4):137–40.
24. Kubo T, Tsuji H, Yamamoto T, Nakahara H, Nakagawa M, Hirasawa Y. Antithrombin III deficiency in a patient with multifocal osteonecrosis. Clin Orthop Relat Res. 2000;378:306–11.
25. Zuo J, Sano H, Yamamoto N, Sakoma Y, Shinozaki N, Itoigawa Y, Omi R, Itoi E. Humeral head osteonecrosis in an adolescent amateur swimming athlete: a case report. Sports Med Arthrosc Rehabil Ther Technol. 2012;4(1):39.
26. Cushner MA, Friedman RJ. Osteonecrosis of the humeral head. J Am Acad Orthop Surg. 1997;5(6):339–46.
27. Cruess RL. Corticosteroid-induced osteonecrosis of the humeral head. Orthop Clin North Am. 1985;16:789–95.
28. Sakai T, Sugano N, Nishii T, Miki H, Ohzono K, Yoshikawa H. Bone scintigraphy screening for osteonecrosis of the shoulder in patients with non-traumatic osteonecrosis of the femoral head. Skeletal Radiol. 2002;31(11):650–5.
29. L'Insalata JC, Pagnani MJ, Warren RF, Dines DM. Humeral head osteonecrosis: clinical course and radiographic predictors of outcome. J Shoulder Elbow Surg. 1996;5:355–61.
30. Hattrup SJ, Cofield RH. Osteonecrosis of the humeral head: relationship of disease stage, extent, and cause to natural history. J Shoulder Elbow Surg. 1999;8:559–64.
31. LaPorte DM, Mont MA, Mohan V, Pierre-Jacques H, Jones LC, Hungerford DS. Osteonecrosis of the humeral head treated by core decompression. Clin Orthop. 1998;355:254–60.
32. Sakai T, Sugano N, Nishii T, Hananouchi T, Yoshikawa H. Extent of osteonecrosis on MRI predicts humeral head collapse. Clin Orthop Relat Res. 2008;466(5):1074–80.
33. Hernigou P, Flouzat-Lachaniette CH, Roussignol X, Poignard A. The natural progression of shoulder osteonecrosis related to corticosteroid treatment. Clin Orthop Relat Res. 2010;468(7):1809–16.
34. Mont MA, Maar DC, Urquhart MW, Lennox D, Hungerford DS. Avascular necrosis of the humeral head treated by core decompression. A retrospective review. J Bone Joint Surg Br. 1993;75(5):785–8.
35. Hayes JM. Arthroscopic treatment of steroid-induced osteonecrosis of the humeral head. Arthroscopy. 1989;5(3):218–21.
36. Nakagawa Y, Ueo T, Nakamura T. A novel surgical procedure for osteonecrosis of the humeral head: reposition of the joint surface and bone engraftment. Arthroscopy. 1999;15:433–8.
37. Hardy P, Decrette E, Jeanrot C, Colom A, Lortat-Jacob A, Benoit J. Arthroscopic treatment of bilateral humeral head osteonecrosis. Arthroscopy. 2000;16(3):332–5.
38. Brannon JK. Thorough debridement of the humeral head for osteonecrosis. Orthopedics. 2011;34(1):56.
39. Sperling JW, Cofield RH, Rowland CM. Neer hemiarthroplasty and Neer total shoulder arthroplasty in patients fifty years old or less. Long-term results. J Bone Joint Surg Am. 1998;80(4):464–73.
40. Neer 2nd CS, Watson KC, Stanton FJ. Recent experience in total shoulder replacement. J Bone Joint Surg Am. 1982;64(3):319–37.
41. Hattrup SJ, Cofield RH. Osteonecrosis of the humeral head: results of replacement. J Shoulder Elbow Surg. 2000;9(3):177–82.
42. Raiss P, Kasten P, Baumann F, Moser M, Rickert M, Loew M. Treatment of osteonecrosis of the humeral head with cementless surface replacement arthroplasty. J Bone Joint Surg Am. 2009;91(2):340–9.
43. Parsch D, Lehner B, Loew M. Shoulder arthroplasty in nontraumatic osteonecrosis of the humeral head. J Shoulder Elbow Surg. 2003;12(3):226–30.
44. Smith RG, Sperling JW, Cofield RH, Hattrup SJ, Schleck CD. Shoulder hemiarthroplasty for steroid-associated osteonecrosis. J Shoulder Elbow Surg. 2008;17(5):685–8.
45. Feeley BT, Fealy S, Dines DM, Warren RF, Craig EV. Hemiarthroplasty and total shoulder arthroplasty for avascular necrosis of the humeral head. J Shoulder Elbow Surg. 2008;17(5):689–94.

Knee Osteonecrosis

55

Karthik E. Ponnusamy, Savyasachi Thakkar, and Harpal S. Khanuja

55.1 Introduction

Osteonecrosis (ON) of the knee is second to the hip as the most common location [1] and presents in two major forms: spontaneous and secondary ON. Spontaneous ON of the knee (SPONK) was first identified as a separate entity by Ahlback et al. in 1968 [2] with no identifiable cause. Secondary ON is due to identifiable causes most commonly steroids and alcohol. Some authors include arthroscopic-associated ON with secondary causes, while others identify it as a separate disease entity. Despite the different clinical presentations of each of these forms, disease severity is classified using the same systems and treatment algorithms composed of the same approaches.

55.2 Etiology

SPONK does not have a specifically identified etiology. The leading theories are trauma and vascular insufficiency [3]. Trauma refers to insufficiency and microfractures in subchondral bone weakened by osteoporosis [4]. One study found significantly lower bone mineral densities of the femoral neck of SPONK patients than in osteoarthritis; however, they did not find a difference in the densities of the medial femoral condyle or medial tibial plateau [5]. The basis of the vascular theory is that an insult to the blood flow to the condyle leads to edema that hinders blood flow further. This cycle ends with ischemia to the bone [4]. Research has found that intraosseous pressures are higher in the medial condyle of SPONK than in the lateral condyle and also relative to both condyles for patients with osteoarthritis. In cases where revascularization restores blood flow, there is a chance for the lesions to heal as long as collapse has not occurred already [4]. Despite these theories, one pathology study of biopsy samples of bone from SPONK patients found only one sample of 22 had evidence of necrotic bone [6]. There is conflicting data on the cause of SPONK, but insufficiency fractures are the leading theory.

Secondary ON has been shown to be caused by a variety of factors including hematologic/oncologic (e.g., sickle-cell disease), rheumatologic (e.g., systemic lupus erythematosus), infectious disease (e.g., HIV), hyperbarism, metabolic disorders (e.g., Gaucher's disease), steroids, and alcohol [3, 7–9]. Hematologic factors may promote the formation of clots and prevent their lyses and consequently leading to disrupted blood flow and ON. Some studies have found that patients with hereditary hypercoagulable diseases were disproportionately found among patients with ON [9]. Although many rheumatologic diseases are treated with steroids, they have higher than expected rates of ON suggesting that the disease process may predispose patients to develop ON. Infectious disease is also on the differential for ON, and research has found that HIV may lead to it and is associated with the duration of infection and antiretroviral treatment [8]. Although the mechanisms remain unknown, hyperbarism is thought to lead to elevated intracortical pressure and consequently to ON [9]. Many metabolic disorders such as Gaucher's disease can lead to increased intraosseous pressures by altering the composition of the marrow [10].

Steroids have been studied extensively to elucidate the mechanism leading to ON. Although there are reports that total dosing of even 480 mg can lead to ON, it is more commonly seen among patients taking chronic daily doses of at least 20 mg a day [11]. Multiple possible factors have been identified in steroid-induced ON. In vivo studies have demonstrated that prolonged steroid treatment can cause apoptosis of osteoclasts and osteoblasts. At the same time, steroids may prolong osteoclast lifespan leading to greater bone

K.E. Ponnusamy • S. Thakkar
Department of Orthopaedic Surgery,
Johns Hopkins University, Baltimore, MD, USA

H.S. Khanuja (✉)
Department of Orthopaedic Surgery,
Johns Hopkins Bayview Medical center, Johns Hopkins University,
4940 Eastern Avenue, Baltimore, MD 21224, USA
e-mail: paulkhanuja@gmail.com

K.-H. Koo et al. (eds.), *Osteonecrosis*,
DOI 10.1007/978-3-642-35767-1_55, © Springer-Verlag Berlin Heidelberg 2014

resorption. Steroids also divert stromal cells to become adipocytes instead of osteoblasts. Another mechanism is that steroids lead to greater hypercoagulability by affecting endothelial cells and hindering clot lysis. Fat emboli are another possible explanation of disrupting blood flow [9]. After causing disruption of blood flow and death to bone cells, steroids can hinder angiogenesis and prevent bone reparative processes. Genetic research has found that patients with certain forms of the P450 enzyme may be more prone to ON from steroid use. Similar findings have been found for patients with certain varieties of apolipoproteins B and A1 [9]. Alcohol may lead to ON by directly killing osteocytes. Other possible explanation is that it promotes the development of a fatty liver and the risk for fat emboli [9].

The use of mechanical debriders, lasers, and radiofrequency ablation is believed to cause arthroscopic-associated ON [3]. Usually the lesion is in the medial femoral condyle, and the lateral condyle is the second most commonly seen site [10]. It is theorized that a pathologic subchondral fracture leads to edema from a combination of the injury and the arthroscopy fluids [10]. In the case of radiofrequency ablation, it is theorized that thermal energy applied near the cartilage causes damage leading to ON [3]. ON usually presents as a sudden onset of pain 24 weeks after arthroscopy but is reported to range from 4 to 92 weeks [10]. Among arthroscopic-associated ON, there has been one case report of lateral femoral condyle ON [12] months after ACL reconstruction. The authors theorized that a combination of bone bruising to the lateral femoral condyle from the initial trauma in conjunction with the drilling of the femoral tunnel led to intramedullary hemorrhage and disrupted blood flow [7].

These various pathways of bone injury and necrosis may later join together to form a common route for degenerative changes at the knee joint. If new bone formation cannot keep pace with resorption of the damaged bone, the bone may collapse. This collapse may lead to further degenerative changes including deformity and articular cartilage damage. Due to this theorized mechanism, it is thought that bisphosphonates may slow resorption and avoid the collapse [13]. They will be discussed at a later point.

55.3 Epidemiology

SPONK is seen in females in a 3–1 ratio, and it also seen in patients who are older than 60 years old [14, 15]. For patients presenting with medial knee pain, 3.4 % of those greater than 50 years old and 9.4 % of those greater than 65 years old have SPONK [10]. It is most frequently seen in the medial condyle but has been reported to occur in the lateral condyle in up to 8 % of cases [4]. SPONK has also been reported to occur in the medial tibial plateau in 2 % of cases [12].

Secondary ON is generally seen in younger patients, usually younger than 50 years old [13]. Although a variety of causes lead to secondary ON, steroids is the most common etiology and together with alcohol accounts for 90 % of cases [9, 10]. In the femoral head, rates of steroid ON have been reported to range from 16.5 to 31.9 % [16], whereas alcohol has been associated with much lower rates of ON in the femoral head (<0.3 %) [16]. Estimates put the incidence of secondary ON of the knee to be 10 % of hip ON [10]. Shigemura et al. looked for ON in the knee in a population of patients who already had ON of the hip due to alcohol or steroids. They chose this population because of the relative rarity of ON of the knee and often asymptomatic presentation. They found that only 18.3 % of patients with alcohol-induced hip ON also had knee ON, while it was 54.9 % for patients with steroid-induced hip ON [16]. This study also reported that approximately a third of the lesions were located in the femoral lateral condyle, which was the most common location. They also found that ON of the knee was more likely to be seen with bilateral femoral head ON suggesting that ON of the knee occurs in more severe disease [16]. However, most of these ON lesions in the knee were asymptomatic in this population [16]. Sickle-cell patients are reported to have an annual incidence of 3.6 % for knee ON [10].

In one study of arthroscopic-associated ON due to RF ablation, they found a 4 % (2/50) risk of developing ON. The average size of the lesion in these two patients was 27.5 % of the condyle [3]. This estimate may be on the high end, since a large number of arthroscopies are performed each year and ON is a relatively rare complication [10].

55.4 Clinical Findings

Ahlback et al. reported that SPONK patients had a "sudden and violent onset of pain," where patients could identify the exact moment the pain started [2] That moment may be associated with a minor accident [14]. The pain generally continued to persist and often increases in severity. The pain improved when weight bearing was avoided, and worsened with activity. The pain also worsened at night [2, 14]. Night pain has been reported in 21–58 % of patients [17]. Some of the other associated symptoms included stiffness, swelling, and catching. Patients seen more than a year after the development of symptoms often had instability and bowing of the knee. On exam, these patients had localized tenderness to the medial knee especially at the medial femoral condyle [2]. Although the medial femoral condyle is most often associated with SPONK, there are case reports of it occurring in the lateral femoral condyle [4]. They could have an effusion, with a normal to slightly decreased range of motion [2]. Secondary ON has an insidious onset of pain, rather than the sudden onset found in SPONK. Also, it often affects multiple joints (>80 %), is bilateral, and affects multiple locations within the same joint [1, 10, 18].

55.5 Classification Systems

Multiple classification systems have been developed for SPONK. Nonetheless, they have been applied to secondary ON as well. The different systems have many similarities, but none has become the standard for use in ON. As a result, interpreting and comparing literature results can be difficult due to the lack of a common standard.

Soucacos et al. developed a classification system for SPONK based primarily on radiographic findings since clinical findings can be similar across the stages they identified. Stage I (incipient stage) has normal plain radiographs, may have normal MRI, and has positive bone scans. The T2-weighted MRI images can be prognostic in those patients where normal images usually do not progress, while those with abnormalities suggest the disease will worsen. These patients can have symptoms for 6–8 weeks and then may resolve. Usually, these patients progress to the second stage 2–4 months after symptom onset. Stage II has radiographic findings of flattening of the medial femoral condyle. At 3–6 months after symptom onset, the disease can progress to stage III, which is notable for a radiolucent lesion on radiographs. This radiolucent lesion is called a crescent/rim sign and is due to necrosis of the subchondral bone and concurrent articular cartilage damage. By 9–12 months after symptom onset, stage IV develops and it indicates worsened subchondral bone and articular cartilage damage that can cover the entire diameter of the medial condyle [14].

Another classification system for SPONK was modified from the Ficat and Arlet system for femoral head ON by Koshino and reported by Motohashi et al. [19]. This system was based on plain radiographs, where Stage 1, the initial stage, demonstrates no changes on radiographs and the patient has pain. Stage 2 is the avascular stage where radiolucency develops and there is sclerosis nearby it. Once the sclerosis surrounds the radiolucency, stage 3, the developed stage, is reached. Stage 4 is the degenerative stage where osteophytes and sclerosis are seen on both sides of the joint [19].

Aglietti et al. modified and expanded Koshino's classification system to include 5 stages. Stage I remained the same. A new Stage II was developed that is an intermediate of Koshino's Stage 1 and 2 where there is some flattening of the weight-bearing condyle. Aglietti's Stage III is similar to Koshino's Stage 2. Stage IV in Aglietti's system has features of Stage 3 and also had subchondral collapse into a calcified plate. Secondary degenerative signs are apparent in Aglietti's Stage V and Koshino's Stage 4 [20].

Another aspect of classifying lesions is based on the size. Multiple systems have been developed to measure the lesion size, but none has been validated [10]. The ones mentioned below do have research suggesting they can be prognostic of disease progression.

Muheim and Bohne proposed measuring ON lesion sizes by calculating the product of the maximum width of the lesion on the anteroposterior and lateral radiographs [21]. Another approach was taken by Lotke et al., who looked at the anteroposterior radiograph and measured the percentage of the maximum transverse width of the condyle that the lesion occupied [22]. Mont et al. modified the use of the Kerboul angle from the femoral head for use in the knee. An angle with the vertex at the physeal scar and sides corresponding to the sides of the lesion are drawn on the anteroposterior and lateral radiographs. The sum of these angles is calculated to determine the size of the lesion. Small lesions measured <150°, medium lesions measured 151–249°, and large lesions were greater than 250°. Mont et al.'s study found that large lesions had significantly worse outcomes than the medium and small lesions [1].

55.6 Natural History

Soucacos et al. suggests that SPONK progresses along the four stages of their classification system to end in severe degenerative knee arthritis in 9–12 months. In cases of Stage I or II, disease with a small lesion of 0.24 cm^2 the disease may regress and resolve on its own [14]. Lotke et al. reported that small lesions of <45 % of the condylar width or less than 3.5 cm^2 do well with conservative treatment with resolution of symptoms at least initially. It is unknown whether these patients will develop degenerative changes later on. For patients with large lesions of >50 % of the condylar width or >5 cm^2, they continue to get progressively worse leading to end-stage degenerative joint changes [23]. Yates et al. looked at patients with stage I SPONK and found that older patients (68 years old) tended to continue to worsen while younger patients (59 years) tended to have resolution. They report that this was not statistically significant, but suggest that age may be a factor in worse outcomes [17].

55.7 Imaging

In evaluating a patient with new onset of knee pain, the first-line imaging acquired are plain radiographs including standing anteroposterior, flexed posteroanterior, lateral, and sunrise views (Fig. 55.1). Further workup of a patient with suspected ON is MRI versus bone scan. Generally, MRI is the preferred imaging technique because it offers good sensitivity and specificity and it can easily measure lesion sizes

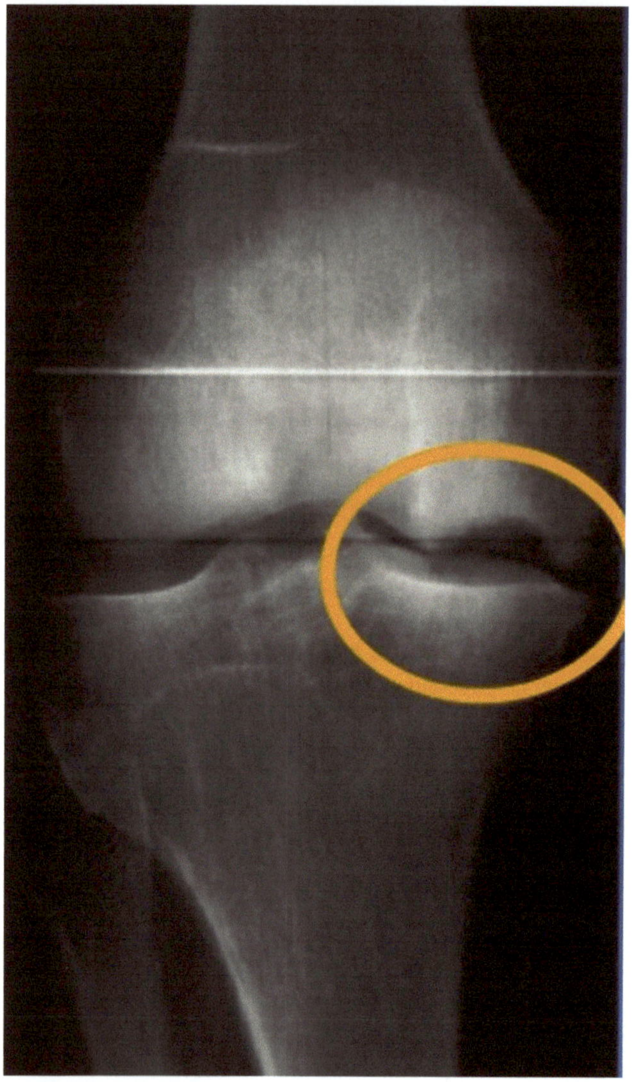

Fig. 55.1 Anteroposterior radiograph of the knee demonstrating a radiolucent (osteonecrosis) lesion (*orange circle*) of the medial femoral condyle with collapse of the weight bearing portion

(Figs. 55.2 and 55.3). In addition, it can evaluate for other diagnosis on the differential including meniscus and ligamentous injuries. Some practitioners prefer bone scintigraphy because it may be more sensitive in detecting marrow edema, but it is not specific for ON. This sensitivity has been contested in the literature with reports suggesting it may not be as sensitive as previously reported [10]. In addition, it is not able to measure lesion sizes.

The initial finding that can first be identified on MRI is bone marrow edema that is not visible on CT or radiographs. MRI's main limitation is that it may not detect an ON lesion for 4–6 weeks after symptom onset. This time frame is called the "window period" [3]. The other limitation of MRI is if it demonstrates bone marrow edema, it may be attributable to other causes including osteochondritis dissecans, bone bruise, or reactive processes [10].

End-stage ON shares many of the radiographic findings of severe osteoarthritis, and cases of ON may be misclassified as osteoarthritis. Fortunately, at that stage treatment is the same for both disease processes [12].

Aratake et al. looked at the use of fluoride PET imaging to evaluate SPONK. They found that fluoride PET scans could detect SPONK and measure lesions with comparative accuracy to radiographs and MRI. Further research will be needed to determine if it or other imaging techniques will provide additional prognostic or diagnostic information [18].

55.8 Diagnosis

The diagnosis of SPONK is heavily based on the history with sudden onset of pain with no identifiable etiology for ON. Secondary ON will have an identifiable cause in the patient's history. Imaging helps confirm the diagnosis, but in the early stages, the findings on imaging are not specific. Osteochondritis dissecans is on the differential, but it is more often found in patients younger than 25 years old and located to a single condyle without affecting other parts of the joint. Also, imaging would demonstrate the separation of articular cartilage with subchondral bone [1]. Other causes of knee pain could include meniscus and ligament injuries that would present with other clinical and imaging findings [10]. Osteoarthritis can have similar symptoms, but it usually has a more chronic and progressive onset of pain.

There are studies being conducted to find additional markers for SPONK such as serum or synovial fluid markers. Synovial levels of chondroitin 6-sulfate have been found to be significantly greater in cases of SPONK than medial compartment osteoarthritis. Studies evaluating serum markers such as bone-specific ALP, osteocalcin, procollagen type I N-terminal propeptide, and C-terminal cross-linking telopeptide did not have any difference between osteoarthritis and SPONK [24]. Further research may be able to identify other markers either in synovial fluid or serum that can help distinguish osteoarthritis from ON. Although with the current treatment options, the clinical utility of distinguishing the two remains to be seen.

55.9 Treatment and Clinical Results

55.9.1 General Principles

Treatment of osteonecrosis of the knee depends on the extent of disease. Early lesions may be treated with nonoperative or joint-preserving techniques. Advanced osteonecrosis may require a joint replacement [25]. Historically, the treatment options for osteonecrosis of the knee include conservative management, arthrotomy with curettage, high tibial

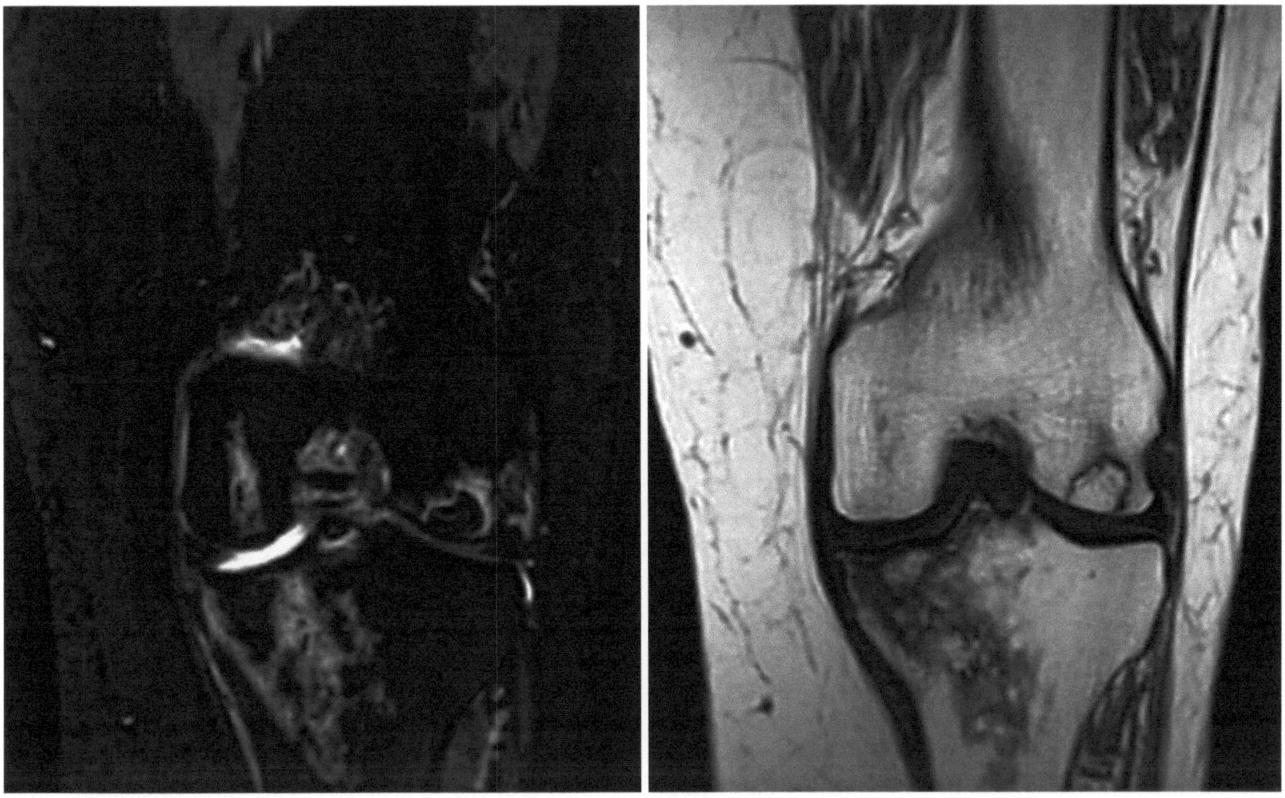

Figs. 55.2 and 55.3 Coronal MRI images suggestive of osteonecrotic regions in the distal femur and the proximal tibia

osteotomy, and arthroplasty [20]. Conservative options include weight loss, analgesics, isometric quadriceps exercises [20], and protected weight-bearing with assistive devices [26]. Traditionally, these options have been reserved for patients with small osteonecrotic lesions with mild symptoms. Muheim and Bohne recommended conservative treatment for patients with small osteonecrotic lesions less than 3.5 cm^2 in area and tibial osteotomy with arthrotomy for those with large osteonecrotic lesions exceeding 5 cm [19, 21]. Initial treatment for patients diagnosed with osteonecrosis involves conservative management for at least 3 months duration [26]. Arthrotomy with curettage is performed in cases with large lesions [20]. These patients have minimal osteoarthritic changes and no significant knee deformity. In cases of significant varus deformity of the knee, high tibial osteotomy may be performed [20]. The ideal correction is to obtain a femorotibial angle of 170° (10° valgus) [20]. Arthroplasty is reserved for large lesions with degenerative changes and possible malalignment of the knee [20].

Modern techniques are also focused on joint-preserving therapies prior to arthroplasty [26]. Patients that remain symptomatic after at least 3 months of conservative management may undergo diagnostic arthroscopy of the affected knee. If diffuse chondral lesions and subchondral collapse are noted, chondroplasty and debridement of loose tissue can be performed 26. If intra-articular pathology such as meniscal lesions is found, appropriate debridement and meniscectomy are performed [26]. After diagnostic or therapeutic arthroscopy, percutaneous core decompression of the osteonecrotic lesion may be performed using a small-diameter drill bit through an extra-articular approach [26]. Focal chondral defects can be treated with osteochondral autologous transfer from less weight-bearing regions of the articular cartilage of the knee [26]. Patients who remain symptomatic despite repeat core decompressions, or who progress to condylar collapse despite joint-preserving surgical treatment, are indicated to undergo total or unicompartmental knee arthroplasty (UKA) [26]. A recent systematic review of the literature between 1999 and 2012 showed that among joint-preserving procedures, core decompression prevented additional surgical treatment in pre-collapse knees with a failure rate of 10.4 %. Autogenous and osteochondral grafts decreased the need for additional surgery in both pre-collapse 0 % and post-collapse knees 10.5 % [27].

55.9.2 Bisphosphonates

Bisphosphonates, such as alendronate, have been used successfully to treat osteonecrosis of the femoral head, as they may prevent bone resorption during the reparative phases of osteonecrosis [25]. Another bisphosphonate, neridronate, is used primarily for the treatment of Paget disease and osteoporosis [25]. Corrado et al. [28] explored the use of this medication as a nonoperative treatment for osteonecrosis of the knee. Their patient had reduced pain and swelling after 2 months of this medication combined with analgesics. Their treatment protocol included 100 mg/day of aspirin, 0.5 μg of calcitriol, and 25 mg/month of intramuscular neridronate. An MRI scan obtained 2 months after initiation of treatment showed decreased bone marrow edema and reduction in the size of the necrotic lesions.

55.9.3 Antitumor Necrosis Factor Alpha (Anti-TNF-Alpha) Agents

Tumor necrosis factor alpha (TNF-alpha) has been identified as the compound that regulates production of interleukin-1 in rheumatoid arthritis which can be treated with anti-TNF-alpha medications such as adalimumab [29, 30]. A case report demonstrates that a 54-year-old man with monoarticular rheumatoid arthritis and osteonecrosis of the left knee, who failed corticosteroids and systemic treatment, was given a 40-mg intra-articular injection of adalimumab, and 1 week later, pain and stiffness resolved and range of motion improved. The patient was given a second injection 15 days later, and an MRI taken 1 month thereafter showed healing of the osteonecrotic lesion [31].

Although the role of anti-TNF-alpha medications in osteonecrosis is not understood, they may affect the cytokines responsible for the osteoclast progenitor cell regulation [29]. In this case, it is difficult to determine whether the change in MRI findings represents resolution of an osteonecrotic lesion or only bony edema associated with degenerative changes [25].

55.9.4 Core Decompression

Jacobs et al. were the first to describe the treatment of osteonecrosis of the knee using core decompression [32]. However, prior to the knee, core decompression was used successfully in the treatment of osteonecrosis of the hip [33]. Marulanda et al. used core decompression and modified the procedure with the percutaneous drilling of 3-mm holes in each of 61 knees (38 patients; average follow-up, 3 years; range, 2–4 years) [34]. They reported a 92 % (56 knees) successful clinical outcome, which they defined as a postoperative Knee Society score of 80 or more points. Two knees with poor outcomes were treated with total knee arthroplasty (TKA) and had postoperative Knee Society scores of 90 and 91 points. Of the remaining three knees with poor outcomes, two were treated with bilateral arthroscopic debridement and one with a bone grafting procedure. At the latest follow-up, however, these three knees were still categorized as having poor outcomes (Knee Society scores <80 points). The authors reported low rates of complications and morbidity with core decompression [34].

55.9.5 Biologic Substitutes

A new technique combines artificial bone grafting and core decompression for selected patients with SPONK [35]. In this study, there were strict primary and secondary indications for identifying which patients were to receive this procedure. Primary indications included a diagnosis of SPONK in the medial femoral condyle and a femorotibial angle between 173° and 179°. A secondary indication was a patient's inability to undergo TKA or high tibial osteotomy because of other diseases. The authors treated 12 patients with this combination approach, which involved decompression and grafting, using a calcium hydroxyapatite ceramic device with an interconnected porous structure (IP-CHA; NEOBONE®, Toshiba Ceramics Company, Tokyo, Japan). The lesions were curetted, and grafting was accomplished with the artificial bone plugs in a mosaicplasty fashion. After an average 2-year follow-up, 12 patients had a statistically significant improvement in the Japanese Orthopedic Association score assessing pain on walking, pain on ascending or descending, range of motion, and joint effusion. MRI scans showed smooth surfaces between the bone graft and the femur in nine (75 %) of 12 patients. There was, however, no histologic evaluation for the presence of osteonecrosis [35]. Larger study groups and long-term follow-up are required before the combination of core decompression (a proven technique) with artificial bone grafting can be considered an option of choice

Adachi et al. described a similar treatment for a patient with corticosteroid-induced osteonecrosis [36]. In addition to building the bony scaffold, clinicians added tissue-engineered cartilage and autologous bone graft. That patient had two large defects, one each on the medial and lateral femoral condyles. Cartilage was harvested from the unaffected knee, and 2.0×106 chondrocytes were extracted, embedded in atelocollagen solution (3 % type I collagen; Koken Co., Ltd., Tokyo, Japan), and allowed to culture for 25 days. The bony defects were grafted using a hydroxyapatite scaffold with interconnected pores, and autologous mesenchymal stem cells harvested and prepared from the iliac crest were added. The tissue-engineered cartilage was used to repair the lesion of the medial femoral condyle; the lateral defect was treated with interconnected porous calcium hydroxyapatite ceramic implants alone. One year after the procedure, the lesions were evaluated arthroscopically. The medial lesion had filled in, whereas the lateral lesion (without the tissue-engineered cartilage) had not. Histologic evaluation showed fibrous and cartilaginous tissue from the medial condyle construct, but it appeared to be deficient in proteoglycans compared with normal cartilage. At the 2-year follow-up, MRI showed smooth congruous tissue covering the medial condyle, and the patient reported a reduction in pain and a full return of function.

These techniques are still early in development. However, they may prove to be useful adjuncts to the current joint-preserving options available.

55.9.6 Arthroplasty

The orthopedic community is excited about the prospects of UKA in osteonecrosis of the knee [26, 37]. Parratte et al. reviewed the records of 30 consecutive patients, seen over 13 years, who had osteonecrosis of the knee and who had been treated with UKA [37]. 21 knees had spontaneous osteonecrosis, and 10 knees had secondary osteonecrosis. Cemented metal-backed prostheses (Miller-Galante; Zimmer, Warsaw, Indiana) were used in all patients. No patients were lost to follow-up, and all showed a statistically significant improvement in postoperative Knee Society Knee and Function scores. At 12-year follow-up, the survival rate for the 31 knees, based on a Kaplan Meier survivorship analysis was 96.7 ± 3 %, with one revision because of aseptic loosening. The revision was a conversion to a TKA that occurred 30 months after the initial surgery, resulted in a knee with no additional complications. The study showed excellent results with this technique, but its findings are limited because it was a retrospective review without a control group [37]. Further refinements in the technique and instrumentation associated with UKA may lead to great strides in the treatment armamentarium for osteonecrosis of the knee.

References

1. Mont MA, Baumgarten KM, Rifai A, Bluemke DA, Jones LC, Hungerford DS. Atraumatic osteonecrosis of the knee. J Bone Joint Surg Am. 2000;82(9):1279–90.
2. Ahlback S, Bauer GC, Bohne WH. Spontaneous osteonecrosis of the knee. Arthritis Rheum. 1968;11(6):705–33.
3. Cetik O, Cift H, Comert B, Cirpar M. Risk of osteonecrosis of the femoral condyle after arthroscopic chondroplasty using radiofrequency: a prospective clinical series. Knee Surg Sports Traumatol Arthrosc. 2009;17(1):24–9.
4. Ohdera T, Miyagi S, Tokunaga M, Yoshimoto E, Matsuda S, Ikari H. Spontaneous osteonecrosis of the lateral femoral condyle of the knee: a report of 11 cases. Arch Orthop Trauma Surg. 2008;128(8):825–31.
5. Akamatsu Y, Mitsugi N, Hayashi T, Kobayashi H, Saito T. Low bone mineral density is associated with the onset of spontaneous osteonecrosis of the knee. Acta Orthop. 2012;83(3):249–55.
6. Mears SC, McCarthy EF, Jones LC, Hungerford DS, Mont MA. Characterization and pathological characteristics of spontaneous osteonecrosis of the knee. Iowa Orthop J. 2009;29:38–42.
7. Shenoy PM, Shetty GM, Kim DH, Wang KH, Choi JY, Nha KW. Osteonecrosis of the lateral femoral condyle following anterior cruciate ligament reconstruction: is bone bruising a risk factor? Arch Orthop Trauma Surg. 2010;130(3):413–6.
8. Nixon SA, O'Brien KK, Rubin G. Nonsurgical management of severe osteonecrosis of the knee in an HIV-positive patient: a case report. Case Rep Infect Dis. 2011;2011:935041.
9. Powell C, Chang C, Gershwin ME. Current concepts on the pathogenesis and natural history of steroid-induced osteonecrosis. Clin Rev Allergy Immunol. 2011;41(1):102–13.
10. Mont MA, Marker DR, Zywiel MG, Carrino JA. Osteonecrosis of the knee and related conditions. J Am Acad Orthop Surg. 2011; 19(8):482–94.
11. Gortz S, De Young AJ, Bugbee WD. Fresh osteochondral allografting for steroid-associated osteonecrosis of the femoral condyles. Clin Orthop Relat Res. 2010;468(5):1269–78.
12. Jung KA, Lee SC, Hwang SH, Kim DS, Kim TK. Spontaneous osteonecrosis of the knee involving both the medial femoral condyle and the medial tibial plateau: report of three cases. Knee Surg Sports Traumatol Arthrosc. 2008;16(8):759–62.
13. Kraenzlin ME, Graf C, Meier C, Kraenzlin C, Friedrich NF. Possible beneficial effect of bisphosphonates in osteonecrosis of the knee. Knee Surg Sports Traumatol Arthrosc. 2010;18(12):1638–44.
14. Soucacos PN, Xenakis TH, Beris AE, Soucacos PK, Georgoulis A. Idiopathic osteonecrosis of the medial femoral condyle. Classification and treatment. Clin Orthop Relat Res. 1997;341: 82–9.
15. Banzer W, Hubscher M, Schikora D. Laser-needle therapy for spontaneous osteonecrosis of the knee. Photomed Laser Surg. 2008; 26(4):301–6.
16. Shigemura T, Nakamura J, Kishida S, et al. The incidence of alcohol-associated osteonecrosis of the knee is lower than the incidence of steroid-associated osteonecrosis of the knee: an MRI study. Rheumatology (Oxford). 2012;51(4):701–6.
17. Yates PJ, Calder JD, Stranks GJ, Conn KS, Peppercorn D, Thomas NP. Early MRI diagnosis and non-surgical management of spontaneous osteonecrosis of the knee. Knee. 2007;14(2):112–6.
18. Aratake M, Yoshifumi T, Takahashi A, Takeuchi R, Inoue T, Saito T. Evaluation of lesion in a spontaneous osteonecrosis of the knee using 18 F-fluoride positron emission tomography. Knee Surg Sports Traumatol Arthrosc. 2009;17(1):53–9.
19. Motohashi M, Morii T, Koshino T. Clinical course and roentgenographic changes of osteonecrosis in the femoral condyle under conservative treatment. Clin Orthop Relat Res. 1991;266:156–61.
20. Aglietti P, Insall JN, Buzzi R, Deschamps G. Idiopathic osteonecrosis of the knee. aetiology, prognosis and treatment. J Bone Joint Surg Br. 1983;65(5):588–97.
21. Muheim G, Bohne WH. Prognosis in spontaneous osteonecrosis of the knee. investigation by radionuclide scintimetry and radiography. J Bone Joint Surg Br. 1970;52(4):605–12.
22. Lotke P, Abend J, Ecker M. The treatment of osteonecrosis of the medial femoral condyle. Clin Orthop Relat Res. 1982;171:109–16.
23. Lotke PA, Ecker ML. Osteonecrosis of the knee. J Bone Joint Surg Am. 1988;70(3):470–3.
24. Berger CE, Kroner A, Kristen KH, Minai-Pour M, Leitha T, Engel A. Spontaneous osteonecrosis of the knee: biochemical markers of bone turnover and pathohistology. Osteoarthritis Cartilage. 2005;13(8):716–21.
25. Goddard MS, Khanuja HS. Osteonecrosis of the knee. Curr Orthop Pract. 2009;20(1):65–72.
26. Duany NG, Zywiel MG, McGrath MS, et al. Joint-preserving surgical treatment of spontaneous osteonecrosis of the knee. Arch Orthop Trauma Surg. 2010;130(1):11–6.
27. Lieberman JR, Varthi AG, Polkowski 2nd GG. Osteonecrosis of the knee – which joint preservation procedures work? J Arthroplasty. 2014;29(1):52–6.

28. Corrado A, Quarta L, Errico S, Cantatore FP. Successful treatment of avascular bone necrosis of the knee with neridronate: a case report. Rheumatol Int. 2007;27(9):891–3.
29. Joosten LA, Helsen MM, Saxne T, van De Loo FA, Heinegard D, van Den Berg WB. IL-1 alpha beta blockade prevents cartilage and bone destruction in murine type II collagen-induced arthritis, whereas TNF-alpha blockade only ameliorates joint inflammation. J Immunol. 1999;163(9):5049–55.
30. Elliott MJ, Maini RN, Feldmann M, et al. Randomised double-blind comparison of chimeric monoclonal antibody to tumour necrosis factor alpha (cA2) versus placebo in rheumatoid arthritis. Lancet. 1994;344(8930):1105–10.
31. Kobak S. Osteonecrosis and monoarticular rheumatoid arthritis treated with intra-articular adalimumab. Mod Rheumatol. 2008;18(3):290–2.
32. Jacobs MA, Loeb PE, Hungerford DS. Core decompression of the distal femur for avascular necrosis of the knee. J Bone Joint Surg Br. 1989;71(4):583–7.
33. Hungerford DS, Zizic TM. II. the treatment of ischemic necrosis of bone in systemic lupus erythematosus. Medicine (Baltimore). 1980;59(2):143–8.
34. Marulanda G, Seyler TM, Sheikh NH, Mont MA. Percutaneous drilling for the treatment of secondary osteonecrosis of the knee. J Bone Joint Surg Br. 2006;88(6):740–6.
35. Deie M, Ochi M, Adachi N, Nishimori M, Yokota K. Artificial bone grafting [calcium hydroxyapatite ceramic with an interconnected porous structure (IP-CHA)] and core decompression for spontaneous osteonecrosis of the femoral condyle in the knee. Knee Surg Sports Traumatol Arthrosc. 2008;16(8):753–8.
36. Adachi N, Ochi M, Deie M, Ishikawa M, Ito Y. Osteonecrosis of the knee treated with a tissue-engineered cartilage and bone implant. A case report. J Bone Joint Surg Am. 2007;89(12):2752–7.
37. Parratte S, Argenson JN, Dumas J, Aubaniac JM. Unicompartmental knee arthroplasty for avascular osteonecrosis. Clin Orthop Relat Res. 2007;464:37–42.

Osteonecrosis of the Talus

56

Kyoung Min Lee, Sung Hun Won, and Moon Seok Park

56.1 Introduction

Osteonecrosis of the talus (ONT) refers to the death of osteocytes and subsequent structural changes leading to talus collapse and secondary ankle joint osteoarthritis. ONT is a rarer disease than osteonecrosis of the femoral head (ONFH); however it is a significant clinical challenge with an uncertain long-term prognosis [1, 2]. In this chapter, we review osteonecrosis of the talus, describing incidence and etiology, blood supply, clinical presentation, diagnostic imaging, classification, and treatment.

56.2 Incidence and Etiology

Epidemiologic studies reporting the incidence and etiology of osteonecrosis of the talus are limited [2]. The major causes of osteonecrosis of the talus are associated with trauma, especially talus fracture [3, 4]. Nontraumatic osteonecrosis is reported as steroid induced [5, 6], resulting from alcohol abuse [6], systemic lupus erythematosus [7], hyperuricemia [8], renal transplantation [9], sickle cell anemia [10, 11], hyperlipidemia [12], and pancreatitis [7]. We report the incidence and etiology of osteonecrosis of the talus divided into "traumatic" and "nontraumatic."

56.2.1 Traumatic Osteonecrosis

The most common causes of osteonecrosis of the talus are traumatic, especially talar neck fracture. Hawkins et al. [3] reported 53 % of talar neck fractures develop osteonecrosis of the talus. They reported that a Hawkins type 1 is a nondisplaced talar neck fracture and has 0–15 % osteonecrosis of the talus risk while type 2 is a talar neck fracture associated with a subluxation or a dislocation of the subtalar joint and has a 20–50 %. Type 3 is a talar neck fracture associated with subluxation or dislocation of the subtalar and ankle joint and has a 90 % risk, and type 4 is a talar neck fracture associated with subluxation or dislocation of the subtalar, ankle, and talonavicular joints and has a 100 % risk of osteonecrosis [3]. Canale and Kelly also reported a high rate of osteonecrosis: 52 % of 71 talar neck fractures [4]. Furthermore, they reported that increased displacement and fracture grading by Hawkins' classification of talar neck fracture were associated with an increased risk of osteonecrosis [4]. Vallier et al. [13] reported that 38 % of 38 patients who underwent surgery of the talar body developed osteonecrosis. Six of these patients, however, had concomitant fractures of talar neck.

56.2.2 Nontraumatic Osteonecrosis

Several nontraumatic causes have been described. Delanois et al. [5] reported that 20 of 24 patients had a history of corticosteroid use. In that study, four patients had a history of regular alcohol use and 16 had immunologic disorders, including systemic lupus erythematosus, scleroderma, diabetes mellitus, and multiple sclerosis. Other disorders that have been associated with osteonecrosis of the talus include hyperlipidemia [12], hyperuricemia [8], renal transplantation [9], sickle cell anemia [10, 11], and pancreatitis [7]. Furthermore, iatrogenic osteonecrosis of the talus also has been reported following hindfoot surgery, such as arthrosis and triple arthrodesis [2] (Table 56.1).

56.3 Blood Supply of the Talus

The blood supply comes mainly from the extraosseous and the intraosseous circulation [14, 15]. The extraosseous circulation, with contributions from the anterior tibial,

K.M. Lee (✉) • S.H. Won • M.S. Park
Department of Orthopaedic Surgery, Seoul National University Bundang Hospital, Seongnam 463-707, South Korea
e-mail: oasis100@empal.com; orthowon@gmail.com; pmsmed@gmail.com

K.-H. Koo et al. (eds.), *Osteonecrosis*,
DOI 10.1007/978-3-642-35767-1_56, © Springer-Verlag Berlin Heidelberg 2014

Table 56.1 Etiological factors associated with osteonecrosis of the talus

Etiology
Traumatic
Talar neck fracture
Talar body fracture
Nontraumatic
Steroids
Alcohol
Systemic lupus erythematosus
Hyperuricemia
Renal transplantation
Sickle cell anemia
Hyperlipidemia
Pancreatitis
Iatrogenic

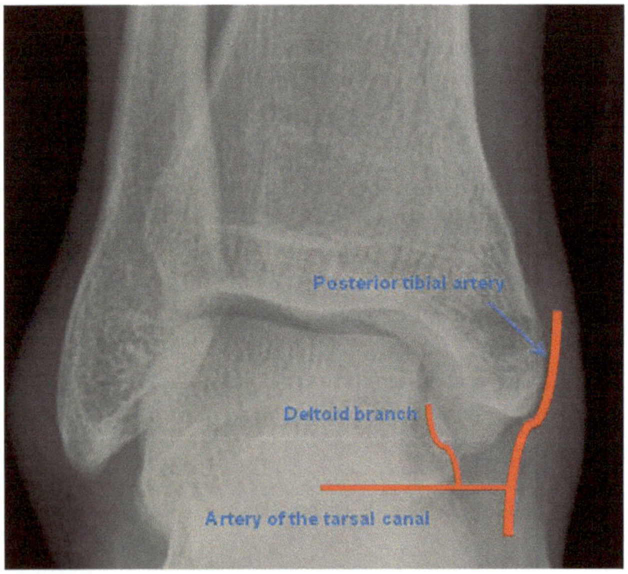

Fig. 56.1 Blood supply of the talus

posterior tibial, and peroneal artery, forms a vascular extraosseous ring around the talar neck and sinus tarsi [14, 15]. The artery of the tarsal canal, a branch of the posterior tibial artery, provides the main blood supply to the body of the talus [16, 17] (Fig. 56.1). Deltoid and posterior tubercle branches from the posterior tibial artery enter the medial talar body and posterior tubercle, respectively [15]. The artery of the sinus tarsi, a branch of the peroneal artery, runs from lateral to medial inferior to the talar neck and eventually anastomoses with the artery of the tarsal canal to form a vascular "sling" beneath the neck of the talus [2]. The dorsalis pedis artery contributes to several branches that enter the talus through the superior neck [16]. The intraosseous anastomoses are variable among individuals and may explain why some patients develop osteonecrosis of talus and while others do not [15, 18]. A complete intraosseous anastomosis between all regions of the talus has been found in 60 % of talar anatomic specimens [14–16]. The talar head has an abundant vasculature, supplied primarily by the anterior tibial artery [14, 16].

56.4 Clinical Presentation

Clinicians should obtain information from patients by careful history taking of trauma, medical history, steroid use, systemic disease, and immunologic disorders. In early precollapse period, patients complain of their ankle pain predominantly [2]. With more advanced disease, articular collapse can lead to mechanical symptoms, such as locking and catching. Physical examination may be unremarkable, especially in early precollapse period. In postcollapse period, however, a joint effusion and joint line tenderness usually can be detected. In severe cases that are characterized by talar dome collapse, range of motion is limited and varus or valgus malalignment may be present [2].

56.5 Diagnostic Imaging

56.5.1 Radiographs

Despite the advent of more advanced imaging modalities, radiographs still play a critical role in the evaluation of osteonecrosis of the talus [2]. The body's response to osteonecrosis is an attempt at repair by means of reossification, revascularization, and resorption of necrotic bone [19]. At initial radiography, necrotic bone and the surrounding viable bone are equal in opacity, and early stages can be missed [20]. As time passes and hyperemia results, healthy bone is resorbed and subsequently becomes osteopenic [20]. Conversely, the lack of blood supply in necrotic bone prevents its resorption, making necrotic bone appear more radiopaque than the surrounding osteopenic bone. At that point, radiographic evidence of osteonecrosis becomes apparent. The opacity of necrotic bone continues to increase as reossification occurs and new bone is laid down over necrotic trabeculae. This process accounts for the typical sclerotic image seen in osteonecrosis of the talus. In addition to reossification, revascularization and resorption also tend to occur around necrotic bone. When these processes occur, a radiolucent rim becomes apparent around the area of osteonecrosis [19, 21]. Radiographs are especially useful following open reduction and internal fixation of displaced talar neck and body fractures [2]. Hawkins' sign is characterized by subchondral osteopenia on anteroposterior or mortise radiographs [3]. Typically, it is present at 6–8 weeks and results from the resorption of subchondral bone in the setting of disuse and a sufficient vascular supply [3]. Canale and Kelly evaluated the reliability of Hawkins' sign at 12 weeks postoperatively in 49 patients [4]. They found that 20 of 26 (77 %) fractures that did not have subchondral osteopenia developed osteonecrosis. However, one of 23 cases that had a positive Hawkins' sign went on to osteonecrosis. Thus Hawkins' sign is a reliable indicator of talar viability and its presence serves as an early negative predictor of osteonecrosis [2–4]. The absence of Hawkins' sign, however, does not confirm osteonecrosis, because it has greater sensitivity than specificity [2–4].

56.5.2 MRI

MR imaging is the most sensitive technique for detecting osteonecrosis of the talus, especially in the early stages [20]. In addition, MR imaging is considered more anatomically detailed and accurate than radiographs and scintigraphy in its ability to identify the extent of talar body involvement [22]. On MR imaging, osteonecrosis of the talus typically is characterized by low signal on T1-weighted images [2]. On T2-weighted images, osteonecrosis produces a mixed and variable appearance that depends on the contents of the avascular region [2]. However, MR imaging non-contrast enhanced is a problem due to the confusing picture of bone edema and ONT having a similar appearance [23]. We recommend MR imaging with contrast such as gadolinium enhancement for accurate diagnosis on early stage of ONT and should be combined with the clinical findings.

56.5.3 Computer Tomography

Computer tomography (CT) scans also reveal characteristic osteonecrosis of the talus patterns and can be used to confirm radiographic findings. The CT arthrogram is a especially helpful method to evaluate the volume and location of the remaining dead bone and associated cartilage damage [23]. Coronal CT of the talus is required for viewing the articular surface of the talar dome to rule out subtle depression, collapse, and fragmentation, especially at preoperative assessment [20] (Fig. 56.2).

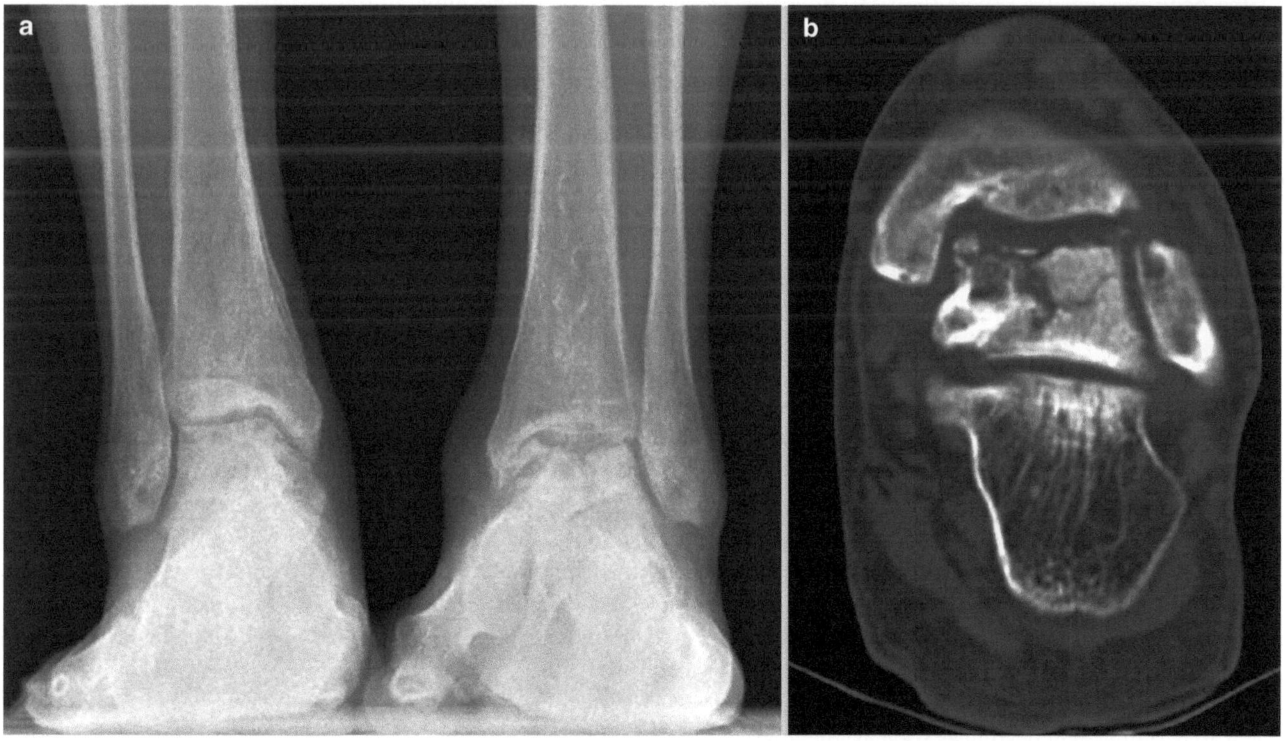

Fig. 56.2 (**a**) Both ankle anteroposterior radiograph while standing of a 33-year-old woman who had a 1-year history of pain in the ankle and loss of motion. She was receiving steroids for systemic lupus erythematosus more than 10 years with 12.5 mg qd. She underwent total hip arthroplasty bilaterally, because of the osteonecrosis of the femoral head. There is a collapse of the talus and joint space narrowing, subchondral sclerosis of the tibia on her left ankle (stage IV osteonecrosis, according to the system of Ficat and Alert modified for the ankle by Mont), and focal radiolucent lesion, subchondral cyst, and subcondral sclerotic change of the talus were shown in her right ankle (stage II). (**b**) Coronal CT scan of the left ankle shows collapse of the articular surface of the talar dome, vertical and horizontal split fracture extending from the talar dome into the talar body. Also there is sclerotic line within the talar body that represents necrotic bone

56.6 Classification

Mont et al. [24] classified osteonecrosis of the talus with the system of Ficat and Arlet, as modified for the ankle. A stage I is characterized by normal radiographs, whereas stage II disease is characterized by cystic or osteosclerotic lesions, normal talar contour, and no subchondral fracture. With stage III disease there is a crescent sign or subchondral collapse, and with type IV disease, arthritic changes are present. The investigators used this staging system as a general guide to treatment and divided cases into either "precollapse disease" (stages I and II) or "postcollapse disease" (stages III and IV).

Thordarson et al. [22] went on to develop a classification system of osteonecrosis that is based on the amount of talar body involvement on MR imaging. Type A has homogeneous signal throughout the body of the talus, type B has signal changes in up to 25 % of the body of the talus, type C has 25–50 %, and type D has more than 50 %. This system was used to guide postoperative weight bearing following open reduction and internal fixation of talar neck fractures. If less than 25 % of the body was involved (type A or B), weight bearing was advanced as tolerated. If more than 25 % of the body was involved (type C of D), protected weight bearing for upward of 6 months was recommended.

56.7 Treatment

56.7.1 Conservative Treatment

The presence of osteonecrosis of the talus before collapse is initially treated nonoperatively. The nonoperative treatment options include applying a short-leg cast, ankle-foot orthosis with analgesics, and no weight bearing [25]. Some previous studies recommend extended non-weight bearing [3, 26]. Others have recommended a patella tendon bearing brace until reconstitution of the talar body is complete [27–29]. However, because the creeping substitution of the talar body can require 36 months to occur, patient compliance is rarely possible for 36 months [1, 30]. Penny et al. [31] reported that weight bearing on sclerotic and osteonecrosis of the talus poses no danger for talar dome collapse and found no relation between poor results with osteonecrosis of the talus and time of non-weight bearing. Therefore, the current consensus is to permit weight bearing as soon as tolerable.

56.7.2 Surgical Treatment

Several treatment options are available for osteonecrosis of the talus. However, surgical treatment options for symptomatic osteonecrosis of the talus are limited. These are core decompression, allograft reconstruction, vascularized autograft reconstruction for early precollapse stage, and arthrodesis and arthroplasty for late postcollapse stage [24, 25, 32–38].

56.7.2.1 For Early Precollapse Stage

Core Decompression

Core decompression is a surgical treatment for the early stage of osteonecrosis. The rationale for core decompression is that it decreases intraosseous pressure and may immediately relieve the associated pain [25]. Mont et al. [24] reported on 17 ankles who had core decompression for symptomatic osteonecrosis of the talus before collapse, with 82 % having an excellent or good outcome. The authors concluded core decompression is a viable method of treatment for symptomatic osteonecrosis of the talus before collapse. Recently Marulanda et al. [39] reported that the percutaneous drilling technique appears to be a satisfactory method for treating osteonecrosis of the talus and is associated with low operative morbidity.

Allograft Reconstruction

Osteonecrosis of the talus involving only the talar dome with ankle joint arthritis can be addressed with fresh osteochondral total ankle allograft transplantation [1]. Gross et al. [33] reported nine cases of osteochondral defects of the talus treated with fresh osteochondral allograft transplantation. All underwent partial talar allograft transplantation and the survival rate at 11 years was six out of nine patients. Jeng et al. [34] reported 29 patients that underwent bipolar osteochondral allograft, including two patients with osteonecrosis of the talus treated, and had 50 % success rate. However, there are no long-term results for talar allograft survival rates.

Vascularized Autograft Reconstruction

Hussl et al. [35] reported use of a vascularized bone graft from the iliac crest for revascularization of the talus in posttraumatic osteonecrosis. Gilbert et al. [36] reported 14 fresh-frozen cadaver lower extremities and were able to identify a consistent blood supply to the distal fibula, cuboid, and cuneiforms I and III with reliable nutrient arteries. The transverse pedicle branch of the proximal lateral tarsal artery reached and supplied the cuboid in every specimen. The first cuneiform was found to be supplied by the middle pedicle branch of the distal medial tarsal artery. Basically, the same is true for the next pedicle of the transverse branch to the third cuneiform off the distal lateral tarsal artery. The fourth potential vascular pedicle was a transverse segment of the anterior lateral malleolar artery to the lateral malleolus. The identification of these new rotational vascular pedicle bone grafts could help to treat osteonecrosis of the talus using a vascularized bone graft. Zhang et al. [37] reported on the curative effect of vascularized bone graft in the treatment of 24 cases, with success rate of 83.3 % at 3–5 years follow-up. There are no long-term results yet.

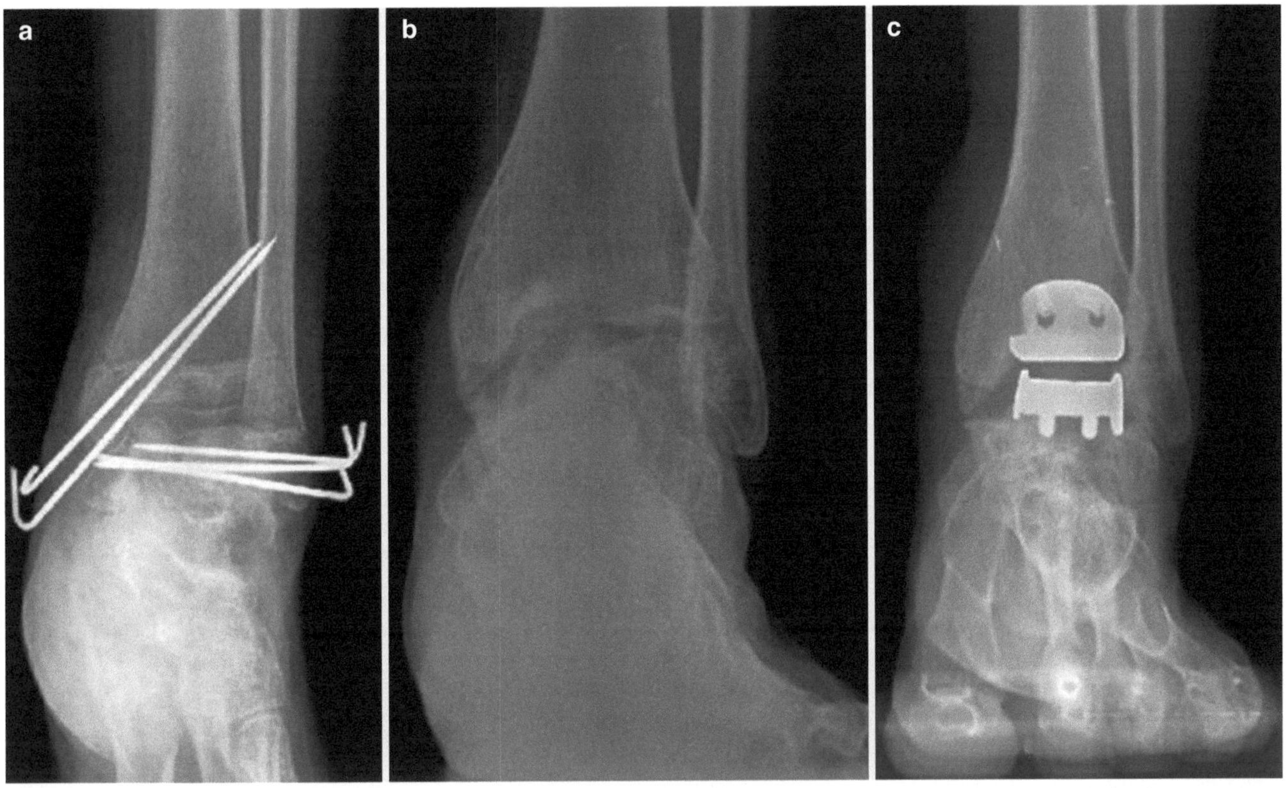

Fig. 56.3 (**a**) Left ankle anteroposterior radiograph of 13-year-old boy who had a talar fracture and a medial malleolar fracture on his left ankle. He underwent open reduction and internal fixation. (**b**) Six years later, his left ankle had a collapse of the talus and joint space narrowing (stage IV osteonecrosis, according to the system of Ficat and Alert modified for the ankle by Mont). (**c**) At 1 year after total ankle arthroplasty, anteroposterior radiograph of the left ankle showed a stable bone-implant interface with no evidence of loosening or subsidence

56.7.2.2 For Late Postcollapse Stage

Arthrodesis

Ankle arthrodesis is a reliable treatment for osteonecrosis of the talus with collapse in cases where symptoms are isolated to the ankle joint [32, 40]. Sufficient talus bone stock following debridement of the osteonecrosis is required for adequate fixation of the ankle joint [1]. Structural defects of the talus are filled with a structural auto- or allograft. Standard fixation for ankle arthrodesis includes multiplanar screws or plate fixation [1]. Prior study report a union rate of 96 % with anterior plate fixation [1]. Antegrade nailing of the ankle joint has been described, but with suboptimal results because of bad fixation in the talus [1]. External fixation has also been used to achieve an ankle fusion [41]. A recent systematic review of intermediate and long-term outcomes of ankle arthrodesis noted that nonunion was observed in 10 % of the patients treated with ankle arthrodesis and 9 % of the arthrodesis group underwent revision [42]. Thus, recently, higher success rates have been achieved using various techniques. Success of ankle arthrodesis also depended on patient factors. Ankle arthrodesis is technically challenging for osteonecrosis of the talus comorbid rheumatoid or osteoarthritis because of the difficulty in achieving well-vascularized bony surfaces for fusion [32]. Frey et al. [43] reported that eight of nine patients showed nonunion. Another study also showed low fusion rate, 38 % in such patients [44]. Therefore ankle arthrodesis is technically demanding and requires a longer period of immobilization for patients with rheumatoid or osteoarthritis compared with other patients [32, 43, 44]. In cases of severe talus collapse, tibiocalcaneal arthrodesis with talectomy and tibiotalocalcaneal arthrodesis were some kind of methods for hindfoot arthrodesis [45]. Tibiocalcaneal arthrodesis was needed to remove the entire talar body, so without structural grafting, this method has poor results because it shortens the leg [45, 46].

Ankle Arthroplasty

Ankle arthroplasty requires a stable and solid bony surface to support the implant over time. Complete debridement of the necrotic bone will often prevent a standard ankle arthroplasty [1]. Historically, osteonecrosis of the talus is accepted as a contraindication of ankle arthroplasty, because of the high rate of talar component subsidence, especially with the Agility prosthesis (Depuy, Warsaw, IN) [47, 48]. However, with the development of newer generations of prostheses that have improved surface coverage of the talus, osteonecrosis of the talus is no longer a contraindication of ankle arthroplasty [49–51] (Fig. 56.3). Ankle arthroplasty is a recent alternative to fusion for osteonecrosis of the talus but long-term outcomes are not yet reported. Harnroongroj and

Vanadurongwan [38] reported satisfactory results of talar body prosthetic replacement in 14 of 16 patients, with average follow-up of 9.5 years. A recent systemic review studies about intermediate and long-term outcomes of total ankle arthroplasty reported that the 5-year implant survival rates ranged from 78 to 85.9 %, the 10-year survival rates were 71–77 %, and the revision rates ranged from 7 to 11.1 %, with the main reason for revisions being aseptic loosening (5.2–28 %) [42]. These studies showed that the 5- and 10-year survival rates were acceptable. However, the failure rate was still high. We recommend that while ankle arthroplasty is one treatment option for osteonecrosis of the talus, clinicians should be careful in selecting the appropriate indications.

56.8 Summary

Despite the development of diagnostic tools and surgical treatment, osteonecrosis of the talus remains a challenging problem for clinicians, because it has unclear and partially understood natural history, pathophysiology, and long-term outcomes of treatment. Further study is necessary to understand this complex disorder fully. However, it is clear that most osteonecrosis of talus is traumatically induced in association with talar neck and body fractures, and other systemic disorders may cause osteonecrosis of the talus. Clinicians should obtain information from patients by careful history taking. Furthermore, it is best treated at early precollapse period with conservative methods such as casts and braces with non-weight bearing. Once prolonged non-weight bearing has failed, another treatment option should be considered, such as core decompression, or bone grafting. At the late postcollapse period, arthrodesis or arthroplasty should be considered.

References

1. Leduc S, Clare MP, Laflamme GY, Walling AK. Posttraumatic avascular necrosis of the talus. Foot Ankle Clin. 2008;13(4):753–65. doi:10.1016/j.fcl.2008.09.004.
2. Chiodo CP, Herbst SA. Osteonecrosis of the talus. Foot and ankle clinics. 2004;9(4):745–55, vi. doi:10.1016/j.fcl.2004.07.002.
3. Hawkins LG. Fractures of the neck of the talus. J Bone Joint Surg Am. 1970;52(5):991–1002.
4. Canale ST, Kelly Jr FB. Fractures of the neck of the talus. Long-term evaluation of seventy-one cases. J Bone Joint Surg Am. 1978;60(2):143–56.
5. Delanois RE, Mont MA, Yoon TR, Mizell M, Hungerford DS. Atraumatic osteonecrosis of the talus. J Bone Joint Surg Am. 1998;80(4):529–36.
6. Harris RD, Silver RA. Atraumatic aseptic necrosis of the talus. Radiology. 1973;106(1):81–3.
7. Baron M, Paltiel H, Lander P. Aseptic necrosis of the talus and calcaneal insufficiency fractures in a patient with pancreatitis, subcutaneous fat necrosis, and arthritis. Arthritis Rheum. 1984; 27(11):1309–13.
8. Miskew DB, Goldflies ML. Atraumatic avascular necrosis of the talus associated with hyperuricemia. Clin Orthop Relat Res. 1980;148:156–9.
9. Stern PJ, Watts HG. Osteonecrosis after renal transplantation in children. J Bone Joint Surg Am. 1979;61(6A):851–6.
10. Mankin HJ. Nontraumatic necrosis of bone (osteonecrosis). N Engl J Med. 1992;326(22):1473–9. doi:10.1056/NEJM199205283262206.
11. Jones Jr JP. Concepts of etiology and early pathogenesis of osteonecrosis. Instr Course Lect. 1994;43:499–512.
12. Harrington KD, Murray WR, Kountz SL, Belzer FO. Avascular necrosis of bone after renal transplantation. J Bone Joint Surg Am. 1971;53(2):203–15.
13. Vallier HA, Nork SE, Benirschke SK, Sangeorzan BJ. Surgical treatment of talar body fractures. J Bone Joint Surg Am. 2003;85-A(9):1716–24.
14. Kelly PJ, Sullivan CR. Blood supply of the talus. Clin Orthop Relat Res. 1963;30:37–44.
15. Mulfinger GL, Trueta J. The blood supply of the talus. J Bone Joint Surg Br. 1970;52(1):160–7.
16. Gelberman RH, Mortensen WW. The arterial anatomy of the talus. Foot Ankle. 1983;4(2):64–72.
17. Peterson L, Goldie I, Lindell D. The arterial supply of the talus. Acta Orthop Scand. 1974;45(2):260–70.
18. Metzger MJ, Levin JS, Clancy JT. Talar neck fractures and rates of avascular necrosis. J Foot Ankle Surg. 1999;38(2):154–62.
19. Morgan A, Kim PS, Christman RA. 2003 William J. Stickel Bronze Award. Radiographic anatomy of the talus. J Am Podiatr Med Assoc. 2003;93(6):449–80.
20. Pearce DH, Mongiardi CN, Fornasier VL, Daniels TR. Avascular necrosis of the talus: a pictorial essay. Radiographics. 2005;25(2): 399–410. doi:10.1148/rg.252045709.
21. Solomon L. Mechanisms of idiopathic osteonecrosis. Orthop Clin North Am. 1985;16(4):655–67.
22. Thordarson DB, Triffon MJ, Terk MR. Magnetic resonance imaging to detect avascular necrosis after open reduction and internal fixation of talar neck fractures. Foot Ankle Int. 1996;17(12): 742–7.
23. Myerson M, Christensen JC, Steck JK, Schuberth JM. Avascular necrosis of the foot and ankle. Foot Ankle Spec. 2012;5(2):128–36. doi:10.1177/1938640012441335.
24. Mont MA, Schon LC, Hungerford MW, Hungerford DS. Avascular necrosis of the talus treated by core decompression. J Bone Joint Surg Br. 1996;78(5):827–30.
25. Horst F, Gilbert BJ, Nunley JA. Avascular necrosis of the talus: current treatment options. Foot Ankle Clin. 2004;9(4):757–73. doi:10.1016/j.fcl.2004.08.001.
26. Adelaar RS, Madrian JR. Avascular necrosis of the talus. Orthop Clin North Am. 2004;35(3):383–95, xi. doi:10.1016/j.ocl.2004.02.010.
27. Comfort TH, Behrens F, Gaither DW, Denis F, Sigmond M. Long-term results of displaced talar neck fractures. Clin Orthop Relat Res. 1985;199:81–7.
28. Grob D, Simpson LA, Weber BG, Bray T. Operative treatment of displaced talus fractures. Clin Orthop Relat Res. 1985;199:88–96.
29. Szyszkowitz R, Reschauer R, Seggl W. Eighty-five talus fractures treated by ORIF with five to eight years of follow-up study of 69 patients. Clin Orthop Relat Res. 1985;199:97–107.
30. Rammelt S, Zwipp H, Gavlik JM. Avascular necrosis after minimally displaced talus fracture in a child. Foot Ankle Int. 2000;21(12):1030–6.
31. Penny JN, Davis LA. Fractures and fracture-dislocations of the neck of the talus. J Trauma. 1980;20(12):1029–37.
32. Urquhart MW, Mont MA, Michelson JD, Krackow KA, Hungerford DS. Osteonecrosis of the talus: treatment by hindfoot fusion. Foot Ankle Int. 1996;17(5):275–82.
33. Gross AE, Agnidis Z, Hutchison CR. Osteochondral defects of the talus treated with fresh osteochondral allograft transplantation. Foot Ankle Int. 2001;22(5):385–91.

34. Jeng CL, Kadakia A, White KL, Myerson MS. Fresh osteochondral total ankle allograft transplantation for the treatment of ankle arthritis. Foot Ankle Int. 2008;29(6):554–60. doi:10.3113/FAI.2008.0554.
35. Hussl H, Sailer R, Daniaux H, Pechlaner S. Revascularization of a partially necrotic talus with a vascularized bone graft from the iliac crest. Arch Orthop Trauma Surg. 1989;108(1):27–9.
36. Gilbert BJ, Horst F, Nunley JA. Potential donor rotational bone grafts using vascular territories in the foot and ankle. J Bone Joint Surg Am. 2004;86-A(9):1857–73.
37. Zhang Y, Liu Y, Jiang Y. Treatment of avascular necrosis of talus with vascularized bone graft. Zhongguo Xiu Fu Chong Jian Wai Ke Za Zhi. 1998;12(5):285–7.
38. Harnroongroj T, Vanadurongwan V. The talar body prosthesis. J Bone Joint Surg Am. 1997;79(9):1313–22.
39. Marulanda GA, McGrath MS, Ulrich SD, Seyler TM, Delanois RE, Mont MA. Percutaneous drilling for the treatment of atraumatic osteonecrosis of the ankle. J Foot Ankle Surg. 2010;49(1):20–4. doi:10.1053/j.jfas.2009.07.004.
40. Kitaoka HB, Patzer GL. Arthrodesis for the treatment of arthrosis of the ankle and osteonecrosis of the talus. J Bone Joint Surg Am. 1998;80(3):370–9.
41. Johnson EE, Weltmer J, Lian GJ, Cracchiolo 3rd A. Ilizarov ankle arthrodesis. Clin Orthop Relat Res. 1992;280:160–9.
42. Haddad SL, Coetzee JC, Estok R, Fahrbach K, Banel D, Nalysnyk L. Intermediate and long-term outcomes of total ankle arthroplasty and ankle arthrodesis. A systematic review of the literature. J Bone Joint Surg Am. 2007;89(9):1899–905. doi:10.2106/JBJS.F.01149.
43. Frey C, Halikus NM, Vu-Rose T, Ebramzadeh E. A review of ankle arthrodesis: predisposing factors to nonunion. Foot Ankle Int. 1994;15(11):581–4.
44. Holt ES, Hansen ST, Mayo KA, Sangeorzan BJ. Ankle arthrodesis using internal screw fixation. Clin Orthop Relat Res. 1991;268: 21–8.
45. Mann RA, Chou LB. Tibiocalcaneal arthrodesis. Foot Ankle Int. 1995;16(7):401–5.
46. Reckling FW. Early tibiocalcaneal fusion in the treatment of severe injuries of the talus. J Trauma. 1972;12(5):390–6.
47. Stamatis ED, Myerson MS. How to avoid specific complications of total ankle replacement. Foot Ankle Clin. 2002;7(4):765–89.
48. Raikin SM, Myerson MS. Avoiding and managing complications of the Agility Total Ankle Replacement system. Orthopedics. 2006;29(10):930–8.
49. Spirt AA, Assal M, Hansen Jr ST. Complications and failure after total ankle arthroplasty. J Bone Joint Surg Am. 2004;86-A(6): 1172–8.
50. Glazebrook MA, Ganapathy V, Bridge MA, Stone JW, Allard JP. Evidence-based indications for ankle arthroscopy. Arthroscopy. 2009;25(12):1478–90. doi:10.1016/j.arthro.2009.05.001.
51. Gougoulias NE, Khanna A, Maffulli N. History and evolution in total ankle arthroplasty. Br Med Bull. 2009;89:111–51. doi:10.1093/bmb/ldn039.

Kienböck's Disease of the Lunate

57

Dawn M. LaPorte and Thomas J. Kim

57.1 Introduction

Osteonecrosis of the lunate or Kienböck's disease is an entity that has been recognized for over a century. It was first described by the Austrian radiologist, Robert Kienböck, and is characterized by progressive pain and dysfunction of the wrist typically without any history of acute trauma. In this chapter, we will discuss the known pathophysiology, clinical evaluation, imaging, and treatments available.

57.2 Anatomy and Pathophysiology

57.2.1 Anatomy

The lunate is located in the center of the proximal carpal row and articulates proximally with the radius and the triangular fibrocartilage complex (TFCC). It articulates distally with the capitate and hamate. Cadaveric studies have shown the blood supply to vary considerably. In one particular study, 80 % of the time the lunate was supplied by both the palmar and dorsal arches, while in the other 20 % of cases, the lunate was supplied from the palmar side alone [1]. The dorsal blood supply is provided by branches of the dorsal intercarpal and radiocarpal arches. The palmar surface of the lunate is supplied by branches of the palmar radiocarpal arch, anterior interosseous artery, and ulnar recurrent artery [2]. This is particularly relevant considering one of the main theories concerning the etiology of the disease process is vascular.

There are several theories concerning the cause of Kienböck's disease. As mentioned, a vascular etiology has been purported as one of the leading possibilities. Several cadaveric studies have been performed which show the vascular intraosseous arborization or branching to vary as does the proportion of volar and dorsal vascular supply [1, 2]. Lunates with limited intraosseous branching or a single arterial blood supply are in theory more vulnerable to avascular necrosis due to the lack of collateral blood flow.

Another proposed cause of osteonecrosis in the lunate is sluggish venous outflow causing an intraosseous compartment syndrome. A cadaveric study identified a dense plexus of veins that exists at the palmar and dorsal periosteal face of the lunate that could potentially be an area where a backflow of venous drainage occurs [3].

A third long-standing theory involves the biomechanics of wrist motion [4, 5]. Necrosis may occur through the compressive forces from the capitate and the radius. Repetitive loads causes microfractures that eventually lead to progressive collapse of the lunate. A predisposition to collapse may be present due to the varying anatomy. An ulnar-negative variant wrist is also thought to be correlated with necrosis of the lunate secondary to the increased height of the radius increasing force transmission across the radiolunate joint [5]. Similarly, decreased radial inclination has also been shown to be associated with lunate necrosis [5, 6].

Systemic conditions that lead to hypercoagulability such as sickle cell anemia, kidney disease, and chronic steroid use may also increase the risk of osteonecrosis through sluggish blood circulation [5, 6].

Although there remains no consensus on the exact etiology of lunate osteonecrosis, it is likely due to a combination of wrist biomechanics, vascular anatomy, and systemic conditions.

57.2.2 Clinical Evaluation

Patients typically present with complaints of dorsal wrist pain and weakness. There is often no history of trauma. Kienböck's disease usually affects adult males from age 20 to 40 years old. It is rarely bilateral and similarly rare in children. On exam, patients may have tenderness upon palpation at the dorsal wrist over the lunate. They may have decreased

D.M. LaPorte (✉) • T.J. Kim
Department of Orthopaedic Surgery, Johns Hopkins University School of Medicine, Baltimore, MD, USA
e-mail: dlaport1@jhmi.edu; tkim62@jhmi.edu

K.-H. Koo et al. (eds.), *Osteonecrosis*,
DOI 10.1007/978-3-642-35767-1_57, © Springer-Verlag Berlin Heidelberg 2014

wrist flexion and extension with pain at the extremes of motion. Grip strength may also be affected and will commonly be noticeably weaker than the unaffected side.

57.2.3 Imaging and Classification

The diagnosis is usually made on plain films and possibly advanced imaging, which form the basis for staging and treatment. Plain radiographs are used to evaluate the lunate as well as important related wrist anatomy, including radial inclination, ulnar variance, carpal height, and radioscaphoid angle.

The classification scheme most commonly used is the Lichtman's classification (Table 57.1). In stage 1, the density and shape of the lunate are normal. A fracture line may be present. Magnetic resonance imaging (MRI) signal changes are present, with diffuse decreased signal on T1 images (Fig. 57.1). In stage 2, lunate sclerosis is seen without changes in shape on plain films (Fig. 57.2). Stage 3 is the most common stage at initial presentation. Collapse of the lunate articular surface is seen. Stage 3 is subdivided into 3-A, which is characterized by lunate collapse with maintained carpal height and alignment, and 3-B, which describes lunate collapse with loss of carpal height, proximal capitate migration, and fixed flexion of the scaphoid (Fig. 57.3). Goldfarb et al. proposed to distinguish stage 3B from 3A using the radioscaphoid angle [7]. Radioscaphoid angles >60° are considered stage 3B. In stage 4, there is lunate collapse along with radiocarpal or midcarpal degenerative changes (Fig. 57.4).

MRI may be useful for the early stages of the disease when no pathology is found on plain films. A decreased T1 signal will commonly be seen. Computed tomography scanning can also be useful to define the lunate collapse seen at later stages.

Table 57.1 Lichtman's classification for Kienböck's disease

Stage 1	No findings on plain films, possible low signal on T1 MRI
Stage 2	Lunate sclerosis evident on plain films
Stage 3a	Collapse of lunate articular surface but with normal carpal height
Stage 3b	Collapse of lunate articular surface and with carpal collapse, fixed scaphoid in flexion, proximal capitate migration
Stage 4	Collapse of lunate with radiocarpal or midcarpal arthritis on plain films

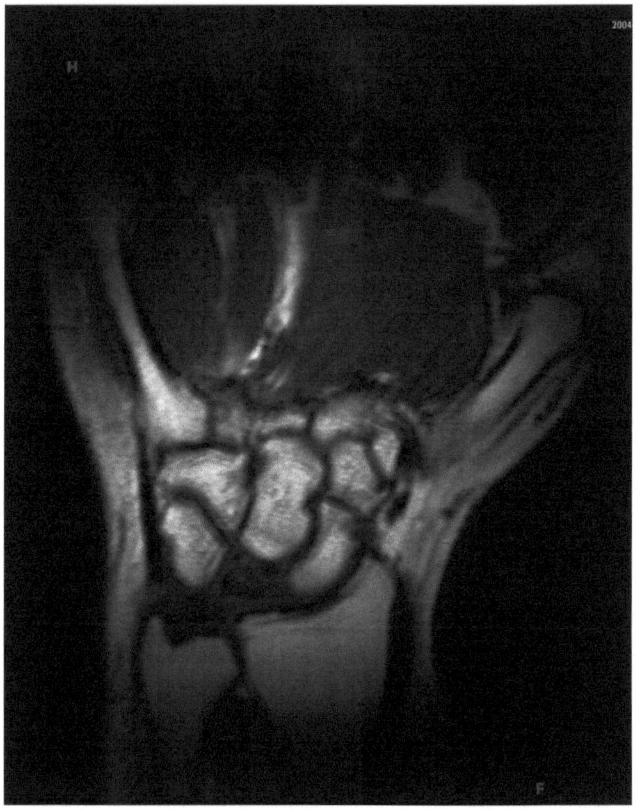

Fig. 57.1 Coronal T1-weighted MRI in a 31-year-old woman with wrist pain. The patient has ulnar-negative variance and low signal is seen in the lunate. Plain radiograph showed no pathology

57.2.4 Treatment

The treatment recommendations for the early stages of this disease remain controversial as do the outcomes. The natural history of lunate osteonecrosis is not clear as there are few limited studies with suboptimal power and study design [8, 9]. A recent systematic review study on nonoperative versus operative treatment showed that in late stages of the disease, nonoperative treatment led to 63 % pain improvement compared to up to 90 % in surgically treated patients [10].

As with most orthopedic conditions, immobilization is the first line of treatment. Studies on conservative treatment have shown that radiographic severity of the disease does not always correlate with severity of symptoms [8, 9]. Thus, patients should be treated according to their symptoms in conjunction with their radiographs rather than by their radiographic disease progression alone. Many patients, including some with advanced radiographic changes, may have limited symptoms or functional limitations. As such, a trial of nonoperative management is recommended in most patients.

In symptomatic patients, after nonoperative measures have failed, surgery is indicated. Surgical options range from arthroscopic debridement, core decompression, osteotomies, to vascularized bone grafting and salvage procedures. Studies have not shown one operative treatment to be significantly superior to another [10].

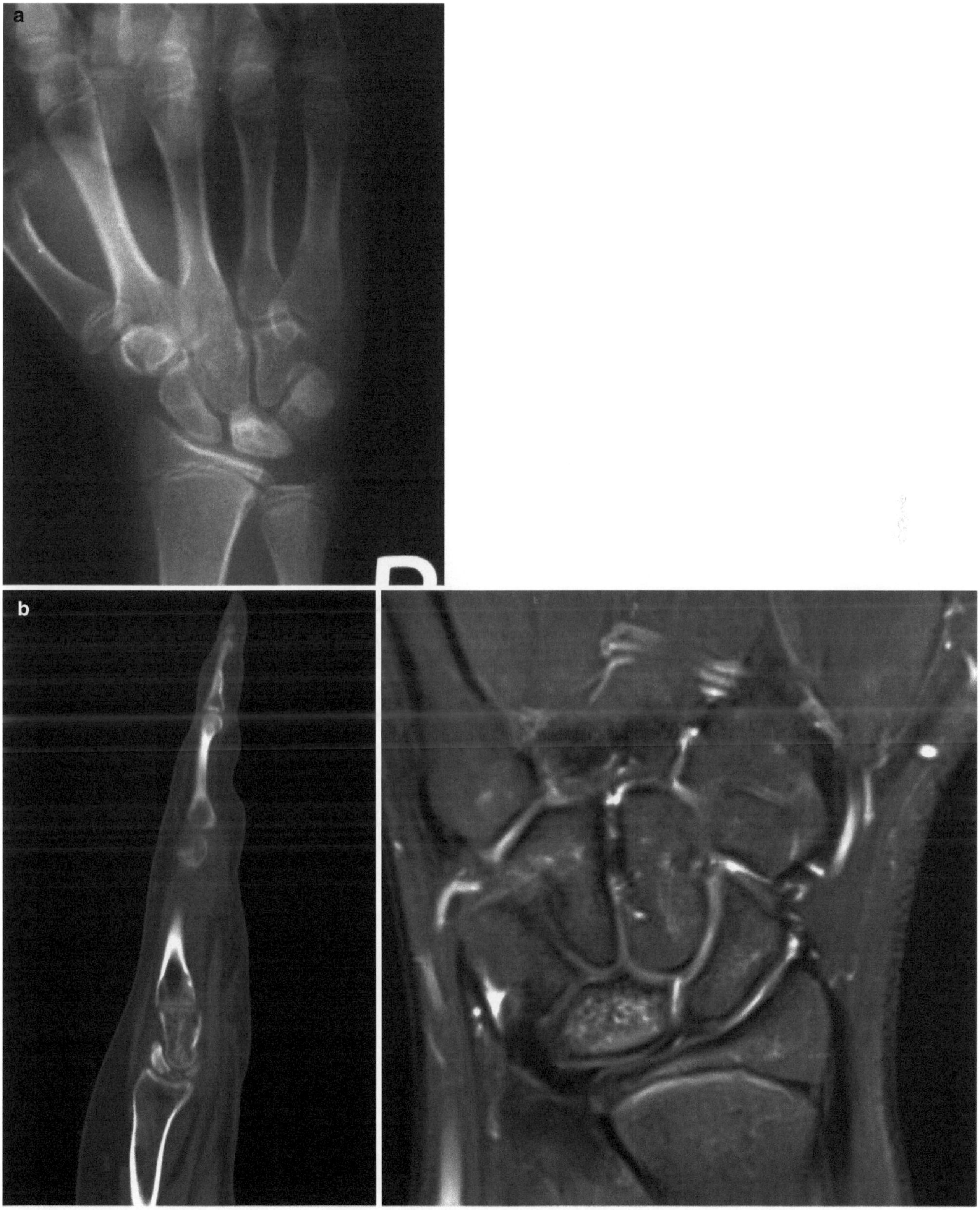

Fig. 57.2 (**a**) PA radiograph of a wrist in a 11-year-old female showing sclerosis of the lunate with no collapse. (**b**) Coronal MRI (fat suppressed proton density) of the same patient showing increased T2 signal in the lunate consistent with possible ischemia and stage 2 Kienbock's disease. (**c**) Coronal T1 weighted image of the same patient showing loss of normal fatty signal in the lunate, consistent with Keinbock's disease. (**d**) Sagittal MRI of the same patient with increased T2 signal in the lunate consistent with possible ischemia and stage 2 Kienbock's disease

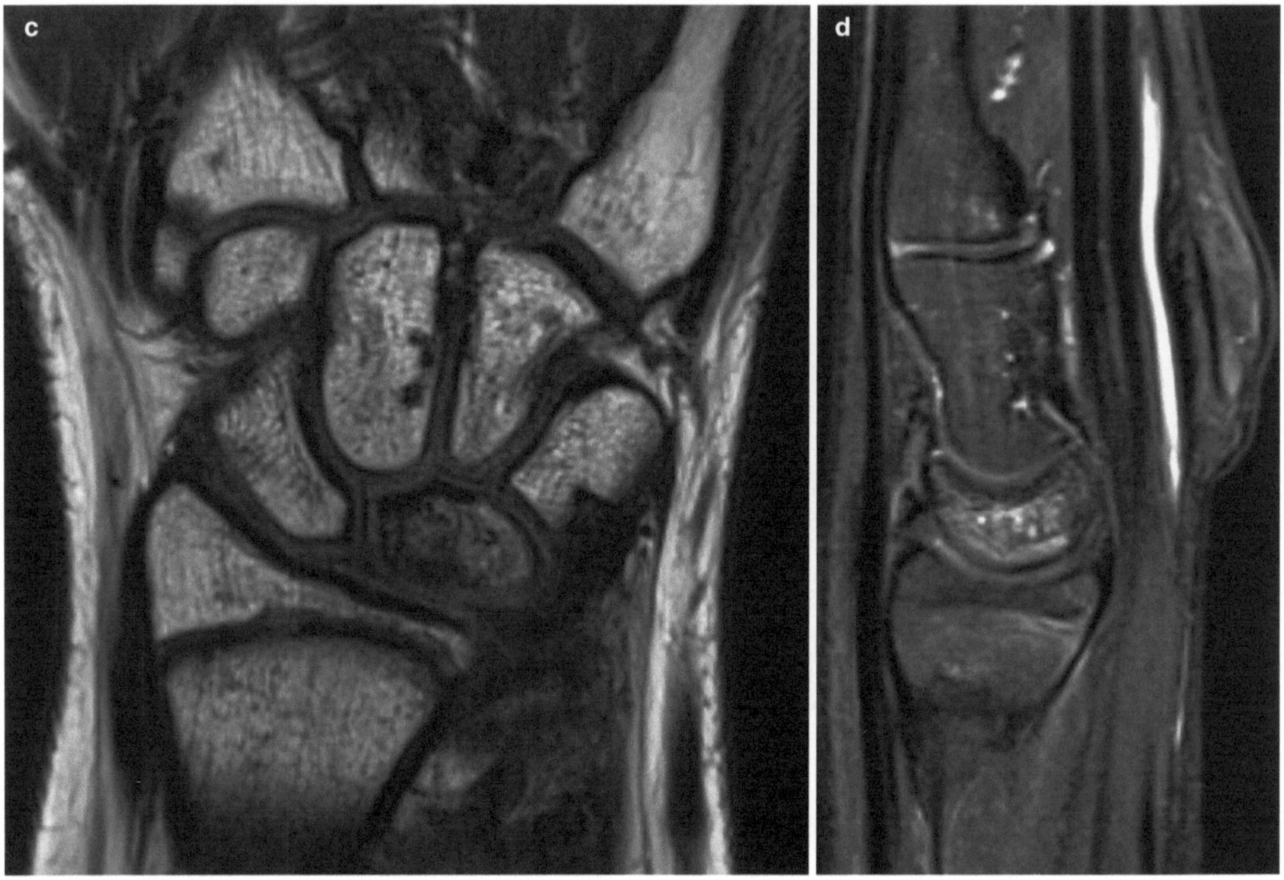

Fig. 57.2 (continued)

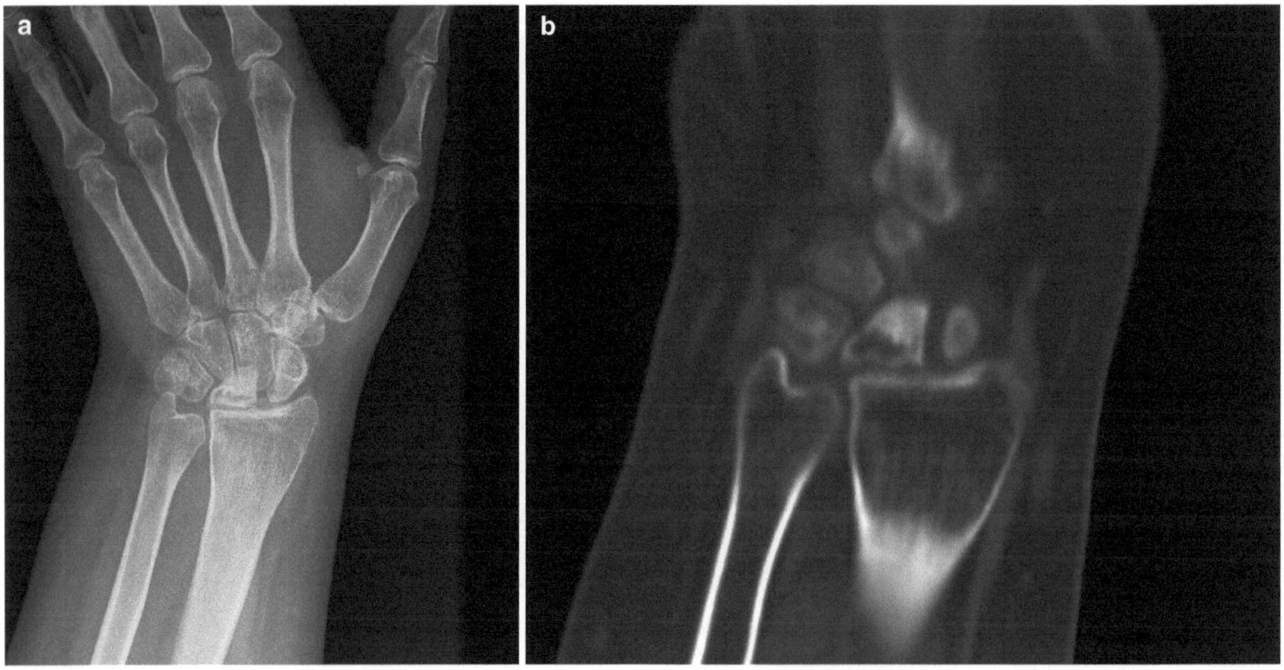

Fig. 57.3 (**a**) PA radiograph of the left wrist in a 20 year-old woman showing sclerosis of the lunate with early collapse, proximal migration of the capitate, and rotation of the scaphoid (Stage 3B). (**b**) Coronal and sagittal CT image of the same wrist showing sclerosis and collapse of the lunate with fracture line through a central lucent area

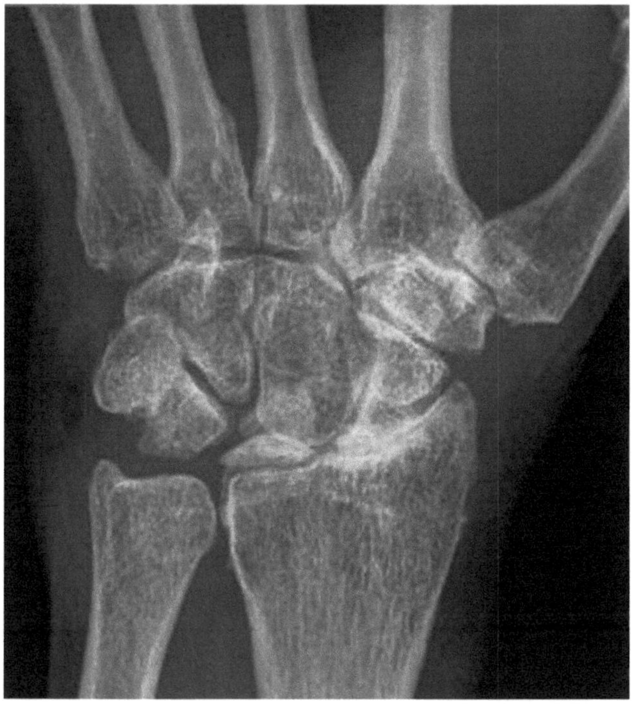

Fig. 57.4 PA radiograph of wrist showing avascular necrosis of the lunate with associated degenerative change

A general algorithm of treatment begins with immobilization with a cast or splint, pins, or an external fixator for up to 12 weeks. This would predominantly apply to patients with minimal symptoms and to symptomatic patients in stage I of the disease. Arthroscopic debridement has been described in early stages with successful symptom relief [6, 11]. Core decompression has also been described in early stages (stages 1-3A) to provide good outcomes [12]. In this procedure, 2×0.5 cm cortical windows are created in the distal radius and ulna, and small curettes are used to decompress the metaphysis.

As the disease progresses to stages 2 and 3, treatment is focused on unloading the lunate and restoring vascularity. In patients with ulnar-negative variance, radial shortening osteotomies or ulnar lengthening procedures can help decrease radiolunate load. Radial shortening procedures are more commonly performed with better reported outcomes compared to ulnar lengthening secondary to higher rates of nonunion in the latter [5, 6, 13, 14]. Radial shortening osteotomy is contraindicated in patients with ulnar neutral or positive variance. Radial wedge or dome osteotomies can be performed in these patients to reduce radial inclination thereby increasing the radiolunate contact surface area. This has been shown to reduce the force across the radiolunate and capitolunate joints [5, 6, 15]. Capitate shortening may also unload the lunate in patients that are ulnar neutral or ulnar positive [16].

Another technique described to unload the lunate consists of selective carpal fusions. These include capitohamate, scaphocapitate, and scaphotrapeziotrapezoid fusions. These techniques have been shown to reduce the load across the radiolunate joint and transfer it to an adjacent joint [5, 6].

Direct revascularization techniques are often selected for stage 2 patients with no lunate collapse but have also been described for patients in stage 3A. Direct revascularization provides implantation of osteoblasts and osteoclasts into the lunate, which promotes primary bone healing. These procedures are often coupled with unloading interventions to allow for revascularization while the lunate is offloaded. A number of different vascularized bone grafts have been described including distal radius, pisiform, dorsal metacarpal, and free vascularized grafts [5, 6].

In the late stages of osteonecrosis (3B-4), it becomes less important to preserve the lunate, and focus is diverted to salvage procedures. Surgical options include lunate excision and interposition arthroplasty, wrist denervation, proximal row carpectomy (PRC), and total wrist arthrodesis. PRC has been shown to be a reliable motion-sparing procedure with good results as long as there are no degenerative changes at the capitate head. PRC is less reliable in patients with stage 4 disease, and thus, total wrist arthrodesis should be considered in stage 4 patients [17].

57.3 Summary and Conclusion

Osteonecrosis of the lunate continues to be an unsolved puzzle, missing the pieces necessary for a complete understanding of the disease process and treatment. It is thought to occur secondary to a combination of vascular insufficiency and biomechanical overloading. Staging is determined by radiographic changes as described by Lichtman et al. [18]. Treatment is dictated by the patient's symptoms and radiographs and includes immobilization, mechanical unloading osteotomies, vascularized bone grafts, proximal row carpectomy, and fusion procedures. No surgical procedure has yet been shown to be vastly superior to another. It is important to recognize the disorder early as it is a progressive disease that in late stages is only able to be treated with salvage procedures.

References

1. Freedman DM, Botte MJ, Gelberman RH. Vascularity of the carpus. Clin Orthop Relat Res. 2001;(383):47–59. Review.
2. Botte MJ, Pacelli LL, Gelberman RH. Vascularity and osteonecrosis of the wrist. Orthop Clin North Am. 2004;35(3):405–21, xi. Review.
3. Pichler M, Putz R. The venous drainage of the lunate bone. Surg Radiol Anat. 2003;24(6):372–6. Epub 2003 Jan 30.

4. Schuind F, Eslami S, Ledoux P. Kienbock's disease. J Bone Joint Surg Br. 2008;90(2):133–9. doi:10.1302/0301-620X.90B2.20112. Review.
5. Lutsky K, Beredjiklian PK. Kienböck disease. J Hand Surg Am. 2012;37(9):1942–52. doi:10.1016/j.jhsa.2012.06.029. Review.
6. Luo J, Diao E. Kienbock's disease: an approach to treatment. Hand Clin. 2006;22:465–73, abstract vi.
7. Goldfarb CA, Hsu J, Gelberman RH, Boyer MI. The Lichtman classification for Kienbock's disease: an assessment of reliability. J Hand Surg. 2003;28A:74–80.
8. Keith PP, Nuttall D, Trail I. Long-term outcome of nonsurgically managed Kienböck's disease. J Hand Surg Am. 2004;29(1): 63–7.
9. Kristensen SS, Thomassen E, Christensen F. Kienböck's disease–late results by non-surgical treatment. A follow-up study. J Hand Surg Br. 1986;11(3):422–5.
10. Innes L, Strauch RJ. Systematic review of the treatment of Kienböck's disease in its early and late stages. J Hand Surg. 2010;35A(713–717):e711–4.
11. Menth-Chiari WA, Poehling GG, Wiesler ER, Ruch DS. Arthroscopic debridement for the treatment of Kienbock's disease. Arthroscopy. 1999;15(1):12–9.
12. Illarramendi AA, Schulz C, De Carli P. The surgical treatment of Kienböck's disease by radius and ulna metaphyseal core decompression. J Hand Surg Am. 2001;26(2):252–60.
13. Salmon J, Stanley JK, Trail IA. Kienböck's disease: conservative management versus radial shortening. J Bone Joint Surg Br. 2000;82(6):820–3.
14. Zenzai K, Shibata M, Endo N. Long-term outcome of radial shortening with or without ulnar shortening for treatment of Kienböck's disease: a 13–25 year follow-up. J Hand Surg Br. 2005;30(2):226–8.
15. Koh S, Nakamura R, Horii E, Nakao E, Inagaki H, Yajima H. Surgical outcome of radial osteotomy for Kienbock's disease—minimum 10 years of follow-up. J Hand Surg. 2003;28A:910–6.
16. Waitayawinyu T, Chin SH, Luria S, Trumble T. Capitate shortening osteotomy with vascularized bone grafting for the treatment of Kienböck's disease in the ulnar positive wrist. J Hand Surg. 2008;33A:1267–73.
17. Croog AS, Stern PJ. Proximal row carpectomy for advanced Kienböck's disease: average 10-year follow-up. J Hand Surg. 2008;33A:1122–30.
18. Lichtman DM, Lesley NE, Simmons SP. The classification and treatment of Kienböck's disease: the state of the art and a look at the future. J Hand Surg. 2010;35E:549–54.

Part XIII

Legg-Calvé-Perthes Disease

58 The Epidemiology and Etiology of Perthes' Disease

Daniel C. Perry

58.1 Introduction

Despite over a century elapsing since the first descriptions of Perthes' disease, the etiological determinants remain unknown. Clues are emerging to help identify these determinants, such as intriguing geographic disease patterns and unexpected longitudinal incidence trends. While genetic tendencies are now generally sought as the answer to unexplained diseases, the absence of concordance in twins and lack of familial clusters suggest that the role of genetics is minimal. Large geographic variations in incidence with "pockets" of disease apparent even within small communities suggest that a major environmental risk factor is likely. The process of identifying the risk factor(s) and mechanism of action continues.

58.2 Descriptive Epidemiology

The foundation of epidemiology is "descriptive epidemiology," which refers to how disease is distributed in a population in terms of person, place, and time. This is one of the most well-documented aspects of Perthes' disease and is fundamental to understanding the etiological determinants.

58.2.1 Person

Perthes' disease affects boys about five times more commonly than girls. It affects individuals at any point between 2 and 14 years old, but the peak age of onset is around 5 years old. The age-of-onset distribution has a marked positive skew, following a lognormal distribution, which means that there is a propensity for the disease to affect younger children rather than older children [1, 2]. This is an unusual distribution in chronic disease and has been likened to incubation period distributions evident in infectious disease epidemiology. This distribution has led to suggestion that, like in an infectious disease outbreak, a single trigger must act at a critical period to produce this finding. Such distributions have been demonstrated in chronic diseases such as childhood leukemia when caused by point exposure to maternal radiation, but not so in idiopathic leukemia of uncertain etiology [3]. This therefore suggests that a critical period exists in hip development, during which exposure to a determinant will initiate the disease process. The age of onset is later among Indian children [4], and it is suggested that the disease may occur earlier in females than males [5, 6]. Such differences may arise due to differing skeletal growth rates and/or variation in the "critical period."

58.2.2 Place

There is marked geographical variation in the frequency of Perthes' disease. A recent systematic review of incidence studies of Perthes' disease used comparable denominator populations to demonstrate international variations (Fig. 58.1) [7]. This review identified large international variation in disease rates, which appeared independently associated with both race and latitude. East Asians appeared least affected by Perthes' disease, with Whites most affected and South Asians in between. There were no robust studies of incidence from countries with a predominantly Black population, which is thought to reflect the near absence of disease among Black individuals. After adjusting for race, every 10° further from the equator resulted in an increase in the incidence of the disease by almost 50 %, suggesting that race alone does not explain the international distribution.

Within countries there is also a marked variation in incidence. This has most clearly been demonstrated in the UK, using a large database of general practice data enumerating

D.C. Perry
Warwick Orthopaedics, Warwick Medical School, Coventry CV4 7AL, UK
e-mail: danperry@doctors.org.uk

K.-H. Koo et al. (eds.), *Osteonecrosis*,
DOI 10.1007/978-3-642-35767-1_58, © Springer-Verlag Berlin Heidelberg 2014

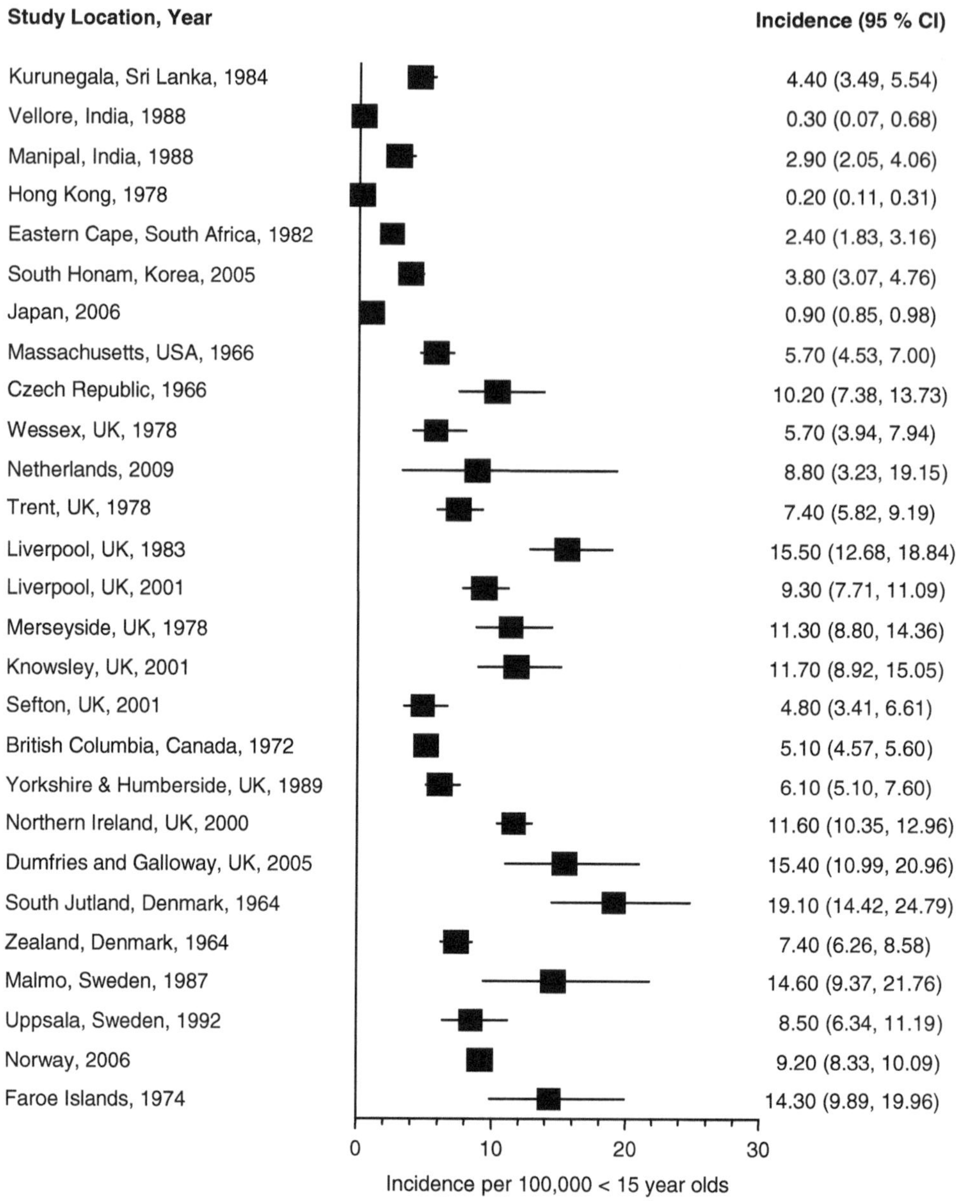

Fig. 58.1 Regional incidence of Perthes' disease per 100,000 children aged <15 years, 1964–2009. Studies are ordered by latitude. *CI* confidence interval, *IR* incidence rate, *UK* United Kingdom, *US* United States (Reproduced with permission from Perry et al. [7])

8 % of the population [8]. A profound North–south gradient was identified, with Perthes' disease rates in the North more than double those in the South, with graduated rates in between (Fig. 58.2).

Even when looking at the lowest levels of UK geography (the Super Output Area (SOA), each unit of which encompasses around 1,500 individuals), rates of Perthes' disease have varied significantly within towns and cities [9]. In fact, all levels of UK administrative geography demonstrate large differences in Perthes' disease incidence rates between areas. Similar variations in incidence have also been demonstrated within other countries, such as India and Norway [2, 4].

Understanding the factors that may influence these geographic patterns is crucial to help identify the disease determinants. Within the UK the geographic patterns observed have been consistently associated with patterns of socioeconomic deprivation, at all geographic levels [8–16]. At the national level, the map of Perthes' disease distribution is an almost identical pattern to that seen in many diseases of deprivation, such as cardiovascular disease and all-cause mortality [17]. At the local level, SOA deprivation quintiles closely correlate with the Perthes' disease incidence rates [9] (Table 58.1). Individual deprivation measures (i.e. recording parental occupation) add support to the association with deprivation [10, 15], and this robust association has also been demonstrated to be apparent outside the UK [18]. The strength and magnitude of the association is such that few other childhood diseases demonstrate such a striking association.

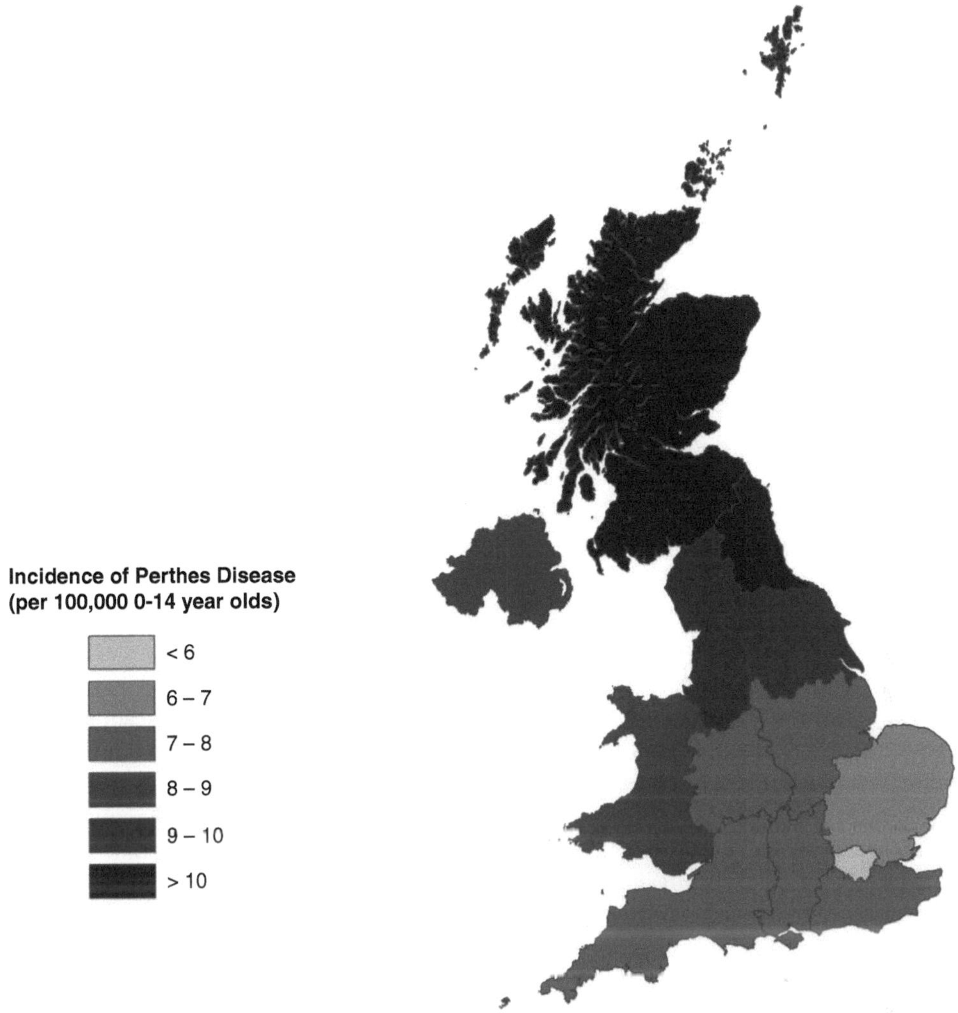

Fig. 58.2 Geographic illustration of the incidence of Perthes' disease by English Strategic Health Authority, Wales, Scotland, and Northern Ireland (Reproduced with permission from Perry et al. [8], Wiley and Sons)

Table 58.1 Incidence of Perthes' disease by Index Multiple Deprivation 2007 Quintile at SOA level, Merseyside, UK 1996–2009

Quintile	Incidence	95 % CI
5 (most deprived)	11.5	9.0–14.5
4	11.7	9.1–14.9
3	7.0	4.9–9.8
2	6.3	4.3–8.9
1 (least deprived)	3.8	2.3–6.0

Reproduced with permission from Perry et al. [9])

However, despite the strength of the deprivation association, it does not appear to offer an explanation to the international distribution of Perthes' disease. Affluent parts of Northern Europe are shown to have high rates of disease compared to less affluent areas such as India. Similarly, while race is clearly important, it does not explain the entire observed difference in disease rates. The independent association of latitude is interesting, particularly as these latitude associations have been demonstrated in other diseases, such as multiple sclerosis and heart disease, which are believed to be a consequence of sunlight exposure and vitamin D synthesis [19, 20]. This may offer future avenues of exploration.

58.2.3 Time

Few studies have measured the influence of time on disease incidence. A study from Dortmund, Germany, between 1924 and 1960 demonstrated fluctuations in case numbers following periods of economic recession [19]. However, uncertainties in case ascertainment and the denominator population raised doubts to the validity of this observation.

More recent studies using several databases from the UK have investigated Perthes' disease incidence over a period of up to 35 years [8, 9, 11, 14]. All of these studies have demonstrated a significant gradual decline in the incidence of Perthes' disease. These declines were most rapid in the most deprived regions. The size and trend of this decline was similar to general markers of population well-being over this period, such as infant mortality and sudden infant death syndrome [21, 22].

58.3 Analytical Epidemiology

The descriptive studies have indicated that the key etiological determinant is intertwined with deprivation and appears to act at a single vulnerable period. The purpose of analytical epidemiology is to develop the hypotheses generated by descriptive studies and anecdotal observation. The objective is to refine the timing of the critical period, to identify additional associations that may enhance understanding of the determinant, and to test specific hypotheses of potential determinants and their mechanism of action.

58.3.1 Growth and Stature

Studies have consistently demonstrated anthropometric abnormalities among affected children. The most detailed of such study was a large cross-sectional study of 232 children from three centers in the UK [23]. This demonstrated a subtle global growth disturbance in affected individuals with a normal head size, yet increasing growth restriction more distally along limbs – a pattern of dysmorphism described as "rostral sparing" (Fig. 58.3). A later study sought to determine if the growth restriction was a true disease phenomena or a function of deprivation [24]. This was achieved by comparing anthropometric markers with siblings of affected children, therefore matching for urban deprivation and family tendencies. This study of 38 cases and 49 sibling controls demonstrated a clear growth restriction most notable in the feet of affected children.

The dysmorphic growth seen was similar to that of intrauterine growth restriction, with head size preserved at the expense of other body parameters. This suggested that there may be an abnormality evident with shape and size from birth and potentially arising in the prenatal period.

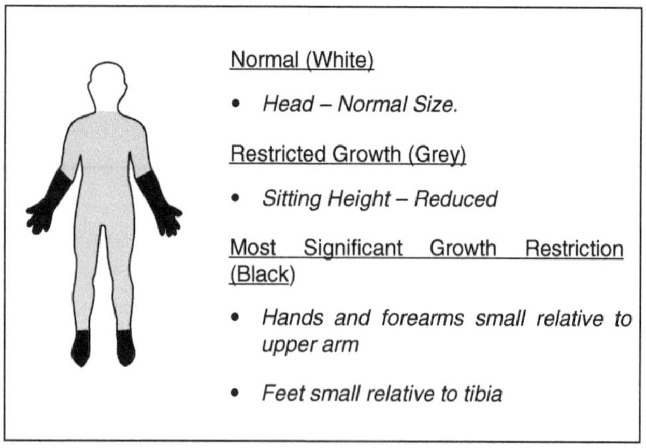

Fig. 58.3 Pattern of abnormal growth in Perthes' disease (Reproduced with permission from Perry et al. [25])

58.3.2 Birth Measures

Birth weight is difficult to study as it is complicated by the number of confounding factors such as gestational age, deprivation, and parental smoking. Numerous studies have sought to quantify this association, but no consistent association has been identified [2, 26, 27]. The most comprehensive study to investigate this used the Swedish Inpatient Register which concluded that, after adjusting for confounding, birth weights less than 1,500 g had an association with Perthes' disease (OR 3.5 95 % CI 1.1–10.8) [28]. The width of the confidence intervals reflects the paucity of cases within this group (9 of 731 cases). It is possible that unmeasured confounders may be apparent, such as steroids used for neonatal chronic lung disease, which may explain this association. It does therefore seem apparent that no major association with birth weight exists.

58.3.3 Congenital Malformations

A possible indication of prenatal exposures may be the presence of congenital malformations. A 1971 study identified an association between with both inguinal hernias and genitourinary malformations, with the frequency of inguinal hernia being eight times the expected number among individuals with Perthes' disease [29]. However, the patient group was selected from a specialized clinic in a tertiary center, and therefore selection bias may have influenced the validity of this finding. Subsequent studies failed to replicate these associations [5, 30] until recently, when large population-based case-control studies confirmed these associations. These studies used the Medical Birth Registry of Norway and the UK General Practice Research Database (GPRD) and confirmed a triad of genitourinary associations including undescended testis, inguinal hernias, and hypospadias, though the magnitude of these was less than previously suggested [2, 31].

These findings are important because they suggest a prenatal component to the disease etiology. The triad of associations identified is also interesting because they are often seen in combination, thought to be caused by altered fetal androgen metabolism [32, 33], which may be important in Perthes' disease, and could explain the strong male disease preponderance of the disease.

58.3.4 Smoking Hypothesis

The association with socioeconomic deprivation, epidemiological similarities with cardiovascular disease, and possible prenatal insult has led to the suggestion that maternal tobacco smoke exposure may be implicated in the disease. Measuring the effects of tobacco smoke exposure is fraught with difficulties, owing to recall bias, parental guilt, and the influence of confounding factors (particularly socioeconomic status). Several studies have investigated this relationship, the most comprehensive of these being a case-control study from the Swedish Inpatient Register [28] and a large case-control study from India [18]. The Swedish study was able to reduce recall bias by using tobacco smoke exposure data collected prior to disease onset, demonstrating a dose-response relationship with a greater risk of Perthes' disease corresponding to a greater degree of tobacco smoke exposure (1–9 cigarettes, OR 1.4 (95 % CI 1.1–1.7); >10 cigarettes, OR 2.0 (95 % CI 1.6–2.6)). The authors considered socioeconomic status as a confounder, although it is unclear how this was measured. The study from India similarly showed an association with tobacco smoke exposure (OR 2.1 (95 % CI 1.3–3.3)), recording current exposure to indoor tobacco smoke as a proxy measure of "lifetime exposure" and adjusting for social class. A tobacco association therefore appears evident, though the effects of bias cannot be completely eliminated, and the effect size is less than that of socioeconomic deprivation suggesting that a different factor confounded by the smoking relationship may be the responsible determinant.

58.3.5 Nutrient Hypothesis

Manganese deficiency has a known association with a disproportionate growth abnormality found in chickens and epiphyseal dysplasia in rats. A case–control study within Liverpool demonstrated the existence of this association among children with Perthes' disease [34], but a later second smaller study failed to replicate this finding [35]. This association therefore remains uncertain.

58.3.6 Coagulopathic Hypothesis

Thrombotic tendencies, such as sickle cell disease, are known to precipitate avascular necrosis of the hip. This has led to widespread belief that Perthes' disease is the result of a primary coagulopathic process. This appears plausible as the pathology of Perthes' disease is avascular necrosis; however, it is difficult to resolve how such a process would solely affect the hip and typically be unilateral.

A series of studies have investigated thrombotic tendencies in Perthes' disease, which were systematically reviewed in 2008 [36]. The review included 475 cases of Perthes' disease, concluding that there were no significant differences in antithrombin activity, protein S or C activity, or antiphospholipid antibodies [34]. There was insufficient data to exclude an association with the factor V Leiden mutation. The only subsequent study to investigate coagulopathies demonstrated a propensity toward factor V Leiden mutations and a raised factor VIII level; however, the study had notable flaws in the study design such that it added little to the earlier review [37]. Studies therefore seem to have excluded a major thrombophilic process in the etiology.

58.3.7 Traumatic Hypothesis

Trauma is one of the oldest etiological theories and was that favored by Georg Perthes in his classic monograph of the disease [38]. Popularity of this theory has been propagated by the anecdotal observations that affected children are "hyperactive" and evidence that their skeleton is underdeveloped for age [39]. It is suggested that a child whose activity level is beyond their bone age may damage the epiphysis precipitating osteonecrosis [40]. Animal studies have offered support to this theory, demonstrating that abnormal loading of the femoral head in rats is associated with hip osteonecrosis [41].

However, confirmation of these anecdotal observations is limited, with only two studies investigating a hyperactive tendency formally. The first used validated questionnaires in 24 children with Perthes' disease, identifying that 8 had a disorder with the attention deficit hyperactivity (ADHD) profile [42]. This study was uncontrolled, comparing the rates of hyperactivity to the expected population level of 3–5 %. The second study used general practice data to identify individuals from 619 cases of Perthes' disease who had sought medical attention for hyperactivity, compared to 2,544 age- and sex-matched population controls [31]. This study found no association with hyperactivity (95 % CI 1.0 (95 % CI 0.5–2.1)). Should a hyperactive tendency exist, then it appears subtle, though could be important in the disease etiology; therefore, further studies are needed using validated and sensitive markers of hyperactive tendencies, which control for confounding factors.

58.3.8 New Insights

Two papers have offered further clues to the etiology of Perthes' disease, which need further development in order to put them into the context of etiological hypotheses. The first looked at long-term comorbidities in a historic cohort of 3,141 individuals diagnosed with Perthes' disease in infancy at a mean of 28 years old, compared to a age-sex-region-matched population cohort [43]. This identified a heightened risk of ischemic heart disease (HR 2.7 (95 % CI 1.2–6.0)), hypertension (HR 3.0 (95 % CI 1.9–4.7)), and anemia (HR 2.9 (95 % CI 1.9–5.4)), suggesting that a generalized vascular phenomenon may be at large, with repercussions later in adulthood. Nevertheless, the cause and effect relationship is unclear, and it may be that osteoarthritis, as a consequence of Perthes' disease, results in impaired cardiovascular fitness and disease. A second study used ultrasound markers of early cardiovascular disease among children with Perthes' disease, demonstrating reduced arterial caliber and blood velocity independent of body composition, suggesting the possibility of generalized vascular phenomena, with potential cardiovascular consequences in adulthood [44]. Both of these therefore suggest that long-term sequelae of Perthes' disease may exist, and further historic cohorts would be useful to investigate this further.

58.4 Discussion

Although a century has passed since Perthes' disease was first described, the etiological determinant remains elusive. There is strong epidemiological evidence that the origin of the disease is environmental, with the disease determinant intertwined with socioeconomic deprivation. It is unknown how socioeconomic deprivation may precipitate osteonecrosis in the infant hip and appears that this is only one manifestation of the disease, with evidence of a global growth disorder characterized by delayed and disproportionate growth. It is unknown when exposure to the disease determinant may act (i.e., the child, the mother, or via an intergenerational epigenetic effect). The decline in incidence appears encouraging, but it remains a debilitating condition throughout the world, particularly in predominantly white non-equatorial regions.

Numerous hypotheses exist to indicate the disease determinants and their mechanism of action, though no consensus exists as to the most likely forerunner. Recent studies suggest that rather than being a disease exclusively of childhood, Perthes' disease may have implications for the long-term vascular health of those affected. Uncovering the determinants of Perthes' disease may therefore offer insights into the nature of other vascular diseases.

References

1. Hall AJ, Barker DJ. The age distribution of Legg-Perthes disease. An analysis using Sartwell's incubation period model. Am J Epidemiol. 1984;120(4):531–6.
2. Wiig O, Terjesen T, Svenningsen S, et al. The epidemiology and aetiology of Perthes' disease in Norway. A nationwide study of 425 patients. J Bone Joint Surg Br. 2006;88(9):1217–23.
3. Armenian HK, Khoury MJ. Age at onset of genetic diseases: an application for Sartwell's model of the distribution of incubation periods. Am J Epidemiol. 1981;113(5):596–605.
4. Joseph B, Chacko V, Rao BS, et al. The epidemiology of Perthes' disease in south India. Int J Epidemiol. 1988;17(3):603–7.
5. Fisher RL. An epidemiological study of Legg-Perthes disease. J Bone Joint Surg Am. 1972;54(4):769–78.
6. Guille JT, Lipton GE, Szöke G, et al. Legg-Calvé-Perthes disease in girls. A comparison of the results with those seen in boys. J Bone Joint Surg Am. 1998;80(9):1256–63.
7. Perry DC, Machin DMG, Pope D, et al. Racial and geographic factors in the incidence of Legg-Calvé-Perthes' disease: a systematic review. Am J Epidemiol. 2012;175(3):159–66.
8. Perry DC, Bruce CE, Pope D, et al. Legg-Calvé-Perthes disease in the UK: geographic and temporal trends in incidence reflecting differences in degree of deprivation in childhood. Arthritis Rheum. 2012;64(5):1673–9.
9. Perry DC, Bruce CE, Pope D, et al. Perthes' disease: deprivation and decline. Arch Dis Child. 2011;96(12):1124–8.
10. Hall AJ, Barker DJ, Dangerfield PH, et al. Perthes' disease of the hip in Liverpool. BMJ. 1983;287(6407):1757–9.
11. Margetts BM, Perry CA, Taylor JF, et al. The incidence and distribution of Legg-Calvé-Perthes' disease in Liverpool, 1982–95. Arch Dis Child. 2001;84(4):351–4.
12. Pillai A, Atiya S, Costigan PS, et al. The incidence of Perthes' disease in Southwest Scotland. J Bone Joint Surg Br. 2005;87(11):1531–5.
13. Kealey WD, Moore AJ, Cook S, et al. Deprivation, urbanisation and Perthes' disease in Northern Ireland. J Bone Joint Surg Br. 2000;82(2):167–71.
14. Perry DC, Bruce CE, Pope D, et al. Perthes' disease of the hip: socioeconomic inequalities and the urban environment. Arch Dis Child. 2012;97(12):1053–7.
15. Hall AJ, Barker DJ. Perthes' disease in Yorkshire. J Bone Joint Surg Br. 1989;71(2):229–33.
16. Barker DJ, Dixon E, Taylor JF, et al. Perthes' disease of the hip in three regions of England. J Bone Joint Surg Br. 1978;60(4):478–80.
17. Walford H, Soljak M, Gordon F, Birger R. CHD prevalence modelling briefing document. London: HM Stationery Office; 2008.
18. Daniel AB, Shah H, Kamath A, et al. Environmental tobacco and wood smoke increase the risk of Legg-Calvé-Perthes disease. Clin Orthop Relat Res. 2011;470(9):2369–75.
19. Johnell O, Borgstrom F, Jonsson B, et al. Latitude, socioeconomic prosperity, mobile phones and hip fracture risk. Osteoporos Int. 2007;18(3):333–7.
20. Hernán MA, Olek MJ, Ascherio A, et al. Geographic variation of MS incidence in two prospective studies of US women. Neurology. 1999;53(8):1711–8.
21. World Development Indicators. World Bank. 2011. Available from http://www.databank.worldbank.org. Accessed 5 Oct 2011.
22. Wood AM, Pasupathy D, Pell JP, et al. Trends in socioeconomic inequalities in risk of sudden infant death syndrome, other causes of infant mortality, and stillbirth in Scotland: population based study. BMJ. 2012;344:e1552.
23. Burwell RG, Dangerfield PH, Hall DJ, et al. Perthes' disease. An anthropometric study revealing impaired and disproportionate growth. J Bone Joint Surg Br. 1978;60(4):461–77.
24. Hall AJ, Barker DJ, Dangerfield PH, et al. Small feet and Perthes' disease. A survey in Liverpool. J Bone Joint Surg Br. 1988;70(4):611–3.
25. Perry DC, Hall AJ. The epidemiology and etiology of Perthes disease. Orthop Clin North Am. 2011;42(3):279–83, v.
26. Wynne-Davies R, Gormley J. The aetiology of Perthes' disease. genetic, epidemiological and growth factors in 310 Edinburgh and Glasgow patients. J Bone Joint Surg Br. 1978;60(1):6–14.
27. Molloy MK, Macmahon B. Birth weight and Legg-Perthes disease. J Bone Joint Surg Am. 1967;49(3):498–506.
28. Bahmanyar S, Montgomery SM, Weiss RJ, et al. Maternal smoking during pregnancy, other prenatal and perinatal factors, and the risk of Legg-Calvé-Perthes disease. Pediatrics. 2008;122(2):e459–64.
29. Catterall A, Lloyd-Roberts G, Wynne-Davies R, et al. Association of Perthes' disease with congenital anomalies of genitourinary tract and inguinal region. Lancet. 1971;297(7707):996–7.

30. Harper PS, Brotherton BJ, Cochlin D, et al. Genetic risks in Perthes' disease. Clin Genet. 1976;10(3):178–82.
31. Perry DC, Bruce CE, Pope D, et al. Comorbidities in Perthes' disease: a case control study using the General Practice Research Database. J Bone Joint Surg Br. 2012;94(12):1684–9.
32. Zhang JF, Yang CJ, Wu T, et al. A two-degree-of-freedom hip exoskeleton device for an immature animal model of exercise-induced Legg-Calvé-Perthes disease. Proc Inst Mech Eng H. 2009;223(8):1059–68.
33. Khuri FJ, Hardy BE, Churchill BM, et al. Urologic anomalies associated with hypospadias. Urol Clin North Am. 1981;8(3):565–71.
34. Hall AJ, Margetts BM, Barker DJ, et al. Low blood manganese levels in Liverpool children with Perthes' disease. Paediatr Perinat Epidemiol. 1989;3(2):131–5.
35. Perry CA, Taylor JF, Nunn A, et al. Perthes' disease and blood manganese levels. Arch Dis Child. 2000;82(5):428.
36. Kenet G, Ezra E, Wientroub S, et al. Perthes' disease and the search for genetic associations: collagen mutations, Gaucher's disease and thrombophilia. J Bone Joint Surg Br. 2008;90(11):1507–11.
37. Vosmaer A, Pereira RR, Koenderman JS, et al. Coagulation abnormalities in Legg-Calvé-Perthes disease. J Bone Joint Surg Am. 2010;92(1):121–8.
38. Perthes G. Uber osteochondritis deformans juvenilis. Arch f Klin Chir. 1913;101:779–807.
39. Cavanaugh LA, Shelton EK, Sutherland R, et al. Metabolic studies in osteochondritis of the capital femoral epiphysis. J Bone Joint Surg Am. 1936;18:957–68.
40. Harrison MH, Burwell RG. Perthes' disease: a concept of pathogenesis. Clin Orthop Relat Res. 1981;156:115–27.
41. Mihara K, Hirano T. Standing is a causative factor in osteonecrosis of the femoral head in growing rats. J Pediatr Orthop. 1998;18(5):665–9.
42. Loder RT, Schwartz EM, Hensinger RN, et al. Behavioral characteristics of children with Legg-Calvé-Perthes disease. J Pediatr Orthop. 1993;13(5):598–601.
43. Hailer YD, Montgomery SM, Ekbom A, et al. Legg-Calve-Perthes disease and risks for cardiovascular diseases and blood diseases. Pediatrics. 2010;125(6):e1308–15.
44. Perry DC, Green DJ, Bruce CE, et al. Abnormalities of vascular structure and function in children with Perthes disease. Pediatrics. 2012;130(1):e126–31.

Legg-Calvé-Perthes Disease: Pathology, Pathophysiology, and Pathogenesis of Deformity

59

Harry K.W. Kim

59.1 Introduction

Femoral head osteonecrosis (FHO) can affect children and adults. While there are similarities between childhood and adult FHO, the differences in the epidemiology, pathology, pathophysiology, pathogenesis of deformity, the natural history, and the outcomes of the childhood and adult FHO are notable. This chapter will focus on the pathology, pathophysiology, and the pathogenesis of femoral head deformity in Legg-Calvé-Perthes disease (LCPD). Furthermore, the differences between childhood and adult FHO will be discussed. A discussion on the differences between the internal structure of the skeletally immature femoral head and the mature femoral head is useful in understanding the differences between childhood and adult FHO.

59.2 Immature and Mature Femoral Head

Children's femoral heads are not just a smaller version of the adult femoral heads. The most apparent difference is that children's femoral heads are growing. Thus, they have an active bone growth, also known as a *modeling* process, in addition to the process of *remodeling* of the already formed bone to adapt to the biomechanical stresses applied to the femoral head from daily activities. Thus, the biological activities of the growing cartilage and bone from the immature femoral head are different from that of the cartilage and bone of the mature femoral head. The marrow content (red marrow vs fatty marrow) of the femoral head [1, 2] and the femoral head vascularity are also changing in the growing femoral head [3–5]. Because of these differences, a disruption of the blood supply to the immature and the mature femoral heads may have different biological implications including the extent of ischemic damage and the potential for repair. It is well known that the age at the onset of LCPD is one of the most consistent prognostic factors with a younger age at onset being associated with a more favorable outcome [6]. This may be explained by greater growth and remodeling potentials remaining in a younger patient. Furthermore, a younger patient would have a smaller bony epiphysis to revascularize and heal compared to an older patient (Fig. 59.1). Along this line of reasoning, the femoral head osteonecrosis in adolescents behave more like adult osteonecrosis in terms of their poor outcome [7, 8] due to the poor healing potential and much larger volume of necrotic bone to revascularize and heal than younger children.

59.2.1 Anatomy and Histology of Immature Femoral Head

The femoral head of a newborn is completely cartilaginous on histological assessment. Furthermore, the cartilage contains vascular canals (also called cartilage canals) where blood vessels are distributed throughout the cartilaginous epiphysis [5, 9]. The vessels provide nutritional support to the cartilaginous structure. Around 4–6 months after birth, a secondary center of ossification (also called bony epiphysis or ossific nucleus) forms via endochondral ossification in the central region of the cartilaginous epiphysis. At the same time, the deep layer of the articular cartilage (also called epiphyseal cartilage) overlying the ossific nucleus becomes established as a spherical growth plate around the secondary center of ossification [10] (Fig. 59.2a). This growth cartilage is responsible for the circumferential growth of the secondary center until a full size of the femoral head is reached. As the secondary center enlarges, the articular cartilage thickness decreases and the cartilage canals regress and disappear [11–13]. In humans, their presence has been observed in

H.K.W. Kim
Center for Excellence in Hip Disorders, Texas Scottish Rite Hospital for Children, 2222 Welborn Street, Dallas, TX 75219, USA

Department of Orthopaedic Surgery, UT Southwestern Medical Center, Dallas, TX, USA
e-mail: harry.kim@tsrh.org

K.-H. Koo et al. (eds.), *Osteonecrosis*,
DOI 10.1007/978-3-642-35767-1_59, © Springer-Verlag Berlin Heidelberg 2014

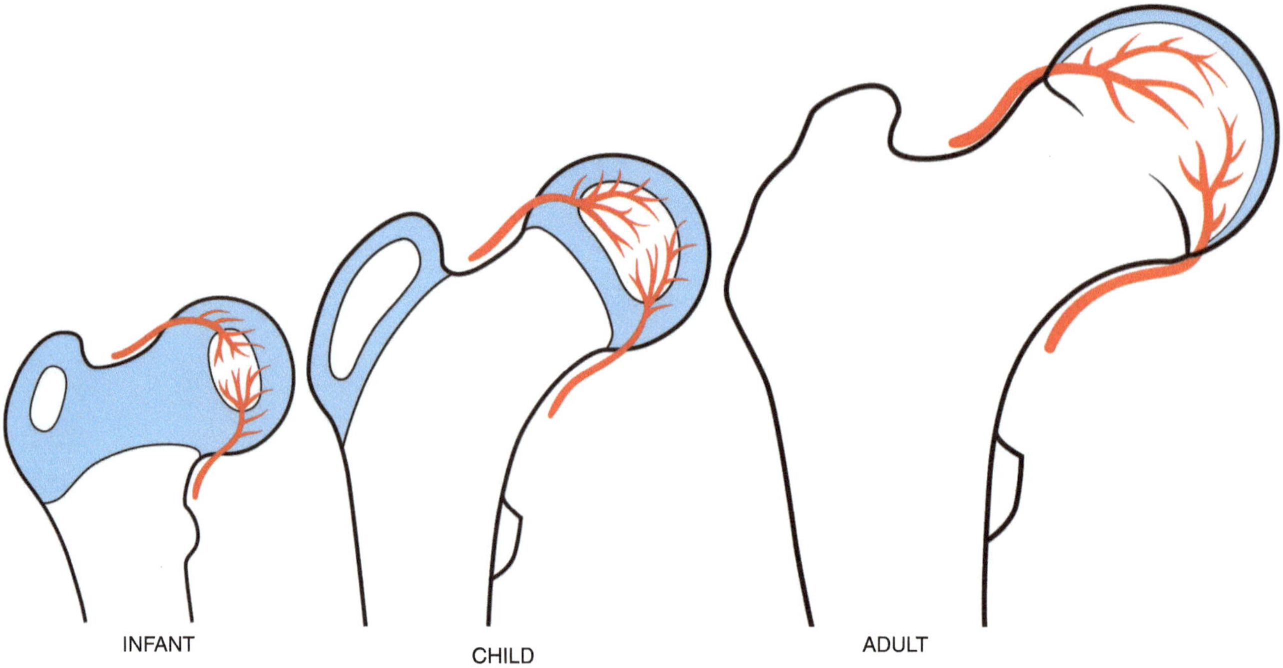

Fig. 59.1 A drawing depicting the developmental changes in the femoral head size, articular cartilage thickness, and epiphyseal vascular anatomy. As the proximal femur matures, the bony epiphysis becomes larger and the cartilage becomes thinner. The blood vessels also do not cross the growth plate cartilage to supply the bony epiphysis. Instead, they enter the cartilaginous epiphysis at the femoral head and neck junction. The onset of ischemic osteonecrosis at an older age would imply less growth and remodeling potentials and a larger bony epiphysis to revascularize and heal (This figure was reproduced with a permission from Texas Scottish Rite Hospital for Children)

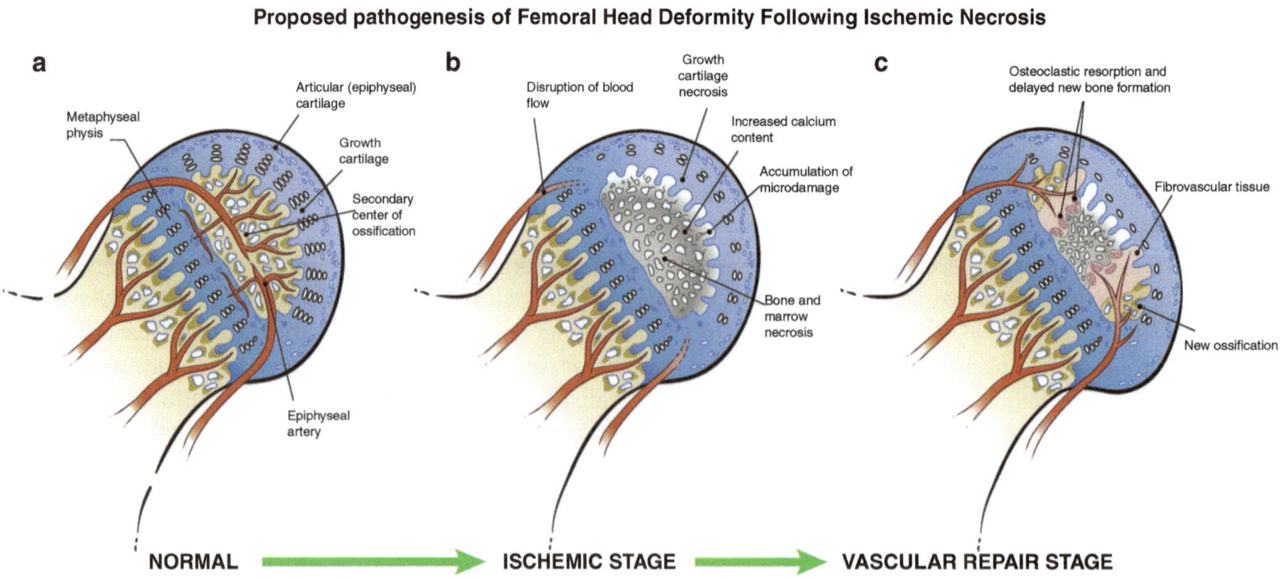

Fig. 59.2 An illustration of the pathological changes observed in the piglet model of ischemic osteonecrosis. (**a**) Normal immature femoral head showing the growth cartilage surrounding the bony epiphysis. This growth cartilage is responsible for the circumferential growth of the epiphysis through endochondral ossification. (**b**) Ischemic injury produces extensive cell death in the bony epiphysis (osteonecrosis) and the deep layer of the articular cartilage (chondronecrosis). The ischemic damage to the deep layer of the cartilage produces a growth arrest of the secondary center. Ischemic osteonecrosis is also associated with an increased calcium content of the necrotic bone, which makes the bone more brittle and more prone to microdamage accumulation with hip joint loading. Subchondral and compaction type fracture seen in the initial stage of LCPD may be a result of microcrack accumulation and mechanical loading. (**c**) Revascularization of the infarcted epiphysis is associated with a predominance of osteoclast-mediated resorption and a delayed bone formation, which further contribute to the femoral head deformity (This figure was reproduced with a permission from Texas Scottish Rite Hospital for Children)

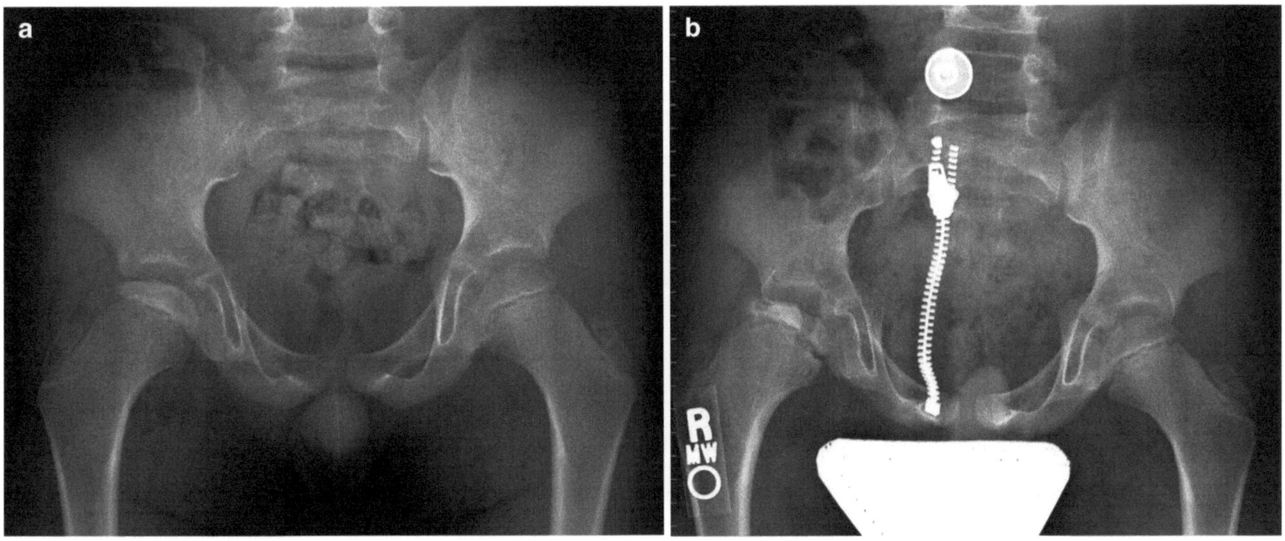

Fig. 59.3 Eight-year-old boy with right hip pain for 5 months. (**a**) AP pelvis radiograph showing a smaller epiphysis due to growth arrest of the epiphysis. Note the increased radiodensity of the epiphysis. The femoral head is in the initial stage of LCPD. (**b**) AP pelvis radiograph obtained 5 months later showing fragmented and resorptive changes in the affected epiphysis with further flattening of the femoral head. Most of the deformity occurs during the stage of fragmentation

early childhood, but it is unclear when they disappear [5]. Since a portion of the articular cartilage is responsible for the growth of the secondary center, the thinning of the cartilage during maturation represents decreasing growth and remodeling potentials of the immature femoral head. At skeletal maturity, the endochondral ossification stops, and the cartilage becomes an adult articular cartilage.

The cessation of endochondral ossification at the femoral head maturity produces histological changes in the subchondral region of the femoral head and, most likely, mechanical changes as well. In the immature femoral head, the subchondral region consists of primary and secondary spongiosa (newly formed immature cancellous bone) due to the ongoing endochondral ossification at the cartilage-bone junction. In the mature femoral head, the subchondral region consists of compact bone (also called subchondral bone plate), and a tidemark forms at the junction of the cartilage and the bone [14]. In the mature femoral head, the nutritional support for the articular cartilage, including its deep layer, is derived mainly from the synovial fluid [15]. In the immature femoral head, the articular cartilage is thicker, and the deep layer of the articular cartilage is dependent on the cartilage canals and the subchondral vascularity for its nutrition [16–19]. Because of this difference, a loss of blood supply to the femoral head in children not only produces a necrotic damage to the bone but also damage to the growth cartilage (chondronecrosis) surrounding the secondary center of ossification as a part of the ischemic damage [20, 21]. The consequence is a growth arrest of the secondary center which is an early radiographic feature of LCPD (Fig. 59.3a). One significant implication of this damage is a potential for growth disturbance of the secondary center once the endochondral ossification is reestablished during healing [17]. Unless the restoration of growth of the secondary center is symmetrical, a further deformity of the femoral head can ensue if the restoration of the growth is asymmetrical (Fig. 59.4). This represents a separate source of deformity from the growth disturbance of the metaphyseal physis which is responsible for the length and the alignment of the femoral neck. The growth disturbance of the metaphyseal physis produces coxa breva (short neck) and coxa vara in LCPD.

59.2.2 Healing Potential of Immature Femoral Head

A further distinction between the immature and the mature femoral head comes from an observation that the superficial layer of the articular cartilage shows evidence of a hypoxic and angiogenic repair response acutely after the induction of ischemic necrosis in a large animal model of LCPD [22]. The levels of hypoxia-inducible factor-1, a master regulator of hypoxic adaptation response, and the vascular endothelial growth factor, a potent angiogenic factor, were significantly increased in the cartilage after the induction of ischemic necrosis in the experimental model of ischemic osteonecrosis [22, 23]. Vascular invasion of the cartilage preceded revascularization of the necrotic bony epiphysis. Thus, the cartilage appears to play an active role in the revascularization process in the immature femoral head from the early stage of the disease process. In contrast, the involvement of the articular cartilage in the adult femoral head osteonecrosis

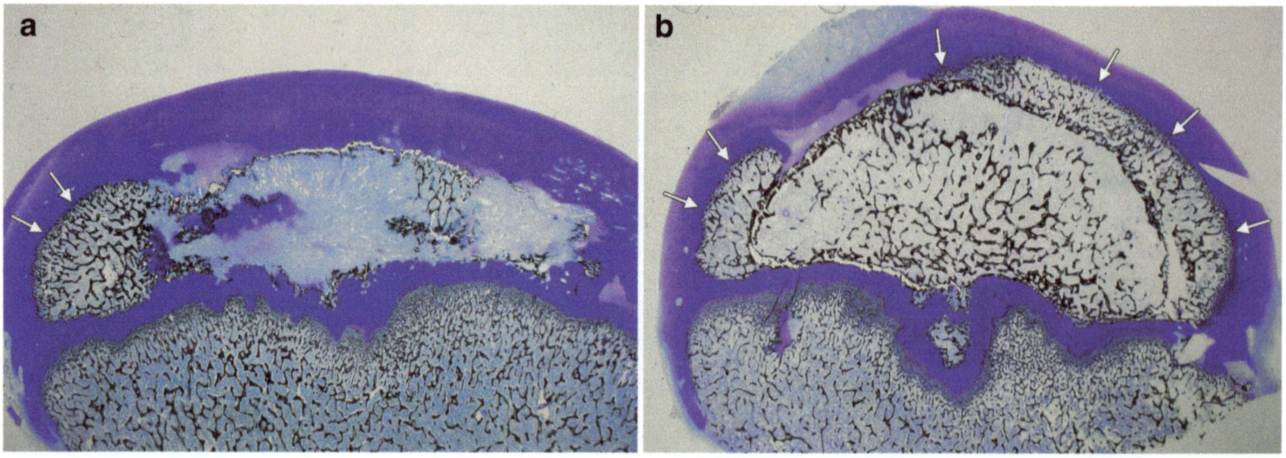

Fig. 59.4 Photomicrographs of the piglet model of ischemic osteonecrosis of the femoral head. (**a**) A deformed femoral head with restoration of endochondral ossification occurring only at the periphery of the epiphysis (*arrows*). This asymmetric restoration of epiphyseal growth will promote a deformed femoral head. (**b**) A spherical femoral head with restoration of endochondral ossification occurring all around the affected epiphysis (*arrows*). This symmetrical restoration of epiphyseal growth will promote a spherical growth

is thought to be a late feature of joint degeneration and osteoarthritis [24–26]. Since the adult articular cartilage derives its nutritional support from the synovial fluid, it is unaffected by the ischemic process in the bone. The cartilage involvement occurs at a later stage when the femoral head collapses and degenerative osteoarthritis ensues. It is also believed that the adult articular cartilage does not play an active role in the repair process. An experimental study suggests that the potential for femoral head healing is greater in younger animals compared to older, immature animals because of robust hypoxic and angiogenic responses from the cartilage [27].

The age of onset of FHO is clearly an important variable that influences the femoral head healing potential. For instance, the majority of children with the onset of LCPD before age 6 is known to heal, remodel, and restore the growth of the necrotic femoral head and have a good outcome (defined as a round femoral head at skeletal maturity) [28]. Older patients with LCPD, however, do not heal and remodel their necrotic femoral heads as well as the younger patients, and their prognosis is guarded [29]. The healing potential of FHO in adolescents is generally poor and their outcomes more closely resemble those of adults than those of younger children [7, 8]. While there are appreciable differences in the morphology and the histology of the immature and adult femoral heads as noted above, the molecular mechanisms responsible for the difference in the healing potential remain unknown. Understanding how the onset of osteonecrosis at different ages or stages in childhood (infantile, toddler, preschool, juvenile, teenager, and adolescence) affects the healing potential and the outcome will be important for developing new treatment strategies to improve the poor outcome observed in older children (after age 8) and adolescents affected with LCPD.

59.2.3 Blood Supply to Immature Femoral Head

In addition to the morphological changes taking place in the femoral head with growth and maturation, the blood supply to the femoral head also changes over time. At birth, the lateral half of the head is supplied by the lateral circumflex artery and the medial half by the medial circumflex artery, which are generally branches of the deep profunda artery from the superficial femoral artery [3, 4]. By 18 months of age, the majority of vessels supplying the femoral epiphysis are from the medial femoral circumflex artery, and no vessels cross the metaphyseal physis. Thus, the femoral neck vessels supplying the secondary center of ossification traverse through the articular cartilage at the junction of the femoral head and neck to gain access to the secondary center of ossification. It has been postulated that the portion of the vessels traversing through the cartilage is at risk for disruption from trauma to the hip joint. By 3 years of age, the medial femoral circumflex supplies the entire proximal femoral epiphysis and the metaphyseal physis. The lateral femoral circumflex supplies the greater trochanter and the trochanteric physis. This leaves the femoral head susceptible to vascular injury particularly at the watershed regions in the lateral and anterior quadrants of the femoral head. An additional predisposing factor for femoral head osteonecrosis is the marginal collateral circulation in the femoral head.

With skeletal maturation, the arrangement of the vasculature within the femoral head changes significantly. The regression and the disappearance of the metaphyseal physis allows the vessels from the femoral neck to supply the femoral head without having to traverse through the articular cartilage (Fig. 59.1). In adults, cadaveric dissection studies have shown that the deep branches or posterosuperior branches of the medial femoral circumflex artery perforate the hip capsule at the level of the superior gemellus and travel up the femoral neck as retinacular vessels and enter the femoral head through vascular foramina at the femoral head and neck junction in the superior region of the neck to provide the majority of the blood supply to the femoral head [30, 31]. These studies have been essential for the development of a safe surgical technique to dislocate the femoral head to visualize and treat various intra-articular hip pathologies in adults without causing FHO.

59.3 Pathology and Pathophysiology

It is generally accepted that a disruption of blood supply to the femoral head is a key pathogenic event associated with the initiation of the disease process. Selective angiography [32–34], bone scintigraphy [35], and perfusion MRI [36] provide evidence of a partial or complete disruption of the blood supply to the femoral head. Histological studies of the biopsy specimens [37] obtained in the early stages of LCPD also show findings consistent with ischemic tissue damage. Furthermore, a disruption of the blood supply to the femoral head in a large animal model produces histopathological and radiographical changes resembling LCPD, including growth arrest of the epiphysis, subsequent fragmented appearance of the epiphysis, and the epiphyseal collapse resembling coxa plana [38].

59.3.1 Histopathological Studies of LCPD

A limited number of histopathological studies on LCPD have been performed. These studies consist of case reports and limited surgical biopsy studies of LCPD patients in the active phase of the disease providing a limited view of the disease which is known to have a wide clinical variability. Only a handful of whole femoral heads have been examined and reported to date [20]. Very little is known about the pathological changes in the preclinical stage of LCPD and the temporal changes that occur within each femoral head over time.

The findings from the limited number of histopathological studies [20, 21, 37, 39–44] can be summarized as follows: LCPD affects the articular cartilage, the bony epiphysis, and, in some cases, the physis and the metaphysis. The articular cartilage damage is observed in the deep layer of the cartilage which is a growth cartilage responsible for the spherical growth of the bony epiphysis. The necrosis in the deep layer of the cartilage produces a cessation of endochondral ossification. This explains why the affected epiphysis is smaller than the unaffected epiphysis in a patient who is growing. Other changes observed in the deep cartilage layer include a separation of the cartilage layer from the underlying subchondral bone, degenerative changes in the cartilage matrix, vascular granulation tissue invasion of the cartilage, and appearance of new accessory ossifications. In the affected bony epiphysis, the necrosis of marrow and bone cells, compression fracture of trabeculae, osteoclastic resorption, fibrovascular granulation tissue invasion of the necrotic head, absence of osteoblasts, empty lacunae in the trabecular bone, and thickened trabeculae have been reported. The metaphyseal growth plate changes are most often seen in the anterior part of the femoral head with focal areas of growth cartilage columns extending below the endochondral ossification line. Since premature growth arrest of the growth plate is seen in about 30 % of patients, it is questionable whether the growth plate damage is a primary feature of LCPD. Another possibility is that the growth plate damage is a result of the mechanical damage from overloading of the femoral head as the mechanical load is transmitted from the compressed, hard necrotic bone to the underlying growth plate. An experimental study in piglets showed that a total disruption of the epiphyseal blood supply does not produce growth arrest in a majority of the animals, suggesting that the metaphyseal growth plate is not dependent on the epiphyseal blood supply [45]. Metaphyseal radiolucent changes are sometimes seen in the early stages of LCPD. The mechanisms responsible for the appearance of these lesions are unclear. Various tissue types have been reported including columns of normal or degenerated cartilage extending down to the metaphysis, fibrocartilage, fat necrosis, vascular proliferation, and focal fibrosis [20]. Some have found an association between the presence of radiolucent metaphyseal changes and poor prognosis while others have not.

59.3.2 Pathophysiology Based on Experimental Studies

The lack of availability of clinical specimens to systematically investigate the pathophysiology of LCPD is a significant hindrance to our understanding of LCPD. To circumvent this obstacle, large animal models have been developed to study the pathophysiology of ischemic osteonecrosis. Of these models, a piglet model of ischemic necrosis has been extensively investigated [17, 38, 45–48]. While the animal model is not a perfect model of LCPD, no perfect model exists currently. The model does provide some new insight about the ischemic bone injury and repair process in the immature femoral head.

Following the induction of ischemic FHO in immature pigs, the earliest histological changes are seen in the marrow space with the death of various cells present, such as the hematopoietic cells, adipocytes, endothelial cells, and stromal cells [17, 49]. Death of osteoblasts lining the trabeculae, osteocytes within the trabecular lacunae, and osteoclasts also takes place in the area of ischemia. The mechanisms of cell death include apoptosis (programmed cell death) as well as necrosis [49]. The appearance of empty lacunae in the trabecular bone, which signifies osteocyte death, is a classic feature of osteonecrosis but a late histological sign taking a few weeks to develop.

Cartilage necrosis (chondronecrosis) is a consistent feature of ischemic injury to the immature femoral head. Induction of ischemic necrosis in the piglet model produces cell death in the growth cartilage surrounding the secondary center (i.e., the deep layer of the articular cartilage) (Fig. 59.2b) [17, 22, 23]. This explains the cessation of endochondral ossification at the growth cartilage-bone junction in the initial stage of LCPD. The other significance is that in order for the epiphyseal growth to resume, the necrotic cartilage has to be repaired and the endochondral ossification reestablished. If the epiphysis becomes deformed over time, the resumption of epiphyseal growth may not be symmetrical. The revascularization and repair of the necrotic cartilage preferentially occur in the periphery of the deformed femoral head and not at the central region. Thus, the reestablished epiphyseal growth may not be spherical as seen in the normal epiphysis and further deformity due to the growth disturbance may occur. In contrast to the growth cartilage in the epiphysis, the metaphyseal physis (the proximal femoral growth plate) is generally spared [45]. In most of the animals, the growth plate did not develop a physeal bar. Endochondral ossification continued following a total disruption of blood flow to the immature femoral head, albeit at a slower rate than the growth plate on the normal side.

In the piglet model of ischemic osteonecrosis, revascularization and healing of the necrotic femoral head come in the form of fibrovascular granulation tissue invasion of the necrotic cartilage and the necrotic marrow space [38]. The new invading vessels arise from the existing vessels on the femoral neck. The angiogenic process is stimulated by increased production of a potent angiogenic factor called the vascular endothelial growth factor (VEGF) which is actively expressed by viable chondrocytes in the superficial region of the articular cartilage [22, 23]. Hypoxia is a potent stimulus for the activation of the hypoxia-inducible factor-1 (HIF-1) which increases VEGF production and angiogenesis. New vessels invade through the cartilage to reach the necrotic secondary center from the periphery of the epiphysis [22]. In general, the invading vessels do not cross the metaphyseal physis.

The fibrovascular granulation tissue consists of inflammatory, mesenchymal (fibroblast-like in appearance), and endothelial cells. In the revascularized regions of the bone, increased presence of osteoclasts is observed with increased osteoclastic resorption of the necrotic bone. The predominance of bone resorption produces a net loss of bone [38]. New bone formation is absent in these areas where the necrotic bone is replaced by a fibrovascular tissue. Radiographic and histological studies of the patients with LCPD also show resorptive changes in the necrotic bone with delayed reossification of the resorbed areas [50]. In LCPD, the resorptive phase of the disease represents the fragmentation stage where radiolucent changes are seen on the radiographs, producing fragmented and resorptive changes in the sclerotic epiphysis (Fig. 59.3b). During the fragmentation stage, most of the deformation of the femoral head takes place indicating that this is the most mechanically vulnerable stage of the disease. As seen in the piglet model, new bone formation (termed reossification in LCPD) does not occur until many months later. Furthermore, the reossification stage is the longest stage of LCPD, especially in the older patients [51].

59.3.3 Pathology of Adult Femoral Head Osteonecrosis

In adult FHO, most of the infarcted region of the femoral head remains necrotic over time with the extent of revascularization and repair taking place being limited to the border of the viable and the necrotic bone, which is called the reparative or hyperemic zone [24–26, 52]. In the reparative zone, a slow healing process described by Phemister as a "creeping substitution" is observed [53]. The term describes the process in which the dead bone is substituted with new bone. In the past, the term "creeping substitution" has been used to describe the repair process in LCPD. However, the application of the term "creeping substitution" to LCPD is incorrect as the repair process in LCPD is staged with resorption occurring first followed by a delay in new bone formation. There is no immediate substitution of the dead bone with the new bone. Instead, the dead bone is substituted to a fibrovascular tissue.

Based on clinical observations, the repair process in adult osteonecrosis appears to be limited if >30 % of the femoral head is involved. Because of the inability to repair a large area of necrosis in adults, the femoral head collapses due to a mechanical failure of the necrotic bone, most often at the junction of the necrotic bone and the reparative zone. A segmental collapse of the necrotic region of the femoral head produces a disruption in the smooth articular surface which leads to the development of premature osteoarthritis.

59.4 Pathogenesis of Femoral Head Deformity

One of the most significant sequelae of LCPD is the development of the femoral head deformity. The experimental studies using the piglet model reveal that the pathogenesis of the femoral head deformity following ischemic osteonecrosis is complex with multiple contributing factors. Mechanical

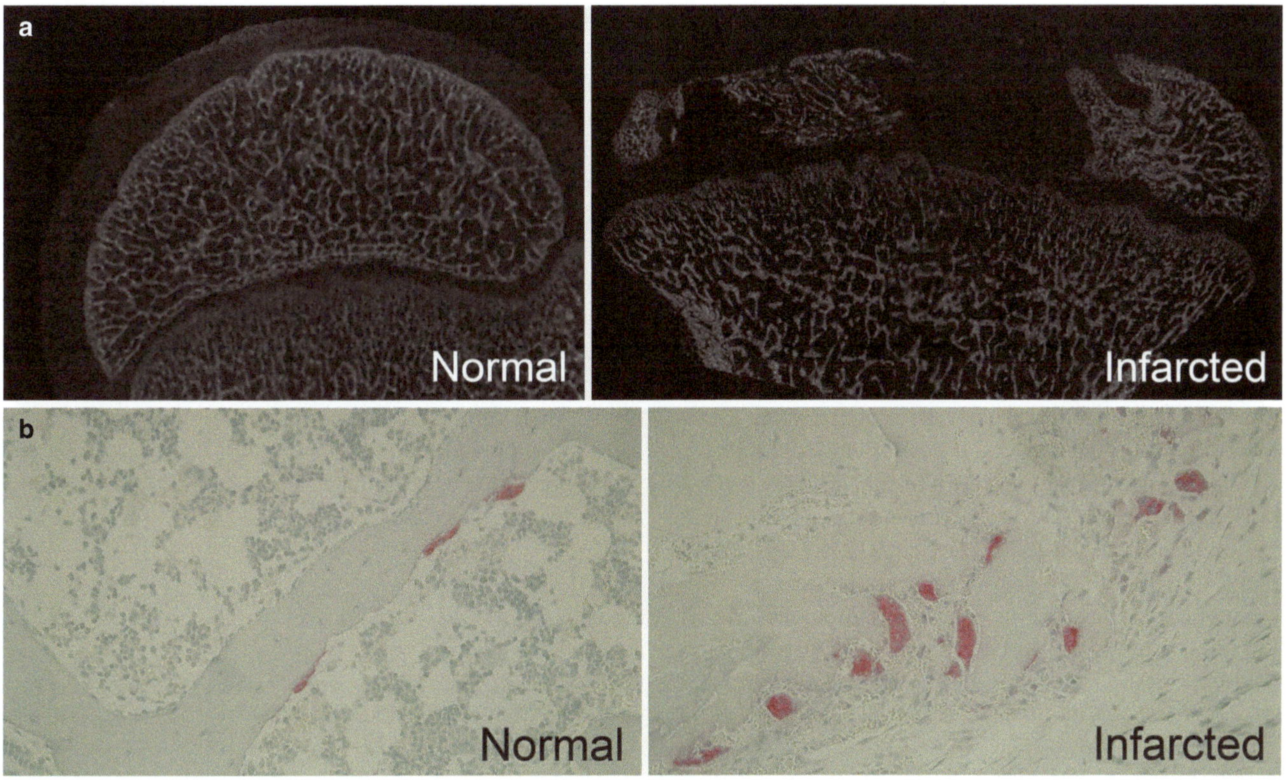

Fig. 59.5 Micro-CT and histological assessments of the piglet model of ischemic osteonecrosis during the vascular repair phase of the model. (**a**) Micro-CT sections reveal increased bone resorption in the infarcted epiphysis compared to the normal. (**b**) Histological assessment showing increased presence of osteoclasts (tartrate-resistant acid phosphatase staining) in the infarcted epiphysis compared to the normal

studies on the piglet model reveal that ischemic osteonecrosis induces a significant mechanical weakening of the immature femoral head [47, 48].

59.4.1 Mechanisms of Deformity in the Avascular Stage

Even in the early stage of the model, significant decreases in the mechanical properties of the infarcted femoral head and its components (articular cartilage and bone) are observed [47, 48]. Further studies undertaken to explain the mechanical weakening revealed that the material and mechanical properties of the trabecular bone are altered following ischemic injury. In the infarcted femoral head, the calcium contents of the calcified cartilage and the subchondral bone are significantly increased compared to the normal femoral head [54]. The change in the calcium content makes the necrotic bone in the subchondral region more brittle and more prone to microcrack development (Fig. 59.2b). A follow-up study indeed showed that the nanoindentation modulus of the necrotic trabeculae was significantly increased in the infarcted femoral heads compared to the contralateral normal femoral heads, making it more brittle [55]. The microcrack density measurement in the subchondral bone was also significantly higher in the infarcted femoral heads. The absence of osteoblasts, osteocytes, and osteoclasts in the necrotic bone due to extensive cell death preclude the detection and the repair of the microcracks that develop with normal daily activities. It is proposed that a subchondral fracture or a compression fracture in the superior aspect of the femoral head develops with normal physiological loading when enough microcracks have accumulated in the early stage of LCPD [56]. The increased calcium content of the necrotic bone may also explain the appearance of increased radiodensity in the early stage of LCPD.

59.4.2 Mechanisms of Deformity in the Vascular Stage

Further collapse of the femoral head occurs in the fragmentation stage of the disease when revascularization and resorption of the necrotic bone take place (Fig. 59.2c). Studies of the piglet model show an imbalance of bone resorption and bone formation. The predominance of osteoclast-mediated bone resorption produces a net bone loss which contributes to the mechanical weakening of the femoral head [38] (Fig. 59.5). Furthermore, inhibition of bone resorption using bisphosphonates or an RANKL inhibitor can decrease the bone loss and improve the preservation of the femoral head shape [57–61]. While few studies on the use of bisphosphonate to treat FHO in non-LCPD patients have been reported [62–64], the efficacy of this treatment for childhood FHO has yet to be investigated with a clinical trial.

59.4.3 Effects of Weight Bearing on Infarcted Femoral Heads

In addition to the pathological repair process occurring within the femoral head, it is also important to consider the external forces acting on the hip joint that produces the deformity. Instrumented total hip replacement studies using an internal strain gauge capable of telemetric transmission of hip contact pressure data in real time have provided valuable information about hip contact pressures associated with normal daily activities. These studies reveal that normal walking or running produces hip contact pressure about 2.5 and 5 times the body weight with each step or each stride, respectively [65, 66]. Greater pressures are generated with a faster speed of walking or running. Other normal activities also produce significant loading of the hip joint. Since children with LCPD in general are very active, the infarcted femoral head is thought to deform when the loading is beyond the mechanical strength of the femoral head to resist deformation. The adverse effect of weight bearing on the infarcted femoral head was shown in an experimental study using the piglet model [67]. In the study, non-weight bearing of the affected hip significantly better preserved the spherical shape of the femoral head. Non-weight bearing treatment, however, increased bone resorption without increasing bone formation. These findings raise some concerns since a loss of compliance to NWB or untimely resumption of full weight bearing may put the femoral head at a risk for collapse due to the increased resorption of the bone and the loss of bone volume in the affected femoral head. These results call for the need to investigate the biological therapeutic strategies to control bone resorption and to stimulate new bone formation to improve the bone healing in LCPD [68–71].

59.5 Summary

Current understanding of LCPD is limited by the unavailability of the tissue samples from various stages of the disease to systematically study its pathophysiology. Limited studies on the histopathology of LCPD indicate ischemic damage to the bony epiphysis and the deep layer of the articular cartilage due to a disruption of the blood supply to the femoral head. Experimental studies using the piglet model reveal that the pathogenesis of femoral head deformity following ischemic osteonecrosis is complex. The necrotic bone has increased calcium content and brittleness, making it more prone to accumulate microcracks. The repair process following the ischemic damage is also pathological with an imbalance of bone resorption and bone formation. The predominance of bone resorption with delayed bone formation weakens the affected bony epiphysis and makes it more susceptible to deformation and collapse during normal daily activities. Growth disturbance of the epiphysis and the age at onset of the disease affect the healing and remodeling potential of the epiphysis. Given the complexity, an osteotomy or a mechanical treatment approach may not adequately address the pathogenesis of the femoral head deformity. More comprehensive approach, which includes specific biological treatments to address the imbalance of bone resorption and bone formation and limited loading of the hip joint during healing, should be investigated.

References

1. Kricun ME. Red-yellow marrow conversion: its effect on the location of some solitary bone lesions. Skeletal Radiol. 1985;14(1):10–9.
2. Waitches G, Zawin JK, Poznanski AK. Sequence and rate of bone marrow conversion in the femora of children as seen on MR imaging: are accepted standards accurate? AJR Am J Roentgenol. 1994;162(6):1399–406.
3. Chung SM. The arterial supply of the developing proximal end of the human femur. J Bone Joint Surg Am. 1976;58(7):961–70.
4. Ogden JA. Changing patterns of proximal femoral vascularity. J Bone Joint Surg Am. 1974;56(5):941–50.
5. Trueta J. The normal vascular anatomy of the human femoral head during growth. J Bone Joint Surg Br. 1957;39-B(2):358–94.
6. Joseph B. Prognostic factors and outcome measures in Perthes disease. Orthop Clin North Am. 2011;42(3):303–15, v–vi. doi:10.1016/j.ocl.2011.03.004. S0030-5898(11)00028-9 [pii].
7. Ippolito E, Tudisco C, Farsetti P. Long-term prognosis of Legg-Calve-Perthes disease developing during adolescence. J Pediatr Orthop. 1985;5(6):652–6.
8. Joseph B, Mulpuri K, Varghese G. Perthes' disease in the adolescent. J Bone Joint Surg Br. 2001;83(5):715–20.
9. Haines RW. Cartilage canals. J Anat. 1933;68(Pt 1):45–64.
10. Ogden JA, Rosenberg LC. Defining the growth plate. In: Uhthoff HK, Wiley JJ, editors. Behavior of the growth plate. New York: Raven Press; 1988. p. 1–15.
11. Hughes LO, Aronson J, Smith HS. Normal radiographic values for cartilage thickness and physeal angle in the pediatric hip. J Pediatr Orthop. 1999;19(4):443–8.
12. Meszaros T, Kery L. Quantitative analysis of the growth of the hip joint. A radiological study. Acta Orthop Scand. 1980;51(2):275–83.
13. Rissech C, Schaefer M, Malgosa A. Development of the femur – implications for age and sex determination. Forensic Sci Int. 2008;180(1):1–9. doi:10.1016/j.forsciint.2008.06.006. S0379-0738(08)00279-X [pii].
14. Madry H, van Dijk CN, Mueller-Gerbl M. The basic science of the subchondral bone. Knee Surg Sports Traumatol Arthrosc. 2010;18(4):419–33. doi:10.1007/s00167-010-1054-z.
15. O'Hara BP, Urban JP, Maroudas A. Influence of cyclic loading on the nutrition of articular cartilage. Ann Rheum Dis. 1990;49(7):536–9.

16. Carlson CS, Meuten DJ, Richardson DC. Ischemic necrosis of cartilage in spontaneous and experimental lesions of osteochondrosis. J Orthop Res. 1991;9(3):317–29. doi:10.1002/jor.1100090303.
17. Kim HK, Su PH, Qiu YS. Histopathologic changes in growth-plate cartilage following ischemic necrosis of the capital femoral epiphysis. An experimental investigation in immature pigs. J Bone Joint Surg Am. 2001;83-A(5):688–97.
18. McKibbin B, Holdsworth FW. The nutrition of immature joint cartilage in the lamb. J Bone Joint Surg Br. 1966;48(4):793–803.
19. Ytrehus B, Andreas Haga H, Mellum CN, Mathisen L, Carlson CS, Ekman S, et al. Experimental ischemia of porcine growth cartilage produces lesions of osteochondrosis. J Orthop Res. 2004;22(6):1201–9. doi:10.1016/j.orthres.2004.03.006. S073602660400066X [pii].
20. Catterall A, Pringle J, Byers PD, Fulford GE, Kemp HB, Dolman CL, et al. A review of the morphology of Perthes' disease. J Bone Joint Surg Br. 1982;64(3):269–75.
21. Milgram JW. Idiopathic osteonecrosis of the juvenile femoral head (Legg-Calve-Perthes disease). Radiologic and histologic pathology of nontumorous diseases of bones and joints. Northbrook: Northbrook Publishing Company; 1990. p. 1093–113.
22. Kim HK, Bian H, Aya-ay J, Garces A, Morgan EF, Gilbert SR. Hypoxia and HIF-1alpha expression in the epiphyseal cartilage following ischemic injury to the immature femoral head. Bone. 2009;45(2):280–8. doi:10.1016/j.bone.2009.03.665. S8756-3282(09)01217-4 [pii].
23. Kim HK, Bian H, Randall T, Garces A, Gerstenfeld LC, Einhorn TA. Increased VEGF expression in the epiphyseal cartilage after ischemic necrosis of the capital femoral epiphysis. J Bone Miner Res. 2004;19(12):2041–8. doi:10.1359/JBMR.040911.
24. Glimcher MJ, Kenzora JE. The biology of osteonecrosis of the human femoral head and its clinical implications: II. The pathological changes in the femoral head as an organ and in the hip joint. Clin Orthop Relat Res. 1979;139:283–312.
25. Glimcher MJ, Kenzora JE. Nicolas Andry award. The biology of osteonecrosis of the human femoral head and its clinical implications: 1. Tissue biology. Clin Orthop Relat Res. 1979;138:284–309.
26. Milgram JW. Osteonecrosis due to trauma and idiopathic causes. Radiologic and histologic pathology of nontumorous diseases of bones and joints. Northbrook: Northbrook Publishing Company; 1990. p. 959–1026.
27. Kim H, Bian H, Aya-ay J, Garces A, Zhang C. Age affects hypoxia and hypoxia-inducible factor-1 (HIF-1) level in the epiphyseal cartilage following ischemic injury to the immature femoral head. J Bone Miner Res. 2009;24(Suppl 1):SU0015.
28. Rosenfeld SB, Herring JA, Chao JC. Legg-Calve-Perthes disease: a review of cases with onset before six years of age. J Bone Joint Surg Am. 2007;89(12):2712–22. doi:10.2106/JBJS.G.00191. 89/12/2712 [pii].
29. Herring JA, Kim HT, Browne R. Legg-Calve-Perthes disease. Part II: Prospective multicenter study of the effect of treatment on outcome. J Bone Joint Surg Am. 2004;86-A(10):2121–34. 86/10/2121 [pii].
30. Gautier E, Ganz K, Krugel N, Gill T, Ganz R. Anatomy of the medial femoral circumflex artery and its surgical implications. J Bone Joint Surg Br. 2000;82(5):679–83.
31. Lavigne M, Kalhor M, Beck M, Ganz R, Leunig M. Distribution of vascular foramina around the femoral head and neck junction: relevance for conservative intracapsular procedures of the hip. Orthop Clin North Am. 2005;36(2):171–6, viii. doi:10.1016/j.ocl.2005.02.002. S0030-5898(05)00010-6 [pii].
32. Atsumi T, Yamano K, Muraki M, Yoshihara S, Kajihara T. The blood supply of the lateral epiphyseal arteries in Perthes' disease. J Bone Joint Surg Br. 2000;82(3):392–8.
33. de Camargo FP, De Godoy Jr RM, Tovo R. Angiography in Perthes' disease. Clin Orthop Relat Res. 1984;191:216–20.
34. Theron J. Angiography in Legg-Calve-Perthes disease. Radiology. 1980;135(1):81–92.
35. Conway JJ. A scintigraphic classification of Legg-Calve-Perthes disease. Semin Nucl Med. 1993;23(4):274–95.
36. Lamer S, Dorgeret S, Khairouni A, Mazda K, Brillet PY, Bacheville E, et al. Femoral head vascularisation in Legg-Calve-Perthes disease: comparison of dynamic gadolinium-enhanced subtraction MRI with bone scintigraphy. Pediatr Radiol. 2002;32(8):580–5. doi:10.1007/s00247-002-0732-5.
37. Jonsater S. Coxa plana; a histo-pathologic and arthrographic study. Acta Orthop Scand Suppl. 1953;12:5–98.
38. Kim HK, Su PH. Development of flattening and apparent fragmentation following ischemic necrosis of the capital femoral epiphysis in a piglet model. J Bone Joint Surg Am. 2002;84-A(8):1329–34.
39. Catterall A, Pringle J, Byers PD, Fulford GE, Kemp HB. Perthes' disease: is the epiphysial infarction complete? J Bone Joint Surg Br. 1982;64(3):276–81.
40. Dolman CL, Bell HM. The pathology of Legg-Calve-Perthes disease. A case report. J Bone Joint Surg Am. 1973;55(1):184–8.
41. Inoue A, Freeman MA, Vernon-Roberts B, Mizuno S. The pathogenesis of Perthes' disease. J Bone Joint Surg Br. 1976;58-B(4):453–61.
42. McKibbin B, Ralis Z. Pathological changes in a case of Perthes' disease. J Bone Joint Surg Br. 1974;56B(3):438–47.
43. Ponseti IV. Legg-Perthes disease; observations on pathological changes in two cases. J Bone Joint Surg Am. 1956;38-A(4):739–50.
44. Ponseti IV, Maynard JA, Weinstein SL, Ippolito EG, Pous JG. Legg-Calve-Perthes disease. Histochemical and ultrastructural observations of the epiphyseal cartilage and physis. J Bone Joint Surg Am. 1983;65(6):797–807.
45. Kim HK, Stephenson N, Garces A, Aya-ay J, Bian H. Effects of disruption of epiphyseal vasculature on the proximal femoral growth plate. J Bone Joint Surg Am. 2009;91(5):1149–58. doi:10.2106/JBJS.H.00654. 91/5/1149 [pii].
46. Kim HK, Skelton DN, Quigley EJ. Pathogenesis of metaphyseal radiolucent changes following ischemic necrosis of the capital femoral epiphysis in immature pigs. A preliminary report. J Bone Joint Surg Am. 2004;86-A(1):129–35.
47. Koob TJ, Pringle D, Gedbaw E, Meredith J, Berrios R, Kim HK. Biomechanical properties of bone and cartilage in growing femoral head following ischemic osteonecrosis. J Orthop Res. 2007;25(6):750–7. doi:10.1002/jor.20350.
48. Pringle D, Koob TJ, Kim HK. Indentation properties of growing femoral head following ischemic necrosis. J Orthop Res. 2004;22(1):122–30. doi:10.1016/S0736-0266(03)00135-9. S0736026603001359 [pii].
49. Kothapalli R, Aya-ay JP, Bian H, Garces A, Kim HK. Ischaemic injury to femoral head induces apoptotic and oncotic cell death. Pathology. 2007;39(2):241–6. doi:10.1080/00313020701230765. 773357195 [pii].
50. Kim HK, Herring JA. Pathophysiology, classifications, and natural history of Perthes disease. Orthop Clin North Am. 2011;42(3):285–95, v. doi:10.1016/j.ocl.2011.04.007. S0030-5898(11)00035-6 [pii].
51. Herring JA, Williams JJ, Neustadt JN, Early JS. Evolution of femoral head deformity during the healing phase of Legg-Calve-Perthes disease. J Pediatr Orthop. 1993;13(1):41–5.
52. Glimcher MJ, Kenzora JE. The biology of osteonecrosis of the human femoral head and its clinical implications: an abridged communication. Clin Orthop Relat Res. 1978;130:47–50.
53. Phemister DB. Treatment of the necrotic head of the femur in adults. J Bone Joint Surg Am. 1949;31A(1):55–66.
54. Hofstaetter JG, Roschger P, Klaushofer K, Kim HK. Increased matrix mineralization in the immature femoral head following ischemic osteonecrosis. Bone. 2010;46(2):379–85. doi:10.1016/j.bone.2009.10.006. S8756-3282(09)01972-3 [pii].
55. Aruwajoye OO, Patel MK, Allen MR, Burr DB, Aswath PB, Kim HK. Microcrack density and nanomechanical properties in the subchondral region of the immature piglet femoral head following

ischemic osteonecrosis. Bone. 2013;52(2):632–9. doi:10.1016/j.bone.2012.07.028. S8756-3282(12)01012-5 [pii].
56. Park SS, Kim HK. Subchondral fracture after ischemic osteonecrosis of the immature femoral head in piglet model. J Pediatr Orthop B. 2011;20(4):227–31. doi:10.1097/BPB.0b013e328346725f. 01202412-201107000-00006 [pii].
57. Aya-ay J, Athavale S, Morgan-Bagley S, Bian H, Bauss F, Kim HK. Retention, distribution, and effects of intraosseously administered ibandronate in the infarcted femoral head. J Bone Miner Res. 2007;22(1):93–100. doi:10.1359/jbmr.060817.
58. Kim HK, Morgan-Bagley S, Kostenuik P. RANKL inhibition: a novel strategy to decrease femoral head deformity after ischemic osteonecrosis. J Bone Miner Res. 2006;21(12):1946–54. doi:10.1359/jbmr.060905.
59. Kim HK, Randall TS, Bian H, Jenkins J, Garces A, Bauss F. Ibandronate for prevention of femoral head deformity after ischemic necrosis of the capital femoral epiphysis in immature pigs. J Bone Joint Surg Am. 2005;87(3):550–7. doi:10.2106/JBJS.D.02192. 87/3/550 [pii].
60. Little DG, McDonald M, Sharpe IT, Peat R, Williams P, McEvoy T. Zoledronic acid improves femoral head sphericity in a rat model of Perthes disease. J Orthop Res. 2005;23(4):862–8. doi:10.1016/j.orthres.2004.11.015. S0736-0266(05)00002-1 [pii].
61. Little DG, Peat RA, McEvoy A, Williams PR, Smith EJ, Baldock PA. Zoledronic acid treatment results in retention of femoral head structure after traumatic osteonecrosis in young Wistar rats. J Bone Miner Res. 2003;18(11):2016–22. doi:10.1359/jbmr.2003.18.11.2016.
62. Kotecha RS, Powers N, Lee SJ, Murray KJ, Carter T, Cole C. Use of bisphosphonates for the treatment of osteonecrosis as a complication of therapy for childhood acute lymphoblastic leukaemia (ALL). Pediatr Blood Cancer. 2010;54(7):934–40. doi:10.1002/pbc.22428.
63. Nguyen T, Zacharin MR. Pamidronate treatment of steroid associated osteonecrosis in young patients treated for acute lymphoblastic leukaemia – two-year outcomes. J Pediatr Endocrinol Metab. 2006;19(2):161–7.
64. Ramachandran M, Ward K, Brown RR, Munns CF, Cowell CT, Little DG. Intravenous bisphosphonate therapy for traumatic osteonecrosis of the femoral head in adolescents. J Bone Joint Surg Am. 2007;89(8):1727–34. doi:10.2106/JBJS.F.00964. 89/8/1727 [pii].
65. Bergmann G, Deuretzbacher G, Heller M, Graichen F, Rohlmann A, Strauss J, et al. Hip contact forces and gait patterns from routine activities. J Biomech. 2001;34(7):859–71. S0021-9290(01)00040-9 [pii].
66. Bergmann G, Graichen F, Rohlmann A. Hip joint loading during walking and running, measured in two patients. J Biomech. 1993;26(8):969–90. 0021-9290(93)90058-M [pii].
67. Kim HK, Aruwajoye O, Stetler J, Stall A. Effects of non-weight-bearing on the immature femoral head following ischemic osteonecrosis: an experimental investigation in immature pigs. J Bone Joint Surg Am. 2013;94(24):2228–37. doi:10.2106/JBJS.L.00300.
68. Kim HK. Pathophysiology and new strategies for the treatment of Legg-Calve-Perthes disease. J Bone Joint Surg Am. 2012;94(7):659–69. doi:10.2106/JBJS.J.01834.
69. Little DG, Kim HK. Potential for bisphosphonate treatment in Legg-Calve-Perthes disease. J Pediatr Orthop. 2011;31 (2 Suppl):S182–8. doi:10.1097/BPO.0b013e318223b541. 01241398-201109001-00014 [pii].
70. Vandermeer JS, Kamiya N, Aya-ay J, Garces A, Browne R, Kim HK. Local administration of ibandronate and bone morphogenetic protein-2 after ischemic osteonecrosis of the immature femoral head: a combined therapy that stimulates bone formation and decreases femoral head deformity. J Bone Joint Surg Am. 2011;93(10):905–13. doi:10.2106/JBJS.J.00716. 93/10/905 [pii].
71. Young ML, Little DG, Kim HK. Evidence for using bisphosphonate to treat Legg-Calve-Perthes disease. Clin Orthop Relat Res. 2012;470(9):2462–75. doi:10.1007/s11999-011-2240-0.

60 Legg-Calvé-Perthes Disease: Diagnosis, Imaging, and Classifications

Benjamin Shore and Harry K.W. Kim

60.1 Introduction

Legg-Calvé-Perthes disease (LCPD) is a self-limited childhood hip disorder of unknown etiology that can produce permanent deformity of the femoral head. Legg of the United States, Calvé of France, and Perthes of Germany independently described the disease in 1910 [1]. The onset of LCPD occurs between 2 and 15 years of age with a peak between 4 and 9 years. Sundt in 1920 reported that boys were four times more likely to have the disease than girls and that 10 % of patients developed bilateral disease [2]. Molloy in 1966 [3] and Catterall in 1981 [4] reported similar findings with bilateral disease occurring in 10–15 % of patients and male-to-female ratio of 4–5:1. The diagnosis of LCPD requires plain radiography and careful history taking as its symptoms and physical findings are nonspecific and it is a diagnosis of exclusion. Other pediatric conditions that produce femoral head osteonecrosis or LCPD-like changes on radiography must be ruled out through history, physical examination, and radiographic assessment.

B. Shore
Department of Orthopaedic Surgery,
Boston Children's Hospital, Harvard Medical School,
Hunnewell 221, 300 Longwood Avenue, Boston, MA 02115, USA
e-mail: benjamin.shore@childrens.harvard.edu

H.K.W. Kim (✉)
Center for Excellence in Hip Disorders,
Texas Scottish Rite Hospital for Children,
2222 Welborn Street, Dallas, TX 75219, USA

Department of Orthopaedic Surgery,
UT Southwestern Medical Center, Dallas, TX, USA
e-mail: harry.kim@tsrh.org

60.2 Diagnosis

60.2.1 Symptoms and Signs

In general, patients suffering from LCPD present with hip (groin), thigh, or knee pain, a mild limp, and a decrease in hip motion which appear in an insidious fashion [5]. This is often first noticed by a parent or teacher. Symptoms are exacerbated by physical activity and alleviated with rest. The pain usually is mild during the early stages of the disease and does not restrict the child from daily activities. Often the limp is more pronounced later in the day if the child has been involved in extended periods of ambulation, running, or jumping.

Commonly the first complaint in children with LCPD is knee pain, leading the unsuspecting physician to obtain radiographs or other imaging of the knee. Wiig reported the results of 425 patients presenting with LCPD, 50 % of children presented with pain in the hip and thigh, 18 % with thigh and knee pain, 14 % with knee only pain, 8 % with pain in all three locations, 1 % in other areas, and 9 % had no pain [6]. Occasionally night pain exists; however, it seems to closely correlate with physical activity from the preceding day.

The patient or parent may recollect an isolated traumatic event that seems to be related with the onset of symptoms. After a few days, these initial symptoms tend to resolve completely. However, because symptoms are aggravated by physical activity, the patient goes through periods of exacerbation and alleviation, with a waxing and waning clinical course. As a result, several months may pass from the onset of symptoms before clinical presentation to a physician's office.

Anecdotal clinical observations suggest that children with LCPD tend to be hyperactive and quite busy. Loder et al. [7] found a 33 % incidence of attention deficit hyperactivity disorder (ADHD) in a small population of children with LCPD,

K.-H. Koo et al. (eds.), *Osteonecrosis*,
DOI 10.1007/978-3-642-35767-1_60, © Springer-Verlag Berlin Heidelberg 2014

much higher than the 3–5 % incidence within the general population. In addition to hyperactivity, many patients have delayed bone ages and appear younger than their chronologic age [8].

60.2.2 Physical Examination

Most patients will have a mild limp, which may be better seen during fast walking. A Trendelenburg gait and a positive Trendelenburg sign may also be present. Accurate assessment of passive hip abduction is a critical aspect of the physical examination for a child with LCPD. For accuracy, it is important to stabilize the pelvis to confirm that leg abduction is coming from the hip joint and not from lateral rotation of the pelvis. Limitation of hip range of motion seems to correlate with the stage of the disease. In the early stages, hip joint synovitis can limit range of motion. Gentle rotation of the affected hip with the leg extended can demonstrate restriction to internal and external rotation, so-called "irritability" of the hip. During the fragmentation stage, the hip motion can decrease significantly and become severely limited due to synovitis and femoral head deformity. The disease process particularly affects hip abduction and rotation. As the disease progresses through the stages of reossification and healing hip motion will improve, unless there is significant femoral head deformity, coxa magna, and flattening which mechanically impinges and hinders motion.

Depending on the duration and severity of the disease, late physical findings may be seen. These include hip flexion and adduction contracture, thigh and calf muscle atrophy, and minor limb length discrepancy (0.5–2 cm). In severe cases, lateralization and deformity of the femoral head during the fragmentation stage can lead to hinge abduction (Fig. 60.1). Clinicians caring for children with LCPD should be aware of hinge abduction and screen for it during regular clinical examination. Hinge abduction is thought to be due to the deformed femoral head abutting against the superior lip of the acetabulum and hinging as the examiner tries to abduct the leg [9–11]. Patients who present with an adduction contracture or complete absence of passive hip abduction during the fragmentation stage of the disease may be suffering from hinge abduction and should be carefully examined both clinically and radiographically. Supine AP pelvis X-ray with maximal abduction of the legs and hip arthrography can help to demonstrate hinge abduction.

60.2.3 Differential Diagnosis

Since LCPD is a diagnosis of exclusion, known causes of juvenile femoral head osteonecrosis or conditions mimicking LCPD must be ruled out (Table 60.1). A careful history should include questions about previous medications to rule out corticosteroid-induced osteonecrosis, previous hip surgery or trauma, and recent trauma. Careful review of family history is important to screen for history of blood disorders (sickle cell disease, coagulopathy, thrombophilia, and thalassemia) and skeletal dysplasias (multiple epiphyseal dysplasias, spondyloepiphyseal dysplasia, Meyer's dysplasia). Physical examination should also include assessment of facial features, spine, skin, and other extremities for skeletal dysplasia or a systemic condition. If there is concern from the medical history, additional lab work can be drawn looking for a low glucocerebrosidase level (Gaucher's disease), a high thyroid-stimulating hormone level (TSH) (hypothyroidism), and other chromosomal abnormalities (Klinefelter's syndrome and trisomy 21). In particular when both hips are affected in synchronous fashion, multiple epiphyseal dysplasia, spondyloepiphyseal dysplasia, and hypothyroidism must be strongly considered as the cause of bilateral epiphyseal changes resembling LCPD (Fig. 60.2).

60.3 Diagnostic Imaging

Several different imaging techniques are available to diagnose LCPD. Each technique has advantages and disadvantages and will be described within this section of the chapter.

60.3.1 Plain Radiography

Plain radiography remains the primary diagnostic assessment tool for LCPD. An anteroposterior (AP) and frog-leg lateral radiograph of the pelvis are used to determine the radiographic stage of the disease (see Waldenström's four stages of disease below), the extent of head involvement and serial progression of the disease. Catterall [4, 12] described a series of classic head at risk signs during the progression of the disease including lateral subluxation, Gage's sign (V-shaped radiolucency in the lateral portion of the epiphysis and/or adjacent metaphysis), calcification lateral to the epiphysis, and horizontal alignment of the growth plate. These are, however, late radiographic signs of a head at risk for having a poor prognosis. Much research effort has been expended to use earlier radiographic features to determine the prognosis and the long-term outcome. Catterall, Salter-Thompson, and lateral pillar classifications described below are such classifications which can be used in the fragmentation stage of the disease to prognosticate outcome, whereas the Stulberg classification is used at the healed stage near or at skeletal maturity. Most of these classifications based on categorizing certain radiographic features are prone to subjectivity and poor to moderate interobserver reliability [13, 14].

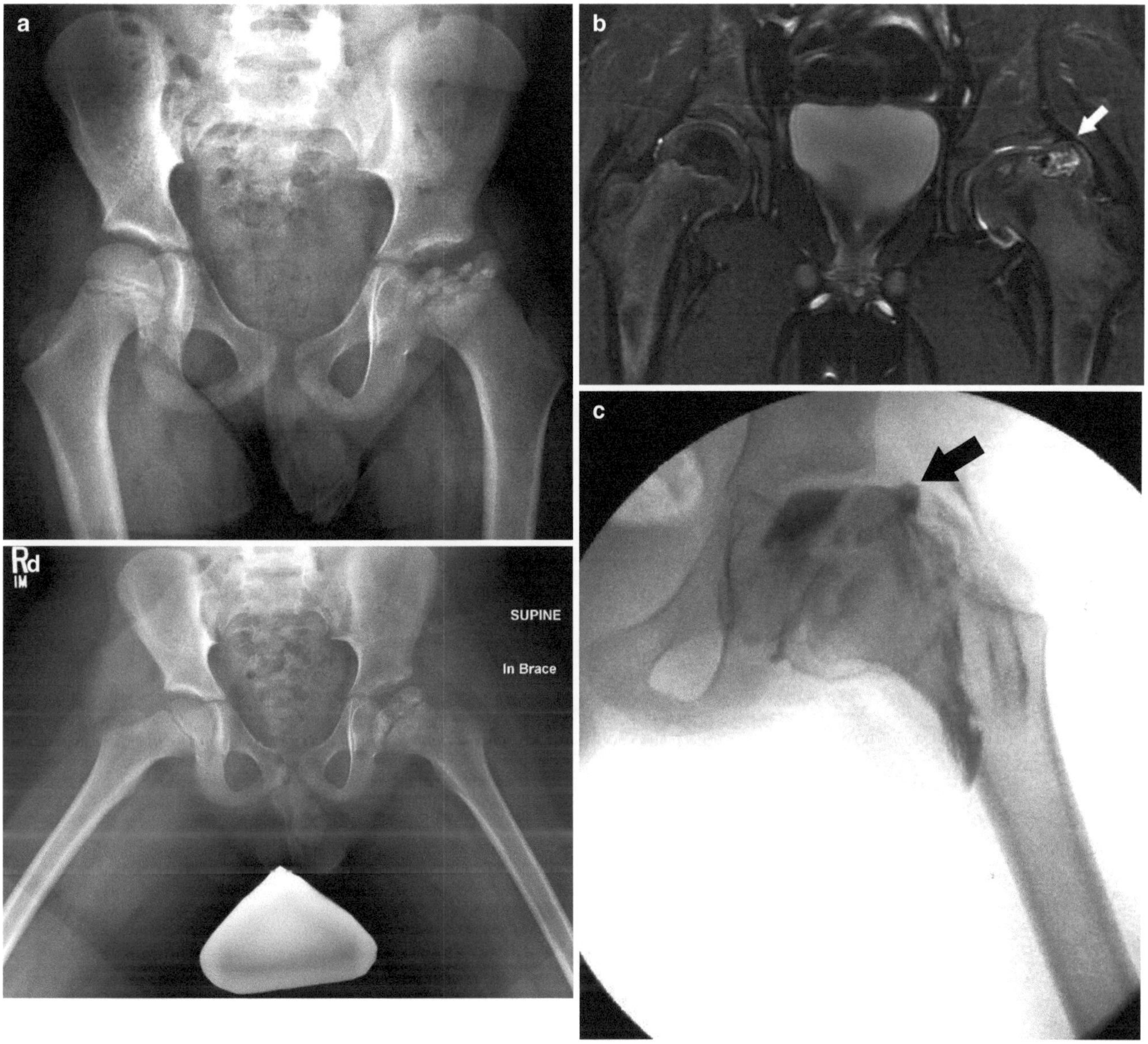

Fig. 60.1 A 7-year-old male complaining of left groin pain and limping for 1 year. This patient was treated in another institution with physiotherapy but no restriction of activities. When the patient presented for a second opinion, he had a very stiff hip with less than 10° of abduction with hips extended. (**a**) AP radiograph showing fragmented and deformed epiphysis on the left side with lateral extrusion. (**b**) MR T2 image showing a depression into the lateral epiphysis by the edge of the acetabulum and the extruded epiphyseal segment impinging of the labrum (*arrow*). (**c**) Hip arthrogram following a percutaneous hip adductor tenotomy showing a bilobed femoral head with a depression in the central portion of the femoral head which is filled with contrast. Other findings are flat, rectangular acetabulum and relief of the labral impingement upon abduction of the leg (*arrow*). This patient was treated with Petrie casts for 6 weeks followed by an A-frame abduction brace for 8 months and weight-bearing restrictions. (**d**) AP pelvis radiograph with the patient in the A-frame brace showing femoral head containment

Although radiography is useful in assessing disease progression, it lacks the sensitivity and specificity needed to demonstrate changes during the early stages of the disease (Fig. 60.3). Radiographic changes consistent with femoral head osteonecrosis may become evident about 3–4 months after their actual onset, and standard radiographic findings may be entirely normal in early symptomatic disease [15–19]. Furthermore, current radiographic classification systems for prognosticating outcomes (Catterall and lateral pillar classifications) have limitations in the early stages, as they cannot be applied until the fragmentation stage of the disease when significant deformity has already occurred. There is a clear need for the development of a more sensitive prognostic indicator to assist in decision making during the early stages of LCPD [20].

Table 60.1 Differential diagnosis of femoral head osteonecrosis and hip pain

Condition	Symptoms/signs	Diagnostic investigations
LCPD	Acute or chronic presentation Insidious onset, intermittent Able to ambulate and participate in sports	Radiographs, MRI
Septic arthritis	Acute pain in hip/knee Acute onset Painful to weight bear Unilateral Systemic symptoms Significantly decreased ROM	Lab: complete cell count, erythrocyte sedimentation rate and C-reactive protein Ultrasound Joint aspiration
Transient synovitis	Acute onset Prior history of viral illness Unilateral Mild systemic symptoms Decreased ROM Improves within 48 h	Lab work: complete cell count, erythrocyte sedimentation rate and C-reactive protein Ultrasound
Sickle cell disease	Anemia or jaundice Pain crisis Splenic sequestration Family history	Hemoglobin electrophoresis Complete cell blood count with differential Genetic testing
Hypothyroid	Unilateral or bilateral hip pain Fatigue and exercise intolerance Course dry hair and skin Cold Intolerance Signs of hypothyroidism	Lab studies: thyroxine (T4) levels and thyroid-stimulating hormone (TSH) Ultrasound thyroid
Multiple epiphyseal dysplasia and other skeletal dysplasias	Joint pain and fatigue Bilateral complaints Waddling gait Deformities in hands and feet Family history	Radiographs/skeletal survey Genetic testing (COL9A2/3 and COMP genes)

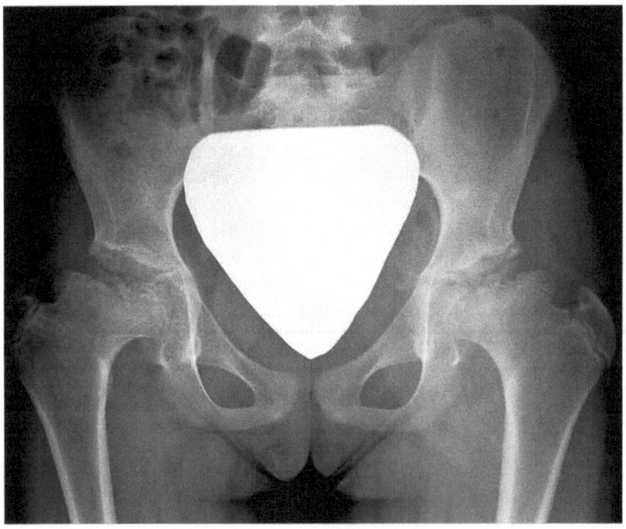

Fig. 60.2 A 10-year-old female complaining of bilateral hip pain. AP radiograph showed epiphyseal fragmentation and resorption along with short, broadened femoral neck and a break in Shenton's line, similar to LCPD. This patient had a family history of multiple epiphyseal dysplasia

60.3.2 Ultrasonography

Ultrasonography can be sometimes used in the early stages of LCPD to demonstrate a joint effusion in a child presenting with a limp. In addition to demonstrating an effusion, ultrasonography has the potential to illustrate the profile of the cartilaginous femoral head and can allow for dynamic examination [21]. Nauman et al. [22] developed a four-stage classification system based on ultrasonography and sonoanatomic criteria for patients with LCPD. Vascular supply to the femoral head has also been demonstrated by Doppler ultrasonography [23] and through microbubble contrast enhancement [24]. Despite these applications for ultrasonography, it is not widely used as a diagnostic tool due to user dependence and unfamiliarity with the techniques.

60.3.3 Scintigraphy

Technetium scanning is a sensitive means of diagnosing LCPD in the early stages before it is evident radiographi-

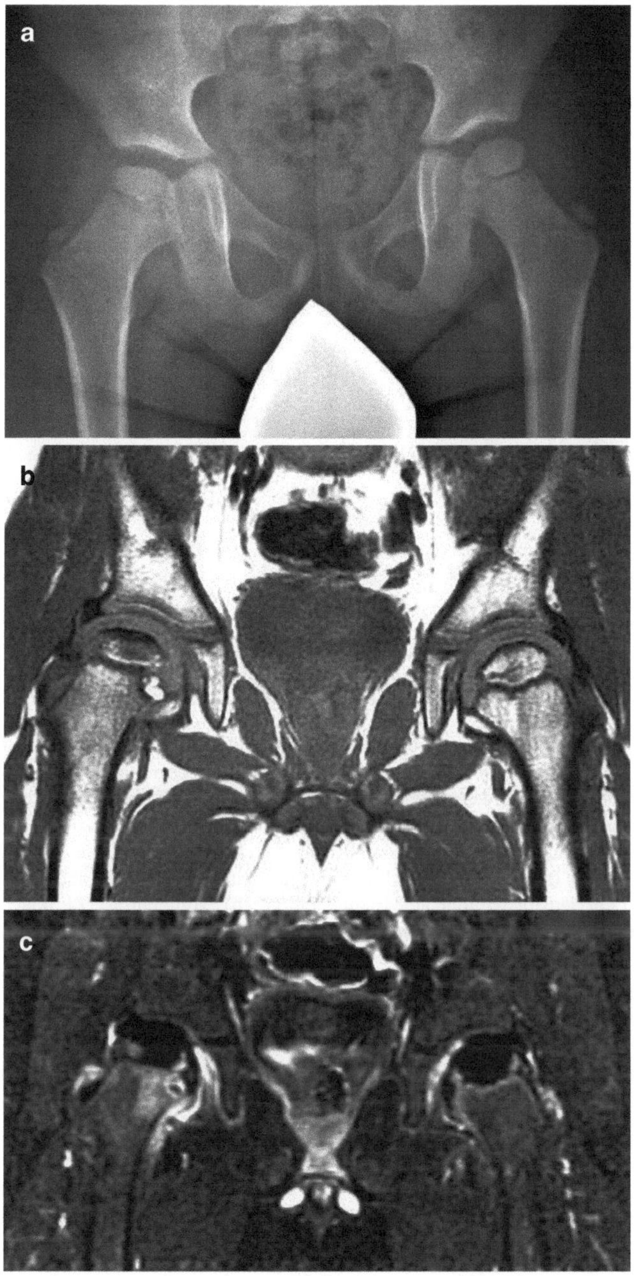

Fig. 60.3 A 5-year-old male complaining of right hip pain for 2 months. (**a**) AP radiograph shows right femoral head in the initial stage of LCPD with increased radiodensity and slight depression of the superior aspect of the epiphysis. (**b**) Non-contrast T1 image showing a noticeable signal decrease in the right epiphysis but no notable decrease in the left epiphysis. (**c**) Contrast-enhanced T1 with subtraction technique showing the loss of blood flow to the right epiphysis and unsuspected loss of blood flow to the left epiphysis not detected on the non-contrast images. This patient became symptomatic on the left side 5 months later and also developed radiographic signs of the initial stage of LCPD on that side

cally. Prior to the availability of magnetic resonance imaging (MRI), bone scan was commonly used to diagnose the condition in the early pre-radiographic stage of the disease. Scintigraphy has also been used to classify the severity of the disease in the early stages, with grade I representing one-fourth epiphyseal involvement and grade IV representing complete involvement [25]. Care must be taken, however, as early bone scan may at times suggest a more severe condition than actually exists.

Revascularization during the stages of LCPD has also been classified using scintigraphy. Conway [26] and Tsao [16] classified revascularization as either recanalization of existing vessel (the type A track or pathway) or neovascularization – new vessel formation (the type B track of pathway). The A pathway is characterized by early appearance of a lateral column formation in the capital femoral epiphysis, indicating uncomplicated, rapid revascularization which can take place over a matter of days. In contrast, the B pathway is characterized by centrally located scintigraphic activity arising from the base of the femoral epiphysis and represents a much slower process of new vessel formation, which occurs over many months to years. This classification scheme precedes radiographic changes by an average of 3 months. Unfortunately it is possible for the healing pattern to change from the A to B pathway, termed the type C pathway. Although rare, this phenomenon makes prognostication difficult [16]. Van Campenhout et al. [27] found a significant correlation between vascularization pattern and the Catterall and lateral pillar classifications. They recommended serial scintigraphy in the early evaluation of the patient with LCPD. However, the application of the classification requires two serial scintigrams and the classification lacks validity regarding tissue confirmation of recanalization and neovascularization. Despite the evidence to suggest its utility, the exposure to ionizing radiation and the inability to provide cross-sectional imaging are significant barriers to current wide spread use of this technique, in particular as MRI has become more accessible.

60.3.4 Computed Tomography

Computed tomography (CT) is able to provide accurate three-dimensional images demonstrating the shape and relationship of the femoral head and acetabulum and provide early diagnosis of bone collapse, curvilinear zones of sclerosis, and subtle changes in bone trabecular pattern [20, 28]. Although a classification scheme exists for patients with LCPD [29], CT is not typically used on a routine basis to evaluate patients with LCPD because of the comparatively high radiation dose [30]. CT may be useful in the later stages of LCPD to differentiate between an area of incomplete reossification within the femoral head and a true osteochondrotic lesion in symptomatic patients [31].

60.3.5 Arthrography

Hip arthrography is utilized to demonstrate the dynamic relationship between acetabulum and femoral head in various leg positions. Often in the early stage of LCPD, an increase in the medial joint space with concomitant lateralization of the femoral head is observed on plain radiographs [32]. Arthrography has demonstrated that this apparent widened medial clear space is due to thickening of the articular cartilage [33].

Hip arthrography is a useful method generally performed in the operating room to assess a patient with moderate to severe limitation of hip range of motion. It can provide reliable information regarding containment of the femoral head within the acetabulum and, specifically, information on loss of hip containment and hinge abduction, in which the femoral head "hinges" out of the acetabulum when the hip is abducted [9]. The degree of reducibility can be determined by the position of the femoral head within the acetabulum without imposing undue pressure on the lateral edge of the acetabulum [34]. Hip adductor tenotomy may be performed based on hip examination and arthrography to improve hip abduction and containment of the femoral head (Fig. 60.1c). Laredo [35] established an arthrographic classification that identifies five types of hips based on femoral head shape and position of the labrum, but this has not been tested prospectively.

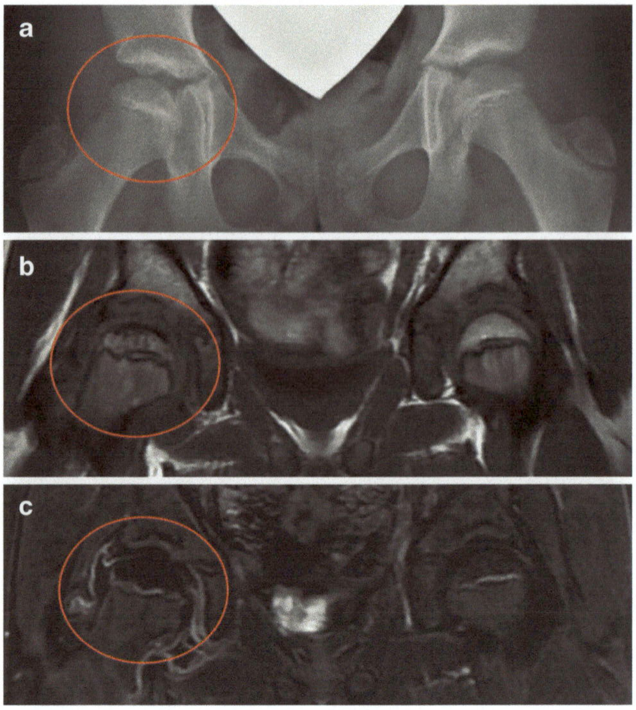

Fig. 60.4 An 11-year-old female with a history of intermittent right hip pain for 2 months prior to the following AP pelvis radiograph (**a**) and MRI showing non-contrast coronal T1 FSE image (**b**) and corresponding contrast-enhanced subtraction image (**c**). (**a**) AP radiograph shows right femoral head (*circle*) is in the initial stage of LCPD (stage I) with slightly smaller ossific nucleus and increased radiodensity without any fragmentation. (**b**) Non-contrast T1 image shows decreased signal in the superior region of the femoral head with spotty areas of decreased signal within the epiphysis. Percent head involvement measured by four observers was 28, 33, 42, and 67 %, showing some interobserver variability. (**c**) Contrast-enhanced subtraction image shows that most of the epiphysis is lacking contrast enhancement (i.e., hypoperfusion). Percent head involvement measured by four observers was 77, 78, 80, and 97 %, showing a larger extent of involvement than depicted by non-contrast imaging. Better interobserver agreement was observed using contrast imaging (From Kim et al. [49])

60.3.6 Magnetic Resonance Imaging

MRI is an accurate imaging modality for the early diagnosis of LCPD. It allows assessment of the extent of femoral head ischemia and provides visualization of the cartilaginous portion of the femoral head and acetabulum. Healing can also be assessed with MRI and can be seen on T1-weighted images as a semilunar, cup-shaped, low-intensity band. The outer zone of the repair tissue is of low intensity in both T1- and T2-weighted images, delineating living from necrotic bone [36–38]. Conventional MRI (non-contrast) has been shown to better delineate the extent of epiphyseal involvement than plain radiography or pinhole scintigraphy [39, 40]. MRI was found to have a diagnostic accuracy of 97–99 %, compared with 88–93 % for radiography and 88–91 % for scintigraphy [41].

The varying modalities of MRI, such as perfusion and diffusion MRI [42, 43], delayed gadolinium-enhanced (dGEMERIC) [44, 45], and dynamic gadolinium-enhanced subtraction (DGS) MRI [46, 47], may offer new insights into the pathophysiology and prognostication of the disorder. Sebag et al. [47] demonstrated the utility of DGS MRI for early detection of epiphyseal ischemia and variations in revascularization patterns. Lamer et al. [46] compared DGS MRI and bone scintigraphy and concluded that there was complete agreement between modalities with DGS MRI being a nonionizing alternative. Several different reperfusion patterns have been identified with DGS MRI, and these patterns mirror those seen with bone scintigraphy. Merlini et al. [42] have compared diffusion-weighted MRI with DGS and concluded that diffusion-weighted MRI can help distinguish between favorable and unfavorable prognosis in LCPD.

In comparison to non-contrast MRI, gadolinium-enhanced MRI provides additional information about the status of blood flow to the affected femoral head. It has been shown to detect changes in bone perfusion in the early stages of LCPD when radiographic changes are not apparent [46]. Non-contrast MRI relies on signal changes from fat present in the epiphysis to detect avascular necrosis. Since it takes weeks to months for the fat to degrade and the signal to decrease, false-negative results from non-contrast MRI have been reported in a handful of early presentation cases [39, 48]. For assessing the extent of femoral head necrosis in the early stages of LCPD, Kim et al. [49] found no correlation when comparing non-contrast and contrast-enhanced MRIs in patients in stage I of LCPD, concluding that these two studies assess two different components of LCPD. Contrast MRI depicting blood flow provided a clearer delineation between perfused and non-perfused regions of the epiphysis and a greater interobserver agreement between four observers compared to non-contrast MRI (Fig. 60.4). A preliminary study also found a correlation between the extent of the epiphyseal perfusion in the early stages of LCPD and the development of femoral head deformity at 2-year follow-up suggesting that contrast-enhanced MRI may provide early prognostic information [50]. Larger and longer follow-up studies are needed to confirm the clinical utility of contrast MRI.

Diffusion-weighted MR imaging has been used to evaluate tissue breakdown following ischemia, especially in acute stroke [51, 52]. This imaging modality has the ability to detect ischemic changes in tissue by measuring microscopic alterations in water mobility. In an animal model, diffusion-weighted MR imaging appeared sensitive to early ischemic changes compared to perfusion MR imaging [53]. Perfusion varies with time from markedly decreased to abnormally increased; however diffusion remains increased after the initial insult [54]. Yoo et al. [43] demonstrated that diffusion-weighted MR imaging was sensitive to epiphyseal changes and could reveal whether there are metaphyseal changes developing that are associated with transphyseal reperfusion to the epiphysis, increased T2–S1 in the metaphysis and focal physeal irregularity in children with LCP. Diffusion-weighted MR imaging provides information regarding epiphyseal and metaphyseal involvement different than that provided by perfusion studies and can therefore may be used as a complimentary tool to evaluate ischemic damage in patients with LCPD.

The role of MRI in the management of LCPD is currently evolving as MRI techniques and our understanding of LCPD evolve. Added advantage of MRI in comparison to CT and bone scan is that it is a nonionizing modality that has the ability to depict and quantify the loss of femoral head sphericity in a three-dimensional model during the early, pre-fragmentation stage of LCPD [55]. The disadvantages of MRI are cost, universal availability, and the duration of the study often requiring sedation for younger children (<8 years).

60.4 Radiographic Classifications and Indices

Radiographic classifications and quantitative indices for LCPD can be divided into three types (Table 60.2): those that define the stage and progression of the disease (e.g., Waldenström staging), those developed to prognosticate outcome during the active stage of the disease (e.g., Catterall and lateral pillar), and those that assess the short-term or longer-term outcome (e.g., deformity index and Stulberg).

60.4.1 Waldenström's Radiographic Staging

Waldenström [56] described four radiographic stages of disease progression: the initial or avascular necrosis stage

Table 60.2 Summary of classifications schemes for LCPD

Classification	Purpose	Components	Radiographic features
Waldenström	Stages of disease progression	1. Initial	1. Increased radiodensity, small ossific nucleus
		2. Fragmentation	2. Fragmentation and radiolucencies of the ossific nucleus due to bone resorption
		3. Reossification	3. Appearance of new bone medial/lateral femoral head
		4. Healed	4. Normal radiodensity of the femoral head
Extrusion index	For prognosis in early fragmentation	Migration percentage	1. Measure amount of femoral extruded lateral to Perkins line on affected hip (A)
	Quantifies degree of extrusion	Normal contralateral hip	2. Measure the width of unaffected femoral head along epiphysis (B)
			3. A/B × 100 = extrusion percentage
Catterall	For prognosis in mid-fragmentation	Group I	1. 25 % involvement
		Group II	2. 50 % involvement
	Categorizes the extent of head involvement	Group III	3. 75 % involvement
		Group IV	4. 100 % involvement
Salter-Thompson	For prognosis in early fragmentation	Type A	1. <50 % femoral head
	Extent of subchondral fracture	Type B	2. >50 % femoral head
Lateral pillar	For prognosis in mid-fragmentation	Group A	1. No loss of lateral pillar height
		Group B	2. Less than 50 % loss of lateral pillar height
	Height of lateral pillar (15–30 % lateral epiphysis)	Group B/C	3. 50 % loss of lateral pillar height
		Group C	4. Greater than 50 % loss of lateral pillar height
Stulberg	For outcome and prognosis at skeletal maturity	Class I	I. Normal hip joint
		Class II	II. Spherical head with large, short neck or dysplastic acetabulum
	Sphericity of femoral head	Class III	III. Nonspherical head (ovoid or mushroom)
		Class IV	IV. Flat head and congruous hip joint
		Class V	V. Flat head and incongruous hip joint

(stage I), fragmentation or resorptive stage (stage II), reossification or healing stage (stage III), and healed stage (stage IV). The radiographic features of each stage are described in the section below. The duration of each stage is variable from one patient to another. Herring et al. [57] found that time from first radiographic evidence of disease to the start of fragmentation had a mean of 6 months (range, 1–14 months), with the fragmentation stage lasting 8 months (range, 2–35 months), and the reossification stage lasting 51 months (range, 2–122 months). The authors noted that the more severe the disease, the longer the duration of each stage, particularly the reossification stage [58].

60.4.2 Modified Waldenström Staging (Elizabethtown)

In 2003, Joseph et al. [59] reported their modification of the Waldenström staging described in 1972 by Canale et al. [60]. The modified staging is referred to as the Elizabethtown classification. Each of the first original three stages described by Waldenström was further subdivided into two substages as stages Ia, Ib, IIa, IIb, IIIa, IIIb, and IV. Stage Ia is the initial stage of the disease, characterized by sclerosis of the epiphysis without any loss of epiphyseal height. In stage Ib the epiphysis is sclerotic and there is slight loss of height of the epiphysis. In this stage the epiphysis is still in a single piece without fragmentation or vertical fracture lines in the epiphysis visible on the AP or frog-lateral views. In stage IIa the epiphysis shows fragmentation and bone resorption seen as radiolucent areas; one or two vertical fissures in the epiphysis are seen in either view. In stage IIb the fragmentation of the epiphysis is advanced and the maximum flattening of the epiphysis is seen. There is no evidence of new bone formation lateral to the fragmented epiphysis. In stage IIIa there is evidence of new bone formation (reossification) at the periphery of the necrotic fragment; the new bone is not of normal radiodensity and covers less than one-third the circumference of the epiphysis. In stage IIIb the new bone is of normal radiodensity and covers more than one-third the circumference of the epiphysis. In stage IV the healing is complete and there is no radiologically identifiable avascular bone. These modifications to the original classification demonstrated good inter- and intra-observer reliability (0.72 and 0.71, respectively) in a review of 610 patients. Joseph et al. [59] calculated the duration of the initial four stages (Ia to IIb) to be approximately 4 months each, and the duration of stages IIIa and IIIb was twice and thrice that of the preceding stages, respectively. The authors found that the greatest amount of epiphyseal extrusion and flattening occurred during late fragmentation, leading the authors to recommend that containment surgery should be performed prior to stage IIb.

60.4.3 Lateral Extrusion Index

Green et al. [61] first described the term epiphyseal extrusion in their study of 200 children with LCPD in 1981. They defined the epiphyseal extrusion as the percentage of affected femoral head lateral to Perkin's line, computed by dividing the amount of involved femoral head that is uncovered by the width of the *opposite* normal femoral head measured at the epiphyseal plate. The authors found that the medial joint space did not correlate well with the degree of epiphyseal extrusion. When the epiphyseal extrusion exceeded 20 %, there was only a 15 % chance of good result regardless of the treatment or Catterall grade. The prognostic value of the epiphyseal extrusion increased when combined with age. Children less than 8 years and extrusion under 20 % had a 56 % chance of good result compared to only 13 % chance of good result when the extrusion was greater than 20 %.

Joseph et al. [59] further reported the prognostic value of epiphyseal extrusion and found a correlation between the degree of epiphyseal extrusion and advanced modified Waldenström stages. The authors found that extrusion increased abruptly during the stage IIb to such an extent that by the time the reossification stage begins (stage IIIa), there is an unacceptable degree of uncovering of the lateral part of the epiphysis in a large proportion of the patients studied. The results of this study further support the notion of greater than 20 % epiphyseal extrusion being associated with the risk of permanent femoral head deformation.

60.4.4 Catterall Classification

The long-term outcome in LCPD is related to the deformity of the femoral head and its congruency within the acetabulum [62, 63]. Three radiographic classification systems, namely, Catterall, Salter-Thompson, and lateral pillar, have been developed as prognosticators of outcome that are to be applied at the stage of fragmentation.

In 1971, Catterall [4, 64] reported that the extent of femoral head involvement based on epiphyseal collapse was an important radiographic predictor of outcome in LCPD. He found that femoral head involvement of <50 % (Catterall groups I and II) was associated with good outcome without specific treatment, whereas involvement >50 % (Catterall III and IV) was associated with poor outcome. While this classification is conceptually intuitive, its clinical application has been hampered by poor interobserver reliability due to the categorical nature of the classification and the need to wait until the mid-fragmentation (stage IIb) when maximal epiphyseal collapse occurs [14, 65, 66]. In addition, interpreting the head at risk signs is difficult [65]. Despite these issues, Catterall's work was instrumental in developing the concept of stratifying patients according to disease severity and attempting to identify reliable prognostic indicators.

60.4.5 Salter-Thompson Classification

In 1984, Salter and Thompson [67] presented a classification based on the extent of subchondral fracture present on the AP and lateral radiographs at the early fragmentation stage (stage 2a). They reported that the extent of subchondral fracture has a prognostic significance. Their classification consisted of two groups: group A (<50 % of head involvement) and group B (>50 % head involvement). One advantage of this classification is that subchondral fractures can be observed during early fragmentation stage, and therefore this classification can be applicable at an earlier time point than the Catterall classification. One major limitation of the classification is that subchondral fracture is only present in about 30 % of patients at the time of presentation and follow-up.

60.4.6 Lateral Pillar Classification

In 1992, Herring et al. [57] published the lateral pillar classification. This was initially based on 93 hips in 86 patients with radiographic follow-up at skeletal maturity. The classification was based on an AP X-ray of the hip, and the greatest involvement within the lateral pillar (15–30 % of lateral epiphysis) was used for the classification, applied as the femoral head enters the fragmentation stage. The initial classification consisted of three groups. Herring et al. made a modification to their existing classification in 2004 [17], adding an intermediate group B/C border, which includes a femoral head with a thin or poorly ossified lateral pillar and with a loss of lateral pillar height of 50 %.

A strong correlation has been reported between the lateral pillar and subsequent outcome [68]. Several studies have demonstrated good results at maturity for group A hips, while group B hips had a good outcome if under 9 years of age, but less favorable if older than 9 years at onset of disease. The majority of the group C patients developed aspherical heads at maturity regardless of age of presentation [57, 68, 69]. Compared to the Catterall classification, the lateral pillar classification system has been found to have a higher interobserver reliability and is a better predictor of final outcome [31, 70–73].

Currently, the most commonly used radiographical classification systems during the active stage of LCPD to prognosticate outcome are the lateral pillar and Catterall classification systems [18, 50, 74]. Because these classification systems are best applied during the stage of maximal fragmentation, the timing poses a dilemma for those patients presenting in earlier stages when the femoral head cannot be accurately classified. Because of the inability to accurately classify severity of disease based on presenting radiographs in the patients who are presenting in the early stage, a common management approach has been to observe the patient until the fragmentation stage before deciding on a surgical treatment. While the "wait-and-classify" approach may prevent unnecessary surgery on patients who would not have needed surgery (Catterall group I and II or lateral pillar A) or those who would not have benefited from it (lateral pillar C), a significant amount of deformity can develop in these patients which may be irreversible. As a result some centers advocate early surgery in older patients (>8 years) rather than waiting for the head to deform, because of the decreased remodeling potential [19, 75]. These controversies highlight the need to develop an earlier prognostic indicator based on a more sensitive imaging modality, such as MRI, to assist with treatment decisions.

60.4.7 Stulberg Classification

Stulberg classification is the current grading system primarily use for determining the long-term radiographic outcome in LCPD [62]. It classifies the hip into one of five classes according to the radiographic appearance at maturity. In contrast to the lateral pillar and the Catterall classifications which are used in the active stage, the Stulberg classification was developed to be used at the healed stage of the disease. This classification can be summarized according to the shape of the femoral head and its congruency to the acetabulum. *Spherical congruency* (classes I and II): 0 and 16 % developed radiographic signs of arthritis at 40-year follow-up, respectively. *Aspherical congruency* (classes III and IV): 58 and 75 % developed signs of arthritis, respectively. *Aspherical* incongruency (class V): 78 % developed signs of arthritis and some before 50 years of age. Shortcomings of this classification are poor reproducibility [76] and categorical subjective measure of outcome rather than a continuous quantitative measure [77]. Modifications to the classification have been made by some authors, such as decreasing the number of categories by combining classes I and II, and Classes IV and V [15], and by using numerical criteria (stage IV – greater than 1 cm in weight-bearing zone) [17] to improve the interobserver reliability (Table 60.3).

60.4.8 Deformity Index

Currently there are few classification systems, which are designed to assess outcome before skeletal maturity. Nelson et al. [78] reported on the *deformity index*, which is measured on plain AP radiographs and applied to patients presenting with *unilateral* disease. The deformity index is a continuous

Table 60.3 Modified Stulberg classification [17]

Class I:	Normal femoral head shape and acetabulum
Class II:	Spherical femoral head with: coxa magna/coxa breva/or acetabular dysplasia. The head fits within 2 mm of a concentric circle on both views
Class III:	Elliptical femoral head (ovoid, mushroom or umbrella, with greater than 2 mm of circular deviation). The head does not fit within 2 mm of a concentric circle on either view
Class IV:	Flattened femoral head (>1 cm in the weight-bearing articular surface) with congruous acetabulum
Class V:	Flattened femoral head with incongruous acetabulum

measure, which incorporates changes in the femoral epiphyseal height and width of the affected femoral head in relation to the contralateral, normal femoral head. The authors reported good inter- and intra-observer reliability. In the study, a deformity index of greater than 0.3 was associated with the development of an aspherical head and predicted Stulberg III or IV hip with a sensitivity of 80 % and specificity of 81 %. At 2 years the authors concluded that the deformity index was a valid and reliable radiological outcome measure for unilateral LCPD. It remains to be seen whether this index proves to be a reliable indicator of outcome by other investigators and in larger prospective studies.

60.4.9 New Quantitative Measures of Deformity and Sphericity

Over the last several decades, many attempts have been made to quantitatively measure the extent of deformation of the femoral head in both the active stage of the disease and during the healing phase [78–81]. One of the limitations of these measurement tools is assessment of deformation only on the anteroposterior radiograph, without assessing deformity on a lateral view [77]. Recently, Shah et al. [77] described a series of quantitative outcome measures (sphericity deviation score, composite femoral congruency arc, and extent of femoral head enlargement) which quantified the shape and size of the femoral head in two views in individuals with healed LCPD. These measures also take into account the femoral-acetabular relationship. In their study, the degree of femoral-acetabular congruency was measured (composite femoral congruency arc) and found to be highest in Stulberg class I hips and lowest in class V hips, with an inverse relationship existing between the sphericity deviation score and the composite femoral congruency arc, indicating that the more aspherical the femoral head, the less congruous the hip. Continuous outcome measures such as the sphericity deviation score have the potential to have a greater interobserver agreement than discrete, categorical outcome measures such as the Stulberg classification. Further studies are needed to reproduce the results reported by the authors and to validate the measures with functional outcome scores.

60.5 Natural History of LCPD

The natural history and prognosis of LCPD is variable. Several authors have proposed a combination of the following three important factors to stratify prognosis of disease: age at onset of the disease, the amount of femoral head involvement, and femoral head coverage [6, 57, 61, 62, 64, 82]. Studies on natural history have tried to account for these risk factors, yet large numbers of patients are needed to make statistical analysis of subgroups meaningful and reliable. The few published long-term studies are limited by small sample size, loss to follow-up and inclusion of patients treated both surgically and nonsurgically [82]. Results from one long-term study from Iowa with a mean follow-up under 40 years have shown that most patients are asymptomatic and remain active despite the presence of femoral head deformity [63]. More recent study with 20-year follow-up, however, showed that 59 % of patients had poor or fair Iowa hip score (score <80), 39 % had pain daily or several times per week, and 44 % had moderate to severe radiographic osteoarthritis [83]. In a long-term study, only 40 % of patients had a good level of function at an average of 47 years of clinical follow-up [84].

Age at diagnosis is strongly related to final outcome, with a better final outcome occurring in younger children [15, 57, 62, 64, 82, 85]. The relationship between femoral head deformity at skeletal maturity and risk of developing osteoarthritis is supported by several studies including the study by Stulberg et al. [62], who demonstrated a higher rate of premature osteoarthritis in those patients with an aspherical femoral head (Stulberg classes III, IV, and V hips). Finally epiphyseal extrusion and reduced femoral head coverage is an important factor in the deformation of the femoral head [59, 61, 64]. Greater than 20 % epiphyseal extrusion indicates a poor prognosis.

60.6 Summary

Legg-Calvé-Perthes disease remains a challenging condition to treat in pediatric orthopedics. Early detection is hampered by insidious, nonspecific presentation and subtle physical findings in the early stage of the disease. As a result, early detection of LCPD prior to the development of femoral head deformity remains one of the challenges for clinicians. Once the diagnosis is suspected, plain radiography is used to confirm the diagnosis and to determine the stage of the disease. Several radiographic classifications have been proposed to determine the prognosis and to assist treatment decision making. However, current radiographic classifications cannot be applied in the early stages of the disease. While several imaging modalities have been described to aid in the diagnosis and prognostication of LCPD, MRI seems to be the most sensitive and promising method to quantify the extent of disease involvement within the bone and cartilage of the femoral head, neck, and acetabulum. With techniques such as fat suppression and gadolinium-enhanced subtraction MRI, MRI sensitivity for early detection of ischemia and delineation of the amount of femoral head necrosis has improved. Recent methods to quantify femoral head perfusion using gadolinium-enhanced MRI have demonstrated good utility in small pilot studies; however, these new tools need to be further validated in prospective, multicentered studies. As our ability to detect early LCPD improves, a new classification may develop to quantify these previously unobserved ischemic changes and correlate the degree of ischemic necrosis with radiographic and functional outcome.

References

1. Skaggs DL, Tolo VT. Legg-Calve-Perthes disease. J Am Acad Orthop Surg. 1996;4(1):9–16.
2. Sundt H. Malum coxae: Calve'-Legg-Perthes. Zentralk Chir. 1920;22:538.
3. Molloy MK, MacMahon B. Incidence of Legg-Perthes disease (osteochondritis deformans). N Engl J Med. 1966;275(18):988–90. doi:10.1056/NEJM196611032751804.
4. Catterall A. Legg-Calve-Perthes syndrome. Clin Orthop Relat Res. 1981;158:41–52.
5. Kim HK. Legg-Calve-Perthes disease. J Am Acad Orthop Surg. 2010;18(11):676–86.
6. Wiig O, Terjesen T, Svenningsen S, Lie SA. The epidemiology and aetiology of Perthes' disease in Norway. A nationwide study of 425 patients. J Bone Joint Surg Br. 2006;88(9):1217–23.
7. Loder RT, Schwartz EM, Hensinger RN. Behavioral characteristics of children with Legg-Calve-Perthes disease. J Pediatr Orthop. 1993;13(5):598–601.
8. Harrison MH, Turner MH, Jacobs P. Skeletal immaturity in Perthes' disease. J Bone Joint Surg Br. 1976;58(1):37–40.
9. Reinker KA. Early diagnosis and treatment of hinge abduction in Legg-Perthes disease. J Pediatr Orthop. 1996;16(1):3–9.
10. Raney EM, Grogan DP, Hurley ME, Ogden MJ. The role of proximal femoral valgus osteotomy in Legg-Calve-Perthes disease. Orthopedics. 2002;25(5):513–7.
11. Yoo WJ, Choi IH, Chung CY, Cho TJ, Kim HY. Valgus femoral osteotomy for hinge abduction in Perthes' disease. Decision-making and outcomes. J Bone Joint Surg Br. 2004;86(5):726–30.
12. Catterall A. Natural history, classification, and x-ray signs in Legg-Calve-Perthes' disease. Acta Orthop Belg. 1980;46(4):346–51.
13. Wiig O, Terjesen T, Svenningsen S. Inter-observer reliability of radiographic classifications and measurements in the assessment of Perthes' disease. Acta Orthop Scand. 2002;73(5):523–30. doi:10.1080/000164702321022794.
14. Ritterbusch JF, Shantharam SS, Gelinas C. Comparison of lateral pillar classification and Catterall classification of Legg-Calve-Perthes' disease. J Pediatr Orthop. 1993;13(2):200–2.
15. Wiig O, Terjesen T, Svenningsen S. Prognostic factors and outcome of treatment in Perthes' disease: a prospective study of 368 patients with five-year follow-up. J Bone Joint Surg Br. 2008;90(10):1364–71. doi:10.1302/0301-620X.90B10.20649.
16. Tsao AK, Dias LS, Conway JJ, Straka P. The prognostic value and significance of serial bone scintigraphy in Legg-Calve-Perthes disease. J Pediatr Orthop. 1997;17(2):230–9.
17. Herring JA, Kim HT, Browne R. Legg-Calve-Perthes disease. Part I: Classification of radiographs with use of the modified lateral pillar and Stulberg classifications. J Bone Joint Surg Am. 2004;86-A(10):2103–20.
18. Lappin K, Kealey D, Cosgrove A. Herring classification: how useful is the initial radiograph? J Pediatr Orthop. 2002;22(4):479–82.
19. Price CT. The lateral pillar classification for Legg-Calve-Perthes disease. J Pediatr Orthop. 2007;27(5):592–3. doi:10.1097/01.bpb.0000279028.74397.02.
20. Dimeglio A, Canavese F. Imaging in Legg-Calve-Perthes disease. Orthop Clin North Am. 2011;42(3):297–302, v. doi:10.1016/j.ocl.2011.04.003.
21. Suzuki S, Awaya G, Okada Y, Ikeda T, Tada H. Examination by ultrasound of Legg-Calve-Perthes disease. Clin Orthop Relat Res. 1987;220:130–6.
22. Naumann T, Kollmannsberger A, Fischer M, Puhl W. Ultrasonographic evaluation of Legg-Calve-Perthes disease based on sonoanatomic criteria and the application of new measuring techniques. Eur J Radiol. 1992;15(2):101–6.
23. Robben SG, Lequin MH, Diepstraten AF, Hop WC, Meradji M. Doppler sonography of the anterior ascending cervical arteries of the hip: evaluation of healthy and painful hips in children. AJR Am J Roentgenol. 2000;174(6):1629–34. doi:10.2214/ajr.174.6.1741629.
24. Doria AS, Guarniero R, Cunha FG, Modena M, De Godoy Jr RM, Luzo C, et al. Contrast-enhanced power Doppler sonography: assessment of revascularization flow in Legg-Calve-Perthes' disease. Ultrasound Med Biol. 2002;28(2):171–82.
25. Fasting OJ, Langeland N, Bjerkreim I, Hertzenberg L, Nakken K. Bone scintigraphy in early diagnosis of Perthes' disease. Acta Orthop Scand. 1978;49(2):169–74.
26. Conway JJ. A scintigraphic classification of Legg-Calve-Perthes disease. Semin Nucl Med. 1993;23(4):274–95.
27. Van Campenhout A, Moens P, Fabry G. Serial bone scintigraphy in Legg-Calve-Perthes disease: correlation with the Catterall and Herring classification. J Pediatr Orthop B. 2006;15(1):6–10.
28. Weisz I, Bialik V, Adler O, Fishman J, Stein H. Some observations on the use of computerised tomography in Legg-Calve-Perthes' disease. Z Kinderchir. 1988;43(6):402–4. doi:10.1055/s-2008-1043493.
29. Moreno P, Cahuzac JP, Pasquie M. Topographic and developmental study of primary osteochondritis of the hip by x-ray computed tomography. Rev Chir Orthop Reparatrice Appar Mot. 1986;72(3):173–82.
30. Jaramillo D. What is the optimal imaging of osteonecrosis, Perthes, and bone infarcts? Pediatr Radiol. 2009;39 Suppl 2:S216–9. doi:10.1007/s00247-009-1151-7.
31. Rowe SM, Yoon TR, Jung ST, Lee KB. Free osteochondral fragment caught in the acetabular fossa in the osteochondritis dissecans after Legg-Calve-Perthes'–disease-report of 2 cases. Acta Orthop Scand. 2003;74(1):107–10. doi:10.1080/00016470310013770.
32. Axer A, Schiller MG. The pathogenesis of the early deformity of the capital femoral epiphysis in Legg-Calve-Perthes syndrome (L.C.P.S.). An arthrographic study. Clin Orthop Relat Res. 1972;84:106–15.
33. Gershuni DH, Axer A, Hendel D. Arthrographic findings in Legg-Calve-Perthes disease and transient synovitis of the hip. J Bone Joint Surg Am. 1978;60(4):457–64.
34. Yoo WJ, Choi IH, Cho TJ, Chung CY, Shin YW, Shin SJ. Shelf acetabuloplasty for children with Perthes' disease and reducible subluxation

of the hip: prognostic factors related to hip remodelling. J Bone Joint Surg Br. 2009;91(10):1383–7. doi:10.1302/0301-620X.91B10.22149.

35. Laredo Filho J. Legg-Perthes-Calve disease: arthrographic classification. Rev Bras Ortop. 1992;27:7–10.
36. Scoles PV, Yoon YS, Makley JT, Kalamchi A. Nuclear magnetic resonance imaging in Legg-Calve-Perthes disease. J Bone Joint Surg Am. 1984;66(9):1357–63.
37. de Sanctis N, Rondinella F. Prognostic evaluation of Legg-Calve-Perthes disease by MRI. Part II: Pathomorphogenesis and new classification. J Pediatr Orthop. 2000;20(4):463–70.
38. de Sanctis N, Rega AN, Rondinella F. Prognostic evaluation of Legg-Calve-Perthes disease by MRI. Part I: The role of physeal involvement. J Pediatr Orthop. 2000;20(4):455–62.
39. Henderson RC, Renner JB, Sturdivant MC, Greene WB. Evaluation of magnetic resonance imaging in Legg-Perthes disease: a prospective, blinded study. J Pediatr Orthop. 1990;10(3):289–97.
40. Uno A, Hattori T, Noritake K, Suda H. Legg-Calve-Perthes disease in the evolutionary period: comparison of magnetic resonance imaging with bone scintigraphy. J Pediatr Orthop. 1995;15(3):362–7.
41. Theissen P, Rutt J, Linden A, Smolarz K, Voth E, Schicha H. The early diagnosis of Perthes disease: the value of bone scintigraphy and magnetic resonance imaging in comparison with x-ray findings. Nuklearmedizin. 1991;30(6):265–71.
42. Merlini L, Combescure C, De Rosa V, Anooshiravani M, Hanquinet S. Diffusion-weighted imaging findings in Perthes disease with dynamic gadolinium-enhanced subtracted (DGS) MR correlation: a preliminary study. Pediatr Radiol. 2010;40(3):318–25. doi:10.1007/s00247-009-1468-2.
43. Yoo WJ, Kim YJ, Menezes NM, Cheon JE, Jaramillo D. Diffusion-weighted MRI reveals epiphyseal and metaphyseal abnormalities in Legg-Calve-Perthes disease: a pilot study. Clin Orthop Relat Res. 2011;469(10):2881–8. doi:10.1007/s11999-011-1931-x.
44. Zilkens C, Holstein A, Bittersohl B, Jager M, Haamberg T, Miese F, et al. Delayed gadolinium-enhanced magnetic resonance imaging of cartilage in the long-term follow-up after Perthes disease. J Pediatr Orthop. 2010;30(2):147–53. doi:10.1097/BPO.0b013e3181cf13e6. 01241398-201003000-00010 [pii].
45. Holstein A, Zilkens C, Bittersohl B, Jager M, Haamberg T, Mamisch TC, et al. Delayed gadolinium-enhanced MRI of cartilage (dGEMRIC) and morphologic MRI of cartilage in the long-term follow-up after Legg-Calve-Perthes disease (LCPD). J Med Imaging Radiat Oncol. 2011;55(3):259–65. doi:10.1111/j.1754-9485.2011.02262.x.
46. Lamer S, Dorgeret S, Khairouni A, Mazda K, Brillet PY, Bacheville E, et al. Femoral head vascularisation in Legg-Calve-Perthes disease: comparison of dynamic gadolinium-enhanced subtraction MRI with bone scintigraphy. Pediatr Radiol. 2002;32(8):580–5. doi:10.1007/s00247-002-0732-5.
47. Sebag G, Ducou Le Pointe H, Klein I, Maiza D, Mazda K, Bensahel H, et al. Dynamic gadolinium-enhanced subtraction MR imaging – a simple technique for the early diagnosis of Legg-Calve-Perthes disease: preliminary results. Pediatr Radiol. 1997;27(3):216–20.
48. Elsig JP, Exner GU, von Schulthess GK, Weitzel M. False-negative magnetic resonance imaging in early stage of Legg-Calve-Perthes disease. J Pediatr Orthop. 1989;9(2):231–5.
49. Kim HK, Kaste S, Dempsey M, Wilkens D. A comparison of non-contrast and contrast-enhanced MRI in the initial stage of Legg-Calve-Perthes disease. Pediatr Radiol. 2013;43(9):1166–73. PubMed PMID: 23478799.
50. Du J, Lu A, Dempsey M, Herring JA, Kim HK. MR perfusion index as a quantitative method of evaluating epiphyseal perfusion in Legg-Calve-Perthes disease and correlation with short-term radiographic outcome: a preliminary study. J Pediatr Orthop. 2013;33(7):707–13. PubMed PMID: 23872796.
51. Chien D, Kwong KK, Gress DR, Buonanno FS, Buxton RB, Rosen BR. MR diffusion imaging of cerebral infarction in humans. AJNR Am J Neuroradiol. 1992;13(4):1097–102; discussion 103–5.
52. Lee LJ, Kidwell CS, Alger J, Starkman S, Saver JL. Impact on stroke subtype diagnosis of early diffusion-weighted magnetic resonance imaging and magnetic resonance angiography. Stroke. 2000;31(5):1081–9.
53. Jaramillo D, Connolly SA, Vajapeyam S, Robertson RL, Dunning PS, Mulkern RV, et al. Normal and ischemic epiphysis of the femur: diffusion MR imaging study in piglets. Radiology. 2003;227(3):825–32. doi:10.1148/radiol.2273011673. 227/3/825 [pii].
54. Menezes NM, Connolly SA, Shapiro F, Olear EA, Jimenez RM, Zurakowski D, et al. Early ischemia in growing piglet skeleton: MR diffusion and perfusion imaging. Radiology. 2007;242(1):129–36. doi:10.1148/radiol.2421050680. 242/1/129 [pii].
55. Pienkowski D, Resig J, Talwalkar V, Tylkowski C. Novel three-dimensional MRI technique for study of cartilaginous hip surfaces in Legg-Calve-Perthes disease. J Orthop Res. 2009;27(8):981–8. doi:10.1002/jor.20909.
56. Waldenstrom H. On coxa plana: osteochondritis deformans coxae juveniles: Legg's disease, maladie de Calve, Perthes Krankreit. Acta Chir Scand. 1922;55:577–90.
57. Herring JA, Neustadt JB, Williams JJ, Early JS, Browne RH. The lateral pillar classification of Legg-Calve-Perthes disease. J Pediatr Orthop. 1992;12(2):143–50.
58. Herring JA, Williams JJ, Neustadt JN, Early JS. Evolution of femoral head deformity during the healing phase of Legg-Calve-Perthes disease. J Pediatr Orthop. 1993;13(1):41–5.
59. Joseph B, Varghese G, Mulpuri K, Narasimha Rao K, Nair NS. Natural evolution of Perthes disease: a study of 610 children under 12 years of age at disease onset. J Pediatr Orthop. 2003;23(5):590–600.
60. Canale ST, D'Anca AF, Cotler JM, Snedden HE. Innominate osteotomy in Legg-Calve-Perthes disease. J Bone Joint Surg Am. 1972;54(1):25–40.
61. Green NE, Beauchamp RD, Griffin PP. Epiphyseal extrusion as a prognostic index in Legg-Calve-Perthes disease. J Bone Joint Surg Am. 1981;63(6):900–5.
62. Stulberg SD, Cooperman DR, Wallensten R. The natural history of Legg-Calve-Perthes disease. J Bone Joint Surg Am. 1981;63(7):1095–108.
63. Gower WE, Johnston RC. Legg-Perthes disease. Long-term follow-up of thirty-six patients. J Bone Joint Surg Am. 1971;53(4):759–68.
64. Catterall A. The natural history of Perthes' disease. J Bone Joint Surg Br. 1971;53(1):37–53.
65. Hardcastle PH, Ross R, Hamalainen M, Mata A. Catterall grouping of Perthes' disease. An assessment of observer error and prognosis using the Catterall classification. J Bone Joint Surg Br. 1980;62-B(4):428–31.
66. Christensen F, Soballe K, Ejsted R, Luxhoj T. The Catterall classification of Perthes' disease: an assessment of reliability. J Bone Joint Surg Br. 1986;68(4):614–5.
67. Salter RB, Thompson GH. Legg-Calve-Perthes disease. The prognostic significance of the subchondral fracture and a two-group classification of the femoral head involvement. J Bone Joint Surg Am. 1984;66:479–89.
68. Herring JA, Kim HT, Browne R. Legg-Calve-Perthes disease. Part II: Prospective multicenter study of the effect of treatment on outcome. J Bone Joint Surg Am. 2004;86-A(10):2121–34.
69. Grzegorzewski A, Bowen JR, Guille JT, Glutting J. Treatment of the collapsed femoral head by containment in Legg-Calve-Perthes disease. J Pediatr Orthop. 2003;23(1):15–9.
70. Aksoy MC, Caglar O, Yazici M, Alpaslan AM. Comparison between braced and non-braced Legg-Calve-Perthes-disease patients: a radiological outcome study. J Pediatr Orthop B. 2004;13(3):153–7.
71. Hall AJ, Margetts BM, Barker DJ, Walsh HP, Redfern TR, Taylor JF, et al. Low blood manganese levels in Liverpool children with Perthes' disease. Paediatr Perinat Epidemiol. 1989;3(2):131–5.

72. Roy DR. Perthes'-like changes caused by acquired hypothyroidism. Orthopedics. 1991;14(8):901–4.
73. Yngve DA, Roberts JM. Acetabular hypertrophy in Legg-Calve-Perthes disease. J Pediatr Orthop. 1985;5(4):416–21.
74. Van Dam BE, Crider RJ, Noyes JD, Larsen LJ. Determination of the Catterall classification in Legg-Calve-Perthes disease. J Bone Joint Surg Am. 1981;63(6):906–14.
75. Little DG. Legg-Calve-Perthes disease: the effect of treatment on outcome. J Bone Joint Surg Am. 2005;87(5):1164–5; author reply -5.
76. Neyt JG, Weinstein SL, Spratt KF, Dolan L, Morcuende J, Dietz FR, et al. Stulberg classification system for evaluation of Legg-Calve-Perthes disease: intra-rater and inter-rater reliability. J Bone Joint Surg Am. 1999;81(9):1209–16.
77. Shah H, Siddesh ND, Pai H, Tercier S, Joseph B. Quantitative measures for evaluating the radiographic outcome of Legg-Calve-Perthes disease. J Bone Joint Surg Am. 2013;95(4):354–61. doi:10.2106/JBJS.L.00172.
78. Nelson D, Zenios M, Ward K, Ramachandran M, Little DG. The deformity index as a predictor of final radiological outcome in Perthes' disease. J Bone Joint Surg Br. 2007;89(10):1369–74. doi:10.1302/0301-620X.89B10.18747.
79. Harry JD, Gross RH. A quantitative method for evaluating results of treating Legg-Perthes syndrome. J Pediatr Orthop. 1987; 7(6):671–6.
80. Lauritzen J. Legg-Calve-Perthes disease. Acta Orthop Scand Suppl. 1975;159:1–137.
81. Meyer J. Legg-Calve-Perthes' disease. Radiological results of treatment and their late clinical consequences. Acta Orthop Scand Suppl. 1977;167:3–131.
82. Terjesen T, Wiig O, Svenningsen S. The natural history of Perthes' disease. Acta Orthop. 2010;81(6):708–14. doi:10.3109/17453674.2010.533935.
83. Larson AN, Sucato DJ, Herring JA, Adolfsen SE, Kelly DM, Martus JE, et al. A prospective multicenter study of Legg-Calve-Perthes disease: functional and radiographic outcomes of nonoperative treatment at a mean follow-up of twenty years. J Bone Joint Surg Am. 2012;999(2):584–92. doi:10.2106/JBJS.J.01073.small.test.
84. McAndrew MP, Weinstein SL. A long-term follow-up of Legg-Calve-Perthes disease. J Bone Joint Surg Am. 1984;66(6):860–9.
85. Ippolito E, Tudisco C, Farsetti P. The long-term prognosis of unilateral Perthes' disease. J Bone Joint Surg Br. 1987;69(2):243–50.

61 Legg-Calvé-Perthes Disease: Treatments

Benjamin D. Martin and Harry K.W. Kim

61.1 Introduction

Legg-Calvé-Perthes disease is a challenging condition to treat. A wide age, variability in the stage of presentation, and the severity of disease, both clinically and radiographically, are diverse making it difficult to apply a standard algorithm to an individual patient who presents to the office. Further complicating this, surgeons often disagree on the treatment for specific patients. Despite all of this, however, there is some evidence to help direct the treatment of LCPD. Current research concerning the biology of the disease and the potential for new treatments is also promising. Even though there is no resounding consensus of the best treatment of LCPD, there is an agreement on the primary goal of treatment – to maintain femoral head sphericity or minimize further deformity if already present. Femoral head deformity while tolerated in the young patient leads to pain, arthritis, and dysfunction in adulthood [1, 2].

61.2 The Concept of Containment

Historically, treatments of LCPD focused on relieving weight bearing via wheelchair or bed rest during a long-term inpatient stay until radiographs showed healing. Attempts were made to develop devices mimicking non-weight bearing in the upright position, such as an ischial seat [3] and the Snyder sling [4]. Over time the concept of containment evolved which is the basis for most current treatments, both operative and nonoperative. The concept is rather simple and was best articulated by Harrison and Menon in 1966 – "if the head is contained within the acetabular cup, then like jelly poured into a mold the head should be the same shape as the cup when it is allowed to come out after reconstitution [5]."

Earliest containment methods focused on abduction casting. Recumbent abduction casting is reported to date back to 1929 by A.O. Parker in Cardiff, Whales [5], but was popularized in a weight-bearing manner by Gordon Petrie in North America [6]. Significant validity was given to the concept of containment with Robert Salter's work using a piglet model [7, 8]. Salter created a Perthes-like condition in immature pigs by occluding the arterial supply to the femoral head. The pigs were divided into three groups – a normal weight-bearing group, a non-weight-bearing group achieved by holding the limb in acute flexion, and a weight-bearing group with the limb abducted in a long leg cast. The abduction, despite weight bearing, seemed to be the most important factor in preventing femoral head deformity.

Over the years the concept of containment has been widely accepted, even though no rigorous scientific evidence supports it. Both nonoperative and operative treatments have been developed in effort to favorably alter the "biological plasticity" of the weak femoral head during the active stage of the disease (i.e., prior to late reossification and healing) by containing it within the acetabulum [8]. Nonoperative options include abduction casting and abduction orthoses, both weight bearing and non-weight bearing. Operative treatments include femoral osteotomy, acetabular procedures, or a combination of both.

Much literature has been dedicated to these treatments, but relatively little investigations have been performed to validate the effectiveness in actually obtaining containment, altering femoral head coverage or relieving mechanical forces. Using gait analysis Rab showed that Petrie casts, abducting and internally rotating the legs, increased the anterior and lateral coverage of the femoral head [9]. The Atlanta

B.D. Martin
Division of Orthopaedic Surgery and Sports Medicine,
Children's National Medical Center,
111 Michigan Avenue, Washington, DC 20010, USA
e-mail: bdmartin@childrensnational.org

H.K.W. Kim (✉)
Center for Excellence in Hip Disorders,
Texas Scottish Rite Hospital for Children,
2222 Welborn Street, Dallas, TX 75219, USA

Department of Orthopaedic Surgery,
UT Southwestern Medical Center, Dallas, TX, USA
e-mail: harry.kim@tsrh.org

K.-H. Koo et al. (eds.), *Osteonecrosis*,
DOI 10.1007/978-3-642-35767-1_61, © Springer-Verlag Berlin Heidelberg 2014

brace, which holds the hips abducted and externally rotated, increased posterior coverage more than lateral. This is not ideal as the anterior and lateral aspect of the head is usually involved. Reporting or calculating "containment" is difficult given that the area of the femoral head in contact with the acetabulum changes with hip motion; thus parts of the head are only "contained" at certain times during gait. Rab developed the "containment index" to describe the percentage of the femoral head that was covered at any point during the gait cycle. The Atlanta brace did increase the percentage of head coverage during the gait cycle while Petrie casts and the Toronto brace did not. However, the Atlanta brace only achieved this in hips with good range of motion. In a stiff or irritable hip, no cast or brace altered the containment index. Rab also showed with computer models that neither a varus femoral osteotomy nor a Salter osteotomy alters the mechanical forces or prevents collapse in an extensively necrotic femoral head that is still spherical in shape [10]. Nevertheless, clinical research suggests that certain "containment" treatments are effective in altering the natural history of Perthes, while others are not, especially if the intervention is instituted early [11, 12].

61.3 Nonoperative Treatments for Legg-Calvé-Perthes Disease

61.3.1 Symptomatic Therapy

Synovitis, especially in the early stages of disease, either is painful or produces involuntary guarding of the hip, resulting in a limp and loss of hip range of motion. Recommended remedies include rest, walking aides such as crutches or a walker, wheelchair, anti-inflammatory medications, and traction. Evidence to support short periods of rest and walking aides is mainly anecdotal but nevertheless seems to provide symptomatic improvement and restore motion. A short course of nonsteroidal anti-inflammatory drugs (NSAIDs) also helps to reduce hip irritability. Due to NSAIDs interference with new bone formation, the long-term use should be avoided whenever possible [13]. A combination of these simple interventions often allows patients to mobilize and avoid missing significant periods of school. Even more important, improving symptoms and restoring range of motion is a prerequisite for containment therapy. Thus, symptomatic treatments are typically the initial steps in the overall treatment plan for LCPD.

Since the active phase of LCPD can last many months, the patient and parents must be educated about the prolonged course of the disease and a longer-term treatment strategy which should be instituted at the early stage of LCPD along with the symptomatic treatments based on the age of the patient, extent of head involvement, and other prognostic and social factors. As a part of a long-term treatment strategy, restriction of high impact activities and restricted weight bearing should be considered in those patients with poor prognosis as we do not have any treatment that can effectively reverse significant femoral head deformity once it occurs.

Certain patients will not respond to symptomatic treatments and alternative means are necessary to restore hip motion. Traction is an effective means to achieve this although it is less commonly used today than in the past. In the past hospital-based traction was used in the USA and Canada; however, this is rather rare now. Home-based traction is safe, tolerated well by patients and families, associated with minimal complications and is cheaper [14]. Skin [15], Russell [16], balanced suspension or "slings and springs" [17, 18] have all been used at different centers. Regardless of locale and the exact type, the most effective position to decrease intra-articular pressure is slight flexion, abduction, and external rotation [16, 19, 20]. Positions of hip extension with either internal or external rotation should be avoided as these positions can lead to intracapsular pressures above systolic pressure [20]. Motion improvement is seen within days [16], with over 60 % of patients achieving greater than 30° of abduction within 13 days [15].

Loss of motion in the early stages of LCPD is typically a result of synovitis and muscle spasm. Restricted motion in the later stages (reossification and healed stages) is often from femoral head deformity and impingement from coxa magna and an overriding greater trochanter. The underlying cause of the restriction of motion is a structural one and the treatment is entirely different.

61.3.2 Nonsurgical Containment Modalities

Nonsurgical modalities to achieve containment include various forms of abduction casting and abduction orthoses. As a prerequisite for the initiation and continuation of treatment, satisfactory motion, especially hip abduction, must be restored and maintained to ensure adequate containment of the femoral head and comfort in the brace or cast. Abduction casting for containment was as an early treatment for LCPD, but most patients were historically restricted to the recumbent position in hospitals to avoid weight bearing. Petrie and Bitenc popularized the use of weight-bearing casts that allowed children to be more active and at home with family [6]. Patients were treated with bed rest or traction until the hip could be abducted to 45°, although some patients required an adductor tenotomy to achieve this motion. Patients were then placed into bilateral long leg casts with two bars holding the legs in 45° of abduction and 5–10° of internal rotation. These casts, now referred to as Petrie casts, were changed every 3–4 months, with a short holiday between casting to ensure knee and ankle range of motion, until the healing stage of LCPD. In the original study, the average time in Petrie casts was 19 months. Of the 60 patients, 60 % had a head with the same radius on both the AP and lateral projections (good result), 31 % had a head that was within 2 mm of the same concentric circle on the two projections (fair result), and 9 % had variations greater than 2 mm on the different views.

With significant alterations to Petrie's original protocol, casting is still a useful treatment modality. As an adjunct to casting, the intraoperative arthrogram is obtained to assess the femoral head cartilaginous contour, acetabular contour, its relationship with the labrum, and its containability at various degrees of abduction. Prolonged casting is impractical and most surgeons cast for 6–12 weeks to restore hip abduction and containment in an irritable hip prior to nonoperative or operative treatment.

A number of weight-bearing orthoses were developed as alternatives to long-term Petrie casting. The braces held the hips in various degrees of abduction and varied in the control of knee motion and hip rotation. The Atlanta Scottish Rite orthosis became one of the more popular braces used in many centers. Initial results were reported to be positive [21–24]; however, follow-up studies failed to prove a benefit [25–30]. In addition, one study indicated that bracing impacted behavior and academic ability more so than surgery [31].

One exception to these poor results, is a recent report on a 25-year experience with an A-frame orthosis [32]. In this retrospective study, 213 patients (240 hips) were treated with a specific protocol focused on maintaining motion via home exercises and an orthosis until reconstitution of the lateral pillar. All patients were in the necrotic or early fragmentation stages. Patients had an examination under anesthesia, adductor tenotomy if hip abduction was less than 35°, followed by Petrie casting for 6 weeks. Patients were then transitioned to a custom A-frame orthoses that maintains the hips abducted such that the femoral head is covered by the acetabulum. This is constructed to hold the hips in internal rotation similar to a Petrie cast. The brace was worn for 20 h/day. Hip and knee range of motion exercises were performed daily, and weight bearing was permitted in the brace. In this study, patients were in the brace for an average of 13 months and the average follow-up was 7.8 years. A modified Stulberg I or II (grade I, normal in appearance; grade II, spherical with mild coxa magna, <5 mm loss of epiphyseal height, and no femoral neck deformity) result was obtained in all lateral pillar A hips, 89 % of lateral pillar B hips, and 67 % of lateral pillar C hips. In other studies, the patients who develop lateral pillar C hips generally had a poor outcome whereas this study showed some improvement even in the lateral pillar C hips. Furthermore, age was not a factor in the outcome within each lateral pillar group and not a single Stulberg V hip was found with this treatment regimen. Some limitations of this study were that 30 % of the hips were in children under 6 years old, which is the age group with more favorable prognosis, and the use of less stringent criteria for a Stulberg II hip [33, 34]. Disadvantages of this form of treatment include the prolonged duration and need for patient compliance over time.

61.4 Surgical Containment

61.4.1 Femoral Varus Osteotomy

A femoral varus osteotomy has been a common surgical containment procedure over the years with literature to support its use [26, 30, 35–43] (Fig. 61.1). As with all containment treatments, adequate motion prior to surgery is a prerequisite. If lateral extrusion of the femoral head is present, reduction of the head within the acetabulum is confirmed with an arthrogram. Hinged abduction is a contraindication to the procedure.

The mechanism by which the varus osteotomy alters the natural history of LCPD is not clear. According to force calculations, reducing the neck-shaft angle from 130° to 110° results in only a 14 % reduction in load across the femoral head [44]. A mathematical model indicated that the compressive forces on the epiphysis is three to four times body weight during normal gait, even after a varus osteotomy [45]. It remains unclear if the osteotomy stimulates or alters the healing process, as studies have conflicting results [12, 38, 46–48]. Potential beneficial effect of varus osteotomy may be a combination of biological effect, alternation of the hip biomechanics, and forced decrease in the activity level as a result of the surgery.

While controversial, femoral osteotomy performed in the initial stage or early fragmentation stage seems to better maintain the sphericity of the femoral head [12, 26, 38, 49]. Axer et al. [49] noted that only 9 % of patients had a poor result if operated on during the initial necrotic stage compared to 14 % during the intermediate fragmentation stage and 56 % treated in late regenerative stage. In a more recent study, 97 patients in different stages of disease were analyzed and the only factor under physician control that altered the femoral head sphericity was timing of surgery [11]. The same group confirmed this is a larger retrospective study of their patient population of 640 patients [38]. A concern previously raised is the possibility of proximal femoral physeal closure if the osteotomy is performed too early in the course of disease [50] and the possibility of operating on a patient with good prognosis who does not need treatment as it is difficult to stratify who needs surgery vs. who does not based on X-rays obtained at the initial stage.

A potential benefit of performing the varus osteotomy in the initial stage of LCPD is bypassing the fragmentation stage

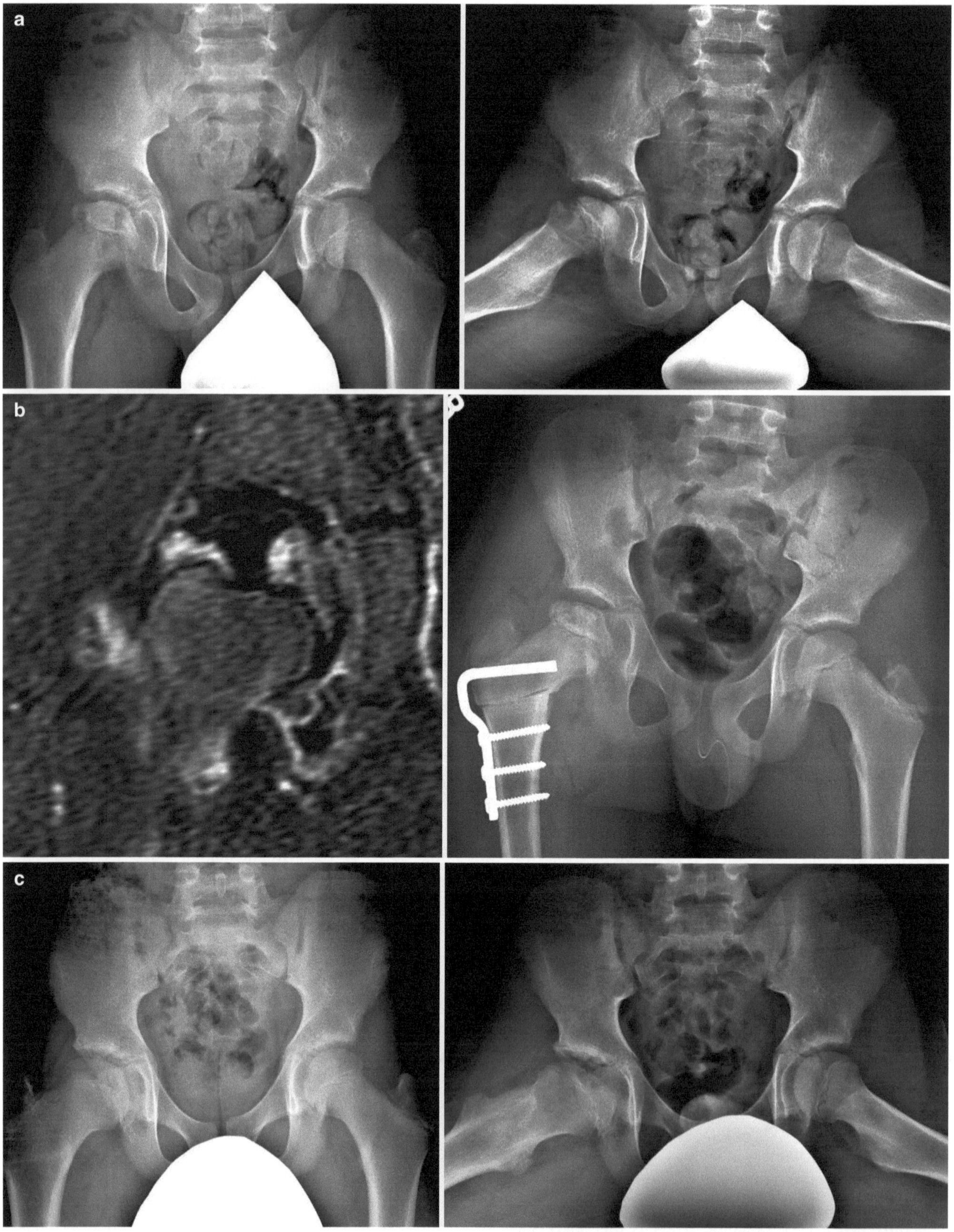

Fig. 61.1 Eleven-year and 7-month-old male with right hip pain for 12 months. (**a**) AP pelvis and frog-leg lateral radiographs showing right hip LCPD in Waldenstrom stage 2A (early fragmentation stage) with some flattening of the superior region of the femoral head. The lateral pillar classification cannot be applied reliably at this stage. (**b**) Gadolinium-enhanced MRI with subtraction technique (perfusion MRI) showing an absence of perfusion in the central and lateral regions of the femoral head (>50 % of epiphysis was hypoperfused). This patient was treated with early femoral varus osteotomy (10–15° varusation) and prolonged toe-touch weight bearing postoperatively. (**c**) AP and frog-leg lateral radiographs obtained 3 years postoperatively. The patient was performing sports activities and symptom free

of disease and shortening the overall duration of disease [38, 49, 51, 52]. This decreases the time the femoral head is fragile and at risk for deformation. Of 314 patients treated with a femoral varus osteotomy, 34 % bypassed the stage of fragmentation compared to only 1 of 40 who were treated nonoperatively [38]. It is important to note that the postoperative regimen included a prolonged duration of non-weight bearing (personal communication from the senior author). The results from this study do contradict older reports that femoral osteotomy does not alter the rate of disease progression [48] but the timing of intervention and postoperative regimen may have been very different between these studies. Incomplete or "biologic" osteotomies have also been attempted without effect on the duration of disease [46, 47].

Some concerns raised about femoral varus osteotomy are the reduction of the abductor lever arm which can potentially worsen a limp, shortening of the affected limb, and worsening of the overriding greater trochanter and lateral impingement. These potential problems are dependent on the amount of varusation and the functional state of the proximal femoral physis. Unfortunately the minimum amount of varus necessary to be effective in altering the natural history of LCPD is not known. It is important to contain the lateral pillar of the head under the acetabulum, and a patient in a later stage of disease with greater femoral head deformity may need more varus than a patient in the initial stage of disease with minimal deformity. The femoral neck-shaft angle does remodel after varus osteotomy [53–55] in about 65 % of the patients with most improvement occurring in the first 2–3 years [56]. However, this is dependent on the health of the proximal femoral physis, which is difficult to predict using plain radiography and some patients simply do not remodel at all [55, 57]. A recent study of patients who had varus osteotomy in the early stage of LCPD found that larger degrees of varus angulation was not associated with better Stulberg outcomes leading the authors to recommend a mild to moderate 10–15° varus osteotomy when performed in the early stage of LCPD [55].

Some surgeons advocate performing an epiphysiodesis of the greater trochanter at the time of femoral varus osteotomy or at the time of hardware removal if it is planned within the first postoperative year [43]. The goal is to avoid a relative trochanteric overgrowth after a varus osteotomy, especially if a growth arrest or disturbance of the proximal femoral physis is present. The beneficial role of the trochanteric epiphysiodesis and the optimal timing of the procedure is not clearly defined at this time.

Complications of femoral varus osteotomy include excessive proximal femoral varus, failure of varus angulation to remodel, limb shortening, limp, overriding greater trochanter with lateral impingement, and widened appearance of the hips and fracture after hardware removal [54]. If the hardware is to be removed, it should be done at 6 months or later [58].

61.4.2 Pelvic Osteotomy

Salter's innominate osteotomy was initially developed for the treatment of congenital hip dislocations [59]. Salter applied this treatment to LCPD to surgically contain the femoral head when extrusion was present [60]. This was analogous to treating a dysplastic hip with residual subluxation. He used this operation in children over 6 years old with moderate to severe involvement and loss of containment. Contraindications included patients with femoral head deformity on arthrogram and significant limitation of motion [61]. Threaded pins were used to avoid postoperative casting and generally removed at 6 weeks postoperatively [18]. Patients were allowed full weight bearing and activities at 6 weeks once the osteotomy healed. Salter and other authors have reported improved outcome with the osteotomy over the natural history of LCPD [18, 61].

Proposed advantages of Salter's innominate osteotomy are that it does not alter the length of the hip abductor muscles nor shorten the limb as with a varus femoral osteotomy. In general, the functional advantage of the Salter's osteotomy over the femoral osteotomy is difficult to demonstrate, but in severe cases where physeal closure is expected, the Salter's osteotomy leads to a smaller leg length discrepancy [62]. Theoretically, the Salter's osteotomy can lengthen the limb, leading some surgeons to modify the osteotomy by recessing the distal fragment into the intact ilium [63]. Complications of the Salter osteotomy include loss of acetabular position, failure of fixation, decreased range of motion, and impingement. Recent recognition of a high prevalence of acetabular retroversion in patients with LCPD has raised a concern about performing an osteotomy that may further contribute to the acetabular mal-orientation and femoroacetabular impingement [64–66]. The validity of this concern remains unclear. Iatrogenic hinged abduction can occur if the Salter does not completely contain the femoral head [67].

61.4.3 Combined Osteotomies and Triple Pelvic Osteotomy

For severe disease, some have recommended a combined femoral varus and Salter osteotomy to maximize the coverage of the necrotic femoral head while balancing the disadvantages of each operation [68–72]. The amount of varus can be minimized to avoid limb shortening and abductor weakness. The Salter osteotomy correction does not have to be as large decreasing the risk of impingement. The clinical merit of the combined osteotomy approach compared to single femoral or pelvic osteotomy has yet to be determined.

The triple pelvic osteotomy has also been used in the treatment of LCPD [71, 73–76]. The goal is to provide an adequate femoral head coverage, while avoiding a femoral osteotomy. More coverage can be obtained, because the acetabulum is completely freed from the remainder of the pelvis [71]. Wenger et al. [71] reported on 40 hips in 39 children, with 42 % of patients having a Stulberg I or II result and 58 % a III, IV, or V. When broken down further, 65 % of lateral pillar B hips and 12 % of C hips had a Stulberg I or II result. Four patients required reoperation, either femoral head osteochondroplasty or valgus osteotomy, for hinged abduction. The radiographic rate of pincer impingement due to over coverage was high [77].

61.4.4 Shelf Acetabuloplasty

The goal of shelf acetabuloplasty is to provide added acetabular coverage over an uncovered femoral head. Originally this was used as a salvage procedure to cover deformed femoral heads with coxa magna, subluxation, or hinged abduction. The indication for this procedure typically occurred in the later stages of disease, and the procedure was therefore used after attempted nonoperative treatment [78]. However, some advocated the use of shelf acetabuloplasty as a primary containment treatment and an alternative to a femoral or innominate osteotomy [79–81]. The proposed benefit of this procedure is that the shelf protects the labrum and stimulates acetabular growth providing femoral head coverage and preventing the development of the femoral head deformity [79, 81, 82].

Various techniques for shelf acetabuloplasty have been reported including a minimally invasive one [79, 83]. Care should be taken to ensure that the graft sits directly on the capsule for the shelf to form appropriately and function as a support. The ideal location is in line with the subchondral bone of the acetabulum. Postoperatively, a spica cast is used and protected weight bearing is recommended while the incorporation of the graft occurs. Complications of the shelf procedure include resorption of the graft (often if placed too high), inadequate coverage, excessive coverage, and impingement.

No prospective study evaluating the shelf procedure for LCPD has been performed. In one study, there was no evidence to indicate that the procedure prevents the development of early osteoarthritis [84].

61.4.5 Hip Arthrodiastasis

Hip arthrodiastasis can be considered as a form of weight relief while allowing limited hip motion. The indications for hip arthrodiastasis and the best time to institute this form of treatment remain unclear. In general, the procedure is reserved for older children with a poor prognosis (typically over 8 years old) or those with significant collapse of the femoral head and a stiff hip. Most reports are small case series [85–87]. A few series reported promising early results with respect to femoral head height during the stage of fragmentation [86, 87]. However, a follow-up study on a set of those patients at skeletal maturity indicated that seven out of ten patients had a Stulberg IV hip [88].

From the available evidence, arthrodiastasis seems to increase hip range of motion and decrease pain. There is no literature to support that it has a beneficial effect on the shape of the femoral head at maturity at this time. Some surgeons believe that it speeds up the rate of healing, but prospective studies have not been performed to support this anecdotal observation. Some limitations of this procedure include pin site infection, loosening, pain that restricts the duration of the treatment, and the need for extensive physiotherapy to gain and maintain hip motion.

61.5 Current Treatment Algorithm for Legg-Calvé-Perthes Disease

61.5.1 Current Best Evidence

Our current treatment algorithm is based on two prospective studies (level 2 evidence) [26, 30] and two meta-analyses with the age at onset of symptoms as a primary factor in decision-making in conjunction with the Waldenström stage, the amount of head necrosis based on perfusion MRI, and the lateral pillar classification if patient presents at the mid-fragmentation stage. Herring et al. [26] reported on 451 hips in 438 patients older than 6 years as a part of a multicenter prospective study. The study was conducted as a "best effort" design such that surgeons chose one of five specific treatments (no treatment, range of motion, brace, innominate osteotomy, or femoral osteotomy) for all his or her patients. Comparisons were made between nonoperative and operative treatments as there were no statistical differences when comparisons were made within each group. For the patients with onset of the disease between age 6 and 8 years, the operative group did not show a statistically significant improvement in the outcome. However, the percent of patients with Stulberg I or II outcomes were higher in the operative groups compared to the range of motion group (Table 61.1). Operative treatment significantly correlated with improved Stulberg outcome in patients over 8 years old with lateral pillar B or B/C hips (Table 61.2). Seventy-three percent of patients over 8 years old in the lateral B group treated surgically had a Stulberg I or II outcome at skeletal maturity compared to only 44 % treated nonoperatively. No difference was found between operative and nonoperative treatment for lateral pillar A or lateral pillar C hips. It is important to note that 115 of the 120 surgically treated hips were operated on during the initial stage or early fragmentation stage, before the lateral pillar classification can be reliably applied

Table 61.1 Outcomes for hips in patients aged 6–8 years at onset in the lateral pillar B and B/C border groups

Group	Total	Stulberg classification I or II	III	IV or IV	p value
Lateral pillar group B, age 6–8 years					
Nonoperative	80	61 (76 %)	17 (21 %)	2 (3 %)	0.99
Operative	43	33 (77 %)	9 (21 %)	1 (2 %)	
Lateral pillar group B/C, age 6–8 years					
Nonoperative	21	6 (29 %)	10 (48 %)	5 (24 %)	0.1
Operative	14	9 (64 %)	4 (29 %)	1 (7 %)	

Reproduced from Herring et al. [26]

Table 61.2 Outcomes for hips in patients older than 8 years at onset in the lateral pillar B and B/C border groups

Group	Total	Stulberg classification I or II	III	IV or IV	p value
Lateral pillar group B, age >8 years					
Nonoperative	62	27 (44 %)	26 (42 %)	9 (15 %)	0.02
Operative	33	24 (73 %)	7 (21 %)	2 (6 %)	
Lateral pillar group B/C, age >8 years					
Nonoperative	15	2 (13 %)	4 (27 %)	9 (60 %)	0.05
Operative	11	0	8 (73 %)	3 (27 %)	

Reproduced from Herring et al. [26]

(i.e., surgeons did not wait to classify before instituting treatment) [89] which makes the interpretation of the results based on the lateral pillar groups difficult.

Wiig et al. [30] performed a nationwide prospective study of 368 patients (all unilateral) treated in Norway. Hips were classified based on a two-group version of the Catterall classification (<50 and >50 % involvement) to improve the interobserver agreement. The lateral pillar classification was also studied. Patients with <50 % involvement were treated with physiotherapy alone. Patients with >50 % involvement were treated with physiotherapy, a Scottish Rite orthosis, or a proximal femoral osteotomy. Surgeons had to choose one of these three treatments for all patients under their care. Children under 6 years of age were included. While the paper did not specifically state the timing of surgery, the patients had femoral varus osteotomy at the mid-fragmentation stage when the lateral pillar classification can be applied (personal communication from Dr. Wiig). Outcomes were based on the Stulberg classification during the healed stage (5-year follow-up) and not at skeletal maturity. Only 15 % had closure of one or both triradiate cartilages and only 14 % had closure of one or both proximal femoral physes. An impressive 97 % of patients returned for follow-up at 5 years. The strongest predictor of outcome was femoral head involvement followed by age. Surgery resulted in statistically significant improvement in the modified Stulberg outcome in patients over 6 years of age with >50 % head involvement (43 % Stulberg I and II) compared to therapy (33 %) and brace treatment (20 %) (Table 61.3). The effect size of the surgery, however, was relatively modest compared to physiotherapy. No stratified analysis of patients between the ages of 6 and 8 was performed. The authors recommended a proximal femoral varus osteotomy for patients over 6 years of age at the time of diagnosis with >50 % head involvement.

Two recent meta-analyses support the results of these two prospective studies [90, 91]. Saran et al. [91] reviewed 14 papers meeting their criteria, which included a total of 1,831 hips. Only proximal femoral and Salter osteotomies were reviewed. Surgery improved femoral head sphericity compared to nonoperative treatment by an odds ratio (OR) of 1.29. For children under 6 years old, surgery was not beneficial (OR 1.02). For children over 6, surgery improved femoral head sphericity by an odds ratio of 2.05. Based on the statistics, surgery seemed to be more beneficial in patients over 8. Despite showing a trend toward improving femoral sphericity, the results did not reach statistical significance when a subgroup analysis was performed on patients aged 6–8.

Nguyen et al. [90] included 23 papers totaling 1,266 hips in a meta-analysis. Patients under 6 years of age were equally likely to have a successful radiographic outcome (Stulberg I or II) with operative or nonoperative treatment. However, the patients under age 6 treated with a pelvic procedure had a five times greater chance of a successful outcome than patients treated with a femoral osteotomy. For the patients over 6 years old, operative treatment was almost twice as likely to result in a successful radiographic outcome. There was no difference between a pelvic or femoral procedure in patients over 6 years of age. No difference in

Table 61.3 The Stulberg outcomes for patients over the age of 6 years old with >50 % of femoral head necrosis

		Stulberg classification		
Group	Total	I or II	III	IV or IV
Physiotherapy	51	17 (33 %)	14 (27 %)	20 (40 %)
Orthosis	25	5 (20 %)	9 (36 %)	11 (44 %)
Varus osteotomy	70	30 (43 %)	32 (46 %)	8 (11 %)[a]

Reproduced from Wiig et al. [30]

[a]The varus osteotomy group showed better Stulberg results compared to the physiotherapy ($p=0.001$) and the orthosis ($p=0.001$) group. There was no difference between the physiotherapy and orthosis groups ($p=0.36$)

outcomes was found between males and females, which contradicts other studies indicating females have a worse prognosis [26].

Surprisingly, these two meta-analyses only shared two articles between them. Some differences in the methodologies of the two studies were as follows. First, slightly different search techniques were used. Second, Saran et al. [91] looked only at femoral and Salter osteotomies, while Nguyen et al. [90] included femoral osteotomy, innominate osteotomy, shelf acetabuloplasty, Chiari osteotomy, and combined procedures (femoral plus pelvic). Interestingly, the prospective study by Wiig et al. [30] was included in both, while the one by Herring et al. [26] was only included in one meta-analysis.

Given the above evidence, we recommend dividing patients based on age of symptom onset into the following groups – less than 6, 6–8, 8–11, and over 11 years of age. For treatment purposes, we consider patients over the age of 11 to have the worst prognosis. Femoral head ischemia in children this age may be more similar to avascular necrosis of the femoral head in adults which has a poor prognosis if a large area of the femoral head is involved [92–94]. In addition to age, we consider the Waldenström stage and lateral pillar classification, if it can be determined. For patients in the initial stage of disease or early fragmentation, when a lateral pillar classification cannot be reliably determined, we use the extent of femoral head necrosis (i.e., hypoperfusion) on a gadolinium-enhanced (perfusion) MRI [95, 96]. In a preliminary study, perfusion MRI has been shown to provide prognostic information about the disease severity in the initial stages of disease (see Chap. 60 on diagnosis, imaging, and classifications). We incorporate age, stage, extent of involvement, range of motion, and social factors to make a shared decision with parents to determine the best treatment course for each patient.

61.5.2 Treatment for Children Under Age 6

It has long been recognized that age correlates with the long-term outcome of Perthes disease [2, 97–100]. The assumption is that a younger patient has more potential to remodel the deformed shape of the femoral head compared to an older patient. Surgery for children under 6 years of age is unlikely to be beneficial as multiple studies have shown no difference between operative and nonoperative treatments [30, 33, 90, 91]. Unfortunately, not all patients in this group are guaranteed a good outcome.

Rosenfeld et al. [34] reported on 188 hips in 172 patients under the age of 6 at onset. The only operative intervention was hip adductor release and/or iliopsoas release in patients treated with a Petrie cast. Eighty-one percent of patients had a Stulberg I or II result at final follow-up and 19 % a Stulberg III or IV. Canavese et al. [33] reported similar results on 166 hips in patients under 6 years of age. Operative treatment was performed on 57 patients, but no difference was noted between those treated operatively and nonoperatively. Overall, 67 % of patients had a Stulberg I or II hip at skeletal maturity and 33 % had a Stulberg III, IV, or V.

We follow these patients with a clinical examination and AP and frog pelvis radiographs every 4 months in the active phase of LCPD. Treatment is focused on pain relief, activity modification, and maintaining good hip range of motion (Fig. 61.2). Short periods of NSAIDs are used when necessary. For significant loss of hip motion and containment, Petrie casting followed by an A-frame brace and activity restrictions are utilized.

61.5.3 Treatment for Children Aged 6–8

Decision-making for patients presenting between the ages of 6 and 8 years old remains a dilemma since the literature has conflicting reports on the success of surgery over nonoperative measures [26, 30, 90, 91]. One prospective study found an increased chance of a Stulberg I or II outcome with a femoral osteotomy [30], while the other found no difference between operative and nonoperative treatments for this age group [26].

For the patients presenting in the initial stage of the disease, our general approach for this age group is to treat nonoperatively, focusing on managing symptoms, maintaining range of motion, and restricting running and jumping activities. For patients with significant decrease in the hip range of motion (hip abduction less than 15–20°), non-weight bearing on the affected limb or home traction is beneficial. If lateral extrusion is present, we perform a hip arthrogram to determine if the hip can be contained with abduction casts. When abduction with or without an adductor tenotomy provides adequate containment, the patient is placed into a Petrie cast for 6 weeks. When the cast is removed, operative containment procedure (femoral osteotomy) or a nonoperative containment using A-frame orthosis [32] is offered. Other options include prolonged weight relief using crutches or wheelchair.

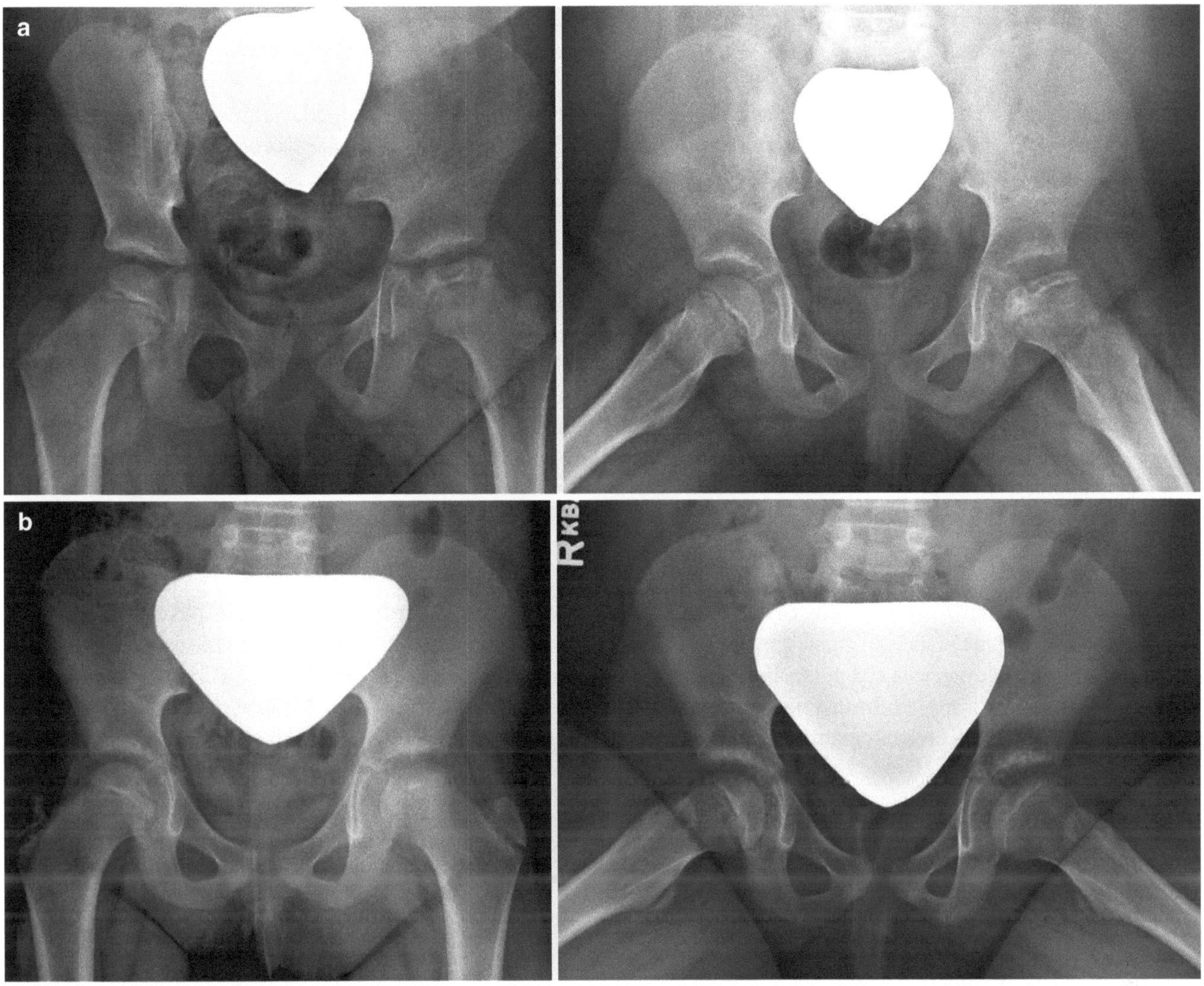

Fig. 61.2 Five-year and 7-month-old female with left hip pain for 1 month. (**a**) AP pelvis and frog-leg lateral radiographs obtained at mid-fragmentation stage showing lateral pillar B hip. This patient was treated symptomatically and with activity restrictions (no running or jumping). (**b**) AP pelvis and frog-leg lateral radiographs obtained 3 years and 6 months later. The patient is doing well with full activities and no symptoms

Perfusion MRI may be useful if surgical treatment is being planned for a patient presenting in the initial or early fragmentation stage of LCPD [96]. Perfusion MRI provides information about the extent of femoral head necrosis in the initial stage when the lateral pillar classification cannot be applied [89]. For patients with >50 % head necrosis (i.e., hypoperfusion), we discuss the option of surgical treatment with families.

For the patients who present in the fragmentation stage, the lateral pillar classification is used to help guide treatment [26]. Lateral pillar A do well without surgery and lateral pillar C hips have poor prognosis regardless of treatment. It is the lateral pillar B and B/C which most likely will benefit from surgical treatment.

While previous strategies to limit weight bearing by bed rest or orthosis have been abandoned [3, 4], there has been a recent revival of the recommendation of non-weight bearing using crutches or wheelchair either as a nonoperative treatment or an integral part of the postoperative protocol. Using an immature pig model, Kim et al. [101] showed that local non-weight bearing after ischemic necrosis of the femoral head resulted in significantly less femoral head deformity than when weight bearing was allowed. This form of treatment is prolonged and requires good compliance. Unfortunately, compliance to non-weight bearing may be a challenge to young, hyperactive patients.

61.5.4 Treatment for Children Aged 8–11

There is a consensus in the literature supporting surgical treatment for patients aged 8–11 years old at onset. Two prospective studies indicate that surgery provides a higher statistical chance of a spherical head at skeletal maturity than nonoperative treatment [26, 30, 90, 91].

The patients who present in the initial stage or early fragmentation stage are a challenge, since the lateral pillar classification cannot be applied reliably to predict the prognosis [89]. Given that operating early provides a better chance at a spherical head [11, 38], we use a perfusion MRI to assess the amount of femoral head necrosis (hypoperfusion). Preliminary studies indicate that perfusion MRI provides an object measure of femoral head involvement and provide information about the prognosis for short-term femoral head deformity [95, 96]. Furthermore, by detecting the patients with good perfusion, this assessment could potentially decrease the number of patients that are "over treated" with surgery. We assume that those with greater than 50 % head involvement have a worse prognosis and may benefit from a surgical treatment. The validity of this assumption needs to be further studied. For those patients with >50 % hypoperfusion at the early stage of LCPD, we recommend a proximal femoral varus osteotomy of 10–15° (Fig. 61.1).

If patients present in the fragmentation stage of LCPD, we stratify treatment based on the lateral pillar classification [26]. Patients with lateral pillar A are treated nonoperatively with symptomatic treatments. Hip arthrogram, possible hip adductor tenotomy, and Petrie casting are considered for patients with lateral pillar C hip with femoral head extrusion (loss of containment) and loss of motion. Following 6 weeks of Petrie casting, prolonged bracing with an A-frame brace [32] (Fig. 61.3) or prolonged non-weight bearing is considered in the lateral pillar C patients to limit additional femoral head deformity [101]. We recommend proximal femoral varus osteotomy for lateral pillar B hips. No cast is applied postoperatively. Some recommend postoperative prolonged non-weight bearing until reossification (Elizabethtown stage IIIb), with unrestricted activity thereafter [12, 101, 102]. Others allow weight bearing after 6 weeks when the osteotomy is typically healed. In the studies by Herring et al. [26] and Wiig et al. [30], a short duration of restricted weight bearing was used with 62 and 43 % patients having Stulberg I or II hips, respectively. If the hip motion is restricted preoperatively, the femoral osteotomy is staged first with a period of rest or Petrie casting to improve hip abduction and to decrease the irritability of the hip joint. Operating on a stiff, irritable hip without staging can lead to persistent stiffness and poor outcome.

61.5.5 Treatment for Children over Age 11

The outcomes for patients over the age of 11 are less predictable and generally poor. These patients have less growth remaining and time to remodel the femoral head. In fact, avascular necrosis in these older children may be similar to the adult form of disease. Multiple epiphyseal drilling [103], core decompression [104, 105], vascularized fibular grafting [106], angular or rotational osteotomy, and arthrodiastasis [85–88] are some of the treatment options. Unfortunately, there is no evidence to support that one treatment is superior to others at this time.

Joseph et al. reviewed 62 patients who presented with the onset of symptoms over the age of 12 years [107]. No patients had a Stulberg I or II result. Three patterns of disease were noted. A late-onset pattern was similar to that seen in younger children in terms of the Waldenström stages. However, remodeling of the femoral head shape did not occur. In the segmental-collapse pattern, early collapse of an involved epiphyseal segment occurred in the weight-bearing area. These hips did not follow the normal Waldenström stages, and the height did not remodel. Eight of ten had a Stulberg III result with two having a Stulberg IV. The destructive pattern was the most severe. After resorption, no reparative process or new bone formation occurred. These hips tended to subluxate as severe deformity developed relatively quickly. Seven patients required hip arthrodesis and one an excisional arthroplasty due to incapacitating pain. From this series it is clear that older patients do not follow the typical pattern of Perthes disease, and most have poor clinical and radiographic results.

The concept of containment is dependent on new bone formation and remodeling after the resorptive phase of osteonecrosis. Therefore, adolescents in this age group probably do not benefit from containment strategies. Treatment should focus on preventing collapse, stimulating revascularization and new bone formation, and preventing deformity before it occurs.

61.6 Treatment for Symptomatic, Healed Legg-Calvé-Perthes

In general, no active treatment is required once the healed stage is reached unless the patient becomes symptomatic. It is important to note that many patients function well as a teenager or an adolescent despite having a significant femoral head deformity. It is worrisome, however, that many patients who develop a Stulberg III, IV, or V hip at skeletal maturity have a high rate of hip pain and radiographic signs of osteoarthritis as young adults [1, 2]. Lateralization of the deformed femoral head with hinge abduction, articular cartilage damage, overriding greater trochanter, unhealed central osteochondral fragment and premature osteoarthritis are some of the potential causes of symptoms at this stage.

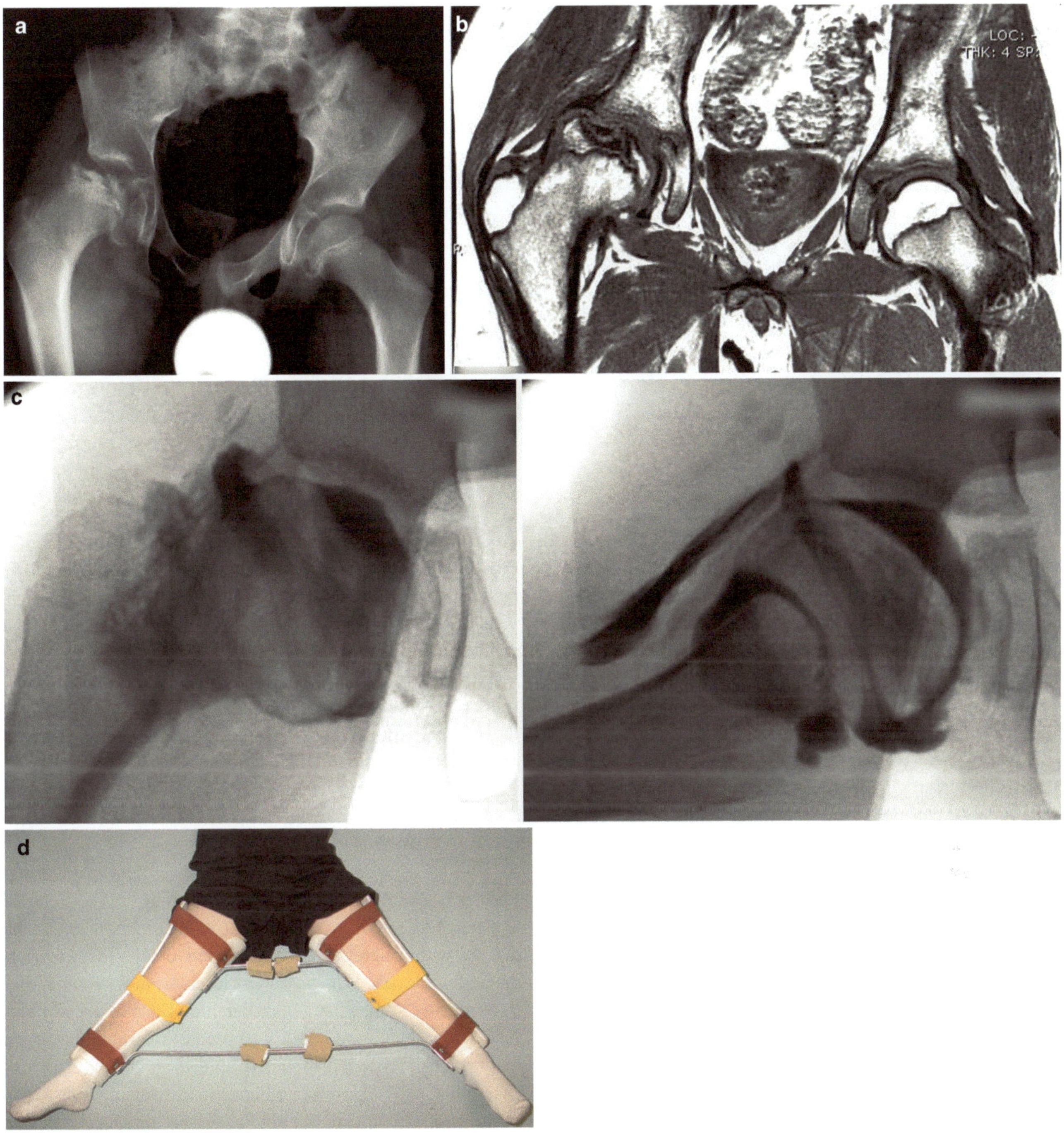

Fig. 61.3 A 10-year-old male complaining of right hip pain for 1 year and 2 months. This patient was treated in another institution with physiotherapy and a period of immobilization. When the patient presented for a second opinion, he had a very stiff hip with adduction and flexion contracture. (**a**) AP radiograph showing fixed adducted position of the right leg, fragmented and deformed epiphysis with lateral extrusion. (**b**) MR T1 image showing the depression in the lateral aspect of the epiphysis by the lateral edge of the acetabulum. (**c**) Hip arthrogram following hip adductor tenotomy showing the depressed portion of the femoral head filled with the contrast. This patient was treated with 6 weeks of Petrie casts followed by A-frame abduction brace (8–12 h/day) for 8 months and weight-bearing restrictions. (**d**) An example of the A-frame abduction orthosis which holds the hips in approximately 30–35° of abduction and slightly internally rotated or neutral position. (**e**) AP and frog-leg lateral radiographs obtained 3 years and 6 months postoperatively (Figures from Kim [126])

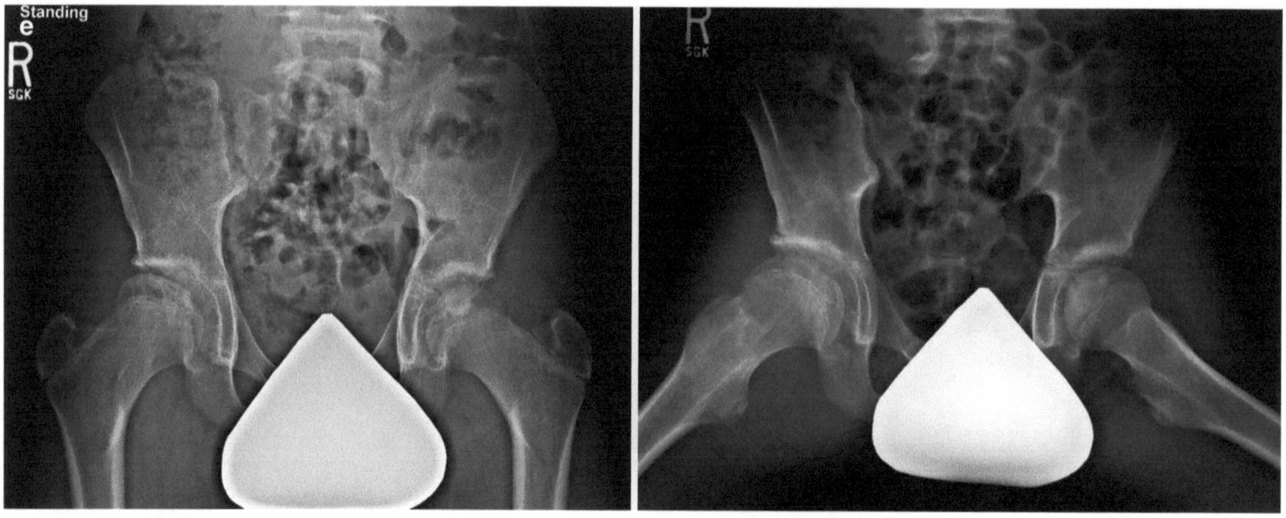

Fig. 61.3 (continued)

Hinged abduction occurs when the deformed femoral head interferes with abduction and the center of rotation is lateralized. The goal of a valgus osteotomy is to redirect the deformed femoral head to increase the congruency of the hip joint. A valgus proximal femoral osteotomy can improve function for patients with hinged abduction [108–110]. Unfortunately, longer follow-up has shown a high rate of failure and need for reoperation [111].

Femoral head asphericity, coxa magna, coxa breva, trochanteric overgrowth, femoral retroversion, and acetabular retroversion can lead to femoroacetabular impingement (FAI) [64, 112–116]. Symptoms are usually related to flexion activities, even simply sitting in a chair for long periods of time. Careful history taking and physical examination along with appropriate imaging studies are needed to further define the source of the symptoms at this stage.

For FAI, conservative treatments include activity modification to avoid high flexion activities, rest, and anti-inflammatory medications. The surgical hip dislocation [117] as described by Professor Ganz has changed the manner in which FAI is treated, especially in situations such as LCPD where a significant deformity is present. This approach allows dynamic inspection of impingement after arthrotomy and femoral head osteochondroplasty is safely performed once the hip is dislocated. A relative femoral neck lengthening with trochanteric advancement may help with external trochanteric impingement and restore length to the hip abductors (Fig. 61.4) [118–120]. A more aggressive procedure, the central head resection has been described as a potential treatment for a saddle-shaped femoral head [120, 121]; however, its indications and efficacy in delaying end-stage osteoarthritis are unknown. To maintain congruency or improve femoral head coverage, a Ganz periacetabular osteotomy can be performed [122].

The only available literature is level IV evidence. These small series indicate that surgical hip dislocation and addressing the abnormal anatomy can improve pain, motion, and function at short term [114, 123–125]. It is unknown whether these interventions will decrease the rate of osteoarthritis or prolong the life of the native hip joint.

61.7 Summary

Perthes is a challenging condition to treat as it affects a wide age range of patients who present at different stages of the disease with different extent of head involvement and different activity levels. With so many variables, the outcome after treatment is somewhat unpredictable. Despite these challenges and our limited ability to predict the outcome, some evidence from recent prospective studies and large retrospective studies provide useful guidance to treatment (Table 61.4). In general, treatment should be based on age, stage of disease, and amount of femoral head involvement. Since the ultimate goal of treatment is to preserve the spherical femoral head shape or to minimize existing deformity, early institution of a treatment plan to proactively decrease the deforming force on the femoral head and to mechanically protect the femoral head via operative or nonoperative means seem reasonable for those groups of patients with poor prognosis or remodeling potential. Multicenter, prospective studies are needed to address the uncertainties and the treatment controversies that are ongoing.

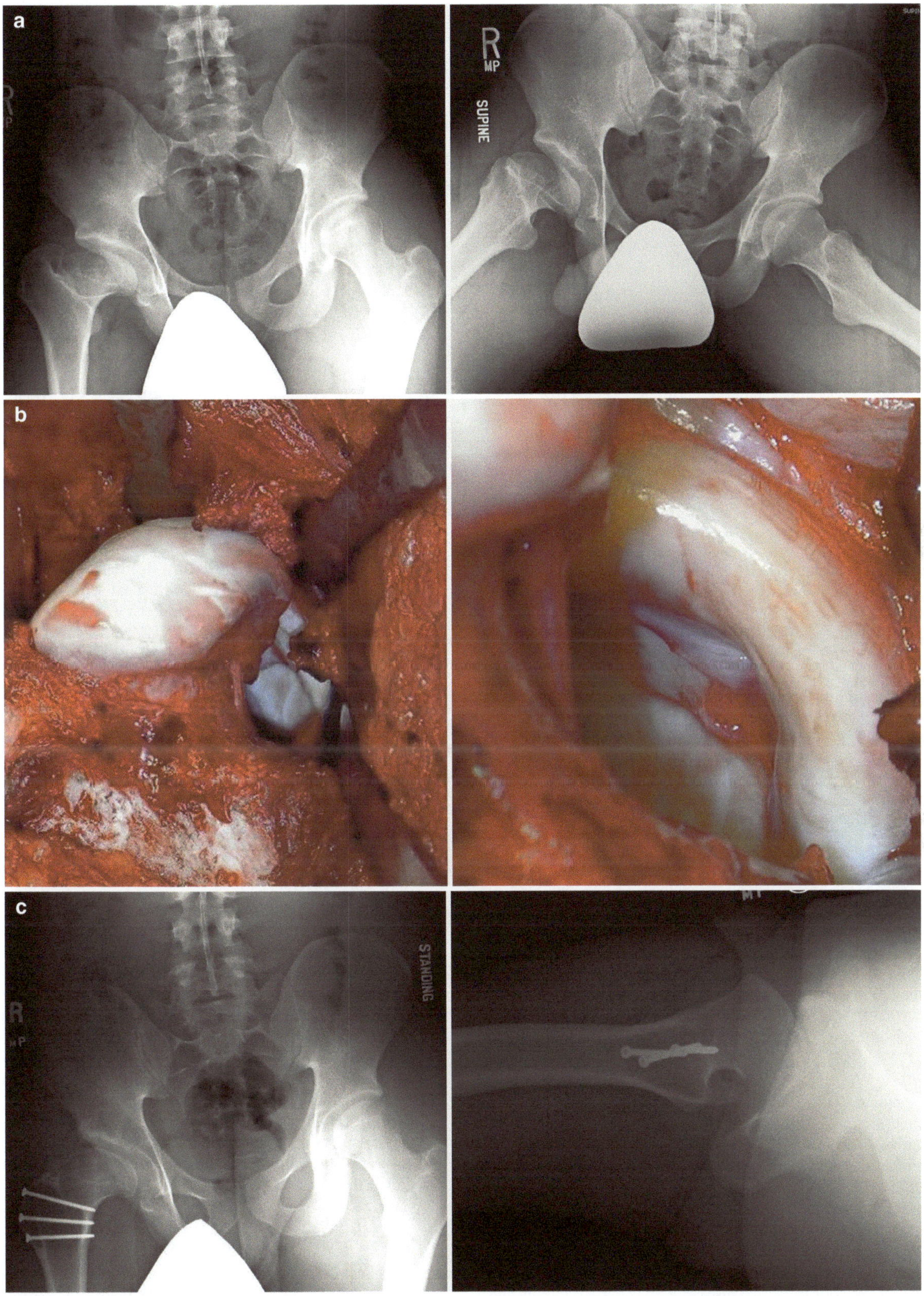

Fig. 61.4 A 17-year-old male with progressive anterior hip pain and a positive impingement sign. (**a**) Preoperative radiographs showing coxa magna, flattened femoral head (Stulberg class IV hip), short neck, overriding greater trochanter, and hanging rope sign. (**b**) Intraoperative photographs obtained at the time of surgical hip dislocation showing deformed, oblong femoral head and labral tear with degenerative changes. The patient was treated with femoral head osteochondroplasty, acetabular resection with labral repair, relative femoral neck lengthening, and greater trochanter advancement distally. (**c**) Two-year follow-up radiographs performed at age 19 (Courtesy of Dr. Daniel J. Sucato, Texas Scottish Rite Hospital for Children, Dallas, TX)

Table 61.4 Current levels of evidence for the various treatment options for LCPD

Age	Treatment	Level of evidence
<6 years old	Nonoperative	Level II
6–8 years old	Nonoperative	Level II
	Varus osteotomy	Level II
	Pelvic osteotomy	Level II
	Combined	Level IV
	Shelf	Level IV
	Arthrodiastasis	Level IV
8–11 years old	Varus osteotomy	Level II
	Pelvic osteotomy	Level II
	Combined	Level IV
	Shelf	Level IV
	Arthrodiastasis	Level IV
>11 years old	Multiple epiphyseal drilling	Level IV

The level II evidence comes from prospective cohort studies. Level IV refers to case series in which there is no control group

References

1. Larson AN, Sucato DJ, Herring JA, Adolfsen SE, Kelly DM, Martus JE, et al. A prospective multicenter study of Legg-Calve-Perthes disease: functional and radiographic outcomes of nonoperative treatment at a mean follow-up of twenty years. J Bone Joint Surg Am. 2012;94(7):584–92. doi:10.2106/JBJS.J.01073.
2. Stulberg SD, Cooperman DR, Wallensten R. The natural history of Legg-Calve-Perthes disease. J Bone Joint Surg Am. 1981;63(7):1095–108.
3. Friberg S. The roentgenological end results after caliper treatment of coxa plana with varying degrees of epiphyseal involvement. Acta Orthop Scand. 1975;46(2):234–45.
4. Snyder CH. A sling for use in Legg-Perthes disease. J Bone Joint Surg Am. 1947;29(2):524–6.
5. Harrison MH, Menon MP. Legg-Calve-Perthes disease. The value of roentgenographic measurement in clinical practice with special reference to the broomstick plaster method. J Bone Joint Surg Am. 1966;48(7):1301–18.
6. Petrie JG, Bitenc I. The abduction weight-bearing treatment in Legg-Perthes' disease. J Bone Joint Surg Br. 1971;53(1):54–62.
7. Salter RB. Experimental and clinical aspects of Perthes' disease. J Bone Joint Surg Br. 1966;48B(2):393–4.
8. Salter RBB, Bell M. The pathogenesis of deformity in Legg-Perthes' disease – an experimental investigation. J Bone Joint Surg Br. 1968;50B(2):436.
9. Rab GT, Wyatt M, Sutherland DH, Simon SR. A technique for determining femoral head containment during gait. J Pediatr Orthop. 1985;5(1):8–12.
10. Rab GT, DeNatale JS, Herrmann LR. Three-dimensional finite element analysis of Legg-Calve-Perthes disease. J Pediatr Orthop. 1982;2(1):39–44.
11. Joseph B, Nair NS, Narasimha Rao K, Mulpuri K, Varghese G. Optimal timing for containment surgery for Perthes disease. J Pediatr Orthop. 2003;23(5):601–6.
12. Joseph B, Varghese G, Mulpuri K, Narasimha Rao K, Nair NS. Natural evolution of Perthes disease: a study of 610 children under 12 years of age at disease onset. J Pediatr Orthop. 2003;23(5):590–600.
13. Vuolteenaho K, Moilanen T, Moilanen E. Non-steroidal anti-inflammatory drugs, cyclooxygenase-2 and the bone healing process. Basic Clin Pharmacol Toxicol. 2008;102(1):10–4. doi:10.1111/j.1742-7843.2007.00149.x.
14. Stevens B, Stockwell M, Browne G, Dent P, Gafni A, Martin R, et al. Evaluation of a home-based traction program for children with congenital dislocated hips and Legg Perthes disease. Can J Nurs Res. 1995;27(4):133–50.
15. Carney BT, Minter CL. Nonsurgical treatment to regain hip abduction motion in Perthes disease: a retrospective review. South Med J. 2004;97(5):485–8.
16. Serlo W, Heikkinen E, Puranen J. Preoperative Russell traction in Legg-Calve-Perthes disease. J Pediatr Orthop. 1987;7(3):288–90.
17. Menelaus MB. Lessons learned in the management of Legg-Calve-Perthes disease. Clin Orthop Relat Res. 1986;209:41–8.
18. Salter RB. The present status of surgical treatment for Legg-Perthes disease. J Bone Joint Surg Am. 1984;66(6):961–6.
19. Kallio P, Ryoppy S. Hyperpressure in juvenile hip disease. Acta Orthop Scand. 1985;56(3):211–4.
20. Vegter J. The influence of joint posture on intra-articular pressure. A study of transient synovitis and Perthes' disease. J Bone Joint Surg Br. 1987;69(1):71–4.
21. Curtis BH, Gunther SF, Gossling HR, Paul SW. Treatment for Legg-Perthes disease with the Newington ambulation-abduction brace. J Bone Joint Surg Am. 1974;56(6):1135–46.
22. Harrison MH, Turner MH, Nicholson FJ. Coxa plana. Results of a new form of splinting. J Bone Joint Surg Am. 1969;51(6):1057–69.
23. Harrison MH, Turner MH, Smith DN. Perthes' disease. Treatment with the Birmingham splint. J Bone Joint Surg Br. 1982;64(1):3–11.
24. Purvis JM, Dimon III JH, Meehan PL, Lovell WW. Preliminary experience with the Scottish Rite Hospital abduction orthosis for Legg-Perthes disease. Clin Orthop Relat Res. 1980;150:49–53.
25. Aksoy MC, Caglar O, Yazici M, Alpaslan AM. Comparison between braced and non-braced Legg-Calve-Perthes-disease patients: a radiological outcome study. J Pediatr Orthop B. 2004;13(3):153–7.
26. Herring JA, Kim HT, Browne R. Legg-Calve-Perthes disease. Part II: prospective multicenter study of the effect of treatment on outcome. J Bone Joint Surg Am. 2004;86-A(10):2121–34.
27. Kamegaya M. Comparative study of Perthes' disease treated by various ambulatory orthoses. Nihon Seikeigeka Gakkai zasshi. 1987;61(7):917–32.
28. Martinez AG, Weinstein SL, Dietz FR. The weight-bearing abduction brace for the treatment of Legg-Perthes disease. J Bone Joint Surg Am. 1992;74(1):12–21.
29. Meehan PL, Angel D, Nelson JM. The Scottish Rite abduction orthosis for the treatment of Legg-Perthes disease. A radiographic analysis. J Bone Joint Surg Am. 1992;74(1):2–12.
30. Wiig O, Terjesen T, Svenningsen S. Prognostic factors and outcome of treatment in Perthes' disease: a prospective study of 368 patients with five-year follow-up. J Bone Joint Surg Br. 2008;90(10):1364–71. doi:10.1302/0301-620X.90B10.20649.
31. Price CT, Day DD, Flynn JC. Behavioral sequelae of bracing versus surgery for Legg-Calve-Perthes disease. J Pediatr Orthop. 1988;8(3):285–7.
32. Rich MM, Schoenecker PL. Management of Legg-Calve-Perthes disease using an a-frame orthosis and hip range of motion: a 25-year experience. J Pediatr Orthop. 2013;33(2):112–99. doi:10.1097/BPO.0b013e318281ab44.
33. Canavese F, Dimeglio A. Perthes' disease: prognosis in children under six years of age. J Bone Joint Surg Br. 2008;90(7):940–5. doi:10.1302/0301-620X.90B7.20691.
34. Rosenfeld SB, Herring JA, Chao JC. Legg-calve-perthes disease: a review of cases with onset before six years of age. J Bone Joint Surg Am. 2007;89(12):2712–22. doi:10.2106/JBJS.G.00191.
35. Axer A. Subtrochanteric osteotomy in the treatment of Perthes' disease: a preliminary report. J Bone Joint Surg Br. 1965;47:489–99.
36. Beer Y, Smorgick Y, Oron A, Mirovsky Y, Weigl D, Agar G, et al. Long-term results of proximal femoral osteotomy in Legg-

Calve-Perthes disease. J Pediatr Orthop. 2008;28(8):819–24. doi:10.1097/BPO.0b013e31818e122b.
37. Friedlander JK, Weiner DS. Radiographic results of proximal femoral varus osteotomy in Legg-Calve-Perthes disease. J Pediatr Orthop. 2000;20(5):566–71.
38. Joseph B, Rao N, Mulpuri K, Varghese G, Nair S. How does a femoral varus osteotomy alter the natural evolution of Perthes' disease? J Pediatr Orthop B. 2005;14(1):10–5.
39. Lloyd-Roberts GC, Catterall A, Salamon PB. A controlled study of the indications for and the results of femoral osteotomy in Perthes' disease. J Bone Joint Surg Br. 1976;58(1):31–6.
40. McElwain JP, Regan BF, Dowling F, Fogarty E. Derotation varus osteotomy in Perthes disease. J Pediatr Orthop. 1985;5(2):195–8.
41. Noonan KJ, Price CT, Kupiszewski SJ, Pyevich M. Results of femoral varus osteotomy in children older than 9 years of age with Perthes disease. J Pediatr Orthop. 2001;21(2):198–204.
42. Terjesen T, Wiig O, Svenningsen S. Varus femoral osteotomy improves sphericity of the femoral head in older children with severe form of Legg-Calve-Perthes disease. Clin Orthop Relat Res. 2012;470(9):2394–401. doi:10.1007/s11999-011-2181-7.
43. Weiner SD, Weiner DS, Riley PM. Pitfalls in treatment of Legg-Calve-Perthes disease using proximal femoral varus osteotomy. J Pediatr Orthop. 1991;11(1):20–4.
44. Heikkinen E, Puranen J. Evaluation of femoral osteotomy in the treatment of Legg-Calve-Perthes disease. Clin Orthop Relat Res. 1980;150:60–8.
45. Rab GT. Containment of the hip: a theoretical comparison of osteotomies. Clin Orthop Relat Res. 1981;154:191–6.
46. Clancy M, Steel HH. The effect of an incomplete interochanteric osteotomy on Legg-Calve-Perthes disease. J Bone Joint Surg Am. 1985;67(2):213–6.
47. Kendig RJ, Evans GA. Biologic osteotomy in Perthes disease. J Pediatr Orthop. 1986;6(3):278–84.
48. Marklund T, Tillberg B. Coxa plana: a radiological comparison of the rate of healing with conservative measures and after osteotomy. J Bone Joint Surg Br. 1976;58(1):25–30.
49. Axer A, Gershuni DH, Hendel D, Mirovski Y. Indications for femoral osteotomy in Legg-Calve-Perthes disease. Clin Orthop Relat Res. 1980;150:78–87.
50. Barnes JM. Premature epiphysial closure in Perthes' disease. J Bone Joint Surg Br. 1980;62-B(4):432–7.
51. Axer A, Schiller MG, Segal D, Rzetelny V, Gershuni-Gordon DH. Subtrochanteric osteotomy in the treatment of Legg-Calve-Perther' syndrome (L.C.P.S.). Acta Orthop Scand. 1973;44(1):31–54.
52. Puranen J, Heikkinen E. Intertrochanteric osteotomy in the treatment of Perthes' disease. Acta Orthop Scand. 1976;47(1):79–88.
53. Evans IK, Deluca PA, Gage JR. A comparative study of ambulation-abduction bracing and varus derotation osteotomy in the treatment of severe Legg-Calve-Perthes disease in children over 6 years of age. J Pediatr Orthop. 1988;8(6):676–82.
54. Karpinski MR, Newton G, Henry AP. The results and morbidity of varus osteotomy for Perthes' disease. Clin Orthop Relat Res. 1986;209:30–40.
55. Kim HK, da Cunha AM, Browne R, Kim HT, Herring JA. How much varus is optimal with proximal femoral osteotomy to preserve the femoral head in Legg-Calve-Perthes disease? J Bone Joint Surg Am. 2011;93(4):341–7. doi:10.2106/JBJS.J.00830.
56. Herceg MB, Cutright MT, Weiner DS. Remodeling of the proximal femur after upper femoral varus osteotomy for the treatment of Legg-Calve-Perthes disease. J Pediatr Orthop. 2004;24(6):654–7.
57. Chiarapattanakom P, Thanacharoenpanich S, Pakpianpairoj C, Liupolvanish P. The remodeling of the neck-shaft angle after proximal femoral varus osteotomy for the treatment of Legg-Calve-Perthes syndrome. J Med Assoc Thai. 2012;95 Suppl 10:S135–41.
58. Schaaf AC, Weiner DS, Steiner RP, Morscher MA, Dicintio MS. Fracture incidence following plate removal in Legg-Calve-Perthes disease: a 32-year study. J Child Orthop. 2008;2(5):381–5. doi:10.1007/s11832-008-0108-y.
59. Salter RB. Innominate osteotomy in the treatment of congenital dislocation and subluxation of the hip. J Bone Joint Surg Br. 1961;43-B(3):518–39.
60. Salter R, Rang M, Bell M. The scientific basis for innominate osteotomy in the treatment of Legg-Perthes disease. Ann Roy Coll Phys Surg Can. 1972;5:62.
61. Salter RB. Legg-Perthes disease: the scientific basis for the methods of treatment and their indications. Clin Orthop Relat Res. 1980;150:8–11.
62. Sponseller PD, Desai SS, Millis MB. Comparison of femoral and innominate osteotomies for the treatment of Legg-Calve-Perthes disease. J Bone Joint Surg Am. 1988;70(8):1131–9.
63. Kalamchi A. Modified Salter osteotomy. J Bone Joint Surg Am. 1982;64(2):183–7.
64. Eijer H, Berg RP, Haverkamp D, Pecasse GA. Hip deformity in symptomatic adult Perthes' disease. Acta Orthop Belg. 2006;72(6):683–92.
65. Ezoe M, Naito M, Inoue T. The prevalence of acetabular retroversion among various disorders of the hip. J Bone Joint Surg Am. 2006;88(2):372–9. doi:10.2106/JBJS.D.02385.
66. Sankar WN, Flynn JM. The development of acetabular retroversion in children with Legg-Calve-Perthes disease. J Pediatr Orthop. 2008;28(4):440–3. doi:10.1097/BPO.0b013e318168d97e.
67. Wenger DR. Selective surgical containment for Legg-Perthes disease: recognition and management of complications. J Pediatr Orthop. 1981;1(2):153–60.
68. Crutcher JP, Staheli LT. Combined osteotomy as a salvage procedure for severe Legg-Calve-Perthes disease. J Pediatr Orthop. 1992;12(2):151–6.
69. Olney BW, Asher MA. Combined innominate and femoral osteotomy for the treatment of severe Legg-Calve-Perthes disease. J Pediatr Orthop. 1985;5(6):645–51.
70. Vukasinovic Z, Slavkovic S, Milickovic S, Siqeca A. Combined salter innominate osteotomy with femoral shortening versus other methods of treatment for Legg-Calve-Perthes disease. J Pediatr Orthop B. 2000;9(1):28–33.
71. Wenger DR, Pring ME, Hosalkar HS, Caltoum CB, Lalonde FD, Bastrom TP. Advanced containment methods for Legg-Calve-Perthes disease: results of triple pelvic osteotomy. J Pediatr Orthop. 2010;30(8):749–57. doi:10.1097/BPO.0b013e3181f5a0de.
72. Craig W, Kramer WG. Combined iliac and femoral osteotomies in Legg-Calve-Perthes syndrome. J Bone Joint Surg Am. 1974;56:1314.
73. Kumar D, Bache CE, O'Hara JN. Interlocking triple pelvic osteotomy in severe Legg-Calve-Perthes disease. J Pediatr Orthop. 2002;22(4):464–70.
74. Poul J, Vejrostova M. Rotational acetabular osteotomy in the treatment of Legg-Calve-Perthes disease. Acta Chir Orthop Traumatol Cech. 2001;68(6):357–62.
75. Vukasinovic Z, Spasovski D, Vucetic C, Cobeljic G, Zivkovic Z, Matanovic D. Triple pelvic osteotomy in the treatment of Legg-Calve-Perthes disease. Int Orthop. 2009;33(5):1377–83. doi:10.1007/s00264-009-0745-x.
76. Wenger DR, Pandya NK. Advanced containment methods for the treatment of Perthes disease: Salter plus varus osteotomy and triple pelvic osteotomy. J Pediatr Orthop. 2011;31(2 Suppl):S198–205. doi:10.1097/BPO.0b013e31822602b0.
77. Hosalkar H, Munhoz da Cunha AL, Baldwin K, Ziebarth K, Wenger DR. Triple innominate osteotomy for Legg-Calve-Perthes disease in children: does the lateral coverage change with time? Clin Orthop Relat Res. 2012;470(9):2402–10.

78. Kruse RW, Guille JT, Bowen JR. Shelf arthroplasty in patients who have Legg-Calve-Perthes disease. A study of long-term results. J Bone Joint Surg Am. 1991;73(9):1338–47.
79. Bowen JR, Guille JT, Jeong C, Worananarat P, Oh CW, Rodriquez A, et al. Labral support shelf arthroplasty for containment in early stages of Legg-Calve-Perthes disease. J Pediatr Orthop. 2011; 31(2 Suppl):S206–11. doi:10.1097/BPO.0b013e31822910ba.
80. Yoo WJ, Choi IH, Cho TJ, Chung CY, Shin YW, Shin SJ. Shelf acetabuloplasty for children with Perthes' disease and reducible subluxation of the hip: prognostic factors related to hip remodelling. J Bone Joint Surg Br. 2009;91(10):1383–7. doi:10.1302/0301-620X.91B10.22149.
81. Yoo WJ, Moon HJ, Cho TJ, Choi IH. Does shelf acetabuloplasty influence acetabular growth and remodeling? Clin Orthop Relat Res. 2012;470(9):2411–20. doi:10.1007/s11999-011-2163-9.
82. Domzalski ME, Glutting J, Bowen JR, Littleton AG. Lateral acetabular growth stimulation following a labral support procedure in Legg-Calve-Perthes disease. J Bone Joint Surg Am. 2006;88(7): 1458–66. doi:10.2106/JBJS.E.00689.
83. Staheli LT, Chew DE. Slotted acetabular augmentation in childhood and adolescence. J Pediatr Orthop. 1992;12(5):569–80.
84. Hsu JE, Baldwin KD, Tannast M, Hosalkar H. What is the evidence supporting the prevention of osteoarthritis and improved femoral coverage after shelf procedure for Legg-Calve-Perthes disease? Clin Orthop Relat Res. 2012;470(9):2421–30. doi:10.1007/s11999-011-2220-4.
85. Hosny GA, El-Deeb K, Fadel M, Laklouk M. Arthrodiastasis of the hip. J Pediatr Orthop. 2011;31(2 Suppl):S229–34. doi:10.1097/BPO.0b013e318223b45a.
86. Maxwell SL, Lappin KJ, Kealey WD, McDowell BC, Cosgrove AP. Arthrodiastasis in Perthes' disease. Preliminary results. J Bone Joint Surg Br. 2004;86(2):244–50.
87. Segev E, Ezra E, Wientroub S, Yaniv M. Treatment of severe late onset Perthes' disease with soft tissue release and articulated hip distraction: early results. J Pediatr Orthop B. 2004;13(3):158–65.
88. Segev E, Ezra E, Wientroub S, Yaniv M, Hayek S, Hemo Y. Treatment of severe late-onset Perthes' disease with soft tissue release and articulated hip distraction: revisited at skeletal maturity. J Child Orthop. 2007;1(4):229–35. doi:10.1007/s11832-007-0046-0.
89. Herring JA, Kim HT, Browne R. Legg-Calve-Perthes disease. Part I: Classification of radiographs with use of the modified lateral pillar and Stulberg classifications. J Bone Joint Surg Am. 2004;86-A(10):2103–20.
90. Nguyen NA, Klein G, Dogbey G, McCourt JB, Mehlman CT. Operative versus nonoperative treatments for Legg-Calve-Perthes disease: a meta-analysis. J Pediatr Orthop. 2012;32(7):697–705. doi:10.1097/BPO.0b013e318269c55d.
91. Saran N, Varghese R, Mulpuri K. Do femoral or salter innominate osteotomies improve femoral head sphericity in Legg-Calve-Perthes disease? A meta-analysis. Clin Orthop Relat Res. 2012;470(9):2383–93. doi:10.1007/s11999-012-2326-3.
92. Cherian SF, Laorr A, Saleh KJ, Kuskowski MA, Bailey RF, Cheng EY. Quantifying the extent of femoral head involvement in osteonecrosis. J Bone Joint Surg Am. 2003;85-A(2):309–15.
93. Ito H, Matsuno T, Omizu N, Aoki Y, Minami A. Mid-term prognosis of non-traumatic osteonecrosis of the femoral head. J Bone Joint Surg Br. 2003;85(6):796–801.
94. Mont MA, Carbone JJ, Fairbank AC. Core decompression versus nonoperative management for osteonecrosis of the hip. Clin Orthop Relat Res. 1996;324:169–78.
95. Du J, Lu A, Dempsey M, Herring JA, Kim HK. MR perfusion index as a quantitative method of evaluating epiphyseal perfusion in Legg-Calve-Perthes disease and correlation with short-term radiographic outcome: a preliminary study. J Pediatr Orthop. 2013;33(7):707–13. doi:10.1097/BPO.0b013e3182a05dc1.
96. Kim HK, Kaste S, Dempsey M, Wilkes D. A comparison of non-contrast and contrast-enhanced MRI in the initial stage of Legg-Calve-Perthes disease. Pediatr Radiol. 2013;43(9):1166–73. doi:10.1007/s00247-013-2664-7.
97. Catterall A. The natural history of Perthes' disease. J Bone Joint Surg Br. 1971;53(1):37–53.
98. Ismail AM, Macnicol MF. Prognosis in Perthes' disease: a comparison of radiological predictors. J Bone Joint Surg Br. 1998;80(2):310–4.
99. McAndrew MP, Weinstein SL. A long-term follow-up of Legg-Calve-Perthes disease. J Bone Joint Surg Am. 1984;66(6): 860–9.
100. Mose K. Methods of measuring in Legg-Calve-Perthes disease with special regard to the prognosis. Clin Orthop Relat Res. 1980;150:103–9.
101. Kim HK, Aruwajoye O, Stetler J, Stall A. Effects of non-weight-bearing on the immature femoral head following ischemic osteonecrosis: an experimental investigation in immature pigs. J Bone Joint Surg Am. 2012;94(24):2228–37. doi:10.2106/JBJS.L.00300.
102. Joseph B, Srinivas G, Thomas R. Management of Perthes disease of late onset in southern India. The evaluation of a surgical method. J Bone Joint Surg Br. 1996;78(4):625–30.
103. Kong SY, Kim HW, Park HW, Lee SY, Lee KS. Effects of multiple drilling on the ischemic capital femoral epiphysis of immature piglets. Yonsei Med J. 2011;52(5):809–17. doi:10.3349/ymj.2011.52.5.809.
104. Herrera-Soto JA, Price CT. Core decompression and labral support for the treatment of juvenile osteonecrosis. J Pediatr Orthop. 2011;31(2 Suppl):S212–6. doi:10.1097/BPO.0b013e318223b4d4.
105. Herrera-Soto JA, Price CT. Core decompression for juvenile osteonecrosis. Orthop Clin North Am. 2011;42(3):429–36. doi:10.1016/j.ocl.2011.04.004.
106. Urbaniak JR, Coogan PG, Gunneson EB, Nunley JA. Treatment of osteonecrosis of the femoral head with free vascularized fibular grafting. A long-term follow-up study of one hundred and three hips. J Bone Joint Surg Am. 1995;77(5):681–94.
107. Joseph B, Mulpuri K, Varghese G. Perthes' disease in the adolescent. J Bone Joint Surg Br. 2001;83(5):715–20.
108. Myers GJ, Mathur K, O'Hara J. Valgus osteotomy: a solution for late presentation of hinge abduction in Legg-Calve-Perthes disease. J Pediatr Orthop. 2008;28(2):169–72. doi:10.1097/BPO.0b013e3181653b13.
109. Raney EM, Grogan DP, Hurley ME, Ogden MJ. The role of proximal femoral valgus osteotomy in Legg-Calve-Perthes disease. Orthopedics. 2002;25(5):513–7.
110. Yoo WJ, Choi IH, Chung CY, Cho TJ, Kim HY. Valgus femoral osteotomy for hinge abduction in Perthes' disease. Decision-making and outcomes. J Bone Joint Surg Br. 2004;86(5): 726–30.
111. Bankes MJ, Catterall A, Hashemi-Nejad A. Valgus extension osteotomy for 'hinge abduction' in Perthes' disease. Results at maturity and factors influencing the radiological outcome. J Bone Joint Surg Br. 2000;82(4):548–54.
112. Eijer H, Podeszwa DA, Ganz R, Leunig M. Evaluation and treatment of young adults with femoro-acetabular impingement secondary to Perthes' disease. Hip Int J Clin Exp Res Hip Pathol Ther. 2006;16(4):273–80.
113. Ganz R, Parvizi J, Beck M, Leunig M, Notzli H, Siebenrock KA. Femoroacetabular impingement: a cause for osteoarthritis of the hip. Clin Orthop Relat Res. 2003;417:112–20. doi:10.1097/01.blo.0000096804.78689.c2.
114. Shore BJ, Novais EN, Millis MB, Kim YJ. Low early failure rates using a surgical dislocation approach in healed Legg-Calve-Perthes disease. Clin Orthop Relat Res. 2012;470(9):2441–9. doi:10.1007/s11999-011-2187-1.

115. Snow SW, Keret D, Scarangella S, Bowen JR. Anterior impingement of the femoral head: a late phenomenon of Legg-Calve-Perthes' disease. J Pediatr Orthop. 1993;13(3):286–9.
116. Tannast M, Hanke M, Ecker TM, Murphy SB, Albers CE, Puls M. LCPD: reduced range of motion resulting from extra- and intraarticular impingement. Clin Orthop Relat Res. 2012;470(9):2431–40. doi:10.1007/s11999-012-2344-1.
117. Ganz R, Gill TJ, Gautier E, Ganz K, Krugel N, Berlemann U. Surgical dislocation of the adult hip a technique with full access to the femoral head and acetabulum without the risk of avascular necrosis. J Bone Joint Surg Br. 2001;83(8):1119–24.
118. Ganz R, Horowitz K, Leunig M. Algorithm for femoral and periacetabular osteotomies in complex hip deformities. Clin Orthop Relat Res. 2010;468(12):3168–80. doi:10.1007/s11999-010-1489-z.
119. Ganz R, Huff TW, Leunig M. Extended retinacular soft-tissue flap for intra-articular hip surgery: surgical technique, indications, and results of application. Instr Course Lect. 2009;58:241–55.
120. Leunig M, Ganz R. Relative neck lengthening and intracapital osteotomy for severe Perthes and Perthes-like deformities. Bull NYU Hosp Jt Dis. 2011;69 Suppl 1:S62–7.
121. Paley D. The treatment of femoral head deformity and coxa magna by the Ganz femoral head reduction osteotomy. Orthop Clin North Am. 2011;42(3):389–99. doi:10.1016/j.ocl.2011.04.006.
122. Ganz R, Klaue K, Vinh TS, Mast JW. A new periacetabular osteotomy for the treatment of hip dysplasias. Technique and preliminary results. Clin Orthop Relat Res. 1988;232:26–36.
123. Albers CE, Steppacher SD, Ganz R, Siebenrock KA, Tannast M. Joint-preserving surgery improves pain, range of motion, and abductor strength after Legg-Calve-Perthes disease. Clin Orthop Relat Res. 2012;470(9):2450–61. doi:10.1007/s11999-012-2345-0.
124. Anderson LA, Erickson JA, Severson EP, Peters CL. Sequelae of Perthes disease: treatment with surgical hip dislocation and relative femoral neck lengthening. J Pediatr Orthop. 2010;30(8):758–66. doi:10.1097/BPO.0b013e3181fcbaaf.
125. Kim YJ, Novais EN. Diagnosis and treatment of femoroacetabular impingement in Legg-Calve-Perthes disease. J Pediatr Orthop. 2011;31(2 Suppl):S235–40. doi:10.1097/BPO.0b013e3182260252.
126. Kim HKW. Legg-Calve-Perthes disease. J Am Acad Orthop Surg. 2010;18:676–86.

Developing Medical Therapy for Legg-Calvé-Perthes' Disease

62

Harry K.W. Kim and David G. Little

62.1 Introduction

Legg-Calvé-Perthes' disease (LCPD) was recognized as a separate disease entity from tuberculosis over 100 years ago by Drs. Legg from the USA [1], Calvé from France [2], and Perthes from Germany [3]. Despite research efforts to improve the knowledge base for this pediatric idiopathic hip disorder, LCPD remains one of the most controversial conditions in pediatric orthopedics. While two prospective multicenter studies [4, 5], meta-analyses [6, 7], and some large retrospective studies [8–10] provide clinically valuable information about the outcomes of current operative and nonoperative treatments for LCPD, the optimal way to treat this condition remains elusive. These studies show that the success rates of current treatments, including a femoral varus osteotomy and the Salter innominate osteotomy, in producing a round femoral head (Stulberg I or II hips) range from 40 to 60 % [4, 5] in those children with the onset of the disease after age 8. These results point to the clinical need to develop more effective treatments including biological treatments to specifically target the pathological processes contributing to the femoral head deformity and the poor bone healing. This chapter discusses the experimental evidence for using bisphosphonate therapy to treat LCPD and the potential limitations of bisphosphonate therapy.

62.2 Rationale for Antiresorptive Therapy

Within the last 10 years, a considerable interest has risen to treat LCPD using a biological approach. This approach stems from recognition that there is a significant biological component to the pathogenesis of the femoral head deformity in the infarcted, immature femoral head [11–13]. This has led to the development of biological treatment concept for LCPD. The biological concept postulates that therapeutically targeting specific biological factors or pathological processes contributing to the pathogenesis of femoral head deformity will decrease the deformity and improve the outcome. An imbalance between bone resorption and bone formation during necrotic bone healing has been identified as one such process in the experimental studies of ischemic osteonecrosis (Fig. 62.1) [12, 14]. Increased osteoclast-mediated bone resorption and delayed new bone formation in the areas of resorption produce a net loss of the trabecular bone in the infarcted femoral head and contribute to its mechanical weakening [12, 13]. Femoral head specimens from the patients with LCPD also show an increased presence of osteoclasts and an absence of osteoblasts in the areas of bone resorption [11, 15]. These findings have led to the hypothesis that an inhibition of osteoclastic resorption using antiresorptive agents, such as bisphosphonate, will preserve the trabecular framework of the necrotic femoral head, minimize the femoral head deformity, and maintain the trabecular scaffold on which new bone formation can occur.

H.K.W. Kim (✉)
Center for Excellence in Hip Disorders,
Texas Scottish Rite Hospital for Children,
2222 Welborn Street, Dallas, TX 75219, USA

Department of Orthopaedic Surgery,
UT Southwestern Medical Center, Dallas, TX, USA
e-mail: harry.kim@tsrh.org

D.G. Little
Department of Orthopaedic Research and Biotechnology,
The Children's Hospital at Westmead and University of Sydney,
Westmead, NSW, Australia

Disclosure
Dr. Kim has previously received research grants from Roche Pharmaceutical (Indianapolis, IN, USA).
Dr. Little has previously received consultancy fees from Novartis Corp (East Hanover, NJ, USA).

K.-H. Koo et al. (eds.), *Osteonecrosis*,
DOI 10.1007/978-3-642-35767-1_62, © Springer-Verlag Berlin Heidelberg 2014

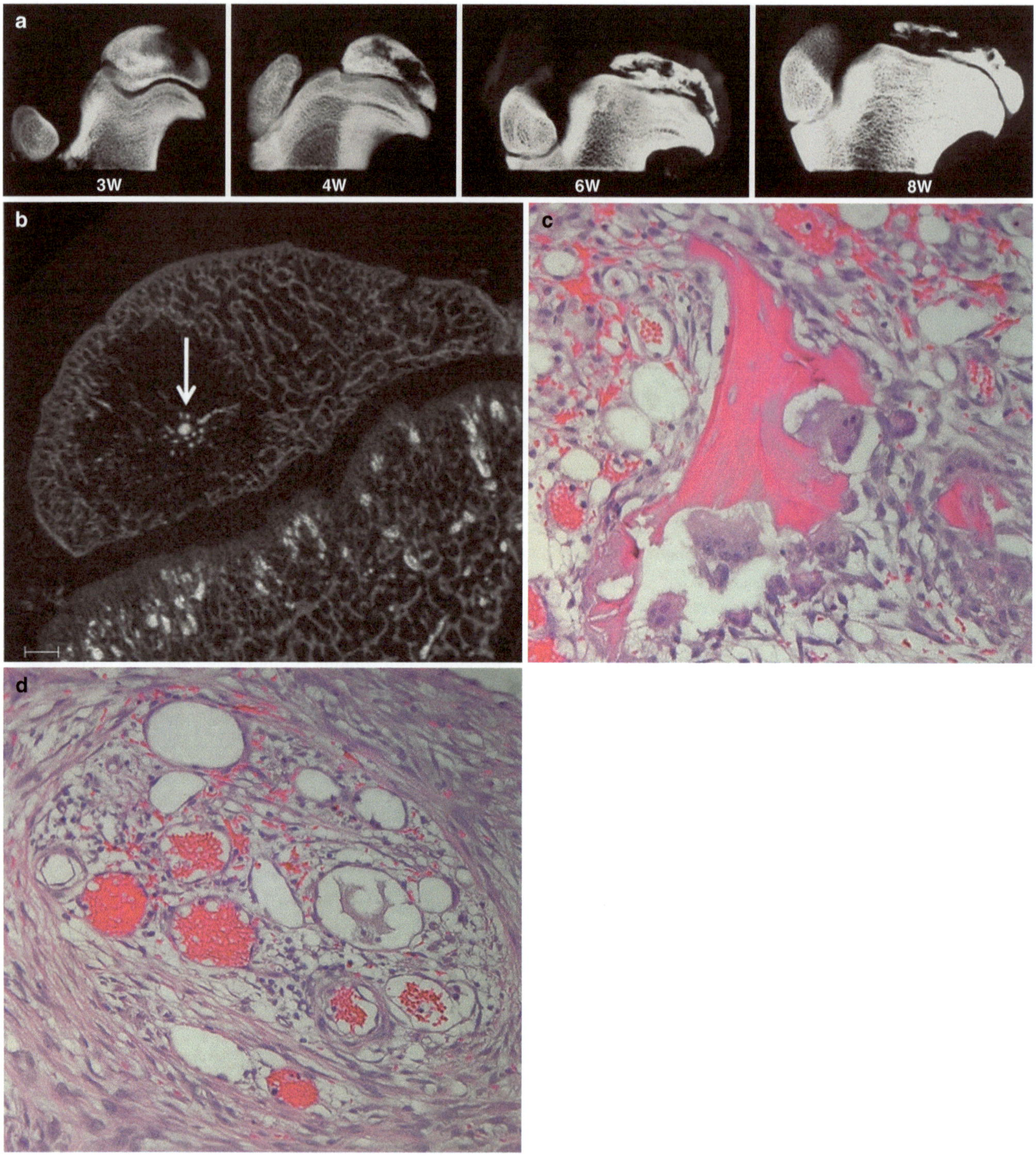

Fig. 62.1 An experimental study of the pathogenesis of femoral head deformity following ischemic osteonecrosis of the immature femoral head in the piglet model. (**a**) Radiographs of the central region of immature femoral heads showing a progression of the femoral head deformity in the piglet model (*w* weeks following the induction of ischemic necrosis). (**b**) A micro-CT image of a central region of the femoral head obtained at 3 weeks postischemia showing a circular area of bone resorption in the necrotic epiphysis. A radiodense, intravascular contrast material (microfil) was infused into the distal aorta before imaging to detect revascularization in the necrotic epiphysis. The *arrow* is pointing to a vessel with multiple small branches within the area of resorption. (**c**) A photomicrograph of a peripheral area of revascularization showing the increased presence of multinucleated cells (osteoclasts) and resorption of the trabecular bone (Hematoxylin and eosin staining, 20×). (**d**) A photomicrograph of a central area of revascularization showing fibrovascular tissue. The resorbed bone was not replaced by new bone (Hematoxylin and eosin staining, 10×) (Figures from Kim [56])

62.3 Bisphosphonate Mechanisms of Action

Bisphosphonates (BPs) are compounds which have a high affinity for bone mineral and are characterized by P–C–P bonds [16, 17]. They have two side chains that affect their binding affinity for minerals and their antiresorptive potency [18]. BPs have been used clinically for over 30 years to treat various metabolic bone disorders in the adult population. Currently, they are also being used in the pediatric population for limited clinical indications such as osteogenesis imperfecta [19]. The older BPs are nonnitrogen-containing compounds (e.g., etidronate and clodronate), whereas the newer BPs are more potent and contain nitrogen (e.g., alendronate, risedronate, pamidronate, ibandronate, and zoledronate). Once taken up by osteoclasts, nonnitrogen BPs produce toxic analogs of ATP that cause osteoclast apoptosis [20]. Nitrogen BPs act by interfering with a prenylation of small GTPase proteins and inhibiting farnesyl pyrophosphatase, an enzyme in the HMG-CoA reductase pathway, which leads to reduced resorptive activity and accelerated apoptosis of the osteoclasts [21]. While BPs have been used to treat osteoporosis, malignancy-induced hypercalcemia, Paget's disease, and other metabolic bone disorders for many years and their clinical efficacy for these indications is well documented, the concept of using BPs to treat femoral head osteonecrosis is relatively new, and the clinical evidence supporting their use for this indication is only slowly emerging.

62.4 Experimental Evidence for Bisphosphonate Therapy

There is consistent evidence demonstrating the protective effects of bisphosphonate therapy on experimentally induced femoral head osteonecrosis. These studies can be divided into small and large animal studies [22–25].

62.4.1 Small Animal Studies

In immature rats, the effects of zoledronic acid (currently the most potent amino-bisphosphonate clinically available) were studied in a surgically induced osteonecrosis model and in spontaneously hypertensive rats that develop a Perthes-like osteonecrosis in 50 % of male animals [24, 25]. In the surgically induced osteonecrosis model, zoledronic acid treatment resulted in significantly greater trabecular bone volume and better preservation of the femoral head shape compared to the saline-treated animals which showed loss of trabecular bone volume and deformation of the femoral head [25]. The best results were obtained when zoledronic acid was administered both prophylactically (i.e., prior to the induction of osteonecrosis) and after the induction of osteonecrosis. These animals were observed to have near complete preservation of the femoral head structure. Interestingly, the animals treated with zoledronic acid after the induction of osteonecrosis also showed new bone formation in the femoral heads albeit less than that of the saline-treated animals. Similarly, treatment of spontaneously hypertensive rats with zoledronic acid increased the bone mineral density and the trabecular bone volume in the femoral head and better preserved the sphericity of the femoral head [24]. These animals also showed new bone formation in the femoral head albeit at a decreased rate than the saline-treated animals. These effects of decreased bone formation are consistent with associated reduction in bone resorption as the two processes are generally coupled.

62.4.2 Large Animal Studies

Similar finding on the inhibition of resorption was obtained using a large animal model of surgically induced osteonecrosis using another bisphosphonate, ibandronate, which is also a potent amino-bisphosphonate [23]. The infarcted femoral heads in the ibandronate-treated animals were significantly better preserved in terms of the femoral head sphericity and the trabecular bone volume. In contrast to the rat study findings, however, the bone formation in the femoral head, as assessed by histology and measurement of the osteoblast surface (%), was significantly decreased in the saline- and the ibandronate-treated animals. The difference between the rat and the piglet studies appears to stem from the rapid remodeling of the necrotic bone and restoration of new bone formation that occurs in the immature rats following osteonecrosis which is not seen in the piglet model. In the rat study, there was an absence of necrotic bone in the saline-treated animals by 6 weeks after the osteonecrosis induction [24]. This finding indicates a rapid removal of the necrotic bone and replacement by new bone which is not seen in the piglet model. The preservation of the necrotic bone following bisphosphonate therapy in the piglet model without new bone formation occurring raises a concern as the necrotic bone preserved by bisphosphonate therapy may eventually fail due to the accumulation of microcracks.

In addition to the immature animal models, bisphosphonate therapy has been shown to increase the bone volume and/or to protect the femoral head from deformity in a mature rat model [26], a rabbit model [27], and a canine model of osteonecrosis [28].

62.4.3 Experimental Studies on Local Intraosseous Bisphosphonate Therapy

It is important to recognize that local bioavailability of bisphosphonate for an avascular bone condition is different from the conditions where blood flow to the bone is not compromised. A radioactive bisphosphonate tracing study in the piglet model of ischemic necrosis showed preferential binding of ^{14}C-ibandronate in the revascularized regions of the infarcted femoral head, whereas binding to the nonvascularized regions of the infarcted head was minimal (Fig. 62.2) [29]. This finding is not surprising since an analog of bisphosphonate, methylene diphosphonate (medronic acid, e.g., technetium MDP), is used as an imaging agent for bone scintigraphy based on its chemical property to selectively localize in the vascularized regions of the bone. After an intravenous or oral administration of bisphosphonate, it is likely that only a very small fraction of the dose actually ends up in the necrotic bone. Because of this uncertainty, multiple dosing regimens are suggested for oral or intravenous administration.

To overcome the limitation associated with a systemic administration, a local intraosseous administration has been investigated as an alternate route for the treatment of femoral head osteonecrosis. In the piglet model of ischemic necrosis, a single injection of ^{14}C-ibandronate directly into the necrotic femoral heads demonstrated a wide distribution of the drug within the necrotic head with good retention at 48 h [22]. Furthermore, a single local injection effectively decreased the femoral head deformity at 8 weeks postischemia induction in the piglet model of ischemic osteonecrosis at a dose that was only 5 % of the systemic dose used in the previous study using the same large animal model (Fig. 62.3).

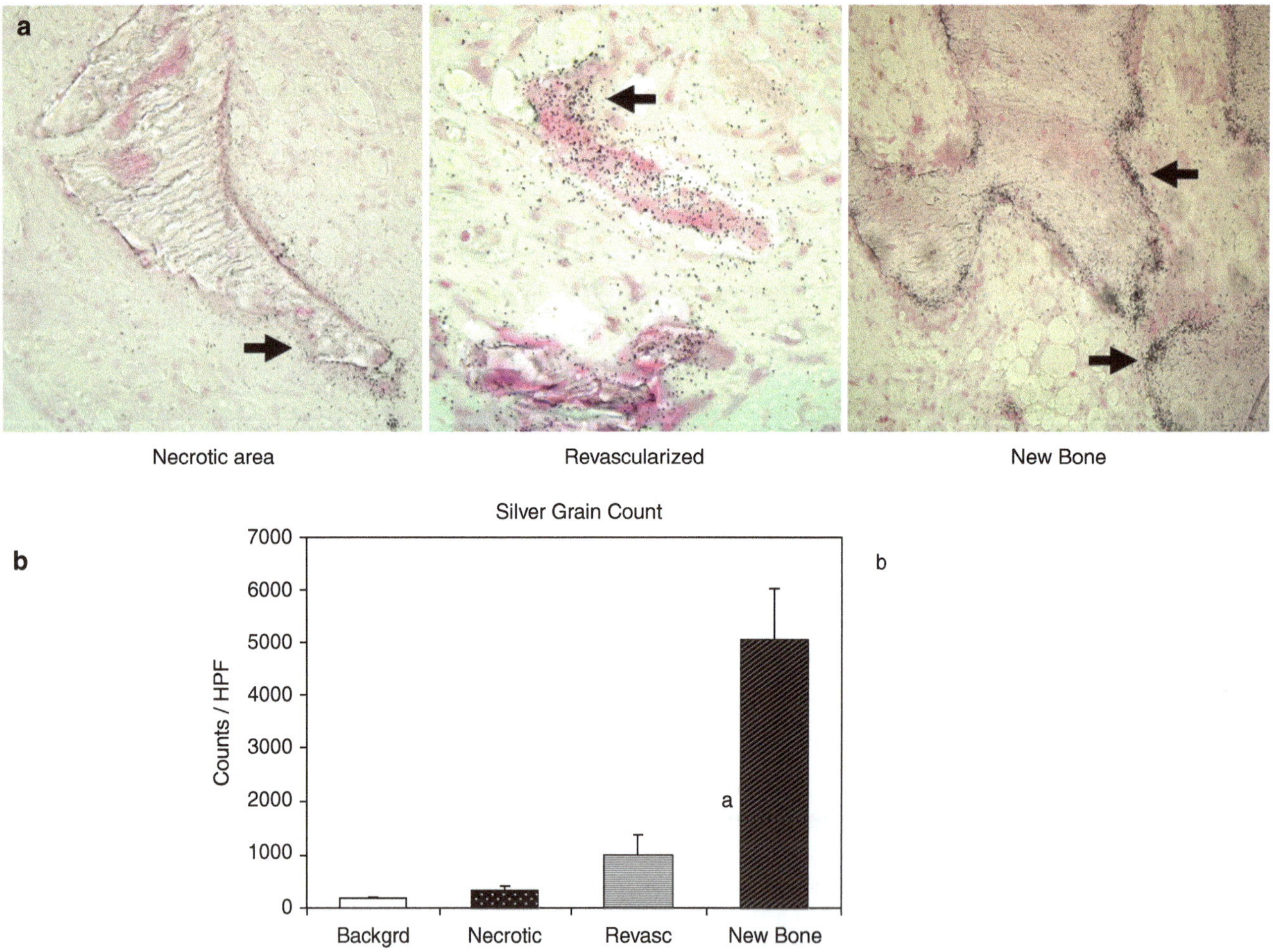

Fig. 62.2 An experimental study of bioavailability of bisphosphonate in the infarcted femoral heads following intravenous administration in immature pigs. (**a**) Autoradiographic images of the three regions (the region of necrotic bone, the region of revascularized marrow space, and the region of newly formed bone) found in the infarcted femoral heads at 6 weeks postischemia induction. ^{14}C-labeled ibandronate was administered intravenously 24 h prior to sacrifice to determine its localization within the necrotic head. *Arrows* indicate the presence of silver grains (indicating ^{14}C radioactivity) on the trabecular surfaces. A dense concentration of the silver grains was present on the newly formed bone but not on the necrotic bone. (**b**) A bar graph of mean silver grain counts obtained from the background and from the three regions found in the infarcted head at 6 weeks. $^{a}p=0.02$ vs. background and $p=0.05$ vs. necrotic region, $^{b}p=0.000001$ vs. all groups (Figures from Kim et al. [29])

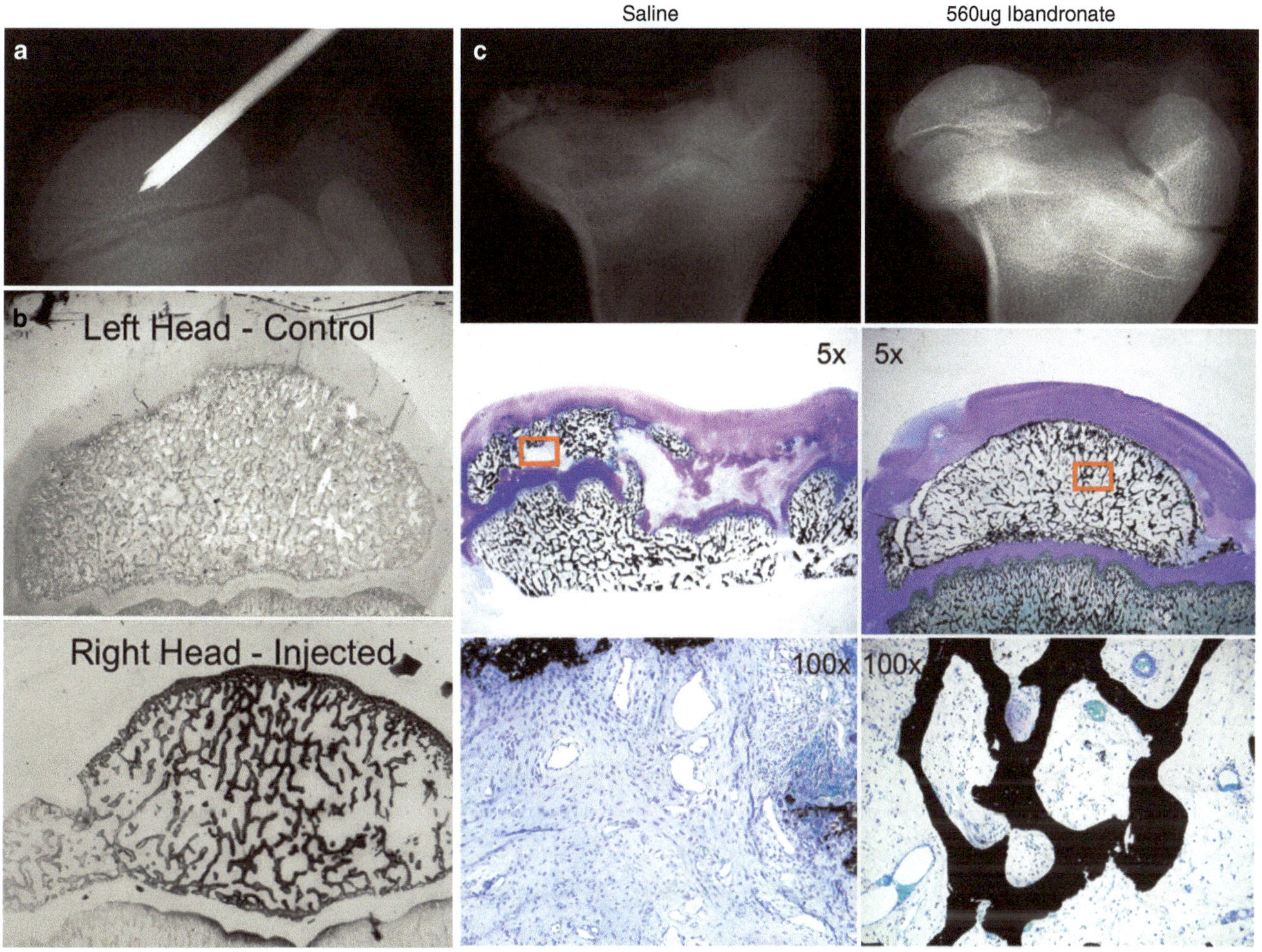

Fig. 62.3 An experimental study on the effects of local intraosseous administration of bisphosphonate in the infarcted femoral heads in immature pigs. (**a**) A radiograph demonstrating an intraosseous needle placed in the central region of the femoral head used to locally deliver bisphosphonate. (**b**) Autoradiographic sections from a control femoral head and an infarcted femoral head injected with ^{14}C-ibandronate. A wide distribution of ^{14}C-ibandronate, marked by diffuse staining of the trabecular bone with black silver grains, is observed in the femoral head following a single intraosseous injection. (**c**) A representative radiograph and photomicrographs obtained from an infarcted femoral head injected with saline (*left*) or 560 μg ibandronate (*right*) 7 weeks before the sacrifice. The femoral head structure and the trabecular bone were significantly better preserved in the ibandronate group compared to the saline group (von Kossa and McNeal's tetrachrome staining) (Figures from Aya-ay et al. [22])

62.4.4 Experimental Studies on Combined Antiresorptive and Bone Anabolic Therapy

An ideal biological treatment for LCPD would be the one that not only controls bone resorption (antiresorptive) but also stimulates new bone formation (bone anabolic). Such treatment will improve the balance of bone resorption and bone formation which is severely perturbed in the fragmentation/resorptive stage of LCPD. While the lack of new bone formation following the administration of bisphosphonate was observed only in the piglet model and not in the rodent studies, the concern has prompted a further study to examine the effects of a combined antiresorptive and anabolic therapy on the femoral head healing following ischemic necrosis using the piglet model [30]. In this study BMP-2 was used as a bone anabolic agent and was administered with ibandronate via a single intraosseous injection into the necrotic femoral heads. In comparison to the control group, the combined therapy group had a significant decrease in the femoral head deformity and the osteoclast number and a significant increase in the trabecular bone volume and the osteoblast surface (Fig. 62.4). In comparison to the local ibandronate treatment group, the combined treatment group also had a significantly higher osteoblast surface, suggesting an increased bone formation as a result of adding BMP-2. One cautionary finding from this study was the presence of heterotopic ossification in the hip joint capsule which was postulated to be due to a leakage of BMP-2 into the joint during and following the local injection procedure. Further studies to determine whether the heterotopic ossification can be prevented by lowering the dose of BMP-2, changing the injection technique, and using another type of BMP are pending.

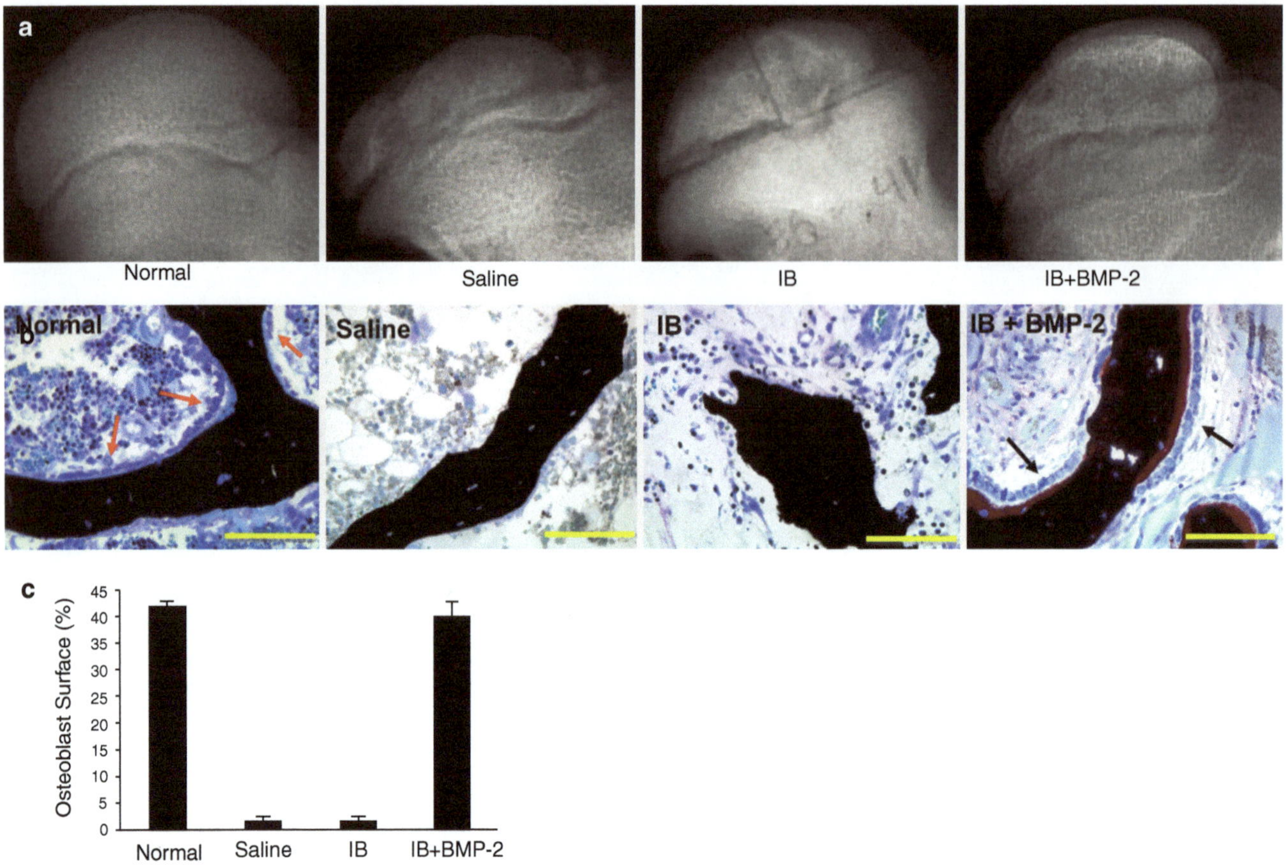

Fig. 62.4 An experimental study on the effects of a combined local bisphosphonate and BMP-2 therapy on the infarcted femoral heads of immature pigs. (**a**) Radiographs of the animals treated with intraosseous saline, ibandronate (IB), or IB plus BMP-2. A single injection of respective agent(s) was rendered 1 week following the induction of ischemic osteonecrosis. (**b**) Photomicrographs showing a presence of osteoblasts on the surface of the trabecular bone in the IB + BMP-2 group. The femoral heads from the saline and the IB groups had a lack of osteoblasts on the trabecular surfaces. (**c**) A bar graph showing significantly greater osteoblast surface (%), an indicator of bone formation, in the IB + BMP-2 group compared to the saline and the IB group (Figures from Vandermeer et al. [30])

62.5 Clinical Evidence

At this time there is no direct clinical evidence to support the use of bisphosphonate therapy to prevent femoral head deformity in LCPD. While the use of bisphosphonate therapy for LCPD has been reported from one center in Australia [31, 32], clinical studies assessing the efficacy of this treatment have not been performed. However, a randomized clinical trial is underway in Australia comparing intravenous administration of zoledronic acid to a standard care (weight-bearing restriction and current treatments) for LCPD (Clinical Trial Registration ACTRN12610000407099). While direct clinical evidence supporting bisphosphonate therapy for LCPD is lacking, a limited number of studies on other forms of childhood femoral head osteonecrosis and adult femoral head osteonecrosis have been reported.

62.5.1 Evidence in Adult Femoral Head Osteonecrosis

In the adult population, at least seven clinical studies on patients treated with bisphosphonate for nontraumatic osteonecrosis of the femoral head are available [33–37]. In general, these studies show some beneficial effects of bisphosphonate therapy on pain, function, and preservation of the femoral head [33–36]. Among these studies, one of them was a randomized clinical trial involving 40 patients (54 hips) with Steinberg IIC and IIIC hips (i.e., pre-collapsed femoral heads with >30 % head involvement on the MRI) [35]. In the study, only 2 out of 29 hips required total hip replacement following oral alendronate therapy (70 mg weekly dosing) for 6 months compared to 19 out of 25 hips in the non-treatment group at the minimum follow-up of 2 years. The short-term results are impressive; however, the authors observed no evidence of reduction or resolution of the necrotic area of the femoral head on radiographs or MRI at the final follow-up suggesting that longer follow-up studies are needed. More recent multicenter, prospective, randomized, double-blinded, placebo-controlled study, however, showed no difference between the alendronate treatment and the placebo group in terms of the radiographic or MRI results at 2-year follow-up [38]. For both groups the rate of total hip replacement at 2-year follow-up was low, 4 out of 32 hips in the alendronate treatment group and 5 out of 33 hips in the placebo group. These low event rates raise the question of whether the patients included in the study had clinically significant femoral head osteonecrosis as the clinical outcome of large femoral head osteonecrosis is generally poor. Further, with this low event rate, it is estimated that a sample size over 200 patients in each group would be required to reach 80 % power.

Among the adult studies, the study by Agarwala et al. had the longest follow-up [34] (up to 8 years). In their clinical series (level 4 evidence) that included 294 patients (395 hips) in Ficat and Arlet stage 1–3, oral alendronate therapy (10 mg daily) produced the best results when the treatment was initiated in the early stage of femoral head osteonecrosis (stage 1). At the mean follow-up of 4 years, 2 % (4 out of 215), 8 % (10 out of 129), and 33 % (17 out of 51) of the patients in stage 1, 2, and 3, respectively, had a total hip replacement. In terms of radiographic progression, 13 % (27 out of 215) of the patients in stage 1 and 56 % (72 out of 129) of the patients in stage 2 had a radiographic evidence of collapse. Major limitations of this study were that the extent of the femoral head involvement was not assessed and no controls were included in the study to determine the efficacy of the treatment.

62.5.2 Evidence in Childhood Femoral Head Osteonecrosis

In children, bisphosphonate therapy has been used to treat LCPD [31, 32], traumatic osteonecrosis [39], and osteonecrosis as a complication of chemotherapy for childhood leukemia and non-Hodgkin lymphoma [40–42]. The numbers of patients treated with bisphosphonate therapy in these studies are small, and the level of evidence is restricted to case reports, case series, or observational studies. The follow-up duration of these studies has also been short. In a small number of patients with LCPD ($n = 17$), the systemic effects of intravenous bisphosphonate have been reported [31]; however, its effect on the preservation of the femoral head has yet to be reported. A prospective case series of traumatic osteonecrosis due to unstable SCFE, hip fracture, or dislocation in adolescents showed that the patients treated with intravenous bisphosphonate (pamidronate or zoledronic acid) did better than expected from historical controls at the minimum follow-up of 2 years [39]. Nine out of 17 patients had a spherical femoral head and 14 out of 17 patients were pain free. The mean Harris hip score, Iowa hip rating, and global PODCI score were 91.2, 92.1, and 91.5, respectively. This study, however, did not have a control group. In an observational study of 17 patients with osteonecrosis as a complication of chemotherapy for childhood leukemia [41], improvements in the pain scores, analgesic requirement, and function were found in the nine patients who received bisphosphonate therapy, while seven of eight patients who did not receive bisphosphonate therapy showed clinical deterioration. A radiographic benefit of the therapy, however, could not be demonstrated. Another small study of childhood leukemic patients found a reduction of pain and increased mobility in four of the six patients treated with pamidronate for 2 years [42]. Pamidronate therapy, however, did not prevent late bone collapse as three of the six patients had a progression and required hip replacement. A more recent study of pediatric oncology patients treated with zoledronate found that only 25 % patients have a spherical femoral head and pain free at the end of treatment, 25 % had hip arthroplasty, and 50 % had ongoing pain and disability that was expected to lead to hip arthroplasty [43].

62.6 Potential Limitations of Bisphosphonate Therapy for LCPD

Potential limitations of bisphosphonate therapy for the treatment of LCPD include no direct mechanical enhancing effect and unknown long-term effects on the growing skeleton. These are in addition to a limited distribution of bisphosphonate in the necrotic bone following oral or intravenous administration and a lack of bone anabolic effect discussed in previous sections.

Experimental studies show that ischemic osteonecrosis of the immature femoral head produces mechanical weakening of the femoral head through weakening of the cartilage and bone [13, 44]. It is unlikely that bisphosphonate therapy will have an immediate effect on restoring the mechanical properties of the necrotic femoral head as the mechanical restoration bone strength will depend on the healing process and new bone formation which will take time. During this time, a protected weight bearing and restriction of activities should be considered even if bisphosphonate therapy is initiated as the femoral head will be mechanically compromised. It is important to note that even with normal activities, considerable hip joint loading occurs [45]. When local non-weight bearing was compare to weight bearing as tolerated in the piglet model of ischemic osteonecrosis, significantly less femoral head deformity was observed in the animals treated with local non-weight bearing [46]. Clinical studies on non-weight bearing, however, are limited, and the results are inconclusive due to study design weaknesses such as a lack of documentation of compliance to non-weight-bearing treatment, retrospective study design, small sample size, and no controls. Since the healing process can be prolonged, especially in older patients with LCPD, a treatment regimen that combines mechanical protection with biological treatments to control bone resorption and to stimulate new bone formation may provide the best long-term results.

In general, severe adverse effects due to bisphosphonate therapy in children are uncommon when the drug is used judiciously [31, 39, 47, 48]. However, one of the unresolved questions is what are the long-term effects of administering repetitive doses of bisphosphonate to a normal growing skeleton? Since LCPD is a self-limiting disease, it is argued that the duration of bisphosphonate therapy required will not be as long as the other conditions that are more chronic in nature, like osteogenesis imperfecta, and the drug may only be required in the initial and resorptive stages of the disease, which would range from 1 to 2 years. It is also argued that if a local administration is used, the exposure of the drug to the rest of the skeleton will be significantly less [22].

Some data on the systemic and skeletal effects of bisphosphonate therapy in children with osteogenesis imperfecta have been reported [49–51]; however, such data on children with normal skeletons are scant. Bisphosphonates have been shown to decrease the long bone growth in some animal studies [23, 52–54] but not in others [55]. The growth inhibition is postulated to be a dose-dependent effect seen in the studies where repeated administration of relatively high dose of bisphosphonate was administered in fast growing animals. In the limited number of clinical studies that are available, the growth inhibition has not been observed [31, 47, 48]. These studies, however, had a relatively small number of patients and a short follow-up to be considered conclusive. In a cohort of 18 children treated for polyostotic fibrous dysplasia with pamidronate for 1.2–9.1 years (median 3.8 years), no significant change in their height Z-scores was observed [48]. A recent review of 17 patients with LCPD treated with zoledronic acid also found maintenance of the height Z-scores over an 18-month period of the study [31].

62.7 Summary

Recent multicenter prospective studies show that current treatments for LCPD produce modest results. These studies clearly demonstrate the need to develop more effective treatments for LCPD to prevent the femoral head deformity and improve the outcome. A pathological repair process marked by an imbalance of bone resorption and bone formation has been recognized as a significant contributor to the pathogenesis of the femoral head deformity. A biological approach using bisphosphonate therapy to inhibit the pathological bone resorption shows improved preservation of the necrotic bone and the femoral head structure. While the results from the experimental studies are promising, well-controlled clinical studies are required to determine the clinical efficacy of this treatment. Further experimental and clinical studies are also needed to delineate the long-term effects of bisphosphonate therapy on the remodeling of the necrotic bone and on the remodeling of the growing skeleton. Potential limitations of bisphosphonate therapy include decreased distribution within the necrotic femoral head with systemic administration, no immediate mechanical protective effect on the necrotic femoral head, and a lack of bone anabolic effect (i.e., stimulation of new bone formation). A combined antiresorptive and bone anabolic approach aimed at preserving the femoral head bone mass while increasing new bone formation is the subject of current experimental investigation.

References

1. Legg AT. An obscure affection of the hip joint. Boston Med Surg J. 1910;162:202–4.
2. Calve J. Sur une forme particulière de pseudo-coxalgie greffée sur des déformations caractéristiques de l'extrémité supérieure du fémur. Rev Chir. 1910;42:54–84.
3. Perthes G. Űber arthritis deformans juvenilis. Deutsche Zeitschr Chir. 1910;107:111–59.
4. Herring JA, Kim HT, Browne R. Legg-Calve-Perthes disease. Part II: prospective multicenter study of the effect of treatment on outcome. J Bone Joint Surg Am. 2004;86-A(10):2121–34. 86/10/2121 [pii].
5. Wiig O, Terjesen T, Svenningsen S. Prognostic factors and outcome of treatment in Perthes' disease: a prospective study of 368 patients with five-year follow-up. J Bone Joint Surg Br. 2008;90(10):1364–71. doi:10.1302/0301-620X.90B10.20649. 90-B/10/1364 [pii].
6. Nguyen NA, Klein G, Dogbey G, McCourt JB, Mehlman CT. Operative versus nonoperative treatments for Legg-Calve-Perthes disease: a meta-analysis. J Pediatr Orthop. 2012;32(7):697–705. doi:10.1097/BPO.0b013e318269c55d. 01241398-201210000-00010 [pii].
7. Saran N, Varghese R, Mulpuri K. Do femoral or salter innominate osteotomies improve femoral head sphericity in Legg-Calve-Perthes disease? A meta-analysis. Clin Orthop Relat Res. 2012;470(9):2383–93. doi:10.1007/s11999-012-2326-3.
8. Canavese F, Dimeglio A. Perthes' disease: prognosis in children under six years of age. J Bone Joint Surg Br. 2008;90(7):940–5. doi:10.1302/0301-620X.90B7.20691. 90-B/7/940 [pii].
9. Joseph B, Rao N, Mulpuri K, Varghese G, Nair S. How does a femoral varus osteotomy alter the natural evolution of Perthes' disease? J Pediatr Orthop B. 2005;14(1):10–5. 01202412-200501000-00002 [pii].
10. Rosenfeld SB, Herring JA, Chao JC. Legg-calve-perthes disease: a review of cases with onset before six years of age. J Bone Joint Surg Am. 2007;89(12):2712–22. doi:10.2106/JBJS.G.00191. 89/12/2712 [pii].

11. Catterall A, Pringle J, Byers PD, Fulford GE, Kemp HB, Dolman CL, et al. A review of the morphology of Perthes' disease. J Bone Joint Surg Br. 1982;64(3):269–75.
12. Kim HK, Su PH. Development of flattening and apparent fragmentation following ischemic necrosis of the capital femoral epiphysis in a piglet model. J Bone Joint Surg Am. 2002;84-A(8):1329–34.
13. Pringle D, Koob TJ, Kim HK. Indentation properties of growing femoral head following ischemic necrosis. J Orthop Res. 2004;22(1):122–30. doi:10.1016/S0736-0266(03)00135-9. S0736026603001359 [pii].
14. Kim HK, Morgan-Bagley S, Kostenuik P. RANKL inhibition: a novel strategy to decrease femoral head deformity after ischemic osteonecrosis. J Bone Miner Res. 2006;21(12):1946–54. doi:10.1359/jbmr.060905.
15. Jonsater S. Coxa plana; a histo-pathologic and arthrographic study. Acta Orthop Scand Suppl. 1953;12:5–98.
16. Fleisch H. Bisphosphonates: mechanisms of action. Endocr Rev. 1998;19(1):80–100.
17. Rodan GA. Mechanisms of action of bisphosphonates. Annu Rev Pharmacol Toxicol. 1998;38:375–88.
18. Russell RG, Xia Z, Dunford JE, Oppermann U, Kwaasi A, Hulley PA, et al. Bisphosphonates: an update on mechanisms of action and how these relate to clinical efficacy. Ann N Y Acad Sci. 2007;1117:209–57. doi:10.1196/annals.1402.089. 1117/1/209 [pii].
19. Speiser PW, Clarson CL, Eugster EA, Kemp SF, Radovick S, Rogol AD, et al. Bisphosphonate treatment of pediatric bone disease. Pediatr Endocrinol Rev. 2005;3(2):87–96.
20. Frith JC, Monkkonen J, Auriola S, Monkkonen H, Rogers MJ. The molecular mechanism of action of the antiresorptive and antiinflammatory drug clodronate: evidence for the formation in vivo of a metabolite that inhibits bone resorption and causes osteoclast and macrophage apoptosis. Arthritis Rheum. 2001;44(9):2201–10.
21. Schmidt A, Rutledge SJ, Endo N, Opas EE, Tanaka H, Wesolowski G, et al. Protein-tyrosine phosphatase activity regulates osteoclast formation and function: inhibition by alendronate. Proc Natl Acad Sci U S A. 1996;93(7):3068–73.
22. Aya-ay J, Athavale S, Morgan-Bagley S, Bian H, Bauss F, Kim HK. Retention, distribution, and effects of intraosseously administered ibandronate in the infarcted femoral head. J Bone Miner Res. 2007;22(1):93–100. doi:10.1359/jbmr.060817.
23. Kim HK, Randall TS, Bian H, Jenkins J, Garces A, Bauss F. Ibandronate for prevention of femoral head deformity after ischemic necrosis of the capital femoral epiphysis in immature pigs. J Bone Joint Surg Am. 2005;87(3):550–7. doi:10.2106/JBJS.D.02192. 87/3/550 [pii].
24. Little DG, McDonald M, Sharpe IT, Peat R, Williams P, McEvoy T. Zoledronic acid improves femoral head sphericity in a rat model of perthes disease. J Orthop Res. 2005;23(4):862–8. doi:10.1016/j.orthres.2004.11.015. S0736-0266(05)00002-1 [pii].
25. Little DG, Peat RA, McEvoy A, Williams PR, Smith EJ, Baldock PA. Zoledronic acid treatment results in retention of femoral head structure after traumatic osteonecrosis in young Wistar rats. J Bone Miner Res. 2003;18(11):2016–22. doi:10.1359/jbmr.2003.18.11.2016.
26. Peled E, Bejar J, Zinman C, Boss JH, Reis DN, Norman D. Prevention of distortion of vascular deprivation-induced osteonecrosis of the rat femoral head by treatment with alendronate. Arch Orthop Trauma Surg. 2009;129(2):275–9. doi:10.1007/s00402-008-0656-0.
27. Hofstaetter JG, Wang J, Yan J, Glimcher MJ. The effects of alendronate in the treatment of experimental osteonecrosis of the hip in adult rabbits. Osteoarthritis Cartilage. 2009;17(3):362–70. doi:10.1016/j.joca.2008.07.013. S1063-4584(08)00248-3 [pii].
28. Bowers JR, Dailiana ZH, McCarthy EF, Urbaniak JR. Drug therapy increases bone density in osteonecrosis of the femoral head in canines. J Surg Orthop Adv. 2004;13(4):210–6. 13-4-4_ftp.pdf?T=open_article,867134 [pii].
29. Kim HK, Sanders M, Athavale S, Bian H, Bauss F. Local bioavailability and distribution of systemically (parenterally) administered ibandronate in the infarcted femoral head. Bone. 2006;39(1):205–12. doi:10.1016/j.bone.2005.12.019. S8756-3282(05)00605-8 [pii].
30. Vandermeer JS, Kamiya N, Aya-ay J, Garces A, Browne R, Kim HK. Local administration of ibandronate and bone morphogenetic protein-2 after ischemic osteonecrosis of the immature femoral head: a combined therapy that stimulates bone formation and decreases femoral head deformity. J Bone Joint Surg Am. 2011;93(10):905–13. doi:10.2106/JBJS.J.00716. 93/10/905 [pii].
31. Johannesen J, Briody J, McQuade M, Little DG, Cowell CT, Munns CF. Systemic effects of zoledronic acid in children with traumatic femoral head avascular necrosis and Legg-Calve-Perthes disease. Bone. 2009;45(5):898–902. doi:10.1016/j.bone.2009.04.255. S8756-3282(09)01579-8 [pii].
32. McQuade M, Houghton K. Use of bisphosphonates in a case of Perthes disease. Orthop Nurs. 2005;24(6):393–8. 00006416-200511000-00003 [pii].
33. Agarwala S, Jain D, Joshi VR, Sule A. Efficacy of alendronate, a bisphosphonate, in the treatment of AVN of the hip. A prospective open-label study. Rheumatology (Oxford). 2005;44(3):352–9. keh481 [pii].
34. Agarwala S, Shah S, Joshi VR. The use of alendronate in the treatment of avascular necrosis of the femoral head: follow-up to eight years. J Bone Joint Surg Br. 2009;91(8):1013–8. doi:10.1302/0301-620X.91B8.21518. 91-B/8/1013 [pii].
35. Lai KA, Shen WJ, Yang CY, Shao CJ, Hsu JT, Lin RM. The use of alendronate to prevent early collapse of the femoral head in patients with nontraumatic osteonecrosis. A randomized clinical study. J Bone Joint Surg Am. 2005;87(10):2155–9. doi:10.2106/JBJS.D.02959. 87/10/2155 [pii].
36. Nishii T, Sugano N, Miki H, Hashimoto J, Yoshikawa H. Does alendronate prevent collapse in osteonecrosis of the femoral head? Clin Orthop Relat Res. 2006;443:273–9. doi:10.1097/01.blo.0000194078.32776.31. 00003086-200602000-00036 [pii].
37. Wang CJ, Wang FS, Yang KD, Huang CC, Lee MS, Chan YS, et al. Treatment of osteonecrosis of the hip: comparison of extracorporeal shockwave with shockwave and alendronate. Arch Orthop Trauma Surg. 2008;128(9):901–8. doi:10.1007/s00402-007-0530-5.
38. Chen CH, Chang JK, Lai KA, Hou SM, Chang CH, Wang GJ. Alendronate in the prevention of collapse of the femoral head in nontraumatic osteonecrosis: a two-year multicenter, prospective, randomized, double-blind, placebo-controlled study. Arthritis Rheum. 2012;64(5):1572–8. doi:10.1002/art.33498.
39. Ramachandran M, Ward K, Brown RR, Munns CF, Cowell CT, Little DG. Intravenous bisphosphonate therapy for traumatic osteonecrosis of the femoral head in adolescents. J Bone Joint Surg Am. 2007;89(8):1727–34. doi:10.2106/JBJS.F.00964. 89/8/1727 [pii].
40. Greggio NA, Pillon M, Varotto E, Zanin A, Talenti E, Palozzo AC, et al. Short-term bisphosphonate therapy could ameliorate osteonecrosis: a complication in childhood hematologic malignancies. Case Rep Med. 2010;2010:206132. doi:10.1155/2010/206132.
41. Kotecha RS, Powers N, Lee SJ, Murray KJ, Carter T, Cole C. Use of bisphosphonates for the treatment of osteonecrosis as a complication of therapy for childhood acute lymphoblastic leukaemia (ALL). Pediatr Blood Cancer. 2010;54(7):934–40. doi:10.1002/pbc.22428.
42. Nguyen T, Zacharin MR. Pamidronate treatment of steroid associated osteonecrosis in young patients treated for acute lymphoblastic leukaemia–two-year outcomes. J Pediatr Endocrinol Metab. 2006;19(2):161–7.
43. Padhye B, Dalla-Pozza L, Little DG, Munns CF. Use of zoledronic acid for treatment of chemotherapy related osteonecrosis in children and adolescents: a retrospective analysis. Pediatr Blood Cancer. 2013;60(9):1539–45. doi:10.1002/pbc.24563.

44. Koob TJ, Pringle D, Gedbaw E, Meredith J, Berrios R, Kim HK. Biomechanical properties of bone and cartilage in growing femoral head following ischemic osteonecrosis. J Orthop Res. 2007;25(6):750–7. doi:10.1002/jor.20350.
45. Bergmann G, Deuretzbacher G, Heller M, Graichen F, Rohlmann A, Strauss J, et al. Hip contact forces and gait patterns from routine activities. J Biomech. 2001;34(7):859–71. S0021-9290(01)00040-9 [pii].
46. Kim HK, Aruwajoye O, Stetler J, Stall A. Effects of non-weight-bearing on the immature femoral head following ischemic osteonecrosis: an experimental investigation in immature pigs. J Bone Joint Surg Am. 2012;94(24):2228–37. doi:10.2106/JBJS.L.00300.
47. Bianchi ML, Cimaz R, Bardare M, Zulian F, Lepore L, Boncompagni A, et al. Efficacy and safety of alendronate for the treatment of osteoporosis in diffuse connective tissue diseases in children: a prospective multicenter study. Arthritis Rheum. 2000;43(9):1960–6.
48. Plotkin H, Rauch F, Zeitlin L, Munns C, Travers R, Glorieux FH. Effect of pamidronate treatment in children with polyostotic fibrous dysplasia of bone. J Clin Endocrinol Metab. 2003;88(10):4569–75.
49. Glorieux FH, Bishop NJ, Plotkin H, Chabot G, Lanoue G, Travers R. Cyclic administration of pamidronate in children with severe osteogenesis imperfecta. N Engl J Med. 1998;339(14):947–52. doi:10.1056/NEJM199810013391402.
50. Zeitlin L, Rauch F, Plotkin H, Glorieux FH. Height and weight development during four years of therapy with cyclical intravenous pamidronate in children and adolescents with osteogenesis imperfecta types I, III, and IV. Pediatrics. 2003;111(5 Pt 1):1030–6.
51. Phillipi CA, Remmington T, Steiner RD. Bisphosphonate therapy for osteogenesis imperfecta. Cochrane Database Syst Rev. 2008(4):CD005088. doi:10.1002/14651858.CD005088.pub2.
52. Camacho NP, Raggio CL, Doty SB, Root L, Zraick V, Ilg WA, et al. A controlled study of the effects of alendronate in a growing mouse model of osteogenesis imperfecta. Calcif Tissue Int. 2001;69(2): 94–101.
53. Lepola VT, Hannuniemi R, Kippo K, Lauren L, Jalovaara P, Vaananen HK. Long-term effects of clodronate on growing rat bone. Bone. 1996;18(2):191–6.
54. Li C, Mori S, Li J, Kaji Y, Akiyama T, Kawanishi J, et al. Long-term effect of incadronate disodium (YM-175) on fracture healing of femoral shaft in growing rats. J Bone Miner Res. 2001; 16(3):429–36.
55. Guy JA, Shea M, Peter CP, Morrissey R, Hayes WC. Continuous alendronate treatment throughout growth, maturation, and aging in the rat results in increases in bone mass and mechanical properties. Calcif Tissue Int. 1993;53(4):283–8.
56. Kim HKW. Pathophysiology and new strategies for the treatment of Legg-Calve-Perthes disease. J Bone Joint Surg Am. 2012;94: 659–69.

63 Corticosteroid-Associated Osteonecrosis in Children

Scott Rosenfeld and Harry K.W. Kim

63.1 Introduction

Corticosteroids are potent anti-inflammatory drugs used to treat various adult and pediatric medical conditions. More than 30 million Americans receive corticosteroids as part of their treatment protocols for acute and chronic illnesses [1, 2]. Use of systemic corticosteroids in children has been most thoroughly studied in patients treated for acute lymphocytic leukemia (ALL), systemic lupus erythematosus (SLE), and renal transplant. In the case of ALL, the addition of corticosteroids to antileukemic protocols has been shown to improve the remission rate [3]. Current treatment protocols characterized by chemotherapy intensified by higher-dose corticosteroids are thought to be partly responsible for improved outcomes in ALL with cure rates ranging from 70 to 90 % [3–7]. In pediatric SLE, long-term survival has improved dramatically as corticosteroids have become the mainstay of treatment [8]. Depending on the specific disease and severity, the length of treatment ranges from days to years to a lifetime of use. As with many medications, chronic use may result in adverse side effects. Such effects of corticosteroids have been described in multiple organ systems including the musculoskeletal system [9]. The specific effect of hypercortisolism on bone was first recognized as a feature of Cushing's disease. Since that time, the cause-effect relationship between corticosteroid treatment and bone disease such as osteoporosis, fractures, and osteonecrosis has become more clearly established [10–12].

S. Rosenfeld
Pediatric Orthopaedic Surgery, Baylor College of Medicine, Texas Children's Hospital, 6701 Fannin St Ste 660, Houston, TX 77030, USA
e-mail: sbrosenf@texaschildrens.org

H.K.W. Kim (✉)
Center for Excellence in Hip Disorders, Texas Scottish Rite Hospital for Children, 2222 Welborn Street, Dallas, TX 75219, USA

Department of Orthopaedic Surgery, UT Southwestern Medical Center, Dallas, TX 75219, USA
e-mail: harry.kim@tsrh.org

63.1.1 Corticosteroids and Bone-Related Side Effects

Various forms of corticosteroids are used in medical and chemotherapy protocols. Each form has unique potencies and durations of treatment. In pediatric conditions, the most commonly prescribed systemic corticosteroids include prednisone, methylprednisolone, and dexamethasone. Dexamethasone has been shown to have enhanced antileukemic effect as compared to prednisone and has become a centerpiece in many ALL treatment protocols [13]. There is conflicting evidence as to whether its increased antileukemic activity also results in increased toxicity and adverse effects. Van Beek et al. found no difference in bone mineral density in ALL survivors treated with dexamethasone or prednisolone [14]. Similarly, Sala et al. found no difference in skeletal toxicity between the two drugs [15]. Other studies, however, have shown increased rates of fractures and osteonecrosis in patients treated with dexamethasone [16, 17]. One of the most severe and debilitating long-term complications of corticosteroid treatment is osteonecrosis. Regardless of the underlying disease or type of corticosteroid, osteonecrosis may result in great morbidity and impairment in survivors of these complex medical problems. Despite increased awareness of the association between osteonecrosis and corticosteroid treatment, the pathophysiology is unclear and treatment efforts have had a modest effect in improving the outcome.

63.2 Epidemiology of Corticosteroid-Associated Osteonecrosis

In adults, corticosteroids have been shown to be the most common cause of nontraumatic osteonecrosis, having that effect in up to 40 % of patients treated [18–20]. The reported incidence of osteonecrosis in pediatric patients treated with corticosteroids ranges between 0.43 and 50 % and is dependent on multiple factors [2, 16, 21–28]. Patient factors such as age, sex, ethnicity, body mass index, underlying disease,

K.-H. Koo et al. (eds.), *Osteonecrosis*,
DOI 10.1007/978-3-642-35767-1_63, © Springer-Verlag Berlin Heidelberg 2014

and genetic polymorphisms have been shown to have variable effects on the incidence of osteonecrosis in children. Incidence is also affected by whether studies report symptomatic patients only or include asymptomatic patients. Additionally, treatment factors such as type of corticosteroid, daily dose, cumulative dose, maximum dose, and route of administration appear to influence the risk of osteonecrosis.

63.2.1 Osteonecrosis in Acute Lymphocytic Leukemia (ALL) Population

The lower range of incidence (0.43–9.3 %) has been shown in various studies reporting on symptomatic osteonecrosis in ALL patients. The Children's Cancer Group reported that the 3-year incidence of osteonecrosis in patients treated for ALL was 9.3 % [22]. In that series, age was an important variable. Only 1 % of patients in the age range of 1–9 years developed osteonecrosis, whereas 14.2 % of patients in the age range of 10–20 years developed osteonecrosis. Additionally, there was a higher rate of osteonecrosis in those patients treated with higher doses of dexamethasone, those that received continuous compared to discontinuous therapy, and those that received double compared to single pulses of corticosteroids. Arico et al. reported their experience with patients treated with the AIEOP-ALL 95 protocol [23]. Their population exhibited a 5-year incidence of osteonecrosis of 1.6 % with higher risk in females and patients older than 10 years. The Childhood Cancer Survivor Study reported long-term follow-up data with an incidence of 0.43 % at 20 years from diagnosis [2]. Older age was also a risk in this group as the incidence was 2.8 % in patients older than 16 years. Other risk factors identified included specific diagnoses (leukemia, lymphoma, and sarcoma) and history of stem cell transplant. Specific corticosteroid protocol is also important as they reported that patients treated with dexamethasone were 30 % more likely to have osteonecrosis than those treated with prednisone. The lower incidence in these studies may be from underestimation of osteonecrosis as a result of the retrospective nature of the study which relied on patient self-reporting of complications. Finally, a prospective study from the Dutch Child Oncology group reported the incidence of symptomatic osteonecrosis to be 6.1 %. This study found increased risk in females, but no difference for type of corticosteroid used [28].

63.2.2 Prevalence of Asymptomatic Osteonecrosis

When MRI is used to diagnose osteonecrosis, the incidence increases in patients treated with corticosteroids for all underlying diseases. MRI is highly sensitive for detecting bone necrosis which improves the ability to diagnose even preclinical and often asymptomatic lesions. Kawedia prospectively screened 364 ALL patients with MRI and found that 54 % had asymptomatic grade 1 osteonecrosis and 17.6 % had symptomatic grades 2–4 lesions [27]. Thus, the overall prevalence of any osteonecrosis in this prospective study was about 72 % using the Total XV protocol for the treatment of ALL. Other MRI screening studies of patients treated for ALL have reported rates of 15 and 38 %, many of which were asymptomatic [24, 29].

Table 63.1 Risk factors for corticosteroid-associated osteonecrosis

1. *Patient specific*
Older age
2. *Disease specific*
Renal failure/transplant
SLE
3. *Corticosteroid specific factors*
Greater individual dose
Greater cumulative dose
Longer duration of therapy
Dexamethasone (vs. prednisone)
Systemic administration

63.2.3 Risk Factors for Corticosteroid-Associated Osteonecrosis

The wide range of incidence of corticosteroid-associated osteonecrosis demonstrates that pathogenesis is likely multifactorial. Several factors specific to the patient, underlying disease, and treatment protocol are commonly reported as risk factors (Table 63.1). Most studies agree that the most important risk factors are older age and sustained large doses of corticosteroid [19, 30].

Age is an important risk factor as 44.6 % of patients older than age 10 years developed symptomatic osteonecrosis as compared to only 10 % in patients less than 10 years old (odds ratio 4.85) in ALL population [27]. Shigemura et al. [31] reported that adolescents and adults with SLE have an increased risk compared to pediatric patients with an odds ratio of 13.3. Nakamura reported incidence in SLE of 6 % in pediatric patients and 49 % in adolescents [21]. In that study, there were no patients under age 14 with osteonecrosis. The reason for this difference can only be speculated. It may be related to more abundant vascular supply in the skeletally immature femoral head allowing for greater collateral circulation and resistance to vascular disruption or a difference in drug kinetics and metabolism related to age. In a follow-up study, Nakamura et al. reported that in the first and fourth months after initiation of corticosteroid treatment, the perfusion to the growth plate and the entire femoral head, respectively, was greater in pediatric patients than in adult patients [32].

The incidence of corticosteroid-associated osteonecrosis has also been shown to vary depending on the underlying disease. This would suggest that the disease itself has an influence on the incidence of osteonecrosis, making it difficult to discern the risk arising from the disease process itself and from the use of corticosteroids in treatment. This is best illustrated in the case of patients with renal insufficiency and transplant. The disease process itself results in renal osteodystrophy which may increase the risk of osteonecrosis whether the patient is being treated with corticosteroids or not [18]. In a prospective MRI study, Shigemura et al. [31] reported that the overall incidence of osteonecrosis was higher in SLE patients than in non-SLE patients (37 % vs. 21 %) regardless of age and that the SLE population had a higher rate of osteonecrosis of the femoral head than other locations. Among pediatric patients specifically, there was no difference between the SLE and non-SLE groups.

In patients treated with allogenic bone marrow transplant for diagnoses such as CML, ALL, AML, and SAA, the incidence of osteonecrosis has been reported to be between 4.3 and 24.2 % [33]. In this patient group, exposure to corticosteroids is the factor most strongly correlated with risk of osteonecrosis [34]. This is likely due to the long-term need for corticosteroid treatment for prevention of graft vs. host disease.

Treatment factors such as type of corticosteroid, daily dose, cumulative dose, maximum dose, and route of administration have been shown to influence incidence of corticosteroid-associated osteonecrosis. For most diseases studied, there is little consensus as to the risks inferred by specific treatment protocols. There appears to be, however, a significant influence on the incidence of osteonecrosis by the underlying disease as well as the corticosteroid type and dosing parameters.

63.2.4 Effects of Dosing, Type, and Route of Administration of Corticosteroids

In studies of pediatric patients treated for ALL, there is an increased incidence of osteonecrosis in patients undergoing chemotherapy utilizing higher cumulative doses of corticosteroids and longer duration of therapy [23, 35, 36]. Mattano et al. [22] reported a 1.4-fold increase in osteonecrosis in patients that underwent two pulses of dexamethasone as compared to those receiving just one. Onset of osteonecrosis is typically within the first few years of therapy suggesting that after the patient reaches a certain posttreatment interval, there is little risk of developing subsequent osteonecrosis [16, 25, 26]. In a 20-year follow-up study of ALL patients, Kadan-Lottick [2] demonstrated that the cumulative incidence continues to increase with time for years after treatment. Sixty-six percent of patients were diagnosed with osteonecrosis between 5 and 20 years after initiation of treatment. There is conflicting evidence as to whether or not the type of corticosteroid used influences the rate of osteonecrosis [15–17]. Pediatric patients in the Childhood Cancer Survivor Study were 30 % more likely to have osteonecrosis if treated with dexamethasone than if treated with prednisone [2]. As far as route of administration, systemic dosing of corticosteroids appears to have the strongest association with osteonecrosis. There are no reported cases of osteonecrosis associated with the use of topical or inhaled steroids alone [37].

Since asthma is a common diagnosis in the pediatric population, the risk of osteonecrosis from inhaled steroids is of particular concern given the possibility for sizeable cumulative doses over time. In a review of the literature, Powell found only four case reports of osteonecrosis related to inhaled steroid use. It is difficult to conclude from this any risk directly related to inhaled agents because all four patients were also treated with oral steroids [37].

Various animal studies have shown associations between dosing and occurrence of osteonecrosis. In a rabbit model, Motomura et al. [38] gave doses of 1, 5, 20, and 40 mg/kg of methylprednisolone which resulted in 0, 42, 70, and 96 % incidence of osteonecrosis, respectively. Yamamoto et al. [39] reported that 43 % of rabbits who received pulsed doses of 20 mg/kg methylprednisolone acetate developed osteonecrosis in multiple sites as compared to those receiving lower doses. Finally, Yang et al. [40] demonstrated that continuous dexamethasone treatment was more osteonecrotic than discontinuous treatment in a mouse model.

63.3 Mechanisms of Corticosteroid-Associated Osteonecrosis

Multiple hypotheses have been proposed regarding the mechanism(s) and pathogenesis of corticosteroid-associated osteonecrosis. Most involve the complex cellular, hematologic, and immunologic effects of corticosteroids including their ability to influence gene transcription involving apoptosis (programmed cell death), immune function, lipid metabolism, and coagulation. These mechanisms alter not only bone cell function and survival but also other cells including vascular endothelial cells. Coagulation factors and lipid metabolism are also affected by corticosteroids. In addition, genetic polymorphisms may affect individual susceptibility to any of the proposed mechanisms. Likely, no single mechanism can be the culprit for such a complex pathogenesis. Instead, it is more likely the result of a multifactorial etiology consisting of variable effects from multiple mechanisms each having different contributions based on the underlying condition and genetic predisposition [18]. Regardless of the complex steps that initiated it, a common pathway in corticosteroid-associated osteonecrosis is cell death and compromised blood flow to the bone. This results in bone necrosis, edema, bone weakening, subchondral fracture, destruction of bony architecture, and femoral head collapse.

63.3.1 Effects on Bone Cells

Corticosteroids have both direct and indirect effects on bone cells (osteoblasts, osteocytes, and osteoclasts). They have the ability to affect both cell proliferation and survival through their interaction with glucocorticoid receptors and their effect on lipid metabolism. Glucocorticoid receptors have been found in osteoblasts, osteocytes, osteoclasts, and chondrocytes both in vitro and in vivo [41–44]. Binding of glucocorticoids to their receptors results in expression or suppression of various transcription factors that act to modulate the mediators of the immune system. This effect on the immune system commonly occurs through the Fas apoptotic pathway. The Fas pathway initiates a caspase cascade resulting in apoptosis of immunogenic cells [45]. This is the basis for the use of steroids as anti-inflammatory agents. Since osteoblasts, osteocytes, and osteoclasts all have glucocorticoid receptors, they too can undergo apoptosis through the activation of this pathway resulting in decreased bone formation and turnover [11, 46]. Steroid-induced bone loss may also be due in part to its seemingly contradictory effect of increasing osteoclast survival [47] through increased tumor necrosis factor (TNF-α) ligand and receptor activator of NF-κB ligand (RANKL) [48]. Repair processes may also be hindered as osteocyte apoptosis can result in disruption of the osteocyte mechanosensory network [49].

63.3.2 Effects on the Vascular System

Glucocorticoids have significant effects on the vascular system architecture and physiology. These effects are mediated by action directly on the vascular endothelial cells as well as on vasoactive substances that balance vascular tone. Corticosteroids can cause direct endothelial cell injury resulting in decreased number of functional microvessels [50, 51]. This may lead to decreased blood flow to the femoral head [52]. PGI_2 is produced mainly by vascular endothelial cells, and damage to these cells decreases the availability of this potent vasodilator and inhibitor of platelet aggregation. This results in increased vascular resistance, increased thrombin, platelet aggregation, thrombosis, and decreased blood flow [1, 53]. The number and function of circulating endothelial progenitor cells have also been shown to be reduced in patients with osteonecrosis, decreasing this system's ability to repair itself [54].

Corticosteroids also affect blood flow by altering the availability of and responsiveness to vasoactive substances. Nitric oxide, endothelin, bradykinin, and prostacyclin are produced by vascular endothelial cells and stimulate contraction and relaxation of vascular smooth muscle. This results in subsequent changes in vascular tone. Corticosteroids can induce overproduction of oxygen free radicals which inactivate and decrease production of nitric oxide. This is further potentiated as corticosteroids decrease the expression of endothelial nitric oxide synthase [55]. Since nitric oxide functions to dilate blood vessels, prevent platelet aggregation, and inhibit monocyte adherence to endothelial cells, its decreased availability may lead to increased vascular resistance and a procoagulant environment [56]. In a series of studies by Drescher et al. [57–59], corticosteroids were shown to affect vasoreactivity by increasing the response of the lateral epiphyseal artery to endothelin-1 (vasoconstrictor) and decreasing the response to bradykinin and the production of prostacyclin (vasodilators). This leads to a cumulative effect of vasoconstriction and decreased blood flow to the femoral head. Similarly, the activity of angiotensin-converting enzyme is increased by dexamethasone leading to increased blood pressure, while the vasodilative effects of the kallikrein-kinin system is suppressed [60].

63.3.3 Effects on Angiogenesis and Repair

Corticosteroids have been shown to affect bone healing after osteonecrosis of the femoral head. Necrotic bone healing is characterized by angiogenesis and migration of new blood vessels into the necrotic segment. Restoration of the blood supply allows further recruitment of inflammatory and repair cells to the necrotic bone which leads to the resorption of the necrotic bone and new bone formation. The repair process is induced by growth factors such as vascular endothelial growth factor (VEGF) as well as through the function of myofibroblastic cells. VEGF acts on endothelial cells to induce angiogenesis [61]. Treatment with corticosteroids can affect the repair process by decreasing the synthesis of VEGF and subsequent inhibition of new capillary growth [62, 63]. Corticosteroids have been shown to inhibit myofibroblastic cell function and suppress collagen production which is necessary for new capillary growth [63, 64]. Further effect of corticosteroids on angiogenesis includes decreased basement membrane turnover through inhibition of plasminogen activators.

63.3.4 Effects on Coagulation Pathways

Various changes in coagulation pathways have been reported to be associated with nontraumatic osteonecrosis. Elements of both thrombophilia and hypofibrinolysis have been demonstrated in pediatric and adult patients with osteonecrosis

[65–68]. Specific abnormalities of coagulation profiles have been observed in patients with nontraumatic osteonecrosis such as resistance to activated protein C, anticardiolipin antibodies, and presence of the Apo (a) phenotype of lipoprotein (a) [69–71]. Other thrombotic disorders such as protein C and S deficiency, antiphospholipid antibodies, lupus anticoagulant, and factor V Leiden have also been associated with femoral head osteonecrosis [70, 72].

The use of glucocorticoids can further alter these coagulation pathways. At high doses, glucocorticoids act to inhibit the fibrinolytic pathway through an increase in activity of plasma plasminogen activator inhibitor (PAI) and decreased tissue plasminogen activator (t-PA) activity [73, 74]. This results in decreased conversion of plasminogen to plasmin and decreased fibrinolysis and increased thrombosis. The subsequent hypofibrinogenolysis is further associated with reduction of femoral head blood flow, a hypercoagulable state, and osteonecrosis [75].

If the use of high dose of corticosteroids had such a systemic effect on clotting function, one would expect there to be a high incidence of end-organ ischemia in addition to osteonecrosis in multiple joints. Instead it has been speculated that clotting dysfunction may be regional. The origin of this regional dysfunction may be related to endothelial cell injury. Endothelial cell damage via direct cytotoxicity and oxygen free radicals in the local vascular bed can activate a regional coagulation cascade [53]. Apoptotic endothelial cells can bind thrombocytes and activate platelets. Additionally, endothelial microparticles, a product of endothelial apoptosis, are increased in patients with osteonecrosis [76]. Procoagulant platelet microparticles and endothelial microparticles can initiate thrombosis through interactions with tissue factor. These locally derived endothelial factors combined with a procoagulant and hypofibrinolytic environment may result in local intravascular coagulation within the femoral head [77].

63.3.5 Effects on Lipid Metabolism

Accumulation of fatty tissue in the femoral head, fat emboli, and the procoagulant effect of adipocyte breakdown particles have all been implicated in the etiology of osteonecrosis. Increased plasma triglyceride and LDL levels as well as increased LDL/HDL ratio have been shown to increase the risk of osteonecrosis [38]. This effect on lipid metabolism seems to begin at the stem cell level. Treatment of pluripotent marrow cell lines with dexamethasone has been shown to push progenitor cells preferentially towards adipose cells over bone forming cells. Increased adipocytogenesis results in fat accumulation in cells [78]. Hence, corticosteroid therapy results in a preferential increase of lipid production and a decrease in bone formation [62]. Increased doses of dexamethasone and greater duration of exposure result in a greater number of adipocytes [79]. This cumulative effect leads to increased fatty deposition into the femoral head [80]. It is postulated that as the amount of intraosseous fat increases, so does the pressure within the femoral head cortex. This increased pressure results in vascular sinusoidal collapse, decreased blood flow, and ultimately ischemia [81]. Such a "compartment syndrome" etiology has been described in hips with osteonecrosis demonstrating increased bone marrow pressure [82]. Corticosteroid administration and hyperlipidemia can also cause increased fat embolization. Fat emboli can result in ischemia either directly by blocking microvascular circulation or indirectly by triggering intravascular coagulation and activation of the complement cascade. The combination of these two effects results in thrombosis and osteonecrosis [83]. Once osteonecrosis occurs, injured local adipocytes release thromboplastin and vasoactive substances, thus continuing the hypercoagulable and ischemic cycle [84]. Lipid-lowering drugs have been shown to alter the intraosseous lipid accumulation in animal models [85].

63.4 Genetic Polymorphisms Associated with Corticosteroid-Associated Osteonecrosis

As most patients treated with corticosteroids for various medical problems do not develop osteonecrosis, it appears that individual host factors likely play a significant role in determining risk. Multiple genetic polymorphisms have been associated with an increased or decreased risk of developing osteonecrosis (Table 63.2). Genes that are involved in coagulation, drug metabolism, and lipid metabolism have been implicated in multiple small studies. Many of the studies have contradicting results highlighting that the true significance of genetic involvement remains unclear. Despite the lack of consistent evidence, it seems reasonable to postulate that genetic variations are likely to affect the susceptibility of the patient. All of the previously described pathogenic mechanisms of corticosteroids may be increased or decreased by each patient's genetic predisposition.

Although strong evidence for the significance of each genetic polymorphism as they relate to the risk of osteonecrosis is lacking, it is generally agreed that these host factors are important. Identification of these genetic variations may improve our understanding of the mechanisms involved in corticosteroid-associated osteonecrosis and lead to more specific treatment options. Furthermore, these polymorphisms could be used as genetic tests to identify patients at greater risk for osteonecrosis should they require corticosteroid treatment. If their medical condition permits and alternative treatment options exist, such patients could be considered for alterations in therapy to lessen the risk of osteonecrosis.

Table 63.2 Genetic polymorphisms associated with osteonecrosis

Gene function	Specific polymorphism	Effect
Coagulation		
PAI-1 [86, 87, 88]	4G polymorphism, SERPINE polymorphism	Hypofibrinolysis
MTHFR [89]	677 C-T mutation	Hyperhomocystinemia and thrombosis
Thymidylate synthase [29]	Low activity 2/2 enhancer repeat genotype	Hyperhomocystinemia and thrombosis
Factor V [90]	Factor V Leiden	Thrombosis
Steroid metabolism		
Multidrug-resistance gene 1 (ABCB1) [91]	3435TT genotype	Increased activity of P-glycoprotein protective against ON
Vitamin D receptor [29]	Fokl start site CC genotype	Increased cellular sensitivity to steroids
Lipid metabolism		
ACP1 and SH3YL1 [27]	rs12714403 and rs4241316	Lower albumin and higher cholesterol
Apolipoprotein B [71]	7623TT allele	Increased in renal transplant patients with ON
Apolipoprotein A1 [92]	A/A substitution at position -75 in promotor	Associated with ON

63.5 Natural History of Corticosteroid-Associated Osteonecrosis

Osteonecrosis associated with corticosteroid use is commonly bilateral and often multifocal. Patients with pain from osteonecrosis in a single joint will often have asymptomatic lesions in other joints (Fig. 63.1) [86]. Studies on patients treated for ALL have reported from 2.2 to 3.4 joints affected per patient [87–89]. In addition to the hip, patients treated with long term or high doses of corticosteroids may develop lesions in the vertebrae, distal femoral condyles, proximal tibia, proximal humerus, ankle, and foot [28, 88, 89]. The effect of corticosteroids on bone is not limited to the epiphysis but may also involve the metaphysis and the diaphysis (Fig. 63.2). Osteonecrosis in these regions may increase the risk of fracture in addition to the joint derangement related to the lesions involving the subchondral bone in the epiphyses. Most studies suggest that symptoms of osteonecrosis of the hip usually begin between 6 months and 4 years after the initiation of corticosteroid therapy [16, 22, 23, 26, 90, 91]. When asymptomatic patients are screened with MRI, changes consistent with osteonecrosis may be seen as early as 7 weeks [27]. Consistent with these findings, osteonecrosis is typically considered an acute effect of corticosteroid therapy. However, one long-term follow-up study on adult survivors of childhood cancers showed that the diagnosis of osteonecrosis may not been made until 5–15 years after beginning therapy [2].

The natural history of corticosteroid-associated osteonecrosis is believed to be dependent on the age of the patient and the size and location of the lesion. Small, asymptomatic lesions found on screening MRI may remain stable or resolve without further damage [24, 87, 92]. Patients with small symptomatic lesions may have improvement of their symptoms over time [25, 91]. Larger lesions involving greater than 30 % of the femoral epiphysis, however, are more likely to progress, leading to collapse and joint arthrosis [93].

Clinical features of corticosteroid-associated osteonecrosis are variable. Most patients diagnosed with small lesions on screening MRI are asymptomatic. In those that are symptomatic, the severity depends on the location and size of the infarcted area and whether femoral head collapse has already occurred or not. Symptoms range from intermittent pain and swelling of the involved joint to severe pain with inability to bear weight. Fifty-seven percent of patients who were long-term survivors of ALL with osteonecrosis reported at least one limitation in activities of daily living including walking, climbing stairs, rising from a chair, putting on pants, reaching to low cupboards, and opening containers [2].

63.6 Treatment

The decision for treatment depends on multiple factors. Unfortunately discontinuing corticosteroid treatment may not be an option for many patients as it remains a vital component of chemotherapy. Symptoms, medical condition, general health, lesion size, location, and collapse of the femoral head all play a role in the treatment decision-making process. In the pediatric population, most patients undergo a prolonged course of nonoperative treatment (Fig. 63.2). Small asymptomatic lesions found on screening MRI are usually treated with observation since these lesions may not progress. As symptoms appear, treatment usually begins with anti-inflammatory medications, physical therapy, decrease weight bearing, and activity modification [86, 87, 94]. Those with more severe pain may require narcotic analgesia. Surgical treatment is aimed at improving pain and preventing progression, femoral head collapse, and joint derangement. There are a plethora of reports in the adult literature on surgical treatment of corticosteroid-associated osteonecrosis. Surgical options in the adult population have included core decompression, osteotomy, free vascularized

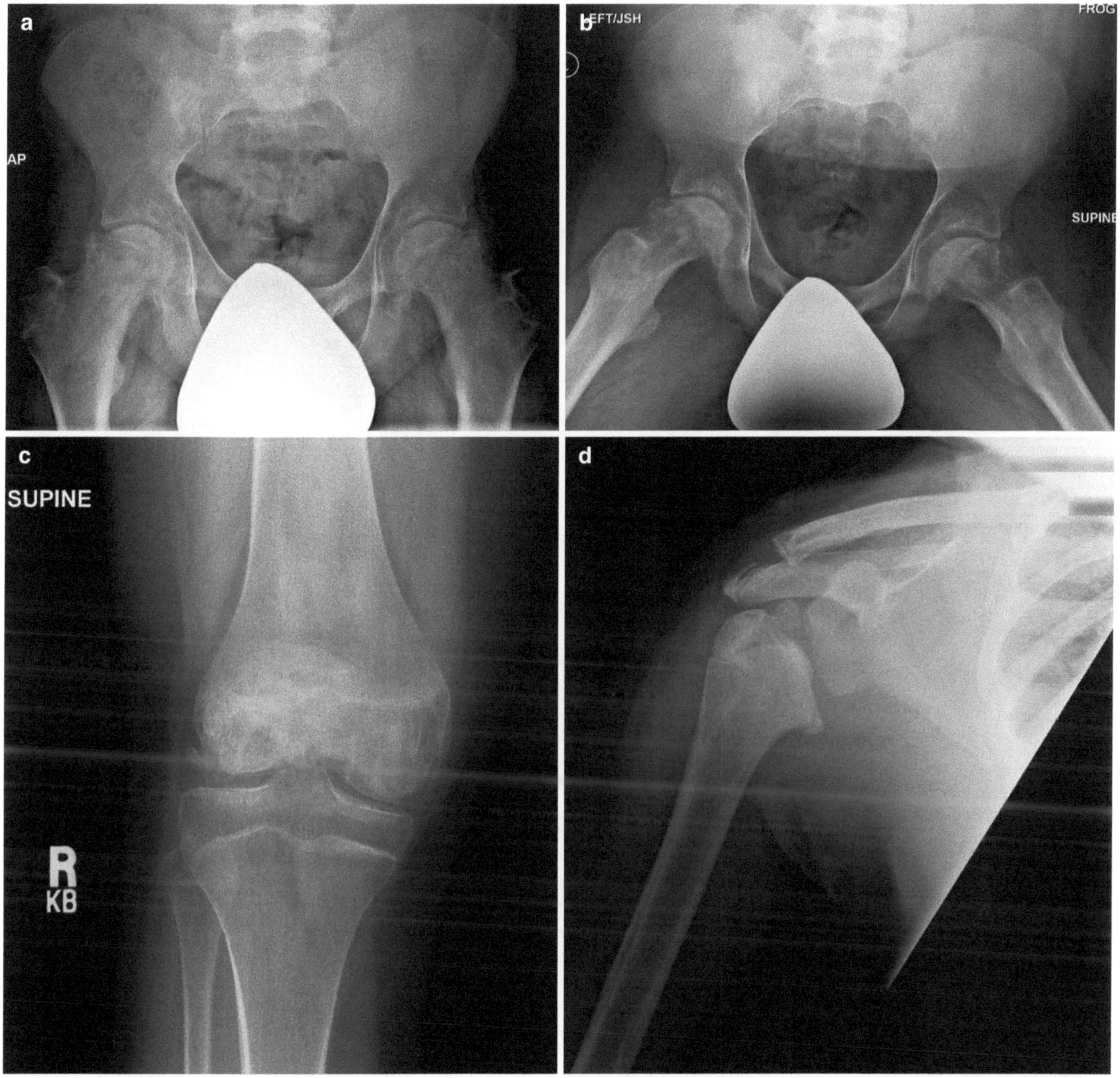

Fig. 63.1 Radiographs of a 15-year-old male with ALL being treated with chemotherapy that includes corticosteroids. The patient had bilateral hip and knee pain and a significant decrease of hip range of motion. This patient presented with some collapse of both femoral heads which limited the options of treatment. (**a**) AP pelvis radiograph showing bilateral femoral head osteonecrosis with increased radiodensity of the femoral heads and some collapse on the lateral aspect of the femoral heads. (**b**) Frog-leg lateral radiograph also showing bilateral femoral head osteonecrosis and some collapse on the anterior aspect of the femoral heads. (**c**) A knee radiograph showing osteonecrosis of both condyles of the distal femur. (**d**) A shoulder radiograph showing osteonecrosis of the humeral head with severe flattening

fibular graft, arthrodesis, and joint replacement. It is important to note that the options of treatment become more limited once the femoral head collapses. This emphasizes the need for early diagnosis and institution of activity and weight-bearing relief to minimize the risk of further femoral head collapse. In adults, core decompression with or without the use of bone graft, bone morphogenic protein, bone marrow, or vascularized fibula graft has been shown to be beneficial in preventing progression of lesions prior to collapse [95–97]. These treatments, however, have not been studied in pediatric population, and nonoperative treatment is the mainstay. There are few reports pertaining to long-term outcomes of these surgical options in children. Furthermore, the use of such surgical treatment options in this specific population presents additional concerns. Drilling across the growth plate for core decompression or multiple epiphyseal drilling risks proximal femoral growth arrest in juvenile patients; however, this is not a significant concern if the patient is near

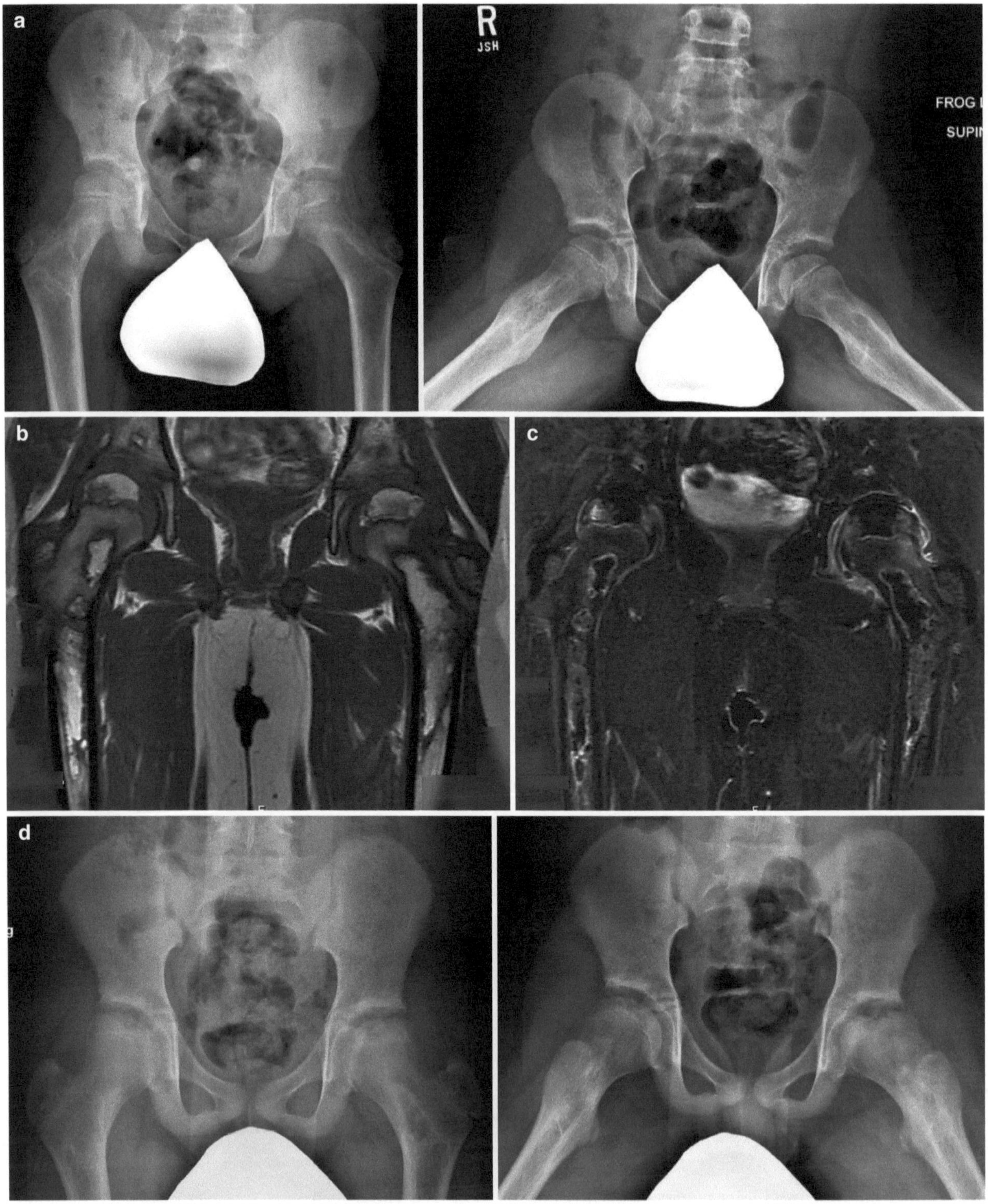

Fig. 63.2 Radiographs and MRIs of a 10-year-old male with ALL being treated with chemotherapy that includes corticosteroids. The patient had bilateral hip and ankle pain. This patient was treated with decreased weight bearing using crutches and wheelchair for long-distance ambulation. For his ankle pain, bilateral ankle foot orthoses (AFO) were prescribed. (**a**) AP pelvis and frog-leg lateral radiographs showing serpentine areas of increased radiodensity in bilateral femoral metaphyses and an area of decreased radiodensity on the proximal diaphysis of left femur. (**b**) Non-contrast T1-weighted MRI showing fat signal changes in the femoral epiphyses, metaphyses, and diaphyses. (**c**) Contrast-enhanced subtraction MRI showing the areas of hypoperfusion (*black*) and hyperperfusion (*white*) in the femoral epiphyses, metaphyses, and the diaphyses. Contrast-enhanced MRI more clearly depicts the areas of necrosis than the non-contrast MRI shown above. (**d**) 3-year follow-up radiographs of the hips showing relatively round femoral heads which are in the late reossification stage. This patient was treated with decreased weight bearing using crutches and wheelchair for long-distance ambulation. At the three year follow up, the patient was asymptomatic, full weight bearing, and participating in activities as tolerates. (**e**) Lateral ankle radiographs obtained at the time of presentation (*left*) showing some collapse of the talar body. A radiograph obtained at 3-year follow-up is shown on the right. At the follow-up, the patient was asymptomatic, full weight bearing, and not requiring AFO

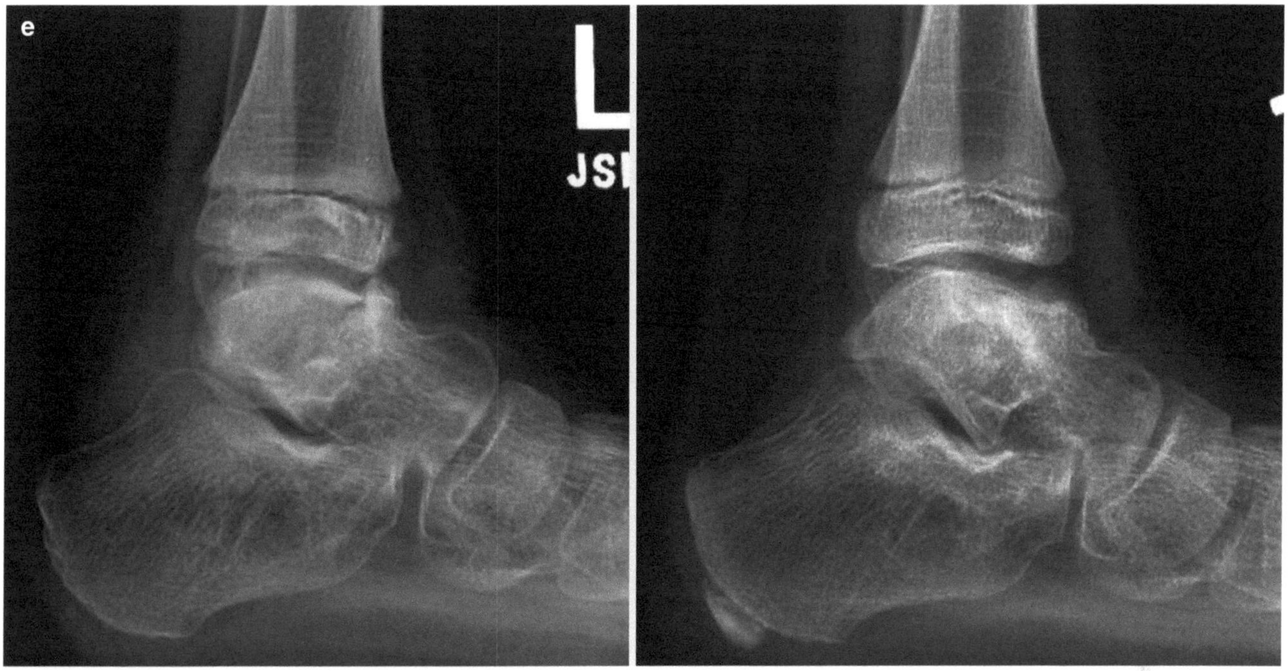

Fig. 63.2 (continued)

skeletal maturity. Arthrodesis is often a poor option in patients with bilateral and multifocal disease. Finally, the finite life span and limited survival of joint replacement prostheses in children make this option less than ideal.

As understanding of the mechanisms of corticosteroid-associated osteonecrosis improves, so do the possibilities of new medical therapies. Treatments with cholesterol-lowering agents, antihypertensives, anticoagulants, and bisphosphonates have all shown promise in animal and adult human studies [98–101]. While there are some case series of pediatric patients treated with bisphosphonate therapy, the safety and efficacy of these medications in children have not yet been determined (see chapter on Development of Medical Therapy for Legg-Calvé-Perthes Disease).

63.7 Summary

Osteonecrosis is well recognized as a serious complication of corticosteroid therapy for various pediatric medical conditions. This is of concern as corticosteroids remain an important component of chemotherapeutic regimens in the treatment of childhood illnesses such as ALL and SLE. In a recent prospective MRI screening study of ALL patients treated with a chemotherapy protocol, 54 % had asymptomatic osteonecrosis and 17.6 % had symptomatic lesions [27]. The majority of patients are likely to be asymptomatic and require no treatment, but many patients will have significant symptoms that affect their ability to participate in routine activities. The potential mechanisms of corticosteroid-associated osteonecrosis include cytotoxicity, coagulopathy, altered lipid metabolism, and effects on vascular tone. It is likely, however, that no single culprit is responsible for the pathogenesis of osteonecrosis. Instead, it is more likely that a combination of multiple corticosteroids induced abnormalities in a patient who is already medically and perhaps genetically susceptible to osteonecrosis. Successful treatment strategies for corticosteroid-associated osteonecrosis in children have yet to be determined. The mainstay of treatment remains analgesic mediations, protected ambulation, and activity modification. Surgical treatments described for adults with corticosteroid-associated osteonecrosis have not been well studied in children. Future treatments may involve medical therapies devised from a more thorough understanding of the pathophysiology of corticosteroid-associated osteonecrosis.

References

1. Kerachian MA, Seguin C, Harvey EJ. Glucocorticoids in osteonecrosis of the femoral head: a new understanding of the mechanisms of action. J Steroid Biochem Mol Biol. 2009;114(3-5):121–8. doi:10.1016/j.jsbmb.2009.02.007. S0960-0760(09)00062-4 [pii].
2. Kadan-Lottick NS, Dinu I, Wasilewski-Masker K, Kaste S, Meacham LR, Mahajan A, et al. Osteonecrosis in adult survivors of childhood cancer: a report from the childhood cancer survivor study. J Clin Oncol. 2008;26(18):3038–45. doi:10.1200/JCO.2007.14.9088.
3. Gaynon PS, Carrel AL. Glucocorticosteroid therapy in childhood acute lymphoblastic leukemia. Adv Exp Med Biol. 1999;457:593–605.
4. Pui CH, Evans WE. Treatment of acute lymphoblastic leukemia. N Engl J Med. 2006;354(2):166–78. doi:10.1056/NEJMra052603.
5. Pui CH, Campana D, Pei D, Bowman WP, Sandlund JT, Kaste SC, et al. Treating childhood acute lymphoblastic leukemia without

cranial irradiation. N Engl J Med. 2009;360(26):2730–41. doi:10.1056/NEJMoa0900386.
6. Silverman LB, Gelber RD, Dalton VK, Asselin BL, Barr RD, Clavell LA, et al. Improved outcome for children with acute lymphoblastic leukemia: results of Dana-Farber Consortium Protocol 91-01. Blood. 2001;97(5):1211–8.
7. Reiter A, Schrappe M, Ludwig WD, Hiddemann W, Sauter S, Henze G, et al. Chemotherapy in 998 unselected childhood acute lymphoblastic leukemia patients. Results and conclusions of the multicenter trial ALL-BFM 86. Blood. 1994;84(9):3122–33.
8. Sallmann S, Fiebig B, Hedrich CM, Heubner G, Gahr M. [Systemic lupus erythematosus in children and adolescents]. Zeitschrift fur Rheumatologie. 2006;65(7):576–8, 80–2, 84–5. doi:10.1007/s00393-006-0115-7.
9. Stanbury RM, Graham EM. Systemic corticosteroid therapy–side effects and their management. Br J Ophthalmol. 1998;82(6):704–8.
10. Sinigaglia L, Mazzocchi D, Varenna M. Bone involvement in exogenous hypercortisolism. J Endocrinol Invest. 2008;31(4):364–70.
11. Weinstein RS, Nicholas RW, Manolagas SC. Apoptosis of osteocytes in glucocorticoid-induced osteonecrosis of the hip. J Clin Endocrinol Metab. 2000;85(8):2907–12.
12. Weinstein RS, Jilka RL, Parfitt AM, Manolagas SC. Inhibition of osteoblastogenesis and promotion of apoptosis of osteoblasts and osteocytes by glucocorticoids. Potential mechanisms of their deleterious effects on bone. J Clin Invest. 1998;102(2):274–82. doi:10.1172/JCI2799.
13. Ito C, Evans WE, McNinch L, Coustan-Smith E, Mahmoud H, Pui CH, et al. Comparative cytotoxicity of dexamethasone and prednisolone in childhood acute lymphoblastic leukemia. J Clin Oncol. 1996;14(8):2370–6.
14. van Beek RD, de Muinck Keizer-Schrama SM, Hakvoort-Cammel FG, van der Sluis IM, Krenning EP, Pieters R, et al. No difference between prednisolone and dexamethasone treatment in bone mineral density and growth in long term survivors of childhood acute lymphoblastic leukemia. Pediatr Blood Cancer. 2006;46(1):88–93. doi:10.1002/pbc.20437.
15. Sala A, Mattano Jr LA, Barr RD. Osteonecrosis in children and adolescents with cancer - an adverse effect of systemic therapy. Eur J Cancer. 2007;43(4):683–9. doi:10.1016/j.ejca.2006.11.002.
16. Strauss AJ, Su JT, Dalton VM, Gelber RD, Sallan SE, Silverman LB. Bony morbidity in children treated for acute lymphoblastic leukemia. J Clin Oncol. 2001;19(12):3066–72.
17. Mattano LA Jr NJ, Devidas M, et al. Increased incidence of osteonecrosis (ON) with a dexamethasone (DEX) induction for high risk acute lymphoblastic leukemia (HR-ALL): a report from the Children's Oncology Group (COG). Blood. 2008;112:A-898.
18. Assouline-Dayan Y, Chang C, Greenspan A, Shoenfeld Y, Gershwin ME. Pathogenesis and natural history of osteonecrosis. Semin Arthritis Rheum. 2002;32(2):94–124.
19. Koo KH, Kim R, Kim YS, Ahn IO, Cho SH, Song HR, et al. Risk period for developing osteonecrosis of the femoral head in patients on steroid treatment. Clin Rheumatol. 2002;21(4):299–303. doi:10.1007/s100670200078.
20. Mankin HJ. Nontraumatic necrosis of bone (osteonecrosis). N Engl J Med. 1992;326(22):1473–9. doi:10.1056/NEJM199205283262206.
21. Nakamura J, Saisu T, Yamashita K, Suzuki C, Kamegaya M, Takahashi K. Age at time of corticosteroid administration is a risk factor for osteonecrosis in pediatric patients with systemic lupus erythematosus: a prospective magnetic resonance imaging study. Arthritis Rheum. 2010;62(2):609–15. doi:10.1002/art.27236.
22. Mattano Jr LA, Sather HN, Trigg ME, Nachman JB. Osteonecrosis as a complication of treating acute lymphoblastic leukemia in children: a report from the Children's Cancer Group. J Clin Oncol. 2000;18(18):3262–72.
23. Arico M, Boccalatte MF, Silvestri D, Barisone E, Messina C, Chiesa R, et al. Osteonecrosis: an emerging complication of intensive chemotherapy for childhood acute lymphoblastic leukemia. Haematologica. 2003;88(7):747–53.
24. Ojala AE, Paakko E, Lanning FP, Lanning M. Osteonecrosis during the treatment of childhood acute lymphoblastic leukemia: a prospective MRI study. Med Pediatr Oncol. 1999;32(1):11–7.
25. Ribeiro RC, Fletcher BD, Kennedy W, Harrison PL, Neel MD, Kaste SC, et al. Magnetic resonance imaging detection of avascular necrosis of the bone in children receiving intensive prednisone therapy for acute lymphoblastic leukemia or non-Hodgkin lymphoma. Leukemia. 2001;15(6):891–7.
26. Burger B, Beier R, Zimmermann M, Beck JD, Reiter A, Schrappe M. Osteonecrosis: a treatment related toxicity in childhood acute lymphoblastic leukemia (ALL)–experiences from trial ALL-BFM 95. Pediatr Blood Cancer. 2005;44(3):220–5. doi:10.1002/pbc.20244.
27. Kawedia JD, Kaste SC, Pei D, Panetta JC, Cai X, Cheng C, et al. Pharmacokinetic, pharmacodynamic, and pharmacogenetic determinants of osteonecrosis in children with acute lymphoblastic leukemia. Blood. 2011;117(8):2340–7. doi:10.1182/blood-2010-10-311969; quiz 556.
28. te Winkel ML, Pieters R, Hop WC, de Groot-Kruseman HA, Lequin MH, van der Sluis IM, et al. Prospective study on incidence, risk factors, and long-term outcome of osteonecrosis in pediatric acute lymphoblastic leukemia. J Clin Oncol. 2011;29(31):4143–50. doi:10.1200/JCO.2011.37.3217.
29. Relling MV, Yang W, Das S, Cook EH, Rosner GL, Neel M, et al. Pharmacogenetic risk factors for osteonecrosis of the hip among children with leukemia. J Clin Oncol. 2004;22(19):3930–6. doi:10.1200/JCO.2004.11.020.
30. Lafforgue P. Pathophysiology and natural history of avascular necrosis of bone. Joint Bone Spine. 2006;73(5):500–7. doi:10.1016/j.jbspin.2006.01.025.
31. Shigemura T, Nakamura J, Kishida S, Harada Y, Ohtori S, Kamikawa K, et al. Incidence of osteonecrosis associated with corticosteroid therapy among different underlying diseases: prospective MRI study. Rheumatology. 2011;50(11):2023–8. doi:10.1093/rheumatology/ker277.
32. Nakamura J, Ohtori S, Watanabe A, Nakagawa K, Inoue G, Kishida S, et al. Recovery of the blood flow around the femoral head during early corticosteroid therapy: dynamic magnetic resonance imaging in systemic lupus erythematosus patients. Lupus. 2012;21(3):264–70. doi:10.1177/0961203311425521.
33. Mattano L. The skeletal remains: porosis and necrosis of bone in the marrow transplantation setting. Pediatr Transplant. 2003;7 Suppl 3:71–5.
34. Fink JC, Leisenring WM, Sullivan KM, Sherrard DJ, Weiss NS. Avascular necrosis following bone marrow transplantation: a case-control study. Bone. 1998;22(1):67–71.
35. Vaidya S, Saika S, Sirohi B, Pai S, Advani S. Avascular necrosis of bone–a complication of aggressive therapy for acute lymphoblastic leukemia. Acta Oncol. 1998;37(2):175–7.
36. Chan-Lam D, Prentice AG, Copplestone JA, Weston M, Williams M, Hutton CW. Avascular necrosis of bone following intensified steroid therapy for acute lymphoblastic leukaemia and high-grade malignant lymphoma. Br J Haematol. 1994;86(1):227–30.
37. Powell C, Chang C, Naguwa SM, Cheema G, Gershwin ME. Steroid induced osteonecrosis: an analysis of steroid dosing risk. Autoimmun Rev. 2010;9(11):721–43. doi:10.1016/j.autrev.2010.06.007.
38. Motomura G, Yamamoto T, Irisa T, Miyanishi K, Nishida K, Iwamoto Y. Dose effects of corticosteroids on the development of osteonecrosis in rabbits. J Rheumatol. 2008;35(12):2395–9.
39. Yamamoto T, Miyanishi K, Motomura G, Nishida K, Iwamoto Y, Sueishi K. Animal models for steroid-induced osteonecrosis. Clin Calcium. 2007;17(6):879–86. doi:CliCa0706879886.
40. Yang L, Boyd K, Kaste SC, Kamdem Kamdem L, Rahija RJ, Relling MV. A mouse model for glucocorticoid-induced osteone-

crosis: effect of a steroid holiday. J Orthop Res. 2009;27(2):169–75. doi:10.1002/jor.20733.

41. Dempster DW, Moonga BS, Stein LS, Horbert WR, Antakly T. Glucocorticoids inhibit bone resorption by isolated rat osteoclasts by enhancing apoptosis. J Endocrinol. 1997;154(3):397–406.
42. Liesegang P, Romalo G, Sudmann M, Wolf L, Schweikert HU. Human osteoblast-like cells contain specific, saturable, high-affinity glucocorticoid, androgen, estrogen, and 1 alpha,25-dihydroxycholecalciferol receptors. J Androl. 1994;15(3):194–9.
43. Yoshioka T, Sato B, Matsumoto K, Ono K. Steroid receptors in osteoblasts. Clin Orthop Relat Res. 1980;148:297–303.
44. Silvestrini G, Mocetti P, Ballanti P, Di Grezia R, Bonucci E. Cytochemical demonstration of the glucocorticoid receptor in skeletal cells of the rat. Endocr Res. 1999;25(1):117–28.
45. Kogianni G, Mann V, Ebetino F, Nuttall M, Nijweide P, Simpson H, et al. Fas/CD95 is associated with glucocorticoid-induced osteocyte apoptosis. Life Sci. 2004;75(24):2879–95. doi:10.1016/j.lfs.2004.04.048.
46. Calder JD, Buttery L, Revell PA, Pearse M, Polak JM. Apoptosis–a significant cause of bone cell death in osteonecrosis of the femoral head. J Bone Joint Surg. 2004;86(8):1209–13.
47. Weinstein RS, Chen JR, Powers CC, Stewart SA, Landes RD, Bellido T, et al. Promotion of osteoclast survival and antagonism of bisphosphonate-induced osteoclast apoptosis by glucocorticoids. J Clin Invest. 2002;109(8):1041–8. doi:10.1172/JCI14538.
48. Bejar J, Peled E, Boss JH. Vasculature deprivation–induced osteonecrosis of the rat femoral head as a model for therapeutic trials. Theor Biol Med Model. 2005;2:24. doi:10.1186/1742-4682-2-24.
49. Zalavras C, Shah S, Birnbaum MJ, Frenkel B. Role of apoptosis in glucocorticoid-induced osteoporosis and osteonecrosis. Crit Rev Eukaryot Gene Expr. 2003;13(2–4):221–35.
50. Jacobs B. Epidemiology of traumatic and nontraumatic osteonecrosis. Clin Orthop Relat Res. 1978;130:51–67.
51. Harper RN, Moore MA, Marr MC, Watts LE, Hutchins PM. Arteriolar rarefaction in the conjunctiva of human essential hypertensives. Microvasc Res. 1978;16(3):369–72.
52. He W, Xu C, Fan Y, Fang B, Li X, Wang H, et al. Effects of the Chinese drugs for activating blood circulation on plasma TXB2 and 6-keto-PGF1alpha contents in rabbits with glucocorticoid-induced femoral head necrosis. J Tradit Chin Med. 2004;24(3):233–7.
53. Kerachian MA, Harvey EJ, Cournoyer D, Chow TY, Seguin C. Avascular necrosis of the femoral head: vascular hypotheses. Endothelium. 2006;13(4):237–44. doi:10.1080/10623320600904211.
54. Feng Y, Yang SH, Xiao BJ, Xu WH, Ye SN, Xia T, et al. Decreased in the number and function of circulation endothelial progenitor cells in patients with avascular necrosis of the femoral head. Bone. 2010;46(1):32–40. doi:10.1016/j.bone.2009.09.001.
55. Wada M, Kumagai K, Murata M, S-Yamashita Y, Shindo H. Warfarin reduces the incidence of osteonecrosis of the femoral head in spontaneously hypertensive rats. J Orthop Sci. 2004;9(6):585–90. doi:10.1007/s00776-004-0829-9.
56. Iuchi T, Akaike M, Mitsui T, Ohshima Y, Shintani Y, Azuma H, et al. Glucocorticoid excess induces superoxide production in vascular endothelial cells and elicits vascular endothelial dysfunction. Circ Res. 2003;92(1):81–7.
57. Drescher W, Bunger MH, Weigert K, Bunger C, Hansen ES. Methylprednisolone enhances contraction of porcine femoral head epiphyseal arteries. Clin Orthop Relat Res. 2004;423:112–7.
58. Drescher W, Li H, Lundgaard A, Bunger C, Hansen ES. Endothelin-1-induced femoral head epiphyseal artery constriction is enhanced by long-term corticosteroid treatment. J Bone Joint Surg Am. 2006;88 Suppl 3:173–9. doi:10.2106/JBJS.F.00773.
59. Drescher W, Varoga D, Liebs TR, Lohse J, Herdegen T, Hassenpflug J, et al. Femoral artery constriction by norepinephrine is enhanced by methylprednisolone in a rat model. J Bone Joint Surg Am. 2006;88 Suppl 3:162–6. doi:10.2106/JBJS.F.00452.
60. Rajashree S, Puvanakrishnan R. Dexamethasone induced alterations in enzymatic and nonenzymatic antioxidant status in heart and kidney of rats. Mol Cell Biochem. 1998;181(1–2):77–85.
61. Yang C, Yang S, Du J, Li J, Xu W, Xiong Y. Vascular endothelial growth factor gene transfection to enhance the repair of avascular necrosis of the femoral head of rabbit. Chin Med J (Engl). 2003;116(10):1544–8.
62. Li X, Jin L, Cui Q, Wang GJ, Balian G. Steroid effects on osteogenesis through mesenchymal cell gene expression. Osteoporos Int. 2005;16(1):101–8. doi:10.1007/s00198-004-1649-7.
63. Harada I. The effects of glucocorticoids on angiogenesis in vitro. Nihon Seikeigeka Gakkai Zasshi. 1992;66(7):763–70.
64. Boss JH. Experimental models of osteonecrosis of the femoral head. J Orthop Sci. 2004;9(5):533–4. doi:10.1007/s00776-004-0817-0.
65. Glueck CJ, Freiberg R, Glueck HI, Henderson C, Welch M, Tracy T, et al. Hypofibrinolysis: a common, major cause of osteonecrosis. Am J Hematol. 1994;45(2):156–66.
66. Glueck CJ, Crawford A, Roy D, Freiberg R, Glueck H, Stroop D. Association of antithrombotic factor deficiencies and hypofibrinolysis with Legg-Perthes disease. J Bone Joint Surg Am. 1996;78(1):3–13.
67. Van Veldhuizen PJ, Neff J, Murphey MD, Bodensteiner D, Skikne BS. Decreased fibrinolytic potential in patients with idiopathic avascular necrosis and transient osteoporosis of the hip. Am J Hematol. 1993;44(4):243–8.
68. Chotanaphuti T, Heebthamai D, Chuwong M, Kanchanaroek K. The prevalence of thrombophilia in idiopathic osteonecrosis of the hip. J Med Assoc Thai. 2009;92 Suppl 6:S141–6.
69. Korompilias AV, Gilkeson GS, Ortel TL, Seaber AV, Urbaniak JR. Anticardiolipin antibodies and osteonecrosis of the femoral head. Clin Orthop Relat Res. 1997;345:174–80.
70. Korompilias AV, Ortel TL, Urbaniak JR. Coagulation abnormalities in patients with hip osteonecrosis. The Orthopedic clinics of North America. 2004;35(3):265–71, vii. doi:10.1016/j.ocl.2004.02.004.
71. Hirata T, Fujioka M, Takahashi KA, Asano T, Ishida M, Akioka K, et al. Low molecular weight phenotype of Apo(a) is a risk factor of corticosteroid-induced osteonecrosis of the femoral head after renal transplant. J Rheumatol. 2007;34(3):516–22.
72. Glueck CJ, Freiberg RA, Boriel G, Khan Z, Brar A, Padda J, et al. The role of the factor V Leiden mutation in osteonecrosis of the hip. Clin Appl Thromb Hemost. 2012;19(5):499–503. doi:10.1177/1076029612449901.
73. Gray E, Thomas S, Mistry Y, Poole S. Inhibition of tissue factor and cytokine release. Haemostasis. 1996;26 Suppl 1:92–5.
74. Minneci PC, Deans KJ, Banks SM, Eichacker PQ, Natanson C. Meta-analysis: the effect of steroids on survival and shock during sepsis depends on the dose. Ann Intern Med. 2004;141(1):47–56.
75. Drescher W, Weigert KP, Bunger MH, Ingerslev J, Bunger C, Hansen ES. Femoral head blood flow reduction and hypercoagulability under 24 h megadose steroid treatment in pigs. J Orthop Res. 2004;22(3):501–8. doi:10.1016/j.orthres.2003.10.002.
76. Kang P, Shen B, Yang J, Pei F. Circulating platelet-derived microparticles and endothelium-derived microparticles may be a potential cause of microthrombosis in patients with osteonecrosis of the femoral head. Thromb Res. 2008;123(2):367–73. doi:10.1016/j.thromres.2008.04.001.
77. Li Y, Chen J, Zhang Z, Wang K, Tong Z, Yan H. The experimental study on treatment of glucocorticoid-induced ischemic necrosis of femoral head by gu fu sheng capsule. J Tradit Chin Med. 2004;24(4):303–7.
78. Cui Q, Wang GJ, Balian G. Steroid-induced adipogenesis in a pluripotential cell line from bone marrow. J Bone Joint Surg Am. 1997;79(7):1054–63.

79. Yin L, Li YB, Wang YS. Dexamethasone-induced adipogenesis in primary marrow stromal cell cultures: mechanism of steroid-induced osteonecrosis. Chin Med J (Engl). 2006;119(7):581–8.
80. Wang GJ, Moga DB, Richemer WG, Sweet DE, Reger SI, Thompson RC. Cortisone induced bone changes and its response to lipid clearing agents. Clin Orthop Relat Res. 1978;130:81–5.
81. Jaffe WL, Epstein M, Heyman N, Mankin HJ. The effect of cortisone on femoral and humeral heads in rabbits. An experimental study. Clin Orthop Relat Res. 1972;82:221–8.
82. Arlet J, Ficat P, Lartigue G, Tran MA. Clinical research on intraosseous pressure in the upper femoral metaphysis and epiphysis in humans. Application to the diagnosis of ischemia and necrosis. Rev Rhum Mal Osteoartic. 1972;39(11):717–23.
83. Jones Jr JP. Fat embolism and osteonecrosis. Orthop Clin North Am. 1985;16(4):595–633.
84. Jones Jr JP, Ramirez S, Doty SB. The pathophysiologic role of fat in dysbaric osteonecrosis. Clin Orthop Relat Res. 1993;296:256–64.
85. Li Z, Zhang N, Yue D. Experimental steroid osteonecrosis in rabbits and pathologic findings. Zhonghua Wai Ke Za Zhi. 1995;33(8):485–7.
86. Vora A. Management of osteonecrosis in children and young adults with acute lymphoblastic leukaemia. Br J Haematol. 2011;155(5):549–60. doi:10.1111/j.1365-2141.2011.08871.x.
87. Bomelburg T, von Lengerke HJ, Ritter J. Aseptic osteonecroses in the treatment of childhood acute leukaemias. Eur J Pediatr. 1989;149(1):20–3.
88. Murphy RG, Greenberg ML. Osteonecrosis in pediatric patients with acute lymphoblastic leukemia. Cancer. 1990;65(8):1717–21.
89. Wei SY, Esmail AN, Bunin N, Dormans JP. Avascular necrosis in children with acute lymphoblastic leukemia. J Pediatr Orthop. 2000;20(3):331–5.
90. Hogler W, Wehl G, van Staa T, Meister B, Klein-Franke A, Kropshofer G. Incidence of skeletal complications during treatment of childhood acute lymphoblastic leukemia: comparison of fracture risk with the General Practice Research Database. Pediatr Blood Cancer. 2007;48(1):21–7. doi:10.1002/pbc.20701.
91. Lackner H, Benesch M, Moser A, Smolle-Juttner F, Linhart W, Raith J, et al. Aseptic osteonecrosis in children and adolescents treated for hemato-oncologic diseases: a 13-year longitudinal observational study. J Pediatr Hematol Oncol. 2005;27(5):259–63.
92. Ojala AE, Lanning FP, Paakko E, Lanning BM. Osteonecrosis in children treated for acute lymphoblastic leukemia: a magnetic resonance imaging study after treatment. Med Pediatr Oncol. 1997;29(4):260–5.
93. Karimova EJ, Rai SN, Howard SC, Neel M, Britton L, Pui CH, et al. Femoral head osteonecrosis in pediatric and young adult patients with leukemia or lymphoma. J Clin Oncol. 2007;25(12):1525–31. doi:10.1200/JCO.2006.07.9947.
94. Scherer A, Engelbrecht V, Krauth KA, Bernbeck B, Reinwand U, Willers R, et al. MRI follow-up study of aseptic osteonecrosis (AON) in children treated with chemotherapy for malignant diseases. Klin Padiatr. 2001;213(2):56–62. doi:10.1055/s-2001-12883.
95. Scully SP, Aaron RK, Urbaniak JR. Survival analysis of hips treated with core decompression or vascularized fibular grafting because of avascular necrosis. J Bone Joint Surg Am. 1998;80(9):1270–5.
96. Steinberg ME. Early diagnosis, evaluation, and staging of osteonecrosis. Instr Course Lect. 1994;43:513–8.
97. Urbaniak JR, Harvey EJ. Revascularization of the femoral head in osteonecrosis. J Am Acad Orthop Surg. 1998;6(1):44–54.
98. Laroche M, Jacquemier JM, Montane de la Roque P, Arlet J, Mazieres B. Nifedipine per os relieves the pain caused by osteonecrosis of the femur head. Rev Rhum Mal Osteoartic. 1990;57(9):669–70.
99. Glueck CJ, Freiberg RA, Sieve L, Wang P. Enoxaparin prevents progression of stages I and II osteonecrosis of the hip. Clin Orthop Relat Res. 2005;435:164–70.
100. Pritchett JW. Statin therapy decreases the risk of osteonecrosis in patients receiving steroids. Clin Orthop Relat Res. 2001;386:173–8.
101. Glueck CJ, McMahon RE, Bouquot JE, Tracy T, Sieve-Smith L, Wang P. A preliminary pilot study of treatment of thrombophilia and hypofibrinolysis and amelioration of the pain of osteonecrosis of the jaws. Oral Surg Oral Med Oral Pathol Oral Radiol Endod. 1998;85(1):64–73.

Part XIV

Animal Models

Animal Models of Corticosteroid-Associated Bone Diseases

64

Lynne C. Jones, Michelle A. Tucci, Azeb Haile, and Dongqing Wang

64.1 Introduction

Osteonecrosis is a disease that is characterized by lesions of dead bone, most frequently detected in the subchondral bone of the convex side of the major diarthrodial joints (hips, knees, shoulders, and talus). High-dose corticosteroid therapy is one major risk factor for osteonecrosis. The pathological appearance of osteonecrosis of the femoral head, however, is fairly consistent regardless of the etiology. Depending on the stage of the disease, this includes evidence of bone marrow edema, lipocyte and bone cell necrosis, fibrosis, creeping substitution (new bone lying on dead bone), and the presence of osteoporosis [1]. Hemorrhage within the bone marrow compartment has also been observed in patient specimens from corticosteroid-associated osteonecrosis [2]. Previous investigators have suggested that corticosteroid-associated osteonecrosis has more rapid progression than other etiologies [1, 3]. The mechanisms involved in the development of osteonecrosis [ON] are difficult to explore from clinical samples as they provide a single snapshot at one time point subsequent to the onset of the disease, usually months after the onset of the disease when the symptoms first appear. While some investigators have used corticosteroid-associated animal models to evaluate different potential treatments [4–6], it is not clear whether the results can be extrapolated to the human condition. A better understanding of the pathophysiological mechanisms is needed.

An animal model of corticosteroid-associated osteonecrosis would allow us to study the pathogenesis, diagnosis, and treatment intervention of this specific etiology. There have been a number of attempts to establish a corticosteroid-associated animal model – primarily focusing on giving different species of animals large doses of corticosteroids such as dexamethasone, prednisolone, and prednisone for various periods of time. Yet, no progressive ON is established with evidence of creeping substitution and subchondral collapse and degenerative joint disease with corticosteroid administration alone. These factors that may confound the development of corticosteroid-associated ON animal models include differences in weight bearing (quadruped vs. bipedal), age, length of treatment, comorbidities, and differences in metabolic pathways. In spite of these differences, these animal models can be used to evaluate the effect of exogenous corticosteroid administration on bone, its vasculature, and other organs. Selected studies used to evaluate the effect of corticosteroid treatment on bone are listed in Table 64.1.

64.2 Defining Osteonecrosis

64.2.1 Definition of Osteonecrosis

How is osteonecrosis defined? There are different perspectives depending on whether you are defining ON clinically or histologically. The distinction between the two relates to lesion size, location, and progression of the pathology. That is, when studying histological slides, one is looking for evidence at the tissue or cellular level as compared to the clinician who is looking at the macroscopic or radiologic level. Steinberg and Steinberg describe ON as "a condition in which a localized area of bone becomes necrotic as a result of cellular injury and death, most frequently due to an interruption to its blood supply" [45]. Bauer, in the early stage of ON, observed hemorrhage, loss of hematopoietic elements, loss

L.C. Jones (✉)
Department of Orthopaedic Surgery, Center for Osteonecrosis Research and Education, Center for Metabolism and Obesity Research, Johns Hopkins University School of Medicine, Baltimore, MD, USA

Johns Hopkins Orthopaedics,
601 N. Caroline St., JHOC 5255, Baltimore, MD 21287, USA
e-mail: ljones3@jhmi.edu

M.A. Tucci
Department of Orthopedic Surgery and Rehabilitation, University of Mississippi Medical Center, Jackson, MS, USA

A. Haile • D. Wang
Department of Orthopaedic Surgery, Center for Metabolism and Obesity Research, Johns Hopkins University School of Medicine, Baltimore, MD, USA

K.-H. Koo et al. (eds.), *Osteonecrosis*,
DOI 10.1007/978-3-642-35767-1_64, © Springer-Verlag Berlin Heidelberg 2014

Table 64.1 Animal models of corticosteroid administration

Animal	Reference	Model description	Observations
Mouse	McLaughlin et al. [7]	BALB/c mice Dexamethasone phosphate daily IP Doses: 1, 5, 10 mg/kg Duration: 2 or 3 weeks	Decreased bone formation rates Decreased trabecular thickness Decreased serum osteocalcin
Mouse	Yang et al. [8]	BALB/cJ mice (4 weeks) Dexamethasone in drinking water Dose: 4 mg/L for the first week, 2 mg/L thereafter Duration: 12 weeks	Osteonecrosis detected in distal femoral epiphysis in 9/21 animals (continuous dose)
Mouse	Wang et al. [9]	BALB/cJ mice (7–9 weeks) Dexamethasone in drinking water Dose: 4 mg/L for the first week, 2 mg/L thereafter Duration: 12 weeks	Osteopenia No significant osteonecrotic lesions
Rat	Wang et al. [10]	5-week-old male Wistar rats 6-Methylprednisolone daily subcutaneous Doses: 2.5, 5, 10, 20 mg/kg Duration: 4 weeks	Endochondral and periosteal bone formation decreased Marked increase in the number of adipocytes in the diaphyseal bone marrow
Rat	Noa et al. [11]	Sprague–Dawley rats Prednisolone daily oral Dose: 6 mg/kg Duration: 80 days	Decreased trabecular bone volume, trabecular thickness, and trabecular number Hypertrophy of bone marrow adipocytes Lipid-laden pluripotential stromal cells in bones
Rat	Murata et al. [12]	SHRSP/Ngsks rats Methylprednisolone acetate one IM injection (17 weeks old) Dose: 20 mg/kg Duration: sacrificed at 19 weeks of age	Model plus steroid resulted in 95.2 % of animals with very early osteonecrosis Swollen adipocytes in bone marrow spaces with partial degeneration/necrosis
Rat	Bekler et al. [13]	Sprague–Dawley rats Created serum disease (serum inj) Methylprednisolone Dose: 40 mg/kg/day for three consecutive days Duration: 2 weeks after last injection	Model + steroid caused development of small areas of necrosis Steroid alone = no osteonecrosis but changes in cellular differentiation in bone marrow
Rat	Kerachian et al. [14]	Hypertensive, Wistar Kyoto, Wistar Furth, SASCO Fisher and Lewis rat Prednisone pellets implanted Dose: 1.82–2.56 mg/kg/day Duration: 90 days	Growth plate disruption with acellular areas in Wistar Kyoto and Wistar Furth rats Apoptotic osteocytes in trabeculae of hypertensive rats The most apoptosis rate was in spontaneous hypertensive rats (+++) and then Wistar Furth (++) and Wistar Kyoto (++)
Rabbits	Fisher et al. [15]	New Zealand white rabbits 30 of 66 rabbits were immature Methylprednisolone (Depo-Medrol) weekly parenterally Dose: 1.5 and 3 mg/kg/day Up to 160 days	Serum lipids increased Pulmonary fat emboli at 3 weeks Extensive osteoporosis Emboli in subchondral bone
Rabbits	Jaffe et al. [16]	New Zealand white rabbits Cortisone acetate Dose: 12.5 mg (daily IM) Duration: up to 9 weeks	Severe subchondral intravascular fat emboli (third week) Osteoporosis (fifth week) No osteonecrosis
Rabbits	Cruess et al. [17]	Adult rabbits Cortisone Dose: 5 mg/kg Duration: up to 60 days	Subchondral vessels packed with lipid material
Rabbits	Wang et al. [18]	New Zealand white rabbits, looked at both immature and mature animals Depo-Medrol (methylprednisolone) IM Dose: 2.7 or 12.25 mg/kg per week Duration: young, up to 12 weeks; older, up to 8 weeks	Immature: increase in marrow fat and increase in fat cell size Fat droplets in the subchondral arterioles Mature: fat cell size increased from 62 to 70 μm. Otherwise similar to immature animals
Rabbits	Gold et al. [19]	New Zealand white rabbits Methylprednisolone acetate (Depo-Medrol) or methylprednisolone succinate IM Dose: .8 mg on alternate days for 8 days .8 daily	Elevated lipid and prostaglandin levels Osteoporosis by 6 weeks Evidence of bone necrosis Fat emboli in second and third weeks Intravascular fat globules

Animal	Reference	Model description	Observations
Rabbits	Warman and Boskey [20]	Rabbits Hydrocortisone acetate Dose: 15 mg/4 kg rabbit Duration: 4 and 9 weeks	Osteoporosis model Elevations in marrow lipid content
Rabbits	Kawai et al. [21]	Female Japanese white rabbits, 3–6 months Methylprednisolone Dose: 4.2 mg/kg weekly Duration: 4 and 8 weeks	Advanced hyperlipidemia at 4 weeks Osteocytes contained small lipid droplets that increased in size compressing nucleus
Rabbits	Warner et al. [22]	Adult New Zealand white rabbits Methylprednisolone Dose: 12.3 mg/week IM Duration: 5–9 weeks	No significant elevation in intramedullary pressure Marked osteoporosis No osteonecrosis
Rabbits	Li et al. [23]	Adult rabbits Hypersensitive vasculitis (serum disease) High-dose corticosteroids	Hemopoietic necrosis Enlargement of fat cells in bone marrow
Rabbits	Yamamoto et al. [24]	Adult male Japanese white rabbits Methylprednisolone (IM) Dose: 20 mg/kg Duration: up to 10 weeks	43 % of the rabbits studied had developed multifocal ON lesions in the femur and/or humerus
Rabbits	Miyanishi et al. [25]	Adult male Japanese white rabbits Methylprednisolone acetate IM Dose: 20 mg/kg Duration: 2 weeks	Osteonecrosis in some animals Bone marrow fat cells larger in rabbits with ON (63.5 μm) than without (53.3 μm)
Rabbits	Motomura et al. [26]	Adult male Japanese white rabbits Methylprednisolone acetate IM Dose: 20 mg/kg Duration: 2 weeks	Incidence of ON is 70 % in steroid-only rabbits
Rabbits	Ichiseki et al. [27]	Japanese white rabbits Methylprednisolone acetate Dose: 4 mg/kg one dose IM Duration: 3, 5, 14 days	ON observed in 7/10 rabbits in S14 group Hematopoietic cell necrosis and fat cell necrosis at 14 days
Rabbits	Wang et al. [28]	Chinese white rabbits Horse serum model Prednisone Dose: IP once/day for 5 days Duration: 3, 7, 21, 35, 49 after last inj	Pathological changes seen 1 and 3 weeks after treatment (model + steroid or steroid alone)
Rabbits	Hu et al. [29]	New Zealand white rabbits Horse serum model Prednisone	Increase of empty osteocyte lacunae and fat cells
Rabbits	Sheng et al. [30]	New Zealand white rabbits LPS inj model Methylprednisolone Dose: 20 mg/kg, three inj IM at a time interval of 24 h Duration: 2 weeks	15 ON+/10 ON– 6 one lesion; 9 had > 1 lesion Increased fat cell density Fat cells larger in the control group More triglyceride formation in ON + group
Rabbits	Kuroda Y, et al. [31]	Japanese white rabbits Vascular occlusion of the capital femoral epiphysis by electrocoagulation 40 mg/kg methylprednisolone Dose: 40 mg/kg IM, once Duration: 4, 8, 12, or 24 weeks	Flattening and loss of sphericity of the femoral head Thinning of the subchondral bone Dead trabecular bone Secondary OA changes 24 weeks, collapse of femoral head reported
Chickens	Cui et al. [32]	Female leghorn chickens Methylprednisolone Dose: 3 mg/kg weekly IM Duration: up to 24 weeks	Serum cholesterol levels increased 4/12 at 12 and 24 weeks showed subchondral destruction and focal necrosis Adipocyte proliferation within 24 h of the inj Number and size of fat cells increased over time

(continued)

Table 64.1 (continued)

Animal	Reference	Model description	Observations
Chicken (leghorn)	Xiao et al. [33]	Leghorn chicken (B) Methylprednisolone (low) 4.2 mg/kg weekly IM (C) Methylprednisolone (high) 6.3 mg/kg weekly IM (D) Dex (1.5 mg/kg) + horse serum weekly IM (E) Dex (2.0 mg/kg) + horse serum weekly IM (F) Dex (2.5 mg/kg) + horse serum weekly IM Duration: 12 weeks	Empty lacuna was higher in group C, E Increase fat cell number and size in B, E, F groups Trabecular bone was broken under cartilage (?) in C, E group
Chicken (broiler)	Wideman et al. [34]	Broilers 0.45–1.5 mg of DEX/kg IM Duration: 28 and 35 days	Growth was inhibited Proximal tibial head necrosis Avascular femoral head necrosis and fatty necrosis of the tibiae(??)
Pigs	Drescher et al. [35]	Immature domestic pigs Methylprednisolone 30 mg/kg IV followed by 5.4 mg/kg/h (megadose)	Reduction in femoral head blood flow
Pigs	Ikeda et al. [36]	Immature female Göttingen minipigs Prednisolone Dose: 0.5 mg/kg BW/day 5 days/week for 26 weeks	Decreased bone formation Did not look at fat cells
Sheep	Lill et al. [37, 38, 39]	Swiss mountain sheep Daily intramuscular injection of 25 mg methylprednisolone, 6 months Ovariectomy Calcium- and vitamin D-restricted diet Malnutrition	BMD decreases 55 % in cancellous bone and 7 % in cortical bone 19 % decrease in trabecular number and 22 % decrease in trabecular thickness
Sheep	Augat et al. [40]	Merino sheep 4–6 years old Subcutaneous injection of 0.6 mg/kg/day prednisolone acetate 5× weekly, 7 months	Significant decrease of cancellous bone volume, trabecular thickness and bone strength Microarchitectural changes in the distal femur and proximal tibia Decreased serum osteocalcin
Ponies	Glade and Krook [41]	Pony foals Dexamethasone IM Dose: 0.5 or 5 mg/100 kg Duration: 3, 8, 11 months	Osteonecrosis in major joints with osteocyte death
Ponies	Nasseri et al. [42]	Adult ponies Dexamethasone IM Dose: 5 mg/100 kg Duration: 4 months	Elevated intraosseous pressures Femoral head contained fat marrow necrosis, marrow edema, and enlarged lipocytes
Emus	Goetz et al. [43]	Groups: Cryoinsult Cryoinsult plus methylprednisolone acetate (5 mg/kg IM) plus ligation of rt. Medial and lateral circumflex arteries Methylprednisolone acetate (5 mg/kg IM) Normal controls Duration: 1 year	Corticosteroids alone caused diffuse, low-grade bony abnormalities in the femoral head Femoral heads of the cryoinsult + corticosteroid + ligation group had the largest amount of high-grade abnormality 2 animals in this group displayed subchondral fracture

Modified from Jones and Allen [44]

of adipocyte nuclei and microvesicular fat, and necrosis of the bone marrow, sometimes accompanied by fibrin deposition [46]. Horvai and Link [47] distinguish the early from late changes: "I. Early changes: necrosis of bone marrow fat and hematopoietic tissue; osteocyte lacunae may be enlarged and empty or normal size with pyknotic nuclei. II. Later changes: ingrowth of granulation tissue from the lesion periphery with layering of new bone over dead trabeculae ("creeping substitution"), which results in formation of a highly collagenized and, later, calcified rim." The use of the term osteonecrosis is further complicated by the finding that osteocyte death may be through apoptosis rather than necrosis [48, 49].

The definition is important when evaluating the animal models of osteonecrosis. Some studies report only the presence of empty lacunae or pyknotic osteocyte nuclei or disruption of the marrow elements as evidence of osteonecrosis.

Bauer et al. raises a major concern stating that this criterion has low sensitivity and low specificity [46]. He expands on this to say that "viable osteocytes often appear shrunken by light microscopy, so nuclear pyknosis is not a reliable sign of osteocyte death in routinely processed, decalcified tissues. Furthermore, osteocyte nuclei may persist in bone after an ischemic event." Furthermore, suboptimal tissue fixation, processing, and staining can also create artifacts that can be misinterpreted [46, 50]. A more stringent definition has been used by several investigators to include the diffuse presence of empty osteocyte lacunae, pyknotic nuclei of ghost osteocytes in the bone trabeculae, and evidence of cellular necrosis within the bone marrow compartment adjacent to the affected bone [8, 24]. With animal models, large lesions, subchondral collapse, or progression of the disease are rarely mentioned.

64.2.2 Perthes Versus Adult

There are a number of distinctions between the radiologic and pathological appearances of the adult form of osteonecrosis and the juvenile form – Legg-Calvé-Perthes disease (also called Perthes disease). These differences relate to the cartilage, growth plate, and distribution of the pathology. Cartilage hypertrophy and malformation are observed in Perthes. In some Perthes patients, there is decreased size of the affected femoral head. The radiographic appearance of the affected femoral head between these two age groups may also be different loss of sphericity associated with subchondral collapse in adult ON and fragmentation of the epiphysis and a misshapened head associated with Perthes patients.

It is not clear as to whether identical pathways are involved in both Perthes and adult osteonecrosis. It appears that there may be differences in the vulnerability of the circulation and bone relating to age [51, 52]. The percentage of children with corticosteroid-associated disease is not as common as adult ON [53, 54]. However, one patient population, children with acute lymphoblastic leukemia receiving high doses of corticosteroids, displays a particularly severe form of ON [55, 56].

A number of animal models have evaluated the effect of corticosteroids on the bony compartment of immature animals. In a study of horse foals, Glade observed slower growth associated with less weight gain [41, 57]. He observed degenerative changes in the growth plates after 3 months of corticosteroid treatment with evidence of retardation of growth plate chondrocytes and irregular penetration of the calcified cartilage by metaphyseal capillaries. By 8 months, the subchondral bone plate was characterized as a "thin distal terminal plate with few supporting trabeculae." After 11 months of treatment, he noted dysplastic hips and ulceration of the cartilage and osteonecrotic lesions in both femoral and humeral heads. Using immature New Zealand white (NZW) rabbits, Wang et al. observed that the femoral and humeral heads were significantly smaller than the untreated controls following treatment with cortisone acetate (15 mg SQ) [18]. They reported that the epiphyseal growth plate was significantly smaller and less active. They found a significantly lower trabecular area fraction (23 %) and a significantly higher percentage of marrow fat (77 %) as compared to the controls (39, 61 %, respectively). An increased accumulation of fat droplets in the subchondral arterioles was noted by the twentieth week of treatment. In a study of immature pigs, Drescher et al. found that high-dose methylprednisolone treatment (100 mg/day) resulted in decreases in total body weight and distinct morphological changes at the interface between the articular cartilage and subchondral bone [58]. They describe a scalloped interface with "cartilaginous projections extended into the subchondral plate." In another study, they found significantly decreased regional blood flow to the femoral head epiphysis, proximal femoral metaphyseal spongiosa, proximal femoral metaphyseal corticalis, and acetabular bone [59].

While mice and rats are now being explored as potential animal models, one caveat is that the epiphyses of mice and rats remain open throughout their life span. So while older rodents may be used in a particular study, it is unclear whether the differences in the morphology and vascularization of the bony region under study may contribute to the pathological findings.

64.2.3 Osteoporosis vs. Osteonecrosis

Numerous investigators have utilized animal models of decreased bone mass to explore osteoporosis, and several outstanding reviews are available [60–66]. Many of these models often use either ovariectomy or orchidectomy of various animal species including mice, rats, monkeys, and sheep [67–74]. Gonadectomy results in bone loss by establishing sex steroid deficiency [75, 76]. Other models have been used to create osteopenia including adrenalectomy (ADX), disuse models (mechanical unloading), diet (e.g., calcium restriction), or administration of various compounds (PTH, RANKL, cyclosporin A) [60]. Ovariectomy models have not only contributed to a better understanding of postmenopausal osteoporosis but have led to a better appreciation of the interaction between glucocorticoids and the musculoskeletal system.

Decreased bone mineral density has been observed in some cases of osteonecrosis clinically [77] as well as in animal models of ON [5, 9, 48, 78, 79]. Osteonecrosis is a well-recognized complication due to glucocorticoid excess. The overall effects of glucocorticoid excess are catabolic in nature. Glucocorticoids inhibit gastrointestinal absorption of calcium as well as increased renal excretion of calcium which can lead to increases in PTH. The increase in PTH can result in an increase in the number of sites undergoing bone remodeling. Glucocorticoids also reduce the level of gonadal hormones which can further augment bone resorption. Glucocorticoids decrease recruitment of osteoblast cells as well as accelerate the apoptosis of both osteoblast and osteocyte cells inhibiting bone remodeling. Due to the many physiological effects of glucocorticoids, the exact mechanism responsible for osteonecrosis remains obscure, whereas osteoporosis due to estrogen loss is straightforward. Lack of estrogen has profound effects on the osteoclast cells. Ovariectomy results in severe cancellous osteopenia in long bone and in the vertebrae of monkeys and rats [80–83]. Ovariectomy results in an increase in the osteoblast-lined perimeter, osteoclast-lined perimeter, and osteoclast size in the long bone of rats [84–86]. In rats, there is a simultaneous increase in the mineral apposition rate and bone formation which suggests chronic high bone turnover. In ovariectomized nonhuman primates, there is also an increase in cancellous bone formation associated with the increase in bone resorption.

Corticosteroid therapy is one of the primary etiological risk factors for both osteoporosis and osteonecrosis. Corticosteroid treatment results in increased osteopenia with decreases in bone mineral density (BMD) and the ratio of bone volume to total volume (BV/TV) [5, 9, 78]. However, exposure to high-dose corticosteroids has also been used to establish animal models which have the characteristic features of early osteonecrosis. So while many investigators have injected high doses of corticosteroids into a number of animals with the hopes of creating a model of osteonecrosis or osteoporosis, it is probably better to call these animal models of high-dose corticosteroid therapy.

As the osteoporosis literature also provides insight to the effect of corticosteroids on bone, this will be discussed later in this manuscript (Sects. 64.3.4 and 64.3.7.3).

64.2.4 Multifactorial Pathogenesis

Both corticosteroid-associated osteonecrosis and osteoporosis are multifactorial diseases. Clearly, there are underlying comorbidities for which the corticosteroids are being administered. In addition, there may be genetic (e.g., inherited coagulopathies) and environmental (e.g., smoking) factors which may predispose an individual to bony sequelae. For this reason, it is not surprising that most, if not all, of the animal models of corticosteroid administration to healthy animals do not develop bony pathology 100 % of the time. In fact, an animal model is considered successful if the incidence exceeds 50 %.

So it is within this framework that we will discuss what we have learned from animal models regarding the effect of corticosteroid treatment on bone and associated tissues.

64.3 Models of Corticosteroid Administration

In order to better understand the effects of corticosteroids on the musculoskeletal system, investigators have injected several species of animals with high doses of corticosteroids for varying periods of time.

64.3.1 Total Body Weight Loss

Many investigators have reported notable weight loss following high-dose corticosteroid administration into various animals [6, 8, 9, 15–18, 21, 22]. This can be associated with a substantial mortality rate depending on the animal model and the dose and duration of corticosteroid treatment [6, 8, 16–18, 22]. This is in contradistinction to the effect in humans where the incidence of weight gain can be greater than 30 % [87]. Furthermore, human osteonecrosis is frequently associated with a cushingoid appearance [88–90]. This difference raises questions about how the weight loss and health status of the animal (e.g., whether they are cachectic) may influence the effect of corticosteroids on bone and bone marrow elements.

64.3.2 Hematological Findings

Evidence of hyperlipidemia following corticosteroid treatment has been reported by a number of studies. Significant elevations in serum cholesterol, triglycerides, and phospholipids have been documented following corticosteroid treatment in various animal models [17, 21, 24]. Others have noted elevated lipid and prostaglandin levels [7, 19].

Yamamoto et al. found that after one injection of methylprednisolone acetate (20 mg/kg) given to Japanese white rabbits, free fatty acids (FFAs), triglycerides, cholesterol, glutamic oxaloacetic transaminase (GOT), and glutamic-pyruvic transaminase (GPT) levels were increased by 1 week with a statistically significant increase by 2 weeks [24]. The levels returned to baseline levels by 6 (GOT and GPT) to 8 (FFAs) weeks. There appeared to be a difference in the triglyceride response between animals diagnosed with ON (remained elevated) compared to those without ON (returned by 8 weeks). Platelet counts and fibrinogen levels decreased significantly at 1 week and then returned to baseline levels.

Kawai et al. studied the effect of repeated injections of methylprednisolone (4.2 mg/kg BW once a week for 4 and 8 weeks) in a rabbit model [21]. After corticosteroid therapy, there was evidence of marked hyperlipidemia and significantly increased values for liver function tests. Cholesterol and triglyceride increased 6.4 and 28.5 times baseline. Phospholipid (3.1×), very low-density lipoprotein (50.5×), and low-density lipoprotein (11.7×) also increased. The liver function tests, GOT and GPT, increased 13.3× and 31.8×, respectively; gamma glutamyl transpeptidase (GGT) increased 8.6 times baseline.

Wang et al. gave high doses of cortisone acetate to immature and mature rabbits for varying periods of time [18]. They noted an increase in serum cholesterol with increasing duration of treatment in both immature and adult animals. In contrast to the previous investigators, Wang et al. did not find significant changes in the serum triglycerides or lipoprotein patterns in either group.

64.3.3 Histopathology of the Liver and Other Organs

Following corticosteroid therapy, many animal studies have reported a fatty metamorphosis of the liver [9, 17, 18, 21, 24]. Yamamoto et al. found evidence of focal necrosis of the liver parenchyma associated with calcification [24]. This group also observed that the liver recovered 10 weeks following one corticosteroid injection. Others have noted an accumulation of fatty droplets in the lungs and kidneys [17, 18]. Wang et al. also reported nephrocalcinosis in the kidneys of several animals [18].

64.3.4 Bone Mass and Histomorphometric Changes

Corticosteroid treatment of healthy animals results in decreased bone mass and related histomorphometric changes in bone [5, 9, 48, 78, 79]. Baofeng et al. injected a group of female NZW rabbits with methylprednisolone succinate (1 mg/kg/day IM) for eight consecutive weeks [78] and noted a significant decrease in trabecular thickness and BV/TV within the lumbar vertebrae along with decreases in maximum load as compared to sham controls. Zhang et al. injected NZW rabbits with dexamethasone (3 mg/kg) twice weekly for either 6 or 12 weeks [5]. In addition to significant decreases in trabecular thickness and BV/TV within the lumbar spine, they observed significant decreases in trabecular number and an increase in trabecular spacing by 6 weeks which decreased further by 12 weeks. Wang et al. evaluated the distal femur of BALB/cJ mice that were administered dexamethasone in the drinking water for 12 weeks [9]. They reported a significant reduction in bone volume fraction (BV/TV) and number of trabeculae with a concomitant increase in trabecular separation. Weinstein et al. implanted pellets subcutaneously which released 0.7 or 2.1 mg/kg/day and evaluated the animals at 27 days [48]. Global (0.7 mg/kg/day) and spinal (2.1 mg/kg/day) bone mineral density (BMD) were significantly decreased, while the hindquarters BMD showed a trend toward decreasing at a much lower level. A substantial decrease (40 %) in vertebral cancellous bone area, trabecular width, bone formation, and turnover was observed. In addition to a dose-dependent decrease in the mineral appositional rate, there was a threefold increase in empty erosion cavities or reversal perimeter, a 26 % decrease in the mineralizing perimeter, and a threefold increase in osteoblast apoptosis in the vertebral cancellous bone of mice receiving the higher dose. In contrast, Eberhardt et al. reported significant bony changes in the proximal femur of a rabbit model injected with methylprednisolone acetate (4 μmol/kg day IM) at day 28 [79]. They found trabecular thinning and increased trabecular separation in the subarticular area of the proximal femur. The subarticular trabecular bone was 50–80 % resorptive in the treated animals and was primarily nonresorptive for the controls. There was evidence of increased osteoclastic resorption and decreased bone formation in the region of interest, and a pattern of tetracycline uptake was suggestive of surface and matrix damage. McLaughlin et al. have also reported decreased bone formation rates in female mice given daily injections of dexamethasone phosphate for 2–3 weeks [7].

64.3.5 The Vasculature and Blood Flow

Boss and Misselevich reported that there is a ubiquitous, intimal thickening of the rabbit veins after an 8-week treatment with methylprednisolone associated with the proliferation of myocyte-derived foam cells [91]. Korompilias et al. evaluated the vessels from animals that had received corticosteroid treatment for 8 months [92]. They observed thrombi in the extraosseous vein of the metaphysis of two steroid-treatment-only rabbits. More extensive vascular pathology occurred when a hypersensitivity reaction was also induced.

Wang and colleagues have observed significantly decreased blood flow to the femoral head of a rabbit model [93, 94]. They also reported increased intraosseous pressures in the femoral head using the same model [95]. Drescher et al. observed decreased bone blood flow to the vertebrae (C6 and L6) in immature pigs [96] and increased flow to the cranial subregion of the femoral head epiphysis [58]. They also found decreased femoral head blood flow following a megadose methylprednisolone infusion (30 mg/kg intravenously as an initial bolus, followed by 5.4 mg/kg/h for further 23 h) in immature pigs [35]. In contrast, other investigators have reported no change in femoral head blood flow or in intraosseous pressure in various corticosteroid-treated animal models [22, 97].

64.3.6 Bone and Bone Marrow

Regarding osteonecrosis of the femoral head in patients, Ficat and Arlet describe a continuum of pathological changes beginning with disruption of bone marrow elements and ending with necrotic lesions and evidence of subchondral collapse [98]. While animal models have attempted to create an animal model that reproduces this natural history, the establishment of a model with collapse and arthrosis has been elusive. However, the majority of these models describe pathological changes which are similar to early-stage osteonecrosis. The early changes may include pre-necrotic plasmostasis, reticular proliferation, hemorrhage, and accumulation of foam cells [98]. This is followed by necrosis of the fatty marrow and then medullary necrosis. Consequently, trabecular lesions can be identified by empty lacunae.

The effect of corticosteroids on bone and bone marrow elements has been studied extensively, as shown in Table 64.1. The histomorphometric alterations reflect the effect of corticosteroids at the cellular level. Changes have been observed in the cells of the bone marrow compartment as well as osteocytes residing in the bone matrix. In most animal models, enlargement of bone marrow adipocytes have been observed following corticosteroid administration [9, 18, 21, 99]. This is often associated with increased numbers of adipocytes [9] and decreased number of hematopoietic cells [9, 21]. Numerous, lipid-laden, pluripotent stromal cells may also be present [91]. Evidence of old and new hemorrhages along with extravasation of red blood cells into the marrow, bone marrow edema, thrombus formation, and marrow necrosis has been observed in the proximal metaphysis and diaphysis [92]. Intravascular fat within the femoral and humeral heads may be evident [16, 17, 19]. Treatment of rabbits for 4 or 9 weeks with hydrocortisone acetate increased cholesterol accumulation in both the cancellous and cortical compartments [77].

Regarding bone cells, most studies have focused on osteocytes. Kawai et al. detected small lipid droplets within osteocyte lacunae in rabbits treated with methylprednisolone (4.2 mg/kg, once a week for 4 or 8 weeks) [21]. Using electron microscopy, they observed that the presence of lipid droplets displaced the nuclei to one side of the lacunae. They concluded that the increased fat depositions resulted in the degeneration and necrosis of osteocytes. Focal osteocytic death in subchondral bone is a frequent consequence of corticosteroid treatment [15, 17, 19, 22]. Gold et al. observed osteocyte death and necrotic debris by 2 weeks following corticosteroid treatment [19]. By 3 weeks, over 20 % of the bone had empty lacunae. After 21–35 days of treatment with cortisone acetate (5 mg/kg), Cruess et al. reported a statistically significant increase in empty osteocyte lacunae (23 %) as compared to controls (10 %) [17]. Weinstein et al. detected apoptosis (TUNEL reactive) of osteoblasts and osteocytes in trabecular bone but not in cortical bone [48].

As discussed previously, the diagnosis of osteonecrosis relates to the presence of empty osteocyte lacunae, pyknotic osteocyte nuclei, and marrow necrosis. Using this criterion, many investigators have evaluated the incidence of osteonecrosis in various animal models. Yamamoto et al. reported that osteonecrosis was prevalent in 43 % of the joints studied 4 weeks after injecting a rabbit model with one dose of methylprednisolone (20 mg/kg IM) [24]. They also found evidence of granulation tissue and appositional bone depending on the number of weeks postinjection. Using the same model, Motomura et al. detected an incidence of 70 % osteonecrosis 2 weeks after the methylprednisolone injection [26]. Yang et al. administered dexamethasone to 4-week-old BALB/cJ mice in the drinking water for up to 12 weeks [8]. The incidence of osteonecrosis ranged from 40 to 45 % in two groups. In a similar study using mature BALB/cJ mice, although increased adipogenesis within the bone marrow compartment of the distal femur was observed, there was no consistent evidence of osteonecrosis [9]. This supports that there may be age-related differences in the response of bone to corticosteroids.

64.3.7 Multifactorial Models

Several investigators have described the pathogenesis of osteonecrosis as multifactorial – using terms such as accumulated stress, multihit, predisposition (genetic or nongenetic), and thresholds. Therefore, it seems reasonable that an animal model of osteonecrosis should incorporate this concept. Perhaps there are animal models that are "predisposed" to develop ON. As corticosteroids are given to individuals to treat some underlying condition, it is realistic for us to evaluate the effect of corticosteroids in animals with features of that underlying condition.

64.3.7.1 Shwartzman Reaction

John Paul Jones, Jr. and others have proposed that intravascular coagulation is an integral mechanism within the pathogenesis of osteonecrosis [100, 101]. One type of animal model has been used to study the effect of corticosteroid therapy in an animal model of the Shwartzman reaction. The Shwartzman reaction is a mechanism of endotoxin (LPS)-mediated tissue injury and can be either systemic or localized [102]; the systemic form is a consequence of widespread intravascular thrombus formation on the surfaces of endothelial cells.

Okazaki et al. injected LPS (2 mg/kg, IV) twice into 10-week-old male Wistar rats and then injected methylprednisolone (20 mg/kg) IM for 3 days [103]. At 1 week, empty lacunae were observed within the trabecular bone of the femoral head. Within the bone marrow, there was a decrease in the number of hematopoietic and fat cells with an increase in cell debris. By week 3, the hematopoietic and fat cells had disappeared, and fibrous tissue had accumulated and formed scar tissue by week 4. Increased levels of IL-1β, IL-2, IL-4, IL-6, IL-10, GM-CSF, IFN-γ, and TNF-α in the blood were observed by week 1. Upregulation of IL-1β was also seen in the liver and kidney. Total plasma cholesterol concentration was increased at 1 and 2 weeks. The investigators propose that the LPS/methylprednisolone-induced osteonecrosis may arise from aberrant activation of the immune system by the TLR4-mediated signaling pathway as well as aberrant lipid metabolism.

Yamamoto et al. established a similar model in New Zealand white rabbits [104]. They compared treatment with LPS alone (100 μg/kg), methylprednisolone alone (20 mg/kg), LPS plus methylprednisolone, and no treatment (controls). A diagnosis of osteonecrosis was determined by the presence of empty lacunae or pyknotic nuclei of osteocytes and bone marrow cell necrosis. They reported a significant increase in the number of cases of osteonecrosis in the metaphysis of the LPS plus corticosteroid group as compared to the LPS alone or corticosteroid alone groups. This increase was also noted in the diaphysis and the epiphyses, although always in animals with metaphyseal ON. Using a similar model in rabbits, Guan and Han [105] found a significantly higher rate of osteonecrosis in the femoral head of animals with both the LPS and corticosteroid treatments (36 %) as compared to the corticosteroid (30 %) and control (17 %) groups. Additionally, they noted significantly elevated serum triglycerides (TGs) and total cholesterol (TC) in the combination group as compared to the other groups at different time periods up to 21 days.

What is the take-home message from these experiments? First, although rare, septic arthritis associated with osteonecrosis does occur [106]. The role of intravascular coagulation within this group remains to be evaluated. Second, corticosteroid treatment exacerbates any effect on bone that a LPS-associated tissue reaction may have. Third, it raises the question of whether aberrant activation of the immune system may play a role in aseptic osteonecrosis.

64.3.7.2 Models Involving Hypersensitivity Reactions

Injections of horse serum have been used to induce a systemic hypersensitivity reaction in animals [33, 107–109]. Two injections of horse serum given 3 weeks apart to adult rabbits may result in the formation of immune complexes within the bone marrow [107]. Matsui et al. observed that corticosteroids augmented the effect of horse serum injections. Furthermore, the incidence of osteonecrosis was notably increased in the combination model (70 % of the animals) [108] as compared to horse serum alone (33 % of the animals) [109]. More animals of the combination group demonstrated the more severe ON in the diaphysis and metaphysic of the proximal femur than either the horse serum-only or corticosteroid-only groups. The bony pathology was associated with intramedullary hemorrhages and vascular lesions including degeneration of the tunica media, loss of smooth muscle cells, and disruption of the internal elastic membrane. As vasculitis is a frequent comorbidity of osteonecrosis, it is reasonable that an animal model should incorporate this into its design [110].

64.3.7.3 Models of Osteoporosis and Corticosteroids

Animal models that evaluate the effects of corticosteroids on osteopenia and osteoporosis can be divided into three categories: models receiving corticosteroid therapy alone (as discussed previously), models that have undergone gonadectomy with and without corticosteroid therapy, and animal models that have undergone adrenalectomy and administered corticosteroid replacement therapy.

Corticosteroid therapy augments the effect of ovariectomy, establishing a more reproducible model of osteoporosis. Using an ovariectomized (OVX) sheep model, Lill and colleagues have evaluated the effect of daily intramuscular injection of methylprednisolone in OVX animals that are placed on a calcium- and vitamin D-restricted diet [37–39]. Corticosteroid treatment increased the bone effects observed with OVX alone. This was further amplified when animals were placed on calcium- and vitamin D-restricted diet. They observed decreases in the bone mineral density of cancellous bone (55 %), cortical bone (7 %), trabecular number (19 %), and trabecular thickness (22 %) in the OVX/corticosteroid/diet group.

Baofeng et al. reported similar findings for a rabbit model of ovariectomy and methylprednisolone (MP) therapy (1 mg/kg/day for 8 weeks starting 2 weeks after OVX); the experiment was terminated at 10 weeks [78]. Regarding bone mineral density (BMD), they found that MP or OVX+MP resulted in statistically significant decreases at 10 weeks as compared to baseline. The decrease in BMD was the greatest for the OVX+MP group (36 %) as compared to the MP (22 %) and OVX (8.5 %) groups. Significant decreases in trabecular thickness and bone volume/total volume were seen for both the MP and OVX+MP group. Significant decreases in trabecular number, trabecular separation, bone surface area/bone volume, and connectivity density were also found for the combination (OVX+MP) group.

Other studies have investigated the effect of corticosteroids on the hypothalamus pituitary axis. Mohamed et al. implanted a tricalcium phosphate drug delivery system to expose a rat model to continuous release of corticosterone for 24 days [111]. They found differences between male and female rats with adrenal atrophy of the zona glomerulosa and hypertrophy of the adrenal medulla in male rats and disorganization of all zones within the adrenal gland with lipohypertrophy in female rats. The hypothalamus pituitary axis can also be disrupted following adrenalectomy (ADX). Li et al. observed that adrenalectomy of male rats resulted in a significantly decreased cancellous bone volume and trends for increased osteoclast and osteoblast surfaces [112]. A dose response was seen with corticosterone treatment in the ADX animals with significant increases in cancellous bone volume and decreases in osteoblast surface, osteoclast surface, and mineralizing surface as compared to untreated placebo and ADX controls. The higher doses of corticosterone (50, 100, 200 mg) were also associated with decreased bone formation rate and longitudinal growth rates.

Do the pathogenesis of osteoporosis and osteonecrosis share common mechanisms? Animal models of osteonecrosis indicate that, depending on the dose and duration, corticosteroid therapy may result in osteopenia. However, factors which trigger the progression to end-stage osteoporosis or osteonecrosis remain to be defined.

64.4 Summary

Animal models have contributed to our understanding of the pathogenesis and natural history of corticosteroid-associated osteonecrosis and osteoporosis. The effects of corticosteroid therapy are both local and systemic. With respect to bone, there may be direct effects on the bone cells as well as bone marrow elements. Hyperlipidemia and increases in intraosseous and extraosseous fat deposits are likely to contribute to the bony pathology. While animal models of corticosteroid treatment alone do not develop the characteristics of advanced osteonecrosis seen in human ON, this may be due to limitations of the animal model (e.g., metabolic differences, quadrupeds) or to the multifactorial nature of this bone disorder. As we learn about the possible genetic predisposition for osteonecrosis, mouse models may be developed that can study the pathogenetic mechanisms involved.

References

1. Chernetsky SG, Mont MA, LaPorte DM, Jones LC, Hungerford DS, McCarthy EF. Pathologic features in steroid and nonsteroid associated osteonecrosis. Clin Orthop Relat Res. 1999;368:149–61.
2. Saito S, Ohzono K, Ono K. Early arteriopathy and postulated pathogenesis of osteonecrosis of the femoral head. The intracapital arterioles. Clin Orthop Relat Res. 1992;277:98–110.
3. Hastings DE, Macnab I. Spontaneous avascular necrosis of the femoral head: a clinical and pathological review. Can J Surg. 1965;8:68–83.
4. Li X, Cui Q, Kao C, Wang GJ, Balian G. Lovastatin inhibits adipogenic and stimulates osteogenic differentiation by suppressing PPARgamma2 and increasing Cbfa1/Runx2 expression in bone marrow mesenchymal cell cultures. Bone. 2003;33(4):652–9.
5. Zhang KJ, Zhang J, Kang ZK, Xue XM, Kang JF, Li YW, et al. Ibandronate for prevention and treatment of glucocorticoid-induced osteoporosis in rabbits. Rheumatol Int. 2012;32(11):3405–11. doi:10.1007/s00296-011-2074-9.
6. Erken HY, Ofluoglu O, Aktas M, Topal C, Yildiz M. Effect of pentoxifylline on histopathological changes in steroid-induced osteonecrosis of femoral head: experimental study in chicken. Int Orthop. 2012;36(7):1523–8. doi:10.1007/s00264-012-1497-6.
7. McLaughlin F, Mackintosh J, Hayes BP, McLaren A, Uings IJ, Salmon P, et al. Glucocorticoid-induced osteopenia in the mouse as assessed by histomorphometry, microcomputed tomography, and biochemical markers. Bone. 2002;30(6):924–30.
8. Yang L, Boyd K, Kaste SC, Kamdem Kamdem L, Rahija RJ, Relling MV. A mouse model for glucocorticoid-induced osteonecrosis: effect of a steroid holiday. J Orthop Res. 2009;27(2):169–75. doi:10.1002/jor.20733.
9. Wang D, Haile A, Jones LC, editors. A MicroCT analysis of trabecular bone structure in a mouse model of glucocorticoid-induced osteonecrosis. San Antonio: Orthopaedic Research Society; 2013.
10. Wang Y, Ohtsuka-Isoya M, Shao P, Sakamoto S, Shinoda H. Effects of methylprednisolone on bone formation and resorption in rats. Jpn J Pharmacol. 2002;90(3):236–46.
11. Noa M, Mendoza S, Mas R, Mendoza N, Leon F. Effect of D-003, a mixture of very high molecular weight aliphatic acids, on prednisolone-induced osteoporosis in Sprague–Dawley rats. Drugs R D. 2004;5(5):281–90.
12. Murata M, Kumagai K, Miyata N, Osaki M, Shindo H. Osteonecrosis in stroke-prone spontaneously hypertensive rats: effect of glucocorticoid. J Orthop Sci. 2007;12(3):289–95. doi:10.1007/s00776-007-1129-y.
13. Bekler H, Uygur AM, Gokce A, Beyzadeoglu T. The effect of steroid use on the pathogenesis of avascular necrosis of the femoral head: an animal model. Acta Orthop Traumatol Turc. 2007;41(1):58–63.
14. Kerachian MA, Harvey EJ, Cournoyer D, Chow TY, Nahal A, Seguin C. A rat model of early stage osteonecrosis induced by glucocorticoids. J Orthop Surg Res. 2011;6:62. doi:10.1186/1749-799X-6-62.
15. Fisher DE, Bickel WH, Holley KE, Ellefson RD. Corticosteroid-induced aseptic necrosis. II. Experimental study. Clin Orthop Relat Res. 1972;84:200–6.
16. Jaffe WL, Epstein M, Heyman N, Mankin HJ. The effect of cortisone on femoral and humeral heads in rabbits. An experimental study. Clin Orthop Relat Res. 1972;82:221–8.
17. Cruess RL, Ross D, Crawshaw E. The etiology of steroid-induced avascular necrosis of bone. A laboratory and clinical study. Clin Orthop Relat Res. 1975;113:178–83.
18. Wang GJ, Sweet DE, Reger SI, Thompson RC. Fat-cell changes as a mechanism of avascular necrosis of the femoral head in cortisone-treated rabbits. J Bone Joint Surg Am. 1977;59(6):729–35.
19. Gold EW, Fox OD, Weissfeld S, Curtiss PH. Corticosteroid-induced avascular necrosis: an experimental study in rabbits. Clin Orthop Relat Res. 1978;135:272–80.
20. Warman M, Boskey AL. Effect of high levels of corticosteroids on the lipids of the long bones of the mature rabbit. Metab Bone Dis Relat Res. 1983;4(5):319–24.
21. Kawai K, Tamaki A, Hirohata K. Steroid-induced accumulation of lipid in the osteocytes of the rabbit femoral head. A histochemical and electron microscopic study. J Bone Joint Surg Am. 1985;67(5):755–63.
22. Warner JJ, Philip JH, Brodsky GL, Thornhill TS. Studies of non-traumatic osteonecrosis. Manometric and histologic studies of the femoral head after chronic steroid treatment: an experimental study in rabbits. Clin Orthop Relat Res. 1987;225:128–40.
23. Li Z, Zhang N, Yue D. Experimental steroid osteonecrosis in rabbits and pathologic findings. Zhonghua Wai Ke Za Zhi. 1995;33(8):485–7.
24. Yamamoto T, Irisa T, Sugioka Y, Sueishi K. Effects of pulse methylprednisolone on bone and marrow tissues: corticosteroid-induced osteonecrosis in rabbits. Arthritis Rheum. 1997;40(11):2055–64. doi:10.1002/1529-0131(199711)40:11<2055::AID-ART19>3.0.CO;2-E.
25. Miyanishi K, Yamamoto T, Irisa T, Yamashita A, Jingushi S, Noguchi Y, et al. Bone marrow fat cell enlargement and a rise in intraosseous pressure in steroid-treated rabbits with osteonecrosis. Bone. 2002;30(1):185–90.
26. Motomura G, Yamamoto T, Miyanishi K, Jingushi S, Iwamoto Y. Combined effects of an anticoagulant and a lipid-lowering agent on the prevention of steroid-induced osteonecrosis in rabbits. Arthritis Rheum. 2004;50(10):3387–91. doi:10.1002/art.20517.
27. Ichiseki T, Matsumoto T, Nishino M, Kaneuji A, Katsuda S. Oxidative stress and vascular permeability in steroid-induced osteonecrosis model. J Orthop Sci. 2004;9(5):509–15. doi:10.1007/s00776-004-0816-1.
28. Wang KZ, Wang CS, Wu YG, Chen H. Changes of vessel in steroid-induced osteonecrosis of femoral head: experimental study of rabbits. Zhonghua Yi Xue Za Zhi. 2006;86(29):2024–7.

29. Hu ZM, Wang HB, Zhou MQ, Yao XS, Ma L, Wang XN. Pathological changes of the blood vessels in rabbit femoral head with glucocorticoid-induced necrosis. Nan Fang Yi Ke Da Xue Xue Bao. 2006;26(6):785–7.
30. Sheng HH, Zhang GG, Cheung WH, Chan CW, Wang YX, Lee KM, et al. Elevated adipogenesis of marrow mesenchymal stem cells during early steroid-associated osteonecrosis development. J Orthop Surg Res. 2007;2:15. doi:10.1186/1749-799X-2-15.
31. Kuroda Y, Akiyama H, Kawanabe K, Tabata Y, Nakamura T. Treatment of experimental osteonecrosis of the hip in adult rabbits with a single local injection of recombinant human FGF-2 microspheres. J Bone Miner Metab. 2010;28(6):608–16. doi:10.1007/s00774-010-0172-5.
32. Cui Q, Wang GJ, Su CC, Balian G. The Otto Aufranc Award. Lovastatin prevents steroid induced adipogenesis and osteonecrosis. Clin Orthop Relat Res. 1997;344:8–19.
33. Xiao CS, Lin N, Lin SF, Wan R, Chen WH. Experimental study on avascular necrosis of femoral head in chickens induced by different glucocorticoides. Zhongguo Gu Shang. 2010;23(3):184–7.
34. Wideman Jr RF, Pevzner I. Dexamethasone triggers lameness associated with necrosis of the proximal tibial head and proximal femoral head in broilers. Poult Sci. 2012;91(10):2464–74. doi:10.3382/ps.2012-02386.
35. Drescher W, Weigert KP, Bunger MH, Ingerslev J, Bunger C, Hansen ES. Femoral head blood flow reduction and hypercoagulability under 24 h megadose steroid treatment in pigs. J Orthop Res. 2004;22(3):501–8. doi:10.1016/j.orthres.2003.10.002.
36. Ikeda S, Morishita Y, Tsutsumi H, Ito M, Shiraishi A, Arita S, et al. Reductions in bone turnover, mineral, and structure associated with mechanical properties of lumbar vertebra and femur in glucocorticoid-treated growing minipigs. Bone. 2003;33(5):779–87
37. Lill CA, Fluegel AK, Schneider E. Sheep model for fracture treatment in osteoporotic bone: a pilot study about different induction regimens. J Orthop Trauma. 2000;14(8):559–65; discussion 65–6.
38. Lill CA, Fluegel AK, Schneider E. Effect of ovariectomy, malnutrition and glucocorticoid application on bone properties in sheep: a pilot study. Osteoporos Int. 2002;13(6):480–6. doi:10.1007/s001980200058.
39. Lill CA, Gerlach UV, Eckhardt C, Goldhahn J, Schneider E. Bone changes due to glucocorticoid application in an ovariectomized animal model for fracture treatment in osteoporosis. Osteoporos Int. 2002;13(5):407–14.
40. Augat P, Schorlemmer S, Gohl C, Iwabu S, Ignatius A, Claes L. Glucocorticoid-treated sheep as a model for osteopenic trabecular bone in biomaterials research. J Biomed Mater Res A. 2003;66(3):457–62. doi:10.1002/jbm.a.10601.
41. Glade MJ, Krook L. Glucocorticoid-induced inhibition of osteolysis and the development of osteopetrosis, osteonecrosis and osteoporosis. Cornell Vet. 1982;72(1):76–91.
42. Nasseri D, Hungerford DS, White KK, Jones LC, editors. Equine model of ischemic necrosis of bone. New Orleans: Orthopaedic Research Society; 1982.
43. Goetz JE, Chung Y-Y, Zimmerman DL, Pederson DR, Conzemius MG, Brown TD. Steroid-induced versus cryoinsult-induced femoral head osteonecrosis: statistical measurement of histologic abnormality focalization. J Musculoskelet Res. 2005;9:161–72.
44. Jones LC, Allen MR. Animal models of osteonecrosis. Clin Rev Bone Miner Metab. 2011;9(1):63–80.
45. Steinberg D, Steinberg M. Osteonecrosis: an overview. Tech Orthop. 2008;23:2–10.
46. Bauer T, McCarthy J, Stulberg B. Osteonecrosis of the femoral head: histologic diagnosis and findings after core biopsy. In: Urbaniak J, Jones JP, editors. Osteonecrosis: etiology, diagnosis, and treatment. Rosemont: American Academy of Orthopaedic Surgeons; 1997. p. 73–9.
47. Horvai A, Link T. Bone and soft tissue pathology. Philadelphia: Saunders; 2012.
48. Weinstein RS, Jilka RL, Parfitt AM, Manolagas SC. Inhibition of osteoblastogenesis and promotion of apoptosis of osteoblasts and osteocytes by glucocorticoids. Potential mechanisms of their deleterious effects on bone. J Clin Invest. 1998;102(2):274–82. doi:10.1172/JCI2799.
49. Zalavras C, Shah S, Birnbaum MJ, Frenkel B. Role of apoptosis in glucocorticoid-induced osteoporosis and osteonecrosis. Crit Rev Eukaryot Gene Expr. 2003;13(2–4):221–35.
50. Fondi C, Franchi A. Definition of bone necrosis by the pathologist. Clin Cases Miner Bone Metab. 2007;4(1):21–6.
51. Launder WJ, Hungerford DS, Jones LH. Hemodynamics of the femoral head. J Bone Joint Surg Am. 1981;63(3):442–8.
52. Eijer H. Towards a better understanding of the aetiology of Legg-Calve-Perthes' disease: acetabular retroversion may cause abnormal loading of dorsal femoral head-neck junction with restricted blood supply to the femoral epiphysis. Med Hypotheses. 2007;68(5):995–7. doi:10.1016/j.mehy.2006.10.011.
53. Hummer Jr CD. Avascular necrosis of the capital femoral epiphysis in a child receiving corticosteroids: a case report. Clin Orthop Relat Res. 1977;125:65–7.
54. Boechat MI, Winters WD, Hogg RJ, Fine RN, Watkins SL. Avascular necrosis of the femoral head in children with chronic renal disease. Radiology. 2001;218(2):411–3.
55. Kawedia JD, Kaste SC, Pei D, Panetta JC, Cai X, Cheng C et al. Pharmacokinetic, pharmacodynamic, and pharmacogenetic determinants of osteonecrosis in children with acute lymphoblastic leukemia. Blood. 2011;117(8):2340–7; quiz 556. doi:10.1182/blood-2010-10-311969.
56. Karimova EJ, Kaste SC. MR imaging of osteonecrosis of the knee in children with acute lymphocytic leukemia. Pediatr Radiol. 2007;37(11):1140–6. doi:10.1007/s00247-007-0579-x.
57. Glade M. Chronic dexamethasone treatment of horse and pony foals. Ithaca: Cornell University; 1980.
58. Drescher W, Li H, Jensen SD, Ingerslev J, Hansen ES, Hauge EM, et al. The effect of long-term methylprednisolone treatment on the femoral head in growing pigs. J Orthop Res. 2002;20(4):662–8. doi:10.1016/S0736-0266(01)00183-8.
59. Drescher W, Schneider T, Becker C, Hobolth J, Ruther W, Hansen ES, et al. Selective reduction of bone blood flow by short-term treatment with high-dose methylprednisolone. An experimental study in pigs. J Bone Joint Surg. 2001;83(2):274–7.
60. Hankenson K, Cavaliere C, Frank R. Animal models of skeletal disease. In: Hau J, Van Hoosier GJ, editors. Handbook of laboratory animal science. 2nd ed. Boca Raton: CRC Press; 2003. p. 183–223.
61. Turner AS. Animal models of osteoporosis–necessity and limitations. Eur Cell Mater. 2001;1:66–81.
62. Turner R, Maran A, Lotinun S, Hefferan T, Evans G, Zhang M, et al. Animal models for osteoporosis. Rev Endocr Metab Disord. 2001;2:117–27.
63. Ochi H, Takeda S. Animal models for bone and joint disease. The genetically-modified mice as a tool for osteoporosis research. Clin Calcium. 2011;21(2):226–32. doi:CliCa1102226232.
64. Miller SC, Bowman BM, Jee WS. Available animal models of osteopenia–small and large. Bone. 1995;17(4 Suppl):117S–23.
65. Thompson DD, Simmons HA, Pirie CM, Ke HZ. FDA guidelines and animal models for osteoporosis. Bone. 1995;17(4 Suppl):125S–33.
66. Kimmel DB. Animal models in osteoporosis research. In: Belezikian JP, Raisz LG, Rodan GA, editors. Principles of bone biology. San Diego: Academic; 2002. p. 1635–55.
67. Oheim R, Amling M, Ignatius A, Pogoda P. Large animal model for osteoporosis in humans: the ewe. Eur Cell Mater. 2012;24:372–85.
68. Turner AS. The sheep as a model for osteoporosis in humans. Vet J. 2002;163(3):232–9.
69. Benghuzzi H, Wilson G, White J, Cason Z, Mohamed A, Cameron JA, et al. The effects of sustained delivery of estrogen and demineralized bone matrix proteins on bone in ovariectomized female rats – biomed 2013. Biomed Sci Instrum. 2013;49:85–93.

70. Edwards MW, Bain SD, Bailey MC, Lantry MM, Howard GA. 17 beta estradiol stimulation of endosteal bone formation in the ovariectomized mouse: an animal model for the evaluation of bone-targeted estrogens. Bone. 1992;13(1):29–34.
71. Jilka RL, Hangoc G, Girasole G, Passeri G, Williams DC, Abrams JS, et al. Increased osteoclast development after estrogen loss: mediation by interleukin-6. Science. 1992;257(5066):88–91.
72. Bagi CM, Mecham M, Weiss J, Miller SC. Comparative morphometric changes in rat cortical bone following ovariectomy and/or immobilization. Bone. 1993;14(6):877–83.
73. Jerome CP, Power RA, Obasanjo IO, Register TC, Guidry M, Carlson CS, et al. The androgenic anabolic steroid nandrolone decanoate prevents osteopenia and inhibits bone turnover in ovariectomized cynomolgus monkeys. Bone. 1997;20(4):355–64.
74. Binkley N, Kimmel D, Bruner J, Haffa A, Davidowitz B, Meng C, et al. Zoledronate prevents the development of absolute osteopenia following ovariectomy in adult rhesus monkeys. J Bone Miner Res. 1998;13(11):1775–82. doi:10.1359/jbmr.1998.13.11.1775.
75. Schot LP, Schuurs AH. Pathophysiology of bone loss in castrated animals. J Steroid Biochem Mol Biol. 1990;37(3):461–5.
76. Thorndike EA, Turner AS. In search of an animal model for postmenopausal diseases. Front Biosci. 1998;3:c17–26.
77. Laroche M, Costa L, Bernard J, Puget J, Constantin A, Cantagrel A, et al. Dual-energy X-ray absorptiometry in osteonecrosis of the femoral head. Rev Rhum Engl Ed. 1998;65(6):393–6.
78. Baofeng L, Zhi Y, Bei C, Guolin M, Qingshui Y, Jian L. Characterization of a rabbit osteoporosis model induced by ovariectomy and glucocorticoid. Acta Orthop. 2010;81(3):396–401. doi:10.3109/17453674.2010.483986.
79. Eberhardt AW, Yeager-Jones A, Blair HC. Regional trabecular bone matrix degeneration and osteocyte death in femora of glucocorticoid- treated rabbits. Endocrinology. 2001;142(3):1333–40.
80. Jerome CP, Kimmel DB, McAlister JA, Weaver DS. Effects of ovariectomy on iliac trabecular bone in baboons (Papio anubis). Calcif Tissue Int. 1986;39(3):206–8.
81. Longcope C, Hoberg L, Steuterman S, Baran D. The effect of ovariectomy on spine bone mineral density in rhesus monkeys. Bone. 1989;10(5):341–4.
82. Bagi CM, Miller SC. Comparison of osteopenic changes in cancellous bone induced by ovariectomy and/or immobilization in adult rats. Anat Rec. 1994;239(3):243–54. doi:10.1002/ar.1092390303.
83. Iwaniec UT, Magee KA, Mitova-Caneva NG, Wronski TJ. Bone anabolic effects of subcutaneous treatment with basic fibroblast growth factor alone and in combination with estrogen in osteopenic ovariectomized rats. Bone. 2003;33(3):380–6.
84. Iwaniec UT, Turner RT. Failure to generate bone marrow adipocytes does not protect mice from ovariectomy-induced osteopenia. Bone. 2013;53(1):145–53. doi:10.1016/j.bone.2012.11.034.
85. Weinstein RS, Chen JR, Powers CC, Stewart SA, Landes RD, Bellido T, et al. Promotion of osteoclast survival and antagonism of bisphosphonate-induced osteoclast apoptosis by glucocorticoids. J Clin Invest. 2002;109(8):1041–8. doi:10.1172/JCI14538.
86. Hietala EL. The effect of ovariectomy on periosteal bone formation and bone resorption in adult rats. Bone Miner. 1993;20(1):57–65.
87. Sarnes E, Crofford L, Watson M, Dennis G, Kan H, Bass D. Incidence and US costs of corticosteroid-associated adverse events: a systematic literature review. Clin Ther. 2011;33(10):1413–32. doi:10.1016/j.clinthera.2011.09.009.
88. Gladman DD, Urowitz MB, Chaudhry-Ahluwalia V, Hallet DC, Cook RJ. Predictive factors for symptomatic osteonecrosis in patients with systemic lupus erythematosus. J Rheumatol. 2001;28(4):761–5.
89. Mont MA, Glueck CJ, Pacheco IH, Wang P, Hungerford DS, Petri M. Risk factors for osteonecrosis in systemic lupus erythematosus. J Rheumatol. 1997;24(4):654–62.
90. Zizic TM, Marcoux C, Hungerford DS, Dansereau JV, Stevens MB. Corticosteroid therapy associated with ischemic necrosis of bone in systemic lupus erythematosus. Am J Med. 1985;79(5):596–604.
91. Boss JH, Misselevich I. Osteonecrosis of the femoral head of laboratory animals: the lessons learned from a comparative study of osteonecrosis in man and experimental animals. Vet Pathol. 2003;40(4):345–54. doi:10.1354/vp.40-4-345.
92. Korompilias AV, Gilkeson GS, Seaber AV, Urbaniak JR. Hemorrhage and thrombus formation in early experimental osteonecrosis. Clin Orthop Relat Res. 2001;386:11–8.
93. Wang GJ, Hubbard SL, Reger SI, Miller ED, Stamp WG. Femoral head blood flow in long-term steroid therapy: study of rabbit model. South Med J. 1983;76(12):1530–2.
94. Wang GJ, Dughman SS, Reger SI, Stamp WG. The effect of core decompression on femoral head blood flow in steroid-induced avascular necrosis of the femoral head. J Bone Joint Surg Am. 1985;67(1):121–4.
95. Wang GJ, Lennox DW, Reger SI, Stamp WG, Hubbard SL. Cortisone-induced intrafemoral head pressure change and its response to a drilling decompression method. Clin Orthop Relat Res. 1981;159:274–8.
96. Drescher W, Li H, Qvesel D, Jensen SD, Flo C, Hansen ES, et al. Vertebral blood flow and bone mineral density during long-term corticosteroid treatment: an experimental study in immature pigs. Spine. 2000;25(23):3021–5.
97. Bouteiller G, Arlet J, Blasco A, Vigoni F, Elefterion A. Is osteonecrosis of the femoral head avascular? Bone blood flow measurements after long-term treatment with corticosteroids. Metab Bone Dis Relat Res. 1983;4(5):313–8.
98. Ficat RA, Arlet J. Ischemia and necroses of bone. Baltimore: Williams and Wilkins; 1980.
99. Jones LC, Hungerford DS. Models of ischemic necrosis of bone. In: Arlet J, Ficat R, Hungerford DS, editors. Bone circulation. Baltimore: William and Wilkins; 1984. p. 30–4.
100. Jones Jr JP. Intravascular coagulation and osteonecrosis. Clin Orthop Relat Res. 1992;277:41–53.
101. Zalavras C, Dailiana Z, Elisaf M, Bairaktari E, Vlachogiannopoulos P, Katsaraki A, et al. Potential aetiological factors concerning the development of osteonecrosis of the femoral head. Eur J Clin Invest. 2000;30(3):215–21.
102. Abbas AK, Lichtman AH, Pober JS. Cellular and molecular immunology. Philadelphia: W.B. Saunders Company; 1991.
103. Okazaki S, Nishitani Y, Nagoya S, Kaya M, Yamashita T, Matsumoto H. Femoral head osteonecrosis can be caused by disruption of the systemic immune response via the toll-like receptor 4 signalling pathway. Rheumatology. 2009;48(3):227–32. doi:10.1093/rheumatology/ken462.
104. Yamamoto T, Hirano K, Tsutsui H, Sugioka Y, Sueishi K. Corticosteroid enhances the experimental induction of osteonecrosis in rabbits with Shwartzman reaction. Clin Orthop Relat Res. 1995;316:235–43.
105. Guan XY, Han D. Role of hypercoagulability in steroid-induced femoral head necrosis in rabbits. J Orthop Sci. 2010;15(3):365–70. doi:10.1007/s00776-010-1452-6.
106. Lee YK, Lee YJ, Ha YC, Kim KC, Koo KH. Septic arthritis of the hip in patients with femoral head osteonecrosis. Arch Orthop Trauma Surg. 2011;131(11):1585–90. doi:10.1007/s00402-011-1334-1.

107. Nakata K, Masuhara K, Nakamura N, Shibuya T, Sugano N, Matsui M, et al. Inducible osteonecrosis in a rabbit serum sickness model: deposition of immune complexes in bone marrow. Bone. 1996;18(6):609–15.
108. Matsui M, Saito S, Ohzono K, Sugano N, Saito M, Takaoka K, et al. Experimental steroid-induced osteonecrosis in adult rabbits with hypersensitivity vasculitis. Clin Orthop Relat Res. 1992;277:61–72.
109. Masuhara M. Animal models of osteonecrosis. In: An Y, Friedman R, editors. Animal models in orthopaedic research. Baco Raton: CRC Press; 1999.
110. Jones JPJ. Risk factors potentially activating intravascular coagulation and causing nontraumatic osteonecrosis. In: Urbaniak J, Jones JPJ, editors. Osteonecrosis: etiology, diagnosis, and treatment. Rosemont: American Academy of Orthopaedic Surgeons; 1997. p. 89–96.
111. Mohamed A, Wilson G, Johnson W, Tucci M, Cameron JA, Cason Z, et al. The effects of sustained delivery of corticosterone on the adrenal gland of male and female rats – biomed 2013. Biomed Sci Instrum. 2013;49:94–100.
112. Li M, Shen Y, Halloran BP, Baumann BD, Miller K, Wronski TJ. Skeletal response to corticosteroid deficiency and excess in growing male rats. Bone. 1996;19(2):81–8.

Animal Models of Bone Necrosis: An Overview

65

Wolf Drescher, Matthias Knobe, Wolfgang Wagner, and Thomas Pufe

65.1 Introduction

65.1.1 Definition and Epidemiology

"Bone necrosis is a disease which causes death of bone and is called 'Osteonecrosis'" [1].

"Death of all the cellular elements of bone indicates osteonecrosis" [2]. Osteonecrosis can be of traumatic or nontraumatic origin [3].

Osteonecrosis accounts for about 10 % of the more than 500,000 total joint replacements performed annually in the United States [3]. The average age of patients receiving total hip replacement for AVN is 38 years with only 20 % of patients being more than 50 years old at the time of operation [4]. Hips are predominantly involved but also the knee, ankle, shoulder, and elbow were shown to be involved. Bilateral involvement of the femoral head in steroid-induced FHN is up to 88.5 % [4]. As osteonecrosis remains a challenge in our daily clinical praxis, animal models of bone necrosis are still important to better understand the mechanism of the disease and to establish better joint-preserving therapies [5].

W. Drescher (✉)
Department of Orthopaedic Surgery, RWTH University Hospital Aachen, Aachen, Germany

Department of Orthopaedic and Spine Surgery, Agaplesion Ev. Bathildis-Hospital, Bad Pyrmont, Germany
e-mail: wdrescher@ukaachen.de

M. Knobe
Department of Traumatology, RWTH University Hospital, Aachen, Germany

W. Wagner
Division for Stem Cell Biology and Cellular Engineering, Helmholtz Institute for Biomedical Engineering, RWTH University Hospital, Aachen, Germany

T. Pufe
Institute of Anatomy and Cell Biology, RWTH University, Aachen, Germany

65.2 The Different Animal Models

65.2.1 The Different Animal Models and Their Mechanisms

65.2.1.1 Mechanical Models of ON

An experimental animal model frequently used to produce temporary femoral head ischemia is that of hip joint tamponade [6]. The intracapsularly running blood supply to the FH epiphysis is impaired by increasing the intra-articular pressure above venous or arterial pressure level. Venous tamponade succeeded in decreasing FH blood flow by 60 % in puppies, but had no influence on FH blood flow in adult dogs [7]. This difference can be explained by the dependence of the immature FH on intracapsularly running blood supply [8].

A model which succeeded in reproducing the histologic characteristics of FHN found in humans is the femoral neck fracture model in miniature swine [9]. A basilar femoral neck osteotomy (simulating a fracture) was created with a 1.5 mm osteotome, reduced, and internally fixed with two 1.6 mm titanium Kirschner wires. Eight weeks postoperatively, the animals were killed and examined. The vasculature supplying the proximal femur of the immature pig was found to be similar to that of humans [10] which makes this model even more viable. The only difference is that the medial circumflex femoral artery is relatively larger compared with the lateral circumflex artery [11].

Also in our first own experimental series, we used an immature porcine model of hip joint tamponade [12]. Surgically, we inserted a plastic cannula into the hip joint via an osseous drill hole through the acetabular bone. This cannula was connected to an infusion bag which was set under 250 mmHg of pressure. Blood flow measurement by radioactively labeled microspheres showed isolated femoral head ischemia on the experimental side.

A further mechanical model is also described in piglets [13]. A ligature is surgically placed around the femoral neck in order to disrupt the blood supply to the femoral head epiphysis.

K.-H. Koo et al. (eds.), *Osteonecrosis*,
DOI 10.1007/978-3-642-35767-1_65, © Springer-Verlag Berlin Heidelberg 2014

65.2.1.2 Fat Cell Hypertrophy and Intraosseous Pressure

Fat cell hypertrophy within the femoral head was found in growing and adult rabbits after methylprednisolone treatment [14]. Growth of fat cells in the intraosseous compartment of the femoral head was suggested to increase intraosseous pressure resulting in sinusoidal compression and thereby to diminish perfusion of FH bone and osteonecrosis. Core decompression resulted in a gradual normalization of femoral head blood flow after steroid treatment in rabbits. Dexamethasone treatment of a pluripotential cell line from mouse bone marrow could be shown to result in differentiation of these cells into fat cells [15].

A single intramuscular methylprednisolone injection 20 mg/kg to male adult Japanese white rabbits produced characteristic histologic signs of femoral and humeral ON [16]. However, osteonecrotic lesions in this model could only be detected in the femoral and humeral diaphysis and metaphysis, not in the femoral or humeral heads. This model was adopted by our group and used to examine the therapeutic effect of either nitric oxide or enoxaparin to prevent the onset of bone necrosis. This is described in another chapter of this textbook.

A combination of the Shwartzman reaction and corticosteroid injections produced femoral and humeral osteonecrotic lesions in male adult New Zealand white rabbits [17]. Rabbits were injected the bacterial endotoxin lipopolysaccharide intravenously twice at an interval of 24 h, followed by three injections of methylprednisolone 20 mg/kg at 24 h intervals. Four weeks after the last injection, the animals were killed.

65.2.2 Own Experimental Studies

65.2.2.1 Megadose Corticosteroid Intravenous Infusion in a Pig Model

The aim of this study was to examine the acute effect of the spinal trauma treatment recommended by NASCIS (methylprednisolone [MP] 30 mg/kg intravenous infusion over 15 min, followed by 45 min break, and 23 h of MP infusion at 5.4 mg/kg/h) on hip perfusion and plasma coagulability in the awake porcine model [18]. Material and methods are as follows: 18 pigs were randomized to MP treatment (n 9) or a placebo-control group (n 9). Regional blood flow of the systematically subdivided femoral head, proximal femur, acetabulum, and soft tissue hip regions was investigated by the radioactive microsphere technique at steady state (phase 1), after the initial bolus infusion (phase 2) and after the completed treatment (phase 3). Plasma coagulability was examined in phases 1 and 3 by determining PT, aPTT, plasma fibrinogen, and AT-III in jugular venous blood. The results are as follows: FH epiphyseal blood flow decreased after the completed steroid infusion (phase 3) in the steroid-treated group, while there was no change in the control group. FH blood flow reduction was global without a tendency to more pronounced blood flow decrease in any subregion. Plasma fibrinogen was significantly higher after 24 h of steroid infusion than in the placebo-control group.

65.2.2.2 Short-Term High-Dose Corticosteroid Treatment in a Pig Model

The aim of this study was to examine the effect of long-term steroid treatment on hip perfusion, histology, and plasma coagulability [19]. Material and methods are as follows: 24 pigs were randomized to 100 mg MP orally per day for 3 months (n 12) or no treatment for 3 months (n 12). After 3 months, regional blood flow of the systematically subdivided femoral head, proximal femur, acetabulum, and soft tissue hip regions was investigated by the radioactive microsphere technique, intraosseous pressure of the FH epiphysis and metaphysis determined, plasma coagulability was monitored by PT, aPTT, AT-III, and plasma fibrinogen in jugular venous blood, and histology of the femoral head was done unilaterally. The results are as follows: Hypercoagulability was found in the steroid-treated group by hyperfibrinogenemia and 50 % shorter aPTT. FH histology revealed osteopenia by decreased trabecular bone volume and a reduced mineralizing bone surface in the steroid-treated group of pigs. The FH epiphysis of the steroid-treated animals showed an irregular cartilage-bone interface with cartilaginous bone defects projecting into the subchondral bone mainly in its cranial part. FH blood flow was higher in the cranial part in the steroid-treated pigs, and unchanged in the other hip regions. Epiphyseal and metaphyseal intraosseous pressure were not different between the experimental groups.

Twenty-four-hour and 2-week high-dose steroid treatment reduced FH blood flow in the immature pig. Twenty-four-hour and 3-month steroid treatment caused hypercoagulability of plasma. FH histology after 3-month steroid treatment revealed no osteonecrosis but subchondral bone defects. A causality between hypercoagulability and the subchondral bone defects could not be shown by this study but is supported by other studies. Reduced bone blood flow and hypercoagulability of plasma may be pathomechanic factors in steroid-induced FHN.

65.3 Summary

Several animal models of bone necrosis have been developed. Models employing mechanical disturbance of femoral head blood flow have been able to mimic human osteonecrosis quite well especially in the pig. However, a good model of corticosteroid-induced bone necrosis remains to be established. To the authors, this seems to be as important as improving knowledge about nontraumatic femoral head necrosis among general practitioners. An early referral of FHN patients – preferably in ARCO stage 1 – to the orthopedic surgeon could probably save more hips.

References

1. ARCO (Association Research Circulation Osseous). Committee on terminology and classification. ARCO News. 1992;4:41–6.
2. Jones Jr JP. Fat embolism, intravascular coagulation, and osteonecrosis. Clin Orthop. 1993;292:294–308.
3. Mankin HJ. Nontraumatic necrosis of bone (osteonecrosis). N Engl J Med. 1992;326(22):1473–9.
4. Mont MA, Hungerford DS. Non-traumatic avascular necrosis of the femoral head. J Bone Joint Surg Am. 1995;77(3):459–74 [see comments].
5. Hauzeur JP, Pasteels JL, Orloff S. Bilateral non-traumatic aseptic osteonecrosis in the femoral head. An experimental study of incidence. J Bone Joint Surg Am. 1987;69(8):1221–5.
6. Ganz R, Luthi U, Rahn B, Perren SM. [Intra-articular pressure rise influencing epiphyseal blood circulation. An experimental model (author's transl)]. Orthopade. 1981;10(1):6–8.
7. Launder WJ, Hungerford DS, Jones LH. Hemodynamics of the femoral head. J Bone Joint Surg Am. 1981;63(3):442–8.
8. Trueta J. The normal vascular anatomy of the human femoral head during growth. J Bone Joint Surg Br. 1957;39(2):358–94.
9. Seiler III JG, Kregor PJ, Conrad III EU, Swiontkowski MF. Posttraumatic osteonecrosis in a swine model. Correlation of blood cell flux, MRI and histology. Acta Orthop Scand. 1996;67(3):249–54.
10. Salter RB, Kostuik J, Dallas S. Avascular necrosis of the femoral head as a complication of treatment for congenital dislocation of the hip in young children: a clinical and experimental investigation. Can J Surg. 1969;12(1):44–61.
11. Fisher III EH, Beck PA, Hoffer MM. Necrosis of the capital femoral epiphysis and medial approaches to the hip in piglets. J Orthop Res. 1991;9(2):203–8.
12. Drescher W, Schneider T, Becker C, Hobolth L, Ruther W, Bunger C, Hansen ES. Reperfusion pattern of the immature femoral head after critical ischemia. Acta Orthop Scand. 1999;70(5):439–45.
13. Kim HK, Aruwajoye O, Stetler J, Stall A. Effects of non-weight-bearing on the immature femoral head following ischemic osteonecrosis: an experimental investigation in immature pigs. J Bone Joint Surg Am. 2012;94(24):2228–37.
14. Wang GJ, Dughman SS, Reger SI, Stamp WG. The effect of core decompression on femoral head blood flow in steroid- induced avascular necrosis of the femoral head. J Bone Joint Surg Am. 1985;67(1):121–4.
15. Cui Q, Wang GJ, Balian G. Steroid-induced adipogenesis in a pluripotential cell line from bone marrow. J Bone Joint Surg Am. 1997;79(7):1054–63.
16. Yamamoto T, Irisa T, Sugioka Y, Sueishi K. Effects of pulse methylprednisolone on bone and marrow tissues: corticosteroid-induced osteonecrosis in rabbits. Arthritis Rheum. 1997;40(11):2055–64.
17. Yamamoto T, Hirano K, Tsutsui H, Sugioka Y, Sueishi K. Corticosteroid enhances the experimental induction of osteonecrosis in rabbits with Shwartzman reaction. Clin Orthop. 1995;316: 235–43.
18. Drescher W, Weigert KP, Bünger MH, Ingerslev J, Bünger C, Hansen ES. Femoral head blood flow reduction and hypercoagulability under 24 h megadose steroid treatment in pigs. J Orthop Res. 2004;22(3):501–8.
19. Drescher W, Schneider T, Becker C, Hobolth J, Rüther W, Hansen ES, Bünger C. Selective reduction of bone blood flow by short-term treatment with high-dose methylprednisolone. An experimental study in pigs. J Bone Joint Surg Br. 2001;83(2):274–7.

Index

A
Acute chest syndrome, 129
Adipogenesis, 255
Alcohol
  epidemiology of alcohol-induced ONFH, 95–96
  interaction with steroid use, 97
  as a risk factor for ONFH, 96–97
Alendronate, 265
Allogeneic stem cells, 287–288
Anatomy
  blodd supply to lunate, 411
  blood supply
    to the femoral head in children, 429
    to the iliac crest, 315
    of the talus, 403–404
  vascular anatomy of the femoral head, 19, 101–102
Animal models, 507
  corticosteroid-associated osteonecrosis, 493
  corticosteroid-induced animal model for ON, 249
  genetically engineered progenitor cells, 262
  Legg-Calvé-Perthes disease, 431
  ligation of vascular supply and deep freezing, 262
  megadose corticosteroid intravenous infusion
    in a pig model, 508
  pathogenesis of ON, 255
  short term high dose corticosteroid treatment
    in a pig model, 508
  steroid-related bone necrosis, 274
Anterior rotational angle, 331
Anticoagulant, 257
Antiphospholipid syndrome, 134
Antiplatelet drug, 250–253
ARCO. *See* Association Research Circulation Osseous (ARCO)
Arlet and Durroux classification, 200
Arterial ring of the femoral neck, 19
Artery of ligamentum teres, 19
Arthroscopic associated ON of knee
Ascending branch of the anterior circumflex artery
    (the arcuate artery), 389
Ascending cervical artery, 19
Aspherical congruency, 445
Association Research Circulation Osseous (ARCO), 4, 220
Autologous spongiosa graft, 273
Autologous stem cells, 287

B
Beta-tricalcium phosphate, 293
Bioactive calcium phosphates, 293
Bisphosphonates, 265
BMES. *See* Bone marrow edema syndrome (BMES)
BMP2 gene therapy, 263
Bone impaction graft, 297
Bone marrow aspirate concentrate (BMAC), 273
Bone marrow edema syndrome (BMES), 146–147, 231, 235
  clinical features and natural course, 235–236
  epidemiology, 235
  MRI, 232
  pathophysiologic relation with osteonecrosis, 237
  pathophysiology, 231–232
  risk factors, 235
Bone morphogenic proteins (BMPs), 261
  angiogenesis, 262
  osteogenesis, 262
Borderline necrosis, 146

C
Caisson's disease, 4, 136–137
Calcar remodeling, 334
Capillaries, types of, 28
Cartilage necrosis, 432
Catterall classification, 444–445
Cement technique, 291
Ceramic fracture, 346
Ceramic on ceramic, 350
Ceramic-on-ceramic articulation, 345
Chemotherapy, 136
Chondronecrosis. *See* Cartilage necrosis
Classification
  Japanese Investigation Committee (JIC), 207–209
  osteonecrosis of the talus, 406
  spontaneous on of knee (SPONK), 397
  University of Pennsylvania, 202
Classification systems, 6–8
  The Association Research Circulation Osseous (ARCO), 7
  Ficat and Arlet, 6–7
  The Japanese Investigation Committee for Avascular
    Necrosis, 7
  Marcus, Enneking and Massam, 7
  The University of Pennsylvania, 7
Coagulation cascade, 72–74
Coagulopathy, 249
Cold lesion, 186
Combined necrotic angle, 8, 211
Conically-threaded monobloc, 345
Containment, 451–452
Conventional total hip arthroplasty, 369–370
Core decompressions, 6, 279, 363
Cortical strut grafting (Phemister), 309

K.-H. Koo et al. (eds.), *Osteonecrosis*,
DOI 10.1007/978-3-642-35767-1, © Springer-Verlag Berlin Heidelberg 2014

Corticosteroid
  and acute lymphocytic leukemia, 480
  bone related side effects, 479
  effects of corticosteroids on osteonecrosis, 91
  epidemiology of corticosteroid associated osteonecrosis, 479–480
  glucocorticoid induced ON in animal models, 82
  hematologic malignancies, 83
  hypercoagulability, 77–78
  kidney transplant patients, 83
  pathogenesis of corticosteroid associated osteonecrosis, 481–482
  prevalence of glucocorticoid induced osteonecrosis, 81–82
  SLE, 82–83
Creeping substitution, 261
Crescent sign, 153, 181

D
Demineralized bone matrix (DBM), 304
Dendritic cells (DC), 29
Dorr's classification, 356
Double-line sign, 184

E
Edge-detection techniques, 359
Endothelial cells (EC), 28
Enoxaparin, 241, 257
Epidemiology
  nontraumatic osteonecrosis in USA, 40–42
  osteonecrosis in Japan, 47
  osteonecrosis in Korea, 52
  osteonecrosis in Taiwan, 57
Epiphyseal arteries, 19
Etiology, of osteonecrosis, 4–5
Exothermic polymerization of the monomer, 292
Extent of necrosis, quantifying, 203
Extracorporeal shock wave therapy (ESWT), 274

F
Fat cell hypertrophy, 508
Fatigue-type fractures, 221
Femoral head osteonecrosis
  clinical features and presentation, 168–170
  etiology of pain, 165
  preradiographic stage, 186
Femoral head resurfacing (FSR), 378
Fibrinolysis, 72
Ficat staging, 200
Fractures, as a etiology of osteonecrosis, 103–104
Free vascularized fibular graft/grafting (FVFG), 10, 321, 363–364
  technique, 322
Freeze-dried irradiated grafts, 301
Fresh-frozen grafts, 301
Full hip resurfacing, 367
Functional bone investigation, 216
Functional exploration of bone, 199
Functional investigation of bone, 5–6
FVFG. *See* Free vascularized fibular graft/grafting (FVFG)

G
Gage's sign, 438
Gaucher's disease, 137
Genetic risk factors
  alcohol-induced osteonecrosis, 64
  glucocorticoid-induced osteonecrosis, 64
  hypercoagulopathy, 63
Genome-wide association study (GWAS), 62
Gluteus minimus pedicle graft, 315

H
Hard on soft bearing, 351
Head at risk signs, 438
Hemiresurfacing, 364–367
Highly cross-linked polyethylene (HXLPE), 355
  third-generation, 355
Highly X-linked polyethylene, 350
Hinged abduction, 453
Hip arthrodiastasis, 456
Histologic criteria of osteonecrosis, 143
3-Hydroxy-3-methylglutaryl coenzyme A (HMG-CoA), 256
Hypercoagulation, 27
Hypofibrinolysis, 75–76

I
IGA. *See* Inferior gluteal artery (IGA)
Iloprost, 273
Imaging
  bone scan, 186
  CT, 185–186
  MRI, 6, 181–182
  PET-CT, 186
  radiography, 179–181
  SPECT, 186
  of total hip replacement, 188–193
Immunoprivileged status, 287–288
Index of necrosis, 8
Inferior gluteal artery (IGA), 19
Insufficiency-type fracture, 221
Intravascular coagulation, 76–77
Intravital microscope (IVM), 30
Ischemic threshold, 77

J
Joint-preserving procedure, 325

K
Kerboul method, 211
Kienböck's disease, 411
  Lichtman's classification, 412

L
Lateral extrusion index, 444
Lateral femoral circumflex artery (LFCA), 24
Lateral pillar classification, 445
Legg-Calve-Perthes disease (LCPD), 263, 427, 437, 451, 469, 497
  anti-resorptive therapy, 469–470
  bisphosphonate/BMP treatment, 263
  combined anti-resorptive and bone anabolic therapy, 473–474
  differential diagnosis, 438
  femoral varus osteotomy, 453–455

natural history, 446
pathology and pathophysiology, 431–432
Lesion volume, with Japanese Investigation Committee, 209
Light bulb procedure, 307
Lipid lowering agents, 249, 255

M
Medial femoral circumflex artery (MFCA), 20
Mesenchymal stem cell introduction, 10
Mesenchymal stem cells (MSCs), 285
Metal on metal, 350
Metaphyseal arteries, 19
Methylmethacrylate, 291
Mevalonate pathway, 266
MFCA. *See* Medial femoral circumflex artery (MFCA)
Modified Kerboul method, 211–212
Multifocal osteonecrosis, 127
location of involvement and clinical features, 384
risk factor, 383
Multiple drilling, 281

N
Natural history
asymptomatic osteonecrosis, 163–164
symptomatic osteonecrosis, 162–163
Natural history of ONFH
Taiwan, 55–56
Necrotic marrow fat, 174
Next-generation sequencing (NGS), 62
Nitrate co-treatment, 274
Non-traumatic ONHH
etiology and pathogenesis, 389–390
Nontraumatic osteonecrosis, 40
Non-vascularized tibial graft, 307

O
Organ transplantation, 134
Osteolysis threshold, 357
Osteonecrosis
definition, 215
of humeral head
adaptation of Ficat-Arlet classification by Cruess, 390
necrotic angle, 391
treatment, 392–393
of the knee
epidemiology, 396
treatment, 398–401
Osteonecrosis of the talus (ONT), 403
talar neck fracture, 403
Osteotomy, proximal femur, 9

P
Pancreatitis, 137
Particle size distribution, 301
Pathologic mechanism of osteonecrosis, 5
Pathology of osteonecrosis, 151–153
Pathomechanism of osteonecrosis, 144–146
Perthes' disease, 419
epidemiology, 419
thombotic tendency, 423
Posterior rotational angle, 332
Posterior rotational osteotomy, 331
Post-traumatic osteonecrosis
incidence, 113–117
risk factor, 113–117
treatment, 119–121
Prevalence of osteonecrosis
Asia, 36–37
Europe, 36
Netherlands, 36
United States, 36
Progression to collapse, risk factors, 162
Pseudopus, 173

Q
Quadratus femoris muscle pedicle graft, 315

R
Radiation, 136
Regional endothelial dysfunctions (RED), 28
Regional migratory osteoporosis (RMO), 237
Reperfusion injury, 29
Resurfacing arthroplasty (RSTHA), 375
indications, 375–376
Risk factors, 136
collapse of femoral head osteonecrosis, 208
developing pain in osteonecrosis, 169–170
Rostral sparing, 422

S
Salter's innominate osteotomy, 455
Salter-Thompson classification, 445
Sandwich type acetabular, 346
Scanning electron microscopy (SEM), 346
Shelf acetabuloplasty, 456
Shwartman reaction, 500–501
Sickle cell disease
evaluation and management, 128
thromboembolic prophylaxis, 129–130
SIF. *See* Subchondral insufficiency fracture (SIF)
Silent hip, 200
SLE. *See* Systemic lupus erythematosus (SLE)
SPECT, 319
Spontaneous ON of the knee (SPONK), 395
epidemiology, 396
etiology, 395–396
natural history, 397
Statin, 256
Stem cell therapy, 273
Stulberg classification, 445
Subchondral insufficiency fracture (SIF), 155–156
Subchondral stress fracture, 221
Subchondral stress fracture of femoral head (SSFFH)
clinical findings, 221–222
differential diagnosis, 225–227
image findings, 222–225
prognosis, 225
treatment, 225
Sugioka operation, 325
Systemic lupus erythematosus (SLE), 209
corticosteroid therapy, 134
hypercoagulopathy, 134

T
Tantalum rod, 364
Templating, 371
Thrombophilia, 74–75
Thrombophilia-hypofibrinolysis, 241
Transient osteoporosis, 156
Transtrochanteric curved varus osteotomy, 339
Transtrochanteric osteotomy, 318, 327
Trapdoor procedure, 307
Traumatic osteonecrosis, 39–40
Trendelenburg gait, 438
Trendelenburg limp, 343
Triple pelvic osteotomy, 455–456

V
Varus angulation, 343
Varus wedge osteotomy, 339
Vascularized bone grafting, 307
Vascularized iliac bone graft (VIBG), 315
  indication, 317

W
Waldenström's radiographic staging, 443–444
Warfarin, 249

FSC
www.fsc.org
MIX
Papier | Fördert gute Waldnutzung
FSC® C083411

Zeitfracht Medien GmbH
Ferdinand-Jühlke-Straße 7
99095 Erfurt, Deutschland
produktsicherheit@kolibri360.de